NURSE'S 3-MINUTE CLINICAL REFERENCE

SECOND EDITION

NURSE'S 3-MINUTE CLINICAL REFERENCE
SECOND EDITION

Wolters Kluwer | Lippincott Williams & Wilkins
Health

Philadelphia · Baltimore · New York · London
Buenos Aires · Hong Kong · Sydney · Tokyo

STAFF

Publisher
Judith A. Schilling McCann, RN, MSN

Editorial Director
H. Nancy Holmes

Clinical Director
Joan M. Robinson, RN, MSN

Art Director
Elaine Kasmer

Editorial Project Manager
Ann E. Houska

Clinical Project Manager
Beverly Ann Tscheschlog, RN, BS

Editor
Jennifer D. Kowalak

Clinical Editor
Maryann Foley, RN, BSN

Copy Editors
Nicholas J. Bilotta, Leslie Dworkin, Jeannine Fielding,
Linda Hager, Laura M. Healy

Digital Composition Services
Diane Paluba (manager), Joyce Rossi Biletz,
Donald G. Knauss

Associate Manufacturing Manager
Beth J. Welsh

Editorial Assistants
Karen J. Kirk, Jeri O'Shea, Linda K. Ruhf

Indexer
Barbara E. Hodgson

The clinical treatments described and recommended in this publication are based on research and consultation with nursing, medical, and legal authorities. To the best of our knowledge, these procedures reflect currently accepted practice. Nevertheless, they can't be considered absolute and universal recommendations. For individual applications, all recommendations must be considered in light of the patient's clinical condition and, before administration of new or infrequently used drugs, in light of the latest package-insert information. The authors and publisher disclaim any responsibility for any adverse effects resulting from the suggested procedures, from any undetected errors, or from the reader's misunderstanding of the text.

© 2008 by Lippincott Williams & Wilkins. All rights reserved. This book is protected by copyright. No part of it may be reproduced, stored in a retrieval system, or transmitted, in any form or by any means—electronic, mechanical, photocopy, recording, or otherwise—without prior written permission of the publisher, except for brief quotations embodied in critical articles and reviews and testing and evaluation materials provided by the publisher to instructors whose schools have adopted its accompanying textbook. Printed in the United States of America. For information, write Lippincott Williams & Wilkins, 323 Norristown Road, Suite 200, Ambler, PA 19002-2756.

N3MCR2011107

Library of Congress Cataloging-in-Publication Data

Nurse's 3-minute clinical reference. — [2nd ed.].
   p. ; cm.
Includes bibliographical references and index.
  1. Nursing—Handbooks, manuals, etc. I. Lippincott Williams & Wilkins. II. Title: Nurse's three-minute clinical reference.
  [DNLM: 1. Clinical Medicine—Handbooks. 2. Nursing Diagnosis—methods—Handbooks. WY 49 N9748 2008]
  RT51.N82 2008
  616.07′5—dc22
ISBN-13: 978-1-58255-670-3 (alk. paper)
ISBN-10: 1-58255-670-9 (alk. paper)   2007031114

Contents

Contributors
and consultants

Lillian Craig, RN, MSN, FNP-C
Adjunct Faculty
Oklahoma Panhandle State University
Goodwell

Laurie Donaghy, RN, CEN
Staff Nurse
Frankford Hospital
Philadelphia

Laura R. Favand, RN, MS, CEN
Chief Nurse
67th Forward Surgical Team
U.S. Army

Susan M. Kilroy, RN, MS
Clinical Nurse Specialist
Massachusetts General Hospital
Boston

Sharon L.G. Lee, RN, MS, APRN, FNP-C, CEN,
   CCRN
Faculty
BryanLGH College of Health
   Sciences/Medical Center
Lincoln, Neb.

Grace G. Lewis, RN, MS, BC
Assistant Professor of Nursing
Georgia Baptist College of Nursing of
   Mercer University
Atlanta

Elizabeth Richards, RN, MSN
Visiting Assistant Professor
Purdue University
West Lafayette, Ind.

Jody Smith, RN, BSN
Nursing Instructor
Del Mar College
Corpus Christi, Tex.

Sheryl Thomas, RN, MSN
Nursing Instructor
Wayne County Community College
Detroit

Elizabeth A. Vincett, RN, BSN, MSN
Registered Nurse Cardiothoracic ICU
   Staff
Pinnacle Health System
Harrisburg, Pa.

Valentina Zamora, RN
Registered Nurse
White Memorial Medical Center
Los Angeles

Foreword

Since the 1999 Institute of Medicine report, "To Err Is Human," health care system leaders have focused more acutely on turning the tide on rising error rates and implementing strategies to ensure patient safety. Although there are improvements in medication packaging and labeling, in medication administration systems, and in avoiding confusion between similar drugs, human factors such as performance and knowledge deficit are cited as the most common cause of adverse drug events. Serious injury and fatality from medication errors is accompanied by the failure to assess and intervene when serious symptoms occur. Errors in assessment, intervention, and the evaluation of care have prompted hospitals to institute expert nurse rapid response teams to provide advice and intervention to the nursing staff when they need direction on the best course of clinical action. However, before the rapid response team arrives, it's incumbent on the nurse to make every effort to access information that could enlighten the clinical situation.

The National Center for Health Statistics reported that in 2004 the fifth leading cause of death in the United States was "unintentional injuries," including all types of medical errors. A serious nursing shortage, higher patient acuity in hospitals, and the growing number of elderly receiving care are only a few of the factors that increase the risk of medical error. Think about your day as a nurse – how many hours do you operate on automatic pilot, relying on past experience and what you believe to be your best clinical judgment to get you through the day? And how often, at the end of a rushed and stressful day, have you wished that you had looked up that disease, drug, or procedure, not only for the patient's safety but for your own peace of mind as well?

Research tells us that most medical error is preventable. Common sense tells us that getting the right information at the right time is the best insurance for delivering safe, quality nursing care. Imagine the security of having the information that you need at your fingertips during the course of caring for patients. *Nurse's 3-Minute Clinical Reference*, 2nd edition, includes the latest information on more than 300 acute and chronic disorders, over 60 treatments, over 80 procedures, and about 150 diagnostic tests that nurses are likely to encounter in practice. The organization and format of the book ensures rapid access to crucial clinical information that will assist with assessment, intervention, and the evaluation of care.

There's no better way to prevent error than to check the knowledge and evidence base in times of uncertainty. Three minutes of information access can make a difference in the health of the patient and in the career of the nurse. The second edition of *Nurse's 3-Minute Clinical Reference* is the book of choice for decision support at the point of care.

Gloria Ferraro Donnelly, RN, PhD, FAAN
Dean and Professor
College of Nursing and Health Professions
Drexel University
Philadelphia

Part I ▷ DISORDERS

Abstract

(see *Types of spontaneous abortion*)

OVERVIEW

Description
- Expelled products of conception from the uterus before fetal viability
- May be spontaneous (miscarriage) (see *Types of spontaneous abortion*)
- May be therapeutic to preserve the mother's mental or physical health in cases of rape, unplanned pregnancy, or medical conditions, such as cardiac dysfunction or fetal abnormality

Pathophysiology
- Abortion may result from fetal, placental, or maternal factors.

FETAL FACTORS
- Abortion usually occurs at 9 to 12 weeks' gestation.
- Abortion may result from defective embryologic development, faulty implantation of the fertilized ovum, or failure of the endometrium to accept the fertilized ovum.

PLACENTAL FACTORS
- Abortion usually occurs at 14 weeks' gestation when the placenta takes over the hormone production necessary to maintain pregnancy.
- Abortion may result from premature separation of a normally implanted placenta, abnormal placental implantation, or abnormal platelet function.

MATERNAL FACTORS
- Abortion usually occurs at 11 to 19 weeks' gestation.

Causes
SPONTANEOUS ABORTION
- Fetal factors
- Placental factors
- Maternal infection
- Severe malnutrition
- Abnormalities of the reproductive organs
- Thyroid gland dysfunction
- Lowered estriol secretion
- Diabetes mellitus
- Trauma
- Surgery that necessitates manipulation of the pelvic organs
- Blood group incompatibility and Rh isoimmunization
- Recreational drug use
- Environmental toxins
- Incompetent cervix

Incidence
- Up to 15% of all pregnancies ending in miscarriage
- About 30% of first pregnancies ending in miscarriage
- At least 75% of miscarriages occurring during the first trimester
- Legally induced abortions increasing in the United States

TYPES OF SPONTANEOUS ABORTION

Depending on clinical findings, a spontaneous abortion (miscarriage) may be threatened or inevitable, incomplete or complete, or missed, habitual, or septic. Here's how the seven types compare.

Threatened abortion
Bloody vaginal discharge occurs during the first half of pregnancy. About 20% of pregnant women have vaginal spotting or actual bleeding early in pregnancy; of these, about 50% abort.

Inevitable abortion
The membranes rupture and the cervix dilates. As labor continues, the uterus expels the products of conception.

Incomplete abortion
The uterus retains part or all of the placenta. Before 10 weeks' gestation, the fetus and placenta usually are expelled together; after the 10th week, they're expelled separately. Because part of the placenta may adhere to the uterine wall, bleeding continues. Hemorrhage is possible because the uterus doesn't contract and seal the large vessels that fed the placenta.

Complete abortion
The uterus passes all the products of conception. Minimal bleeding usually accompanies complete abortion because the uterus contracts and compresses the maternal blood vessels that fed the placenta.

Missed abortion
The uterus retains the products of conception for 2 months or more after the death of the fetus. Uterine growth ceases; uterine size may even seem to decrease. Prolonged retention of the dead products of conception may cause coagulation defects such as disseminated intravascular coagulation.

Habitual abortion
Spontaneous loss of three or more consecutive pregnancies constitutes habitual abortion.

Septic abortion
Infection accompanies abortion. This may occur with spontaneous abortion, but usually results from an illegal abortion or from the presence of an intrauterine device.

Common characteristics
- Pink discharge for several days before cramping
- Scant brown discharge for several weeks before cramping
- Cramps
- Vaginal bleeding

Complications
- Infection
- Hemorrhage
- Anemia
- Coagulation defects
- Disseminated intravascular coagulation
- Psychological issues of loss and failure

ASSESSMENT

History
- Pink discharge for several days or scant brown discharge for several weeks before onset of cramps and increased vaginal bleeding
- Cramps that appear for a few hours, intensify, and occur more frequently
- If entire contents of the uterus expelled, cramps and bleeding may subside
- Continued cramps and bleeding if any contents remain

Physical findings
- Vaginal bleeding
- Cervical dilation
- Passage of nonviable products of conception

Test results
LABORATORY
- Decreased serial levels of serum human chorionic gonadotropin suggests spontaneous abortion.
- Evidence of products of conception is shown by cytologic analysis.
- Levels of serum hemoglobin and hematocrit are decreased due to blood loss.

IMAGING
- Presence or absence of fetal heart tones or empty amniotic sac are revealed by ultrasound examination.

◆ TREATMENT

General
- Accurate evaluation of uterine contents and confirmation of abortion necessary before planning treatment
- Progression of spontaneous abortion unpreventable, except in those cases caused by an incompetent cervix
- Hospitalization to control severe hemorrhage

Diet
- No restrictions; NPO, if surgery is planned

Activity
- Bed rest likely

Medication
- Transfusion with packed red blood cells or whole blood (severe bleeding)
- I.V. oxytocin (stimulates uterine contractions)
- $Rh_o(D)$ immune globulin for Rh-negative female with negative indirect Coombs' test

IF SECOND-TRIMESTER INDUCED ABORTION
- Injection of hypertonic saline solution into amniotic sac
- Injection of prostaglandin into the amniotic sac
- Insertion of a prostaglandin vaginal suppository

PREVENTING SPONTANEOUS ABORTION

To minimize the risk of future spontaneous abortion, emphasize to the pregnant woman the importance of good nutrition and the need to avoid alcohol, cigarettes, and drugs. The couple should also wait for 2 to 3 normal menstrual cycles after spontaneous abortion before attempting conception.

If there's a history of spontaneous abortion, suggest that the patient and her partner have a thorough examination. This may include premenstrual endometrial biopsy, hormone assessment (estrogen and progesterone as well as thyroid, follicle-stimulating, and luteinizing hormones), and hysterosalpingography and laparoscopy to detect anatomic abnormalities. Genetic counseling may also be indicated.

Surgery
- Dilatation and curettage or dilatation and evacuation (D&E), if remnants remain in the uterus
- D&E, if first-trimester induced abortion
- Surgical reinforcement of the cervix (cerclage)

❖ NURSING CONSIDERATIONS

Nursing diagnoses
- Anxiety
- Compromised family coping
- Deficient knowledge (spontaneous abortion)
- Dysfunctional grieving
- Ineffective coping
- Risk for infection

Key outcomes
The patient will:
- communicate feelings about the current situation
- use available support systems, such as family and friends, to aid in coping
- verbalize understanding of current situation and participate in planning her own care
- express feelings of having greater control over the current situation
- demonstrate use of positive coping strategies
- remain free from signs and symptoms of infection.

Nursing interventions
- Do *not* allow bathroom privileges as the patient may expel uterine contents without knowing it.
- Inspect bedpan contents carefully for intrauterine material.
- Save all sanitary pads for evaluation.
- Administer medications, as ordered.
- Provide perineal care.
- Provide emotional support and counseling.
- Encourage expression of feelings.
- Help the patient develop effective coping strategies.

Monitoring
- Amount, color, and odor of vaginal bleeding
- Vital signs
- Intake and output

▶ PATIENT TEACHING

Be sure to cover:
- disorder, diagnosis, and treatment
- vaginal bleeding or spotting
- bleeding that lasts longer than 8 to 10 days or excessive bleeding
- importance of reporting signs of bright red blood immediately
- signs of infection, such as fever and foul-smelling vaginal discharge
- gradual increase of daily activities
- when to return to work (normally within 1 to 4 weeks)
- abstinence from intercourse for 1 to 2 weeks
- prevention of spontaneous abortion (see *Preventing spontaneous abortion*)
- contraceptive information
- avoidance of tampons for 1 to 2 weeks
- importance of follow-up examination.

Discharge planning
- Refer the patient for professional counseling, if indicated.

✷ RESOURCES

Organizations
American College of Obstetricians and Gynecologists: *www.acog.org*
American Society for Reproductive Medicine: *www.asrm.org*
National Abortion Federation: *www.prochoice.org*
National Abortion Rights Action League: *www.naral.org*

Selected references
Cook, R.J., et al., "Legal Abortion for Mental Health Indications," *International Journal of Gynecology and Obstetrics* 95(2):185-90, September 2006.
Taylor, D., et al. "Care for Women Choosing Medication Abortion," *Nurse Practitioner* 29(10):65-70, October 2004.
Wysocki, S. "A Clinician's View of Abortion," *The Nurse Practitioner: The American Journal of Primary Health Care* 28(11):12, November 2003.

Abruptio placentae

● OVERVIEW

Description
- Premature separation of the placenta from the uterine wall
- Usually occurs after 20 weeks' gestation
- Common cause of bleeding during the second half of pregnancy
- Fetal prognosis depends on gestational age and amount of blood lost
- Good maternal prognosis if hemorrhage can be controlled
- Classified according to degree of placental separation and severity of maternal and fetal symptoms (see *Degrees of placental separation in abruptio placentae*)
- Also called *placental abruption*

Pathophysiology
- Spontaneous rupture of blood vessels at the placental bed may be due to lack of resiliency or to abnormal changes in uterine vasculature and may be further complicated by hypertension or by an enlarged uterus that can't contract sufficiently to seal off the torn vessels.
- Consequently, bleeding continues unchecked, possibly shearing off the placenta partially or completely.

Causes
- Exact cause unknown
- Traumatic injury
- Amniocentesis
- Chronic or pregnancy-induced hypertension
- Multiparity
- Short umbilical cord
- Dietary deficiency
- Smoking
- Advanced maternal age
- Pressure on the vena cava from an enlarged uterus
- Diabetes mellitus

Incidence
- Most common in multigravidas, women older than age 35, women with pregnancy-induced hypertension, and women who use cocaine

Common characteristics
- Vaginal bleeding
- Abdominal discomfort
- Abdominal tenderness

Complications
- Hemorrhage
- Shock
- Renal failure
- Disseminated intravascular coagulation (DIC)
- Maternal death
- Fetal death

✳ ASSESSMENT

History
MILD ABRUPTIO PLACENTAE (MARGINAL SEPARATION)
- Mild to moderate vaginal bleeding
- Vague lower abdominal discomfort
- Mild to moderate abdominal tenderness

MODERATE ABRUPTIO PLACENTAE (ABOUT 50% PLACENTAL SEPARATION)
- Continuous abdominal pain
- Moderate dark red vaginal bleeding
- Severe or abrupt onset of symptoms

SEVERE ABRUPTIO PLACENTAE (70% PLACENTAL SEPARATION)
- Abrupt onset of agonizing, unremitting uterine pain
- Moderate vaginal bleeding

Physical findings
MILD ABRUPTIO PLACENTAE
- Fetal monitoring that may indicate uterine irritability
- Strong and regular fetal heart tones

MODERATE ABRUPTIO PLACENTAE
- Vital signs that may indicate impending shock
- Tender uterus that remains firm between contractions
- Barely audible or irregular and bradycardic fetal heart tones
- Labor that usually starts within 2 hours and often proceeds rapidly

SEVERE ABRUPTIO PLACENTAE
- Vital signs that indicate rapidly progressive shock
- Absence of fetal heart tones

DEGREES OF PLACENTAL SEPARATION IN ABRUPTIO PLACENTAE

Placental abruption is classified according to the degree of placental separation from the uterine wall and the extent of hemorrhage.

Mild separation
Internal bleeding between the placenta and uterine wall characterize mild separation.

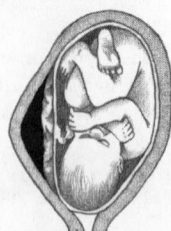

Moderate separation
In moderate separation, external hemorrhage occurs through the vagina.

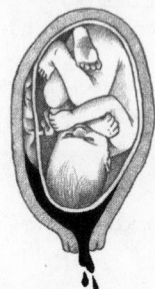

Severe separation
External hemorrhage is also characteristic in severe separation.

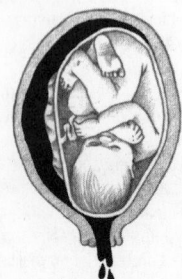

- Tender uterus with boardlike rigidity
- Possible increased uterine size in severe concealed abruptions

Test results

LABORATORY
- Serum hemoglobin and platelet counts are decreased.
- Progression of abruptio placentae and detection of DIC are shown by fibrin split products.

IMAGING
- Pelvic examination under double setup (preparations for an emergency cesarean) and ultrasonography may rule out placenta previa.

◆ TREATMENT

General
- Assessment and management of blood loss
- Delivery of viable infant
- Prevention of coagulation disorders
- If placental separation is severe with no signs of fetal life, vaginal delivery, unless contraindicated by uncontrolled hemorrhage or other complications

 NURSING ALERT Because of possible fetal blood loss through the placenta, a pediatric team should be ready at delivery to assess and treat the neonate for shock, blood loss, and hypoxia.

NURSING ALERT Complications of abruptio placentae require prompt appropriate treatment. With a complication, such as DIC, the patient needs immediate intervention with heparin, platelets, and whole blood, as ordered, to prevent exsanguination.

Diet
- Nothing to eat or drink

Activity
- Bed rest

Medication
- I.V. fluid infusion (by large-bore catheter), as ordered

Surgery
- Cesarean delivery if the fetus is in distress

❖ NURSING CONSIDERATIONS

Nursing diagnoses
- Acute pain
- Anxiety
- Compromised family coping
- Deficient fluid volume
- Deficient knowledge (abruptio placentae)
- Dysfunctional grieving
- Fear
- Ineffective coping
- Ineffective tissue perfusion: Cardiopulmonary

Key outcomes
The patient will:
- express feelings of comfort and decreased pain
- express feelings of decreased anxiety
- seek support systems, such as family, and exhibit adequate coping behaviors
- maintain balanced fluid volume
- demonstrate understanding of situation and treatment measures
- communicate feelings about the situation
- express feelings of decreased fear
- demonstrate effective coping mechanisms
- maintain hemodynamic stability.

Nursing interventions
- Insert indwelling urinary catheter.
- Obtain blood specimens for hemoglobin and hematocrit, coagulation studies, and type and cross-matching, as ordered.
- Provide emotional support during labor.
- Provide information of progress through labor and condition of fetus.
- Encourage verbalization of feelings.
- Help develop effective coping strategies.
- Administer I.V. fluids and blood products, as ordered.

Monitoring
- Maternal vital signs
- Central venous pressure
- Intake and output
- Vaginal bleeding
- Fetal heart rate electronically
- Intake and output
- Progression of labor

▶ PATIENT TEACHING

Be sure to cover:
- disorder, diagnosis, and treatment
- signs of placental abruption
- possibility of an emergency cesarean delivery
- possibility of the delivery of a premature infant
- changes to expect in the postpartum period
- possibility of neonatal death
- factors affecting survival of neonate
- importance of frequent monitoring and prompt management to reduce risk of death.

Discharge planning
- Refer the patient for professional counseling, if necessary.

✴ RESOURCES

Organizations
American College of Obstetricians and Gynecologists: *www.acog.org*
American Society for Reproductive Medicine: *www.asrm.org*

Selected references
Grossman, N.B. "Blunt Trauma in Pregnancy," *American Family Physician* 70(7):1303-310, October 2004.
Korby, J. "Abruprio Placentae," *Nursing2004* 32(4):96, February 2004.

Acceleration-deceleration injuries

● OVERVIEW

Description
- Injury resulting from sharp hyperextension and flexion of the neck that damages muscles, ligaments, disks, and nerve tissue
- Excellent prognosis; symptoms usually subsiding with symptomatic treatment
- Also called *whiplash*

Pathophysiology
- Unexpected force causes the head to jerk back and then forward.
- The bones of the neck snap out of position, causing injury.
- Irritated nerves can interfere with blood flow and transmission of nerve impulses.
- Pinched nerves can affect certain body part functions.

Causes
- Motor vehicle accidents
- Sports accidents
- Falls

Risk factors
- Absence of head restraint in automobile
- Osteoporosis
- Driving under the influence of alcohol or drugs

Incidence
- 1,000,000 cases each year in the United States

Common characteristics
- Nuchal rigidity
- Neck muscle asymmetry

Complications
- Temporomandibular disorder

✳ ASSESSMENT

History
- Moderate to severe pain in the anterior and posterior neck
- Dizziness
- Headache
- Back pain

Physical findings
- Neck muscle asymmetry
- Gait disturbances
- Rigidity or numbness in the arms
- Pain at the exact location of the injury or with range of motion

Test results
IMAGING
- Full cervical spine X-rays rule out cervical fracture.

◆ TREATMENT

General
- Soft cervical collar to protect cervical spine
- Ice packs
- Physical therapy

Diet
- No restrictions

Activity
- Limited activity during first 72 hours after injury
- Limited neck movement
- No strenuous activities, such as lifting and contact sports

Medication
- Oral analgesics (acetaminophen, nonsteroidal anti-inflammatory drugs)

Surgery
- Surgical stabilization (in severe cervical acceleration-deceleration injuries)

✿ NURSING CONSIDERATIONS

Nursing diagnoses
- Acute pain
- Anxiety
- Deficient knowledge (neck and spinal injury)
- Impaired physical mobility
- Risk for posttrauma syndrome

Key outcomes
The patient will:
- articulate factors that intensify pain
- develop effective coping mechanisms
- verbalize understanding of how to modify behavior accordingly
- attain the highest degree of mobility possible
- state feelings and fears.

Nursing interventions
- Provide protection of the spine during all care.
- Administer medications, as ordered.
- Apply a soft cervical collar.

Monitoring
- Level of pain
- Response to medications
- Complications
- Neurologic status

▶ PATIENT TEACHING

Be sure to cover:
- activity restrictions
- proper application of soft cervical collar
- medication administration, dosage, and possible adverse effects
- instructions regarding driving and the use of alcohol while on opioids.

✳ RESOURCES

Organizations
American Academy of Neurology: *www.aan.com*
Southern California Orthopedic Institute: *www.scoi.com*

Selected references
Atlas of Pathophysiology, 2nd ed. Philadelphia: Lippincott Williams & Wilkins, 2005.
Oman, K., et al., eds. *Emergency Nursing Secrets,* 2nd ed. St. Louis: Mosby, 2007.
O'Shea, R.A. *Principles and Practice of Trauma Nursing.* Philadelphia: Elsevier, 2006.

Acquired immunodeficiency syndrome and human immunodeficiency virus

● OVERVIEW

Description
- Marked by progressive failure of the immune system
- Patients becoming susceptible to opportunistic infections, unusual cancers, and other abnormalities that define acquired immunodeficiency syndrome (AIDS)
- Human immunodeficiency virus (HIV) type I, a retrovirus, primary cause of AIDS
- Transmission of HIV occurring through contact with infected blood or body fluids and associated with identifiable high-risk behaviors

Pathophysiology
- HIV strikes helper T cells bearing the CD4 antigen.
- The antigen serves as a receptor for the retrovirus and lets it enter the cell.
- After invading a cell, HIV replicates, leading to cell death, or becomes latent.
- HIV infection leads to profound pathology, either directly, through destruction of CD4 cells, other immune cells, and neuroglial cells, or indirectly, through the secondary effects of CD4 T-cell dysfunction and resultant immunosuppression.

Causes
- Infection with HIV, a retrovirus

Incidence
- Exact numbers difficult to determine as average time between exposure to the virus and diagnosis of AIDS is 8 to 10 years, but shorter and longer incubation times on record
- An estimated 850,000 to 950,000 United States residents living with HIV infection
- About 40,000 new HIV infections each year; about 70% males and 30% females
- More than one-half of those newly infected younger than age 25

Common characteristics
- May be asymptomatic for years

Complications
- Repeated opportunistic infections
- Neoplasms
- Premalignant diseases
- Organ-specific syndrome

✳ ASSESSMENT

History
- After a high-risk exposure and inoculation, a mononucleosis-like syndrome, then possibly asymptomatic for years
- In latent stage, only sign of HIV infection is laboratory evidence of seroconversion

Physical findings
- Persistent generalized adenopathy
- Nonspecific symptoms (weight loss, fatigue, night sweats, fevers)
- Neurologic symptoms resulting from HIV encephalopathy
- Opportunistic infection or cancer

  ✳ AGE-RELATED CONCERN Children show a higher incidence of bacterial infections.

Test results
LABORATORY
- CD4 T-cell count of at least 200 cells/ml confirms HIV infection.
- Presence of HIV antibodies indicate HIV infection.

◆ TREATMENT

General
- Variety of therapeutic options for opportunistic infections (leading cause of morbidity and mortality in patients infected with HIV)
- Disease-specific therapy for a variety of neoplastic and premalignant diseases and organ-specific syndromes
- Symptom management

Diet
- Balanced, nutritious

Activity
- Regular exercise, as tolerated
- Adequate rest periods

Medication
- Immunomodulatory agents
- Anti-infective agents
- Antineoplastic agents

PRIMARY THERAPY
- Protease inhibitors
- Nucleoside reverse transcriptase inhibitors
- Nonnucleoside reverse transcriptase inhibitors

PREVENTING HIV TRANSMISSION

- Health care workers and the public are advised to use precautions in all situations that risk exposure to blood, body fluids, and secretions. Diligently practicing standard precautions can prevent the inadvertent transmission of human immunodeficiency virus (HIV), hepatitis B, hepatitis C, and other infectious diseases that are transmitted by similar routes.
- Educate the patient and his family members, sexual partners, and friends about disease transmission and prevention of extending the disease to others.
- Inform the patient not to donate blood, blood products, organs, tissue, or sperm.
- If the patient uses I.V. drugs, caution him not to share needles.
- Inform the patient that high-risk sexual practices for HIV transmission are those that exchange body fluids, such as vaginal or anal intercourse without a condom.
- Discuss safe sexual practices, such as hugging, petting, mutual masturbation, and protected sexual intercourse. Abstaining is also the most protective method of not transmitting the disease.
- Advise the female patient of childbearing age to avoid pregnancy. Explain that an infant may become infected before birth, during delivery, or during breast-feeding.

Nursing diagnoses

- Activity intolerance
- Compromised family coping
- Disturbed body image
- Fatigue
- Hopelessness
- Imbalanced nutrition: Less than body requirements
- Impaired skin integrity
- Ineffective coping
- Ineffective sexuality patterns
- Powerlessness
- Risk for deficient fluid volume
- Risk for infection
- Social isolation

Key outcomes

The patient will:
- perform activities of daily living without fatigue
- seek support systems and exhibit adequate coping behaviors
- verbalize feelings about changed body image
- express feelings of energy and decreased fatigue
- develop adequate coping mechanisms and support systems
- express feelings and concerns
- consume required caloric intake
- exhibit improved or healed wounds or lesions
- demonstrate effective coping skills
- voice feelings about changes in sexual identity and social response to disease, and follow safer sex practices
- express feelings of having greater control over the current situation
- have balanced intake and output
- remain free from signs and symptoms of infection
- maintain social interaction to the extent possible.

Nursing interventions

- Recognize that a diagnosis of AIDS is profoundly distressing. Coping with an altered body image, the emotional burden of serious illness, and the threat of death may overwhelm the patient.
- Avoid glycerin swabs for mucous membranes. Use normal saline or bicarbonate mouthwash for daily oral rinsing.

- Ensure adequate fluid intake during episodes of diarrhea.
- Provide meticulous skin care, especially in the debilitated patient.
- Encourage the patient to maintain as much physical activity as he can tolerate. Make sure his schedule includes time for exercise and rest.

Monitoring

- Fever, noting any pattern, and signs of skin breakdown, cough, sore throat, and diarrhea
- Swollen, tender lymph nodes
- Laboratory values
- Calorie intake
- Progression of lesions in Kaposi's sarcoma
- Opportunistic infections or signs of disease progression (see *Preventing HIV transmission*)

▶ **PATIENT TEACHING**

Be sure to cover:
- medication administration, dosage, and possible adverse effects
- importance of informing potential sexual partners and health care workers of HIV infection
- signs of impending infection and the importance of seeking immediate medical attention
- symptoms of AIDS dementia and its stages and progression.

Discharge planning

- Refer the patient with AIDS to hospice care, as indicated.

✹ **RESOURCES**

Organizations

Center for AIDS Prevention Studies: *www.caps.ucsf.edu*
Centers for Disease Control and Prevention: *www.cdc.gov*

Selected references

Jones, S.G. "A Step-By-Step Approach to HIV/AIDS," *The Nurse Practitioner: The American Journal of Primary Health Care* 31(6):26-39, June 2006.

Kasper, D.L., et al., eds. *Harrison's Principles of Internal Medicine*, 16th ed. New York: McGraw-Hill Book Co., 2005.

Oyeyemi, A., et al. "Caring for Patients Living with AIDS: Knowledge, Attitude, and Global Levels of Comfort," *Journal of Advanced Nursing* 53(2):196-204, January 2006.

Acute poststreptococcal glomerulonephritis

● OVERVIEW

Description
- Follows a streptococcal infection of the respiratory tract or, less often, a skin infection such as impetigo
- Up to 95% of children and 70% of adults fully recovering
- In elderly patients, possible progression to chronic renal failure within months
- Relatively common
- Also called *acute glomerulonephritis*

Pathophysiology
- Antigen-antibody complexes are produced in response to group A beta-hemolytic streptococcus infection.
- Entrapment and collection of antigen-antibody complexes occurs in the glomerular capillary membranes.
- Inflammatory damage results, impeding glomerular function.
- Immune complement may further damage the glomerular membrane.
- Damaged and inflamed glomeruli lose the ability to be selectively permeable.
- Red blood cells (RBCs) and proteins then filter through as the glomerular filtration rate decreases.
- Uremic poisoning may result.

Causes
- Untreated group A beta-hemolytic streptococcal infection, especially of the respiratory tract

Risk factors
- Impetigo

Incidence
- Occurs most commonly in boys ages 3 to 7, but can occur at any age

Common characteristics
- Oliguria
- Fluid overload

Complications
- Progressive deterioration of renal function

✳ ASSESSMENT

History
- Untreated respiratory streptococcal infection 1 to 3 weeks earlier
- Decreased urination
- Smoky or coffee-colored urine
- Fatigue
- Dyspnea and orthopnea

Physical findings
- Oliguria
- Mild to moderate periorbital edema
- Mild to severe hypertension
- Bibasilar crackles (with heart failure)

Test results
LABORATORY
- Abnormal blood values include electrolyte imbalances; elevated blood urea nitrogen (BUN) and creatinine levels; decreased serum protein levels; the presence of RBCs, white blood cells, mixed cell casts, and protein in the urine that indicate renal failure; and high levels of fibrin-degradation products and C3 protein.

  ✴ **AGE-RELATED CONCERN** Proteinuria in an elderly patient usually isn't as pronounced as in a younger patient.
- Antistreptolysin-O titers are elevated (in 80% of patients); streptozyme and anti-DNase B titers are elevated; and serum complement levels are low, which verifies recent streptococcal infection.
- Throat culture reveals group A beta-hemolytic streptococci.

IMAGING
- Kidney-ureter-bladder X-rays reveal bilateral kidney enlargement.

DIAGNOSTIC PROCEDURES
- Renal biopsy or assessment of renal tissue confirms diagnosis.

◆ TREATMENT

General
- Correction of electrolyte imbalances (possible dialysis)

Diet
- Fluid restriction
- High in calories
- Low-protein, sodium, potassium

Activity
- Bed rest

Medication
- Antibiotics, if appropriate
- Loop diuretics, such as metolazone or furosemide

NURSING CONSIDERATIONS

Nursing diagnoses
- Acute pain
- Decreased cardiac output
- Excess fluid volume
- Fatigue
- Imbalanced nutrition: Less than body requirements
- Impaired gas exchange
- Impaired physical mobility
- Risk for infection
- Risk for injury

Key outcomes
The patient will:
- report increased comfort and decreased pain
- maintain adequate cardiac output
- maintain fluid balance
- express feelings of energy and decreased fatigue
- consume required caloric intake
- maintain adequate ventilation
- perform activities of daily living within confines of disorder
- remain free from signs and symptoms of infection
- remain free from injury.

Nursing interventions
- Administer medications, as ordered.
- Encourage verbalization.
- Provide support.

Monitoring
- Vital signs
- Electrolyte values, serum creatinine, and BUN levels
- Urine creatinine clearance test results
- Intake and output
- Daily weight

PATIENT TEACHING

Be sure to cover:
- disorder, diagnosis, and treatment
- importance of follow-up examinations to monitor renal function
- medication administration, dosage, and possible adverse effects.

Discharge planning
- Refer the patient to resources for information and support.

RESOURCES

Organizations
American Association of Kidney Patients: *www.aakp.org*
National Institute of Diabetes & Digestive & Kidney Diseases: *www.niddk.nih.gov*

Selected references
Diseases, 4th ed. Philadelphia: Lippincott Williams & Wilkins, 2006.
Hahn, R.G., et al. "Evaluation of Poststreptococcal Illness," *American Family Physician* 71(10):1949-954, May 2005.

Acute pyelonephritis

● OVERVIEW

Description
- One of the most common renal diseases
- Usually occurs mainly in the interstitial tissue and renal pelvis and occasionally in the renal tubules
- Affects one or both kidneys
- Good prognosis; extensive permanent damage rare
- Also called *acute infective tubulointerstitial nephritis*

Pathophysiology
- Infection spreads from the bladder to ureters to the kidneys, commonly through vesicoureteral reflux.
- Vesicoureteral reflux may result from congenital weakness at the junction of the ureter and bladder.
- Bacteria refluxed to intrarenal tissues may create colonies of infection within 24 to 48 hours.
- Female anatomy allows for higher incidence of infection.

Causes
- Bacterial infection of the kidneys

Risk factors
- Urinary procedures that involve instrumentation such as cystoscopy
- Hematogenic infection, such as septicemia
- Sexually active women
- Pregnant women
- Neurogenic bladder
- Obstructive disease
- Renal diseases

Incidence
- More common in women than in men
- Community-acquired cases in 15 per 100,000 annually
- Hospital-acquired cases in 7 per 10,000 annually

Common characteristics
- Pain over one or both kidneys
- Urinary urgency and frequency
- Dysuria
- Nocturia

Complications
- Renal calculi
- Renal failure
- Renal abscess
- Septic shock
- Chronic pyelonephritis

✳ ASSESSMENT

History
- Pain over one or both kidneys
- Urinary urgency and frequency
- Burning during urination
- Dysuria, nocturia, hematuria
- Anorexia, vomiting, diarrhea
- General fatigue
- Symptoms that develop rapidly over a few hours or a few days

Physical findings
- Pain on flank palpation
- Cloudy urine
- Ammonia-like or fishy odor to urine
- Fever of 102° F (38.9° C) or higher
- Shaking chills

Test results
LABORATORY
- Pyuria, significant bacteriuria, low specific gravity and osmolality, slightly alkaline urine pH, or proteinuria, glycosuria, and ketonuria (less frequent) are revealed by urinalysis and culture and sensitivity testing.
- White blood cell count, neutrophil count, and erythrocyte sedimentation rate are elevated.

IMAGING
- Kidney-ureter-bladder radiography reveals calculi, tumors, or cysts in the kidneys and urinary tract.
- Excretory urography shows asymmetrical kidneys, possibly indicating a high frequency of infection.

◆ TREATMENT

General
- Identification and correction of predisposing factors to infection, such as obstruction and calculi
- Short courses of therapy for uncomplicated infections

Diet
- No restrictions
- Increased fluid intake

Activity
- No restrictions

Medication
- Antibiotics
- Urinary analgesics, such as phenazopyridine

❖ NURSING CONSIDERATIONS

Nursing diagnoses
- Acute pain
- Deficient knowledge (acute pyelonephritis)
- Excess fluid volume
- Fatigue
- Impaired physical mobility
- Impaired urinary elimination
- Ineffective tissue perfusion: Renal
- Risk for infection

Key outcomes
The patient will:
- report increased comfort and decreased pain
- verbalize understanding of disorder and treatment
- maintain fluid balance
- express feelings of energy and decreased fatigue
- perform activities of daily living within the confines of the disorder
- maintain urine specific gravity within the designated limits
- identify risk factors that exacerbate decreased tissue perfusion and modify lifestyle appropriately
- remain free from signs and symptoms of infection.

Nursing interventions
- Administer medication, as ordered.

Monitoring
- Vital signs
- Intake and output
- Characteristics of urine
- Pattern of urination
- Daily weight
- Renal function studies

▶ PATIENT TEACHING

Be sure to cover:
- disorder, diagnosis, and treatment
- avoidance of bacterial contamination by wiping the perineum from front to back after bowel movements (for women)
- proper technique for collecting a clean-catch urine specimen
- medication administration, dosage, and possible adverse effects
- routine checkup with a history of urinary tract infections
- signs and symptoms of recurrent infection.

✳ RESOURCES

Organizations
American Association of Kidney Patients: *www.aakp.org*
National Institute of Diabetes & Digestive & Kidney Diseases: *www.niddk.nih.gov*

Selected references
Diseases, 4th ed. Philadelphia: Lippincott Williams & Wilkins, 2006.
Ramakirshnan, K., and Scheid, D.C. "Diagnosis and Management of Acute Pyelonephritis in Adults," *American Family Physician* (71)5:933-42, March 2005.

Acute respiratory distress syndrome

● OVERVIEW

Description
- Form of pulmonary edema; may be difficult to recognize
- Hallmark sign: hypoxemia despite increased supplemental oxygen
- Four-stage syndrome; can rapidly progress to intractable and fatal hypoxemia
- In patients who recover, little or no permanent lung damage
- May coexist with disseminated intravascular coagulation (DIC)
- Also known as *shock, stiff, white, wet,* or *Da Nang lung* and *ARDS*

Pathophysiology
- Increased permeability of the alveolocapillary membranes allows fluid to accumulate in the lung interstitium, alveolar spaces, and small airways, causing the lung to stiffen.
- Ventilation is impaired, reducing oxygenation of pulmonary capillary blood.
- Elevated capillary pressure increases interstitial and alveolar edema.
- Alveolar closing pressure then exceeds pulmonary pressures, resulting in closure and collapse of the alveoli.

Causes
- Indirect or direct lung trauma (most common)
- Anaphylaxis
- Aspiration of gastric contents
- Diffuse pneumonia (especially viral)
- Drug overdose
- Idiosyncratic drug reaction
- Inhalation of noxious gases
- Near-drowning
- Oxygen toxicity
- Coronary artery bypass grafting
- Hemodialysis
- Leukemia
- Acute miliary tuberculosis
- Pancreatitis
- Thrombotic thrombocytopenic purpura
- Uremia
- Venous air embolism

Incidence
- In patients with three concurrent causes, 85% probability of developing ARDS

Common characteristics
- Shortness of breath
- Dry cough with thick, frothy sputum
- Bloody, sticky secretions

Complications
- Metabolic acidosis
- Respiratory acidosis
- Cardiac arrest

✳ ASSESSMENT

History
- Dyspnea, especially on exertion

Physical findings
STAGE I
- Shortness of breath, especially on exertion
- Normal to increased respiratory and pulse rates
- Diminished breath sounds
STAGE II
- Respiratory distress
- Use of accessory muscles
- Pallor, anxiety, and restlessness
- Dry cough with thick, frothy sputum
- Bloody, sticky secretions
- Cool, clammy skin
- Tachycardia and tachypnea
- Elevated blood pressure
- Basilar crackles
STAGE III
- Breathing rate more than 30 breaths/minute
- Tachycardia with arrhythmias
- Labile blood pressure
- Productive cough
- Pale, cyanotic skin
- Crackles and rhonchi possible
STAGE IV
- Acute respiratory failure with severe hypoxia
- Deteriorating mental status
- May become comatose
- Pale, cyanotic skin
- Lack of spontaneous respirations
- Bradycardia with arrhythmias
- Hypotension
- Metabolic and respiratory acidosis

Test results
LABORATORY
- Arterial blood gas (ABG) analysis initially shows a reduced partial pressure of arterial oxygen (PaO_2) (less than 60 mm Hg) and a decreased partial pressure of arterial carbon dioxide ($PaCO_2$) (less than 35 mm Hg).
- ABG analysis later shows increased $PaCO_2$ (more than 45 mm Hg) and decreased bicarbonate levels (less than 22 mEq/L) and decreased PaO_2 despite oxygen therapy.
- Gram stain and sputum culture and sensitivity show infectious organism.
- Blood cultures reveal infectious organisms.
- Toxicology tests show drug ingestion.
- Serum amylase is increased in pancreatitis.
IMAGING
- Chest X-rays may show early bilateral infiltrates; in later stages, a ground-glass appearance and, eventually, "whiteouts" of both lung fields.
DIAGNOSTIC PROCEDURES
- Pulmonary artery catheterization may show a pulmonary artery wedge pressure of 12 to 18 mm Hg.

◆ TREATMENT

General
- Treatment of the underlying cause
- Correction of electrolyte and acid-base imbalances

FOR MECHANICAL VENTILATION
- Target low tidal volumes; use of increased respiratory rates
- Target plateau pressures less than or equal to 40 cm H_2O

Diet
- Fluid restriction
- Tube feedings
- Parenteral nutrition

Activity
- Bed rest

Medication
- Humidified oxygen
- Bronchodilators
- Diuretics

FOR MECHANICAL VENTILATION
- Sedatives
- Opioids
- Neuromuscular blocking agents
- Short course of high-dose corticosteroids, if fatty emboli or chemical injury
- Sodium bicarbonate, if severe metabolic acidosis
- Fluids and vasopressors, if hypotensive
- Antimicrobials, if nonviral infection

Surgery
- Possible tracheostomy

❖ NURSING CONSIDERATIONS

Nursing diagnoses
- Anxiety
- Decreased cardiac output
- Fatigue
- Fear
- Imbalanced nutrition: Less than body requirements
- Impaired gas exchange
- Impaired physical mobility
- Ineffective tissue perfusion: Cardiopulmonary
- Risk for impaired skin integrity
- Risk for infection

Key outcomes
The patient will:
- express feelings of increased comfort and decreased pain
- maintain adequate cardiac output
- express feelings of energy and decreased fatigue
- verbalize feelings of anxiety and fear
- consume required caloric intake
- maintain a patent airway
- maintain joint mobility and range of motion (ROM)
- maintain hemodynamic stability
- maintain skin integrity
- remain free from signs and symptoms of infection.

Nursing interventions
- Administer medication, as ordered.
- Maintain a patent airway.
- Ensure adequate humidification.
- Use strict sterile technique.
- Reposition the patient often.
- Consider prone positioning for alveolar recruitment.
- Administer tube feedings and parenteral nutrition, as ordered.
- Allow periods of uninterrupted sleep.
- Perform passive range-of-motion exercises.
- Provide meticulous skin care.
- Reposition the endotracheal tube, if used for mechanical ventilation, from side to side every 24 hours.
- Provide emotional support.
- Provide alternative communication means.

Monitoring
- Vital signs
- Hemodynamics
- Intake and output
- Respiratory status
- Mechanical ventilator settings
- Sputum characteristics
- Level of consciousness
- Breath sounds
- Daily weight
- ABG results
- Pulse oximetry
- Cardiac rate and rhythm
- Serum electrolyte results
- Response to treatment
- Complications, such as cardiac arrhythmias, DIC, GI bleeding, infection, malnutrition, and pneumothorax
- Nutritional status

NURSING ALERT Because positive end-expiratory pressure (PEEP) may lower cardiac output, check for hypotension, tachycardia, and decreased urine output. To maintain PEEP, suction only as needed.

▶ PATIENT TEACHING

Be sure to cover:
- disorder, diagnosis, and treatment
- medication administration, dosage, and possible adverse effects
- when to notify the physician
- complications to report, such as GI bleeding, infection, and malnutrition
- approximate recovery time.

Discharge planning
- Refer the patient to a pulmonary rehabilitation program, if indicated.

✳ RESOURCES

Organizations
ARDS Clinical Network: *www.ardsnet.org*
National Heart, Lung and Blood Institute: *www.nhlbi.nih.gov*

Selected references
Kane, C., and Galanes, S. "Adult Respiratory Distress Syndrome," *Critical Care Nursing Quarterly* 27(4): 325-35, October-December 2004.

Kayyal, A., et al. "Critical Care Extra: Informing Practice: The Use of Corticosteroids in ARDS," *AJN* 106(9):72KK-72OO, September 2006.

Pruitt, B. "Take an Evidence-based Approach to Treating Acute Lung Injury," *Nursing2006 Critical Care* 1(1):44-51, January 2006.

Taylor, H. "ARDS Diagnosis and Management: Implications for the Critical Care Nurse," *Dimensions of Critical Care Nursing* 24(5):197-207, September-October 2005.

White, M. "Proning for ARDS Makes a Comeback," *Nursing2005* 35(4):32cc1-32cc2, April 2005.

Acute respiratory failure

● OVERVIEW

Description
- Results from the inability of the lungs to adequately maintain arterial oxygenation or eliminate carbon dioxide
- Considered life-threatening

Pathophysiology
- If respiratory failure is primarily hypercapnic, it's the result of inadequate alveolar ventilation.
- If respiratory failure is primarily hypoxemic, it's the result of inadequate exchange of oxygen between the alveoli and capillaries.
- Many people have a combined hypercapnic and hypoxemic respiratory failure.

Causes
- Any condition that increases the work of breathing and decreases the respiratory drive of patients with chronic obstructive pulmonary disease
- Respiratory tract infection
- Bronchospasm
- Accumulated secretions secondary to cough suppression
- Ventilatory failure
- Gas exchange failure
- Central nervous system depression
- Myocardial infarction (MI)
- Heart failure
- Pulmonary emboli
- Airway irritants
- Endocrine or metabolic disorders
- Thoracic abnormalities

Incidence
- Occurs in patients with hypercapnea and hypoxemia
- Occurs in patients who have an acute deterioration in arterial blood gas (ABG) values

Common characteristics
- Rapid breathing
- Restlessness
- Anxiety
- Depression
- Lethargy
- Agitation
- Confusion

Complications
- Tissue hypoxia
- Chronic respiratory acidosis
- Metabolic alkalosis
- Respiratory and cardiac arrest

✳ ASSESSMENT

History
PRECIPITATING EVENTS
- Infection
- Accumulated pulmonary secretions secondary to cough suppression
- Trauma
- MI
- Heart failure
- Pulmonary emboli
- Exposure to irritants
- Myxedema
- Metabolic acidosis

Physical findings
- Cyanosis of the oral mucosa, lips, and nail beds
- Yawning and use of accessory muscles
- Pursed-lip breathing
- Nasal flaring
- Ashen skin
- Rapid breathing
- Cold, clammy skin
- Asymmetrical chest movement
- Decreased tactile fremitus over an obstructed bronchi or pleural effusion
- Increased tactile fremitus over consolidated lung tissue
- Hyperresonance
- Diminished or absent breath sounds
- Wheezes, in asthma
- Rhonchi, in bronchitis
- Crackles, in pulmonary edema

Test results
LABORATORY
- ABG analysis reveals hypercapnea and hypoxemia.
- Increased serum white blood cell count is increased in bacterial infections.
- Serum hemoglobin and hematocrit show decreased oxygen-carrying capacity.
- Serum electrolyte results reveal hypokalemia and hypochloremia.
- Blood cultures, Gram stain, and sputum cultures show the pathogen. (See *Identifying respiratory failure.*)

IMAGING
- Chest X-rays may show underlying pulmonary diseases or conditions, such as emphysema, atelectasis, lesions, pneumothorax, infiltrates, and effusions.

DIAGNOSTIC PROCEDURES
- Electrocardiography may show arrhythmias, cor pulmonale, and myocardial ischemia.
- Pulse oximetry may show decreased arterial oxygen saturation.
- Pulmonary artery catheterization may show pulmonary or cardiovascular causes of acute respiratory failure.

◆ TREATMENT

General
- Mechanical ventilation with an endotracheal or a tracheostomy tube
- High-frequency ventilation, if the patient doesn't respond to conventional mechanical ventilation

Diet
- Fluid restriction with heart failure

Activity
- As tolerated

Medication
- Cautious oxygen therapy to increase partial pressure of arterial oxygen
- Antacids
- Histamine-receptor antagonists, as ordered
- Antibiotics
- Bronchodilators
- Corticosteroids
- Positive inotropic agents
- Vasopressors
- Diuretics

Surgery
- Possible tracheostomy

❖ NURSING CONSIDERATIONS

Nursing diagnoses
- Anxiety
- Fatigue
- Fear
- Imbalanced nutrition: Less than body requirements
- Impaired gas exchange
- Impaired skin integrity
- Impaired verbal communication
- Ineffective breathing pattern
- Ineffective coping
- Ineffective tissue perfusion: Cardiopulmonary

Key outcomes
The patient will:
- express feelings of comfort and decreased anxiety
- express feelings of energy and decreased fatigue
- verbalize feelings of anxiety and fear
- consume required caloric intake
- maintain a patent airway
- maintain skin integrity
- develop alternate means of communication to express self
- maintain adequate ventilation
- cope effectively
- maintain hemodynamic stability.

Nursing interventions
- Administer medication, as ordered.
- Orient the patient frequently.
- Administer oxygen, as ordered.
- Maintain a patent airway.
- Encourage pursed-lip breathing.
- Encourage the use of an incentive spirometer.
- Reposition the patient every 1 to 2 hours.

IDENTIFYING RESPIRATORY FAILURE

Use these measurements to identify respiratory failure:
- vital capacity less than 15 cc/kg
- tidal volume less than 3 cc/kg
- negative inspiratory force under –25 cm H_2O
- respiratory rate more than twice the normal rate
- diminished partial pressure of arterial oxygen despite increased fraction of inspired oxygen
- elevated partial pressure of arterial carbon dioxide with pH lower than 7.25.

- Help clear the patient's secretions with postural drainage and chest physiotherapy.
- Assist with or perform oral hygiene.
- Position the patient for comfort and optimal gas exchange.
- Maintain normothermia.
- Schedule care to provide frequent rest periods.

IF THE PATIENT REQUIRES MECHANICAL VENTILATION
- Obtain blood samples for ABG analysis, as ordered.
- Suction the trachea, as needed, after hyperventilation and hyperoxygenation.
- Provide humidification.
- Secure tube properly.
- Prevent infection.
- Prevent tracheal erosion.
- Measure cuff pressure every 8 hours.
- Prevent skin breakdown.
- Reposition endotracheal tubing from side to side, and retape as needed.
- Help the patient communicate.

Monitoring
- Vital signs
- Intake and output
- Serum electrolyte and complete blood count results
- Daily weight
- Cardiac rate and rhythm
- Respiratory status
- Breath sounds
- Oxygen saturation levels
- ABG results
- Chest X-ray results
- Complications
- Sputum quality, consistency, and color
- Signs and symptoms of infection

IF THE PATIENT REQUIRES MECHANICAL VENTILATION
- Ventilator settings
- Cuff pressures
- Complications of mechanical ventilation
- Complications of endotracheal intubation
- Endotracheal tube position and patency
- Signs and symptoms of stress ulcers

▶ PATIENT TEACHING

Be sure to cover:
- disorder, diagnosis, and treatment
- medication administration, dosage, and possible adverse effects
- when to notify the physician
- effects of smoking
- communication techniques, if intubated
- signs and symptoms of respiratory infection.

Discharge planning
- Refer the patient to a smoking-cessation program, if applicable.

✻ RESOURCES

Organizations
National Lung Health Education Program: www.nlhep.org

Selected references
Guyton, A.C., and Hall, J.E. *Textbook of Medical Physiology,* 11th ed. Philadelphia: W.B. Saunders Co., 2006.

Paus-Jenssen, E.S., et al. "The Use of Noninvasive Ventilation in Acute Respiratory Failure at a Tertiary Care Center," *Chest* 126(1):165-72, July 2004.

Simmons, P., and Simmons, M. "Informed Nursing Practice: The Administration of Oxygen to Patients with COPD," *Medical Surgical Nursing* 13(2):82-85, April 2004.

Age-related macular degeneration

● OVERVIEW

Description
- Pigmentary changes in the macula
- Associated with vision loss
- May be atrophic, also called involutional or dry
- May be exudative, also called hemorrhagic or wet
- May be retinal pigment epithelial detachment, also called wet
- No cure for atrophic form

Pathophysiology
- Pathologic changes occur primarily in the retinal pigment epithelium, Bruch's membrane, and choriocapillaries in the macular region that result from the hardening and obstruction of retinal arteries.

ATROPHIC FORM
- Deterioration of retinal pigment epithelium occurs due to aging.
- Waste accumulation causes eventual degeneration of light sensitive cells.
- Thinning of the epithelium, with eventual vision loss, occurs as the retinal epithelium detaches and becomes atrophic.

EXUDATIVE FORM
- New blood vessels form in the choroid.
- These vessels project through abnormalities in Bruch's membrane, invading the macular space underneath the retinal epithelium and obscuring central vision. (See *Understanding wet macular degeneration*.)
- These vessels leak fluid in the retinal pigment epithelium, thus increasing the incidence of blurred vision.

RETINAL PIGMENT EPITHELIAL DETACHMENT
- Fluid leaks from the choroids under the retinal pigment epithelium without appearance of new blood vessels in the choroid.
- Fluid then collects under the retinal pigment epithelium, appearing as a bump or blisterlike area.
- Eventually, new blood vessels develop leading to exudative macular degeneration.

Causes
- Age-related degenerative changes
- Genetic in origin
- Injury
- Inflammation
- Infection

Incidence
- Commonly affects both eyes
- Leading cause of blindness in the United States
- Irreversible central vision loss in at least 10% of elderly people
- Atrophic form in about 70% of cases

Common characteristics
- Distorted central vision
- Progressive worsening

Complications
- Blindness
- Nystagmus

✴ ASSESSMENT

History
- Sees blank spot in the center of a page (scotoma) while reading
- Central vision blurs intermittently and has gradually worsened
- Straight lines appear distorted
- Letters appear broken up

Physical findings
- Tiny yellowish spots (drusen) beneath retina

Test results
IMAGING
- Optical coherence tomography may identify and show areas of thinning or thickening of the retina and fluid in or under the retinal pigment epithelium.

DIAGNOSTIC PROCEDURES
- Indirect ophthalmoscopy may show changes in the macular region of the fundus.
- Fluorescein angiography may show leaking vessels in subretinal neovascular net.
- Amsler grid test may detect visual distortion.

◆ TREATMENT

General
- Laser treatment, if leaking blood vessels have developed away from the fovea
- Lutein, vitamins C and E, and beta-carotene (under investigation)

Diet
- High in vitamins A, C, and E; beta-carotene; and zinc

UNDERSTANDING WET MACULAR DEGENERATION

With wet macular degeneration, new blood vessels form in the choroids, invading the space under the retinal pigment epithelium. Fluid then leaks from the vessels, causing blurred vision.

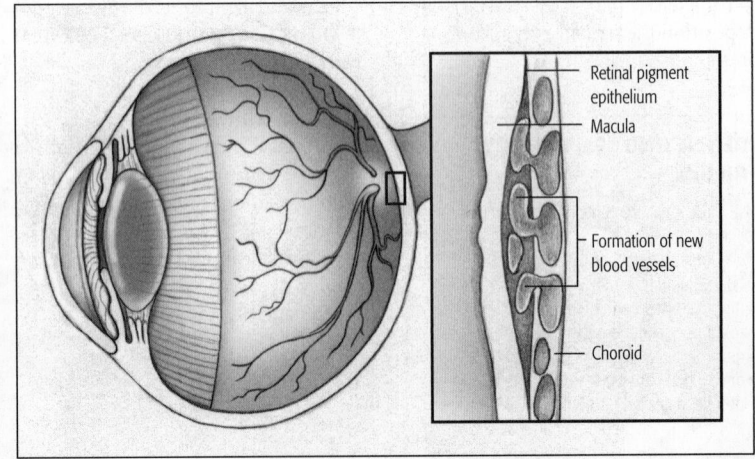

Activity

- Restrictions based on visual acuity

Medication

- Zinc supplements
- Anti-vascular endothelial growth factor (anti-VEGF)

Surgery

- In exudative form, argon laser photocoagulation to slow the progression of severe visual loss
- When vessels are located directly under the fovea, photodynamic therapy (use of cold laser and I.V. light sensitizing drug) to close off abnormal blood vessels without harming macula

❖ NURSING CONSIDERATIONS

Nursing diagnoses

- Deficient knowledge (macular degeneration)
- Disturbed sensory perception: Visual
- Fear
- Risk for injury
- Social isolation

Key outcomes

The patient will:
- verbalize understanding of the condition and treatment
- maintain visual function or adapt as necessary
- express feelings and concerns
- sustain no harm or injury
- maintain social interaction to the extent possible.

Nursing interventions

- Help the patient to obtain optical aids such as magnifiers.
- Offer the patient emotional support.
- Encourage expression of fears and concerns.

Monitoring

- Visual acuity

▶ PATIENT TEACHING

Be sure to cover:
- ways to modify the home environment for safety
- affects on peripheral vision.

Discharge planning

- Refer the patient to the American Foundation for the Blind or Associated Services for the Blind, as indicated.

✷ RESOURCES

Organizations

American Academy of Ophthalmology: *www.eyenet.org*
American Foundation for the Blind: *www.afb.org*
National Eye Institute: *www.nei.nih.gov*

Selected references

Kennedy, M.S. "News: Growing Older, Seeing Less: Blindness and Visual Impairment are on the Rise in Older Americans," *AJN* 104(7):21, July 2004.
Seppa, N. "Blindness Hazard: Gene Variation Tied to Macular Degeneration," *Science News* 167(11):163, March 2005.

Alcoholism

● OVERVIEW

Description
- Chronic disorder of uncontrolled intake of alcoholic beverages
- Interferes with physical and mental health, social and familial relationships, and occupational responsibilities

Pathophysiology
- Alcohol is soluble in water and lipids and permeates all body tissues.
- Liver metabolizes 90% of alcohol absorbed and is the most severely affected organ; hepatic steatosis followed by hepatic fibrosis is evident days after heavy drinking.
- Laennec's cirrhosis may develop after inflammatory response (alcoholic hepatitis) or in absence of inflammation, as a consequence of direct activation of lipocytes (Ito cells).
- Lactic acidosis and excess uric acid is promoted; gluconeogenesis, B-oxidation of fatty acids, and the Krebs cycle is opposed; and hypoglycemia and hyperlipidemia develop.
- Toxicity of cells occurs through reduction of mitochondrial oxygenation utilization, depletion of deoxyribonucleic acid, and other actions.

Causes
- Biological factors
- Psychological factors
- Sociocultural factors

Risk factors
- Male gender
- Low socioeconomic status
- Family history
- Depression
- Anxiety
- History of other substance abuse disorders

Incidence
- Affects all social and economic groups
- Ten percent of population accounting for 50% of all alcohol consumed
- About 13% of all adults older than age 18 suffering from alcohol abuse or dependence
- Males two to five times more likely to abuse alcohol than females

- Occurs at all stages of the life cycle, beginning as early as elementary school age
- ✸ AGE-RELATED CONCERN Prevalence of drinking is highest between ages 21 and 34, but current statistics show that up to 19% of 12- to 17-year-olds have serious drinking problems. Research also suggests that alcoholism affects 2% to 10% of adults older than age 60.

Common characteristics
- May hide or deny addiction
- May temporarily manage to maintain a functional lifestyle

Complications
- Cardiomyopathy
- Pneumonia
- Cirrhosis
- Esophageal varices
- Pancreatitis
- Alcoholic dementia
- Wernicke's encephalopathy
- Seizure disorder
- Depression
- Multiple substance abuse
- Hypoglycemia
- Leg and foot ulcers

✳ ASSESSMENT

History
- Need for daily or episodic alcohol use for adequate function
- Inability to discontinue or reduce alcohol intake
- Episodes of anesthesia or amnesia during intoxication
- Episodes of violence during intoxication
- Interference with social and familial relationships and occupational responsibilities
- Malaise, dyspepsia, mood swings or depression, and an increased incidence of infection
- Untreated injuries

Physical findings
- Poor personal hygiene
- Unusually high tolerance for sedatives and opioids
- Signs of nutritional deficiency
- Secretive behavior
- Physical complications
- Withdrawal signs and symptoms
- Major motor seizures

Test results
- Diagnosis is based on *DSM-IV-TR* criteria findings

DSM-IV-TR criteria
- A diagnosis is confirmed when the patient meets at least three of these signs and symptoms:
  - more alcohol ingested than intended
  - persistent desire or efforts to diminish alcohol use
  - excessive time spent obtaining alcohol
  - frequent intoxication or withdrawal symptoms
  - impairment of social, occupational, or recreational activities
  - continued alcohol consumption despite knowledge of a social, psychological, or physical problem that's caused or exacerbated by alcohol use
  - marked tolerance
  - characteristic withdrawal symptoms
  - alcohol used to relieve or avoid withdrawal symptoms
  - persistent symptoms for at least 1 month or recurrence over a longer time.

LABORATORY

- Blood alcohol tests show levels of at least 0.10% weight/volume (200 mg/dl).
- Serum electrolyte levels are abnormal.
- Serum ammonia levels are abnormal.
- Serum amylase levels are increased.
- Urine toxicology may show abuse of other drugs.
- Liver function studies are abnormal.

◆ TREATMENT

Immediate
- Supportive respiration
- Prevention of aspiration of vomitus
- Fluid replacement
- I.V. glucose
- Correction of hypothermia or acidosis
- Treatment for trauma, infection, or GI bleeding

Long-term
- Total abstinence
- Detoxification, rehabilitation, and aftercare program
- Supportive counseling
- Individual, group, or family psychotherapy
- Ongoing support groups

Diet
- Balanced with adequate vitamins

Activity
- No restrictions
- Safety precautions, including preventing aspiration of vomitus
- Seizure precautions

Medication
- Anticonvulsants
- Antiemetics
- Antidiarrheals
- Tranquilizers, particularly benzodiazepines
- Naltrexone
- Antipsychotics
- Daily oral disulfiram
- Vitamin supplements

❖ NURSING CONSIDERATIONS

Nursing diagnoses
- Anxiety
- Bathing or hygiene self-care deficit
- Compromised family coping
- Dressing or grooming self-care deficit
- Dysfunctional family processes: Alcoholism
- Imbalanced nutrition: Less than body requirements
- Impaired social interaction
- Risk for injury
- Risk for other-directed violence

Key outcomes
The patient (or family) will:
- verbalize feelings of anxiety and fear
- demonstrate improved hygiene and other self-care measures
- express feelings and concerns
- demonstrate improved grooming and other self-care measures
- express understanding of the disorder and treatment modality, as will his family
- consume required caloric intake
- engage in appropriate social interactions with others
- remain free from injury
- inflict no harm upon others.

Nursing interventions
- Institute seizure precautions.
- Administer medications, as ordered.
- Orient the patient to reality.
- Maintain a calm environment, minimizing noise and shadows.
- Avoid restraints, unless necessary for protection.
- Use a nonthreatening approach.

Monitoring
- Mental status
- Vital signs
- Safety measures
- Nutritional and hydration status

▶ PATIENT TEACHING

Be sure to cover:
- disorder, diagnosis, and treatment
- alcohol abstinence
- plan for relapse
- medication administration, dosage, and possible adverse effects.

Discharge planning
Refer the patient to:
- rehabilitation program
- social services
- support services.

✹ RESOURCES

Organizations
Al-Anon: *www.al-anon.org*
Al-Ateen: *www.alateen.org*
Alcoholics Anonymous: *www.alcoholics-anonymous.org*
National Association for Children of Alcoholics: *www.nacoa.net*

Selected references
Blondell, R.D. "Ambulatory Detoxification of Patients with A Lethal Dependence," *American Family Physician* 71(3):495-502, February 2005.

Diagnostic and Statistical Manual of Mental Disorders, Text Revision, 4th ed. Washington, D.C.: American Psychiatric Association, 2000.

"Drug News: Monthly Injection Approved for Alcoholism," *Nursing2006* 36(8):31, August 2006.

Risser, N., and Murphym, M. "Literature Review: Acomprosate Therapy for Alcoholism," *The Nurse Practitioner: The American Journal of Primary Health Care* 30(3):62, March 2005.

Allergic rhinitis

● OVERVIEW

Description
- Inhaled airborne allergens that trigger an immune response of the upper airways in susceptible people
- Seasonal allergic rhinitis: immunoglobulin (Ig) E-mediated type I hypersensitivity response to an environmental antigen (allergen) in a genetically susceptible person
- Perennial allergic rhinitis: inhaled allergens that provoke antigen responses, producing signs and symptoms year-round

Pathophysiology
- The body's immune system overresponds to common allergens in the nose.
- Antibodies attach to mast cells, which release several chemicals, including histamine, which cause dilation of blood vessels, skin redness, and swollen membranes in the nose.

Causes
SEASONAL ALLERGIC RHINITIS
- Tree pollens (in spring)
- Grass and weed pollens (in summer)
- Weed pollens (in fall)
- Mold spores (occasionally, in summer and fall)
PERENNIAL ALLERGIC RHINITIS
- House dust and dust mites
- Molds
- Animal dander
- Tobacco smoke
- Processed materials or industrial chemicals

Incidence
- Affects more than 20 million Americans
- Most prevalent in young children and adolescents, but can affect anyone at any age

Common characteristics
- Swollen nasal membranes

Complications
- Secondary sinus and middle ear infections
- Nasal polyps

✳ ASSESSMENT

History
SEASONAL ALLERGIC RHINITIS
- Paroxysmal sneezing, profuse watery rhinorrhea
- Nasal obstruction or congestion
- Pruritus of the nose and eyes
- Headache or sinus pain
- Itchy throat, malaise, and fever
PERENNIAL ALLERGIC RHINITIS
- Chronic and extensive nasal obstruction or stuffiness

Physical findings
SEASONAL ALLERGIC RHINITIS
- Pale, cyanotic, edematous nasal mucosa
- Red and edematous eyelids and conjunctivae
- Excessive lacrimation
PERENNIAL ALLERGIC RHINITIS
- Nasal polyps
- Dark circles may appear under the eyes (allergic shiners)

Test results
LABORATORY
- High number of eosinophils is revealed in sputum and nasal secretions.
- IgE levels are normal or elevated, possibly linked to seasonal overproduction of interleukin-4 and -5 (involved in the allergic inflammatory process).

◆ TREATMENT

General
- Elimination of environmental antigens, if possible

Diet
- No restrictions
- Increased fluid intake to loosen secretions

Activity
- Activity restriction in areas of allergen exposure

Medication
- Antihistamines
- Intranasal corticosteroids
- Nasal decongestants
LONG-TERM MANAGEMENT
- Immunotherapy or desensitization with injections of allergen extracts administered preseasonally, coseasonally, or perennially

✦ NURSING CONSIDERATIONS

Nursing diagnoses
- Acute pain
- Deficient knowledge (allergic rhinitis)
- Impaired skin integrity
- Ineffective airway clearance
- Ineffective breathing pattern
- Ineffective health maintenance
- Risk for infection

Key outcomes
The patient (or family) will:
- express feelings of comfort and decreased pain
- verbalize understanding of the condition and treatment measures
- maintain skin integrity
- maintain a patent airway
- maintain effective breathing pattern
- maintain current health status
- remain free from signs and symptoms of infection.

Nursing interventions
- Implement measures to relieve signs and symptoms and increase the patient's comfort.
- Increase fluid intake to loosen secretions.
- Elevate the head of the bed and provide humidification to ease breathing.

⬙ **NURSING ALERT** Before desensitization injections, assess the patient's symptoms. After giving the injection, observe him for 30 minutes to detect adverse reactions, including anaphylaxis and severe localized erythema. Make sure that epinephrine and emergency resuscitation equipment are readily available.

Monitoring
- Compliance with the prescribed drug regimen
- Changes in control of signs and symptoms as well as indications of drug misuse

▶ PATIENT TEACHING

Be sure to cover:
- importance of calling the physician if the patient experiences a delayed reaction to the desensitizing injections
- reduction of environmental exposure to airborne allergens
- skin protectant applications
- possible lifestyle changes, such as relocation to a pollen-free area either seasonally or year-round, in severe and resistant allergic rhinitis
- medication administration, dosage, and possible adverse effects.

✸ RESOURCES

Organizations
Asthma and Allergy Foundation of America: *www.aafa.org*
National Institute of Allergies and Infectious Diseases: *www.governmentguide.com/ams*
Quarterly public service newsletter, hosted by a board-certified allergist/immunologist: *www.allergyasthma.com*

Selected references
Gelfan, E.W. "Pediatric Allergic Rhinitis: Factors Affecting Treatment Choice," *Ear Nose & Throat Journal* 84(3):163-68, March 2005.

Hayden, M.L. "Allergic Rhinitis: Proper Management Benefits Concomitant Diseases," *The Nurse Practitioner: The American Journal of Primary Health Care* (29)12:26-37, December 2004.

Hayden, M.L. "Ask the Expert: The Itching 'Runny' Sneezy Misery of Allergic Rhinitis,'" *Nursing Made Incredibly Easy* 3(2):64, March-April 2005.

Kasper, D.L., et al., eds. *Harrison's Principles of Internal Medicine*, 16th ed. New York: McGraw-Hill Book Co., 2005.

Alzheimer's disease

● OVERVIEW

Description
- Degenerative disorder of the cerebral cortex (especially the frontal lobe)
- Poor prognosis
- No cure or definitive treatment

Pathophysiology
- The disorder results from a genetic abnormality on chromosome 21.
- Brain damage is caused by a genetic substance (amyloid).
- Brain tissue reflects three distinguishing features: neurofibrillary tangles, neuritic plaques, and granulovascular degeneration.

Causes
- Unknown

Risk factors
NEUROCHEMICAL
- Deficiencies of neurotransmitters
ENVIRONMENTAL
- Aluminum and manganese
- Trauma
- Genetic abnormality on chromosome 21
- Slow-growing central nervous system viruses

Incidence
- Severe form in patients over age 65
- Mild to moderate dementia in 12% of patients

Common characteristics
- Gradual loss of recent and remote memory
- Loss of sense of smell
- Flattening of affect and personality
- Difficulty with learning new information
- Deterioration in personal hygiene
- Inability to concentrate
- Increasing difficulty with abstraction and judgment
- Impaired communication
- Loss of coordination
- Inability to write or speak
- Nocturnal awakenings
- Signs of anxiety
- Loss of eye contact and fearful look
- Acute confusion, agitation, obsessive-compulsive behavior

Complications
- Injury from violent behavior, wandering, or unsupervised activity
- Pneumonia and other infections
- Malnutrition and dehydration

✱ ASSESSMENT

History
- History obtained from a family member or caregiver
- Insidious onset; initial changes almost imperceptible
- Forgetfulness and subtle memory loss
- Recent memory loss
- Difficulty learning and remembering new information
- General deterioration in personal hygiene
- Inability to concentrate
- Tendency to perform repetitive actions and experience restlessness
- Negative personality changes (irritability, depression, paranoia, hostility)
- Nocturnal awakening
- Disorientation
- Suspicious and fearful of imaginary people and situations
- Misperceives own environment
- Unable to identify objects and people
- Complains of stolen or misplaced objects
- Labile emotions
- Mood swings, sudden angry outbursts, and sleep disturbances

Physical findings
- Impaired sense of smell (usually an early symptom)
- Impaired stereognosis
- Gait disorders
- Tremors
- Loss of recent memory
- Positive snout reflex
- Organic brain disease in adults
- Urinary or fecal incontinence
- Seizures

Test results
- Diagnosed by exclusion; tests are performed to rule out other diseases.
- Positive diagnosis is made on autopsy.

IMAGING
- Position emission tomography reveals metabolic activity of the cerebral cortex.
- Computed tomography scan shows excessive and progressive brain atrophy.
- Magnetic resonance imaging rules out intracranial lesions.
- Cerebral blood flow studies reveal abnormalities in blood flow to the brain.

DIAGNOSTIC PROCEDURES
- Cerebrospinal fluid analysis shows chronic neurologic infection.

OTHER
- EEG evaluates the brain's electrical activity and may show slowing of the brain waves in late stages of the disease.
- Neuropsychologic tests may show impaired cognitive ability and reasoning.

◆ TREATMENT

General
- Hyperbaric oxygen

Diet
- Avoidance of coffee, tea, cola, and chocolate

Activity
- No restrictions; as tolerated

Medication
- Cerebral vasodilators
- Psychostimulators
- Antidepressants
- Anticholinesterase agents
- Anxiolytics
- Neurolytics
- Vitamin E

✤ NURSING CONSIDERATIONS

Nursing diagnoses
- Bathing or hygiene self-care deficit
- Compromised family coping
- Constipation
- Dressing or grooming self-care deficit
- Feeding self-care deficit
- Imbalanced nutrition: Less than body requirements
- Impaired verbal communication
- Ineffective coping
- Risk for infection
- Risk for injury
- Toileting self-care deficit

Key outcomes
The patient (or his family) will:
- perform self-care activities related to bathing and hygiene
- use support systems and develop adequate coping behaviors
- have normal bowel movements
- perform self-care activities related to dressing and grooming
- consume required daily caloric intake
- develop alternate means of communication to express oneself
- demonstrate effective coping skills
- remain free from signs and symptoms of infection
- remain free from injury
- perform self-care activities related to toileting.

Nursing interventions
- Provide an effective communication system.
- Use soft tones and a slow, calm manner when speaking to the patient.
- Allow the patient sufficient time to answer questions.
- Protect him from injury.
- Provide rest periods.
- Provide an exercise program.
- Encourage independence.
- Tell the patient to avoid coffee, tea, cola, and chocolate.
- Offer frequent toileting.
- Assist with hygiene and dressing.
- Administer medication, as ordered.

Monitoring
- Response to medication
- Fluid intake and nutrition status
- Safety

▶ PATIENT TEACHING

Be sure to cover:
- disease process
- exercise regimen
- limitation of foods on the plate
- importance of cutting food and providing finger foods, if indicated
- use of plates with rim guards, built-up utensils, and cups with lids
- independence.

Discharge planning
- Refer family members to Alzheimer's Association.

✳ RESOURCES

Organizations
National Institutes of Health: *www.nih.gov*
Welcome to the Alzheimer's Association: *www.alz.org*

Selected references
Diseases, 4th ed. Philadelphia: Lippincott Williams & Wilkins, 2006.
Handbook of Pathophysiology, 2nd ed. Philadelphia: Lippincott Williams & Wilkins, 2005.
Sixsmith, A. "New Technologies to Support Independent Living and Quality of Life for People with Dementia," *Alzheimer's Care Quarterly* 7(3):194-202, July-September 2006.
Taylor, R, "Alzheimer's Disease Experienced," *Alzheimer's Care Quarterly* 6(2):85-98, April-June 2005.
Warchol, K. "Facilitating Functional and Quality of Life Potential: Strength-based Assessment and Treatment for All Stages of Dementia," *Topics in Geriatric Rehabilitation* 22(3):212-27, July-September 2006.

Amyotrophic lateral sclerosis

● OVERVIEW

Description
- Most common motor neuron disease of muscular atrophy
- Chronic, progressive, and debilitating disease that's invariably fatal (no cure)
- Also known as *Lou Gehrig's disease*

Pathophysiology
- An excitatory neurotransmitter accumulates to toxic levels.
- Motor units no longer innervate.
- Progressive degeneration of axons cause loss of myelin.
- Progressive degeneration of upper and lower motor neurons occurs, resulting in progressive degeneration of motor nuclei in the cerebral cortex and corticospinal tracts.

Causes
- Exact cause unknown
- Inherited as an autosomal dominant trait in 10% of patients
- Virus that creates metabolic disturbances in motor neurons
- Immune complexes such as those formed in autoimmune disorders

PRECIPITATING FACTORS THAT CAUSE ACUTE DETERIORATION
- Severe stress, such as myocardial infarction
- Traumatic injury
- Viral infections
- Physical exhaustion

Incidence
- Three times more common in men than in women
- Affects people ages 40 to 70

Common characteristics
- Muscle weakness
- Atrophy
- Fasciculations

Complications
- Respiratory tract infections
- Complications of physical immobility

✳ ASSESSMENT

History
- Mental function intact
- Family history of amyotrophic lateral sclerosis (ALS)
- Asymmetrical weakness first noticed in one limb
- Easy fatigue and easy cramping in the affected muscles

Physical findings
- Location of the affected motor neurons
- Severity of the disease
- Fasciculations in the affected muscles
- Progressive weakness in muscles of the arms, legs, and trunk
- Brisk and overactive stretch reflexes
- Difficulty talking, chewing, swallowing, and breathing
- Shortness of breath and occasional drooling

Test results
LABORATORY
- Cerebrospinal fluid reveals increased protein.

IMAGING
- Computed tomography scan rules out other disorders.

DIAGNOSTIC PROCEDURES
- Muscle biopsy discloses atrophic fibers.

OTHER
- EEG rules out other disorders.
- Electromyography shows the electrical abnormalities of involved muscles.
- Nerve conduction studies appear normal.

◆ TREATMENT

General
- Rehabilitative measures

Diet
- May need tube feedings

Activity
- No restrictions; as tolerated

Medication
- Muscle relaxants
- Dantrolene
- Baclofen
- I.V. or intrathecal administration of thyrotropin-releasing hormone

NURSING CONSIDERATIONS

Nursing diagnoses
- Anticipatory grieving
- Anxiety
- Bathing or hygiene self-care deficit
- Compromised family coping
- Dressing or grooming self-care deficit
- Feeding self-care deficit
- Imbalanced nutrition: Less than body requirements
- Impaired physical mobility
- Impaired verbal communication
- Ineffective airway clearance
- Ineffective breathing pattern
- Ineffective coping
- Risk for impaired skin integrity
- Risk for infection

Key outcomes
The patient will:
- demonstrate adaptive coping behaviors
- verbalize feelings of anxiety and fear
- perform self-care activities related to bathing and hygiene
- develop adequate coping mechanisms and support systems
- perform self-care activities related to dressing and grooming
- perform self-care activities related to feeding
- consume required caloric intake
- maintain joint mobility and range of motion (ROM)
- develop alternate means of communication to express oneself
- maintain a patent airway and adequate ventilation
- maintain effective breathing pattern
- seek support systems and exhibit adequate coping behaviors
- maintain skin integrity
- remain free from signs and symptoms of infection.

Nursing interventions
- Provide emotional and psychological support.
- Teach the patient about active exercises and ROM exercises.
- Promote independence.
- Teach about meticulous skin care.
- Turn and reposition the patient frequently.
- Administer ordered medication.
- Teach how to perform deep-breathing and coughing exercises.
- Provide airway and respiratory management.
- Promote nutrition.
- Teach about swallowing regimens and aspiration precautions.

Monitoring
- Muscle weakness
- Respiratory status
- Speech
- Swallowing ability
- Skin integrity
- Nutritional status
- Response to treatment
- Complications
- Signs and symptoms of infection

MODIFYING THE HOME FOR A PATIENT WITH ALS

To help the patient with amyotrophic lateral sclerosis live safely at home, follow these guidelines:

- Explain basic safety precautions, such as keeping stairs and pathways free from clutter; using nonskid mats in the bathroom and in place of loose throw rugs; keeping stairs well lit; installing handrails in stairwells and the shower, tub, and toilet areas; and removing electrical and telephone cords from traffic areas.
- Discuss the need for rearranging the furniture, moving items in or out of the patient's care area, and obtaining such equipment as a hospital bed, a commode, or oxygen equipment.
- Recommend devices to ease the patient's and caregiver's work, such as extra pillows or a wedge pillow to help the patient sit up, a draw sheet to help him move up in bed, a lap tray for eating, or a bell for calling the caregiver.
- Help the patient adjust to changes in the environment. Encourage independence.
- Advise the patient to keep a suction machine handy to reduce the fear of choking due to secretion accumulation and dysphagia. Teach him to suction himself.

PATIENT TEACHING

Be sure to cover:
- disorder, diagnosis, and treatment
- swallowing therapy regimen
- medication administration, dosage, and adverse effects
- safety in the home. (See *Modifying the home for a patient with ALS.*)

Discharge planning
- Refer the patient to a local ALS support group.

RESOURCES

Organizations
ALS Association: *www.alsa.org*
National Institutes of Health: *www.nih.gov*

Selected references
Diseases, 4th ed. Philadelphia: Lippincott Williams & Wilkins, 2006.
Handbook of Pathophysiology, 2nd ed. Philadelphia: Lippincott Williams & Wilkins, 2005.
Palmieri, R.L. "Taking Aim at Amyotrophic Lateral Sclerosis," *Nursing2005* 35(11):32hn1-32hn2, November 2005.
Stuban, S. "Critical Care Extra: Living, Not Dying with ALS: Confounding the Predictions of Lou Gehrig Disease," *AJN* 104(5):72KK-72Q, May 2004.

Anaphylaxis

● OVERVIEW

Description
- Dramatic, acute atopic reaction
- Marked by sudden onset of rapidly progressive urticaria and respiratory distress
- More severe the sooner signs and symptoms appear after exposure to antigen
- Severe reactions: may initiate vascular collapse, leading to systemic shock and, possibly, death

Pathophysiology
- After initial exposure to an antigen, the immune system produces specific immunoglobulin (Ig) antibodies in the lymph nodes. Helper T cells enhance the process.
- The antibodies (IgE) then bind to membrane receptors located on mast cells and basophils.
- After the body reencounters the antigen, the IgE antibodies, or cross-linked IgE receptors, recognize the antigen as foreign; this activates the release of power chemical mediators.
- IgG or IgM enters into the reaction and activates the release of complement factors.

Causes
- Systemic exposure to sensitizing drugs, foods, insect venom, or other specific antigens

Incidence
- Most common anaphylaxis-causing antigen is penicillin, which induces a reaction in 1 to 4 of every 10,000 patients treated

Common characteristics
- Apprehension and anxiety

Complications
- Respiratory obstruction
- Systemic vascular collapse
- Death

✳ ASSESSMENT

History
- Immediately after exposure, complaints of a feeling of impending doom or fright and exhibiting apprehension, restlessness, cyanosis, cool and clammy skin, erythema, edema, tachypnea, weakness, sweating, sneezing, dyspnea, nasal pruritus, and urticaria
- Angioedema that may cause a "lump" in the patient's throat
- Dyspnea and complaints of chest tightness

Physical findings
- Hives
- Hoarseness or stridor and wheezing
- Severe abdominal cramps, nausea, and diarrhea
- Urinary urgency and incontinence
- Dizziness, drowsiness, headache, restlessness, and seizures
- Hypotension and shock; sometimes, angina and cardiac arrhythmias

Test results
- No tests are required to identify anaphylaxis. The patient's history and signs and symptoms establish the diagnosis.

LABORATORY
- Skin testing may help to identify a specific allergen.

◆ TREATMENT

General
- Patent airway
- Cardiopulmonary resuscitation, if cardiac arrest occurs

Diet
- Nothing by mouth, until stable

Activity
- Bed rest, until stable

Medication
- *Immediate* injection of epinephrine 1:1,000 aqueous solution; 0.1 to 0.5 ml S.C. for mild signs and symptoms
- Corticosteroids
- Diphenhydramine I.V.
- Volume expander infusions, as needed
- Vasopressors
- Norepinephrine
- Dopamine
- Aminophylline I.V.

Nursing diagnoses
- Anxiety
- Decreased cardiac output
- Deficient fluid volume
- Impaired gas exchange
- Impaired skin integrity
- Ineffective breathing pattern
- Powerlessness

Key outcomes
The patient will:
- express feelings of decreased anxiety
- maintain normal cardiac output and normal heart rate
- maintain adequate fluid volume
- maintain a patent airway and adequate ventilation
- maintain skin integrity
- exhibit effective breathing pattern
- express feelings of improved control over the situation.

Nursing interventions
- Provide supplemental oxygen and prepare to help insert an artificial airway.
- Insert a peripheral I.V. line.
- Continually reassure the patient, and explain all tests and treatments.
- If the patient undergoes skin or scratch testing, monitor for signs of a serious allergic response. Keep emergency resuscitation equipment readily available.

◈ **NURSING ALERT** If a patient must receive a drug to which he's allergic, prevent a severe reaction by making sure he receives careful desensitization with gradually increasing doses of the antigen or with advance administration of corticosteroids. Closely monitor the patient during testing and have resuscitation equipment and epinephrine readily available.

Monitoring
- Vital signs
- Adverse reactions from radiographic contrast media
- Respiratory status
- Serious allergic response after skin or scratch testing
- Neurologic status
- Response to treatment
- Complications

Be sure to cover:
- risk for delayed symptoms and the importance of reporting them immediately
- avoidance of exposure to known allergens
- importance of carrying an anaphylaxis kit whenever he's outdoors and how to familiarize himself with the kit and use it before the need arises
- medical identification.

Organizations
American Academy of Allergy, Asthma and Immunology: *www.aaaai.org*
The Food Allergy & Anaphylaxis Network: *www.foodallergy.org*
Mayo Clinic Allergy and Asthma Center: *www.mayoclinic.com*

Selected references
Burns, A. "Anaphylaxis," *Nursing2004* 34(3):88, March 2004.
Kasper, D.L., et al., eds. *Harrison's Principles of Internal Medicine*, 16th ed. New York: McGraw-Hill Book Co., 2005.
Scarlett, C. "Anaphylaxis," *Journal of Infusion Nursing* 29(1):39-44, January-February 2006.

Anemia, aplastic

Description
- May be fatal; results from injury to or destruction of stem cells in bone marrow or the bone marrow matrix
- Causes pancytopenia (anemia, leukopenia, thrombocytopenia) and bone marrow hypoplasia

Pathophysiology
- The disorder usually develops when damaged or destroyed stem cells inhibit red blood cell (RBC) production.
- Although less common, it may develop when damaged bone marrow microvasculature creates an unfavorable environment for cell growth and maturation.

Causes
- Result of adverse drug reactions
- Immunologic factors; severe disease, especially hepatitis; viral infection, especially in children; and preleukemic and neoplastic infiltration of bone marrow
- Congenital hypoplastic anemia, also known as anemia of Blackfan and Diamond, that develops between ages 2 and 3 months and Fanconi's syndrome, between birth and age 10
- May also be idiopathic

Incidence
- More common in children and young adults

Common characteristics
- Pallor and ecchymoses

Complications
- Hemorrhage
- Infection
- Heart failure

History
- Signs and symptoms of anemia, or signs of thrombocytopenia

Physical findings
- Pallor, ecchymosis, petechiae, or retinal hemorrhage
- Alterations in level of consciousness, weakness, and fatigue
- Bibasilar crackles, tachycardia, and a gallop murmur
- Fever, oral and rectal ulcers, and sore throat
- Nausea
- Decreased hair and skin quality

Test results
LABORATORY
- RBCs account for 1 million/mm³ or less, usually with normochromic and normocytic cells (although macrocytosis [larger-than-normal erythrocytes] and anisocytosis [excessive variation in erythrocyte size] may exist); absolute reticulocyte count is very low.
- Serum iron levels (unless bleeding occurs), are elevated, but total iron-binding capacity is normal or slightly reduced.
- Serum platelet and white blood cell counts are decreased.

DIAGNOSTIC PROCEDURES
- Bone marrow biopsies performed at several sites may yield a dry tap or show severely hypocellular or aplastic marrow, with a varying amount of fat, fibrous tissue, or gelatinous replacement; absence of tagged iron and megakaryocytes; and depression of erythroid elements.

General
- Elimination of any identifiable cause
- Vigorous supportive measures, such as packed RBCs, platelets, and experimental histocompatibility antigen-matched leukocyte transfusions
- Respiratory support with oxygen in addition to blood transfusions
- Bone marrow transplantation (for severe aplasia and patients who need constant RBC transfusions)
- Prevention of infection ranging from frequent hand washing to filtered airflow

Diet
- No restrictions
- Foods high in nutritional value

Activity
- Isolation procedures, if neutropenic

Medication
- Antibiotics
- Corticosteroids
- Marrow-stimulating agents, such as androgens; antilymphocyte globulin (experimental); and immunosuppressant agents
- Granulocyte colony-stimulating factor, granulocyte-macrophage colony-stimulating factor, and erythropoietic stimulating factor

❖ NURSING CONSIDERATIONS

Nursing diagnoses
- Activity intolerance
- Acute pain
- Decreased cardiac output
- Fatigue
- Impaired gas exchange
- Impaired physical mobility
- Ineffective thermoregulation
- Ineffective tissue perfusion: Cardiopulmonary, cerebral
- Risk for infection

Key outcomes
The patient will:
- state the need to increase activity level gradually
- express feelings of comfort and decreased pain
- maintain normal cardiac output
- express feelings of energy and decreased fatigue
- exhibit adequate ventilation
- maintain joint mobility and range of motion
- remain normothermic
- maintain vital signs within prescribed limits during activity
- remain free from signs and symptoms of infection.

Nursing interventions
- Help the patient to prevent or manage hemorrhage, infection, adverse effects of drug therapy, and blood transfusion reaction.
- If the patient's platelet count is low (less than 20,000/mm^3), prevent hemorrhage by avoiding I.M. injections and suggesting the use of an electric razor and a soft toothbrush. Apply pressure to venipuncture sites until bleeding stops.
- Help prevent infection by washing hands thoroughly before entering the patient's room, by making sure the patient is receiving a nutritious diet, and by encouraging meticulous mouth and perianal care.
- Make sure throat, urine, nasal, stool, and blood cultures are done regularly and correctly to check for infection.
- If the patient has a low hemoglobin level, which causes fatigue, schedule frequent rest periods. Administer oxygen therapy, as needed.
- Ensure a comfortable environmental temperature.
- If blood transfusions are necessary, assess for transfusion reactions.

Monitoring
- Blood studies in patients receiving anemia-inducing drugs
- Early detection of bleeding

▶ PATIENT TEACHING

Be sure to cover:
- avoidance of contact with potential sources of infection, such as crowds, soil, and standing water that can harbor organisms
- disorder, diagnosis, and treatment
- medication administration, dosage, and possible adverse effects
- normal lifestyle with appropriate restrictions until remission occurs (for the patient who doesn't require hospitalization).

Discharge planning
- Refer the patient to the Aplastic Anemia Foundation of America for additional information and assistance.

✱ RESOURCES

Organizations
Aplastic Anemia Foundation of America: *www.aplastic.org*
National Institutes of Health: *www.nih.gov*

Selected references
Holcomb, S.S. "Recognizing and Managing Anemia," *The Nurse Practitioner; The American Journal of Primary Health Care* 30(12):16-31, December 2005.
Kasper, D.L., et al., eds. *Harrison's Principles of Internal Medicine*, 16th ed. New York: McGraw-Hill Book Co., 2005.
McPhee, S. J., et al. *Current Medical Diagnosis and Treatment*. New York: McGraw-Hill Book Co., 2007.

Anemia, folic acid (folate) deficiency

● OVERVIEW

Description
- Common, slowly progressive megaloblastic anemia
- Caused by deficiency of the vitamin, folate

Pathophysiology
- When folic acid stores in the body are low or the diet is deficient in folic acid, the bone marrow produces large red blood cells or megaloblasts resulting in anemia.

Causes
- Alcohol abuse
- Poor diet
- Impaired absorption from small intestine
- Bacteria competing for available folic acid
- Excessive cooking of foods, which destroys the available nutrient
- Limited storage capacity in infants
- Prolonged drug therapy with such drugs as anticonvulsants, estrogens, and methotrexate
- Increased folic acid requirements during pregnancy, during rapid growth periods in infancy, during childhood and adolescence because of consumption of folate-poor cow's milk, and in patients with neoplastic diseases and some skin diseases such as exfoliative dermatitis

Incidence
- Most prevalent in infants, adolescents, pregnant and lactating women, alcoholics, elderly people, and people with malignant or intestinal diseases

Common characteristics
- Progressive fatigue
- Systemic signs of anemia

Complications
- In pregnant women, increased risk for giving birth to a neonate with a neural tube defect

✳ ASSESSMENT

History
- May reveal severe, progressive fatigue, the hallmark of folic acid deficiency

Physical findings
- Shortness of breath, palpitations, diarrhea, nausea, anorexia, headaches, forgetfulness, and irritability
- Weakness and light-headedness
- Generalized pallor and jaundice
- May appear wasted or malnourished
- Cheilosis and glossitis

Test results
LABORATORY
- Folic acid deficiency anemia and pernicious anemia are distinguished by the Schilling test and a therapeutic trial of vitamin B_{12} injections.
- Reticulocyte count is decreased, mean corpuscular volume is increased, platelets are abnormal, serum folate levels are less than 4 mg/ml, and macrocytosis is present.

◆ TREATMENT

General
- Elimination of contributing causes

Diet
- Well-balanced (see *Foods high in folic acid content*)

Activity
- No restrictions
- Frequent rest periods

Medication
- Supplements of folic acid given orally or parenterally
- Vitamin supplementation (women, planning to become pregnant, should begin at least 3 months before conception)
- Blood transfusions in severe cases

FOODS HIGH IN FOLIC ACID CONTENT

Folic acid (pteroylglutamic acid, folacin) is found in most body tissues, where it acts as a coenzyme in metabolic processes involving 1-carbon transfer. It's essential for formation and maturation of red blood cells and for synthesis of deoxyribonucleic acid. Although body stores are comparatively small (about 70 mg), this vitamin is plentiful in most well-balanced diets. However, because folic acid is water-soluble and heat-labile, it's easily destroyed by cooking. Also, about 20% of folic acid intake is excreted unabsorbed. Insufficient daily folic acid intake (less than 50 mcg/day) usually induces folic acid deficiency within 4 months. Below is a list of foods high in folic acid content.

Food	mcg/100 g
Asparagus spears	109
Beef liver	294
Broccoli spears	54
Collards (cooked)	102
Mushrooms	24
Oatmeal	33
Peanut butter	57
Red beans	180
Wheat germ	305

Nursing diagnoses

- Activity intolerance
- Deficient fluid volume
- Delayed growth and development
- Diarrhea
- Imbalanced nutrition: Less than body requirements
- Impaired gas exchange
- Impaired oral mucous membranes

Key outcomes

The patient will:

- state the need to increase activity level gradually
- maintain adequate fluid balance
- express understanding of norms for growth and development
- have normal bowel movements
- consume required caloric intake
- maintain adequate ventilation and oxygenation
- exhibit improved or healed wounds or lesions.

Nursing interventions

- Plan activities, while also allowing for rest periods, and necessary diagnostic tests to conserve energy.
- Advise the patient to report signs and symptoms of decreased perfusion to vital organs (dyspnea, chest pain, dizziness).
- If the patient has glossitis, emphasize the importance of good oral hygiene.
- Ask the dietitian to give the patient nonirritating foods because a sore mouth and tongue make eating painful. If these symptoms make talking difficult, supply a pad and pencil or some other aid to facilitate communication.
- To ensure accurate Schilling test results, make sure that all urine excreted over a 24-hour period is collected and that the specimens remain uncontaminated by bacteria.
- Provide a well-balanced diet, including foods high in folate, such as dark green leafy vegetables, organ meats, eggs, milk, oranges, bananas, dry beans, and whole-grain breads.

Monitoring

- Vital signs
- Fluid and electrolyte balance

Be sure to cover:

- importance of a well-balanced diet high in folic acid
- daily folic acid requirements and the need to keep taking the supplements even when the patient begins to feel better
- importance of guarding against infections and to report signs of infection promptly.

Organizations

Iron Disorders Institute: *www.irondisorders.org*
Mayo Clinic: *www.mayohealth.org*

Selected references

Kasper, D.L., et al., eds. *Harrison's Principles of Internal Medicine*, 16th ed. New York: McGraw-Hill Book Co., 2005.

Koren, G. "Low-Carb Diets and Folic Acid Intake," *OB/GYN News* 39(16):9 August 2004.

McPhee, S.J., et al. *Current Medical Diagnosis and Treatment*. New York: McGraw-Hill Book Co., 2007.

Anemia, iron deficiency

● OVERVIEW

Description
- Stems from an inadequate supply of iron for optimal formation of red blood cells (RBCs)
- Produces smaller (microcytic) cells with less color on staining (hypochromia)

Pathophysiology
- Body stores of iron, including plasma iron, decrease.
- Transferrin, which binds with and transports iron, also decreases.
- Insufficient body stores of iron lead to a depleted RBC mass and to a decreased hemoglobin concentration, which results in decreased oxygen-carrying capacity of the blood. (See *Iron absorption and storage.*)

Causes
- Inadequate dietary intake of iron
- Iron malabsorption
- Blood loss secondary to drug-induced GI bleeding or due to heavy menses, hemorrhage from trauma, GI ulcers, malignant tumors, and varices
- Pregnancy
- Intravascular hemolysis-induced hemoglobinuria or paroxysmal nocturnal hemoglobinuria
- Mechanical erythrocyte trauma caused by a prosthetic heart valve or vena cava filter

Incidence
- Common disease worldwide
- Affects 10% to 30% of the adult population of the United States
- Most prevalent among premenopausal women, infants, children, adolescents, alcoholics, and elderly people

Common characteristics
- Fatigue
- Systemic signs of anemia

Complications
- Infection
- Pneumonia

 AGE-RELATED CONCERN In a child, iron deficiency anemia can cause pica, which may lead to eating lead-based paint and can result in lead poisoning.

- Over-replacement of oral or I.M. iron supplements, which can affect the liver, heart, pituitary glands, and joints

✳ ASSESSMENT

History
- Can persist for years without signs and symptoms
- Fatigue, inability to concentrate, headache, and shortness of breath (especially on exertion) that may not develop until long after iron stores and circulating iron become low
- Increased frequency of infections and pica—an uncontrollable urge to eat strange things, such as clay, starch, ice and, in children, lead
- Menorrhagia
- Dysphagia
- Vasomotor disturbances, numbness and tingling of the extremities, and neuralgic pain

Physical findings
- Red, swollen, smooth, shiny, and tender tongue (glossitis)
- Corners of the mouth eroded, tender, and swollen (angular stomatitis)
- Spoon-shaped, brittle nails
- Tachycardia

IRON ABSORPTION AND STORAGE

Iron is essential to erythropoiesis and is abundant throughout the body. Two-thirds of total-body iron is found in hemoglobin; the other third, mostly in the reticuloendothelial system (liver, spleen, and bone marrow), with small amounts in muscle, serum, and body cells.

Adequate dietary ingestion of iron and recirculation of iron released from disintegrating red blood cells maintain iron supplies. The duodenum and upper part of the small intestine absorb dietary iron. Such absorption depends on gastric acid content, the amount of reducing substances (ascorbic acid, for example) present in the alimentary canal, and dietary iron intake. If iron intake is deficient, the body gradually depletes its iron stores, causing decreased hemoglobin levels and, eventually, signs and symptoms of iron deficiency anemia.

Test results
LABORATORY
- Serum hemoglobin (males, less than 12 g/dl; females, less than 10 g/dl) are low or mean corpuscular hemoglobin is decreased (in severe anemia).
- Serum hematocrit is low (males, less than 47 ml/dl; females, less than 42 ml/dl).
- Serum iron levels with high binding capacity are low.
- Serum ferritin levels are low.
- Serum RBC count with microcytic and hypochromic cells is low (in early stages, RBC count may be normal, except in infants and children).

DIAGNOSTIC PROCEDURES
- Bone marrow studies reveal depleted or absent iron stores (done by staining) as well as normoblastic hyperplasia.
- GI studies, such as guaiac stool tests, barium swallow and enema, endoscopy, and sigmoidoscopy, rule out or confirm the diagnosis of bleeding causing the iron deficiency.

◆ TREATMENT

General
- Determination of underlying cause

Diet
- Nutritious, nonirritating foods

Activity
- No restrictions
- Planned rest periods

Medication
- Oral preparation of iron or a combination of iron and ascorbic acid
- I.M. iron in rare cases
- Total-dose I.V. infusions of supplemental iron for pregnant and elderly patients with severe disease

❖ NURSING CONSIDERATIONS

Nursing diagnoses
- Activity intolerance
- Delayed growth and development
- Fatigue
- Imbalanced nutrition: Less than body requirements
- Impaired gas exchange
- Impaired oral mucous membranes
- Ineffective tissue perfusion: Cardiopulmonary, cerebral

Key outcomes
The patient will:
- state an understanding of the need to increase activity level gradually
- express understanding of norms for growth and development
- express feelings of energy and decreased fatigue
- maintain weight without further loss
- maintain adequate ventilation
- exhibit improved or healed wounds or lesions
- maintain vital signs within prescribed limits during activity.

Nursing interventions
- Note the patient's signs or symptoms of decreased perfusion to vital organs.
- Provide oxygen therapy, as necessary.
- Assess the family's dietary habits for iron intake, noting the influence of childhood eating patterns, cultural food preferences, and family income on adequate nutrition.
- Ask the dietitian to give the patient nonirritating foods.
- As ordered, administer analgesics for headache and other discomfort.
- Evaluate the patient's drug history. Certain drugs, such as pancreatic enzymes and vitamin E, can interfere with iron metabolism and absorption; aspirin, steroids, and other drugs can cause GI bleeding.
- Provide frequent rest periods to decrease physical exhaustion. Plan activities so that the patient has sufficient rest between them.
- If the patient receives iron I.V., monitor the infusion rate carefully and observe for an allergic reaction.
- Use the Z-track injection method when administering iron I.M. to pre-

vent skin discoloration, scarring, and irritating iron deposits in the skin.
- Provide good nutrition and meticulous care of I.V. sites.

Monitoring
- Vital signs
- Compliance with prescribed iron supplement therapy
- Iron replacement overdose (see *Recognizing iron overdose*)

▶ PATIENT TEACHING

Be sure to cover:
- disorder, diagnosis, and treatment
- possible complications
- dangers of lead poisoning, especially if the patient reports pica
- importance of not stopping therapy even if the patient feels better
- absorption interference with milk or antacid of iron supplementation
- increased absorption with vitamin C
- avoidance of staining teeth by drinking liquid supplemental iron through a straw
- when to report adverse effects of iron therapy
- basics of a nutritionally balanced diet
- protection against infections because a weakened condition may increase susceptibility
- when to report signs of infection
- need for regular checkups
- compliance with prescribed treatment.

RECOGNIZING IRON OVERDOSE

Excessive iron replacement is demonstrated when such signs and symptoms as diarrhea, fever, severe stomach pain, nausea, and vomiting occur.

Notify the physician promptly when these signs and symptoms occur and administer prescribed treatments. For this acute condition, treatment includes chelation therapy, vigorous I.V. fluid replacement, gastric lavage, possible whole-bowel irrigation, and supplemental oxygen.

✸ RESOURCES

Organizations
Iron Disorders Institute: *www.irondisorders.org*
Mayo Clinic: *www.mayohealth.org*

Selected references
Holcomb, S. "Recognizing and Managing Anemia," *The Nurse Practitioner: The American Journal of Primary Health Care* 30(12):16-31, December 2005.

Kasper, D.L., et al., eds. *Harrison's Principles of Internal Medicine*, 16th ed. New York: McGraw-Hill Book Co., 2005.

McPhee, S.J., et al. *Current Medical Diagnosis and Treatment.* New York: McGraw-Hill Book Co., 2007.

Anemia, pernicious

● OVERVIEW

Description
- Characterized by decreased gastric production of hydrochloric acid and deficiency of intrinsic factor, essential for vitamin B_{12} absorption
- Deficiency of vitamin B_{12} that causes serious neurologic, psychological, gastric, and intestinal abnormalities
- Also known as *Addison's anemia*

Pathophysiology
- An inherited autoimmune response may cause gastric mucosal atrophy and resultant decreased hydrochloric acid and intrinsic factor production, a substance normally secreted by the parietal cells of the gastric mucosa.
- Intrinsic factor deficiency impairs vitamin B_{12} absorption.
- Vitamin B_{12} deficiency inhibits the growth of all cells, particularly red blood cells (RBCs), leading to insufficient and deformed RBCs with poor oxygen-carrying capacity.

Causes
- Genetic predisposition
- Secondary pernicious anemia that results from partial removal of the stomach
- Chronic gastric inflammation

Incidence
- In the United States, most common in New England and the Great Lakes region because of ethnic concentration
- Also common in Northern Europeans of fair complexion
- Rare in children, Blacks, and Asians
- Onset typically between ages 50 and 60; incidence increasing with advancing age

Common characteristics
- Weakness
- Beefy red, sore tongue
- Systemic signs of anemia

Complications
- Heart failure with severe anemia
- Myocardial ischemia
- Paralysis
- Psychotic behavior
- Loss of sphincter control of bowel and bladder
- Peptic ulcer disease

✳ ASSESSMENT

History
- Characteristic triad of symptoms: weakness; a beefy red, sore tongue; and numbness and tingling in the extremities
- May also complain of nausea, vomiting, anorexia, weight loss, flatulence, diarrhea, and constipation
- Peripheral numbness and paresthesia
- Light-headedness
- Headache
- Diplopia and blurred vision
- Taste
- Tinnitus

Physical findings
- Lips, gums, and tongue that appear markedly bloodless
- Slightly jaundiced sclera and pale to bright yellow skin
- Tachycardia
- Systolic murmur
- Enlarged liver and spleen
- Weakness in the extremities
- Disturbed position sense
- Lack of coordination
- Impaired fine finger movement
- Loss of bowel and bladder control
- Impotence (in males)
- Irritable, depressed, delirious, and ataxic
- Memory loss
- Positive Babinski's and Romberg's signs
- Optic muscle atrophy

Test results
LABORATORY
- Complete blood count reveals decreased hemoglobin levels (4 to 5 g/dl), decreased RBC count, and increased mean corpuscular volume (under 120 mm³); because larger-than-normal RBCs each contain increased amounts of hemoglobin, mean corpuscular hemoglobin concentration is also increased; white blood cell and platelet counts may be low with large, malformed platelets; serum vitamin B_{12} tests may show levels less than 0.1 µg/ml; serum lactate dehydrogenase tests may show elevated serum lactate dehydrogenase levels.

DIAGNOSTIC PROCEDURES
- Bone marrow studies reveal erythroid hyperplasia with increased numbers of megaloblasts but few normally developing RBCs.
- Gastric analysis shows an absence of free hydrochloric acid after histamine or pentagastrin injection.
- The Schilling test may reveal a urinary excretion of less than 3% in the first 24 hours in patients with pernicious anemia; it may also reveal normal excretion of vitamin B_{12} when repeated with intrinsic factor added.

◆ TREATMENT

General
- Based on underlying cause

Diet
- Well-balanced, including foods high in vitamin B_{12}
- Sodium and fluid restriction for heart failure

Activity
- If anemia causes extreme fatigue, bed rest until hemoglobin increases

Medication
- Early I.M. vitamin B_{12} replacement
- Maintenance levels (monthly) of vitamin B_{12} doses, after the patient's condition improves

❖ NURSING CONSIDERATIONS

Nursing diagnoses
- Activity intolerance
- Fatigue
- Imbalanced nutrition: Less than body requirements
- Impaired gas exchange
- Impaired oral mucous membranes
- Impaired physical mobility
- Ineffective tissue perfusion: Cardio-pulmonary
- Risk for infection
- Risk for injury

Key outcomes
The patient will:
- state his understanding of the need to increase activity level gradually
- express feelings of energy and decreased fatigue
- consume required caloric intake
- maintain adequate ventilation
- exhibit improved or healed wounds or lesions
- maintain joint mobility and range of motion
- modify lifestyle to minimize risk for decreased tissue perfusion
- remain free from signs and symptoms of infection
- remain free from injury.

Nursing interventions
- If the patient has severe anemia, plan activities, rest periods, and necessary diagnostic tests to conserve his energy.
- To ensure accurate Schilling test results, make sure that all urine excreted over a 24-hour period is collected.
- Provide a well-balanced diet, including foods high in vitamin B_{12}.
- Institute safety precautions to prevent falls.

Monitoring
- Vital signs
- Mental and neurologic status

▶ PATIENT TEACHING

Be sure to cover:
- protection against infections and when to report signs of infection
- when to report signs and symptoms of decreased perfusion to vital organs and symptoms of neuropathy
- avoidance of irritating foods
- avoidance of exposure to extreme heat or cold on the extremities
- continuation of vitamin B_{12} replacement even after symptoms subside
- proper injection techniques
- observance of and when to report confusion and irritability
- prevention of pernicious anemia, by taking vitamin B_{12} supplements, in patients who have had extensive gastric resections or who follow strict vegetarian diets.

✳ RESOURCES

Organizations
Mayo Clinic: *www.mayohealth.org*
National Institutes of Health: *www.nih.gov*

Selected references
Holcomb, S. "Recognizing and Managing Anemia," *The Nurse Practitioner: The American Journal of Primary Health Care* 30(12):16-31, December 2005.

Kasper, D.L., et al., eds. *Harrison's Principles of Internal Medicine*, 16th ed. New York: McGraw-Hill Book Co., 2005.

McPhee, S.J., et al. *Current Medical Diagnosis and Treatment*. New York: McGraw-Hill Book Co., 2007.

Anemia, sickle cell

OVERVIEW

Description
- Congenital hemolytic disease that results from a defective hemoglobin (Hb) molecule (HbS) that causes red blood cells (RBCs) to become sickle shaped
- Impairs circulation, resulting in chronic ill health (fatigue, dyspnea on exertion, swollen joints), periodic crises, long-term complications, and premature death
- No cure

Pathophysiology
- The abnormal HbS found in the patient's RBCs becomes insoluble whenever hypoxia occurs.
- The RBCs become rigid, rough, and elongated, forming a crescent or sickle shape.
- Sickling can produce hemolysis (cell destruction).
- The altered cells accumulate in capillaries and smaller blood vessels, making the blood more viscous.
- Normal circulation is impaired, causing pain, tissue infarctions, and swelling.

Causes
- Homozygous inheritance of the HbS-producing gene (defective Hb gene from each parent)

Incidence
- Most common in tropical Africans and in people of African descent
- About 1 in 10 blacks carrying the abnormal gene; if two such carriers have offspring, each child has 1-in-4 chance of developing the disease
- Occurs in one in every 500 blacks in the United States
- Also occurs in Puerto Rico, Turkey, India, the Middle East, and the Mediterranean area

Common characteristics
- Chronic fatigue
- Intense pain due to vascular occlusion in a sickling episode
- Frequent bacterial infections due to involvement of spleen
- Systemic signs of anemia

Complications
- Chronic obstructive pulmonary disease
- Heart failure
- Retinopathy
- Nephropathy

ASSESSMENT

History
- Asymptomatic until after age 6 months
- Chronic fatigue
- Unexplained dyspnea or dyspnea on exertion
- Joint swelling
- Aching bones
- Chest pain
- Ischemic leg ulcers
- Increased susceptibility to infection
- Pulmonary infarctions and cardiomegaly

Physical findings
- Jaundice or pallor
- May appear small in stature for age
- Delayed growth and puberty
- Spiderlike body build (narrow shoulders and hips, long extremities, curved spine, and barrel chest) in adult
- Tachycardia
- Hepatomegaly and, in children, splenomegaly
- Systolic and diastolic murmurs
- Sleepiness with difficulty awakening
- Hematuria
- Pale lips, tongue, palms, and nail beds
- Body temperature over 104° F (40° C) or a temperature of 100° F (37.8° C) that persists for 2 or more days

IN PAINFUL CRISIS
- Most common crisis and hallmark of the disease; usually appears periodically after age 5, characterized by severe abdominal, thoracic, muscle, or bone pain and, possibly, increased jaundice, dark urine, and a low-grade fever

IN APLASTIC CRISIS
- Pallor, lethargy, sleepiness, dyspnea, possible coma, markedly decreased bone marrow activity, and RBC hemolysis

IN ACUTE SEQUESTRATION CRISIS
- Occurs in infants between ages 8 months and 2 years; causes lethargy, pallor and, if untreated, progresses to hypovolemic shock and death

IN HEMOLYTIC CRISIS
- Liver congestion and hepatomegaly

Test results
LABORATORY
- Stained blood smear shows sickle cells and Hb electrophoresis shows HbS. (Electrophoresis should be done on umbilical cord blood samples at birth to provide sickle cell disease screening for all neonates at risk.)
- RBC count is low, white blood cell and platelet counts are elevated, erythrocyte sedimentation rate is decreased, and serum iron levels are increased.
- Complete blood count (CBC) reveals decreased RBC survival and reticulocytosis and normal or low Hb levels.

IMAGING
- A lateral chest X-ray detects the characteristic "Lincoln log" deformity. (This spinal abnormality develops in many adults and some adolescents with sickle cell anemia, leaving the vertebrae resembling logs that form the corner of a cabin.)

DIAGNOSTIC PROCEDURES
- Corkscrew or comma-shaped vessels in the conjunctivae are detected by an ophthalmoscopic examination.

TREATMENT

General
- Avoidance of extreme temperatures
- Avoidance of stress

Diet
- Well-balanced
- Adequate amounts of folic acid-rich foods
- Adequate fluid intake

Activity
- Bed rest with crises
- As tolerated

Medication
- Vaccines, such as polyvalent pneumococcal vaccine and *Haemophilus influenzae* B vaccine
- Anti-infectives
- Analgesics
- Iron supplements

- Transfusion of packed RBCs, if Hb level decreases suddenly or if condition deteriorates rapidly
- Sedation and administration of analgesics, blood transfusion, oxygen therapy, and large amounts of oral or I.V. fluids, in an acute sequestration crisis

❖ NURSING CONSIDERATIONS

Nursing diagnoses
- Acute pain
- Deficient knowledge (sickle cell anemia)
- Delayed growth and development
- Disturbed body image
- Fatigue
- Hyperthermia
- Impaired gas exchange
- Impaired tissue integrity
- Ineffective tissue perfusion: Peripheral
- Risk for deficient fluid volume

Key outcomes
The patient will:
- express feelings of comfort and decreased pain
- verbalize understanding of disorder and treatment measures
- demonstrate age-appropriate skills and behaviors to the extent possible
- verbalize feelings about changes in body image
- express feelings of energy and decreased fatigue
- exhibit a temperature within an acceptable range
- exhibit adequate ventilation
- maintain normal skin color and temperature
- maintain normal peripheral pulses
- maintain balanced fluid volume where input equals output.

Nursing interventions
- Encourage the patient to talk about his fears and concerns.
- If a male patient develops sudden, painful priapism, reassure him that such episodes are common and have no permanent harmful effects.
- Ensure that the patient receives adequate amounts of folic acid-rich foods, such as leafy green vegetables.
- Encourage adequate fluid intake.

- Apply warm compresses, warmed thermal blankets, and warming pads or mattresses to painful areas of the patient's body, unless he has neuropathy.
- Administer analgesics and antipyretics, as necessary.
- When cultures demonstrate the presence of infection, administer antibiotics, as ordered.
- Administer prophylactic antibiotics, as ordered.
- Use strict sterile technique when performing treatments.
- Encourage bed rest with the head of the bed elevated to decrease tissue oxygen demand.
- Administer oxygen, as needed.
- Administer blood transfusions, as ordered.
- If the patient requires general anesthesia for surgery, help ensure that he receives adequate ventilation to prevent hypoxic crisis.

Monitoring
- Vital signs
- Intake and output
- CBC and other laboratory study results

▶ PATIENT TEACHING

Be sure to cover:
- avoidance of tight clothing that restricts circulation
- conditions that provoke hypoxia, such as strenuous exercise, vasoconstricting medications, cold temperatures, unpressurized aircraft, and high altitude
- importance of normal childhood immunizations, meticulous wound care, good oral hygiene, regular dental checkups, and a balanced diet as safeguards against infection
- need for prompt treatment of infection
- need to increase fluid intake to prevent dehydration, which can cause increased blood viscosity; tell parents to encourage a child to drink more fluids other than milk, especially in the summer
- reassurance that the adolescent will grow and mature
- symptoms of vaso-occlusive crisis
- need for hospitalization in a vaso-occlusive crisis in which I.V. fluids, par-

enteral analgesics, oxygen therapy, and blood transfusions may be necessary
- need to inform all health care providers that the patient has this disease before undergoing any treatment, especially major surgery
- pregnancy and the disease
- balanced diet, including folic acid supplements during pregnancy.

Discharge planning
- Refer parents of children with sickle cell anemia for genetic counseling to answer their questions about the risk to future offspring.
- Refer other family members for genetic counseling to determine if they're heterozygote carriers.
- If necessary, refer the patient for psychological counseling to help him cope.
- Refer women with sickle cell anemia for birth control counseling.

✷ RESOURCES

Organizations
Sickle Cell Disease Association of America: www.sicklecelldisease.org
U.S. Food and Drug Administration: www.fda.gov

Selected references
Kasper, D.L., et al., eds. *Harrison's Principles of Internal Medicine*, 16th ed. New York: McGraw-Hill Book Co., 2005.
Perry, V. "Myths & Facts: About Sickle Cell Disease," *Nursing2005* 35(12): 27, December 2005.
Platt, A., and Beasley, J. "Puzzled about Sickle Cell Disease?" *Nursing Made Incredibly Easy* 3(6):60-64, November-December 2005

Anemia, sideroblastic

⬤ OVERVIEW

Description
- Group of heterogenous disorders with a common defect that causes failure to use iron in hemoglobin synthesis despite the availability of adequate iron stores
- Can be acquired or hereditary; the acquired form, in turn, can be primary or secondary

Pathophysiology
- Normoblasts fail to use iron to synthesize hemoglobin.
- Iron is deposited in the mitochondria of normoblasts, rather than in the hemoglobin molecules.
- Iron toxicity can cause organ damage.

Causes
- Hereditary form possibly due to a rare genetic defect on the X chromosome
- Acquired form possibly secondary to ingestion of or exposure to toxins, such as alcohol and lead, or to drugs, such as isoniazid and chloramphenicol
- Complication of neoplastic and inflammatory diseases, such as lymphoma, rheumatoid arthritis, lupus erythematosus, multiple myeloma, tuberculosis, and severe infections
- In primary acquired form, cause unknown

Incidence
- Most prevalent in young males; females are carriers, but usually show no signs of disorder
- Appears to be transmitted by X-linked inheritance
- Primary acquired form most common in elderly people, but occasionally develops in young people

Common characteristics
- Anorexia and fatigue
- Systemic signs of anemia

Complications
- Severe cardiac, hepatic, splenic, and pancreatic disease
- Acute myelogenous leukemia

✳ ASSESSMENT

History
- May reveal anorexia, fatigue, weakness, dizziness, and dyspnea

Physical findings
- Pale skin and oral mucous membranes
- Slight jaundice
- Petechiae or bruises
- Enlarged lymph nodes
- Hepatosplenomegaly

Test results
LABORATORY
- Red blood cell (RBC) indices show erythrocytes to be hypochromic or normochromic and slightly macrocytic; RBC precursors may be megaloblastic, with anisocytosis (abnormal variation in RBC size) and poikilocytosis (abnormal variation in RBC shape).
- Vitamin B_{12} and folic acid levels are normal unless combined anemias are present.
- Serum reticulocyte count is low because young cells die in the marrow.

DIAGNOSTIC PROCEDURES
- Ringed sideroblasts on microscopic examination of bone marrow aspirate stained with Prussian blue dye confirms the diagnosis. (See *Ringed sideroblast.*)

RINGED SIDEROBLAST

Electron micocroscopy shows large iron deposits in the mitochondria that surround the nucleus, forming the characteristic ringed sideroblast.

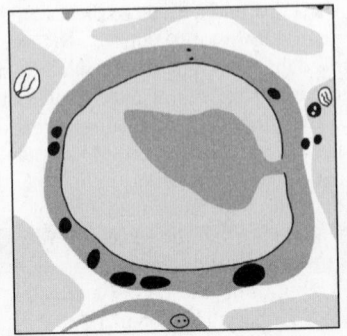

◆ TREATMENT

General
- Treatment dependent on underlying cause; for example, in acquired secondary form, causative drug or toxin removed
- Phlebotomy

Diet
- Nutritious
- No restrictions

Activity
- Frequent rest periods

Medication
IN HEREDITARY SIDEROBLASTIC ANEMIA
- High doses of pyridoxine
IN PRIMARY ACQUIRED ANEMIA
- Transfusion or high doses of androgens
IN CHRONIC IRON OVERLOAD
- Deferoxamine

Nursing diagnoses
- Decreased cardiac output
- Fatigue
- Impaired oral mucous membranes
- Impaired skin integrity
- Risk for infection
- Risk for injury

Key outcomes
The patient will:
- maintain adequate cardiac ouput
- express feelings of energy and decreased fatigue
- show improvement or healing in wounds or lesions
- maintain skin integrity
- remain free from signs and symptoms of infection
- remain free from injury.

Nursing interventions
- Provide frequent rest periods. Plan activities and diagnostic tests so the patient can rest in between.
- Institute safety measures to prevent falls.
- Administer medications, as ordered.
- Provide comfort measures; have the patient perform relaxation techniques to facilitate coping.
- Administer ordered blood transfusions. Notify the physician if signs of a transfusion reaction occur.
- If the patient has jaundice or pruritus, provide meticulous skin care.
- Inquire about possible exposure to lead in the home (especially for children) or on the job.

Monitoring
- Vital signs
- Complications
- Response to treatment
- Signs and symptoms of neuropathy
- Signs and symptoms of decreased perfusion

Be sure to cover:
- prescribed treatment and possible complications
- importance of continuing prescribed therapy, even after the patient begins to feel better
- precautions for parents about house paint and not allowing children to eat paint chips because of the possibility of lead
- recognition of and when to report adrenergic adverse effects, if androgens are used as part of the treatment
- phlebotomy (if scheduled)
- recognition of and when to report signs and symptoms of heart failure
- need for proper hygiene and other measures to guard against infections and when to report signs and symptoms of infection.

Discharge planning
- Identify patients who abuse alcohol and refer them for appropriate therapy.

Organizations
Iron Disorders Institute: *www.irondisorders.org*
Mayo Clinic: *www.mayohealth.org*

Selected references
Kasper, D.L., et al., eds. *Harrison's Principles of Internal Medicine*, 16th ed. New York: McGraw-Hill Book Co., 2005.
McPhee, S. J., et al. *Current Medical Diagnosis and Treatment*. New York: McGraw-Hill Book Co., 2007.

Aneurysm, abdominal aortic

● OVERVIEW

Description
- Abnormal dilation in the arterial wall
- Generally occurs in the aorta between the renal arteries and iliac branches
- Can be fusiform (spindle-shaped), saccular (pouchlike), or dissecting

Pathophysiology
- Focal weakness occurs in the tunica media layer of the aorta.
- The tunica intima and tunica adventitia layers begin to stretch outward due to degenerative changes.
- Blood pressure within the aorta progressively weakens vessel walls and enlarges the aneurysm.

Causes
- Arteriosclerosis or atherosclerosis (95%)
- Trauma
- Syphilis; other infections

Incidence
- Seven times more common in hypertensive men than in women
- Most common in whites ages 50 to 80

Common characteristics
- Ninety-eight percent located in the infrarenal aorta
- Most develop at bifurcations

Complications
- Hemorrhage
- Shock
- Dissection

✳ ASSESSMENT

History
- Asymptomatic until the aneurysm enlarges and compresses surrounding tissue
- Syncope when aneurysm ruptures
- When clot forms and bleeding stops, may again be asymptomatic or have abdominal pain because of bleeding into the peritoneum

Physical findings
INTACT ANEURYSM
- Gnawing, generalized, steady abdominal pain
- Lower back pain unaffected by movement
- Gastric or abdominal fullness
- Sudden onset of severe abdominal pain or lumbar pain with radiation to flank and groin

RUPTURED ANEURYSM
- Into the peritoneal cavity, severe, persistent abdominal and back pain
- Into the duodenum, GI bleeding with massive hematemesis and melena
- May note a pulsating mass in the periumbilical area: don't palpate
- Mottled skin; poor distal perfusion
- Decreased level of consciousness
- Diaphoresis
- Hypotension
- Tachycardia
- Oliguria
- Distended abdomen
- Ecchymosis or hematoma in the abdominal, flank, or groin area
- Paraplegia if aneurysm rupture reduces blood flow to the spine
- Systolic bruit over the aorta
- Tenderness over affected area
- Absent peripheral pulses distally

Test results
IMAGING
- Abdominal ultrasonography or echocardiography can determine the size, shape, and location of the aneurysm.
- Anteroposterior and lateral abdominal X-rays can detect aortic calcification, which outlines the mass, at least 75% of the time.
- Computed tomography scan can visualize aneurysm's effect on nearby organs.
- Aortography shows condition of vessels proximal and distal to the aneurysm and extent of aneurysm; aneurysm diameter may be underestimated because it shows only the flow channel and not the surrounding clot.

◆ TREATMENT

General
- If aneurysm is small and asymptomatic, surgery delayed
- Careful control of hypertension
- Fluid and blood replacement

Diet
- Weight reduction, if appropriate
- Low-fat

Activity
- No restrictions unless surgery

Medication
- Beta-adrenergic blockers
- Antihypertensives
- Analgesics
- Antibiotics

Surgery
- Resection of large aneurysms or those that produce symptoms
- Bypass procedures for poor perfusion distal to aneurysm

✤ NURSING CONSIDERATIONS

Nursing diagnoses
- Acute pain
- Anxiety
- Decreased cardiac output
- Deficient fluid volume
- Impaired gas exchange
- Impaired physical mobility
- Impaired skin integrity
- Ineffective tissue perfusion: Cardio-pulmonary, renal

Key outcomes
The patient will:
- express feelings of increased comfort and decreased pain
- express feelings of decreased anxiety
- maintain adequate cardiac output
- maintain adequate urine output (output equivalent to intake)
- maintain adequate ventilation
- maintain optimal mobility within the confines of the disorder
- maintain skin integrity
- maintain palpable pulses distal to the aneurysm site and hemodynamic stability.

Nursing interventions
IN A NONACUTE SITUATION
- Allow the patient to express his fears and concerns and identify effective coping strategies.
- Offer the patient and family members psychological support.
- Before elective surgery, weigh the patient, insert an indwelling urinary catheter and an I.V. line, and assist with insertion of the arterial line and pulmonary artery catheter to monitor hemodynamic balance.
- Give prophylactic antibiotics, as ordered.

IN AN ACUTE SITUATION
- Insert an I.V. line with at least a 14G needle to facilitate blood replacement.
- As ordered, obtain blood samples for ordered laboratory tests.
- Administer ordered medication.

◈ **NURSING ALERT** Be alert for signs of rupture, which may be immediately fatal. If rupture does occur, get the patient to surgery immediately. Medical antishock trousers may be used while transporting him to surgery.

AFTER SURGERY
- Assess peripheral pulses for graft failure or occlusion.
- Watch for signs of bleeding retroperitoneally from the graft site.
- Maintain blood pressure in prescribed range with fluids and medications.

◈ **NURSING ALERT** Assess for severe back pain, which can indicate that the graft is tearing.
- Have the patient cough, or suction the endotracheal tube, as needed.
- Provide frequent turning, and assist with ambulation as soon as he's able.

Monitoring
- Cardiac rhythm and hemodynamics
- Vital signs, intake and hourly output, neurologic status, and arterial blood gas levels
- Respirations and breath sounds at least every hour
- Daily weight
- Fluid status
- Nasogastric intubation for patency, amount, and type of drainage
- Signs and symptoms of renal failure
- Abdominal dressings
- Wound site for infection

▶ PATIENT TEACHING

Be sure to cover:
- surgical procedure and the expected postoperative care
- importance of taking all medications as prescribed and carrying a list of medications at all times, in case of an emergency
- physical activity restrictions until medically cleared by the physician
- need for regular examination and ultrasound checks to monitor progression of the aneurysm, if surgery wasn't performed.

✳ RESOURCES

Organizations
American Heart Association: *www.americanheart.org*
National Heart, Lung and Blood Institute: *www.nhlbi.nih.gov*

Selected references
Alspach, J., ed. *AACN Core Curriculum for Critical Care Nursing*, 6th ed. Philadelphia: W.B. Saunders Co., 2006.
Beese-Bjurstrom, S. "Hidden Danger: Aortic Aneurysms and Dissections," *Nursing2004* 34(2):36-42, February 2004.
Dambro, M.R. *Griffith's Five-Minute Clinical Consult.* Philadelphia: Lippincott Williams & Wilkins, 2006.
Gendreau-Webb, R. "Is it a Kidney Stone or Abdominal Aortic Aneurysm?" *Nursing2006* 36(5 Suppl): 22-24, Spring 2006.

Aneurysm, thoracic aortic

● OVERVIEW

Description
- Abnormal widening of the ascending, transverse, or descending part of the aorta
- May be saccular (outpouching), fusiform (spindle-shaped), or dissecting
- Occurs in about 60% of patients, is usually an emergency, and has a poor prognosis

Pathophysiology
- The condition results in a circumferential or transverse tear of the aortic wall intima, usually within the medial layer.

Causes
- Atherosclerosis
- Blunt chest trauma
- Bacterial infections, usually at an atherosclerotic plaque
- Coarctation of the aorta
- Syphilis infection
- Rheumatic vasculitis

Risk factors
- Cigarette smoking
- Hypertension

Incidence
- Ascending thoracic aorta most common site
- Occurs predominantly in men younger than age 60 who have coexisting hypertension
- Descending thoracic aortic aneurysms most common in younger patients who have had chest trauma

Common characteristics
- Asymptomatic until dissection

Complications
- Cardiac tamponade
- Dissection

✳ ASSESSMENT

History
- Asymptomatic until aneurysm expands and begins to dissect
- Sudden pain and possibly syncope

Physical findings
- Pallor, diaphoresis, dyspnea, cyanosis, leg weakness, or transient paralysis
- Abrupt onset of intermittent neurologic deficits
- Abrupt loss of radial and femoral pulses and right and left carotid pulses
- Increasing area of flatness over the heart, suggesting cardiac tamponade and hemopericardium

IN DISSECTING ASCENDING ANEURYSM
- Pain with a boring, tearing, or ripping sensation in the thorax or the right anterior chest; may extend to the neck, shoulders, lower back, and abdomen
- Pain most intense at onset
- Murmur of aortic insufficiency, a diastolic murmur
- Pericardial friction rub (if hemopericardium present)
- Blood pressure possibly normal or significantly elevated, with a large difference in systolic blood pressure between the right and left arms

IN DISSECTING DESCENDING ANEURYSM
- Sharp, tearing pain located between the shoulder blades that usually radiates to the chest
- Carotid and radial pulses present and equal bilaterally
- Systolic blood pressure equal
- May detect bilateral crackles and rhonchi if pulmonary edema is present

IN DISSECTING TRANSVERSE ANEURYSM
- Sharp, boring, and tearing pain that radiates to the shoulders
- Hoarseness, dyspnea, throat pain, dysphagia, and a dry cough

Test results
LABORATORY
- Hemoglobin levels are normal or decreased from blood loss caused by a leaking aneurysm.

IMAGING
- Posteroanterior and oblique chest X-rays show widening of the aorta and mediastinum.
- Aortography shows lumen of the aneurysm and its size and location.
- Magnetic resonance imaging and computed tomography scan help confirm and locate the presence of aortic dissection.

DIAGNOSTIC PROCEDURES
- Electrocardiography helps rule out the presence of myocardial infarction.
- Echocardiography may help identify dissecting aneurysm of the aortic root.
- Transesophageal echocardiography can be used to measure the aneurysm in the ascending and descending aorta.

◆ TREATMENT

General
- I.V. fluids and whole blood transfusions, if needed

Diet
- Weight reduction, if appropriate
- Low-fat

Activity
- No restrictions unless surgery

Medication
- Beta-adrenergic blockers
- Antihypertensives
- Negative inotropic agents
- Analgesics
- Antibiotics

Surgery
- Surgical resection with a Dacron or Teflon graft replacement

◆ NURSING CONSIDERATIONS

Nursing diagnoses

- Acute pain
- Anxiety
- Decreased cardiac output
- Hopelessness
- Ineffective breathing pattern
- Ineffective tissue perfusion: Cardio-pulmonary, renal
- Risk for deficient fluid volume
- Risk for infection

Key outcomes

The patient will:
- express feelings of comfort and decreased pain
- express feelings of decreased anxiety
- maintain adequate cardiac output and hemodynamic stability
- express feelings of hope
- maintain an effective breathing pattern
- maintain tissue perfusion and oxygenation
- maintain adequate fluid volume
- remain free from signs and symptoms of infection.

Nursing interventions

- In a nonemergency situation, allow him to express his fears and concerns and identify and use effective coping strategies.
- Offer the patient and family psychological support.
- Give analgesics to relieve pain, as ordered.

AFTER REPAIR OF THORACIC ANEURYSM

- Maintain blood pressure in prescribed range with fluids and medication.
- Administer analgesics, as ordered.
- After stabilization of vital signs, encourage and assist the patient in turning, coughing, and deep breathing.
- Help the patient walk as soon as he's able.
- Assist the patient with range-of-motion leg exercises.

Monitoring

- Vital signs and hemodynamics
- Chest tube drainage
- Heart and lung sounds
- Ordered laboratory tests
- Distal pulses
- Level of consciousness and pain
- Signs of infection
- I.V. therapy and intake and output

◈ **NURSING ALERT** After surgical repair, monitor for signs that resemble those of the initial dissecting aneurysm, suggesting a tear at the graft site.

▶ PATIENT TEACHING

Be sure to cover:
- disorder, diagnosis, and treatment
- procedure and expected postoperative care, if surgery is scheduled
- compliance with antihypertensive therapy, including the need for such drugs and the expected adverse effects
- monitoring of blood pressure
- when to call the physician if the patient has sharp pain in the chest or back of the neck.

Discharge planning

- Refer the patient to a smoking-cessation program, if indicated.

✱ RESOURCES

Organizations

American Heart Association: *www.americanheart.org*
The Aneurysm Center—Heartcenter Online for Patients: *www.heartcenteronline.com*

Selected references

lspach, J., ed. *AACN Core Curriculum for Critical Care Nursing*, 6th ed. Philadelphia: W.B. Saunders Co., 2006.

Kasper, D.L., et al., eds. *Harrison's Principles of Internal Medicine*, 16th ed. New York: McGraw-Hill Book Co., 2005.

Kline, D.G. "Thoracic Aortic Aneurysm," *Journal of Cardiovascular Nursing* 20(4):245-50, July-August 2005.

Wung, S., and Aouizerat, B. "Newly Mapped Gene for Thoracic Aortic Aneurysm and Dissection," *Journal of Cardiovascular Nursing* 19(6):409-16, November-December 2004.

Aneurysm, ventricular

● OVERVIEW

Description
- An outpouching, almost always of the left ventricle, that produces ventricular wall dysfunction
- May develop within days to weeks after myocardial infarction (MI) or may be delayed for years

Pathophysiology
- When MI destroys a large muscular section of the left ventricle, necrosis reduces the ventricular wall to a thin sheath of fibrous tissue.
- Under intracardiac pressure, the thin sheath stretches and forms a separate noncontractile sac (aneurysm).
- Abnormal muscle wall movement accompanies ventricular aneurysm.
- During systolic ejection, the abnormal muscle wall movements cause the remaining normally functioning myocardial fibers to increase the force of contraction to maintain stroke volume and cardiac output.
- At the same time, a portion of the stroke volume is lost to passive distention of the noncontractile sac.

Causes
- MI

Incidence
- Occurs in about 20% of patients after MI

Common characteristics
- Occurs after MI

Complications
- Ventricular arrhythmias
- Cerebral embolization
- Heart failure

✳ ASSESSMENT

History
- Previous MI
- Dyspnea
- Fatigue

Physical findings
- Edema
- Visible or palpable systolic precordial bulge
- Distended neck veins, if heart failure is present
- Irregular peripheral pulse rhythm
- Arrhythmias such as premature ventricular contractions
- Pulsus alternans
- Double, diffuse, or displaced apical impulse
- Gallop rhythm
- Crackles and rhonchi

Test results
IMAGING
- Two-dimensional echocardiography demonstrates abnormal motion in the left ventricular wall.
- Left ventriculography reveals left ventricular enlargement, with an area of akinesia or dyskinesia (during cineangiography) and diminished cardiac function.
- Chest X-rays may disclose an abnormal bulge distorting the heart's contour if the aneurysm is large; X-rays may be normal if the aneurysm is small.
- Noninvasive nuclear cardiology scan may indicate the site of infarction and suggest the area of aneurysm.

DIAGNOSTIC PROCEDURES
- Electrocardiography may show persistent ST-T wave elevations.

◆ TREATMENT

General
- Dependent on the size of the aneurysm and the presence of complications
- May require only routine medical examination to follow the patient's condition
- May require aggressive measures, such as cardioversion, defibrillation, and endotracheal intubation

Diet
- Weight reduction, if appropriate
- Low-fat

Activity
- No restrictions, unless surgery

Medication
- Antiarrhythmics
- Cardiac glycosides
- Diuretics
- Fluid and electrolyte replacement
- Analgesics
- Antihypertensives
- Nitrates
- Anticoagulation

Surgery
- Embolectomy
- Aneurysmectomy with myocardial revascularization

❖ NURSING CONSIDERATIONS

Nursing diagnoses
- Activity intolerance
- Anxiety
- Decreased cardiac output
- Excess fluid volume
- Fatigue
- Fear
- Impaired gas exchange
- Ineffective breathing pattern
- Ineffective tissue perfusion: Cardio-pulmonary
- Risk for infection

Key outcomes
The patient will:
- carry out activities of daily living without excess fatigue or exhaustion
- express feelings of decreased anxiety
- maintain adequate cardiac output
- maintain adequate fluid balance
- express feelings of increased energy and decreased fatigue
- express feelings of decreased fear
- maintain adequate ventilation
- maintain an effective breathing pattern
- maintain hemodynamic stability
- remain free from signs and symptoms of infection.

Nursing interventions
- Administer medications, as ordered.
- Prepare for surgery, if indicated.

NURSING ALERT Be alert for sudden changes in sensorium that may indicate cerebral embolization and for any signs that suggest renal failure or MI.
- Provide psychological support for the patient and family members.

Monitoring
IN HEART FAILURE
- Vital signs and heart sounds
- Cardiac rhythm, especially for ventricular arrhythmias
- Intake and output and fluid and electrolyte balance
- Blood urea nitrogen and serum creatinine levels

AFTER SURGERY
- Pulmonary artery catheter pressures
- Signs and symptoms of infection
- Type and amount of chest tube drainage

▶ PATIENT TEACHING

Be sure to cover:
- disorder, diagnosis, and treatment
- medication administration, dosage, and possible adverse effects
- when to notify the physician
- expected postoperative care, if the patient is scheduled to undergo resection
- monitoring pulse irregularity and rate changes.

Discharge planning
Refer the patient (or family) to a:
- community-based cardiopulmonary resuscitation training program.
- weight-reduction program, if indicated.
- smoking-cessation program, if indicated.

✳ RESOURCES

Organizations
American Heart Association:
www.americanheart.org
The Aneurysm Center—Heartcenter Online for Patients:
www.heartcenteronline.com

Selected references
Chulay, M., et al. *AACN Essentials of Critical Care Nursing.* New York: McGraw-Hill Medical, 2006.

Kasper, D.L., et al., eds. *Harrison's Principles of Internal Medicine*, 16th ed. New York: McGraw-Hill Book Co., 2005.

The Merck Manual of Diagnosis & Therapy, 18th ed. Whitehouse Station, N.J.: Merck & Co., Inc., 2006.

Ankylosing spondylitis

● OVERVIEW

Description
- Primarily affects sacroiliac, apophyseal, and costocervical joints and adjacent ligamentous or tendinous attachments to bone
- Usually occurs as a primary disorder; may occur secondary to Reiter's syndrome, psoriatic arthritis, or inflammatory bowel disease
- Also called *rheumatoid spondylitis* or *Marie-Strümpell disease*

Pathophysiology
- The disorder begins in the sacroiliac joint, gradually progresses to the lumbar, thoracic, and cervical spine.
- Bone and cartilage deterioration leads to fibrous tissue formation and eventual fusion of the spine or peripheral joints.

Causes
- Unknown
- Familial tendency
- Initial inflammation may result from immune system activation by bacterial infection

Incidence
- Affects men 2 to 3 times more often than women
- Overlooked or missed in women as they have more peripheral joint involvement

Common characteristics
- Symptoms can unpredictably remit, exacerbate, or arrest at any stage

Complications
- Atlantoaxial subluxation
- Deposits of amyloid material in the kidneys, which may lead to renal impairment or failure

✳ ASSESSMENT

History
- Intermittent low back pain most severe in the morning or after inactivity and relieved by exercise
- Mild fatigue, fever, anorexia, and weight loss
- May describe pain in shoulders, hips, knees, and ankles
- Pain over the symphysis pubis, which may lead to its being mistaken for pelvic inflammatory disease (see *Detecting spondylitis in women*)

Physical findings
- Stiffness or limited motion of the lumbar spine
- Pain and limited chest expansion
- Kyphosis
- Iritis
- Warmth, swelling, or tenderness of affected joints
- Small joints, such as toes, possibly becoming sausage-shaped
- Aortic murmur caused by regurgitation
- Cardiomegaly
- Upper lobe pulmonary fibrosis, which mimics tuberculosis, that may reduce vital capacity to 70% or less of predicted volume

Test results
- A diagnosis of primary ankylosing spondylitis requires meeting established criteria. (See *Diagnosing primary ankylosing spondylitis.*)

LABORATORY
- HLA antigen typing test shows serum findings that include HLA-B27 in about 95% of patients with primary ankylosing spondylitis and up to 80% of patients with secondary disease.
- Serum rheumatoid factor tests show the absence of rheumatoid factor, which helps to rule out rheumatoid arthritis, which has similar symptoms.
- Serum alkaline phosphate and creatine kinase tests show slightly elevated erythrocyte sedimentation rate, serum alkaline phosphate levels, and creatine kinase levels in active disease.
- Serum immunoglobulin profile shows elevated serum IgA levels.

IMAGING
- X-ray studies define characteristic changes, such as bilateral sacroiliac involvement (the hallmark of the disease); blurring of the joints' bony margins in early disease; patchy sclerosis with superficial bony erosions; eventual squaring of vertebral bodies; and "bamboo spine" with complete ankylosis.

◆ TREATMENT

General
- Good posture; stretching and deep-breathing exercises
- If appropriate, braces and lightweight supports
- Heat, warm showers, baths, ice, and nerve stimulation

Diet
- Nutritious
- No restrictions

Activity
- As tolerated

Medication
- Nonsteroidal anti-inflammatory drugs

Surgery
- Hip replacement surgery, with severe hip involvement
- Spinal wedge osteotomy, with severe spinal involvement

DETECTING SPONDYLITIS IN WOMEN

Because ankylosing spondylitis seldom occurs in women, the disorder may be easily overlooked. Typically, if a woman's symptoms include pelvic pain, diagnosticians suspect pelvic inflammatory disease rather than ankylosing spondylitis. That's one reason to assess carefully if the female patient has apparent pelvic inflammatory disease but culture results identify no apparent cause. In compiling a thorough health and social history, investigate a possible family history of ankylosing spondylitis. Otherwise, misdiagnosis can lead to unwarranted invasive tests and treatments and cause the patient needless anxiety related to contracting a sexually transmitted disease.

NURSING CONSIDERATIONS

Nursing diagnoses
- Activity intolerance
- Chronic pain
- Disturbed body image
- Fatigue
- Impaired gas exchange
- Impaired physical mobility
- Powerlessness
- Risk for injury

Key outcomes
The patient will:
- express feelings of increased energy
- express feelings of comfort and decreased pain
- verbalize feelings about changes in body image
- report a decrease in fatigue
- maintain adequate ventilation and oxygenation
- maintain optimal mobility within the confines of the disorder
- recognize limitations imposed by illness and express feelings about these limitations
- identify factors that increase the potential for injury.

Nursing interventions
- Keep in mind the patient's limited range of motion (ROM) when planning self-care tasks and activities.
- Offer support and reassurance.
- Give analgesics, as ordered.
- Apply heat locally and massage as indicated.
- Have the patient perform active ROM exercises.
- Pace periods of exercise and rest to help the patient achieve comfortable energy levels and lung oxygenation.
- If treatment includes surgery, ensure proper body alignment and positioning.
- Involve other caregivers, such as a social worker, visiting nurse, and dietitian.

Monitoring
- Mobility and comfort level
- Respiratory status
- Heart sounds

PATIENT TEACHING

Be sure to cover:
- avoidance of physical activity that places stress on the back such as lifting heavy objects
- importance of standing upright; sitting upright in a high, straight-backed chair; and avoiding leaning over a desk
- importance of sleeping in a prone position on a hard mattress and avoiding using pillows under the neck or knees
- avoidance of prolonged walking, standing, sitting, or driving
- regular stretching and deep-breathing exercises; swimming on a regular basis, if possible
- measurement of patient's height every 3 to 4 months to detect kyphosis
- nutrition and weight maintenance.

Discharge planning
Refer the patient to:
- physical therapy, as needed
- the Spondylitis Association of America or the Arthritis Foundation for additional support and information.

RESOURCES

Organizations
Arthritis Foundation: *www.arthritis.org*
Spondylitis Association of America: *www.spondylitis.org*

Selected references
Kasper, D.L., et al., eds. *Harrison's Principles of Internal Medicine*, 16th ed. New York: McGraw-Hill Book Co., 2005.
Kataria, R.K., and Brent, L.H., "Spondyloarthropathies," *American Family Physician* 69(12):2853-860, June 2004.
The Merck Manual of Diagnosis & Therapy, 18th ed. Whitehouse Station, N.J.: Merck & Co., Inc., 2006.

DIAGNOSING PRIMARY ANKYLOSING SPONDYLITIS

The following are the diagnostic criteria for primary ankylosing spondylitis. For a reliable diagnosis, the patient must meet:
- criterion 7 and any one of criteria 1 through 5 *or*
- any five of criteria 1 through 6 if he doesn't have criterion 7.

Seven criteria
1. Axial skeleton stiffness of at least 3 months' duration relieved by exercise
2. Lumbar pain that persists at rest
3. Thoracic cage pain of at least 3 months' duration that persists at rest
4. Past or current iritis
5. Decreased lumbar range of motion
6. Decreased chest expansion (age-related)
7. Bilateral, symmetrical sacroiliitis demonstrated by radiographic studies

Anorexia nervosa

● OVERVIEW

Description
- Self-imposed starvation resulting from a distorted body image and an intense and irrational fear of gaining weight
- Actual loss of appetite, which is rare
- May occur simultaneously with bulimia nervosa

Pathophysiology
- Decreased calorie intake depletes body fat and protein stores.
- Estrogen deficiency occurs (in women) due to lack of lipid substrate for synthesis, causing amenorrhea.
- Testosterone levels fluctuate (in men) and decreased erectile function and sperm count occurs.
- Ketoacidosis occurs from increased use of fat as energy fuel.

Causes
- Exact cause unknown
- Social attitudes that equate slimness with beauty
- Subconscious effort to exert personal control over life or to protect oneself from dealing with issues surrounding sexuality
- Elaborate food preparation and eating rituals
- Pressure to achieve
- Dependence and independence issues
- Stress due to multiple responsibilities
- History of sexual abuse

Risk factors
- Low self-esteem
- Compulsive personality
- High achievement goals

Incidence
- Five to 10% of the population; more than 90% of those affected are females

  ✺ **AGE-RELATED CONCERN** Anorexia nervosa occurs primarily in adolescents and young adults but also may affect older women and, occasionally, males.

Common characteristics
- Preoccupation with body size
- Tendency to describe self as "fat"
- Dissatisfaction with a particular aspect of physical appearance
- Compulsive exercising
- Self-induced vomiting
- Laxative or diuretic abuse
- Limits or restricts food intake; eats small portions (see *Criteria for hospitalizing patients with anorexia*)

Complications
- Death
- Suicide
- Electrolyte imbalances
- Malnutrition
- Dehydration
- Esophageal erosion, ulcers, tears, and bleeding
- Tooth and gum erosion and dental caries
- Decreased left ventricular muscle mass and chamber size
- Decreased cardiac output
- Hypotension
- Electrocardiogram (ECG) changes
- Heart failure
- Sudden death
- Increased susceptibility to infection
- Amenorrhea
- Anemia

✳ ASSESSMENT

History
- 15% or greater weight loss for no organic reason
- Morbid dread of being fat
- Compulsion to be thin
- Angry disposition
- Tendency to minimize weight loss
- Ritualistic
- Amenorrhea
- Infertility
- Loss of libido
- Fatigue
- Sleep alterations
- Intolerance to cold
- Constipation or diarrhea

Physical findings
- Hypotension
- Bradycardia
- Emaciated appearance
- Skeletal muscle atrophy
- Loss of fatty tissue
- Atrophy of breast tissue
- Blotchy or sallow skin
- Lanugo on the face and body
- Dryness or loss of scalp hair
- Calluses of the knuckles
- Abrasions and scars on the dorsum of the hand
- Dental caries
- Oral or pharyngeal abrasions
- Painless salivary gland enlargement
- Bowel distention
- Slowed reflexes

Test results
- Diagnosis is based on *DSM-IV-TR* criteria findings.

DSM-IV-TR criteria
These criteria must be documented:
- refusal to maintain or achieve normal weight for age and height
- intense fear of gaining weight or becoming fat, even though underweight
- disturbance in perception of body weight, size, or shape
- in females, absence of at least three consecutive menstrual cycles when otherwise expected to occur.

LABORATORY
- Hemoglobin level, platelet count, and white blood cell count are low.
- Bleeding time is prolonged.
- Erythrocyte sedimentation rate is decreased.
- Serum creatinine, blood urea nitrogen, uric acid, cholesterol, total protein, albumin, sodium, potassium, chloride, calcium, and fasting blood glucose levels are low.
- In severe starvation states, alanine aminotransferase and aspartate aminotransferase levels are elevated.
- Serum amylase levels are elevated.
- In females, levels of serum luteinizing hormone and follicle-stimulating hormone are decreased.
- Triiodothyronine levels are decreased.
- Urinalysis shows dilute urine.

DIAGNOSTIC PROCEDURES
- ECG may show nonspecific ST interval, T-wave changes, and prolonged PR interval; ventricular arrhythmias also may be present.

◆ TREATMENT

General
- Behavior modification
- Curtailed activity for cardiac arrhythmias
- Group, family, or individual psychotherapy

Diet
- Balanced with a normal eating pattern
- Hyperalimentation

Activity
- Gradual increase in physical activity when weight gain and stabilization occur

Medication
- Vitamin and mineral supplements

❖ NURSING CONSIDERATIONS

Nursing diagnoses
- Chronic low self-esteem
- Constipation
- Delayed growth and development
- Disturbed body image
- Imbalanced nutrition: Less than body requirements

Key outcomes
The patient will:
- express positive feelings about self
- regain normal bowel function
- express understanding of norms for growth and development
- acknowledge change in body image
- achieve and maintain expected body weight.

Nursing interventions
- Support the patient's efforts to achieve target weight.
- Negotiate an adequate food intake with the patient.

Monitoring
- Vital signs
- Intake and output
- Electrolyte and complete blood count levels
- Weight on a regular schedule
- Activity for compulsive exercise

◆ **NURSING ALERT** Monitor the patient for 1 hour postprandial to ensure no self-induced vomiting.

▶ PATIENT TEACHING

Be sure to cover:
- nutrition
- importance of keeping a food journal
- avoidance of discussions about food between the patient and family members.

Discharge planning
- Refer the patient to support services.

✹ RESOURCES

Organizations
American Anorexia Bulimia Association:
www.aabainc.org
National Association of Anorexia Nervosa and Associated Disorders:
www.anad.org
Overeaters Anonymous:
www.overeatersanonymous.org

Selected references
Diagnostic and Statistical Manual of Mental Disorders, Text Revision, 4th ed. Washington, D.C.: American Psychiatric Association, 2000.
Hayman, L., and Callister, L.C. "Toward Evidence-Based Practice: Understanding Women's Journey of Recovering from Anorexia Nervosa," *MCN: The American Journal of Maternal/Child Nursing* 30(4):274, July-August 2005.
Nix, S. *William's Basic Nutrition and Diet Therapy,* 11th ed. St. Louis: Mosby–Year Book, Inc., 2005.

CRITERIA FOR HOSPITALIZING PATIENTS WITH ANOREXIA

Patients with anorexia can be successfully treated on an outpatient basis. But if the patient displays any of the signs listed below, hospitalization is mandatory:
- rapid weight loss equal to 15% or more of normal body mass
- persistent bradycardia (50 beats/minute or less)
- hypotension with a systolic reading less than or equal to 90 mm Hg
- hypothermia (core body temperature less than or equal to 97° F ([36.1° C])
- presence of medical complications, suicidal ideation
- persistent sabotage or disruption of outpatient treatment—resolute denial of condition and the need for treatment.

Anthrax

Description

- An acute bacterial infection that occurs most commonly in herbivorous animals; humans showing greater resistance to anthrax than these animals
- Also known as a potential agent for use in bioterrorism and biological warfare; classified as a Category A biological disease
- Human cases: classified as either agricultural or industrial
- In humans, occurs in three forms, depending on the mode of transmission: cutaneous (most common form), inhalation (woolsorters' disease), and GI
- Cutaneous: with treatment, mortality rate less than 1%; without treatment, mortality rate 20%
- Inhalation: even with treatment, usually fatal
- GI: even with treatment, death occurring in 25% to 60% of cases
- No screening test for anthrax

Pathophysiology

- *Bacillis anthracis* is an encapsulated, chain-forming, aerobic, gram-positive rod that forms oval spores; spores are hardy and can survive for years under adverse conditions.
- *B. anthracis,* an extracellular pathogen, evades phagocytosis, invades the bloodstream, and multiplies rapidly.
- In cutaneous anthrax, spores enter the body through abraded or broken skin or by biting flies; the spores germinate within hours, the vegetative cells multiply, and anthrax toxin is produced.
- In inhalation anthrax, spores are deposited directly into the alveoli and phagocytized by macrophages; some are carried to and germinate in mediastinal nodes. This may result in overwhelming bacteremia, hemorrhagic mediastinitis, and secondary pneumonia.
- In GI anthrax, primary infection can occur in the intestine by organisms that survive passage through the stomach; acute inflammation of the intestinal tract results.

Causes

- Bacterial infection with *B. anthracis*

HUMAN CASES

- Contact with infected animals or contaminated animal products
- Insect bites
- Inhalation
- Ingestion

AGRICULTURAL CASES

- Contact with animals that have anthrax
- Bites of contaminated or infected flies
- Consumption of contaminated meat

INDUSTRIAL CASES

- Animal hides
- Goat's hair
- Wool
- Bones

Risk factors

- Laboratory and industrial workers at risk for occupational exposure

Incidence

- Occurs worldwide
- Most common in developing countries
- Most common in domestic herbivores, including sheep, cattle, horses, and goats, and wild herbivores
- Estimates of 20,000 to 100,000 cases per year
- Approximately 95% of human anthrax are cutaneous form; about 5% are inhalation form; GI anthrax rare

Common characteristics

- History of exposure to *B. anthracis* spores
- Clinical manifestation dependent on form of anthrax

IN CUTANEOUS ANTHRAX

- Painless ulcers associated with vesicles and edema
- Contact with animals or animal products

Complications

- Septicemia
- Hemorrhagic mediastinitis
- Pneumonia
- Respiratory failure
- Hemorrhagic thoracic lymphadenitis
- Meningitis
- Death

History

IN CUTANEOUS ANTHRAX

- Contact with animals or animal products
- Painless ulcer
- Mild or no constitutional symptoms

IN INHALATIONAL ANTHRAX

- Initial prodromal flulike symptoms:
  - Malaise; dry cough
  - Mild fever; chills
  - Headache; myalgia
  - Severe respiratory distress
  - Chest pain

IN GI ANTHRAX

- Nausea; vomiting
- Decreased appetite
- Fever
- Abdominal pain
- Vomiting blood
- Severe bloody diarrhea

Physical findings

IN CUTANEOUS ANTHRAX

- Initially, a small, papular, pruritic lesion that resembles an insect bite
- Lesion that develops into a vesicle in 1 to 2 days
- Lesion that finally becomes a small, painless ulcer with a necrotic center, surrounded by nonpitting edema
- Smaller secondary vesicles that may surround some lesions
- Lesions that are generally located on exposed areas of the skin
- Painful, regional, nonspecific lymphadenitis

IN INHALATIONAL ANTHRAX

- Increasing fever
- Dyspnea; stridor
- Hypoxia; cyanosis
- Hypotension; shock

IN GI ANTHRAX

- Fever
- Rapidly developing ascites

Test results

LABORATORY

- Gram stain, direct fluorescent antibody staining, and culture show presence of *B. anthracis.*
- Blood cultures show presence of *B. anthracis.*
- Cerebrospinal fluid analysis reveals presence of *B. anthracis.*

- Complete blood count shows polymorphonuclear leukocytosis in severe disease.
- Serum antibody test reveals the presence of the specific antibody to *B. anthracis*.

IMAGING
- Chest X-ray may show symmetric mediastinal widening in hemorrhagic mediastinitis.

◆ TREATMENT

General
- Initiated as soon as exposure to anthrax is suspected to prevent anthrax infection; early treatment and, possibly, death

Diet
- Solids and liquids, as tolerated
- Adequate fluid intake

Activity
- As tolerated

Medication
- Antibiotics
- Oxygen, as needed

Surgery
- May be necessary for such complications as hemorrhagic mediastinitis

❖ NURSING CONSIDERATIONS

Nursing diagnoses
- Anxiety
- Diarrhea
- Fear
- Imbalanced nutrition: Less than body requirements
- Impaired physical mobility
- Ineffective breathing pattern
- Risk for deficient fluid volume

Key outcomes
The patient will:
- verbalize feelings of anxiety
- regain normal bowel function
- verbalize feelings of fear
- maintain adequate nutrition and hydration
- maintain joint mobility and range of motion
- maintain effective ventilation
- exhibit balanced intake and output.

Nursing interventions
- Administer medications, as ordered.
- Maintain patent airway and adequate ventilation.
- Report any case of anthrax in either livestock or humans to the local board of health.
- Maintain standard precautions.
- Encourage verbalization of fears and concerns.
- Provide adequate hydration.
- Provide a well-balanced diet.
- Help the patient to develop effective coping mechanisms.
- Provide adequate rest periods.

Monitoring
- Vital signs
- Intake and output
- Respiratory status
- Neurologic status
- Cardiovascular status
- Skin lesions
- GI status
- Complications
- Response to treatment
- Progression of infection

▶ PATIENT TEACHING

Be sure to cover:
- disorder, diagnosis, and treatment
- medication administration, dosage, and possible adverse effects
- when to notify the physician
- anthrax prevention.

 NURSING ALERT An anthrax vaccine is available but, due to limited supplies, it's now administered only to U.S. military personnel and isn't for routine civilian use.

✳ RESOURCES

Organizations
Centers for Disease Control and Prevention: *www.cdc.gov*
National Center for Infectious Diseases: *www.cdc.gov/ncidod/diseases/cjd/bse_cjd_qa.htm*

Selected references
"Clinical Rounds: How to Identify Inhalation Anthrax," *Nursing2004* 34(10):34-35, October 2004.

Godyn, J.J., et al. "Cutaneous Anthrax: Conservative or Surgical Treatment," *Advances in Skin and Wound Care: The Journal for Prevention and Healing* 19(3):146-50, April 2005.

Kimmel, S.R., et al. "Vaccines and Bioterrorism: Smallpox and Anthrax," *Journal of Family Practice* 52(1 Suppl):556-61, January 2003.

Aortic insufficiency

● OVERVIEW

Description
- Valvular dysfunction that causes back flow of blood into the heart
- Also called *aortic regurgitation (AR)*

Pathophysiology
- Blood flows back into the left ventricle during diastole, causing increased left ventricular (LV) diastolic pressure.
- This results in volume overload, dilation and, eventually, hypertrophy of the left ventricle.
- Excess fluid volume also eventually results in increased left atrial pressure and increased pulmonary vascular pressure.

Causes
- Rheumatic fever
- Primary disease of the aortic valve leaflets, the wall or the aortic root, or both
- Hypertension
- Infective endocarditis
- Trauma
- Idiopathic valve calcification
- Aortic dissection
- Aortic aneurysm
- Connective tissue diseases

Incidence
- Occurs most commonly among males
- When associated with mitral valve disease, more common among females

Common characteristics
- Typically asymptomatic until 4th or 5th decade of life
- Orthopnea
- Paroxysmal nocturnal dyspnea
- Exertional dyspnea

Complications
- Left-sided heart failure
- Pulmonary edema
- Myocardial ischemia

✳ ASSESSMENT

History
- Exertional dyspnea, orthopnea, paroxysmal nocturnal dyspnea
- Sensation of a forceful heartbeat, especially in supine position
- Angina, especially nocturnal
- Fatigue
- Palpitations, head pounding
- Symptoms of heart failure, in late stages

Physical findings
- Corrigan's pulse (jerky carotid pulse)
- Bisferious pulse (arterial pulse with palpable peaks)
- Water-hammer pulse (bounding and forceful)
- Pulsating nail beds and Quincke's sign
- Wide pulse pressure
- Diffuse, hyperdynamic apical impulse, displaced laterally and inferiorly
- Systolic thrill at base or suprasternal notch
- S_3 gallop with increased LV end-diastolic pressure
- High frequency, blowing early-peaking, diastolic decrescendo murmur best heard with the patient sitting leaning forward and in deep fixed expiration (see *Identifying the murmur of aortic insufficiency*)
- Austin Flint murmur
- Head bobbing with each heartbeat
- Tachycardia, peripheral vasoconstriction, and pulmonary edema if severe AR

Test results
IMAGING
- Chest X-rays may show LV enlargement and pulmonary vein congestion.
- Echocardiography may show LV enlargement, increased motion of the septum and posterior wall, thickening of valve cusps, prolapse of the valve, flail leaflet, vegetations, or dilation of the aortic root.

DIAGNOSTIC PROCEDURES
- Electrocardiography shows sinus tachycardia, left axis deviation, LV hypertrophy, and left atrial hypertrophy in severe disease.
- Cardiac catheterization shows presence and degree of AR, LV dilation and function, and coexisting coronary artery disease.

◆ TREATMENT

General
- Periodic noninvasive monitoring of AR and LV function with echocardiogram
- Medical control of hypertension

Diet
- Low-sodium

Activity
- Planned periodic rest periods to avoid fatigue

Medication
- Cardiac glycosides
- Diuretics
- Vasodilators
- Antihypertensives
- Antiarrhythmics
- Infective endocarditis prophylaxis

◉ **NURSING ALERT** Avoid using beta-adrenergic blockers due to negative inotropic effects.

Surgery
- Valve replacement

IDENTIFYING THE MURMUR OF AORTIC INSUFFICIENCY

A high-pitched, blowing decrescendo murmur that radiates from the aortic valve area to the left sternal border characterizes aortic insufficiency.

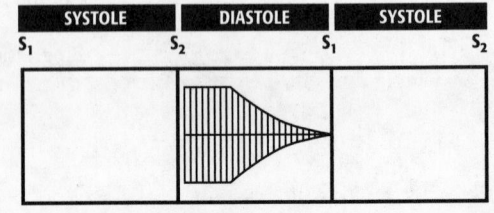

SYSTOLE		DIASTOLE		SYSTOLE	
S_1		S_2		S_1	S_2

❖ NURSING CONSIDERATIONS

Nursing diagnoses
- Activity intolerance
- Decreased cardiac output
- Excess fluid volume
- Fatigue
- Impaired gas exchange
- Impaired physical mobility
- Ineffective coping
- Ineffective tissue perfusion: Cardio-pulmonary

Key outcomes
The patient will:
- carry out activities of daily living without excess fatigue or decreased energy
- maintain cardiac output, demonstrate hemodynamic stability, and not develop arrhythmias
- maintain adequate fluid balance
- express feelings of energy and decreased fatigue
- maintain adequate ventilation
- maintain optimal mobility within the confines of the disorder
- demonstrate effective coping skills
- maintain tissue perfusion and oxygenation.

Nursing interventions
- Administer medications, as ordered.
- If the patient needs bed rest, stress its importance; provide a bedside commode.
- Alternate periods of activity and rest.
- Allow the patient to express his concerns about the effects of activity restrictions on his responsibilities and routines.
- Keep the patient's legs elevated while he sits in a chair.
- Place the patient in an upright position, if necessary, and administer oxygen.
- Keep the patient on a low-sodium diet. Consult a dietitian.
- Following surgery, watch for hypotension, arrhythmias, and thrombus formation.

Monitoring
- Signs and symptoms of heart failure
- Pulmonary edema
- Adverse reactions to drug therapy
- Complications

AFTER SURGERY
- Vital signs and cardiac rhythm
- Heart tones
- Chest tube drainage
- Neurologic status
- Arterial blood gas levels
- Intake and output; daily weights
- Blood chemistry studies, prothrombin time, and International Normalized Ratio values
- Chest X-ray results
- Pulmonary artery catheter pressures

▶ PATIENT TEACHING

Be sure to cover:
- disorder, diagnosis, and treatment
- medication administration, dosage, and possible adverse effects
- when to notify the physician
- periodic rest periods in his daily routine
- leg elevation whenever the patient sits
- dietary restrictions
- signs and symptoms of heart failure
- importance of consistent follow-up care
- monitoring of pulse rate and rhythm
- blood pressure control.

Discharge planning
Refer the patient to:
- an outpatient cardiac rehabilitation program, if indicated
- a smoking-cessation program, if indicated
- a weight-reduction program, if indicated.

✹ RESOURCES

Organizations
American Heart Association: *www.americanheart.org*
Mayo Health Clinic: *www.mayohealth.org*

Selected references
Goldman, L., and Ausiello, D. *Cecil Textbook of Medicine,* 22nd. Philadelphia: W.B. Saunders Co., 2004.

Kasper, D.L., et al., eds. *Harrison's Principles of Internal Medicine,* 16th ed. New York: McGraw-Hill Book Co., 2005.

Kinney, M.R., et al. *AACN Essentials of Critical Care Nursing.* New York: McGraw-Hill Medical, 2006.

The Merck Manual of Diagnosis & Therapy, 18th ed. Whitehouse Station, N.J.: Merck & Co., Inc., 2006.

Aortic stenosis

● OVERVIEW

Description
- Narrowing of the aortic valve
- Classified as either acquired or rheumatic

Pathophysiology
- Stenosis of the aortic valve results in impedance to forward blood flow.
- The left ventricle requires greater pressure to open the aortic valve.
- This added workload increases myocardial oxygen demands.
- Diminished cardiac output reduces coronary artery blood flow, which results in left ventricular (LV) hypertrophy and failure.

Causes
- Idiopathic fibrosis and calcification
- Congenital aortic bicuspid valve
- Rheumatic fever
- Atherosclerosis

Risk factors
- Diabetes mellitus
- Hypercholesterolemia

Incidence
- Possibly asymptomatic until ages 50 to 70, even though stenosis has been present since childhood
- Occurs primarily in males (about 80%)

Common characteristics
- Long latent period
- Classic triad of angina pectoris, syncope, and dyspnea

Complications
- Left-sided heart failure
- Right-sided heart failure
- Infective endocarditis
- Cardiac arrhythmias, especially atrial fibrillation
- Sudden death

✱ ASSESSMENT

History
- May be asymptomatic
- Dyspnea on exertion
- Angina
- Exertional syncope
- Fatigue
- Palpitations
- Paroxysmal nocturnal dyspnea

Physical findings
- Small, sustained arterial pulses that rise slowly
- Distinct lag between carotid artery pulse and apical pulse
- Orthopnea
- Prominent jugular vein *a* waves
- Peripheral edema
- Diminished carotid pulses with delayed upstroke
- Apex of the heart possibly displaced inferiorly and laterally
- Suprasternal thrill

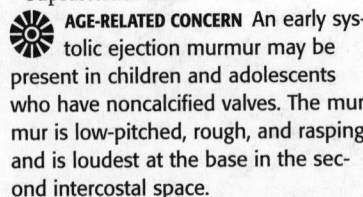 **AGE-RELATED CONCERN** An early systolic ejection murmur may be present in children and adolescents who have noncalcified valves. The murmur is low-pitched, rough, and rasping and is loudest at the base in the second intercostal space.

- Split S_2 that develops as stenosis becomes more severe
- Prominent S_4
- Harsh, rasping, mid-to late-peaking systolic murmur that's best heard at the base and commonly radiates to carotids and apex (see *Identifying the murmur of aortic stenosis*)

Test results
IMAGING
- Chest X-ray shows valvular calcification, LV enlargement, pulmonary vein congestion and, in later stages, left atrial, pulmonary artery, right atrial, and right ventricular enlargement.
- Echocardiography shows decreased valve area, increased gradient, and increased LV wall thickness.

DIAGNOSTIC PROCEDURES
- Cardiac catheterization shows increased pressure gradient across the aortic valve, increased LV pressures, and presence of coronary artery disease.

OTHER
- Electrocardiography may show LV hypertrophy, atrial fibrillation, or other arrhythmia.

◆ TREATMENT

General
- Periodic noninvasive evaluation of the severity of valve narrowing
- Life-long treatment and management of congenital aortic stenosis

Diet
- Low-sodium
- Low-fat, low-cholesterol

Activity
- Planned rest periods

Medication
- Cardiac glycosides
- Antibiotic infective endocarditis prophylaxis

⬙ **NURSING ALERT** The use of diuretics and vasodilators may lead to hypotension and inadequate stroke volume.

Surgery
- In adults, valve replacement after they become symptomatic with hemodynamic evidence of severe obstruction
- Percutaneous balloon aortic valvuloplasty
- In children without calcified valves, simple commissurotomy under direct visualization
- In patients younger than age 5, Ross procedure

Nursing diagnoses
- Activity intolerance
- Decreased cardiac output
- Excess fluid volume
- Fatigue
- Impaired gas exchange
- Impaired physical mobility
- Ineffective coping
- Ineffective tissue perfusion: Cardiopulmonary

Key outcomes
The patient will:
- carry out activities of daily living without excess fatigue or decreased energy
- maintain cardiac output, demonstrate hemodynamic stability, and not develop arrhythmias
- maintain adequate fluid balance
- express feelings of energy and decreased fatigue
- maintain adequate ventilation
- maintain optimal mobility within the confines of the disorder
- demonstrate effective coping skills
- maintain tissue perfusion and oxygenation.

Nursing interventions
- Stress importance of bed rest. Provide a bedside commode.
- Alternate periods of activity and rest.
- Allow the patient to voice concerns about the effects of activity restrictions.
- Keep the patient's legs elevated while he sits in a chair.
- Place the patient in an upright position and administer oxygen, as needed.
- Maintain a low-sodium diet. Consult with a dietitian.
- Allow the patient to express his fears and concerns.
- Administer medications, as ordered.

Monitoring
- Vital signs
- Intake and output
- Signs and symptoms of heart failure
- Signs and symptoms of progressive aortic stenosis
- Daily weight
- Arrhythmias

- Respiratory status

IF THE PATIENT HAS SURGERY
- Signs and symptoms of thrombus formation
- Hemodynamics
- Arterial blood gas results
- Blood chemistry results
- Chest X-ray results

▶ PATIENT TEACHING

Be sure to cover:
- disorder, diagnosis, and treatment
- medication administration, dosage, and possible adverse effects
- when to notify the physician
- periodic rest in the patient's daily routine
- leg elevation whenever the patient sits
- dietary and fluid restrictions
- importance of consistent follow-up care
- signs and symptoms of heart failure
- infective endocarditis prophylaxis
- pulse rate and rhythm
- monitoring for atrial fibrillation and other arrhythmias.

Discharge planning
Refer the patient to:
- a weight-reduction program, if indicated.
- a smoking-cessation program, if indicated.

✵ RESOURCES

Organizations
American Heart Association: *www.americanheart.org*
Mayo Health Clinic: *www.mayohealth.org*

Selected references
Dambro, M.R. *Griffith's Five-Minute Clinical Consult 2006.* Philadelphia: Lippincott Williams & Wilkins, 2006.
Goldman, L., and Ausiello, D. *Cecil Textbook of Medicine,* 22nd ed. Philadelphia: W.B. Saunders Co., 2004.
Kasper, D.L., et al., eds. *Harrison's Principles of Internal Medicine,* 16th ed. New York: McGraw-Hill Book Co., 2005.
The Merck Manual of Diagnosis & Therapy, 18th ed. Whitehouse Station, N.J.: Merck & Co., Inc., 2006.

IDENTIFYING THE MURMUR OF AORTIC STENOSIS

A low-pitched, harsh crescendo-decrescendo murmur that radiates from the aortic valve area to the carotid artery characterizes aortic stenosis.

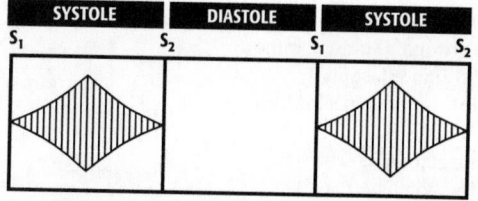

Appendicitis

Description
- Most common major abdominal surgical disease
- Inflammation of the vermiform appendix
- If left untreated, gangrene and perforation developing within 36 hours, leading to death

Pathophysiology
- Mucosal ulceration triggers inflammation, which temporarily obstructs the appendix.
- This obstruction causes mucus outflow, increasing pressure in the distended appendix; the appendix then contracts.
- Bacteria multiply and inflammation and pressure increase, restricting blood flow and causing thrombus and abdominal pain.

Causes
- Foreign body
- Neoplasm
- Mucosal ulceration
- Fecal mass
- Stricture
- Barium ingestion
- Viral infection

Risk factors
- Adolescent male

Incidence
- Can occur at any age; however, majority of cases occur between ages 11 to 20
- Affects both sexes equally; however, between puberty and age 25, more prevalent in men

Common characteristics
- Abdominal pain
- Anorexia
- Vomiting

Complications
- Peritonitis (most common)
- Wound infection
- Intra-abdominal infection
- Fecal fistula
- Intestinal obstruction
- Incisional hernia
- Death

History
- Abdominal pain that's initially generalized, then localizes in the right lower abdomen (McBurney's point)
- Anorexia
- Nausea, vomiting

Physical findings
- Low-grade fever, tachycardia
- Adjusts posture to decrease pain
- Guarding
- Normoactive bowel sounds, with possible constipation or diarrhea
- Rebound tenderness and spasm of the abdominal muscles
- Rovsing's sign
- Psoas sign
- Obturator sign
- Absent abdominal tenderness or flank tenderness with retrocele or pelvic appendix

Test results
LABORATORY
- White blood cell count is moderately elevated, with increased numbers of immature cells.
IMAGING
- Abdominal or transvaginal ultrasound show appendiceal inflammation.
- Barium enema reveals nonfilling appendix.
- Abdominal computed tomography scan demonstrates suspected perforation or abscess.

General
- If an abscess is suspected, surgery delayed until antibiotic therapy has been initiated

Diet
- Nothing by mouth (NPO) until after surgery, then gradual return to regular diet

Activity
- Early postoperative ambulation

Medication
- I.V. fluids
- Analgesics
- Antibiotics preoperatively and if peritonitis develops

Surgery
- Appendectomy

Nursing diagnoses
- Acute pain
- Imbalanced nutrition: Less than body requirements
- Impaired skin integrity
- Ineffective tissue perfusion: GI
- Risk for deficient fluid volume
- Risk for infection

Key outcomes
The patient will:
- express feelings of comfort and decreased pain
- maintain calorie requirement
- maintain skin integrity
- maintain adequate GI tissue perfusion
- maintain normal fluid volume
- remain free from signs and symptoms of infection.

Nursing interventions
- Maintain NPO status until surgery is performed.
- Administer I.V. fluids.
- Avoid administering analgesics until the diagnosis is confirmed.
- Avoid administering cathartics or enemas that may rupture appendix.
- Place the patient in Fowler's position to decrease pain.

◆ **NURSING ALERT** Never apply heat to the right lower abdomen; this can cause the appendix to rupture.
- Administer prescribed preoperative medication.

Monitoring
AFTER SURGERY
- Vital signs
- Intake and output
- Pain relief
- Bowel sounds, passing of flatus, or bowel movements
- Wound healing

Be sure to cover:
- disorder, diagnosis, and treatment
- preoperative teaching
- possible complications
- appropriate wound care
- medication administration, dosage, and possible adverse effects
- postoperative activity limitations.

Organizations
National Digestive Diseases Information Clearinghouse: *www.niddk.nih.gov/health/digest/nddic.htm*

Selected references
Grover, S. *Blueprints Pocket Gastroenterology*, Philadelphia: Lippincott Williams & Wilkins, 2007.

Handbook of Diseases, 3rd ed. Philadelphia: Lippincott Williams & Wilkins, 2004.

McPhee, S.J., et al. *Current Medical Diagnosis and Treatment.* New York: McGraw-Hill Book Co., 2007.

Arterial occlusive disease

● OVERVIEW

Description
- An obstruction or narrowing of the lumen of the aorta and its major branches
- May affect arteries including the carotid, vertebral, innominate, subclavian, femoral, iliac, renal, mesenteric, and celiac arteries
- Prognosis dependent on location of the occlusion and the development of collateral circulation that counteracts reduced blood flow

Pathophysiology
- The narrowing leads to interrupted blood flow, usually to the legs and feet.
- During times of increased activity or exercise, blood flow to surrounding muscles is unable to meet the metabolic demand, which results in pain in affected areas.

Causes
- Atherosclerosis
- Immune arteritis
- Embolism
- Thrombosis
- Thromboangiitis obliterans
- Raynaud's disease
- Fibromuscular disease
- Atheromatous debris (plaques)
- Indwelling arterial catheter
- Direct blunt or penetrating trauma

Risk factors
- Smoking
- Hypertension
- Dyslipidemia
- Diabetes mellitus
- Advanced age

Incidence
- More common in males than in females; usually over age 50
- Higher incidence in patients with diabetes
- Arteries in lower extremities more commonly affected

Common characteristics
- Intermittent claudication
- Decreased temperature in extremities
- Numbness or paresthesias

Complications
- Severe ischemia
- Skin ulceration
- Gangrene
- Limb loss

✳ ASSESSMENT

History
- One or more risk factors
- Family history of vascular disease
- Intermittent claudication
- Rest pain
- Poor-healing wounds or ulcers
- Impotence
- Dizziness or near syncope
- Transient ischemic attack symptoms

Physical findings
- Trophic changes of involved extremity
- Diminished or absent pulses in extremity
- Presence of ischemic ulcers
- Pallor with elevation of extremity
- Dependent rubor
- Arterial bruit
- Hypertension
- Pain
- Pallor
- Pulselessness distal to the occlusion
- Paralysis and paresthesia occurring in the affected extremity
- Poikilothermy

Test results
IMAGING
- Arteriography shows type, location, and degree of obstruction, and the establishment of collateral circulation.
- Ultrasonography and plethysmography show decreased blood flow distal to the occlusion.
- Doppler ultrasonography shows a relatively low-pitched sound and a monophasic waveform.
- Electroencephalography and computed tomography scan may show the presence of brain lesions.

OTHER
- Segmental limb pressures and pulse volume measurements show the location and extent of the occlusion.
- Ophthalmodynamometry shows the degree of obstruction in the internal carotid artery.

- Electrocardiogram may show presence of cardiovascular disease.

◆ TREATMENT

General
- Elimination of smoking
- Hypertension, diabetes, and dyslipidemia control
- Foot and leg care
- Weight control

Diet
- Low-fat

Activity
- Regular walking program

Medication
- Antiplatelets
- Lipid-lowering agents
- Hypoglycemic agents
- Antihypertensives
- Thrombolytics
- Anticoagulation

Surgery
- Embolectomy
- Endarterectomy
- Atherectomy
- Laser angioplasty
- Endovascular stent placement
- Percutaneous transluminal angioplasty
- Laser surgery
- Patch grafting
- Bypass graft
- Lumbar sympathectomy
- Amputation
- Bowel resection

❖ NURSING CONSIDERATIONS

Nursing diagnoses
- Activity intolerance
- Chronic pain
- Impaired physical mobility
- Impaired skin integrity
- Ineffective coping
- Ineffective tissue perfusion: Peripheral
- Risk for infection

Key outcomes
The patient will:
- carry out activities of daily living without excess fatigue or exhaustion
- report increased comfort and decreased pain
- maintain joint mobility and range of motion
- maintain skin integrity
- demonstrate effective coping skills
- maintain normal peripheral pulses and collateral circulation
- remain free from signs or symptoms of infection.

Nursing interventions
FOR CHRONIC ARTERIAL OCCLUSIVE DISEASE
- Use preventive measures, such as minimal pressure mattresses, heel protectors, a foot cradle, or a footboard.
- Avoid using restrictive clothing such as antiembolism stockings.
- Administer medications, as ordered.
- Allow the patient to express fears and concerns.
FOR PREOPERATIVE CARE DURING AN ACUTE EPISODE
- Assess the patient's circulatory status.
- Administer analgesics, as needed.
- Administer heparin or thrombolytics, as ordered.
- Wrap the patient's affected foot in soft cotton batting, and reposition it frequently to prevent pressure on any one area.
- Strictly avoid elevating or applying heat to the affected leg.
FOR POSTOPERATIVE CARE
- Watch the patient closely for signs of hemorrhage.
- In mesenteric artery occlusion, connect a nasogastric tube to low intermittent suction.

- Provide analgesics, as ordered.
- Assist with early ambulation, but don't allow the patient to sit for an extended period.
- If amputation has occurred, check the stump carefully for drainage and note and record its color and amount and the time.
- Elevate the stump, as ordered.

Monitoring
- Signs and symptoms of fluid and electrolyte imbalance and renal failure
- Signs and symptoms of stroke
- Vital signs
- Intake and output
- Distal pulses
- Neurologic status
- Bowel sounds

▶ PATIENT TEACHING

Be sure to cover:
- disorder, diagnosis, and treatment
- medication administration, dosage, and possible adverse effects
- when to notify the physician
- dietary restrictions
- regular exercise program
- foot care
- signs and symptoms of graft occlusion
- signs and symptoms of arterial insufficiency and occlusion
- avoidance of wearing constrictive clothing, crossing legs, or wearing garters
- smoking cessation
- risk factor modification
- avoidance of temperature extremes.

Discharge planning
Refer the patient to:
- a physical and occupational therapist, as indicated.
- a podiatrist for foot care, as needed.
- an endocrinologist for strict glucose control, as indicated.
- a smoking-cessation program, as indicated.

✳ RESOURCES

Organizations
American Heart Association: *www.americanheart.org*
Mayo Health Clinic: *www.mayohealth.org*

Selected references
Day, M.W., "Acute Peripheral Arterial Occlusion," *Nursing2004* 34(1):88, January 2004.
Kasper, D.L., et al., eds. *Harrison's Principles of Internal Medicine*, 16th ed. New York: McGraw-Hill Book Co., 2005.
The Merck Manual of Diagnosis & Therapy, 18th ed. Whitehouse Station, N.J.: Merck & Co., Inc., 2006.

Asbestosis

● OVERVIEW

Description
- Characterized by diffuse interstitial pulmonary fibrosis resulting from prolonged exposure to airborne asbestos particles
- Also causes pleural plaques and mesotheliomas of the pleura and the peritoneum
- May develop years (about 15 to 20) after regular exposure to asbestos ceases
- A form of pneumoconiosis

Pathophysiology
- Inhaled asbestos fibers travel down the airway and penetrate respiratory bronchioles and alveolar walls.
- Mucus production and goblet cells are stimulated to protect the airway and aid in expectoration.
- Fibers become encased in a brown, iron-rich, proteinlike sheath, called asbestosis bodies.
- Chronic irritation by the fibers continues, causing edema of the airways.
- Fibrosis develops in response to the chronic irritation.

Causes
- Prolonged inhalation of asbestos fibers from industries, such as mining and milling, construction, fireproofing, and textile
- Exposure to production of paints, plastics, and brake and clutch linings
- Exposure to fibrous dust shaken off workers' clothing
- Exposure to fibrous dust or waste piles from nearby asbestos plants

Incidence
- Commonly occurs between ages 40 to 75
- Affects males more than females

Common characteristics
- Dyspnea
- Dry cough
- Recurrent respiratory tract infections

Complications
- Pulmonary fibrosis
- Respiratory failure
- Pulmonary hypertension
- Cor pulmonale

✱ ASSESSMENT

History
- Exposure to asbestos fibers
- Exertional or rest dyspnea
- Cough
- Chest pain
- Recurrent respiratory tract infections

Physical findings
- Tachypnea
- Clubbing of the fingers
- Characteristic dry crackles in the lung bases

Test results
LABORATORY
- Arterial blood gas analysis shows decreased partial pressures of arterial oxygen and carbon dioxide.

IMAGING
- Chest X-rays may show fine, irregular, and linear diffuse infiltrates; a honey-comb or ground-glass appearance to lungs; and pleural thickening and pleural calcification, bilateral obliteration of costophrenic angles, and an enlarged heart with "shaggy" border.

OTHER
- Pulmonary function tests may show decreased vital capacity, forced vital capacity (FVC), and total lung capacity; decreased or normal forced expiratory volume in 1 second (FEV_1); a normal ratio of FEV_1 to FVC; and reduced diffusing capacity for carbon monoxide.

◆ TREATMENT

General
- Controlled coughing and postural drainage with chest percussion and vibration

Diet
- At least 3 L of fluids daily
- Salt restriction
- High-calorie, high-protein

Activity
- As tolerated

Medication
- Inhaled mucolytics
- Supplemental oxygen
- Diuretics
- Cardiac glycosides
- Antibiotics

Surgery
- Lung transplantation, in severe cases

❖ NURSING CONSIDERATIONS

Nursing diagnoses
- Anxiety
- Deficient knowledge (asbestosis)
- Fatigue
- Fear
- Imbalanced nutrition: Less than body requirements
- Impaired gas exchange
- Ineffective breathing pattern
- Interrupted family processes

Key outcomes
The patient will:
- express feelings of decreased anxiety
- verbalize understanding of disorder and treatment
- identify measures to prevent or reduce fatigue
- express feelings of decreased fear
- maintain adequate calorie intake
- maintain adequate ventilation
- maintain effective breathing pattern
- express understanding of the disorder and treatment modality, as will his family.

Nursing interventions
- Administer medication, as ordered.
- Provide supportive care.
- Provide chest physiotherapy.
- Provide high-calorie, high-protein foods.
- Offer small, frequent meals.
- Encourage oral fluid intake.
- Provide frequent rest periods.

Monitoring
- Vital signs
- Intake and output
- Daily weight
- Respiratory status
- Breath sounds
- Sputum production
- Mentation
- Complications

▶ PATIENT TEACHING

Be sure to cover:
- disorder, diagnosis, and treatment
- medication administration, dosage, and possible adverse effects
- transtracheal catheter care, if applicable
- prevention of infection
- signs and symptoms of infection
- influenza and pneumococcus immunizations
- home oxygen therapy, if required
- importance of follow-up care
- chest physiotherapy
- high-calorie, high-protein diet
- adequate oral fluid intake
- energy conservation techniques.

Discharge planning
- Refer the patient to a smoking-cessation program, if indicated.

✴ RESOURCES

Organizations
Asbestos Institute:
  www.asbestos-institute.ca/main.html
National Institute for Occupational Safety and Health:
  www.cdc.gov/maso/nioshfs.htm

Selected references
American Thoracic Society. "Diagnosis and Initial Management of Nonmalignant Diseases Related to Asbestos," *American Journal of Respiratory and Critical Care Medicine* 170(6):691-715, September 2004.

Kasper, D.L., et al., eds. *Harrison's Principles of Internal Medicine*, 16th ed. New York: McGraw-Hill Book Co., 2005.

Asphyxia

● OVERVIEW

Description
- Condition of insufficient oxygen and accumulating carbon dioxide in the blood and tissues
- Leads to cardiopulmonary arrest and is fatal without prompt treatment

Pathophysiology
- Normal respirations are impeded, causing insufficient oxygen intake, accumulation of carbon dioxide, hypoxemia, and inadequate tissue perfusion.

Causes
- Narcotic abuse
- Respiratory muscle paralysis
- Airway obstruction
- Aspiration
- Pulmonary edema
- Near drowning
- Tumor
- Strangulation
- Trauma to airway
- Carbon monoxide poisoning
- Smoke inhalation

Incidence
- Can occur at any age

Common characteristics
- Altered respirations
- Changes in level of consciousness
- Cardiac arrest

Complications
- Neurologic damage
- Death

✳ ASSESSMENT

History
- Cause of asphyxia apparent
- Signs and symptoms vary

Physical findings
- Anxiousness or agitation
- Confusion
- Dyspnea
- Prominent neck muscles
- Wheezing and stridor
- Altered respiratory rate
- Little or no air movement
- Intercostal rib retractions
- Pale skin
- Cyanosis in mucous membranes, lips, and nail beds
- Erythema and petechiae on the upper chest (trauma)
- Mucous membranes cherry-red (carbon monoxide poisoning)
- Decreased or absent breath sounds

Test results
LABORATORY
- Arterial blood gas (ABG) analysis reveals decreased partial pressure of arterial oxygen (less than 60 mm Hg) and increased partial pressure of arterial carbon dioxide (more than 50 mm Hg).
- Toxicology tests show drugs, chemicals, or abnormal hemoglobin level.
IMAGING
- Chest X-rays may detect a foreign body, pulmonary edema, or atelectasis.
- Bronchoscopy may also locate foreign body.
- Pulmonary function tests may indicate respiratory muscle weakness.

◆ TREATMENT

General
- Established airway and ventilation
- Treatment of underlying cause

Diet
- Nothing by mouth until able to protect airway

Activity
- Based on outcome of interventions

Medication
- Oxygen

Surgery
- Tumor removal

Nursing diagnoses

- Decreased cardiac output
- Impaired gas exchange
- Ineffective airway clearance
- Ineffective breathing pattern
- Risk for aspiration
- Risk for suffocation

Key outcomes

The patient will:

- maintain acceptable cardiac output
- maintain adequate ventilation and oxygenation
- maintain a patent airway
- maintain an effective breathing pattern
- remain free from signs and symptoms of aspiration
- demonstrate knowledge of safety measures to prevent suffocation.

Nursing interventions

- Perform abdominal thrust, if obstruction is present.
- Maintain patent airway.
- Begin cardiopulmonary resuscitation, if necessary.
- Insert a nasogastric tube or an Ewald tube for lavage (for poisoning).
- Administer medications, as ordered.
- Reassure the patient and family members.
- Ensure I.V. access.

Monitoring

- ABG levels, pulse oximetry
- Respiratory status
- Cardiac status
- Vital signs
- Neurologic status

Be sure to cover:

- cause of asphyxia (with patient and family members, discuss measures to prevent recurrence, if appropriate)
- safety measures if the victim is a child.

Discharge planning

Refer the patient to:

- proper authorities if criminal intent was involved.
- resource and support services, if appropriate.

Organizations

American Academy of Neurology: *www.aan.com*

Selected references

Diseases, 4th ed. Philadelphia: Lippincott Williams & Wilkins, 2006.

Jenkins, J.I., and Braen, G.R. *Manual of Emergency Medicine,* 5th ed. Philadelphia: Lippincott Williams & Wilkins, 2005.

Klein, C.A., "Prenatal Asphyxia Requires Immediate Response," *Nurse Practitioner* 29(5):10, May 2004.

Asthma

Description

- Involves episodic, reversible airway obstruction resulting from bronchospasms, increased mucus secretions, and mucosal edema
- Signs and symptoms ranging from mild wheezing and dyspnea to life-threatening respiratory failure
- Signs and symptoms of bronchial airway obstruction possibly persisting between acute episodes
- A chronic reactive airway disorder

Pathophysiology

- Tracheal and bronchial linings overreact to various stimuli, causing episodic smooth-muscle spasms that severely constrict the airways.
- Mucosal edema and thickened secretions further block the airways.
- Immunoglobulin (Ig) E antibodies, attached to histamine-containing mast cells and receptors on cell membranes, initiate intrinsic asthma attacks.
- When exposed to an antigen such as pollen, the IgE antibody combines with the antigen. On subsequent exposure to the antigen, mast cells degranulate and release mediators.
- The mediators cause the bronchoconstriction and edema of an asthma attack.
- During an asthma attack, expiratory airflow decreases, trapping gas in the airways and causing alveolar hyperinflation.
- Atelectasis may develop in some lung regions.
- The increased airway resistance initiates labored breathing.

Causes

- Sensitivity to specific external allergens or from internal, nonallergenic factors

IN EXTRINSIC ASTHMA (ATOPIC ASTHMA)

- Pollen
- Animal dander
- House dust or mold
- Kapok or feather pillows
- Food additives containing sulfites and any other sensitizing substance

IN INTRINSIC ASTHMA (NONATOPIC ASTHMA)

- Emotional stress
- Genetic factors

IN BRONCHOCONSTRICTION

- Hereditary predisposition
- Sensitivity to allergens or irritants such as pollutants
- Viral infections
- Drugs, such as aspirin, beta-adrenergic blockers, and nonsteroidal anti-inflammatory drugs
- Tartrazine
- Psychological stress
- Cold air
- Exercise

Incidence

- Can strike at any age; about half of all patients under age 10; affects twice as many boys as girls
- About one-third experience onset between ages 10 and 30
- About one-third share disease with at least one immediate family member
- Can coexist (intrinsic and extrinsic asthma) in many asthmatics

Common characteristics

- Wheezing
- Shortness of breath, feelings of suffocation
- Tightness in chest
- Extrinsic asthma beginning in children; commonly accompanied by other manifestations of atopy

Complications

- Status asthmaticus
- Respiratory failure
- Death

History

- Irritants, severe respiratory tract infections (especially in adults), emotional stress, fatigue, endocrine changes, temperature and humidity variations, and exposure to noxious fumes possibly preceding instrinsic asthma attacks
- Dramatic onset with severe, multiple symptoms; or insidious onset, with gradually increasing respiratory distress
- Sudden onset of dyspnea and wheezing and tightness in the chest accompanied by a cough that produces thick, clear, or yellow sputum

Physical findings

- Visibly dyspneic
- Ability to speak only a few words before pausing for breath
- Use of accessory respiratory muscles
- Diaphoresis
- Increased anteroposterior thoracic diameter
- Hyperresonance
- Tachycardia; tachypnea; mild systolic hypertension
- Inspiratory and expiratory wheezes
- Prolonged expiratory phase of respiration
- Diminished breath sounds
- Cyanosis, confusion, and lethargy indicate the onset of life-threatening status asthmaticus and respiratory failure

Test results

LABORATORY

- Arterial blood gas (ABG) analysis reveals hypoxemia.
- Serum IgE levels are increased from an allergic reaction.
- Complete blood count with differential shows increased eosinophil count.

IMAGING

- Chest X-rays may show hyperinflation with areas of focal atelectasis.

DIAGNOSTIC PROCEDURES

- Pulmonary function studies may show decreased peak flows and forced expiratory volume in 1 second, low-normal or decreased vital capacity, and increased total lung and residual capacities.
- Skin testing may identify specific allergens.
- Bronchial challenge testing shows the clinical significance of allergens identified by skin testing.

OTHER

- Pulse oximetry measurements may show decreased oxygen saturation.

TREATMENT

General
- Avoidance of precipitating factors
- Desensitization to specific antigens
- Prompt treatment of status asthmaticus to prevent progression to fatal respiratory failure

Diet
- Fluid replacement

Activity
- As tolerated

Medication
- Bronchodilators
- Corticosteroids
- Histamine antagonists
- Leukotriene antagonists
- Anticholinergic bronchodilators
- Low-flow oxygen
- Antibiotics
- Heliox trial (before intubation)
- I.V. magnesium sulfate (controversial)

NURSING ALERT The patient with increasingly severe asthma that doesn't respond to drug therapy is usually admitted for treatment with corticosteroids, epinephrine, and sympathomimetic aerosol sprays. He may require endotracheal intubation and mechanical ventilation.

USING A METERED-DOSE INHALER

When instructing your patient about proper metered-dose inhaler (MDI) use, include the following points:
- Shake the MDI well before use.
- Exhale normally. Then place the mouthpiece in your mouth and close your lips around it.
- Begin slow, steady inspirations through the mouth until your lungs feel full.
- While inhaling slowly, squeeze firmly on the MDI to deliver the dose while continuing to breathe in one deep steady breath, not several shallow ones.
- Hold the breath for several seconds before exhaling.
- Exhale slowly through pursed lips.
- Gargle with normal saline solution, if desired.

Note: When using an extender or a spacer device, follow the same routine as above, with the MDI mouthpiece inserted in one end of the spacer and the other end placed in the mouth. Many spacers are equipped with a small whistle that sounds if the dose is being inhaled too fast.

NURSING CONSIDERATIONS

Nursing diagnoses
- Anxiety
- Deficient knowledge (asthma)
- Fear
- Impaired gas exchange
- Ineffective airway clearance
- Ineffective breathing pattern

Key outcomes
The patient will:
- report feelings of comfort and decreased anxiety
- verbalize understanding of disorder and treatment
- verbalize feelings of fear
- maintain adequate ventilation and oxygenation
- maintain a patent airway
- maintain an effective breathing pattern.

Nursing interventions
- Administer medication, as ordered.
- Place the patient in high Fowler's position.
- Encourage pursed-lip and diaphragmatic breathing.
- Administer prescribed humidified oxygen.
- Adjust oxygen according to the patient's vital signs and ABG values.
- Anticipate intubation and mechanical ventilation.
- Perform postural drainage and chest percussion, if tolerated.
- Suction an intubated patient, as needed.
- Treat the patient's dehydration with I.V. or oral fluids, as tolerated.
- Anticipate bronchoscopy or bronchial lavage.
- Keep the room temperature comfortable.
- Use an air conditioner or a fan in hot, humid weather.

Monitoring
- Vital signs
- Intake and output
- Severity of asthma
- Signs and symptoms of theophylline toxicity
- Breath sounds
- ABG results
- Pulmonary function test results
- Pulse oximetry
- Complications of corticosteroids
- Level of anxiety

PATIENT TEACHING

Be sure to cover:
- disorder, diagnosis, and treatment
- medication administration, dosage, and possible adverse effects
- when to notify the physician
- avoidance of known allergens and irritants
- metered-dose inhaler use (see *Using a metered-dose inhaler*)
- pursed-lip and diaphragmatic breathing
- peak flow meter
- effective coughing techniques
- adequate hydration.

Discharge planning
- Refer the patient to a local asthma support group.

RESOURCES

Organizations
American Academy of Allergy, Asthma and Immunology: *www.aaaai.org*
Asthma and Allergy Foundation of America: *www.aafa.org*
Global Institute for Asthma: *www.ingasthma.com*
National Asthma Education and Prevention Program: *www.nhlbi.nih.gov/about/naepp*

Selected references
Holcomb, S.S. "Asthma Update 2005: Guidelines for Pregnant Women," *Dimensions of Critical Care Nursing* 24(6):263-66, November-December 2005.
Mintz, M. "Asthma Update: Part 1. Diagnosis, Monitoring, and Prevention of Disease Progression," *American Family Physician* 70(5):893-98, September 2004.
Murphy, K.R., et al. "Asthma: Helping Patients Breathe Easier," *Nurse Practitioner* 29(10):38-55, October 2004.
Pruitt, B., and Jacobs, M. "Caring for a Patient with Asthma," *Nursing2005* 35(2):48-51, February 2005.

Atrial fibrillation

● OVERVIEW

Description
- Rhythm disturbance of the atria
- Characterized by an irregularly irregular cardiac rate and rhythm (see *Recognizing atrial fibrillation*)

Pathophysiology
- Rapid discharges from numerous ectopic foci occur in the atria, leading to erratic and uncoordinated atrial rhythm.

Causes
- Hypertension
- Myocardial infarction
- Pulmonary embolism
- Heart failure
- Cardiomyopathy
- Hypersympathetic state associated with acute alcohol ingestion
- Pericarditis
- Hyperthyroidism
- Valvular disease
- Cardiothoracic surgery

Incidence
- More common in patients older than age 70
- Affects men more than women

Common characteristics
- Irregularly irregular cardiac rhythm

Complications
- Transient ischemic attacks
- Stroke
- Heart failure
- Thromboembolism

✳ ASSESSMENT

History
- May be symptomatic
- Palpitations
- Fatigue
- Dyspnea
- Chest pain
- Syncope

Physical findings
- Irregular pulse
- Possible tachycardia
- Hypotension
- Signs of heart failure
- Respiratory distress

Test results
LABORATORY
- Cardiac enzymes show myocardial damage.
- Thyroid function studies reveal hyperthyroidism.
- Complete blood count, if history of recent blood loss, reveals anemia.

IMAGING
- Chest X-ray may determine if pulmonary edema is present.
- Echocardiogram or transesophageal echocardiography may help to identify valvular disease, left ventricular dysfunction, and atrial clots.

DIAGNOSTIC PROCEDURES
- Electrocardiogram may indicate irregular rhythm.
- Holter monitor may diagnose paroxysmal atrial fibrillation.

◆ TREATMENT

General
- Possible electrical cardioversion
- Control of ventricular rate
- Atrial fibrillation suppression pacemaker
- Ablation

Diet
- Sodium restriction, if indicated
- Low-fat, if indicated
- Fluid restriction, if indicated

Activity
- Planned rest periods, as needed

Medication
- Calcium channel blockers
- Beta-adrenergic blockers
- Antiarrhythmics
- Cardiac glycosides
- Anticoagulation

RECOGNIZING ATRIAL FIBRILLATION

The following rhythm strip shows atrial fibrillation.

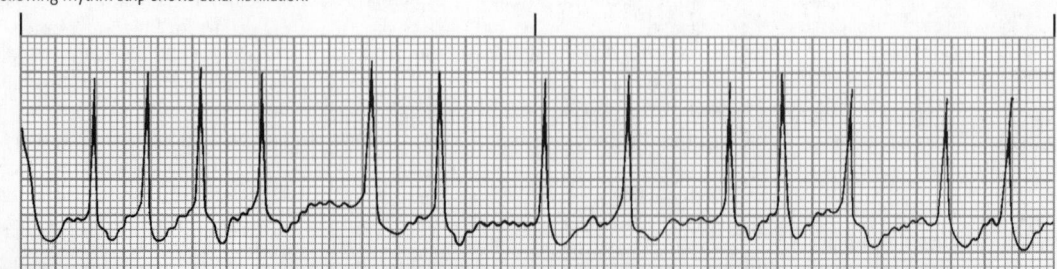

- Rhythm: irregular
- Rate: atrial – indiscernible; ventricular – 130 beats/minute
- P wave: absent; replaced by fine fibrillatory waves
- PR interval: indiscernible
- QRS complex: 0.08 second
- T wave: indiscernible
- QT interval: unmeasurable
- Other: none

NURSING CONSIDERATIONS

Nursing diagnoses
- Activity intolerance
- Anxiety
- Fatigue
- Noncompliance: Medication regimen

Key outcomes
The patient will:
- report ways to reduce activity intolerance
- identify effective coping mechanisms to manage anxiety
- report feelings of energy and decreased fatigue
- verbalize understanding of medication regimen.

Nursing interventions
- Administer medications, as ordered.
- Encourage the patient and family members to talk about feelings and concerns.
- Plan rest periods.

Monitoring
- Vital signs at rest and after physical activity
- Signs and symptoms of embolism
- Intake and output
- Daily weight
- Abnormal bleeding

PATIENT TEACHING

Be sure to cover:
- disorder, diagnosis, and treatment
- medication administration, dosage, and possible adverse effects
- when to notify the physician
- instructions on how to monitor pulse
- anticoagulation precautions
- abnormal bleeding
- signs and symptoms of embolic events.

RESOURCES

Organizations
American Heart Association: *www.americanheart.org*
St. Jude Medical Center: *www.aboutatrialfibrillation.com*

Selected references
Dambro, M.R., ed. *Griffith's Five-Minute Clinical Consult 2006.* Philadelphia: Lippincott Williams & Wilkins, 2006.
Holten, K.B. "How Should We Manage Newly Diagnosed Atrial Fibrillation?" *Journal of Family Practice* 53(8):641-43, August 2004.
Weiss, E.M., et al. "Atrial Fibrillation Treatment Options and Caveats," *AACN Advanced Critical Care* 15(3):362-76, July-September 2004.
Yee, C.A., "Atrial Fibrillation: The Ruthless Irregular Rhythm," *Nursing Critical Care* 1(5):30-37, September 2006.

Attention deficit hyperactivity disorder

● OVERVIEW

Description
- Behavioral problem characterized by difficulty focusing attention, engaging in quiet passive activities, or both
- May have attention deficit without hyperactivity

Pathophysiology
- Alleles of dopamine genes may alter dopamine transmission in the neural networks.
- During fetal development, bouts of hypoxia and hypotension could selectively damage neurons located in some of the critical regions of the anatomical networks.

Causes
- Underlying causes unknown
- Limited evidence of a genetic component
- May result from altered neurotransmitter levels in the brain

Risk factors
- Family history
- History of learning disability
- Mood or conduct disorder

Incidence
- Present at birth, but diagnosis before age 4 or 5 is difficult; some patients not diagnosed until adulthood
- Occurs in 3% to 5% of school-age children
- Affects males three times more than females

Common characteristics
- Impulsive behavior
- Inattentiveness
- Disorganization in school
- Tendency to jump quickly from one partly completed project, thought, or task to another
- Difficulty meeting deadlines and keeping track of school or work tools and materials

Complications
- Emotional and social complications
- Poor nutrition

✳ ASSESSMENT

History
- Characterized as a fidgeter and a day-dreamer
- Appears inattentive and lazy
- Performs sporadically at school or work

Physical findings
SYMPTOMS OF INATTENTION
- Makes careless mistakes
- Struggles to sustain attention
- Fails to finish activities
- Difficulty with organization
- Avoids tasks that require sustained mental effort
- Distracted or forgetful
SYMPTOMS OF HYPERACTIVITY
- Fidgets
- Unable to sit for sustained period
- Difficulty playing quietly
- Talks excessively
SYMPTOMS OF IMPULSIVITY
- Interrupts
- Can't wait patiently

Test results
- Diagnosis is based on *DSM-IV-TR* criteria findings.

DSM-IV-TR criteria
These criteria confirm a diagnosis:
- six symptoms or more from the inattention and/or hyperactivity-impulsivity categories
- symptoms present for at least 6 months
- symptoms evident before age 7
- impairment present in two or more settings
- symptoms aren't accounted for by another mental disorder.■
Complete psychological, medical, and neurologic evaluations rule out other problems; specific tests include continuous performance test, behavior rating scales, and learning disability.

◆ TREATMENT

General
- Education regarding the nature and effect of the disorder
- Behavior modification
- External structure
- Supportive psychotherapy

Diet
- Elimination of sugar, dyes, and additives

Activity
- Monitor for safety

Medication
- Stimulants
- Tricyclic antidepressants
- Mood stabilizers
- Beta-adrenergic blockers

Nursing diagnoses
- Compromised family coping
- Impaired social interaction
- Ineffective family therapeutic regimen management

Key outcomes
The patient (or family) will:
- seek out supportive services and demonstrate positive coping strategies
- demonstrate effective social interaction skills in one-on-one and group settings
- report improvement in family and social interactions.

Nursing interventions
- Set realistic expectations and limits (due to easy frustration).
- Maintain a calm and consistent manner.
- Keep all instructions short and simple — make one-step requests.
- Provide praise, rewards, and positive feedback whenever possible.
- Provide diversional activities suited to a short attention span.

Monitoring
- Activity level
- Nutritional status
- Adverse drug reactions
- Response to treatment
- Complications

Be sure to cover:
- behavior therapy
- reinforcement of good behavior
- realistic expectations
- medication administration, dosage, and possible adverse effects
- nutrition.

Discharge planning
- Refer the patient to family therapy.

Organizations
ADD helpline: *www.addhelpline.org*
Children and Adults with ADD: *www.chadd.org*
National Center for Learning Disabilities: *www.ncld.org*

Selected references
Diagnostic and Statistical Manual of Mental Disorders, Text Revision, 4th ed. Washington, D.C.: American Psychiatric Association, 2000.

McDonnell, M.A., and Dougherty, M. "Righting a Troubled Course. Diagnosing and Treating ADHD in Adults," *Advance for Nurse Practitioners* 13(8):53-56, August 2005.

Wolraich, M.I., et al. "Teachers' Screening for Attention Deficit/Hyperactivity Disorder: Comparing Multinational Samples on Teacher Ratings of ADHD," *Journal of Abnormal Child Psychology* 31(4):445-55, August 2003.

Autistic disorder

● OVERVIEW

Description
- Severe, pervasive developmental disorder
- Degree of impairment varies
- Usually apparent before age 3
- Poor prognosis
- Sometimes called *Kanner's autism*

Pathophysiology
- Defects in the central nervous system (CNS) that may arise from prenatal complications

Causes
- Exact cause unknown
- Defects in CNS from prenatal complications such as rubella
- Nutritional deficiency
- Disease possibly caused or triggered by immunizations

Risk factors
- High-risk pregnancy

Incidence
- Affects 4 to 5 children per 10,000 births
- Four to five times more likely in males than in females, usually the firstborn male

Common characteristics
- Unresponsive to social contact
- Gross deficit in intelligence and language development
- Ritualistic and compulsive behavior
- Restricted capacity for developmentally appropriate activities and interests
- Bizarre response to the environment

Complications
- Epileptic seizures
- Depression

DURING STRESS
- Catatonic phenomena
- Undifferentiated psychotic state

✳ ASSESSMENT

History
- Becomes rigid or flaccid when held
- Cries when touched
- Shows little or no interest in human contact

Physical findings
- Delayed smiling response
- Severe language impairment
- Lack of socialization and imaginative play
- Echolalia
- Pronoun reversal
- Bizarre or self-destructive behavior
- Extreme compulsion for sameness
- Abnormal reaction to sensory stimuli
- Cognitive impairment
- Eating, drinking, and sleeping problems
- Mood disorders

Test results
- Diagnosis is based on *DSM-IV-TR* criteria findings.

DSM-IV-TR criteria
At least six of these 12 characteristics must be present, including at least two items from the first section, one from the second, and one from the third.
- Qualitative impairment in social interaction:
  - impaired nonverbal behavior
  - absence of peer relationships
  - failure to seek or share enjoyment, interests, or achievements
  - lack of social or emotional reciprocity.
- Qualitative impairment in communication:
  - delay or lack of language development
  - failure to initiate or sustain conversation
  - idiosyncratic or repetitive language
  - lack of appropriate imaginative play.
- Restricted repetitive and stereotyped patterns of behavior, interests, and activities:
  - abnormal preoccupation with a restricted pattern of interest
  - inflexible routines or rituals
  - repetitive motor mannerisms
  - preoccupation with parts of objects.
- The diagnostic criteria also include delays or abnormal functioning in at least one of these areas before age 3:
  - social interaction and language skills
  - symbolic or imaginative play.

◆ TREATMENT

General
- Structured treatment plan
- Behavioral techniques
- Pleasurable sensory and motor stimulation

Diet
- No restrictions

Activity
- No restrictions
- Monitor for safety

Medication
- Haloperidol

❖ NURSING CONSIDERATIONS

Nursing diagnoses
- Delayed growth and development
- Disabled family coping
- Impaired verbal communication
- Interrupted family processes
- Risk for injury
- Risk for self-directed violence
- Social isolation

Key outcomes
The patient (or family) will:
- as much as possible, demonstrate age-appropriate skills and behaviors
- seek support systems and exhibit adequate coping behaviors
- develop alternate means of communication to express self
- identify and contact available resources, as needed
- practice safety measures and take safety precautions in the home
- refrain from harming self
- interact with family or friends.

Nursing interventions
- Institute safety measures when appropriate.
- Provide positive reinforcement.
- Encourage development of self-esteem.
- Encourage self-care.
- Prepare the child for change by telling him about it.
- Assist family members to develop strong one-on-one relationships with the patient.

Monitoring
- Response to treatment
- Complications
- Adverse drug reactions
- Patterns of behavior
- Nutritional status
- Social interaction
- Communication skills

▶ PATIENT TEACHING

Be sure to cover:
- physical care for the child's needs
- importance of identifying signs of excessive stress and coping skills.

Discharge planning
- Refer to resource and support services.

✳ RESOURCES

Organizations
Autism Society of America: *www.autism-society.org*
Center for the Study of Autism: *www.autism.org*
National Alliance for Autism Research: *www.naar.org*

Selected references
Corsello, C.M. "Early Intervention in Autism," *Infants and Young Children* 18(2):74-85, April-June 2005.
Diagnostic and Statistical Manual of Mental Disorders, Text Revision, 4th ed. Washington, D.C.: American Psychiatric Association, 2000.
Johnson, T. "Dietary Considerations in Autism: Identifying a Reasonable Approach," *Topics in Clinical Nutrition* 21(3):212-25, July-September 2005.
Mohr, W.K. *Psychiatric-Mental Health Nursing,* 6th ed. Philadelphia: Lippincott Williams & Wilkins, 2006.
Schumann, C.M., et al., "The Amygdala is Enlarged in Children But Not Adolescents with Autism; the Hippocampus is Enlarged at All Ages," *Journal of Neuroscience* 24(28):6392-401, July 2004.

Avian flu

● OVERVIEW

Description
- Infectious, contagious disease caused by the highly pathogenic influenza A (H5Nl) virus
- Carried in the intestines of wild birds worldwide without causing sickness, but highly contagious and deadly to domesticated birds (chickens, ducks, turkeys)
- In humans, caused by contact with infected poultry or contaminated surfaces
- Ongoing close monitoring of human infection and transmission due to concern over potential global outbreak in humans or influenza pandemic
- Also called *bird flu*

Pathophysiology
- After attaching to the host cell, viral ribonucleic acid enters the cell and uses host components to replicate its genetic material and protein, which are then assembled into new virus particles.
- Newly produced viruses burst forth to invade other healthy cells. (See *A closer look at the avian flu virus.*)
- Viral invasion destroys host cells, impairing respiratory defenses (especially the mucociliary transport system) and predisposing the patient to secondary bacterial infection.

Causes
- H5Nl virus
- Isolated reports of human-to-human transmission

Risk factors
- Direct or close contact with infected poultry or contaminated surfaces

Incidence
- Over 100 human cases reported since 1997, mostly by viruses of the H5 and H7 subtypes (H5Nl, H7N7, H7N3)

Common characteristics
- Flulike symptoms
- Signs and symptoms of upper respiratory infection such cough, fever, and sore throat

Complications
- Conjunctivitis
- Pneumonia
- Acute respiratory distress
- Viral pneumonia
- Sepsis
- Organ failure
- Death

✳ ASSESSMENT

History
- Direct contact with infected poultry or contaminated surfaces

Physical findings
- Fever
- Cough (dry or productive)
- Sore throat
- Difficulty breathing
- Diarrhea
- Runny nose
- Headache
- Muscle aches
- Malaise

Test results
LABORATORY
- Viral culture by polymerase chain reaction positive for H5Nl virus.

IMAGING
- None

Diagnostic procedures
- None

◆ TREATMENT

General
- Fluid and electrolyte replacements
- Oxygen and assisted ventilation, if indicated

Diet
- Increased fluid intake

Activity
- Rest periods, as needed

Medications
- Antiviral medications: oseltamavir (Tamiflu) and zanamavir (Relenza)

  ⬣ **NURSING ALERT** The avian flu virus, H5N1, has shown resistance to amantadine and rimantadine, two other antiviral agents used to treat influenza.
- Acetaminophen or aspirin
- Guaifenesin (Hytuss) or expectorant
- Antibiotics
- Vaccine (currently under investigation)

A CLOSER LOOK AT THE AVIAN FLU VIRUS

An electron microscope reveals the avian flu virus to have a rough, outer protein coat that appears speckled.

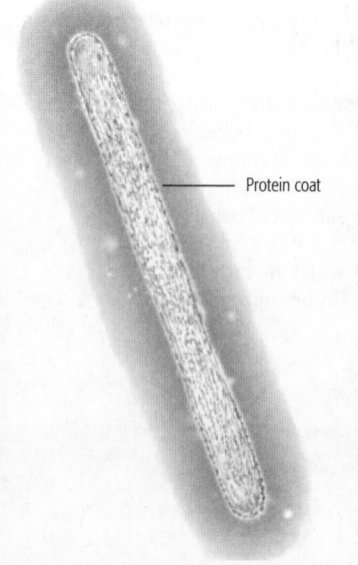

Protein coat

NURSING CONSIDERATIONS

Nursing diagnoses
- Acute pain
- Fatigue
- Hyperthermia
- Ineffective breathing pattern
- Risk for deficient fluid volume
- Risk for infection

Key outcomes
The patient will:
- express feelings of increased comfort and decreased pain
- report increased energy level
- maintain a normal temperature
- maintain respiratory rate of within 5 breaths/minute of baseline
- maintain adequate fluid volume
- remain free from signs and symptoms of infection.

Nursing interventions
- Give prescribed drugs.
- Follow standard precautions.
- Administer oxygen therapy, if warranted.
- Administer fluid therapy, as indicated.
- Notify local health authorities, as indicated.

Monitoring
- Temperature
- Signs and symptoms of dehydration
- Respiratory status, including respiratory rate and breath sounds
- Response to treatment

PATIENT TEACHING

Be sure to cover:
- the disorder, diagnosis, and treatment
- importance of increased fluids to prevent dehydration
- signs and symptoms of infection.
- Reiterate the importance of follow-up care.

RESOURCES

Organizations
Centers for Disease Control and Prevention: *www.cdc.gov*
National Institutes of Health: *www.nlm.nih.gov*
U.S. Department of Agriculture: *www.usda.gov*
World Health Organization: *www.who.int/en*

Selected references
Gani, R. "Potential Impact of Antiviral Drug Use During Influenza Pandemic," *Emerging Infectious Diseases* 11(9):1355-362, September 2005.
Henley, E. "The Growing Threat of Avian Influenza," *Journal of Family Practice* 54(5):442-44, May 2005.

Basal cell carcinoma

● OVERVIEW

Description
- Slow-growing, destructive skin tumor
- Two major types: noduloulcerative and superficial
- Most common malignant tumor that affects whites (see *Identifying basal cell carcinoma*)

Pathophysiology
- Although the pathogenesis is uncertain, some experts hypothesize that it originates when undifferentiated basal cells become carcinomatous instead of differentiating into sweat glands, sebum, and hair.

Causes
- Prolonged sun exposure (90% of tumors occur on sun-exposed areas of the body)

Risk factors
- Arsenic ingestion
- Radiation exposure
- Burns
- Immunosuppression
- Vaccinations a rare possibility

Incidence
- Usually occurs in people over age 40
- Most prevalent in blond, fair-skinned men

Common characteristics
- Lesion found on face, head, neck, and back
- Five warning signs, including:
  - an open sore
  - a reddish patch
  - a shiny bump
  - a pink growth
  - a scarlike area.

Complications
- Disfiguring lesions of the eyes, nose, and cheeks

✳ ASSESSMENT

History
- Odd-looking skin lesion
- Prolonged exposure to the sun

Physical findings
- Lesions characterized as small, smooth, pinkish, and translucent papules (early-stage noduloulcerative)
- Telangiectatic vessels cross surface and lesions may be pigmented
- Lesions becoming enlarged with depressed centers and firm and elevated borders (also called rodent ulcers)
- Multiple oval or irregularly shaped, lightly pigmented plaques on chest or back
- Head and neck showing waxy, sclerotic, yellow to white plaques without distinct borders

Test results
DIAGNOSTIC PROCEDURES
- Incisional or excisional biopsy and histologic study may help to determine the tumor type and histologic subtype.
OTHER
- All types of basal cell epitheliomas are diagnosed by clinical appearance.

IDENTIFYING BASAL CELL CARCINOMA

The illustration below shows an enlarged nasal nodule in basal cell carcinoma. Note its depressed center and firm, elevated border.

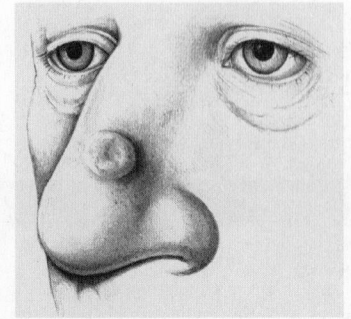

◆ TREATMENT

General
- Dependent on the size, location, and depth of the lesion
- Irradiation, if the tumor location requires it; preferred for elderly or debilitated patients who might not tolerate surgery
- Cryotherapy

Diet
- Well-balanced; no restrictions

Activity
- Restricted sun exposure

Medication
- Chemotherapy, such as topical fluorouracil and topical corticosteroids

Surgery
- Curettage and electrodesiccation
- Microscopically controlled surgical excision of lesion (after removal of large lesions, skin grafting may be required)
- Chemosurgery

Nursing diagnoses
- Anxiety
- Chronic low self-esteem
- Disturbed body image
- Fear
- Imbalanced nutrition: Less than body requirements
- Impaired skin integrity
- Ineffective coping
- Risk for infection

Key outcomes
The patient (or family) will:
- identify effective coping mechanisms to manage anxiety
- express positive feelings about self
- verbalize feelings about changed body image
- verbalize feelings of anxiety and fear
- maintain adequate nutrition and hydration
- exhibit improved or healed lesions or wounds
- demonstrate effective coping mechanisms
- remain free from signs and symptoms of infection.

Nursing interventions
- Encourage verbalization and provide support.
- Provide appropriate wound care.

Monitoring
- Complications of treatment
- Response to treatment
- Signs and symptoms of infection
- Wound healing
- Skin surveillance for additional lesions

Be sure to cover:
- need for frequent, small, high-protein meals
- appropriate skin care
- avoidance of excessive sun exposure and use of a strong sunscreen or sunshade to protect the skin.

Discharge planning
- Refer the patient to resource and support services.

Organizations
American Cancer Society: *www.cancer.org*
Guide to Internet Resources for Cancer: *www.cancerindex.org*
National Cancer Institute: *www.cancer.gov*

Selected references
Atlas of Pathophysiology, 2nd ed. Philadelphia: Lippincott Williams & Wilkins, 2005.

Casciato, D.A. *Manual of Clinical Oncology,* 5th ed. Philadelphia: Lippincott Williams & Wilkins, 2005.

Colvett, K.T., et al. "Atypical Presentation of Metastatic Basal Cell Carcinoma," *Southeastern Medical Journal* 97(3):305-07, March 2004.

Marin-Gutzke, M., et al. "Basal Cell Carcinoma in Childhood After Radiation Therapy: Case Report and Review," *Annals of Plastic Surgery* 53(6):593-95, December 2004.

National Cancer Institute, National Institutes of Health. *SEER Cancer Statistics Review* [Online]. Available: *seer.cancer.gov/Publications.*

Netscher, D.T., and Spira, M. "Basal Cell Carcinoma: An Overview of Tumor Biology and Treatment," *Plastic & Reconstructive Surgery* 113(5):74e-94e, April 2004.

Bell's palsy

● OVERVIEW

Description
- Impulses from the seventh cranial nerve blocked
- Rapid onset
- Subsides spontaneously in 80% to 90% of patients
- Complete recovery in 1 to 8 weeks
- Recovery possibly delayed in elderly people
- Partial recovery: contractures may develop on the paralyzed side of the face
- May recur on the same or the opposite side of the face

Pathophysiology
- Inflammatory reaction occurs around the seventh cranial nerve (motor innervation of the facial muscles), usually at the internal auditory meatus.
- Unilateral facial weakness or paralysis results.

Causes
- Unknown
- Ischemia
- Viral disease, such as herpes simplex or herpes zoster
- Local traumatic injury
- Autoimmune disease
- Lyme disease
- Tumor
- Bacterial infections such as meningitis

Incidence
- Affects all age-groups
- Most common between ages 20 to 60

Common characteristics
- Unilateral face weakness
- Aching at jaw angle
- Drooping mouth
- Distorted and loss of taste
- Impaired ability to fully close eye on affected side
- Tinnitus

Complications
- Corneal ulceration and blindness
- Impaired nutrition secondary to paralysis of the lower face
- Long-term psychosocial problems

✳ ASSESSMENT

History
- Pain occurring on the affected side around the angle of the jaw or behind the ear for a few hours or days before the onset of weakness
- Difficulty chewing on the affected side
- Difficulty speaking clearly

Physical findings
- Mouth droops on affected side (see *Facial paralysis in Bell's palsy*)
- Smooth-appearing forehead
- Distorted taste perception
- Unable to raise eyebrow, smile, show teeth, or puff out cheek
- Ability to close eye on the weak side markedly impaired
- Eye rolls upward (Bell's phenomenon) when attempting to close the eye
- Excessive tearing

Test results
- Diagnosis is based on clinical presentation.

◆ TREATMENT

General
- Elimination of source of damage to nerve immediately
- Oral hygiene maintenance
- Eye protection such as sunglasses
- Hearing protection
- Moist heat

Diet
- As tolerated

Activity
- As tolerated

Medication
- Oral corticosteroids
- Analgesics
- Saline eye drops

Surgery
- Possible exploration of the facial nerve

FACIAL PARALYSIS IN BELL'S PALSY

Unilateral facial paralysis characterizes Bell's palsy. The paralysis produces a distorted appearance and an inability to wrinkle the forehead, close the eyelid, smile, show the teeth, or puff out the cheek on the affected side.

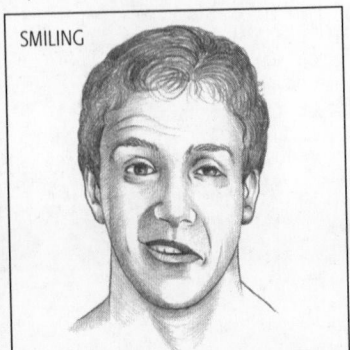

SMILING

❖ NURSING CONSIDERATIONS

Nursing diagnoses
- Acute pain
- Anxiety
- Disturbed body image
- Imbalanced nutrition: Less than body requirements
- Ineffective role performance
- Interrupted family processes
- Situational low self-esteem

Key outcomes
The patient will:
- experience increased comfort and relief from pain
- express feelings of decreased anxiety
- verbalize feelings about changed body image
- consume an adequate number of calories daily
- express feelings about diminished capacity to perform usual roles
- report improvement in family interactions
- state positive feelings about self.

Nursing interventions
- Provide psychological support.
- Apply moist heat to the affected side of the face.
- Massage the patient's face with a gentle upward motion.
- Provide a facial sling.
- If the patient had surgery, provide preoperative and postoperative care.
- Administer medication, as ordered.

Monitoring
- Response to medications
- Signs and symptoms of peptic ulceration, pancreatitis, or other GI adverse effects of prednisone
- Nutritional status

▶ PATIENT TEACHING

Be sure to cover:
- disorder, diagnosis, and treatment
- medication administration, dosage, and possible adverse effects
- protection of affected eye
- exercises of the facial muscles
- nutritional management program.

✹ RESOURCES

Organizations
National Institutes of Health: *www.nih.gov*
WebMD: *www.webmd.com*

Selected references
Ashtekar, C.S., et al. "Do We Need to Give Steroids in Children with Bell's Palsy?," *Emergency Medical Journal* 22(7):505-07, July 2005.

Diseases, 4th ed. Philadelphia: Lippincott Williams & Wilkins, 2006.

Handbook of Pathophysiology, 2nd ed. Philadelphia: Lippincott Williams & Wilkins, 2005.

Kanoh, N. et al. "Nocturnal Onset and Development of Bell's Palsy," *Laryngoscope* 115(1):99-100, January 2005.

Benign prostatic hyperplasia

● OVERVIEW

Description
- Prostate gland enlarges sufficiently to compress urethra, causing overt urinary obstruction
- Depending on the size of prostate, age and health of patient, and extent of obstruction, may be treated surgically or symptomatically
- Referred to as *BPH*

Pathophysiology
- Changes occur in periurethral glandular tissue.
- As the prostate enlarges, it may extend into bladder.
- Compression or distortion of prostatic urethra obstructs urine outflow.
- BPH may cause a diverticulum musculature, retaining urine.

Causes
- Unknown
- Recent evidence suggesting a possible link with hormonal activity

Risk factors
- Age
- Intact testes

Incidence
- 80% of all men older than age 40
- 95% of all men older than age 80

Common characteristics
- Changes in voiding patterns and urine stream

Complications
- Urinary stasis, urinary tract infection (UTI), or calculi
- Bladder wall trabeculation
- Detrusor muscle hypertrophy
- Bladder diverticula and saccules
- Urethral stenosis
- Hydronephrosis
- Paradoxical (overflow) incontinence
- Acute or chronic renal failure
- Acute postobstructive diuresis

✳ ASSESSMENT

History
- Decreased urine stream caliber and force
- Interrupted urinary stream
- Urinary hesitancy and frequency
- Difficulty starting urination
- Nocturia, hematuria
- Dribbling, incontinence
- Urine retention

Physical findings
- Visible midline mass above the symphysis pubis
- Distended bladder
- Enlarged prostate

Test results
LABORATORY
- Elevated blood urea nitrogen and serum creatinine levels suggest impaired renal function.
- Bacterial count exceeds $100,000/mm^3$, revealing hematuria, pyuria, and UTI.

IMAGING
- Excretory urography may indicate urinary tract obstruction, hydronephrosis, calculi or tumors, and bladder filling and emptying defects.

DIAGNOSTIC PROCEDURES
- Cystourethroscopy determines the best surgical intervention and shows prostate enlargement, bladder wall changes, calculi, and raised bladder.

◆ TREATMENT

General
- Prostatic massages
- Sitz baths
- Regular sexual intercourse

Diet
- Short-term fluid restriction (prevents bladder distention)

Activity
- After surgery, avoiding lifting, performing strenuous exercises, and taking long automobile rides for at least 1 month
- No sexual intercourse for several weeks after discharge

Medication
- Antibiotics, if infection present
- Alpha-1-adrenergic blockers such as terazosin
- Finasteride (Proscar)

Surgery
- For relief of acute urine retention, hydronephrosis, severe hematuria, and recurrent UTI or for palliative relief of intolerable symptoms
- Suprapubic (transvesical) prostatectomy
- Perineal prostatectomy
- Retropubic (extravesical) prostatectomy
- Transurethral resection
- Balloon dilatation, ultrasound needle ablation, and use of stents

Nursing diagnoses
- Acute pain
- Deficient knowledge (BPH)
- Disturbed body image
- Impaired urinary elimination
- Risk for infection
- Sexual dysfunction

Key outcomes
The patient will:
- express feelings of comfort and decreased pain
- verbalize understanding of disorder and treatment
- verbalize feelings about changed body image
- demonstrate skill in managing urinary elimination
- remain free from signs and symptoms of infection
- express feelings about potential or actual changes in sexual activity.

Nursing interventions
- Administer medication, as ordered.
- Avoid giving tranquilizers, alcohol, antidepressants, or anticholinergics (can worsen the obstruction).
- Provide I.V. therapy, as ordered.

Monitoring
- Vital signs
- Intake and output
- Daily weight

⬥ **NURSING ALERT** Watch for signs of postobstructive diuresis, characterized by polyuria exceeding 2 L in 8 hours and excessive electrolyte losses. Although usually self-limiting, it can result in vascular collapse and death if not promptly treated.

AFTER PROSTATIC SURGERY
- Pain control
- Catheter function and drainage
- Signs of infection

Be sure to cover:
- disorder, diagnosis, and treatment
- signs of UTI that should be reported
- when to seek medical care (fever, unable to void, or passing bloody urine).

Organizations
American Association of Kidney Patients: *www.aakp.org*
National Institute of Diabetes & Digestive & Kidney Diseases: *www.niddk.nih.gov*

Selected references
Diseases, 4th ed. Philadelphia: Lippincott Williams & Wilkins, 2006.
Gilchrist, K.L. "Twin Perils of Prostate Health," *Nursing Made Incredibly Easy* 3(6):30-42, November-December 2005.
McPhee, S.J., et al., eds. *Current Medical Diagnosis and Treatment,* New York: McGraw-Hill Book Co., 2007.

Bipolar disorder

OVERVIEW

Description
- Affective disorder marked by severe pathologic mood swings from hyperactivity and euphoria to sadness and depression
- Cyclothymia, a variant of bipolar disorder: numerous episodes of hypomania and depressive symptoms too mild to meet criteria for major depression or bipolar disorder (see *Cyclothymic disorder*)
- Manic episodes: emerge over a period of days to weeks, but onset within hours is possible
- Untreated episodes: can last weeks or as long as 8 to 12 months, with some having an unremitting course
- Rapid cycling: occurs when four or more episodes of either depression or mania occur in a given year and occurs in 15% of all patients, almost all women
- Results in difficulties in work performance and psychosocial functioning (in approximately half of all patients)

Pathophysiology
- Mood swings may involve membrane changes in sodium- and potassium-activated adenosine triphosphatase, involving disordered intracellular signals.

Causes
- Exact cause unknown
- Autosomal dominant inheritance found in genetic studies (possible link to an X chromosome disorder)
- May be triggered by death, separation, and divorce
- Imbalances in the biochemistry that controls food (biochemical) imbalances

Risk factors
- Family history
- Drug abuse

Incidence
- Affects 3 million people in the United States
- Equally common in women and men
- Depressive episodes more prevalent in women
- Manic episodes more prevalent in men

- Higher among relatives of affected patients than in the general population
- **AGE-RELATED CONCERN** Age of onset is usually between ages 20 and 35, but 35% of patients experience onset between ages 35 and 60.

Common characteristics
MANIC PHASE
- Accelerated speech
- Frequent changes of topic
- Flight of ideas

DEPRESSIVE PHASE
- Loss of self-esteem
- Overwhelming inertia
- Social withdrawal
- Feelings of hopelessness
- Apathy or self-reproach
- Suicidal thoughts

BIPOLAR II DISORDER
- Meets all the diagnostic criteria for a manic episode
- May experience recurrent depressions, separated by periods of mild activation and increased energy

Complications
- Emotional and social consequences
- Sexually transmitted disease
- Exhaustion
- Nutritional deficits
- Sleep disturbances
- Suicide

ASSESSMENT

History
- Sleeping and eating disturbances
- Exhibits expansive, grandiose, sometimes irritable, mood alternating with symptoms of depression

Physical findings
MANIA
- Increased psychomotor activity
- Excessive social extroversion
- Impulsive actions
- Impaired judgment
- Delusions
- Paranoid thinking
- Limited attention span
- Inflated sense of self-esteem
- Rapid responses to external stimuli

DEPRESSION
- Slow speech and response
- No obvious disorientation or intellectual impairment
- Psychomotor retardation
- Lethargy
- Low muscle tone
- Weight loss
- Slowed gait

Test results
- Diagnosis is based on *DSM-IV-TR* criteria findings.

DSM-IV-TR criteria
A diagnosis is confirmed when the patient meets the criteria established for a manic or hypomanic episode:
- experiences a distinct period of abnormally and persistently elevated, expansive, or irritable mood
- during the mood disturbance, at least three of these symptoms must persist (four, if the mood is only irritable) and be present to a significant degree:
  - inflated self-esteem or grandiosity
  - decreased need for sleep
  - excessive talking
  - flight of ideas
  - easily distracted
  - psychomotor agitation
  - excessive involvement in dangerous activities
  - symptoms don't meet criteria for a mixed episode
  - impairment in occupational function, usual social activities, or relations with others severe enough to

require hospitalization to prevent harm to self or others
– substance or medical conditions aren't present.

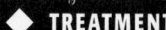 TREATMENT

General
- Group and individual therapy

Diet
- No restrictions

Activity
- Monitor activity when in manic phase

Medication
- Lithium
- Antipsychotics
- Valproic acid
- Carbamazepine
- Antidepressants

CYCLOTHYMIC DISORDER

A chronic mood disturbance of at least 2 years' duration, cyclothymic disorder involves numerous episodes of hypomania or depressive symptoms that aren't of sufficient severity or duration to qualify as a major depressive episode.

In the hypomanic phase, the patient may experience insomnia; hyperactivity; inflated self-esteem; increased productivity and creativity; overinvolvement in pleasurable activities, including an increased sexual drive; physical restlessness; and rapid speech. Depressive symptoms may include insomnia, feelings of inadequacy, decreased productivity, social withdrawal, loss of libido, loss of interest in pleasurable activities, lethargy, depressed speech, and crying.

A number of medical disorders (for example, endocrinopathies, such as Cushing's disease, stroke, brain tumors, head trauma, and drug overdose) can produce a similar pattern of mood alteration. These organic causes must be ruled out before making a diagnosis of cyclothymic disorder.

⚜ NURSING CONSIDERATIONS

Nursing diagnoses
- Disturbed personal identity
- Impaired social interaction
- Ineffective coping
- Ineffective role performance
- Situational low self-esteem

Key outcomes
The patient will:
- express positive feelings about self
- demonstrate effective social interaction skills
- identify effective coping techniques
- express feelings about diminished capacity to perform usual roles
- voice feelings related to self-esteem.

Nursing interventions
FOR THE MANIC PATIENT
- Encourage activities that require gross motor movements.
- Assist with personal hygiene; encourage responsibility for personal care.
- Protect from overstimulation.
- Set realistic goals and limits for the patient's behavior.
- Provide diversional activities suited to a short attention span.
- Reorient to reality.
- Avoid power struggles.

FOR THE DEPRESSED PATIENT
- Avoid overwhelming expectations.
- Allow increased time for activities and responses.
- Provide a structured routine.
- Promote interaction with others.
- Encourage verbalization; provide support.
- Institute safety measures.
- Encourage physical activity.

Monitoring
- Patterns of behavior
- Response to treatment
- Social interaction
- Complications
- Adverse drug reactions
- Nutritional status

▶ PATIENT TEACHING

Be sure to cover:
- disorder, diagnosis, and treatment
- medication administration, dosage, and possible adverse effects
- importance of continuing the prescribed medication regimen.

Discharge planning
- Refer the patient to support services.

✳ RESOURCES

Organizations
American Psychiatric Association: *www.helping.apa.org*
National Alliance for the Mentally Ill: *www.nami.org*
National Depressive and Manic-Depressive Association: *www.ndmda.org*
National Mental Health Association: *www.nmha.org*

Selected references
Diagnostic and Statistical Manual of Mental Disorders, Text Revision, 4th ed. Washington, D.C.: American Psychiatric Association, 2000.
Murphy, K., "Managing the Ups and Downs of Bipolar Disorder," *Nursing2006* 36(10):58-63, October 2006.
Murphy, K., "The Separate Reality of Bipolar Disorder and Schizophrenia," *Nursing Made Incredibly Easy* 3(3):6-18, May-June 2005.
Schapiro, N.A., "Bipolar Disorders in Children and Adolescents," *Journal of Pediatric Health Care* 19(3):131-41, May-June 2005.
Swann, A.C., et al. "Psychosis in Mania: Specificity of Its Role in Severity and Treatment Response," *Journal of Clinical Psychiatry* 65(6):825-29, June 2004.

Bladder cancer

● OVERVIEW

Description
- Most common cancer of the urinary tract
- Transitional cell carcinomas: account for about 90% of bladder cancers and arise from the transitional epithelium of mucous membranes (they may result from malignant transformation of benign papillomas)
- Less common bladder tumors: adenocarcinomas, epidermoid carcinomas, squamous cell carcinomas, sarcomas, tumors in bladder diverticula, and carcinoma in situ

Pathophysiology
- Benign or malignant tumors may develop on the bladder wall surface or grow within the wall and quickly invade underlying muscles.

Causes
- Exact cause unknown
- Associated with chronic bladder irritation and infection in people with renal calculi, indwelling urinary catheters, chemical cystitis caused by cyclophosphamide, and pelvic irradiation

Risk factors
- Certain environmental carcinogens, such as 2-naphthylamine, tobacco, nitrates, and coffee
- Occupational exposure to carcinogens

Incidence
- Most prevalent in people over age 50
- More common in men than in women
- Occurs more commonly in densely populated industrial areas

Common characteristics
- Asymptomatic in early stages for 25% of patients
- Gross, painless, intermittent hematuria, with or without clots (first sign)
- Suprapubic pain after voiding most often associated with invasive lesions
- Bladder irritability
- Urinary frequency
- Nocturia
- Dribbling

Complications
- Bone metastases
- Problems resulting from tumor invasion of contiguous viscera

✱ ASSESSMENT

History
- Gross, painless, intermittent hematuria, often with clots
- Suprapubic pain after voiding, which suggests invasive lesions
- Bladder irritability, urinary frequency, nocturia, and dribbling
- Flank pain that may indicate an obstructed ureter

Physical findings
- Gross hematuria
- Flank tenderness if ureteral obstruction present

Test results
LABORATORY
- Complete blood count helps to detect anemia.
- Urinalysis detects blood and malignant cells in the urine.

IMAGING
- Excretory urography can identify a large, early-stage tumor or an infiltrating tumor; delineate functional problems in the upper urinary tract; assess hydronephrosis; and detect rigid deformity of the bladder wall.
- Retrograde cystography evaluates bladder structure and integrity; also helps confirm a bladder cancer diagnosis.
- Bone scan can detect metastases.
- Computed tomography scan can define the thickness of the involved bladder wall and disclose enlarged retroperitoneal lymph nodes.
- Ultrasonography can find metastases in tissues beyond the bladder and can distinguish a bladder cyst from a bladder tumor.

DIAGNOSTIC PROCEDURES
- Cystoscopy and biopsy confirm bladder cancer diagnosis; if the test results show cancer cells, further studies will determine the cancer stage and treatment.

OTHER
- Bimanual examination may be performed during a cystoscopy if the patient has received an anesthetic; this helps to determine whether the bladder is fixed to the pelvic wall.

◆ TREATMENT

General
- Therapy dependent on cancer's stage and the patient's lifestyle, other health problems, and mental outlook

Diet
- No restrictions

Activity
- Initially postoperatively, no heavy lifting and contact sports
- After recovery, no restrictions

Medication
- Intravesical chemotherapy, such as thiotepa, doxorubicin, and mitomycin
- Attenuated bacille Calmette-Guérin vaccine live

Surgery
- Transurethral resection (cystoscopic approach) and fulguration (electrically)
- Segmental bladder
- Radical cystectomy
- Ureterostomy, nephrostomy, continent vesicostomy (Kock pouch), ileal bladder, and ureterosigmoidostomy

Nursing diagnoses
- Acute pain
- Anxiety
- Disabled family coping
- Disturbed body image
- Fear
- Impaired skin integrity
- Impaired urinary elimination
- Ineffective coping
- Risk for infection
- Sexual dysfunction

Key outcomes
The patient will:
- express feelings of comfort and decreased pain
- express feelings of decreased anxiety
- seek support systems and exhibit adequate coping behaviors
- verbalize feelings about changed body image
- verbalize feelings of anxiety and fear
- maintain skin integrity
- demonstrate skill in managing urinary elimation
- exhibit adequate coping mechanisms
- remain free from signs of infection
- voice feelings about potential or actual changes in sexual activity.

Nursing interventions
- Provide support and encourage verbalization.
- Administer medications, as ordered.
- Provide preoperative teaching; discuss procedure and postoperative course.

Monitoring
- Wound site
- Postoperative complications
- Intake and output
- Pain control

Be sure to cover:
- disorder, diagnosis, and treatment
- stoma care
- skin care and evaluation
- avoidance of heavy lifting and contact sports (postoperatively with a urinary stoma)
- encouragment of participation in usual athletic and physical activities.

Discharge planning
- Refer the patient to resource and support services.
- Before discharge, arrange for follow-up home nursing care.
- Refer the patient to an enterostomal therapist.

Organizations
American Cancer Society: *www.cancer.org*
Guide to Internet Resources for Cancer: *www.cancerindex.org*
National Cancer Institute: *www.nci.org*
National Institute of Diabetes & Digestive & Kidney Diseases: *www.niddk.nih.gov*
United Ostomy Association, Inc: *www.uoa.org*

Selected references
Atlas of Pathophysiology, 2nd ed. Philadelphia: Lippincott Williams & Wilkins, 2005.

Burkhard, F.C., et al. "Continent Urinary Diversion," *Critical Reviews in Oncology/Hematology* 57(3):255-64, March 2006.

McGrath, M., et al. "Hormonal and Reproductive Factors and the Risk of Bladder Cancer in Women," *American Journal of Epidemiology* 63(3):236-44, November 2005.

National Cancer Institute, National Institutes of Health. *SEER Cancer Statistics Review* [Online]. Available: *www.seer.cancer.gov/Publications.*

Vogelzang, N., et al. *Comprehensive Textbook of Genitourinary Oncology*, 3rd ed. Lippincott Williams & Wilkins, 2006.

Blood transfusion reaction

Description
- Accompanies or follows I.V. administration of blood components
- Mediated by immune or nonimmune factors
- Severity ranging from mild to severe

Pathophysiology
- A hemolytic reaction follows the transfusion of mismatched blood.
- Recipient's antibodies, immunoglobulin (Ig) G or IgM, attach to donor red blood cells (RBCs), leading to widespread clumping and destruction of recipient's RBCs.
- Transfusion with Rh-incompatible blood triggers a less serious reaction, known as Rh isoimmunization, within several days to 2 weeks. (See *Understanding the Rh system.*)
- A febrile nonhemolytic reaction—the most common type of reaction—develops when cytotoxic or agglutinating antibodies in the recipient's plasma attack antigens on transfused lymphocytes, granulocytes, or plasma cells.

Causes
- Transfusion with incompatible blood

Incidence
- Mild reactions occurring in 1% to 2% of transfusions

Common characteristics
- Mild to severe fever: hallmark of a febrile nonhemolytic reaction that begins at the start of transfusion or within 2 hours after its completion

Complications
- Bronchospasm
- Acute tubular necrosis leading to acute renal failure
- Anaphylactic shock
- Vascular collapse
- Disseminated intravascular coagulation

History
- Reaction occurring within a few minutes or hours after transfusion begins
- Chills, nausea, vomiting, chest tightness, and chest and back pain

Physical findings
- Fever, tachycardia, and hypotension
- Dyspnea and apprehension
- Urticaria and angioedema
- Wheezing
- In a surgical patient, blood oozing from mucous membranes or the incision site
- In a hemolytic reaction, fever, an unexpected decrease in serum hemoglobin level, frank blood in urine, and jaundice

Test results
LABORATORY
- Serum hemoglobin levels are decreased.
- Serum bilirubin levels and indirect bilirubin levels are elevated.
- Urinalysis reveals hemoglobinuria.
- Indirect Coombs' test or serum antibody screen is positive for serum anti-A or anti-B antibodies.
- Prothrombin time is increased and fibrinogen levels are decreased.
- Blood urea nitrogen and serum creatinine levels are increased.

General
- Immediate cessation of transfusion
- Dialysis, if acute tubular necrosis occurs

Diet
- As tolerated

Activity
- Bed rest

Medication
- Osmotic or loop diuretics
- I.V. normal saline solution
- I.V. vasopressors
- Epinephrine
- Diphenhydramine
- Corticosteroids
- Mannitol or furosemide
- Antipyretics

❖ NURSING CONSIDERATIONS

Nursing diagnoses
- Acute pain
- Anxiety
- Decreased cardiac output
- Impaired gas exchange
- Impaired tissue integrity
- Powerlessness
- Risk for imbalanced body temperature
- Risk for injury

Key outcomes
The patient will:
- express feelings of comfort and relief from pain
- verbalize measures to reduce his anxiety level
- maintain adequate cardiac output
- maintain adequate ventilation and oxygenation
- exhibit reduced redness, swelling, and pain at the site of impaired tissue
- express feelings of control over his well-being
- maintain a normal body temperature
- remain free from injury.

Nursing interventions
- Maintain a patent I.V. line with normal saline solution.
- Insert an indwelling urinary catheter.
- Report early signs of complications.
- Cover the patient to ease chills.
- Administer supplemental oxygen, as needed.
- Document the transfusion reaction on the patient's chart, noting the duration of the transfusion and the amount of blood absorbed.
- Make sure you know and follow your facility's blood transfusion policy and procedure.

◈ **NURSING ALERT** Double-check the patient's name, identification number, ABO group, and Rh status before administering blood. If you find any discrepancy, don't administer the blood. Notify the blood bank immediately and return the unopened unit.

Monitoring
- Intake and output
- Vital signs
- Signs of shock
- Laboratory results

▶ PATIENT TEACHING

Be sure to cover:
- transfusion reaction
- type of transfusion after recovery.

✳ RESOURCES

Organizations
American Association of Blood Banks: *www.aabb.org*
Centers for Disease Control and Prevention: *www.cdc.gov*

Selected references
Kaspar, D.L., et al., eds. *Harrison's Principles of Internal Medicine*, 16th ed. New York: McGraw-Hill Book Co., 2005.
The Merck Manual of Diagnosis & Therapy, 18th ed. Whitehouse Station, N.J.: Merck & Co., Inc., 2006.
Sapatnekar, S., et al. "Acute Hemolytic Transfusion Reaction in a Pediatric Patient Following Transfusion of Apheresis Platelets," *Journal of Clinical Apheresis* 20(4):225-29, December 2005.
Young, J. "Transfusion Reaction," *Nursing 2000* 30(12):33, December 2000.

UNDERSTANDING THE RH SYSTEM

The Rh system contains more than 30 antibodies and antigens. Of the world's population, about 85% are Rh positive, which means that their red blood cells carry the D or Rh antigen. The rest of the population is Rh negative and don't have this antigen.

Effects of sensitization
When an Rh-negative person receives Rh-positive blood for the first time, he becomes sensitized to the D antigen but shows no immediate reaction to it. If he receives Rh-positive blood a second time, he experiences a massive hemolytic reaction.

For example, an Rh-negative mother who delivers an Rh-positive baby is sensitized by the baby's Rh-positive blood. During her next Rh-positive pregnancy, her sensitized blood will cause a hemolytic reaction in the fetal circulation.

Preventing sensitization
To prevent the formation of antibodies against Rh-positive blood, an Rh-negative mother should receive $Rh_o(D)$ immune globulin (human) (RhoGAM) I.M. within 72 hours after delivering an Rh-positive baby.

Body dysmorphic disorder

● OVERVIEW

Description
- Preoccupation with an imagined (or, if present, slight) defect in physical appearance
- Characterized by patient's belief that he's hideous or grotesque despite reassurance from others that he looks fine
- Thinks about the defect for at least 1 hour each day

Pathophysiology
- Biological theories for body dysmorphic disorder include a genetic predisposition, adolescent stressors, or imbalanced levels of serotonin or other chemicals in the brain.
- The psychological theory for body dysmorpic disorder is low self-esteem, resulting in the tendency to judge oneself almost exclusively by appearance.

Causes
- Exact cause unknown
- Biological or psychological theories
- Perfectionism and heightened perception about appearance causing increased focus on every perceived imperfection or slight abnormality

Incidence
- Affects 1% to 2% of the general population in the United States; however, may be underestimated because the disorder frequently goes undiagnosed
- Chronic condition with age of onset usually in the late teens (average age 17); affects males and females equally

Common characteristics
- Perception of a defect, such as skin imperfections, absence of or excessive hair, or size or shape of a body part
- Distorted view of self
- Significant distress due to perceived defect

Complications
- Obsessive-compulsive disorder
- Major depression
- Social phobia
- Suicide

✳ ASSESSMENT

History
- Preoccupation with imagined (or, if present, slight) defect in physical appearance
- Thinks about defect for at least 1 hour daily

Physical findings
Suspect body dysmorphic disorder in patient who reports or exhibits any of these behaviors:
- often checks reflection in the mirror, or avoids mirrors
- frequently compares appearance against that of others
- frequently examines the appearance of other people
- tries to cover the perceived defect with clothing, makeup, or a hat or by changing posture
- seeks corrective treatment, such as surgery or dermatologic therapy, to eradiate the perceived defect
- constantly seeks reassurance from others about the perceived flaw, or, conversely, tries to convince others of its repulsiveness
- performs long grooming rituals, such as repeatedly combing or cutting hair or applying makeup or cover-up creams
- picks at the skin or squeezes pimples or blackheads for hours
- frequently touches the perceived problem area
- measures the body part that's repulsive
- displays anxiety and self-consciousness
- feels acute distress over appearance, causing functional impairment
- avoids social situations where the perceived defect may be exposed
- has difficulty maintaining relationships with peers, family, and spouse
- performs poorly in school, work, or takes frequent sick days
- has low self-esteem
- has suicidal thoughts or behaviors.

Test results
- Diagnosis is based on *DSM-IV-TR* criteria findings

DSM-IV-TR criteria
The patient must meet all three criteria
- Patient is preoccupied with an imagined defect in appearance; if a slight physical abnormality actually is present, concern over it is markedly excessive.
- Preoccupation causes clinically significant distress or impairment in social, occupational, or other important areas of functioning.
- Preoccupation isn't better explained by another mental disorder, such as anorexia nervosa.

◆ TREATMENT

General
- Enhancement of self-esteem
- Reduction of preoccupation with perceived flaw
- Elimination of harmful effects of compulsive behaviors
- Cognitive-behavioral group therapies
- Behavioral methods (aversion therapy, thought stopping, and implosion therapy)

Diet
- No restrictions or recommendations

Activity
- No restrictions or recommendations

Medication
- Selective serotonin reuptake inhibitors
- Tricyclic antidepressants

Surgery
- None

❖ NURSING CONSIDERATIONS

Nursing diagnoses
- Chronic low self-esteem
- Disturbed body image
- Disturbed personal identity
- Impaired social interaction
- Ineffective coping
- Ineffective health maintenance
- Risk for suicide
- Social isolation

Key outcomes
The patient will:
- voice feelings related to self-esteem
- express positive feelings about self
- establish a firm, positive sense of personal identity
- exhibit effective social interaction skills
- identify effective and ineffective coping mechanisms
- maintain a state of wellness
- not harm self
- maintain family and peer relationships.

Nursing interventions
- Approach the patient unhurriedly.
- Keep the patient's physical health in mind.
- Provide an accepting, nonjudgmental attitude.
- Let the patient see that you're aware of her behavior.
- Give the patient time to carry out ritualistic behavior.
- Impose reasonable demands.
- Set reasonable limits.
- Identify insight and improved behavior and offer praise.
- Engage the patient in activities that create positive accomplishments.
- Help the patient devise new ways to solve problems.
- Listen attentively and offer feedback.
- Monitor the patient for desired effect of medications, as appropriate.

Monitoring
- Patterns of behavior
- Response to treatment, including medications
- Social interaction

▶ PATIENT TEACHING

Be sure to cover:
- active diversions, such as whistling or humming to divert the patient's attention away from unwanted thoughts
- new ways to solve problems and develop more effective coping skills by setting limits on unacceptable behavior
- use of appropriate techniques to relieve stress, loneliness, and isolation
- importance of follow-up care.

Discharge planning
- Refer the patient to appropriate support services.

✷ RESOURCES

Organizations
American Psychiatric Association:
www.psych.org
National Mental Health Association:
www.nmha.org

Selected references
Castle, D.J., & Rossell, S.L. "An Update on Body Dysmorphic Disorder," *Current Opinion in Psychiatry* 19(1):74-78, January 2006.

Diagnostic and Statistical Manual of Mental Disorders, Text Revision, 4th ed., Washington, D.C.: American Psychiatric Association, 2000.

Metules, T. "Cosmetic Surgery: Is It Really Right for Your Patient?" *RN* 68(3):32acl-5, March 2005.

Nettina, S.M. *Lippincott Manual of Nursing Practice,* 8th ed. Philadelphia: Lippincott Williams & Wilkins, 2006.

Botulism

● OVERVIEW

Description
- Life-threatening paralytic illness
- Results from an exotoxin produced by the gram-positive, anaerobic bacillus *Clostridium botulinum*
- Occurs as botulism food poisoning, wound botulism, and infant botulism
- Mortality rate about 25%, with death most commonly caused by respiratory failure during the first week of illness
- Onset within 24 hours signaling critical and potentially fatal illness

Pathophysiology
- Endotoxin acts at the neuromuscular junction of skeletal muscle, preventing acetylcholine release and blocking neural transmission, eventually resulting in paralysis.

Causes
- Eating improperly preserved foods

Risk factors
- Honey contaminated with *C. botulinum* spores (see *Infant botulism*)

Incidence
- Occurs worldwide
- Affects adults more than children

Common characteristics
- Signs appearing 12 to 36 hours after ingestion of contaminated food; however possible delay of up to 8 days before symptoms appear
- Signs ranging in severity and can mimic other illnesses, especially neurologic disorders

Complications
- Respiratory failure
- Paralytic ileus
- Death

✳ ASSESSMENT

History
- Consumption of home-canned food 12 to 36 hours before onset of symptoms
- Vertigo
- Sore throat
- Weakness
- Nausea and vomiting
- Constipation or diarrhea
- Diplopia
- Blurred vision
- Dysarthria
- Dysphagia
- Dyspnea

Physical findings
- Ptosis
- Dilated, nonreactive pupils
- Oral mucous membranes that appear dry, red, and crusted
- Abdominal distention with absent bowel sounds
- Descending weakness or paralysis of muscles in the extremities or trunk
- Deep tendon reflexes that may be intact, diminished, or absent
- Unexplained postural hypotension
- Urinary retention
- Photophobia

Test results
LABORATORY
- Mouse bioassay detects toxin that's found in the patient's serum, stool, or gastric contents.
DIAGNOSTIC PROCEDURES
- Electromyogram shows diminished muscle action potential after a single supramaximal nerve stimulus.

◆ TREATMENT

General
- Early tracheotomy and ventilatory assistance in respiratory failure
- Nasogastric suctioning

Diet
- Total parenteral nutrition

Activity
- Bed rest

Medication
- I.V. or I.M. administration of botulinum antitoxin

INFANT BOTULISM

Infant botulism, which usually afflicts infants between 3 and 20 weeks old, is often associated with a history of honey ingestion. This disorder can produce floppy infant syndrome, which is characterized by constipation, a feeble cry, a depressed gag reflex, and an inability to suck. The infant also exhibits a flaccid facial expression, ptosis, and ophthalmoplegia—the result of cranial nerve deficits.

As the disease progresses the infant develops generalized weakness, hypotonia, areflexia, and a sometimes-striking loss of head control. Respiratory arrest occurs in almost half of affected infants.

Intensive supportive care allows most infants to recover completely. Antitoxin therapy isn't recommended because of the risk of anaphylaxis.

✤ NURSING CONSIDERATIONS

Nursing diagnoses
- Acute pain
- Imbalanced nutrition: Less than body requirements
- Impaired physical mobility
- Impaired swallowing
- Impaired verbal communication
- Ineffective airway clearance
- Ineffective breathing pattern
- Risk for injury

Key outcomes
The patient will:
- express feelings of comfort and reduced pain
- maintain adequate daily calorie requirements
- return to his usual mobility level
- swallow without pain or difficulty
- demonstrate effective communication skills
- maintain a patent airway
- maintain tissue perfusion and cellular oxygenation
- remain free from injury.

Nursing interventions
- Obtain history of food intake for the past several days.
- Obtain family history of similar symptoms and food intake.
- Administer I.V. fluids, as ordered.

🔷 **NURSING ALERT** Immediately report all cases of botulism to the local board of health.

Monitoring
- Neurologic status
- Cardiac and respiratory function
- Cough and gag reflexes
- Input and output
- Arterial blood gas levels

▶ PATIENT TEACHING

Be sure to cover:
- disorder, diagnosis, and treatment
- proper techniques in processing and preserving foods
- never tasting food from a bulging can or one with a peculiar odor
- sterilizing utensils by boiling what came in contact with suspected food
- not feeding honey to infants (can be fatal if contaminated).

✴ RESOURCES

Organizations
Centers for Disease Control and Prevention (CDC): www.cdc.gov
Harvard University Consumer Health Information: www.intelihealth.com
National Health Information Center: www.health.gov/nhic
National Library of Medicine: www.nlm.nih.gov
National Organization for Rare Disorders: www.rarediseases.org

Selected references
Cherrington, M. "Botulism: Update and Review," *Seminars in Neurology* 24(2):155-63, June 2004.
Gupta, A. et al. "Adult Botulism Type F in the United States, 1981-2002," *Neurology* 65(11):1694-700, December 2005.
Kaspar, D.L., et al., eds. *Harrison's Principles of Internal Medicine*, 16th ed. New York: McGraw-Hill Book Co., 2005.
Sieradzan, K.A., "Wound Botulism," *Practical Neurology* 5(1):46-51, February 2005.
Walker, B. "Combating Infection: Beating Botulism," *Nursing2004* 34(6):74, June 2004.

Brain cancer

● OVERVIEW

Description
- Growths within the intracranial space; tumors of the brain tissue, meninges, pituitary gland, and blood vessels
- In adults: most common tumor types are gliomas and meningiomas, which usually occur above the covering of the cerebellum, or supratentorial tumors
- In children: most common tumor types are astrocytomas, medulloblastomas, ependymomas, and brain stem gliomas
- Most common cause of cancer death in children

Pathophysiology
- Brain cancer is classified based on histology or grade of cell malignancy.
- The central nervous system changes through invasion and destruction of tissues and by secondary effect — mainly compression of the brain, cranial nerves, and cerebral vessels; cerebral edema; and increased intracranial pressure (ICP).

Causes
- Cause unknown

Risk factors
- Preexisting cancer

Incidence
- Slightly more common in men than in women
- Gliomas, meningiomas, and schwannomas have overall incidence of 4.5 per 100,000
- Can occur at any age; however in adults, incidence highest between ages 40 and 60
- Most occur in children before age 1 or between ages 2 and 12

Common characteristics
- Increased ICP
- Headache
- Decreased motor strength and coordination
- Seizures
- Altered vital signs
- Nausea and vomiting
- Papilledema

Complications
- Radiation encephalopathy

LIFE-THREATENING COMPLICATIONS FROM INCREASED ICP
- Coma
- Respiratory or cardiac arrest
- Brain herniation

✳ ASSESSMENT

History
- Insidious onset
- Headache
- Nausea and vomiting

Physical findings
SIGNS AND SYMPTOMS OF INCREASED ICP
- Vision disturbances
- Weakness, paralysis
- Aphasia, dysphagia
- Ataxia, incoordination
- Seizure

Test results
IMAGING
- Skull X-rays, brain scan, computed tomography scan, magnetic resonance imaging, and cerebral angiography all confirm presence of tumor.

DIAGNOSTIC PROCEDURES
- Tissue biopsy confirms presence of tumor.

OTHER
- Lumbar puncture shows increased cerebrospinal fluid (CSF) pressure, which reflects increased ICP, increased protein levels, decreased glucose levels and, occasionally, tumor cells in CSF.

◆ TREATMENT

General
- Specific treatments dependent on tumor's histologic type, radiosensitivity, and location

Diet
- No restrictions unless swallowing impaired

Activity
- Ability possibly altered based on neurologic status

Medication
- Chemotherapy such as nitrosoureas
- Steroids
- Antacids and histamine-receptor antagonists
- Anticonvulsants

Surgery
FOR GLIOMA
- Resection by craniotomy
- Radiation therapy and chemotherapy follow resection

FOR LOW-GRADE CYSTIC CEREBELLAR ASTROCYTOMA
- Surgical resection

FOR ASTROCYTOMA
- Repeated surgeries, radiation therapy, and shunting of fluid from obstructed CSF pathways

FOR OLIGODENDROGLIOMA AND EPENDYMOMA
- Surgical resection and radiation therapy

FOR MEDULLOBLASTOMA
- Surgical resection
- Possibly, intrathecal infusion and methotrexate or another antineoplastic drug

FOR MENINGIOMA
- Surgical resection, including dura mater and bone

FOR SCHWANNOMA
- Microsurgical technique

✿ NURSING CONSIDERATIONS

Nursing diagnoses
- Activity intolerance
- Acute pain
- Anxiety
- Bathing or hygiene self-care deficit
- Decreased intracranial adaptive capacity
- Disturbed body image
- Disturbed sensory perception: All
- Fear
- Hopelessness
- Impaired physical mobility
- Ineffective breathing pattern
- Ineffective coping
- Ineffective role performance
- Powerlessness

Key outcomes
The patient will:
- maintain optimal mobility within the confines of the disorder
- verbalize feelings of comfort and decreased pain
- express feelings of decreased anxiety
- resume self-care activities to the highest level possible within the limitations of the illness
- exhibit signs of maintaining adequate cerebral perfusion
- express feelings about changed body image
- maintain optimal functioning within the limits of the visual impairment
- verbalize feelings and fears about the condition
- make decisions about his care, as appropriate
- maintain muscle strength and joint mobility at the highest possible level
- maintain respiratory rate within 5 breaths/minute of baseline
- demonstrate positive coping mechanism
- recognize limitations imposed by illness and express feelings about them
- express feelings of control over his well-being.

Nursing interventions
- Maintain a patent airway.
- Take steps to protect the patient's safety.
- Administer medication.

- After supratentorial craniotomy, elevate the head of the bed about 30 degrees.
- After infratentorial craniotomy, keep the patient flat for 48 hours.
- As appropriate, instruct the patient to avoid Valsalva's maneuver and isometric muscle contractions when moving or sitting up in bed.
- Consult with occupational, speech, and physical therapists.
- Provide emotional support.

Monitoring
- Neurologic status
- Vital signs
- Wound site
- Postoperative complications

▶ PATIENT TEACHING

Be sure to cover:
- disorder, diagnosis, and treatment
- signs of infection or bleeding that may result from chemotherapy
- adverse effects of chemotherapy treatments and actions that may alleviate them
- early signs of tumor recurrence.

Discharge planning
- Consult with occupational and physical therapy staff for postdischarge care plan.
- Refer the patient to resource and support services.

✷ RESOURCES

Organizations
American Brain Tumor Association: *www.abta.org*
American Cancer Society: *www.cancer.org*
Guide to Internet Resources for Cancer: *www.cancerindex.org*
National Cancer Institute: *www.nci.org*

Selected references
Atlas of Pathophysiology, 2nd ed. Philadelphia: Lippincott Williams & Wilkins, 2005.
Graham, C.A,. and Cloughesy, T.F. "Brain Tumor Treatment: Chemotherapy and Other New Developments," *Seminars in Oncology Nursing* 20(4)260-72, November 2004.
Loghlin, M., and Levin, V.A. "Headache Related to Brain Tumors," *Current Treatment Options in Neurology* 8(1):21-32, January 2006.
Lovely, M.P., "Symptom Management of Brain Tumor Patients," *Seminars in Oncology Nursing* 20(4):273-83, November 2004.
National Cancer Institute, National Institutes of Health. *SEER Cancer Statistics Review* [Online]. Available: *www.seer.cancer.gov/Publications.*

Breast cancer

● OVERVIEW

Description
- Along with lung cancer, leading killer of women ages 35 to 54
- Early detection and treatment key to promising prognosis
- Most reliable breast cancer detection method: regular breast self-examination, followed by immediate professional evaluation of any abnormality (theoretically, slow-growing breast cancer may take up to 8 years to become palpable at ⅜″ or 1 cm)
- With adjunctive therapy, 10-year survival of 70% to 75% of women with negative nodes, compared with 20% to 25% of women with positive nodes

Pathophysiology
- Breast cancer spreads by way of the lymphatic system and the bloodstream through the right side of the heart to the lungs and to the other breast, chest wall, liver, bone, and brain.

CLASSIFICATION
- Adenocarcinoma (ductal)—arising from the epithelium
- Intraductal—developing within the ducts (includes Paget's disease)
- Infiltrating—occurring in the breast's parenchymal tissue
- Inflammatory (rare)—growing rapidly and causing overlying skin to become edematous, inflamed, and indurated
- Lobular carcinoma in situ—involving the lobes of glandular tissue
- Medullary or circumscribed—enlarging tumor with rapid growth rate

Causes
- Unknown

Risk factors
- Family history of breast cancer, particularly first-degree relatives, including mother, sister, maternal grandmother, and maternal aunt
- Positive tests for genetic mutations (*BRCA1*)
- Being older than age 45 and premenopausal
- Long menstrual cycles
- Early onset of menses, late menopause
- Nulliparous or first pregnancy after age 30
- High-fat diet
- Endometrial or ovarian cancer
- History of unilateral breast cancer
- Radiation exposure
- Estrogen therapy
- Antihypertensive therapy
- Alcohol and tobacco use
- Preexisting fibrocystic disease

Incidence
- Strikes about 10% of all women
- May develop any time after puberty, but most common after age 50
- Seldom occurs in men

Common characteristics
- Lump or mass in the breast (see *Breast tumor sources and sites*)
- Breast pain
- Change in symmetry or size of breast
- Change in skin, such as thickening, scaly skin around the nipple, dimpling, edema, or ulceration
- Nipple discharge

Complications
- Distant metastasis
- Infection
- Central nervous system effects
- Respiratory effects

✱ ASSESSMENT

History
- Detection of a painless lump or mass in the breast
- Change in breast tissue
- History of risk factors

Physical findings
- Clear, milky, or bloody nipple discharge, nipple retraction, scaly skin around the nipple, and skin changes, such as dimpling, or inflammation
- Arm edema
- Hard lump, mass, or thickening of breast tissue
- Lymphadenopathy

Test results
LABORATORY
- Alkaline phosphatase levels and liver function uncover distant metastases.
- Hormonal receptor assay determines whether the tumor is estrogen- or progesterone-dependent; also guides decisions to use therapy that blocks the action of the estrogen hormone that supports tumor growth.

IMAGING
- Mammography can reveal a tumor that's too small to palpate.
- Ultrasonography can distinguish between a fluid-filled cyst and solid mass.
- Chest X-rays can pinpoint metastases in the chest.
- Scans of the bone, brain, liver, and other organs can detect distant metastases.

DIAGNOSTIC PROCEDURES
- Fine-needle aspiration and excisional biopsy provide cells for histologic examination, which may confirm the diagnosis.

BREAST TUMOR SOURCES AND SITES

About 90% of all breast tumors arise from the epithelial cells lining the ducts. About half of all breast cancers develop in the breast's upper outer quadrant—the section containing the most glandular tissue.

The second most common cancer site is the nipple, where all the breast ducts converge.

The next most common site is the upper inner quadrant, followed by the lower outer quadrant and, finally, the lower inner quadrant.

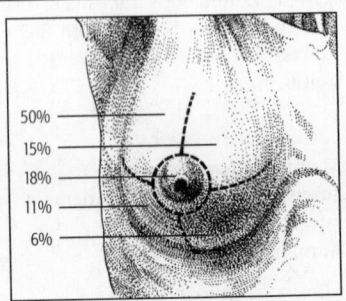

50%
15%
18%
11%
6%

◆ TREATMENT

General
- Treatment usually dependent on the stage and type of disease, woman's age and menopausal status, and disfiguring effects of surgery
- May include any combination of surgery, radiation, chemotherapy, and hormone therapy

Diet
- No restrictions

Activity
- May need arm stretching exercises after surgery

Medication
- Chemotherapy, such as a combination of drugs including cyclophosphamide, fluorouracil, methotrexate, doxorubicin, vincristine, paclitaxel, and prednisone
- Regimen of cyclophosphamide, methotrexate, and fluorouracil, which is used in premenopausal and postmenopausal women
- Antiestrogen therapy such as tamoxifen
- Hormonal therapy including antiestrogen agents, progesterone, androgen, or antiandrogen aminoglutethimide therapy

Surgery
- Lumpectomy
- Partial, total, or modified radical mastectomy

Other
- Primary radiation therapy
- Preoperative breast irradiation

♣ NURSING CONSIDERATIONS

Nursing diagnoses
- Acute pain
- Anxiety
- Disturbed body image
- Energy field disturbance
- Fear
- Imbalanced nutrition: Less than body requirements
- Impaired physical mobility
- Impaired skin integrity
- Ineffective coping
- Ineffective role performance
- Risk for infection

Key outcomes
The patient will:
- express feelings of comfort and decreased pain
- express feelings of decreased anxiety
- express feelings about changed body image
- express increased sense of well-being
- use situational supports to reduce fear
- maintain adequate nutritional intake
- maintain optimal muscle strength and joint range of motion
- maintain skin integrity
- demonstrate adequate coping behaviors
- recognize limitations imposed by illness and express feelings about these limitations
- remain free from signs and symptoms of infection.

Nursing interventions
- Provide information about the disease process, diagnostic tests, and treatment.
- Administer medication, as ordered.

Monitoring
- Wound site
- Postoperative complications
- Vital signs
- Intake and output
- White blood cell count
- Pain control
- Psychological status

▶ PATIENT TEACHING

Be sure to cover:
- all procedures and treatments
- optimal positioning
- activities or exercises that promote healing
- breast self-examination
- risks and signs and symptoms of recurrence
- avoidance of venipuncture or blood pressure monitoring on the affected arm.

Discharge planning
- Refer the patient to local and national support groups.

✷ RESOURCES

Organizations
American Cancer Society: *www.cancer.org*
Guide to Internet Resources for Cancer: *www.cancerindex.org*
National Cancer Institute: *www.nci.org*

Selected references
Adebamowo, C.A., et al. "Dietary Patients and the Risk of Breast Cancer," *Annals of Epidemiology* 15(10):789-95, November 2005.

Atlas of Pathophysiology, 2nd ed. Philadelphia: Lippincott Williams & Wilkins, 2005.

Knopf, M.T., and Sun, Y. "A Longitudinal Study of Symptoms and Self Care Activities in Women Treated with Primary Radiotherapy for Breast Cancer," *Cancer Nursing* 28(3):210-18, May-June 2005.

Leadbeater, M., "A Nurse-Led E-mail Service for Breast Cancer Information," *Nursing Times* 101(39):36-38, September-October 2005.

National Cancer Institute, National Institutes of Health. *SEER Cancer Statistics Review* [Online]. Available: *www.seer.cancer.gov/Publications.*

Perreault, A., and Bourbonnais, F.F. "The Experience of Suffering as Lived by Women with Breast Cancer," *International Journal of Palliative Nursing* 11(10):510, 512-19, October 2005.

Bronchiectasis

Description
- Characterized by abnormal dilation of the bronchi and destruction of the bronchial walls
- Results from conditions associated with repeated damage to bronchial walls and with abnormal mucociliary clearance, causing a breakdown of supporting tissue adjacent to the airways
- Can occur throughout the tracheobronchial tree, or may be confined to one segment or lobe
- Usually bilateral and involves the basilar segments of the lower lobes
- Occurs in three forms: cylindrical (fusiform), varicose, and saccular (cystic)

Pathophysiology
- Hyperplastic squamous epithelium, denuded of cilia, replace ulcerated columnar epithelia.
- Abscess formation occurs, involving all layers of the bronchial walls, which produces inflammatory cells and fibrous tissues, resulting in dilation and narrowing of the airways.
- Sputum stagnates in the dilated bronchi and leads to secondary infection, characterized by inflammation and leukocytic accumulations.
- Additional debris collects in the bronchi and occludes them.
- Building pressure from the retained secretions induces mucosal injury.
- Extensive vascular proliferation of bronchial circulation occurs and produces frequent hemoptysis.

Causes
- Mucoviscidosis
- Immune disorders
- Recurrent bacterial respiratory tract infections
- Complications of measles, pneumonia, pertussis, or influenza
- Obstruction with recurrent infection
- Inhalation of corrosive gas
- Repeated aspiration of gastric juices
- Congenital anomalies (rare) such as bronchomalacia
- Various rare disorders such as immotile cilia syndrome

Incidence
- Affects people of both sexes and all ages
- Dramatically decreased incidence over the past 20 years due to the availability of antibiotics to treat acute respiratory infections
- Incidence highest among Inuit populations in the northern hemisphere and the Maoris of New Zealand

Common characteristics
- Chronic, productive cough
- Dyspnea

Complications
- Chronic malnutrition
- Amyloidosis
- Right-sided heart failure
- Cor pulmonale

History
- Frequent bouts of pneumonia
- Coughing up blood or blood-tinged sputum
- Chronic cough that produces copious, foul-smelling, mucopurulent secretions
- Dyspnea
- Weight loss
- Malaise

Physical findings
- Sputum possibly showing a cloudy top layer, a central layer of clear saliva, and a heavy, thick, purulent bottom layer
- Clubbed fingers and toes
- Cyanotic nail beds
- Dullness over affected lung fields, if pneumonia or atelectasis present
- Diminished breath sounds
- Inspiratory crackles during inspiration over affected area
- Occasional wheezes

Test results
LABORATORY
- Sputum culture and Gram stain show predominant pathogens.
- Complete blood count reveals anemia and leukocytosis.
IMAGING
- Computed tomography scan shows bronchiectasis.
- Bronchography shows location and extent of disease.
- Chest X-rays show peribronchial thickening, atelectatic areas, and scattered cystic changes.
DIAGNOSTIC PROCEDURES
- Bronchoscopy may show the source of secretions or the bleeding site in hemoptysis.
- Pulmonary function studies show decreased vital capacity, expiratory flow, and hypoxemia.
OTHER
- A sweat electrolyte test may show cystic fibrosis as the underlying cause.

◆ TREATMENT

General
- Postural drainage and chest percussion
- Bronchoscopy to remove secretions

Diet
- Well-balanced, high-calorie
- Adequate hydration

Activity
- As tolerated

Medication
- Antibiotics
- Bronchodilators
- Oxygen

Surgery
FOR POOR PULMONARY FUNCTION
- Segmental resection
- Bronchial artery embolization
- Lobectomy
- Surgical removal of the affected lung portion

♣ NURSING CONSIDERATIONS

Nursing diagnoses
- Anxiety
- Fatigue
- Imbalanced nutrition: Less than body requirements
- Impaired gas exchange
- Ineffective airway clearance
- Ineffective breathing pattern
- Risk for infection

Key outcomes
The patient will:
- identify strategies to reduce anxiety
- utilize energy conservation techniques
- maintain adequate nutrition and hydration
- maintain adequate ventilation and oxygenation
- maintain a patent airway
- maintain an effective breathing pattern
- remain free from signs and symptoms of infection.

Nursing interventions
- Administer medications, as ordered.
- Provide supportive care.
- Administer oxygen, as needed.
- Perform chest physiotherapy.
- Provide a warm, quiet, comfortable environment.
- Alternate rest and activity periods.
- Provide well-balanced, high-calorie meals.
- Offer small, frequent meals.
- Provide adequate hydration.
- Provide frequent mouth care.

Monitoring
- Vital signs
- Intake and output
- Respiratory status
- Breath sounds
- Sputum production
- Pulse oximetry
- Arterial blood gas results
- Complications
- Chest tube drainage after surgery

▶ PATIENT TEACHING

Be sure to cover:
- disorder, diagnosis, and treatment
- medication administration, dosage, and possible adverse effects
- when to notify the physician
- proper disposal of secretions
- infection control techniques
- frequent rest periods
- preoperative and postoperative instructions, if surgery is required
- postural drainage and percussion
- coughing and deep-breathing techniques
- avoidance of air pollutants and people with known upper respiratory tract infections
- immunizations
- balanced, high-protein diet
- small, frequent meals
- avoidance of milk products
- adequate hydration.

Discharge planning
- Refer the patient to a smoking-cessation program, if indicated.

✳ RESOURCES

Organizations
American Association for Respiratory Care: *www.aarc.org*
American Lung Association: *www.lungusa.org*
National Heart, Lung and Blood Institute: *www.nhlbi.nih.gov*

Selected references

Kaspar, D.L., et al., eds. *Harrison's Principles of Internal Medicine*, 16th ed. New York: McGraw-Hill Book Co., 2005.

Pryor, J.A. "Physical Therapy for Adults with Bronchiectasis," *Clinical Pulmonary Medicine* 11(4):205-09, July 2005.

Weycker, D., et al. "Prevalence and Economic Burden of Bronchiectasis," *Clinical Pulmonary Medicine* 12(4):205-09, July 2005.

Bronchitis, chronic

● OVERVIEW

Description
- Form of chronic obstructive pulmonary disease
- Characterized by excessive production of tracheobronchial mucus with a cough for at least 3 months each year for 2 consecutive years
- Severity linked to amount of cigarette smoke or other pollutants inhaled and inhalation duration
- Respiratory tract infections that typically exacerbate the cough and related symptoms
- Few patients with chronic bronchitis develop significant airway obstruction

Pathophysiology
- The disorder results in hypertrophy and hyperplasia of the bronchial mucous glands, increased goblet cells, ciliary damage, squamous metaplasia of the columnar epithelium, and chronic leukocytic and lymphocytic infiltration of bronchial walls.
- Additional effects include widespread inflammation, airway narrowing, and mucus within the airways—all producing resistance in the small airways and, in turn, a severe ventilation-perfusion imbalance. (See *What happens in chronic bronchitis*.)

Causes
- Cigarette smoking
- Possible genetic predisposition
- Environmental pollution
- Organic or inorganic dusts and noxious gas exposure

Incidence
- Occurs in about 20% of men
- Children of parents who smoke at higher risk

Common characteristics
- Long-time smoker
- Frequent upper respiratory tract infections
- Productive cough

Complications
- Cor pulmonale
- Pulmonary hypertension
- Right ventricular hypertrophy
- Acute respiratory failure

✴ ASSESSMENT

History
- Long-time smoker
- Frequent upper respiratory tract infections
- Productive cough
- Exertional dyspnea
- Cough, initially prevalent in winter, but gradually becoming year-round
- Increasingly severe coughing episodes
- Worsening dyspnea

Physical findings
- Cough producing copious gray, white, or yellow sputum
- Cyanosis, also called a "blue bloater"
- Accessory respiratory muscle use
- Tachypnea
- Substantial weight gain
- Pedal edema
- Neck vein distention
- Wheezing
- Prolonged expiratory time
- Rhonchi

Test results
LABORATORY
- Arterial blood gas analysis shows decreased partial pressure of oxygen and normal or increased partial pressure of carbon dioxide.
- Sputum culture reveals the number microorganisms and neutrophils.

IMAGING
- Chest X-ray may show hyperinflation and increased bronchovascular markings.

DIAGNOSTIC PROCEDURES
- Pulmonary function tests show increased residual volume, decreased vital capacity and forced expiratory flow, and normal static compliance and diffusing capacity.

OTHER
- Electrocardiography may show atrial arrhythmias; peaked P waves in leads II, III, and aV_F; and right ventricular hypertrophy.

WHAT HAPPENS IN CHRONIC BRONCHITIS

In chronic bronchitis, irritants inhaled for a prolonged period inflame the tracheobronchial tree. The inflammation leads to increased mucus production and a narrowed or blocked airway.

As inflammation continues, the mucus-producing goblet cells undergo hypertrophy, as do the ciliated epithelial cells that line the respiratory tract. Hypersecretion from the goblet cells blocks the free movement of the cilia, which normally sweep dust, irritants, and mucus from the airways.

As a result, the airway stays blocked, and mucus and debris accumulate in the respiratory tract.

CROSS SECTION OF NORMAL BRONCHIAL TUBE

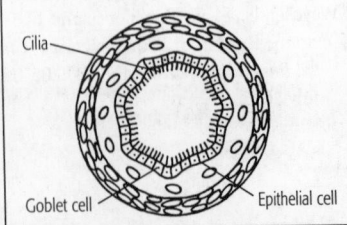

NARROWED BRONCHIAL TUBE IN CHRONIC BRONCHITIS

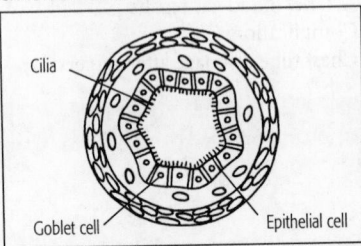

◆ TREATMENT

General
- Smoking cessation
- Avoidance of air pollutants
- Chest physiotherapy
- Ultrasonic or mechanical nebulizer treatments

Diet
- Adequate fluid intake
- High-calorie, protein-rich

Activity
- As tolerated with frequent rest periods

Medication
- Oxygen
- Antibiotics
- Bronchodilators
- Corticosteroids
- Diuretics

Surgery
- Tracheostomy in advanced disease

❖ NURSING CONSIDERATIONS

Nursing diagnoses
- Anxiety
- Fatigue
- Imbalanced nutrition: Less than body requirements
- Impaired gas exchange
- Ineffective breathing pattern
- Ineffective coping
- Risk for infection

Key outcomes
The patient will:
- identify strategies to reduce anxiety
- utilize energy conservation techniques
- maintain adequate nutrition and hydration
- maintain adequate ventilation and oxygenation
- maintain a patent airway
- maintain an effective breathing pattern
- demonstrate effective coping behaviors
- remain free from signs and symptoms of infection.

Nursing interventions
- Administer medication, as ordered.
- Encourage expression of fears and concerns.
- Include the patient and family members in care decisions.
- Perform chest physiotherapy.
- Provide a high-calorie, protein-rich diet.
- Offer small, frequent meals.
- Encourage energy-conservation techniques.
- Ensure adequate oral fluid intake.
- Provide frequent mouth care.
- Encourage daily activity.
- Provide diversional activities as appropriate.
- Provide frequent rest periods.

Monitoring
- Vital signs
- Intake and output
- Sputum production
- Respiratory status
- Breath sounds
- Daily weight
- Edema
- Response to treatment

▶ PATIENT TEACHING

Be sure to cover:
- disorder, diagnosis, and treatment
- medication administration, dosage, and possible adverse effects
- when to notify the physician
- infection control practices
- influenza and pneumococcus immunizations
- home oxygen therapy, if required
- postural drainage and chest percussion
- coughing and deep-breathing exercises
- inhaler use
- high-calorie, protein-rich meals
- adequate hydration
- avoidance of inhaled irritants
- prevention of bronchospasm.

Discharge planning
- Refer the patient to a smoking-cessation program, if indicated.

✳ RESOURCES

Organizations
American Association of Respiratory Care *www.aarc.org*
American Lung Association *www.lung-usa.org*
Mayo Foundation for Medical Education and Research: *www.mayohealth.org*
National Heart, Lung and Blood Institute: *www.nhlbi.nih.gov*

Selected references
Donner, C.F. "Acute Exacerbation of Chronic Bronchitis: Need for an Evidence-Based Approach," *Pulmonary Pharmocology & Therapeutics* 19(Suppl 1)4-10, December 2005.

Hu, J., and Meek, P. "Health-Related Quality of Life in Individuals with Chronic Obstructive Pulmonary Disease," *Heart & Lung* 34(6):415-22, November-December 2005.

Willemse, B., et al. "High Cessation Rates of Cigarette Smoking in Subjects With and Without COPD," *Chest* 128(5):3685-687, November 2005.

Bulimia nervosa

● OVERVIEW

Description
- Eating binges followed by feelings of guilt, humiliation, and self-deprecation
- Self-induced vomiting, the use of laxatives or diuretics, or strict dieting or fasting to overcome the effects of the binges
- Seldom incapacitating

Pathophysiology
- Decreased caloric intake depletes body fat and protein stores.
- Purging behavior leads to loss of fluid and electrolytes, causing imbalances.
- Estrogen deficiency occurs (in women) due to lack of lipid substrate for synthesis, causing amenorrhea.
- Testosterone levels fluctuate (in men) and decreased erectile function and sperm count occurs.
- Ketoacidosis occurs from increased use of fat as energy fuel.

Causes
- Exact cause unknown
- Family disturbance or conflict
- Sexual abuse
- Maladaptive learned behavior
- Struggle for control or self-identity
- Cultural overemphasis on physical appearance
- Parental obesity

Incidence
- Affects nine females for every one male
- Between 1% and 3% of adolescent and young women meet the diagnostic criteria; 5% to 15% have some symptoms of the disorder

✸ **AGE-RELATED CONCERN** Bulimia has been found to begin in adolescence or early adulthood.

Common characteristics
- Strongly associated with depression
- Can occur simultaneously with anorexia nervosa
- More prone to psychoactive substance abuse
- Hyperactivity
- Peculiar eating habits or rituals
- Frequent weighing
- Perceived by others as a "perfect" student, mother, or career woman
- Distinguished for participation in competitive activities

Complications
- Dental caries
- Erosion of tooth enamel
- Parotitis
- Gum infections
- Electrolyte imbalances
- Dehydration
- Arrhythmias
- Cardiac failure
- Sudden death
- Esophageal tears
- Gastric ruptures
- Mucosal damage to intestine
- Suicide

✳ ASSESSMENT

History
- Episodic binge eating
- Continues eating until abdominal pain, sleep, or the presence of another person interrupts it
- Preferred food usually sweet, soft, and high in calories and carbohydrates
- Exaggerated sense of guilt
- Depression
- Childhood trauma
- Parental obesity
- Unsatisfactory sexual relationships

Physical findings
- Thin or slightly overweight with use of diuretics, laxatives, vomiting, and exercise
- Abdominal and epigastric pain
- Amenorrhea
- Painless swelling of the salivary glands
- Hoarseness
- Throat irritation or lacerations
- Calluses of the knuckles or abrasions and scars on the dorsum of the hand

Test results
- Diagnosis is based on *DSM-IV-TR* criteria findings

DSM-IV-TR criteria
Diagnosis of bulimia nervosa can be confirmed when these criteria are met, on average, twice a week for 3 months:
- recurrent episodes of binge eating
- repeated inappropriate behaviors to prevent weight gain.

Test results
LABORATORY
- Serum electrolyte studies shows elevated bicarbonate, decreased potassium, and decreased sodium levels.

OTHER
- The Beck Depression Inventory may identify coexisting depression.

◆ TREATMENT

General
- Inpatient or outpatient psychotherapy
- Self-help groups
- Drug rehabilitation

Diet
- Balanced
- Monitoring of eating pattern

Activity
- Monitoring of activity

Medication
- Antidepressants

❖ NURSING CONSIDERATIONS

Nursing diagnoses
- Anxiety
- Chronic low self-esteem
- Constipation
- Deficient fluid volume
- Disturbed body image
- Disturbed sleep pattern
- Imbalanced nutrition: Less than body requirements
- Ineffective coping
- Social isolation

Key outcomes
The patient will:
- identify strategies to reduce anxiety
- express positive feelings about self
- have regular bowel elimination patterns
- maintain adequate fluid balance
- acknowledge change in body image
- verbalize feeling well rested
- display appropriate eating patterns, including regular, nutritious meals
- demonstrate effective coping behaviors
- interact with family or friends.

Nursing interventions
- Supervise mealtime and for a specified period after meals, usually up to 1 hour.
- Set a time limit for each meal.
- Provide a pleasant, relaxed environment for eating.
- Use behavior modification techniques.
- Establish a food contract, specifying the amount and type of food to be eaten at each meal.
- Encourage verbalization and provide support.

Monitoring
- Suicide potential
- Elimination patterns
- Eating patterns
- Complications
- Response to treatment

▶ PATIENT TEACHING

Be sure to cover:
- importance of keeping a food journal
- risks of laxative, emetic, and diuretic abuse
- assertiveness training
- medication administration, dosage, and possible adverse effects.

Discharge planning
- Refer the patient to support services.

✳ RESOURCES

Organizations
American Anorexia Bulimia Association: *www.aabainc.org*
National Association of Anorexia Nervosa and Associated Disorders: *www.anad.org*
Overeaters Anonymous: *www.overeatersanonymous.org*

Selected references
Diagnostic and Statistical Manual of Mental Disorders, Text Revision, 4th ed. Washington, D.C.: American Psychiatric Association, 2000.
Harris, M. et al. "Health Matters: Helping Teenagers with Eating Disorders," *Nursing2004* 34(10):24-25, October 2004.
McFarlane, T.L., et al. "Beliefs and Expectations Regarding Etiology, Treatment and Outcome in Bulimia Nervosa," *Eating and Weight Disorders* 10(3):187-92, September 2005.
Olson, A.F. "Outpatient Management of Electrolyte Imbalances Associated with Anorexia Nervosa and Bulimia Nervosa," *Journal of Infusion Nursing* 28(2):118-22, March-April 2005.
Wolfe, B.F. "Reproductive Health in Women with Eating Disorders," *Journal of Obstetric, Gynecologic, and Neonatal Nursing* 34(2):255-63, March-April 2005.

Burns

● OVERVIEW

Description
- Heat or chemical injury
- May be permanently disfiguring and incapacitating
- May be partial thickness or full thickness

Pathophysiology
SUPERFICIAL PARTIAL THICKNESS (FIRST-DEGREE BURNS)
- Injury is limited to epidermis and is not life-threatening.

DEEP, PARTIAL THICKNESS (SECOND-DEGREE BURNS)
- Epidermis and some dermis is destroyed.
- Thin-walled and fluid-filled blisters develop.
- As blisters break, nerve endings become exposed to air, resulting in pain.
- Barrier function of the skin is lost.

FULL THICKNESS (THIRD- AND FOURTH-DEGREE BURNS)
- Every body system and organ is affected.
- Injury extends into the subcutaneous tissue layer, damaging muscle, bone, and interstitial tissues.
- Interstitial fluids collect, resulting in edema.
- An immediate immunologic response occurs.
- Wound sepsis is a threat.
- Injury is usually painless.

Causes
- Residential fires
- Motor vehicle accidents
- Improper use or handling of matches
- Improperly stored gasoline
- Space heater or electrical malfunctions
- Improper handling of firecrackers
- Scalding accidents
- Child or elder abuse
- Contact, ingestion, inhalation, or injection of acids, alkali, or vesicants
- Contact with faulty electrical wiring
- Contact with high-voltage power lines
- Chewing electric cords
- Friction or abrasion
- Sun exposure

Incidence
- Affects more than 2 million people each year, resulting in 70,000 hospitalizations and 20,000 specialized burn unit admissions

Common characteristics
SUPERFICIAL PARTIAL THICKNESS
- Localized pain
- Erythema
- Blanching
- Chills
- Headache
- Nausea and vomiting

DEEP, PARTIAL THICKNESS
- Thin-walled, fluid-filled blisters
- Mild to moderate pain
- White, waxy appearance of damaged area

FULL THICKNESS
- Pale, white, brown, or black leathery tissue
- Visible thrombosed vessels
- No blister formation
- Painless

ELECTRICAL BURNS
- Silver colored, raised area at contact site
- Smoke inhalation and pulmonary damage
- Singed nasal hair

MUCOSAL BURNS
- Sores in mouth or nose
- Voice changes
- Coughing, wheezing
- Darkened sputum

Complications
- Respiratory complications
- Sepsis
- Hypovolemic shock
- Anemia
- Malnutrition
- Multisystem organ dysfunction

✳ ASSESSMENT

History
- Cause of burn revealed
- Preexisting medical conditions

Physical findings
- Depth, size, and severity of the burn assessed
- Major—more than 10% of the patient's body surface area (BSA); more than 20% of a child's
- Moderate—on 3% to 10% of a patient's BSA; 10% to 20% of a child's
- Minor—less than 3% of a patient's BSA; 10% in a child
- Respiratory distress and cyanosis
- Edema
- Alteration in pulse rate, strength, and regularity
- Stridor, wheezing, crackles, and rhonchi
- S_3, or S_4, gallop or murmur
- Hypotension

Test results
LABORATORY
- Arterial blood gas levels show evidence of smoke inhalation and, possibly, decreased alveolar function and hypoxia.
- Complete blood count shows decreased hemoglobin level and hematocrit if blood loss occurs.
- Electrolytes are abnormal due to fluid losses and shifts.
- Blood urea nitrogen is increased with fluid losses.
- In children, glucose is decreased due to limited glycogen storage.
- Urinalysis shows myoglobinuria and hemoglobinuria.
- Carboxyhemoglobin is increased.

DIAGNOSTIC PROCEDURES
- Electrocardiogram may show ischemia, injury, or arrhythmias especially in electrical burns.
- Fiber-optic bronchoscopy may show edema of the airways.

◆ TREATMENT

General
- Stop the burn process
- Secured airway
- Prevention of hypoxia
- Administration of lactated Ringer's solution through a large-bore I.V. line (see *Fluid replacement after a burn*)
  - Adult: maintain a urine output of 30 to 50 ml/hour
  - Child under 66 lb (30 kg): maintain urine output at 1 ml/kg/hour
- Insertion of nasogastric tube and Foley catheter
- Wound care

Diet
- Nothing by mouth until severity of burn is established
- High-protein, high-calorie
- Increased hydration
- Total parenteral nutrition if unable to take food by mouth

Activity
- Limitation based on extent and location of burn
- Physical therapy

Medication
- Booster of tetanus toxoid
- Analgesics
- Antibiotics
- Antianxiety agents

Surgery
- Loose tissue and blister debridement
- Escharotomy
- Skin grafting

FLUID REPLACEMENT AFTER A BURN

The commonly used Parkland formula is a guideline for fluid replacement for patients with burns. Variations may be made dependent on the patient's response to treatment.

Parkland formula:

$$4 \text{ ml/kg body weight} \times \% \text{ body surface area burned.}$$

Over 24 hours, give one-half of the total amount of solution over the first 8 hours and the rest of the solution over the next 16 hours.

♣ NURSING CONSIDERATIONS

Nursing diagnoses
- Acute pain
- Anxiety
- Decreased cardiac output
- Deficient fluid volume
- Disturbed body image
- Imbalanced nutrition: Less than body requirements
- Impaired gas exchange
- Impaired skin integrity
- Ineffective airway clearance
- Ineffective coping
- Ineffective protection
- Ineffective tissue perfusion: Peripheral
- Risk for infection
- Risk for posttrauma syndrome

Key outcomes
The patient will:
- achieve pain relief with analgesia or other measures
- express feelings of decreased anxiety
- maintain adequate cardiac output
- maintain fluid volume within the acceptable range
- express feelings about changed body image
- maintain daily calorie requirements
- maintain adequate ventilation
- have wounds and incisions that appear clean, pink, and free from purulent drainage
- maintain a patent airway
- demonstrate effective coping behaviors
- verbalize methods to prevent burns
- exhibit signs of adequate peripheral perfusion
- remain free from signs and symptoms of infection
- express feelings and fears about the traumatic event.

Nursing interventions
- Apply immediate, aggressive burn treatment.
- Use strict sterile technique.
- Remove clothing that's still smoldering.
- Remove the patient's rings and other constricting items.
- Perform appropriate wound care.
- Provide adequate hydration.
- Weigh the patient daily.

- Encourage verbalization and provide support.

Monitoring
- Vital signs
- Respiratory status
- Signs of infection
- Intake and output
- Hydration and nutritional status

▶ PATIENT TEACHING

Be sure to cover:
- information about the injury, diagnosis, and treatment
- appropriate wound care
- medication administration, dosage, and possible adverse effects
- a dietary plan
- signs and symptoms of complications.

Discharge planning
Refer the patient to:
- rehabilitation, if appropriate.
- psychological counseling, if necessary.
- resource and support services.

✴ RESOURCES

Organizations
American Academy of Dermatology: *www.aad.org*
American Burn Association: *www.ameriburn.org*
National Center for Injury Prevention and Control: *www.cdc.ncipc*

Selected references
Anwar, M.U., et al. "Smoking, Substance Abuse, Psychiatric History, and Burns: Trends in Adult Patients," *Journal of Burn Care & Rehabilitation* 26(6):493-501, November-December 2005.

Atlas of Pathophysiology, 2nd ed. Philadelphia: Lippincott Williams & Wilkins, 2005.

Burd, A., and Noronha, F. "What's New in Burns Trauma?" *Surgical Practice* 9(4):126-36, November 2005.

Cinat, M.E., and Carson, J.G. "Burns and Motor Vehicle Crashes," *Topics in Emergency Medicine* 28(1):56-67, January-March 2006.

Candidiasis

Description
- Mild, superficial fungal infection
- Can lead to severe disseminated infections and fungemia in immunocompromised patient, transplant recipient, burn patient, low-birth-weight neonate, or patient receiving hyperalimentation
- Prognosis varies, depending on patient's resistance
- Also known as *candidosis* and *moniliasis*

Pathophysiology
- Change in the patient's resistance to infection, his immunocompromised state, and antibiotic use permit the sudden proliferation of *Candida albicans.*

Causes
- In most cases, infection with *C. albicans* or *C. tropicalis*

Risk factors
- Maternal vaginitis present during vaginal delivery
- Preexisting diabetes mellitus, cancer, or immunosuppressant illness
- Immunosuppressant drug use
- Radiation
- Aging
- Irritation from dentures
- I.V. or urinary catheterization
- Drug abuse
- Total parenteral nutrition
- Surgery
- Use of antibiotics
- Use of corticosteroids

Incidence
- Affects 14% of immunocompromised patients
- Affects men and women equally
- Can occur at any age

Common characteristics
- Causative fungi that infect the nails (paronychia), skin (diaper rash), or mucous membranes, especially the oropharynx (thrush), vagina (vaginitis), esophagus, and GI tract (see *Identifying thrush*)
- Systemic infection that predominates among drug abusers and diabetic and immunosuppressed patients

Complications
- Dissemination with organ failure of the kidneys, brain, GI tract, eyes, lungs, and heart

---

IDENTIFYING THRUSH

Candidiasis of the oropharyngeal mucosa (thrush) causes cream-colored or bluish white pseudomembranous patches on the tongue, mouth, or pharynx (as shown). Fungal invasion may extend to circumoral tissues.

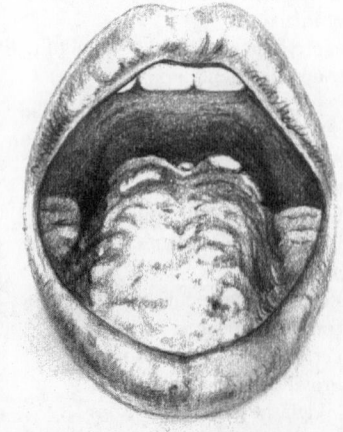

History
- Underlying illness
- Recent course of antibiotic or antineoplastic therapy
- Drug abuse
- Hyperalimentation

Physical findings
- Skin — scaly, erythematous, papular rash, possibly covered with exudate and erupting in breast folds, between fingers, and at the axillae, groin, and umbilicus
- Nails — red, swollen, darkened nailbeds; occasionally, purulent discharge; possible separation from the nailbed
- Esophageal mucosa — occasionally, scales in the mouth and throat
- Vaginal mucosa — white or yellow discharge, with local excoriation; white or gray raised patches on vaginal walls, with local inflammation
- Oropharyngeal mucosa — cream-colored or bluish white lacelike patches of exudate on the tongue, mouth, or pharynx that reveal bloody engorgement when scraped
- Lungs — hemoptysis, cough; coarse breath sounds in the infected lung fields
- Kidneys — flank pain, dysuria, hematuria, cloudy urine with casts
- Brain — headache, nuchal rigidity, seizures, focal neurologic deficits
- Eyes — blurred vision, orbital or periorbital pain, exudate, floating scotomata, and lesions with a white, cotton-ball appearance seen during ophthalmoscopy
- Endocardium — chest pain and arrhythmias
- Systemic — septic shock

Test results
LABORATORY
- Fungal serological panel shows the presence of the candidal organism.

General
- Treatment of predisposing condition

Diet
- No restrictions unless oral infection
- With oral infection, spicy food only as tolerated

Activity
- No restrictions

Medication
- Antifungals
- Amphotericin B
- Topical anesthetics

Surgery
- Abscess drainage; surgically or percutaneously

Nursing diagnoses
- Acute pain
- Impaired oral mucous membrane
- Impaired skin integrity
- Risk for aspiration
- Sexual dysfunction

Key outcomes
The patient will:
- express increased comfort and decreased pain
- exhibit intact oral mucous membranes
- maintain skin integrity
- exhibit no signs of aspiration
- express feelings about potential or actual changes in sexual activity.

Nursing interventions
- Observe standard precautions.
- Administer medications, as ordered.
- Provide a nonirritating mouthwash to loosen tenacious secretions and a soft toothbrush to avoid irritation.
- Observe high-risk patients daily for patchy areas, irritation, sore throat, oral and gingival bleeding, and other signs of superinfection.
- Assess the patient for underlying systemic causes.

Monitoring
- Vital signs
- Intake and output
- Blood urea nitrogen, serum creatinine, and urine blood and protein levels
- Potassium levels

Be sure to cover:
- disorder, diagnostic tests, and treatment
- good oral hygiene practices
- (for a woman in her third trimester of pregnancy) the need for examination for vaginitis to protect her neonate from thrush infection at birth.

Organizations
Centers for Disease Control and Prevention: *www.cdc.gov*
Harvard University Consumer Health Information: *www.intelihealth.com*
National Health Information Center: *www.health.gov/nhic/*
National Library of Medicine: *www.nlm.nih.gov*

Selected references
Kasper, D.L. et al., eds. *Harrison's Principles of Internal Medicine,* 16th ed. New York: McGraw-Hill Book Co., 2005.

Spellberg, B.J., et al. "Current Treatment Strategies for Disseminated Candidiasis," *Clinical Infectious Diseases* 42(2):244-51, January 2006.

Theroux, R. "Factors Influencing Women's Decisions to Self-Treat Vaginal Symptoms," *Journal of the American Academy of Nursing Practitioners* 17(4):156-62, April 2005.

Cardiac tamponade

● OVERVIEW

Description
- Rapid increase in intrapericardial pressure
- Impaired diastolic filling of the heart

Pathophysiology
- Progressive accumulation of fluid in the pericardial sac causes compression of the heart chambers.
- Compression of the heart chambers obstructs blood flow into the ventricles and reduces the amount of blood pumped out with each contraction.
- With each contraction more fluid accumulates, decreasing cardiac output.

Causes
- May be idiopathic
- Effusion in cancer, bacterial infections, tuberculosis and, rarely, acute rheumatic fever
- Trauma
- Hemorrhage from nontraumatic cause
- Viral, postirradiation, or idiopathic pericarditis
- Acute myocardial infarction
- Chronic renal failure
- Drug reaction
- Connective tissue disorders
- Cardiac catheterization
- Cardiac surgery

Incidence
- More common in males
- Occurs with 2% of penetrating chest traumas

Common characteristics
- Systemic hypotension
- Muffled heart sounds
- Jugular vein distention

Complications
- Cardiogenic shock
- Death

✳ ASSESSMENT

History
- Presence of one or more causes
- Dyspnea
- Shortness of breath
- Chest pain

Physical findings
- Vary with volume of fluid and speed of fluid accumulation
- Diaphoresis
- Anxiety and restlessness
- Pallor or cyanosis
- Neck vein distention
- Edema
- Rapid, weak pulses; tachycardia
- Hepatomegaly
- Decreased arterial blood pressure
- Increased central venous pressure
- Pulsus paradoxus
- Narrow pulse pressure
- Muffled heart sounds

Test results
IMAGING
- Chest X-rays show slightly widened mediastinum and enlargement of the cardiac silhouette.

DIAGNOSTIC PROCEDURES
- Electrocardiography may show low voltage complexes in the precordial leads.
- Hemodynamic monitoring shows equalization of mean right atrial, right ventricular diastolic, pulmonary capillary wedge pressure, and left ventricular diastolic pressures.
- Echocardiography may show an echo-free space, indicating fluid accumulation in the pericardial sac.

◆ TREATMENT

General
- Pericardiocentesis (possible)

Diet
- As tolerated

Activity
- Bed rest with leg elevation

Medication
- Intravascular volume expansion
- Inotropic agents
- Oxygen

Surgery
- Pericardiocentesis
- Pericardial window
- Subxiphoid pericardiotomy
- Complete pericardectomy
- Thoracotomy

♣ NURSING CONSIDERATIONS

Nursing diagnoses
- Activity intolerance
- Acute pain
- Anxiety
- Decreased cardiac output
- Deficient fluid volume
- Impaired gas exchange
- Ineffective tissue perfusion: Cardio-pulmonary
- Risk for infection

Key outcomes
The patient will:
- maintain hemodynamic stability
- express feelings of increased comfort and decreased pain
- identify positive methods for reducing anxiety
- maintain adequate cardiac output
- remain free of arrhythmias
- maintain adequate fluid volume
- maintain adequate ventilation and oxygenation
- maintain adequate cardiopulmonary perfusion
- remain free from signs of infection.

Nursing interventions
- Administer medications, as ordered.
- Provide reassurance.
- Assist with pericardiocentesis, if necessary.
- Infuse I.V. solutions, as ordered.
- Administer oxygen therapy, as needed.
- Maintain the chest drainage system, if used.

Monitoring
- Vital signs
- Intake and output
- Signs and symptoms of increasing tamponade
- Arrhythmias
- Hemodynamic stability
- Arterial blood gas levels
- Heart and breath sounds
- Complications

▶ PATIENT TEACHING

Be sure to cover:
- disorder, diagnostic tests, and treatment
- medication administration, dosage, and possible adverse effects
- when to notify the physician
- preoperative and postoperative care
- emergency procedures.

✳ RESOURCES

Organizations
American Heart Association: *www.americanheart.org*
National Heart, Lung and Blood Institute: *www.nhlbi.nih.gov*

Selected references
Kasper, D.L., et al., eds. *Harrison's Principles of Internal Medicine,* 16th ed. New York: McGraw-Hill Book Co., 2005.
The Merck Manual, 18th ed. Whitehouse Station, N.J.: Merck and Co., Inc., 2006.
Shatzer, M., and Castor, A. "How Transthoracic Echocardiography Detects Cardiac Tamponade," *Nursing* 34(3):73-74, March 2004.
Wade, C.R., et al. "Postoperative Nursing Care of the Cardiac Transplant Recipient," *Critical Care Nursing Quarterly* 27(1):17-28, January-March, 2004.

Cardiomyopathy, dilated

● OVERVIEW

Description
- Disease of the heart muscle fibers
- Also called *congestive cardiomyopathy*

Pathophysiology
- Extensively damaged myocardial muscle fibers reduce contractility of left ventricle.
- As systolic function declines, cardiac output falls.
- The sympathetic nervous system is stimulated to increase heart rate and contractility.
- When compensatory mechanisms can no longer maintain cardiac output, the heart begins to fail.

Causes
- Viral or bacterial infections
- Hypertension
- Peripartum syndrome related to toxemia
- Ischemic heart disease
- Valvular disease
- Drug hypersensitivity
- Chemotherapy
- Cardiotoxic effects of drugs or alcohol

Incidence
- Most commonly affects middle-aged men but can occur in any age group

Common characteristics
- Dyspnea on exertion
- Dry cough at night

Complications
- Intractable heart failure
- Arrhythmias
- Emboli

✳ ASSESSMENT

History
- Possible history of a disorder that can cause cardiomyopathy
- Gradual onset of shortness of breath, orthopnea, dyspnea on exertion, paroxysmal nocturnal dyspnea, fatigue, dry cough at night, palpitations, and vague chest pain

Physical findings
- Peripheral edema
- Jugular vein distention
- Ascites
- Peripheral cyanosis
- Clubbing
- Tachycardia even at rest and pulsus alternans in late stages
- Hepatomegaly and splenomegaly
- Narrow pulse pressure
- Irregular rhythms, diffuse apical impulses, pansystolic murmur
- S_3 and S_4 gallop rhythms
- Pulmonary crackles
- Dilated cardiomyopathy that may need to be differentiated from other types of cardiomyopathy (see *Assessment findings in cardiomyopathies*)

Test results

IMAGING
- Angiography results are used to rule out ischemic heart disease.
- Chest X-rays demonstrate moderate to marked cardiomegaly and possible pulmonary edema.
- Echocardiography may reveal ventricular thrombi, global hypokinesis, and the degrees of left ventricular dilation and dysfunction.
- Gallium scans may be used to identify patients with dilated cardiomyopathy and myocarditis.

DIAGNOSTIC PROCEDURES
- Cardiac catheterization can show left ventricular dilation and dysfunction, elevated left ventricular and, often, right ventricular filling pressures, and diminished cardiac output.
- Transvenous endomyocardial biopsy may be useful in some patients to determine the underlying disorder.
- Electrocardiography is used to rule out ischemic heart disease.

ASSESSMENT FINDINGS IN CARDIOMYOPATHIES

Type	Assessment findings
DILATED CARDIOMYOPATHY	• Generalized weakness, fatigue • Chest pain, palpitations • Syncope • Tachycardia • Narrow pulse pressure • Pulmonary congestion, pleural effusions • Neck vein distention, peripheral edema • Paroxysmal nocturnal dyspnea, orthopnea, dyspnea with exertion
HYPERTROPHIC CARDIOMYOPATHY	• Angina, palpitations • Syncope • Orthopnea, dyspnea with exertion • Pulmonary congestion • Loud systolic murmur • Life-threatening arrhythmias • Sudden cardiac arrest
RESTRICTIVE CARDIOMYOPATHY	• Generalized weakness, fatigue • Bradycardia • Dyspnea • Neck vein distention, peripheral edema • Liver congestion, abdominal ascites

TREATMENT

General
- For cardiomyopathy caused by alcoholism, cessation of alcohol ingestion

✴ **AGE-RELATED CONCERN** A woman of childbearing age with dilated cardiomyopathy should avoid pregnancy.

Diet
- Low-sodium diet supplemented by vitamin therapy

Activity
- Rest

Medication
- Cardiac glycosides
- Diuretics
- Angiotensin-converting enzyme inhibitors
- Oxygen
- Anticoagulants
- Vasodilators
- Antiarrhythmics
- Beta-adrenergic blockers

Surgery
- Heart transplantation
- Possible cardiomyoplasty

NURSING CONSIDERATIONS

Nursing diagnoses
- Activity intolerance
- Anxiety
- Decreased cardiac output
- Deficient knowledge (dilated cardiomyopathy)
- Dysfunctional family processes: Alcoholism
- Excess fluid volume
- Fatigue
- Hopelessness
- Impaired gas exchange
- Impaired physical mobility
- Ineffective breathing pattern
- Ineffective tissue perfusion: Cardiopulmonary

Key outcomes
The patient will:
- verbalize strategies to reduce anxiety level
- maintain adequate cardiac output and hemodynamic stability
- recognize and accept limitations of chronic illness and changes in lifestyle
- develop no complications of excess fluid volume
- express feelings of increased energy and decreased fatigue
- participate in decision-making as appropriate
- maintain adequate ventilation and oxygenation
- maintain joint mobility and range of motion
- maintain adequate cardiopulmonary perfusion
- resume and maintain as many former roles as possible.

Nursing interventions
- Alternate periods of rest with required activities of daily living.
- Provide active or passive range-of-motion exercises.
- Consult with the dietitian to provide a low-sodium diet.
- Administer oxygen, as needed.
- Check serum potassium levels for hypokalemia, especially if therapy includes cardiac glycosides.
- Offer support and let the patient express his feelings.
- Allow the patient and his family members to express their fears and concerns and help them identify effective coping strategies.

Monitoring
- Vital signs
- Hemodynamics
- Intake and output
- Daily weights
- Signs and symptoms of progressive heart failure

PATIENT TEACHING

Be sure to cover:
- disorder, diagnostic tests, and treatment
- medication administration, dosage, and possible adverse effects
- when to notify the physician
- sodium and fluid restriction
- signs and symptoms of worsening heart failure.

Discharge planning
- Refer family members to community cardiopulmonary resuscitation classes.

RESOURCES

Organizations
Mayo Health Clinic: *www.mayohealth.org*
National Heart, Lung and Blood Institute: *www.nhlbi.nih.gov*

Selected references
Dambro, M.R. *Griffith's 5-Minute Clinical Consult 2006.* Philadelphia: Lippincott Williams & Wilkins, 2006.
Kasper, D.L., et al., eds. *Harrison's Principles of Internal Medicine,* 16th ed. New York: McGraw-Hill Book Co., 2005.
Marooka, T., et al. "An Appropriate Indication for the Initiation of Beta-Blocker Therapy in Dilated Cardiomyopathy," *Cardiology* 105(1):61-66, 2006.
The Merck Manual, 18th ed. Whitehouse Station, N.J.: Merck and Co., Inc., 2006.
Professional Guide to Diseases, 8th ed. Philadelphia: Lippincott Williams & Wilkins, 2005.

Cardiomyopathy, hypertrophic

● OVERVIEW

Description
- Primary disease of cardiac muscle
- Also known as *idiopathic hypertrophic subaortic stenosis, hypertrophic obstructive cardiomyopathy,* and *muscular aortic stenosis*

Pathophysiology
- The hypertrophied ventricle becomes stiff, noncompliant, and unable to relax during ventricular filling.
- Ventricular filling time is reduced as compensation to tachycardia.
- Reduced ventricular filling leads to low cardiac output.

Causes
- Transmission by autosomal dominant trait (about one-half of all cases)
- Associated with hypertension

Incidence
- More common in men and in blacks
- Affects 5 to 8 per 100,000 in the United States

Common characteristics
- Left ventricular hypertrophy
- Disproportionate, asymmetrical thickening of the intraventricular septum and free wall of the left ventricle

Complications
- Pulmonary hypertension
- Heart failure
- Ventricular arrhythmias

✳ ASSESSMENT

History
- Generally, no visible clinical features until disease is well advanced
- Atrial dilation and, sometimes, atrial fibrillation, that abruptly reduce blood flow to left ventricle
- Possible family history of hypertrophic cardiomyopathy
- Orthopnea and dyspnea on exertion
- Anginal pain, palpitations
- Fatigue
- Syncope, even at rest

Physical findings
- Rapidly rising carotid arterial pulse possible
- Pulsus biferiens
- Double or triple apical impulse, possibly displaced laterally
- Bibasilar crackles if heart failure is present
- Harsh systolic murmur heard after S_1 at the apex near the left sternal border
- S_4 also possibly audible

Test results
IMAGING
- Chest X-rays may show a mild to moderate increase in heart size.
- Thallium scan usually reveals myocardial perfusion defects.

DIAGNOSTIC PROCEDURES
- Echocardiography shows left ventricular hypertrophy and a thick, asymmetrical intraventricular septum in obstructive hypertrophic cardiomyopathy, whereas hypertrophy affects various ventricular areas in nonobstructive hypertrophic cardiomyopathy.
- Cardiac catheterization reveals elevated left ventricular end-diastolic pressure and, possibly, mitral insufficiency.
- Electrocardiography usually shows left ventricular hypertrophy, ST-segment and T-wave abnormalities, Q waves in leads II, III, aV_F, and in V_4 to V_6 (due to hypertrophy, not infarction), left anterior hemiblock, left axis deviation, and ventricular and atrial arrhythmias.

◆ TREATMENT

General
- Cardioversion for atrial fibrillation

Diet
- Low-fat, low-salt
- Fluid restriction
- Avoidance of alcohol

Activity
- Variable limitations
- Bed rest possible

Medication
- Beta-adrenergic blockers
- Calcium channel blockers
- Amiodarone, unless atrioventricular block exists
- Antibiotic prophylaxis

 NURSING ALERT Nitrates, digoxin, angiotensin-converting enzyme inhibitors, and other beta-adrenergic blockers are contraindicated.

Surgery
- Ventricular myotomy alone or combined with mitral valve replacement
- Pacemaker insertion
- Implantable cardioverter-defibrillator
- Heart transplantation

❖ NURSING CONSIDERATIONS

Nursing diagnoses
- Activity intolerance
- Acute pain
- Decreased cardiac output
- Deficient knowledge (hypertrophic cardiomyopathy)
- Fatigue
- Excess fluid volume
- Ineffective coping
- Risk for infection

Key outcomes
The patient will:
- express feelings of increased comfort and decreased pain
- maintain adequate cardiac output and hemodynamic stability
- demonstrate understanding of condition and treatment
- carry out activities of daily living (ADLs) without excess fatigue or decreased energy
- develop no complications of excess fluid volume
- develop adequate coping mechanisms
- remain free of signs and symptoms of infection.

Nursing interventions
- Alternate periods of rest with required ADLs and treatments.
- Provide personal care, as needed, to prevent fatigue.
- Provide active or passive range-of-motion exercises.

◈ **NURSING ALERT** If propranolol is to be discontinued, don't stop the drug abruptly; doing so may cause rebound effects, resulting in myocardial infarction or sudden death.

- Offer support and let the patient express his feelings.
- Allow the patient and family members to express their fears and concerns and identify effective coping strategies.

Monitoring
- Vital signs
- Hemodynamics
- Intake and output

▶ PATIENT TEACHING

Be sure to cover:
- that propranolol can cause depression and the need to notify the physician if symptoms occur
- instructions to take medication, as ordered
- need to notify any physician caring for him that he shouldn't be given nitroglycerin, digoxin, or diuretics because they can worsen obstruction
- the need for antibiotic prophylaxis before dental work or surgery to prevent infective endocarditis
- warnings against strenuous activity, which may precipitate syncope or sudden death
- need to avoid Valsalva's maneuver or sudden position changes.

Discharge planning
- Refer family members to community cardiopulmonary resuscitation classes.

✴ RESOURCES

Organizations
Mayo Health Clinic: *www.mayohealth.org*
National Heart, Lung and Blood Institute: *www.nhlbi.nih.gov*

Selected references
Graham-Cryan, M.A., et al. "Obstructive Hypertrophic Cardiomyopathy," *Progress in Cardiovascular Nursing* 19(4):133-40, Fall 2004.

Ivens, E. "Hypertrophic Cardiomyopathy," *Heart, Lung and Circulation* 13(Suppl 3):S48-55, 2004.

Kasper, D.L., et al., eds. *Harrison's Principles of Internal Medicine*, 16th ed. New York: Mc-Graw-Hill Book Co., 2005.

The Merck Manual of Diagnosis & Therapy, 18th ed. Whitehouse Station, N.J.: Merck & Co., Inc., 2006.

Professional Guide to Diseases, 8th ed. Philadelphia: Lippincott Williams & Wilkins, 2005.

Carpal tunnel syndrome

● OVERVIEW

Description
- Compression of median nerve in the wrist
- Most common nerve entrapment syndrome
- Affects people who move their wrists continuously
- May pose a serious occupational health problem

Pathophysiology
- The median nerve controls motions in the forearm, wrist, and hand and supplies sensation to the index, middle, and ring fingers.
- Compression of the median nerve interrupts normal function. (See *The carpal tunnel*.)

Causes
- Exact cause unknown
- Repetitive wrist motions involving excessive flexion or extension
- Dislocation
- Acute sprain that may damage the median nerve
- Amyloidosis
- Edema-producing conditions
- Gout
- Tumors

Risk factors
- Diabetes
- Pregnancy
- Alcoholism
- Hypothyroidism
- Renal failure

Incidence
- Most common in women between ages 30 and 60

Common characteristics
- Weakness, pain, burning, numbness, and tingling in both hands
- Paresthesia that affects thumb, forefinger, middle finger, and half of 4th finger
- Inability to clench fist
- Atrophic nails
- Dry and shiny skin

Complications
- Tendon inflammation
- Compression

THE CARPAL TUNNEL

The carpal tunnel is clearly visible in this palmar view and cross section of a right hand. Note the median nerve, flexor tendons of fingers, and blood vessels passing through the tunnel on their way from the forearm to the hand.

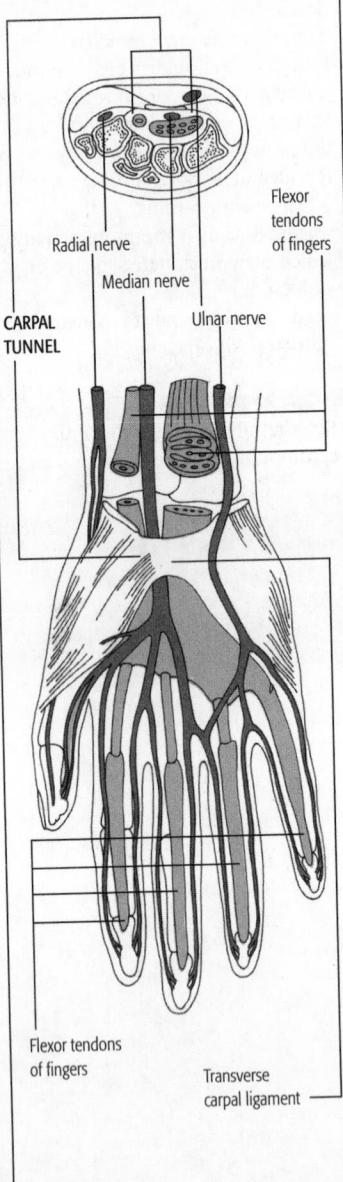

Flexor tendons of fingers

Radial nerve

Median nerve

CARPAL TUNNEL

Ulnar nerve

Flexor tendons of fingers

Transverse carpal ligament

- Neural ischemia
- Permanent nerve damage with loss of movement and sensation

✱ ASSESSMENT

History
- Occupation or hobby requiring strenuous or repetitive use of the hands
- Condition that causes swelling in carpal tunnel structures
- Weakness, pain, burning, numbness, or tingling that occurs in one or both hands
- Paresthesia that worsens at night and in the morning
- Pain that spreads to the forearm and, in severe cases, as far as the shoulder
- Pain that can be relieved by:
  - shaking hands vigorously
  - dangling the arms at sides

Physical findings
- Inability to make a fist
- Fingernails that may be atrophied, with surrounding dry, shiny skin

Test results
IMAGING
- Electromyography shows a median nerve motor conduction delay of more than 5 milliseconds.
- Digital electrical stimulation shows median nerve compression by measuring the length and intensity of stimulation from the fingers to the median nerve in the wrist.

OTHER
- Compression test result supports the diagnosis.

General
- Conservative initially:
  - Splinting the wrist for 1 to 2 weeks
  - Possible occupational changes
  - Correction of any underlying disorder

Diet
- No restrictions

Activity
- As tolerated

Medication
- Nonsteroidal anti-inflammatory drugs (NSAIDs)
- Corticosteroids
- Vitamin B complex

Surgery
- Decompression of the nerve
- Neurolysis

Nursing diagnoses
- Anxiety
- Chronic pain
- Impaired physical mobility
- Ineffective role performance
- Self care deficit (dressing/grooming, bathing/hygiene)

Key outcomes
The patient will:
- identify measures to reduce anxiety
- express feelings of increased comfort and decreased pain
- maintain muscle strength
- maintain joint mobility and range of motion
- continue to function in usual roles as much as possible
- perform activities of daily living.

Nursing interventions
- Promote self-care and allow adequate time.
- Administer analgesics, as ordered.

Monitoring
- Response to analgesia
- After surgery, vital signs
- Color, sensation, and motion of the affected hand

Be sure to cover:
- splint application
- hand exercises in warm water
- medication administration, dosage, and possible adverse effects
- avoidance of NSAIDs in pregnancy.

Discharge planning
- Refer the patient for occupational counseling if a job change is necessary.

Organizations
National Institutes of Health: *www.nih.gov*
The Paget Foundation: *www.paget.org*
WebMD: *www.webmd.com*

Selected references
Callandro, P., et al. "Distribution of Paresthesia in Carpal Tunnel Syndrome Reflects the Degree of Nerve Damage at Wrist," *Clinical Neurophysiology* 118(1):228-31, January 2006.

Diseases, 4th ed., Philadelphia: Lippincott Williams & Wilkins, 2006.

Handbook of Pathophysiology, 2nd ed. Philadelphia: Lippincott Williams & Wilkins, 2005.

Hopp, P.T., et al. "Carpal Tunnel Syndrome—The Role of Psychosocial Factors in Recovery," *AAOHN Journal* 52(11):458-60, November 2005.

Kent, V.P. "PathoPuzzle: Taking the Puzzle out of Carpal Tunnel Syndrome," *Nursing Made Incredibly Easy,* 4(2):4-5, March-April 2006.

Cataract

● OVERVIEW

Description
- Opacity of the lens or lens capsule of the eye
- Common cause of gradual vision loss
- Commonly affects both eyes
- Traumatic cataracts usually unilateral

Pathophysiology
- The clouded lens blocks light shining through the cornea.
- Images cast onto the retina are blurred.
- A hazy image is interpreted by the brain.

Causes
- Classified according to cause

SENILE CATARACTS
- Chemical changes in lens proteins in elderly patients

CONGENITAL CATARACTS
- Inborn errors of metabolism
- Maternal rubella infection during the first trimester
- Congenital anomaly
- Genetic causes (usually autosomal dominant)
- Recessive cataracts that may be sex-linked

TRAUMATIC CATARACTS
- Foreign bodies causing aqueous or vitreous humor to enter lens capsule

COMPLICATED CATARACTS
- Uveitis
- Glaucoma
- Retinitis pigmentosa
- Retinal detachment
- Diabetes
- Hypoparathyroidism
- Atopic dermatitis
- Ionizing radiation or infrared rays

TOXIC CATARACTS
- Drug or chemical toxicity:
  - ergot
  - dinitrophenol
  - naphthalene
  - phenothiazines

Incidence
- Most prevalent in people over age 70

Common characteristics
- Painless, gradual vision loss
- Glare
- Milky-white pupil

Complications
- Complete vision loss

POSSIBLE COMPLICATIONS OF SURGERY
- Loss of vitreous
- Wound dehiscence
- Hyphema
- Pupillary block glaucoma
- Retinal detachment
- Infection

✱ ASSESSMENT

History
- Painless, gradual vision loss
- Glare, especially from headlights with night driving
- Poor reading vision
- Better vision in dim light than in bright light (central opacity)

Physical findings
- Milky-white pupil on inspection with a penlight
- Grayish-white area behind the pupil (advanced cataract)
- Absence of red reflex is lost (mature cataract)

Test results

DIAGNOSTIC PROCEDURES
- Indirect ophthalmoscopy reveals a dark area in the normally homogeneous red reflex.
- Slit-lamp examination confirms lens opacity.
- Visual acuity test result establishes the degree of vision loss.

◆ TREATMENT

General
- Before surgery, eyeglasses and contact lenses that may help to improve vision
- Sunglasses in bright light and lamps that provide reflected lighting rather than direct lighting, thus decreasing glare and aiding vision

Diet
- No restrictions

Activity
- Restricted according to vision loss

Medication

FOR CATARACT REMOVAL
- Nonsteroidal anti-inflammatory drugs
- Short-acting local anesthetic
- Mydriatics
- Corticosteroids
- Antibiotics

Surgery
- Lens extraction and implantation of intraocular lens
- Extracapsular cataract extraction
- Intracapsular cataract extraction
- Phacoemulsification

NURSING CONSIDERATIONS

Nursing diagnoses
- Anxiety
- Deficient knowledge (cataract removal)
- Disturbed sensory perception: Visual
- Risk for infection
- Risk for injury

Key outcomes
The patient will:
- voice feelings and concerns
- express understanding of the disorder
- regain visual function
- remain free of harm or injury
- remain free from signs and symptoms of infection.

Nursing interventions
- Perform routine postoperative care.
- Assist with early ambulation.
- Apply an eye shield or eye patch postoperatively, as ordered.

Monitoring
- Vital signs
- Visual acuity
- Complications of surgery

PATIENT TEACHING

Be sure to cover:
- need to avoid activities that increase intraocular pressure, such as straining with coughing, bowel movements, or lifting
- need to abstain from sexual intercourse until he receives physician's approval
- proper instillation of ophthalmic ointment or drops.

  NURSING ALERT If the patient has increased eye discharge, sharp eye pain that's unrelieved by analgesics, or deterioration in vision, instruct him to notify his physician immediately.

RESOURCES

Organizations
American Academy of Ophthalmology: *www.eyenet.org*
National Eye Institute: *www.nei.nih.gov*

Selected references
Robman, L., and Taylor, H. "External Factors in the Development of Cataracts," *Eye* 19(10):1074-1082, October 2005.
Stava, C., et al. Cataracts Among Cancer Survivors. *American Journal of Clinical Oncology* 28(6):603-08, December 2005.

Cellulitis

● OVERVIEW

Description
- Acute infection of the dermis and subcutaneous tissue
- May follow damage to the skin, such as a bite or wound
- Prognosis usually good with timely treatment
- With other comorbidities, such as diabetes, increased risk of developing or spreading cellulitis

Pathophysiology
- A break in skin integrity almost always precedes infection.
- As the offending organism invades the compromised area, it overwhelms the defensive cells, including the neutrophils, eosinophils, basophils, and mast cells, that normally contain and localize the inflammation.
- As cellulitis progresses, the organism invades tissue around the initial wound site.

Causes
- Bacterial infections, usually by Staphylococcus aureus and Group A beta-hemolytic streptococci
- Fungal infections
- Extension of a skin wound or ulcer
- Furuncles or carbuncles

Risk factors
- Venous and lymphatic compromise
- Edema
- Diabetes mellitus
- Underlying skin lesion
- Prior trauma

Incidence
- Occurs most commonly in the lower extremities
- Affects males and females equally

✹ **AGE-RELATED CONCERN** Perianal cellulitis occurs more commonly in children, especially boys.

Common characteristics
- Tenderness
- Pain
- Erythema
- Warmth
- Edema

Complications
- Sepsis
- Deep vein thrombosis
- Progression of cellulitis
- Local abscesses
- Thrombophlebitis
- Lymphangitis

✹ **AGE-RELATED CONCERN** Cellulitis of the lower extremity is more likely to develop into thrombophlebitis in an elderly patient.

✱ ASSESSMENT

History
- Presence of one or more risk factors
- Tenderness
- Pain at the site and possibly surrounding area
- Erythema and warmth
- Edema
- Possible fever, chills, malaise

Physical findings
- Erythema with indistinct margins
- Fever
- Warmth and tenderness of the skin
- Regional lymph node enlargement and tenderness
- Lymphatic streaking

Test results
LABORATORY
- White blood cell count shows mild leukocytosis.
- Erythrocyte sedimentation rate shows mild elevation.
- Culture and gram stain may show the offending organism.

◆ TREATMENT

General
- Immobilization and elevation of the affected extremity
- Moist heat

Diet
- Well-balanced

Activity
- Possible bed rest with severe infection

Medication
- Antibiotics
- Topical antifungals
- Analgesics

Surgery
- Tracheostomy, for severe cellulitis of head and neck
- Abscess drainage
- Amputation (with gas-forming cellulitis [gangrene])

✣ NURSING CONSIDERATIONS

Nursing diagnoses
- Acute pain
- Ineffective health maintenance
- Fear
- Risk for impaired skin integrity
- Risk for infection
- Risk for injury

Key outcomes
The patient will:
- express feelings of increased comfort and decreased pain
- maintain optimum health status
- verbalize feelings and concerns
- remain free from skin breakdown and signs and symptoms of infection
- avoid injury.

Nursing interventions
- Administer medications, as ordered.
- Elevate affected extremity.
- Apply moist heat, as ordered.
- Encourage a well-balanced diet.
- Encourage adequate fluid intake.
- Encourage verbalization of feelings and concerns.
- Institute safety precautions.

Monitoring
- Vital signs
- Pain
- Edema
- Laboratory results
- Signs and symptoms of infection
- Complications
- Cellulitis progression

▶ PATIENT TEACHING

Be sure to cover:
- disorder, diagnostic tests, and treatment
- medication administration, dosage, and possible adverse effects
- when to notify the physician
- warm compresses
- complications
- signs and symptoms of infection
- prevention of injury and trauma
- infection control
- signs and symptoms of deep vein thrombosis.

Discharge planning
- Refer the patient for management of diabetes mellitus as indicated.

✳ RESOURCES

Organizations
American Academy of Dermatology: *www.aad.org*
American Diabetes Association: *www.diabetes.org*
Dermatology Foundation: *www.dermfnd.org*

Selected references
Barza, M. "Noninfectious Causes of Cellultis," *Annals of Internal Medicine* 143(8):614, October 2005.
Donald, M., et al. "Emergency Department Management of Home Intravenous Antibiotic Therapy for Cellulitis," *Emergency Medicine Journal* 22(10):715-17, October 2005.

Cerebral contusion

OVERVIEW

Description
- Ecchymosis of brain tissue that results from severe blow to the head
- Most commonly occurs in frontal and temporal lobes

Pathophysiology
- Trauma to the head causes tearing or twisting of the structures and blood vessels of the brain.
- Scattered hemorrhages form over the surface, disrupting and, possibly, prolonging return of function.

Causes
- Acceleration-deceleration or coup-contrecoup injuries
- Trauma to the head

Risk factors
- Unsteady gait
- Participation in contact sports
- Receiving anticoagulant therapy

Incidence
- Occurs at any age

Common characteristics
- Change in level of consciousness
- Hypotension
- Dizziness
- Headache
- Nausea and vomiting
- Pupil changes
- Hemiparesis
- Memory loss or forgetfulness
- Seizure

Complications
- Increased intracranial pressure
- Intracranial hemorrhage
- Hematoma
- Tentorial herniation

ASSESSMENT

History
- Head injury or motor vehicle accident
- Loss of consciousness

Physical findings
- Unconscious patient: pale and motionless; altered vital signs
- Conscious patient: drowsy or easily disturbed
- Scalp wound
- Possible involuntary evacuation of bowel and bladder
- Hemiparesis

Test results
IMAGING
- Computed tomography scan shows areas of damage.
- Magnetic resonance imaging denotes areas of damage.
- Electroencephalography helps confirm diagnosis.
- Cerebral angiography aids in confirming diagnosis.

TREATMENT

General
- Establishing a patent airway
- Administration of I.V. fluids
- Minimization of environmental stimuli

Diet
- Nothing by mouth until fully conscious

Activity
- Based on neurologic status
- Initially, bed rest
- Avoidance of contact sports

Medication
- Nonopioid analgesics
- Anticonvulsants
- Antibiotics
- Corticosteroids

Surgery
- Craniotomy
- Suturing

Nursing diagnoses
- Acute pain
- Anxiety
- Decreased intracranial adaptive capacity
- Disturbed sensory perception: Kinesthetic, tactile
- Impaired verbal communication
- Risk for acute confusion
- Risk for imbalanced fluid volume
- Risk for infection
- Risk for injury
- Risk for posttrauma syndrome

Key outcomes
The patient will:
- express feelings of increased comfort and decreased pain
- use support systems to assist with anxiety
- maintain a stable neurologic state
- maintain optimal functioning within limits of kinesthetic and tactile impairments
- use effective means of communicating
- exhibit an alert level of consciousness
- maintain adequate fluid volume
- remain free from signs and symptoms of infection and avoid injury
- express fears and feelings about traumatic event.

Nursing interventions
- Perform neurologic examinations.
- Maintain a patent airway.
- Administer medication, as ordered (no aspirin).
- Protect from injury.

Monitoring
- Vital signs
- Neurologic status
- Cerebrospinal fluid (CSF) leakage

Be sure to cover:
- need to avoid coughing, sneezing, or blowing the nose until after recovery
- observation for CSF drainage
- how to detect and report mental status changes
- signs and symptoms of infection.

Discharge planning
- Refer the patient to a neurologist for follow-up, as indicated.

Organizations
American Academy of Neurology: *www.aan.com*
Brain Injury Society: *www.bisociety.org*
Head Injury Hotline: *www.headinjury.com*
Med Help International: *www.medhelp.org*

Selected references
Nolan, S. "Traumatic Brain Injury: A Review," *Critical Care Nursing Quarterly* 28(2):188-94, April-June 2005.

Rigg, J.L., et al. "Corticosteroids in TBI: Is the Story Closed?" *Journal of Head Trauma Rehabilitation* 21(3):285-88, May-June 2006.

Zink, E.K. et al. "Managing Traumatic Brain Injury," *Nursing2006* 35(9):36-43, September 2005.

Cerebral palsy

● OVERVIEW

Description

- Most common crippling disease in children
- Comprises several neuromuscular disorders
- Results from prenatal, perinatal, or postnatal central nervous system (CNS) damage
- Three types (sometimes occur in mixed forms):
  - spastic (affecting about 70% of children with cerebral palsy)
  - athetoid (affecting about 20%)
  - ataxic (affecting about 10%)
- Minimal or severely disabling motor impairment
- Associated defects:
  - seizures
  - speech disorders
  - mental retardation
- Variable prognosis

Pathophysiology

- A lesion or an abnormality occurs in the early stages of brain development.
- Structural and functional defects occur, impairing motor or cognitive function.
- Defects may not be distinguishable until months after birth.

Causes

- Conditions that result in cerebral anoxia, hemorrhage, or other CNS damage

PRENATAL CAUSES

- Rh factor incompatibility
- ABO blood type incompatibility
- Maternal infection (especially rubella in the first trimester)
- Maternal diabetes
- Irradiation
- Anoxia
- Toxemia
- Malnutrition
- Abnormal placental attachment
- Isoimmunization

PERINATAL CAUSES

- Trauma during delivery
- Depressed maternal vital signs from general or spinal anesthesia
- Asphyxia from the cord wrapping around the neck
- Prematurity
- Prolonged or unusually rapid labor
- Multiple births (neonates born last in a multiple birth have an especially high rate of cerebral palsy)

POSTNATAL CAUSES

- Infections, such as meningitis and encephalitis
- Head trauma
- Poisoning
- Any condition that results in cerebral thrombus or embolus

Incidence

- Highest in premature neonates and in those who are small for gestational age
- Slightly more common in boys than in girls
- Occurs more commonly in whites

Common characteristics

- Excessive lethargy or irritability
- High-pitched cry
- Poor head control
- Weak sucking reflex
- Delayed motor development
- Abnormal head circumference
- Abnormal postures
- Abnormal reflexes
- Abnormal muscle tone and performance

Complications

- Seizure disorders
- Speech, vision, and hearing problems
- Language and perceptual deficits
- Mental retardation (in up to 40% of patients)
- Dental problems
- Respiratory difficulties
- Poor swallowing and gag reflexes

✱ ASSESSMENT

History

- Maternal or patient history revealing possible cause (see *When to suspect cerebral palsy*)

Physical findings

- Child with retarded growth and development
- Difficulty chewing and swallowing

SPASTIC CEREBRAL PALSY

- Underdevelopment of affected limbs
- Characteristic scissors gait
- Walks on toes
- Crosses one foot in front of the other
- Hyperactive deep tendon reflexes
- Increased stretch reflexes
- Rapid alternating muscle contraction and relaxation
- Muscle weakness
- Contractures that occur in response to manipulation of muscles

ATHETOID CEREBRAL PALSY

- Involuntary movements
- Grimacing
- Wormlike writhing
- Dystonia
- Sharp jerks that impair voluntary movement
- Involuntary facial movements (speech difficult)

ATAXIC CEREBRAL PALSY

- Lack of leg movement during infancy
- Wide gait when child begins to walk
- Disturbed balance
- Incoordination (especially of the arms)
- Hypoactive reflexes
- Nystagmus
- Muscle weakness
- Tremors

Test results

IMAGING

- Computed tomography scan and magnetic resonance imaging may show structural abnormalities of the brain such as cerebral atrophy.
- EEG may show the source of seizure activity.

WHEN TO SUSPECT CEREBRAL PALSY

Early detection is essential for effective treatment and requires careful clinical observation during infancy and precise neurologic assessment. Suspect cerebral palsy whenever a neonate:

- has difficulty sucking or keeping the nipple or food in his mouth
- seldom moves voluntarily or has arm or leg tremors with voluntary movement
- crosses his legs when lifted from behind rather than pulling them up or bicycling like a normal neonate
- has legs that are hard to separate, making diaper changing difficult
- persistently uses only one hand or, as he gets older, uses his hands well but not his legs.

◆ TREATMENT

General
- Braces or splints
- Special appliances, such as adapted eating utensils and low toilet seat with arms

Diet
- No restrictions

Activity
- Range-of-motion (ROM) exercises
- Prescribed exercises to maintain muscle tone

Medication
- Anticonvulsants
- Muscle relaxants
- Antianxiety agents

Surgery
- Orthopedic surgery
- Neurosurgery

♣ NURSING CONSIDERATIONS

Nursing diagnoses
- Chronic low self-esteem
- Deficient knowledge (cerebral palsy)
- Delayed growth and development
- Disturbed body image
  Disturbed sensory perception: Kinesthetic
- Imbalanced nutrition: Less than body requirements
- Impaired physical mobility
- Impaired swallowing
- Interrupted family processes
- Risk for impaired parenting
- Risk for impaired skin integrity

Key outcomes
The patient will:
- express positive feelings about self
- demonstrate knowledge of the condition
- achieve age-appropriate growth and development milestones
- consume calorie requirements daily
- maintain joint mobility and ROM
- maintain optimal level of functioning within limitations

- swallow without pain or aspiration
- identify realistic goals with parents
- remain free of skin breakdown.

Nursing interventions
- Speak slowly and distinctly.
- Give all care in an unhurried manner.
- Allow participation in care decisions.
- Provide a diet with adequate calories. Stroking the throat may aid swallowing.
- Provide frequent mouth and dental care.
- Apply braces.
- Provide skin care.
- Massage the area under the brace daily.
- Perform prescribed exercises to maintain muscle tone.
- Care for associated hearing and vision disturbances, as necessary.
- Postoperatively, give analgesics, as ordered.

Monitoring
- Pain relief
- Seizure activity
- Speech
- Visual and auditory acuity
- Respiratory status
- Swallowing function
- Reflexes
- Nutritional status
- Skin integrity
- Motor development
- Muscle strength

▶ PATIENT TEACHING

Be sure to cover:
- medication administration, dosage, and possible adverse effects
- daily skin inspection and daily massage
- need to place food far back in patient's mouth to facilitate swallowing
- need to chew food thoroughly
- drinking through a straw
- sucking lollipops to develop muscle control
- proper nutrition
- opportunities for learning, such as summer camps or Special Olympics.

Discharge planning
- Refer family members to community support groups such as the local chapter of the United Cerebral Palsy Association.

✳ RESOURCES

Organizations
American Academy of Pediatrics:
www.aap.org
National Institutes of Health: *www.nih.gov*
United Cerebral Palsy Association:
www.ucpa.org

Selected references
Handbook of Pathophysiology, 2nd ed. Philadelphia: Lippincott Williams & Wilkins, 2005.
Livinec, F., et al. "Prenatal Risk Factors for Cerebral Palsy in Very Preterm Singletons and Twins," *Obstetrics and Gynecology* 105(6):1341-347, June 2005.
Professional Guide to Diseases, 8th ed. Philadelphia: Lippincott Williams & Wilkins, 2005.

Cervical cancer

● OVERVIEW

Description
- Third most common cancer of the female reproductive system
- Classified as either preinvasive or invasive
- Preinvasive cancer: curable in 75% to 90% of patients with early detection and proper treatment
- Invasive cancer: squamous cell carcinoma (95% of cases); adenocarcinoma (5% of cases)

Pathophysiology
PREINVASIVE CANCER
- Preinvasive cancer ranges from minimal cervical dysplasia, in which the lower third of the epithelium contains abnormal cells, to carcinoma in situ, in which the full thickness of epithelium contains abnormally proliferating cells.

INVASIVE CANCER
- Cancer cells penetrate the basement membrane and can spread directly to contiguous pelvic structures or disseminate to distant sites by way of lymphatic routes.

Causes
- Unknown

Risk factors
- Human papillomavirus (HPV)
- Frequent intercourse at a young age (under age 16)
- Multiple sexual partners
- Multiple pregnancies
- Bacterial or viral venereal infections

Incidence
- Typically occurs between ages 30 and 50; rarely, under age 20

Common characteristics
- Abnormal vaginal bleeding

Complications
- Renal failure
- Distant metastasis
- Vaginal stenosis
- Ureterovaginal or vesicovaginal fistula
- Proctitis
- Cystitis
- Bowel obstruction

✳ ASSESSMENT

History
- One or more risk factors present

PREINVASIVE CANCER
- No symptoms or other clinical changes

INVASIVE CANCER
- Abnormal vaginal bleeding or discharge
- Gradually increasing flank pain

Physical findings
- Vaginal discharge
- Postcoital bleeding
- Irregular bleeding

Test results
IMAGING
- Lymphangiography, cystography, and organ and bone scans all may show metastasis.

DIAGNOSTIC PROCEDURES
- Papanicolaou (Pap) test shows abnormal cells, and colposcopy shows the source of the abnormal cells seen on the Pap test.
- Cone biopsy is performed if endocervical curettage is positive.
- Vira Pap test (under investigation) permits examination of the specimen's deoxyribonucleic acid structure to detect HPV.

◆ TREATMENT

General
- Accurate clinical staging used to determine type of treatment

Diet
- Well-balanced; as tolerated

Activity
- No restrictions

Medication
- Multidrug chemotherapy regimens

Surgery
PREINVASIVE LESIONS
- Total excisional biopsy
- Cryosurgery
- Laser destruction
- Conization, followed by frequent Pap test follow-ups
- Hysterectomy (rare)

INVASIVE SQUAMOUS CELL CARCINOMA
- Radical hysterectomy and radiation therapy (internal, external, or both)
- Pelvic exenteration (rare; may be performed for recurrent cervical cancer)

❖ NURSING CONSIDERATIONS

Nursing diagnoses
- Acute pain
- Anxiety
- Fear
- Impaired physical mobility
- Impaired skin integrity
- Ineffective coping
- Ineffective sexuality patterns
- Risk for infection
- Sexual dysfunction

Key outcomes
The patient will:
- report feelings of decreased pain and anxiety
- verbalize concerns and fears related to diagnosis
- maintain joint mobility and range of motion
- remain free from signs and symptoms of skin breakdown
- demonstrate effective coping strategies
- resume appropriate safe sexual activity patterns to fullest extent possible
- remain free from signs and symptoms of infection
- express feelings and perceptions with her partner about changes in sexual performance.

Nursing interventions
- Encourage verbalization and provide support.
- Administer medication, as ordered.

Monitoring
- Vital signs
- Complications
- Pain control
- Vaginal discharge
- Renal status
- Response to treatment

▶ PATIENT TEACHING

Be sure to cover:
- disorder, diagnostic tests, and treatment
- importance of follow-up care
- how treatment won't radically alter the patient's lifestyle or prohibit sexual intimacy
- medication administration, dosage, and possible adverse effects.

Discharge planning
- Refer the patient to resource and support services.

✳ RESOURCES

Organizations
American Cancer Society: *www.cancer.org*
Guide to Internet Resources for Cancer: *www.cancerindex.org*
National Cancer Institute: *www.nci.nih.gov*

Selected references
Atlas of Pathophysiology, 2nd ed. Philadelphia: Lippincott Williams & Wilkins, 2005.

Bertram, C.C. "Evidence for Practice: Oral Contraception and Risk of Cervical cancer," *Journal of the American Academy of Nurse Practitioners* 16(10):455-61, October 2004.

Schmiedeskamp, M.R., and Kockler, D.R. "Human Papillomavirus Vaccines," *Annals of Pharmacotherapy* 40(7-8):1344-352, July-August 2006.

Schneier, A., and Hertel, H. "Surgical and Radiographic Staging in Patients with Cervical Cancer," *Current Opinion in Obstetrics & Gynecology* 16(1):11-18, February 2004.

Suprasert, P., et al. "Radical Hysterectomy for Stage IIB Cervical Cancer: A Review," *Intenational Journal of Gynecological Cancer* 15(6):995-1001, November-December 2005.

Chlamydia

Description
- Infection that results in cervicitis in women, urethritis in men, and lymphogranuloma venereum in both sexes
- Most common sexually transmitted disease (STD) in the United States
- Trachoma inclusion conjunctivitis: seldom occurs in United States, but is leading cause of blindness in developing countries

Pathophysiology
- Chlamydial infections are transmitted by direct contact (such as sexual), producing local inflammatory action as the result of infection.
- Endometritis and salpingitis occur as the organism ascends the genitourinary tract.

Causes
- Transmission of *Chlamydia trachomatis*, by sexual contact (oral, anal, or vaginal)
- Neonate infection caused by transport through the birth canal of infected mother

Risk factors
- Multiple sex partners or new sex partner
- Unprotected sex
- Coinfection with another STD

Incidence
- Approximately 4 million cases reported annually

✸ AGE-RELATED CONCERN Chlamydial infections have a 10% incidence among sexually active adolescent girls.

Common characteristics
- Primarily follows vaginal or rectal intercourse or oral-genital contact with an infected person
- Signs and symptoms appear late in the course of disease
- Sexual transmission of organism occurs unknowingly

Complications
- Infertility
- Pelvic inflammatory disease
- Urethral and rectal strictures
- Perihepatitis
- Cervical cancer

History
- Unprotected sexual contact with an infected person
- Previous STD

Physical findings
- Two-thirds of patients asymptomatic

FEMALE
- Pelvic or abdominal pain
- Dyspareunia
- Cervical erosion
- Mucopurulent discharge
- Dysuria
- Urinary frequency

MALE
- Dysuria
- Urinary frequency
- Pruritus
- Urethral discharge (copious and purulent)
- Meatal erythema
- Severe scrotal pain

LYMPHOGRANULOMA VENEREUM
- Painless vesicle or nonindurated ulcer, 2 to 3 mm in diameter, on the glans or shaft of the penis; on the labia, vagina, or cervix; or in the rectum
- Enlarged inguinal lymph nodes
- Regional nodes that appear as series of bilateral buboes

- Untreated, buboes may rupture and form sinus tracts that discharge thick, yellow, granular secretion

Test results
LABORATORY
- Swab culture of the infection site shows *C. trachomatis*. (See *Chlamydia trachomatis.*)
- Culture of aspirated blood, pus, or cerebrospinal fluid establishes epididymitis, prostatitis, and lymphogranuloma venereum.
- Serologic studies reveal previous exposure.
- Enzyme-linked immunosorbent assay shows *C. trachomatis* antibody.

CHLAMYDIA TRACHOMATIS

In chlamydial infections, microscopic examination reveals *C. trachomatis*, a unicellular parasite with a rigid cell wall.

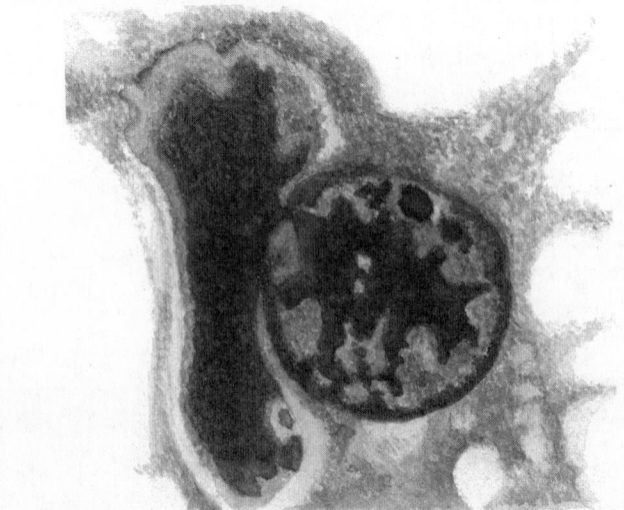

General
- Symptomatic treatment

Diet
- No restrictions

Activity
- Abstinence from sexual activity until infection resolved

Medication
- Antibiotics

Nursing diagnoses
- Acute pain
- Deficient knowledge (STDs and transmission)
- Impaired skin integrity
- Impaired urinary elimination
- Ineffective sexuality patterns
- Sexual dysfunction
- Situational low self-esteem

Key outcomes
The patient will:
- express feelings of increased comfort and decreased pain
- verbalize knowledge of STDs and modes of transmission
- exhibit improved or healed lesions or wounds
- maintain fluid balance, with intake equal to output
- voice feelings about changes in sexuality and potential or actual changes in sexuality
- express concern about self-concept, self-esteem, and body image.

Nursing interventions
- Use standard precautions.
- Check the neonate of an infected mother for signs of infection.
- Administer medications, as ordered.
- Provide appropriate skin care.
- If required in your state, report cases of chlamydial infection to the local board of health for follow-up on sexual contacts.

Monitoring
- Response to treatment
- Adverse effects of medication
- Complications

Be sure to cover:
- disorder, diagnostic tests, and treatment
- good hand-washing techniques
- abstinence from intercourse or use of condoms
- importance of getting tested for the human immunodeficiency virus
- dealing with long-term risks and complications from infection
- transmission of infection
- prevention of STDs
- importance of follow-up care.

Discharge planning
- Refer the patient to support services.

Organizations
Centers for Disease Control and Prevention: *www.cdc.gov*
Harvard University Consumer Health Information: *www.intelihealth.com*
National Health Information Center: *www.health.gov/nhic*
National Library of Medicine: *www.nlm.nih.gov*

Selected references
Kasper, D.L., et al., eds. *Harrison's Principles of Internal Medicine*, 16th ed. New York: McGraw-Hill Book Co., 2005.
Mpiga, P., and Ravaorinoro, M., "Chlamydia Trachomatis Persistence: An Update," *Microbiological Research* 161(1):9-19, January 2006.

Cholelithiasis, cholecystitis, and related disorders

● OVERVIEW

Description
CHOLELITHIASIS
- Leading biliary tract disease
- Formation of calculi (gallstones) in the gallbladder
- Prognosis usually good with treatment, unless infection occurs

CHOLECYSTITIS
- Related disorder that arises from formation of gallstones
- Gallbladder becoming acutely or chronically inflamed
- Usually caused by a gallstone lodged in the cystic duct
- Acute form most common during middle age
- Chronic form most common among elderly persons
- Prognosis good with treatment

CHOLEDOCHOLITHIASIS
- Related disorder that arises from formation of gallstones
- Partial or complete biliary obstruction due to gallstones lodged in the common bile duct
- Prognosis good, unless infection occurs

CHOLANGITIS
- Related disorder that arises from formation of gallstones
- Infected bile duct
- Commonly associated with choledocholithiasis
- Nonsuppurative cholangitis: usually responds rapidly to antibiotic treatment
- Suppurative cholangitis: poor prognosis unless surgery to correct obstruction and drain infected bile is performed promptly

GALLSTONE ILEUS
- Related disorder that arises from formation of gallstones
- Obstruction of the small bowel by a gallstone
- Most common in elderly persons
- Prognosis good with surgery

Pathophysiology
- Calculi formation in the biliary system causes obstruction.
- Obstruction of hepatic duct leads to intrahepatic retention of bile; increased release of bilirubin into the bloodstream occurs.
- Obstruction of cystic duct leads to inflammation of the gallbladder; increased gallbladder contraction and peristalsis occurs.
- Obstruction of bile causes impairment of digestion and absorption of lipids.

Causes
- Calculi formation; type of disorder that develops dependent on where in the gallbladder or biliary tract the calculi collect
- Acute cholecystitis also a result of conditions that alter gallbladder's ability to fill or empty (trauma, reduced blood supply to the gallbladder, prolonged immobility, chronic dieting, adhesions, prolonged anesthesia, and opioid abuse)

Risk factors
- High-calorie, high-cholesterol diet
- Associated with obesity
- Elevated estrogen levels from oral contraceptive use, postmenopausal hormone-replacement therapy, or pregnancy
- Diabetes mellitus, ileal disease, hemolytic disorders, hepatic disease (cirrhosis), or pancreatitis
- Rapid weight loss

Incidence
- Occur during middle age
- Six times more common in women between ages 20 and 50
- Affect men and women equally after age 50, increasing with each succeeding decade

Common characteristics
- Epigastric or right upper quadrant abdominal pain
- Nausea, vomiting
- Low-grade fever

Complications
CHOLELITHIASIS
- Cholangitis
- Cholecystitis
- Choledocholithiasis
- Gallstone ileus

CHOLECYSTITIS
- Gallbladder complications, such as empyema, hydrops or mucocele, and gangrene
- Chronic cholecystitis and cholangitis

CHOLEDOCHOLITHIASIS
- Cholangitis
- Obstructive jaundice
- Pancreatitis
- Secondary biliary cirrhosis

CHOLANGITIS
- Septic shock
- Death

GALLSTONE ILEUS
- Bowel obstruction

✳ ASSESSMENT

History
- May produce no symptoms (even when X-rays reveal gallstones)
- Acute cholelithiasis, acute cholecystitis, and choledocholithiasis producing symptoms of classic gallbladder attack

GALLBLADDER ATTACK
- Sudden onset of severe steady or aching pain in the midepigastric region or the right upper abdominal quadrant
- Pain radiating to the back, between the shoulder blades or over the right shoulder blade, or just to the shoulder area
- Ocurs after eating a fatty meal or a large meal after fasting for an extended time
- Occurs in the middle of the night
- Nausea, vomiting, and chills
- Low-grade fever
- History of milder GI symptoms that preceded the acute attack: indigestion, vague abdominal discomfort, belching, and flatulence after eating meals or snacks rich in fats

Physical findings
GALLBLADDER ATTACK
- Severe pain
- Pallor
- Diaphoresis
- Low-grade fever (high in cholangitis)
- Exhaustion
- Jaundice (chronic)
- Dark-colored urine and clay-colored stools
- Tachycardia
- Tenderness over the gallbladder, which increases on inspiration (Murphy's sign)

- Palpable, painless, sausagelike mass (calculus-filled gallbladder without ductal obstruction)
- Hypoactive bowel sounds

Test results

LABORATORY
- Blood studies may reveal elevated levels of serum alkaline phosphatase, lactate dehydrogenase, aspartate aminotransferase, icteric index, and total bilirubin; white blood cell count is slightly elevated during cholecystitis attack.

IMAGING
- Plain abdominal X-rays show gallstones if they contain enough calcium to be radiopaque; X-rays are also helpful in identifying porcelain gallbladder, limy bile, and gallstone ileus.
- Ultrasonography of the gallbladder confirms cholelithiasis in most patients and distinguishes between obstructive and nonobstructive jaundice; calculi as small as 2 mm can be detected.
- Oral cholecystography confirms the presence of gallstones, although this test is gradually being replaced by ultrasonography.
- Technetium-labeled iminodiacetic acid scan of the gallbladder indicates cystic duct obstruction and acute or chronic cholecystitis if the gallbladder can't be seen.

DIAGNOSTIC PROCEDURES
- Percutaneous transhepatic cholangiography—imaging performed under fluoroscopic guidance—supports the diagnosis of obstructive jaundice and is used to visualize calculi in the ducts.

◆ TREATMENT

General
- Endoscopic retrograde cholangiopancreatography to visualize and remove calculi
- Lithotripsy

Diet
- Low-fat
- Nothing by mouth if surgery required

Activity
- As tolerated
- Avoidance of heavy lifting or contact sports for 6 weeks after surgery

Medication
- Gallstone dissolution therapy
- Vitamin supplements
- Bile salts
- Analgesics
- Antispasmodics
- Anticholinergics
- Antiemetics
- Antibiotics

Surgery
- Most common treatment for gallbladder and duct disease
- May include cholecystectomy (laparoscopic or abdominal), cholecystectomy with operative cholangiography, choledochostomy, or exploration of the common bile duct

❖ NURSING CONSIDERATIONS

Nursing diagnoses
- Acute pain
- Deficient knowledge (cholelithiasis, cholecystitis)
- Imbalanced nutrition: Less than body requirements
- Ineffective tissue perfusion: GI
- Risk for deficient fluid volume
- Risk for infection

Key outcomes
The patient will:
- express feelings of increased comfort and decreased pain
- verbalize understanding of the disorder
- achieve adequate caloric and nutritional intake
- maintain adequate GI perfusion
- maintain fluid volume within acceptable parameters
- remain free of signs and symptoms of infection.

Nursing interventions
- Administer medication, as ordered.

Monitoring
- Vital signs
- Intake and output
- Pain control

AFTER SURGERY
- Signs and symptoms of bleeding, infection, or atelectasis
- Wound site
- Drain function and drainage
- Bowel function
- T-tube patency and drainage

▶ PATIENT TEACHING

Be sure to cover:
- disorder, diagnostic tests, and treatment
- how to breathe deeply, cough, expectorate, and perform leg exercises that are necessary after surgery
- dietary modifications
- medication administration, dosage, and possible adverse effects.

✴ RESOURCES

Organizations
Digestive Disease National Coalition: *www.ddnc.org*
National Digestive Diseases Information Clearinghouse: *www.niddk.nih.gov/health/digest/nddic.htm*

Selected references
Diseases, 4th ed. Philadelphia: Lippincott Williams & Wilkins, 2006.
Knaja, R.J., and Greer, L.A. "Manifestations of Chronic Disease During Pregnancy," *JAMA* 295(21):2751-757, December 2005.
Lammert, F., and Sauerbruch, T. "Mechanisms of Disease: The Genetic Epidemiology of Gallbladder Stones," *National Clinical Practice Gastroenterology and Hepatology* 2(9):432-33, September 2005.

Chronic fatigue and immune dysfunction syndrome

OVERVIEW

Description
- Characterized by prolonged overwhelming fatigue
- Also called *chronic fatigue syndrome, chronic Epstein-Barr virus, myalgic encephalomyelitis,* and *Yuppie flu*

Pathophysiology
- Infectious agents or environmental factors trigger an abnormal immune response and hormonal alterations.

Causes
- Precise cause unknown
- May result from cytomegalovirus, herpes simplex virus types 1 and 2, human herpesvirus 6, Inoue-Melnick virus, human adenovirus 2, enteroviruses, measles virus, or a retrovirus that resembles human T-cell lymphotropic virus type II
- May also result from overactive immune system

Risk factors
- Genetic predisposition
- Age
- Hormonal balance
- Neuropsychiatric factors
- Sex
- Previous illness
- Stressful environment

Incidence
- Affects people of all ages, occupations, and income levels
- More common in women than in men or children, especially women under age 45
- Has been observed as sporadic and epidemic

  AGE-RELATED CONCERN Chronic fatigue and immune dysfunction syndrome is most prevalent among professionals in their 20s and 30s.

Common characteristics
- Suggests viral illness in some cases
- Characterized by incapacitating fatigue
- Waxing and waning symptoms
- Severely debilitating and can last for months or years
- Depression and anxiety after the syndrome's onset
- Fever

- Pharyngitis
- Lymphadenopathy

Complications
- Social and occupational impairment

ASSESSMENT

History
- Characteristic complaints of prolonged, overwhelming fatigue (see *Diagnostic criteria in chronic fatigue syndrome*)

Physical findings
- Myalgia
- Cognitive dysfunction

Test results
LABORATORY
- Lymphocyte differential reveals reduced natural killer cell cytotoxicity, abnormal CD4:CD8 T-cell ratios, and mild lymphocytosis.
- Immunoglobulin profile shows decreased immunoglobulin subclasses.
- Immune complex profile reveals circulating immune complexes.
- Antimicrosomal antibody testing reveals increased levels of antimicrosomal antibodies.

DIAGNOSTIC CRITERIA IN CHRONIC FATIGUE SYNDROME

Chronic fatigue is defined by the presence of both:
- New or onset of relapsing fatigue that isn't the result of ongoing exertion, isn't alleviated by rest, and results in reduced occupational, educational, social, or personal activities or efforts
- Four or more of the following symptoms, occurring for 6 months or more:
  — self-reported impairment in short-term memory or concentration
  — sore throat
  — tender cervical or axillary nodes
  — muscle pain
  — multiple joint pain without redness or swelling
  — headaches of a new pattern or severity
  — nonrefreshing sleep
  — postexertional malaise lasting 24 hours or longer

TREATMENT

General
- Supportive care
- Psychiatric evaluation
- Behavioral therapy
- Massage therapy
- Chiropractic and therapeutic touch

Diet
- Well-balanced diet high in vitamins and minerals

Activity
- Frequent rest periods, as needed
- Avoidance of strenuous activities

Medication
- Nonsteroidal anti-inflammatory drugs
- Antidepressants
- Antihistamines
- Anxiolytics
- Stimulants

❖ NURSING CONSIDERATIONS

Nursing diagnoses
- Activity intolerance
- Fatigue
- Ineffective coping
- Ineffective role performance
- Powerlessness
- Situational low self-esteem

Key outcomes
The patient will:
- verbalize importance of balancing activity with rest
- verbally report having an increased energy level
- identify appropriate coping strategies
- express feelings about diminished capacity to perform usual roles
- recognize limitations imposed by illness and express feelings about these limitations
- voice feelings related to positive self-esteem
- participate in self-care and decision-making process.

Nursing interventions
- Provide emotional support.
- Begin a graded exercise program.

Monitoring
- Response to treatment
- Adverse effects of medication
- Complications

▶ PATIENT TEACHING

Be sure to cover:
- need to decrease activities when fatigue is greatest
- need to avoid bed rest, which has no proven therapeutic value
- medication administration, dosage, and possible adverse effects
- appropriate activity planning.

Discharge planning
- Refer the patient to support services.

✳ RESOURCES

Organizations
Centers for Disease Control and Prevention: *www.cdc.gov*
CFIDS Association of America: *www.cfids.org*
Harvard University Consumer Health Information: *www.intelihealth.com*
National Health Information Center: *www.health.gov/nhic/*
National Library of Medicine: *www.nlm.nih.gov*

Selected references
Kasper, D.L., et al., eds. *Harrison's Principles of Internal Medicine,* 16th ed. New York: McGraw-Hill Book Co., 2005.
Mandell, G.L., et al. *Principles and Practice of Infectious Diseases*, 6th ed. New York: Churchill Livingstone Inc., 2005.
Shaver, J.L. "Fibromyalgia Syndrome in Women," *The Nursing Clinics of North America* 39(1):194-204, viii. March 2004.
Viner, R., et al. "Outpatient Rehabilitative Treatment of Chronic Fatigue Syndrome," *Archives of Disease in Childhood* 89(7)615-19, July 2004.

Cirrhosis

 OVERVIEW

Description
- Chronic hepatic disease
- Several types

Pathophysiology
- Diffuse destruction and fibrotic regeneration of hepatic cells occurs.
- Necrotic tissue yields to fibrosis.
- Liver structure and normal vasculature are altered.
- Blood and lymph flow are impaired.
- Hepatic insufficiency occurs.

Causes
LAËNNEC'S OR MICRONODULAR CIRRHOSIS (ALCOHOLIC OR PORTAL CIRRHOSIS)
- Chronic alcoholism
- Malnutrition

POSTNECROTIC OR MACRONODULAR CIRRHOSIS
- Complication of viral hepatitis
- Possible after exposure to such liver toxins as arsenic, carbon tetrachloride, and phosphorus

BILIARY CIRRHOSIS
- Prolonged biliary tract obstruction or inflammation

IDIOPATHIC CIRRHOSIS (CRYPTOGENIC)
- Sarcoidosis
- Chronic inflammatory bowel disease

Risk factors
- Alcoholism
- Toxins
- Biliary obstruction
- Hepatitis
- Metabolic disorders

Incidence
- Tenth most common cause of death in the United States
- Most common among those ages 45 to 75

Common characteristics
- Abdominal pain
- Pruritus
- Jaundice
- Ascites

Complications
- Portal hypertension
- Bleeding esophageal varices
- Hepatic encephalopathy
- Hepatorenal syndrome
- Death

✱ ASSESSMENT

History
- Chronic alcoholism
- Malnutrition
- Viral hepatitis
- Exposure to liver toxins such as arsenic
- Prolonged biliary tract obstruction or inflammation

IN EARLY STAGE
- Vague signs and symptoms
- Abdominal pain
- Diarrhea, constipation
- Fatigue
- Nausea, vomiting
- Muscle cramps

WITH DISEASE PROGRESSION
- Chronic dyspepsia
- Constipation
- Pruritus
- Weight loss
- Bleeding tendency, such as frequent nosebleeds, easy bruising, and bleeding gums
- Hepatic encephalopathy

Physical findings
- Telangiectasis on the cheeks
- Spider angiomas on the face, neck, arms, and trunk
- Gynecomastia
- Umbilical hernia
- Distended abdominal blood vessels
- Ascites
- Testicular atrophy
- Menstrual irregularities
- Palmar erythema
- Clubbed fingers
- Thigh and leg edema
- Ecchymosis
- Anemia
- Jaundice
- Palpable, large, firm liver with a sharp edge (early finding)
- Enlarged spleen
- Asterixis
- Slurred speech, paranoia, hallucinations

Test results
LABORATORY
- Liver enzyme levels are elevated, such as alanine aminotransferase, aspartate aminotransferase, total serum bilirubin, and indirect bilirubin; total serum albumin and protein levels are decreased; prothrombin time is prolonged; hemoglobin, hematocrit, and serum electrolyte levels are decreased; vitamins A, C, and K are deficient.
- Urine levels of bilirubin and urobilinogen are increased; fecal urobilinogen levels are increased.
- Elevated ammonia levels are elevated

IMAGING
- Abdominal X-rays show liver and spleen size and cysts or gas in the biliary tract or liver; liver calcification; and massive ascites.
- Computed tomography and liver scans are used to determine liver size, identify liver masses, and visualize hepatic blood flow and obstruction
- Radioisotope liver scans show liver size, blood flow, or obstruction.

DIAGNOSTIC PROCEDURES
- Liver biopsy is the definitive test for cirrhosis, revealing hepatic tissue destruction and fibrosis.
- Esophagogastroduodenoscopy reveals bleeding esophageal varices, stomach irritation or ulceration, and duodenal bleeding and irritation.

◆ TREATMENT

General
- Removal or alleviation of underlying cause
- Paracentesis
- Esophageal balloon tamponade
- Sclerotherapy
- I.V. fluids
- Blood transfusion

Diet
- Restricted sodium consumption
- Restricted fluid intake
- No alcohol
- Nutritional supplements

Activity
- Frequent rest periods as needed

Medication
- Vitamins
- Antacids
- Potassium-sparing diuretics
- Beta-adrenergic blockers and vasopressin
- Ammonia detoxicant
- Antiemetics

Surgery
- May be required to divert ascites into venous circulation; if so, peritoneovenous shunt is used
- Portal-systemic shunt
- Transplantation

❖ NURSING CONSIDERATIONS

Nursing diagnoses
- Activity intolerance
- Excess fluid volume
- Hopelessness
- Imbalanced nutrition: Less than body requirements
- Risk for deficient fluid volume
- Risk for impaired skin integrity
- Risk for injury

Key outcomes
The patient will:
- perform activities of daily living without fatigue or exhaustion
- maintain adequate fluid balance
- participate in care and decisions
- maintain caloric intake ,as required
- remain free of injury and skin breakdown and injury.

Nursing interventions
- Administer I.V. fluids and blood products, as ordered.
- Administer medications, as ordered.
- Encourage verbalization and provide support.
- Provide appropriate skin care.

Monitoring
- Vital signs
- Complete blood count, electrolytes
- Hydration and nutritional status
- Abdominal girth
- Weight
- Bleeding tendencies
- Skin integrity
- Changes in mentation, behavior

▶ PATIENT TEACHING

Be sure to cover:
- disorder, diagnostic tests, and treatment
- over-the-counter medications that may increase bleeding tendencies
- dietary modifications
- need to avoid infections and abstain from alcohol
- need to avoid sedatives and acetaminophen (Tylenol) (hepatotoxic)
- importance of high-calorie and moderate- to high-protein diet and small, frequent meals.

Discharge planning
- Refer the patient to Alcoholics Anonymous, if appropriate.

✱ RESOURCES

Organizations
Alcoholics Anonymous:
  www.alcoholicsanonymous.org
American Liver Foundation:
  www.liverfoundation.org
Digestive Disease National Coalition:
  www.ddnc.org
National Digestive Diseases Information Clearinghouse:
  www.niddk.nih.gov/health/digest/nddic.htm
National Institute of Diabetes and Digestive and Kidney Disorders:
  www.niddk.nih.gov

Selected references
Diseases, 4th ed. Philadelphia: Lippincott Williams & Wilkins, 2006.

Kasper, D.L., et al., eds. *Harrison's Principles of Internal Medicine,* 16th ed. New York: McGraw-Hill Book Co., 2005.

McNally, P. *GI/Liver Secrets,* 3rd ed. Philadelphia: Hanley & Belfus, 2006.

Randi, G., et al. "History of Cirrhosis and Risk of Digestive Tract Neoplasms," *Annals of Oncology* 16(9):1551-555, September 2005.

Clostridium difficile infection

● OVERVIEW

Description
- Gram-positive anaerobic bacterium often resulting in antibiotic-associated diarrhea
- Symptoms ranging from asymptomatic carrier states to severe pseudomembranous colitis caused by exotoxins—toxin A (enterotoxin), toxin B (cytotoxin)
- Within 14 to 30 days of treatment, recurrence with the same organism possible in 10% to 20% of cases; beyond 30 days, recurrence may be relapse or reinfection of *Clostridium difficile*

Pathophysiology
- Antibiotics may trigger toxin production.
- Toxin A mediates alteration in fluid secretion, enhances inflammation, and causes leakage of albumin from the postcapillary venules.
- Toxin B causes damage and exfoliation to the superficial epithelial cells and inhibits adenosine diphosphate ribosylation of Rho proteins.
- Both toxins cause electrophysiologic alterations of colonic tissue.

Causes
- Antibiotics that disrupt the bowel flora
- Enemas and intestinal stimulants
- Transmission from infected person
- Some antiviral and antifungal agents

Risk factors
- Contaminated equipment and surfaces
- Antibiotic therapy
- Abdominal surgery
- Antineoplastic agents that have an antibiotic activity
- Immunocompromised state

Incidence
- Occurs more commonly in those in nursing homes and day-care facilities
- One of the most common nosocomial infections

Common characteristics
- Watery, foul-smelling diarrhea

Complications
- Electrolyte abnormalities
- Hypovolemic shock
- Toxic megacolon
- Colonic perforation
- Peritonitis
- Sepsis
- Hemorrhage

✳ ASSESSMENT

History
- History of recent antibiotic therapy
- Abdominal pain
- Cramping

Physical findings
- Soft, unformed, or watery diarrhea (more than 3 stools in a 24-hour period) that may be foul smelling or grossly bloody
- Tenderness
- Fever

Test results
LABORATORY
- Cell cytotoxin test shows toxins A and B.
- Enzyme immunoassay identifies *C. difficile*; slightly less sensitive than cell cytotoxin test but has a turnaround time of only a few hours.
- Stool culture identifies *C. difficile*.

◆ TREATMENT

General
- Withdrawal of causative antibiotic

Diet
- Well-balanced
- Increased fluid intake, if appropriate

Activity
- No restriction
- Rest periods, if fatigued

Medication
- Metronidazole
- Vancomycin
- If relapse occurred and previous treatment was metronidazole, low-dose vancomycin
- Combination of vancomycin and rifampin
- Experimental treatments involving the administration of yeast *Saccharomyces boulardii* with metronidazole or vancomycin and biologic vaccines to restore the normal GI flora
- Lactobacillus
- Cholestyramine

✤ NURSING CONSIDERATIONS

Nursing diagnoses
- Acute pain
- Activity intolerance
- Hyperthermia
- Imbalanced nutrition: Less than body requirements
- Impaired skin integrity
- Risk for deficient fluid volume

Key outcomes
The patient will:
- verbalize increased comfort and decreased pain
- perform activities of daily living without exhaustion or excess fatigue
- exhibit a body temperature within acceptable parameters
- maintain normal electrolyte levels
- exhibit improved or healed lesions or wounds
- maintain adequate fluid volume.

Nursing interventions
- Administer medication as ordered.
- Use contact precautions for those with active diarrhea.
- Wash your hands with an antiseptic soap after direct contact with the patient or his immediate environment.
- Make sure reusable equipment is disinfected before it's used on another patient.

Monitoring
- Vital signs
- Intake and output
- Complications
- Serum electrolytes
- Hydration status
- Adverse effects of medication
- Response to treatment
- Amount and characteristics of stools

▶ PATIENT TEACHING

Be sure to cover:
- disorder, diagnostic tests, and treatment
- good hand-washing techniques
- proper disinfection of contaminated clothing or household items
- adequate fluid intake
- signs and symptoms of dehydration
- medication administration, dosage, and possible adverse effects
- complications and when to notify the physician
- perirectal skin care
- prevention of bacteria spread.

✴ RESOURCES

Organizations
Centers for Disease Control and Prevention: *www.cdc.gov*
Harvard University Consumer Health Information: *www.intelihealth.com*
National Health Information Center: *www.health.gov/nhic*
National Institute of Allergy and Infectious Diseases: *www.niaid.nih.gov*
National Library of Medicine: *www.nlm.nih.gov*

Selected references
Kasper, D.L., et al., eds. *Harrison's Principles of Internal Medicine,* 16th ed. New York: McGraw-Hill Book Co., 2005.
Mandell, G.L., et al. *Principles and Practice of Infectious Diseases*, 6th ed. New York: Churchill Livingstone Inc., 2005.
Starr, J. "*Clostridium Difficile* Associated Diarrhoea: Diagnosis and Treatment," *British Medical Journal* 331(7515):498-501, September 2005.
Tonna, L., and Welsby, P.D. "Pathogenesis and Treatment of *Clostridium Difficile* Infection," *Postgraduate Medical Journal* 81(956):367-69, June 2005.

Cold injuries

● OVERVIEW

Description
- Includes localized injuries (frostbite) and systemic injuries (hypothermia)
- Frostbite: superficial or deep; can lead to gangrene
- Hypothermia: core body temperature below 95° F (35° C)

Pathophysiology
- Cold temperature causes ice crystals to form within and around tissue cells.
- Cell membranes rupture and enzymatic activities are interrupted.
- Histamine is released.
- Aggregation of red blood cells results.

Causes
- Prolonged exposure to freezing temperatures
- Prolonged exposure to cold, wet environments
- Administration of large amounts of cold blood

Risk factors
- Lack of insulating body fat
- Substance abuse
- Cardiac disease
- Poverty, homelessness
- Cold water immersion

Incidence
- More common among men

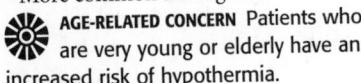 **AGE-RELATED CONCERN** Patients who are very young or elderly have an increased risk of hypothermia.

Common characteristics
FROSTBITE
- Initial coldness
- Stinging, burning, throbbing
- Numbness, followed by complete loss of sensation
- Loss of fine muscle dexterity
- Loss of large muscle dexterity
- Severe joint pain

HYPOTHERMIA
- Severe shivering, slurred speech, and amnesia
- Unresponsive, with peripheral cyanosis and muscle rigidity
- Shock
- Cardiopulmonary arrest

Complications
- Renal failure
- Rhabdomyolysis
- Avascular necrosis
- Gangrene
- Severe infection
- Aspiration pneumonia
- Cardiac arrhythmias
- Hypoglycemia or hyperglycemia
- Metabolic acidosis
- Pancreatitis

✳ ASSESSMENT

History
- Burning, numbness, tingling, and itching
- Paresthesia and stiffness while the part is still frozen
- Burning pain when the part thaws

Physical findings
FROSTBITE
- Superficial—swollen, with a mottled, blue-gray skin color
- Deep—white or yellow until it's thawed; then it turns purplish blue
- Edema, skin blisters, and necrosis
- Skin immobility
- Presence or absence of associated peripheral pulses

HYPOTHERMIA
- Mild—severe shivering, slurred speech, and amnesia
- Moderate—unresponsive, with peripheral cyanosis and muscle rigidity
- Severe—appears dead, with no palpable pulse and no audible heart sounds

Test results
LABORATORY
- Complete blood count and coagulation profile may show blood loss related to clotting abnormalities.
- Serum amylase levels are elevated.
- Serum glucose may show hypoglycemia or hyperglycemia.
- Liver function studies may show hepatic failure.
- Serum adrenocorticotropic hormone levels are elevated.
- Elevated serum thyroid-stimulating hormone levels are elevated.
- White blood cell count is elevated.
- Arterial blood gas levels show acid-base derangements and hypoxia.
- Serum electrolytes show electrolyte derangements.

IMAGING
- Technetium pertechnetate scanning shows perfusion defects, deep tissue damage, and nonviable bone.
- Doppler and plethysmographic studies locate pulses and show extent of frostbite.

◆ TREATMENT

General
FROSTBITE
- Rapid rewarming of injured part
- Whirlpool treatments

HYPOTHERMIA
- Supportive measures
- Cardiopulmonary resuscitation
- Administration of oxygen
- Endotracheal intubation with controlled ventilation
- I.V. fluids
- Treatment metabolic acidosis

Diet
FROSTBITE
- No restriction

HYPOTHERMIA
- Nothing by mouth until fully alert
- Warm fluids to drink

Activity
FROSTBITE
- Active range-of-motion (ROM) exercises
- Elevation of extremity after rewarming

HYPOTHERMIA
- Rest until rewarmed

Medication
FROSTBITE
- Tetanus toxoid
- Antibiotics

HYPOTHERMIA
- Antiarrhythmics, as needed

Surgery
- Fasciotomy or amputation for extensive tissue damage

✿ NURSING CONSIDERATIONS

Nursing diagnoses
- Acute pain
- Anxiety
- Decreased cardiac output
- Hypothermia
- Impaired gas exchange
- Impaired physical mobility
- Impaired skin integrity
- Ineffective tissue perfusion: Cardiopulmonary, peripheral
- Risk for disuse syndrome
- Risk for infection

Key outcomes
The patient will:
- express feelings of increased comfort and decreased pain
- express feelings of decreased anxiety
- maintain adequate cardiac output
- experience a return of body temperature to normal
- maintain adequate ventilation
- attain the highest degree of mobility possible within the confines of the injury
- regain skin integrity
- exhibit signs of adequate cardiopulmonary and peripheral perfusion
- maintain muscle strength and tone and joint ROM
- remain free from signs and symptoms of infection.

Nursing interventions
FROSTBITE
- Remove constrictive clothing and jewelry.
- Perform rewarming measures.
- Administer medications, as ordered.

  ◈ **NURSING ALERT** Never rub the injured area because this can aggravate tissue damage. Don't rupture any blebs.

HYPOTHERMIA
- Maintain airway, breathing, and circulation.
- Perform rewarming measures.
- Perform supportive measures, as needed.

Monitoring
- Core body temperature
- Vital signs
- Cardiac status
- Peripheral vascular circulation

▶ PATIENT TEACHING

Be sure to cover:
- disorder, diagnostic tests, and treatment
- measures to avoid hypothermia
- complications and when to notify the physician.

Discharge planning
- Refer the patient to resource and support services.

✳ RESOURCES

Organizations
National Center for Injury Prevention and Control: *www.cdc.gov/ncipc/ncipchm.htm*
National Institutes of Health: *www.nih.gov*

Selected references
Davies, A. "Nursing a Patient with Frostbite," *Nursing Times* 101(46):52-54, November 2005.

McGillion, R. "Frostbite: Case Report, Practical Summary of ED Treatment," *Journal of Emergency Nursing* 31(5):500-502, October, 2005.

Neno, R. "Hypothermia: Assessment, Treatment and Prevention," *Nursing Standard* 19(20):47-52, January-February 2005.

Wolfson, A.B., et al. *Harwood-Nuss' Clinical Practice of Emergency Medicine*, 4th ed. Philadelphia: Lippincott Williams & Wilkins, 2005.

Colorectal cancer

● OVERVIEW

Description
- Malignant tumors of colon or rectum that are almost always adenocarcinomas (about half are sessile lesions of rectosigmoid area; all others are polypoid lesions)
- Slow progression
- Five-year survival rate 50%; potentially curable in 75% of patients if early diagnosis allows resection before nodal involvement
- Second most common visceral neoplasm in United States and Europe

Pathophysiology
- Most lesions of the large bowel are moderately differentiated adenocarcinomas.
- Tumors tend to grow slowly and remain asymptomatic for long periods of time.
- Tumors in the sigmoid and descending colon undergo circumferential growth and constrict the intestinal lumen.
- At diagnosis, tumors in the ascending colon are usually large and are palpable on physical examination.

Causes
- Unknown

Risk factors
- Intake of excessive saturated animal fat
- Diseases of the digestive tract
- Age over 40
- History of ulcerative colitis
- Familial polyposis
- Family history of colon cancer
- High-protein, low-fiber diet

Incidence
- Equally distributed between men and women
- Greater in areas of higher economic development

Common characteristics
- Changes in bowel habits
- Symptoms of direct extension to bladder, prostate, ureters, vagina, or sacrum
- Symptoms of local obstruction

Complications
- Abdominal distention and intestinal obstruction as tumor growth encroaches on abdominal organs
- Anemia

✳ ASSESSMENT

History
- Right colon tumors: no signs and symptoms in early stages because stool is liquid in that part of colon
- Black, tarry stools
- Abdominal aching, pressure, or dull cramps
- Weakness
- Diarrhea, anorexia, obstipation, weight loss, and vomiting
- Rectal bleeding
- Intermittent abdominal fullness
- Rectal pressure
- Urgent need to defecate on arising

Physical findings
- Abdominal distention or visible masses
- Enlarged abdominal veins
- Enlarged inguinal and supraclavicular nodes
- Abnormal bowel sounds
- Abdominal masses (right side tumors usually feel bulky; tumors of transverse portion more easily detected)
- Generalized abdominal tenderness

Test results
LABORATORY
- Fecal occult blood test may show blood in stools, a warning sign of rectal cancer
- Carcinoembryonic antigen permits patient monitoring before and after treatment to detect metastasis or recurrence.

IMAGING
- Excretory urography verifies bilateral renal function and allows inspection for displacement of the kidneys, ureters, or bladder by a tumor pressing against these structures.
- Barium enema studies use a dual contrast of barium and air and allow the location of lesions that aren't detectable manually or visually. Barium examination shouldn't precede colonoscopy or excretory urography because barium sulfate interferes with these tests.
- Computed tomography scan allows better visualization if a barium enema yields inconclusive results or if metastasis to the pelvic lymph nodes is suspected.

DIAGNOSTIC PROCEDURES
- Proctoscopy or sigmoidoscopy permits visualization of the lower GI tract. It can detect up to 66% of colorectal cancers.
- Colonoscopy permits visual inspection and photography of the colon up to the ileocecal valve and provides access for polypectomies and biopsies of suspected lesions.

OTHER
- Digital rectal examination can be used to detect almost 15% of colorectal cancers; specifically, it can be used to detect suspicious rectal and perianal lesions.

◆ TREATMENT

General
- Radiation preoperatively and postoperatively to induce tumor regression

Diet
- High fiber

Activity
- After surgery, avoidance of heavy lifting and contact sports
- After recovery, no restrictions

Medication
- Chemotherapy for metastasis, residual disease, or recurrent inoperable tumor
- Analgesics

Surgery
- Resection or right hemicolectomy for advanced disease; may include resection of the terminal segment of the ileum, cecum, ascending colon, and right half of the transverse colon with corresponding mesentery
- Right colectomy that includes the transverse colon and mesentery corresponding to midcolic vessels, or segmental resection of the transverse colon and associated midcolic vessels

- Resection usually limited to the sigmoid colon and mesentery
- Anterior or low anterior resection (newer method, using a stapler, allows for much lower resections than previously possible)
- Abdominoperineal resection and permanent sigmoid colostomy

❖ NURSING CONSIDERATIONS

Nursing diagnoses
- Acute pain
- Anxiety
- Constipation
- Deficient fluid volume
- Diarrhea
- Disabled family coping
- Disturbed body image
- Fear
- Imbalanced nutrition: Less than body requirements
- Impaired oral mucous membrane
- Impaired skin integrity
- Ineffective coping
- Risk for infection
- Sexual dysfunction

Key outcomes
The patient will:
- express feelings of increased comfort and decreased pain
- express feelings of decreased anxiety
- have soft, formed stools that are easy to pass
- maintain normal fluid volume
- resume a regular elimination pattern
- express a positive feeling about self
- verbalize fears and concerns relating to the diagnosis and condition
- maintain adequate nutrition and hydration
- have mucous membraines that remain intact
- maintain skin integrity
- demonstrate adaptive coping behaviors
- remain free from infection and other complications
- verbalize feelings about potential or actual changes in sexual activity.

Nursing interventions
- Provide support and encourage verbalization.
- Administer medications, as ordered.

Monitoring
- Stools
- Diet

POSTOPERATIVE
- Vital signs
- Intake and output
- Hydration and nutritional status
- Electrolyte levels
- Wound site
- Postoperative complications
- Bowel function
- Pain control
- Psychological status

▶ PATIENT TEACHING

Be sure to cover:
- disorder, diagnostic tests, and treatment
- stoma care
- avoidance of heavy lifting
- need for keeping follow-up appointments
- risk factors and signs of reoccurrence.

Discharge Planning
- Refer the patient to resource and support services.

✴ RESOURCES

Organizations
American Cancer Society: *www.cancer.org*
Guide to Internet Resources for Cancer: *www.cancerindex.org*
National Cancer Institute: *www.nci.nih.gov*
United Ostomy Association, Inc: *www.uoa.org*

Selected references
Abraham, J. *Bethesda Handbook of Clinical Oncology.* Phialdelphia: Lippincott Williams & Wilkins, 2005.
Atlas of Pathophysiology, 2nd ed. Philadelphia: Lippincott Williams & Wilkins, 2005.
Viale, P.H., et al. "Advanced Colorectal Cancer: Current Treatment and Nursing Management with Economic Considerations," *Clinical Journal of Oncology Nursing* 9(5):541-52, October 2005.
Wiles, G.M. "Therapeutic Options in the Management of Colon Cancer: 2005 Update," *Clinical Journal of Oncology Nursing* 9(1):31-44, February 2005.

Compartment syndrome

Description

- Condition involving the muscle tissue, nerves and blood vessels of a compartment (the space within each layer of fascia that separate groups or muscles)
- Classified as acute or chronic (see *Understanding chronic compartment syndrome*)
- Most commonly affects an extremity, such as the arm or leg, or foot

Pathophysiology

- The confined space inside the layer of fascia experiences an increase in pressure due to an increase in volume or constriction.
- The increased pressure leads to decreased perfusion from a rise in venous pressure, resulting in capillary collapse.

UNDERSTANDING CHRONIC COMPARTMENT SYNDROME

Chronic compartment syndrome is commonly associated with vigorous exercise or intense muscle use. It's believed to result when tissue pressure increases from tight thickened fascia, muscle swelling and hypertrophy, or pressure applied externally, such as with taping or casting. Like acute compartment syndrome, the increased pressure leads to compromised tissue perfusion resulting in ischemia to muscles and nerves.

Typically patients with chronic compartment syndrome report recurrent severe pain and tightness of the area, usually the leg or foot, with an activity, such as running. This sensation disappears when the patient stops the activity, only to reappear on resuming the activity. Palpation reveals significant hardening of the area. The patient will also complain of pain when the area is passively stretched. There may be weakness with muscle testing, numbness of the affected nerves, and changes in gait.

Testing of the pressures of the compartment before and after exercise is considered the gold standard for diagnosis. The only definitive cure for this condition is a decompressive fasciotomy of the compartment. However, patients may opt to live with this condition either by eliminating or limiting the causative activity, or they may elect conservative treatment with rest, modifications in training regimens, and deep massage.

- As the capillaries collapse, blood flow and oxygen delivery ceases causing hypoxia.
- Hypoxia causes the release of vasoactive substances in an attempt to increase endothelial permeabililty.
- Fluid loss through the capillaries occurs further increasing the pressure within the compartment
- Lack of oxygen delivery causes anaerobic metabolism to take over, lowering the tissue pH
- Tissue necrosis occurs and if pressure is not decreased, loss of the extremity is possible.

Causes

- Crush injuries
- Hemorrhage, trauma
- Burns
- Bites (envenomation)
- Fractures
- Casts, splints
- Use of military antishock trousers (MAST)
- Hemorrhage from a large vessel injury
- Malfunctioning sequential compression devices
- Muscle tear

Incidence

- Most commonly involves the anterior distal compartment of the lower extremity
- Estimated 30% of extremities to develop compartment syndrome after vascular injury

Common characteristics

- Severe pain
- Swelling and pallor
- Hardening of the area
- Weakness of the affected part

Complications

- Nerve damage
- Infection
- Reperfusion injury
- Loss of limb
- Death

History

- Recent injury to area
- Severe pain or burning in area, increased with passive stretching and out of proportion to the injury
- Weakness in affected area
- Complaints of tense feeling in area
- Paresthesia

Physical findings

- Swelling
- Pallor
- Shiny skin with hardness on palpation of affected area
- Diminished peripheral pulses
- Slowed capillary refill

Test results

LABORATORY

- Urinalysis may be positive for blood but show no evidence of red blood cells suggesting myoglobin in the urine.
- Complete blood cell count may reveal anemia, which exacerbates muscle ischemia.
- Serum myoglobin and creatine kinase levels are increased, indicating muscle necrosis.

IMAGING

- Extremity X-rays may show fracture pattern, soft tissue injury, or evidence of occult fractures.
- Computed tomography and magnetic resonance imaging scanning may aid in determining evidence of increased pressure in the compartment.

DIAGNOSTIC PROCEDURES

- Direct measurement of intracompartmental pressure (considered the gold standard for diagnosis) reveals elevated pressure in the compartment.
- Doppler ultrasonography aids in determining arterial blood flow and ruling out deep vein thrombosis.

◆ TREATMENT

General
- Removal of constriction if present, such as bivalving a cast, removing dressings
- Hyperbaric oxygen therapy to promote hyperoxic vasoconstriction which reduces swelling and edema and promotes local blood flow and oxygenation.

Diet
- No restrictions

Activity
- Bed rest with extremity placed at heart level

Medication
- Antivenom if due to bite
- Anagelsics
- Mannitol (to reduce compartment pressures and decrease risk of reperfusion injury)

Surgery
- Emergency fasciotomy

❖ NURSING CONSIDERATIONS

Nursing diagnoses
- Acute pain
- neffective tissue perfusion, peripheral
- Impaired sensory perception, kinesthetic, tactile
- Impaired physical mobility
- Anxiety
- Fear
- Deficient knowledge
- Risk for injury
- Risk for infection (post-fasciotomy)

Key outcomes
The patient will:
- report feelings of pain relief
- maintain optimal functioning within limits of kinesthetic and tactile impairment
- achieve highest degree of mobility possible within the confines of the injury
- demonstrate positive coping strategies for anxiety relief

- verbalize feelings related to diagnosis and condition
- demonstrate understanding of condition and treatment
- remain free of injury
- remain free of signs and symptoms of infection.

Nursing interventions
- Provide proper positioning of affected area as ordered.

> **NURSING ALERT** Don't elevate the patient's limb above the level of the heart because doing so would decrease arterial blood flow, which would increase the ischemia.

- Give prescribed analgesics as indicated.
- Provide wound care.
- Protect patient from injury.
- Administer intravenous fluids as ordered.
- Prepare the patient for fasciotomy if indicated.

AFTER FASCIOTOMY
- Provide postoperative care as appropriate.
- Perform wound care including dressing changes as indicated.
- Assist with rehabilitation program.

Monitoring
- Neurovascular status
- Pain
- Vital signs
- Skin appearance and integrity

AFTER FASCIOTOMY
- Hemodynamic status
- Wound and dressings
- Neurovascular status

▶ PATIENT TEACHING

Be sure to cover:
- disorder, diagnostic tests, and treatment
- procedures involved in reducing pressure
- methods to evaluate neurovascular status
- how to assess skin integrity
- signs and symptoms of infection
- danger signs and symptoms to report
- importance of follow-up

Discharge planning
- Assist with arrangements for rehabilitation, such as exercise regimen
- Refer the patient for home health care if appropriate

✳ RESOURCES

Organizations
American Academy of Orthopedic Surgeons: *www.aaos.org*
American Academy of Podiatric Sports Medicine: *www.apsm.org*
American Orthopedic Association: *www.aoassn.org*
The American Orthopedic Society for Sports Medicine: *www.sportsmed.org*

Selected references
Handbook of Pathophysiology, 2nd edition. Philadelphia: Lippincott Williams & Wilkins, 2005.
Paula, Richard. "Compartment Syndrome, Extremity." eMedicine, June 22, 2006. Available at: *http://www.emedicine. com/emerg/top[ic739.htm.* Accessed 10/26/06.
Smeltzer, S.C. et al. *Brunner and Suddarth's Textbook of Medical-Surgical Nursing*, 11th edition. Philadelphia: Lippincott Williams & Wilkins, 2007.
Wallace, S. "Compartment Syndrome, Lower Extremity." eMedicine, March 3, 2004. Available at: *www.emedicine.com/ orthoped/topic596.htm.* Accessed 10/26/06.

Concussion

● OVERVIEW

Description
- Acceleration-deceleration injury
- Blow to the head forceful enough to jostle the brain and make it strike the skull
- Causes temporary (less than 48 hours) neural dysfunction

Pathophysiology
- Concussion causes diffuse soft tissue damage.
- Inflammation occurs.
- Structural damage is usually minimal.

Causes
- Trauma to the head

Incidence
- More than 2 million instances of concussion per year in the United States
- May occur in up to 20% of football players
- More common in males than females
- Most commonly affects those ages 15 to 24

Common characteristics
- Short-term loss of consciousness
- Nausea and vomiting
- Dizziness
- Retrograde amnesia
- Erratic behavior

Complications
- Seizures
- Persistent vomiting
- Intracranial hemorrhage (rare)

✳ ASSESSMENT

History
- Trauma to head
- Short-term loss of consciousness
- Vomiting
- Antegrade and retrograde amnesia
- Change in level of consciousness (LOC)
- Dizziness
- Nausea
- Severe headache

Physical findings
- Tenderness or hematomas on skull palpation

Test results
IMAGING
- Computed tomography scan and magnetic resonance imaging help to rule out fractures and more serious injuries.

◆ TREATMENT

General
- Observation for changes in mental status

Diet
- No restriction
- Clear liquids if vomiting occurs

Activity
- Bed rest initially
- Avoidance of contact sports until fully recovered

Medication
- Nonopioid analgesics

❖ NURSING CONSIDERATIONS

Nursing diagnoses
- Acute pain
- Anxiety
- Decreased intracranial adaptive capacity
- Ineffective coping
- Risk for deficient fluid volume
- Risk for injury
- Risk for acute confusion
- Risk for posttrauma syndrome

Key outcomes
The patient will:
- express feelings of increased comfort and decreased pain
- state feelings of decreased anxiety
- maintain stable neurologic status
- demonstrate appropriate coping strategies
- maintain adequate fluid volume
- identify factors that increase the potential for injury
- respond appropriately to questions and commands
- recover or be rehabilitated from physical injuries to the extent possible.

Nursing interventions
- Administer medications as ordered and avoid narcotics that may decrease LOC.

Monitoring
- Vital signs
- Neurologic status
- Pain

▶ PATIENT TEACHING

Be sure to cover:
- the injury, diagnostic tests, and treatments
- nonnarcotic analgesics for a headache and avoidance of products containing aspirin
- change in LOC or projectile vomiting requires a return to the hospital
- signs and symptoms of increased intracranial pressure.

Discharge planning
- Arrange for continued observation at home. (See *What to look for after a concussion.*)

WHAT TO LOOK FOR AFTER A CONCUSSION

Before the patient's discharge, follow these teaching guidelines. Instruct the caregiver to awaken the patient every 2 hours through the night and to ask his name and whether he can identify the caregiver.

Advise the caregiver to return the patient to the facility immediately if he is difficult to arouse, is disoriented, or has a headache, forceful or constant vomiting, blurred vision, changes in personality, abnormal eye movements, a staggering gait, or twitching. If the patient is a child, explain to the parents that some children have no apparent ill effects immediately after a concussion but may grow lethargic or somnolent a few hours later. Teach the patient the signs of postconcussion syndrome— headache, vertigo, anxiety, personality changes, memory loss, and fatigue. Explain that these signs may persist for several weeks.

✳ RESOURCES

Organizations
American Academy of Neurology: *www.aan.com*
Brain Injury Society: *www.bisociety.org*
Head Injury Hotline: *www.headinjury.com*
Med Help International: *www.medhelp.org*

Selected references
Collins, M. et al. "New Developments in the Management of Sports Concussion," *Current Opinion in Orthopedics* 15(2):100-107, April 2004.
Moser, R.S. et al. "Prolonged Effects of Concussion in High School Athletes," *Neurosurgery* 57(2):300-306, August, 2005.
Nolan, S. "Traumatic Brain Injury: A Review," *Critical Care Nursing Quarterly* 28(2):188-94, April-June 2005.

Conjunctivitis

● OVERVIEW

Description
- Inflammation of palpebral or bulbar conjunctiva
- Characterized by hyperemia of the conjunctiva
- Usually spreads rapidly from one eye to the other
- Usually benign and self-limiting
- Seldom affects vision
- If chronic, may signal degenerative changes or damage from repeated acute attacks
- Acute bacterial conjunctivitis (pink eye) usually lasting about 2 weeks
- Other viral conjunctival infections lasting 2 to 3 weeks

Pathophysiology
- Conjunctivitis is an inflammatory response of the conjunctiva that usually begins in one eye and may rapidly spread to the other eye.
- Vernal conjunctivitis is associated with a severe form of immunoglobulin E–mediated mast cell hypersensitivity reaction.

Causes
- Allergens
- Bacteria
- Viruses
- Chemical irritations
- Transmission by contaminated towels, washcloths, or one's own hand
- Systemic diseases, such as erythema multiforme and thyroid disease
- Candidal infection

Incidence
- Most common eye disorder in the Western Hemisphere
- Responsible for about 30% of all eye complaints

Common characteristics
- Redness
- Edema
- Pain
- Lacrimation

Complications
- Tic
- Corneal infiltrates
- Corneal ulcers
- Eye loss

✳ ASSESSMENT

History
- Eye pain
- Photophobia
- Burning, itching, and sensation of a foreign body in the eye
- Sore throat and fever, in children

Physical findings
- Conjunctival hyperemia
- Discharge
- Tearing
- Crust of sticky, mucopurulent discharge (in bacterial conjunctivitis)
- Profuse, purulent discharge (in gonococcal conjunctivitis)
- Copious tearing and minimal discharge (in viral conjunctivitis)
- Conjunctival papillae (in vernal conjunctivitis) (see *Conjunctival papillae*)
- Ipsilateral preauricular lymph node enlargement (in viral conjunctivitis)

Test results
LABORATORY
- Culture and sensitivity tests may identify the bacterial pathogen.
- Stained smears of conjunctival scrapings may show mostly monocytes with viral conjunctivitis; polymorphonuclear cells (neutrophils) predominate with bacterial conjunctivitis; and eosinophils predominate with allergic conjunctivitis.

◆ TREATMENT

General
- Dependent on cause
- Warm compresses

Diet
- No restrictions

Activity
- No restrictions

Medication
- Antibiotics
- Antivirals
- Corticosteroids
- Histamine-1 receptor antagonists
- Oral antihistamines

CONJUNCTIVAL PAPILLAE

If you see papillae in the conjunctiva of the upper eyelid, your patient may have vernal (allergic) conjunctivitis. These cobblestone bumps are the telltale sign. They result from swollen lymph tissue within the conjunctival membrane.

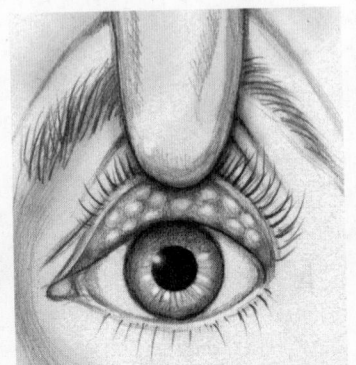

✤ NURSING CONSIDERATIONS

Nursing diagnoses
- Anxiety
- Disturbed sensory perception: Visual
- Ineffective health maintenance
- Risk for infection
- Risk for injury

Key outcomes
The patient will:
- report feeling less anxious
- regain visual function
- maintain current health status
- remain free from signs of infection or injury.

Nursing interventions
- Apply warm compresses.
- Apply therapeutic ointment or eye-drops, as ordered.
- Avoid irrigating the eye to prevent the spread of infection.
- Notify public health officials if culture results identify *Neisseria gonorrhoeae*.
- Obtain culture specimens before antibiotic therapy.

Monitoring
- Response to treatment
- Signs and symptoms of complications
- Adverse reactions
- Visual acuity

▶ PATIENT TEACHING

Be sure to cover:
- proper hand-washing techniques
- need to avoid sharing washcloths, towels, and pillows
- instillation of eyedrops and ointments
- medication administration, dosgae, and possible adverse effects
- completing the prescribed antibiotics
- methods for preventing disease transmission if conjunctivitis is caused by a sexually transmitted organism
- importance of avoiding chemical irritants
- importance of follow-up care.

◈ **NURSING ALERT** Caution the patient to avoid rubbing the infected eye to prevent the spread of infection to the other eye or to other people.

✱ RESOURCES

Organizations
American Academy of Ophthalmology: *www.eyenet.org*
National Institute of Allergy and Infectious Diseases: *www.niaid.nih.gov*

Selected references
Bonini, S. "Allergic Conjunctivitis: The Forgotten Disease," *Chemical Immunology and Allergy* 91:110-20, 2006.
Khan, J. "Eye Know It's Red," *Lancet* 366(9496):1583, October-November 2005.
Professional Guide to Diseases, 8th ed. Philadelphia: Lippincott Williams & Wilkins, 2005.

Corneal abrasion

● OVERVIEW

Description
- Scratch on the epithelial surface of the cornea
- With appropriate treatment, good prognosis usually

Pathophysiology
- Superficial abrasions don't involve the Bowman's membrane.
- Deep abrasions penetrate the Bowman's membrane.

Causes
- Foreign bodies embedded under eyelid
- Contact lenses
- Chemicals
- Fingernails
- Hair brushes
- Tree branches
- Dust

Incidence
- Common
- Affects males and females equally

Common characteristics
- Pain
- Erythema
- Feeling of "something in the eye"

Complications
- Corneal erosion
- Corneal ulceration
- Permanent vision loss
- Secondary infection

✳ ASSESSMENT

History
- Eye trauma
- Prolonged contact lens wear
- Sensation of "something in the eye"
- Sensitivity to light
- Decreased visual acuity
- Eye pain

Physical findings
- Redness
- Increased tearing
- Possibly a foreign object embedded under the eyelid, uncovered by eyelid eversion
- Disruption of corneal surface

Test results
DIAGNOSTIC PROCEDURES
- Fluorescein staining of the injured area of the cornea appears green when illuminated.
- Slit-lamp examination discloses the depth of the abrasion.

◆ TREATMENT

General
- Removal of foreign body
- Eye irrigation
- Warm compresses
- Eye patch for 24 hours

Diet
- No restrictions

Activity
- Eye protection with potentially dangerous activities

Medication
- Antibiotic eyedrops or ointment

Surgery
- Surgical repair of corneal lacerations by an ophthalmologist

✤ NURSING CONSIDERATIONS

Nursing diagnoses
- Acute pain
- Disturbed sensory perception: Visual
- Fear
- Ineffective health maintenance
- Risk for injury

Key outcomes
The patient will:
- express feelings of increased comfort and decreased pain
- regain visual function
- verbalize feelings and concerns
- maintain current health status
- sustain no harm or injury.

Nursing interventions
- Use a flashlight to inspect the cornea.
- Check visual acuity before treatment begins.
- If a foreign body is present, irrigate the eye with 0.9% sodium chloride solution.
- Administer prescribed antibiotics and cycloplegics as ordered.
- Instill topical anesthetics as ordered.

◈ **NURSING ALERT** Never give the patient topical anesthetic drops for self-administration. Abuse of this medication can delay healing, especially if the patient rubs the numb eye, further injuring it.

Monitoring
- Visual acuity
- Response to treatment

◈ **NURSING ALERT** Pulse oximeter probes should be applied to the middle, ring, or, preferably, little finger, but never the index finger, to minimize the likelihood of corneal abrasion, especially as patients emerge from anesthesia.

▶ PATIENT TEACHING

Be sure to cover:
- healing process
- proper instillation of antibiotic eye-drops
- effects of untreated corneal infection
- need to wear safety glasses in the workplace, if appropriate
- contact lens care and instructions for wear.

✳ RESOURCES

Organizations
American Academy of Ophthalmology: *www.eyenet.org*
National Eye Institute: *www.nei.nih.gov*

Selected references
Nettina, S.M. *Lippincott Manual of Nursing Practice,* 8th ed. Philadelphia: Lippincott Williams & Wilkins, 2006.
Professional Guide to Diseases, 8th ed. Philadelphia: Lippincott Williams & Wilkins, 2005.
Thyagarajan, S.K. et al. "An Audit of Corneal Abrasion Management Following the Introduction of Local Guidelines in an Accident and Emergency Department," *Emergency Medicine Journal* 23(7):526-29, July 2006.

Coronary artery disease

● OVERVIEW

Description
- Results from narrowing of coronary arteries over time due to atherosclerosis
- Primary effect: loss of oxygen and nutrients to myocardial tissue because of diminished coronary blood flow

Pathophysiology
- Fatty, fibrous plaques narrow the coronary artery lumina, reducing the blood volume that flows through them, leading to myocardial ischemia.
- As atherosclerosis progresses, luminal narrowing is accompanied by vascular changes that impair the ability of the diseased vessel to dilate. This can lead to tissue injury or necrosis.
- Oxygen deprivation forces the myocardium to shift from aerobic to anaerobic metabolism, leading to accumulation of lactic acid and reduction of cellular pH.
- The combination of hypoxia, reduced energy availability, and acidosis rapidly impairs left ventricular function.
- The strength of contractions in the affected myocardial region is reduced as the fibers shorten inadequately, resulting in less force and velocity.
- Wall motion is abnormal in the ischemic area, resulting in less blood being ejected from the heart with each contraction.

Causes
- Atherosclerosis
- Dissecting aneurysm
- Infectious vasculitis
- Syphilis
- Congenital defects
- Coronary artery spasm

Risk factors
- Family history
- High cholesterol level
- Smoking
- Diabetes
- Hormonal contraceptives
- Obesity
- Sedentary lifestyle
- Stress
- Increased homocystine levels

Incidence
- Occurs after age 40
- Men eight times more susceptible than premenopausal women
- Positive family history increasing risk
- White men more susceptible than nonwhite men; nonwhite women more susceptible than white women
- Occurs in approximately 11 million Americans

Common characteristics
- Angina

Complications
- Arrhythmias
- Myocardial infarction (MI)
- Heart failure

✳ ASSESSMENT

History
- Angina that may radiate to the left arm, neck, jaw, or shoulder blade
- Commonly occurs after physical exertion but may also follow emotional excitement, exposure to cold, or a large meal
- May develop during sleep, waking the patient
- Nausea
- Vomiting
- Fainting
- Sweating
- Stable angina (predictable and relieved by rest or nitrates)
- Unstable angina (increases in frequency and duration and is more easily induced and generally indicates extensive or worsening disease and, untreated, may progress to MI)
- Crescendo angina (effort-induced pain that occurs with increasing frequency and with decreasing provocation)
- Prinzmetal's or variant angina pectoris (severe non-effort-produced pain that occurs at rest without provocation)

Physical findings
- Cool extremities
- Xanthoma
- Arteriovenous nicking of the eye
- Obesity
- Hypertension
- Positive Levine sign (holding fist to chest)
- Decreased or absent peripheral pulses

Test results
IMAGING
- Myocardial perfusion imaging with thallium 201 during treadmill exercise shows ischemic areas of the myocardium, visualized as "cold spots."
- Pharmacologic myocardial perfusion imaging in arteries with stenosis shows decrease in blood flow proportional to the percentage of occlusion.
- Multiple-gated acquisition scanning demonstrates cardiac wall motion and reflects injury to cardiac tissue.
- Coronary angiography reveals the location and degree of coronary artery stenosis or obstruction, collateral circulation, and the condition of the artery beyond the narrowing.
- Stress echocardiography may show abnormal wall motion.

DIAGNOSTIC PROCEDURES
- Electrocardiography may be normal between anginal episodes. During angina, it may show ischemic changes.
- Exercise testing may be performed to detect ST-segment changes during exercise, indicating ischemia, and to determine a safe exercise prescription.
- Cardiac catheterization reveals occluded vessels.

◆ TREATMENT

General
- Stress reduction techniques essential, especially if known stressors precipitate pain
- Lifestyle modifications, such as smoking cessation and maintaining ideal body weight (see *Preventing coronary artery disease*)

Diet
- Low-fat and low-sodium

Activity
- Restrictions possible
- Regular exercise

Medication

- Aspirin
- Nitrates
- Beta-adrenergic blockers
- Calcium channel blockers
- Antiplatelets
- Antilipemics
- Antihypertensives
- Estrogen replacement therapy

Surgery

- Coronary artery bypass graft
- "Keyhole" or minimally invasive surgery
- Angioplasty
- Endovascular stent placement
- Laser angioplasty
- Atherectomy

❖ NURSING CONSIDERATIONS

Nursing diagnoses

- Activity intolerance
- Acute pain
- Anxiety
- Decreased cardiac output
- Disturbed body image
- Imbalanced nutrition: More than body requirements
- Impaired gas exchange
- Ineffective denial
- Ineffective role performance
- Ineffective sexuality patterns
- Ineffective tissue perfusion: Cardiopulmonary

PREVENTING CORONARY ARTERY DISEASE

Because coronary artery disease is so widespread, prevention is important. Dietary restrictions aimed at reducing the intake of calories (in obesity) and of salt, fats, and cholesterol minimize the risk, especially when supplemented with regular exercise. Abstention from smoking and reduction of stress are also essential.

Other preventive actions include control of hypertension (with diuretics or sympathetic beta blockers), control of elevated serum cholesterol or triglyceride levels (with antilipemics such as HMG-reductase inhibitors, including atorvastatin [Lipitor], pravastatin [Pravachol] or simvastatin [Zocor]), and measures to minimize platelet aggregation and the danger of blood clots (with aspirin, for example).

Key outcomes

The patient will:

- state the importance of balancing activity, as tolerated, with rest periods
- express feelings of increased comfort and decreased pain
- verbalize strategies to reduce anxiety
- maintain adequate cardiac output
- express concern about self-concept, esteem, and body image
- plan menus for prescribed diet
- maintain adequate ventilation and oxygenation
- recognize and accept needed lifestyle changes
- verbalize feelings about how the chronic condition affects roles and responsibilities
- identify measures to maintain sexual function, as tolerated
- maintain hemodynamic stability.

Nursing interventions

- Ask the patient to grade the severity of his pain on a scale of 1 to 10.
- Keep nitroglycerin available for immediate use. Instruct the patient to call immediately whenever he feels pain and before taking nitroglycerin.
- Perform vigorous chest physiotherapy and guide the patient in pulmonary self-care.

Monitoring

- Vital signs
- Intake and output
- Anginal episodes
- Abnormal bleeding and distal pulses following intervention procedures
- Breath sounds
- Chest tube drainage, after surgery
- Cardiac rate and rhythm

▶ PATIENT TEACHING

Be sure to cover:

- avoidance of activities that precipitate episodes of pain
- effective coping mechanisms to deal with stress
- need to follow the prescribed drug regimen
- low-sodium and low-calorie diet
- (after PTCA) recurrent angina symptoms or that rotational ablation may signal reocclusion

---

- importance of regular, moderate exercise
- reassurance that the patient can resume sexual activity.

Discharge planning

Refer the patient to:

- a weight-loss program, if needed
- a smoking-cessation program if needed
- a cardiac-rehabilitation program, if indicated.

✸ RESOURCES

Organizations

American Heart Association: *www.americanheart.com*
Mayo Health Clinic: *www.mayohealth.org*

Selected references

Casey, P.F. "Markers of Myocardial Injury and Dysfunction," *AACN Clinical Issues* 15(4):547-57. October-December 2004.

Coats, A.J. "Advances in the Non-Drug, Non-Surgical, Non-Device Management of Chronic Heart Failure," *International Journal of Cardiology* 100(1):1-4, April 2005.

Kasper, D.L., et al., eds. *Harrison's Principles of Internal Medicine,* 16th ed. New York: McGraw-Hill Book Co., 2005.

Price, J.A. "Management and Prevention of Cardiovascular Disease in Women," *The Nursing Clinics of North America* 39(4):873-84, xi, December 2004.

Professional Guide to Diseases, 8th ed. Philadelphia: Lippincott Williams & Wilkins, 2005.

Creutzfeldt-Jakob disease

● OVERVIEW

Description
- Rapidly progressive prion disease that attacks the central nervous system (CNS) and is always fatal
- Not transmitted by normal casual contact (although iatrogenic transmission can occur)
- Typical duration of Creutzfeldt-Jakob disease (CJD) 4 months
- New variant of CJD (nvCJD) that emerged in Europe in 1996 (see *Understanding nvCJD*)
- No cure and progression can't be slowed

Pathophysiology
- CJD is caused by the abnormal accumulation or metabolism of prion proteins.
- These modified proteins are resistant to proteolytic digestion and aggregate in the brain to produce rodlike particles.
- The accumulation of these modified cellular proteins results in neuronal degeneration and spongiform changes in brain tissue.

Causes
- Familial or genetically inherited form
- Sporadic form of unknown etiology
- Iatrogenic or acquired form due to inadvertent exposure to CJD-contaminated equipment or material as a result of brain surgery, corneal grafts, or use of human pituitary-derived growth hormones or gonadotropin

Incidence
- Approximately 1 case in 1 million people worldwide annually
- Most cases sporadic, accounting for approximately 85% of all cases
- Approximately 5% to 15% of cases familial, with an autosomal dominant pattern of inheritance
- Usually affects individuals over age 55; median age of death in the United States is 68
- Affects men and women of diverse ethnic backgrounds
- Most cases in Libya, North Africa, and Slovakia

Common characteristics
- Rapidly progressive dementia
- Prominent myoclonus

Complications
- Severe, progressive dementia
- CNS abnormalities
- Death

✳ ASSESSMENT

History
- Mood changes
- Emotional lability
- Poor concentration
- Lethargy
- Impaired judgment
- Memory loss
- Involuntary muscle movements
- Vision disturbances or other types of hallucinations
- Gait disturbances

Physical findings
- Dementia
- Myoclonus
- Spasticity
- Agitation
- Tremor
- Clumsiness
- Ataxia
- Hypokinesis and rigidity
- Hyperreflexia

Test results
LABORATORY
- Cerebral spinal fluid (CSF) immunoassay may show abnormal protein species.
- CSF analysis may show mildly elevated protein level.

IMAGING
- Computed tomography scan and magnetic resonance imaging of the brain may show evidence of generalized cortical atrophy.

DIAGNOSTIC PROCEDURES
- EEG may show typical changes in brain wave activity.
- Brain biopsy may show spongiform changes.

OTHER
- Autopsy of brain tissue allows definitive diagnosis.

◆ TREATMENT

General
- No specific treatment
- Palliative care to make the patient comfortable and to ease symptoms

Diet
- Well-balanced
- Adequate fluid intake

Activity
- As tolerated

Medication
- Amantadine

Surgery
- Possible brain biopsy for diagnosis

Nursing diagnoses

- Anxiety
- Anticipatory grieving
- Disabled family coping
- Disturbed thought processes
- Fear
- Imbalanced nutrition: Less than body requirements
- Impaired physical mobility
- Impaired social interaction
- Ineffective coping
- Risk for injury
- Social isolation

Key outcomes

The patient will:

- report feeling less anxious
- express feelings related to grief, anger, and sorrow, appropriately
- verbalize feelings of fear
- maintain adequate nutritional status
- maintain activity level to extent possible
- maintain social interaction to the extent possible
- demonstrate effective coping strategies
- remain free from injury.

Nursing interventions

- Assist the patient and family members through the grieving process.
- Institute standard precautions.
- Encourage verbalization of concerns and fears.
- Encourage involvement of patient and family in care decisions.

Monitoring

- Vital signs
- Intake and output
- Neurologic status
- Mental status

Be sure to cover:

- disorder, diagnostic tests, and supportive treatment
- prevention of disease transmission
- effective coping strategies
- safety precautions.

Discharge planning

- Refer the patient and family members to CJD support groups.
- Refer the patient for hospice care, as appropriate.

Organizations

Centers for Disease Control and Prevention: *www.cdc.gov*

National Center for Infectious Diseases: *www.cdc.gov/ncidod/index.htm*

National Prion Disease Pathology Surveillance Center: *www.cjdsurveillance.com*

Selected references

Bosque, P. "Molecular Types of Creutzfeld-Jakob Disease: The Stranger Diversity of Prions," *Neurology* 65(10)1520-521, November 2005.

Smith-Rathgate, B. "Creutzfeldt-Jakob Disease: Diagnosis and Nursing Care Issues," *Nursing Times* 101(20):52-53, May 2005.

Sperling, R., et al. "Creutzfeldt-Jakob Disease in the Obstetric Patient," *Journal of Obstetric, Gynecologic, and Neonatal Nursing* 34(5):546-50, September-October 2005.

UNDERSTANDING nvCJD

Like conventional Creutzfeldt-Jakob disease (CJD), new variant CJD (nvCJD) is a rare, fatal neurodegenerative disease. Most cases have been reported in the United Kingdom. NvCJD is most likely caused by exposure to bovine spongiform encephalopathy (BSE), a fatal brain disease in cattle also known as mad cow disease. Ingestion of beef products from cattle with BSE is the most probable route of exposure.

NvCJD affects patients at a much younger age (under 55) than CJD and the duration of the illness is much longer (14 months).

Regulations have been established in Europe to control outbreaks of BSE in cattle and to prevent contaminated meat from entering the food supply. NvCJD and its relationship with BSE are still being explored by the Centers for Disease Control and Prevention and World Health Organization.

Croup

● OVERVIEW

Description
- Viral infection that causes severe inflammation and obstruction of the upper airway
- Childhood disease manifested by acute laryngotracheobronchitis (most commonly), laryngitis, acute spasmodic laryngitis, and febrile rhinitis
- Incubation period about 3 to 6 days; contagious while febrile
- Recovery usually complete

Pathophysiology
- Viral invasion of the laryngeal mucosa leads to inflammation, hyperemia, edema, epithelial necrosis, and shedding.
- This leads to irritation and cough, reactive paralysis and continuous stridor, or collapsible supraglottic or inspiratory stridor and respiratory distress.
- A thin fibrinous membrane covers the mucosa of the epiglottis, larynx, and trachea. (See *How croup affects the upper airways.*)

Causes
- Parainfluenza viruses
- Adenoviruses
- Respiratory syncytial virus
- Influenza viruses
- Measles viruses
- Bacteria (pertussis and diphtheria)

Incidence
 AGE-RELATED CONCERN Occurs mainly in children ages 3 months to 3 years
- Affects boys more commonly than girls
- Usually occurs in winter

ACUTE SPASMODIC LARYNGITIS
AGE-RELATED CONCERN Affects children between ages 1 and 3, particularly those with allergies

Common characteristics
- Sharp, barklike, or brassy cough
- Hoarse or muffled vocal sounds

Complications
- Airway obstruction
- Respiratory failure
- Dehydration
- Ear infection
- Pneumonia
- Hypoxia
- Hypercapnia

✱ ASSESSMENT

History
- Recent upper respiratory infection

LARYNGOTRACHEOBRONCHITIS
- Fever and breathing problems that usually occur at night
- Difficulty exhaling

LARYNGITIS IN CHILDREN
- Mild sore throat
- Cough
- Rarely, marked hoarseness
- No respiratory distress

LARYNGITIS IN INFANTS
- Respiratory distress

ACUTE SPASMODIC LARYNGITIS
- Mild to moderate hoarseness
- Nasal discharge
- Characteristic cough and noisy inspiration
- Anxiety
- Increased dyspnea
- Transient cyanosis

Physical findings
- Use of accessory muscles
- Nasal flaring
- Barklike cough
- Hoarse, muffled vocal sounds
- Inspiratory stridor
- Diminished breath sounds

LARYNGOTRACHEOBRONCHITIS
- Edema of bronchi and bronchioles
- Decreased breath sounds
- Expiratory rhonchi
- Scattered crackles

LARYNGITIS
- Suprasternal and intercostal retractions
- Inspiratory stridor
- Dyspnea
- Diminished breath sounds
- Severe dyspnea and exhaustion in later stages

ACUTE SPASMODIC LARYNGITIS
- Labored breathing with retractions
- Clammy skin
- Rapid pulse rate

HOW CROUP AFFECTS THE UPPER AIRWAYS

In croup, inflammatory swelling and spasms constrict the larynx, thereby reducing airflow. This cross-sectional drawing (from chin to chest) shows the upper airway changes caused by croup. Inflammatory changes almost completely obstruct the larynx (which includes the epiglottis) and significantly narrow the trachea.

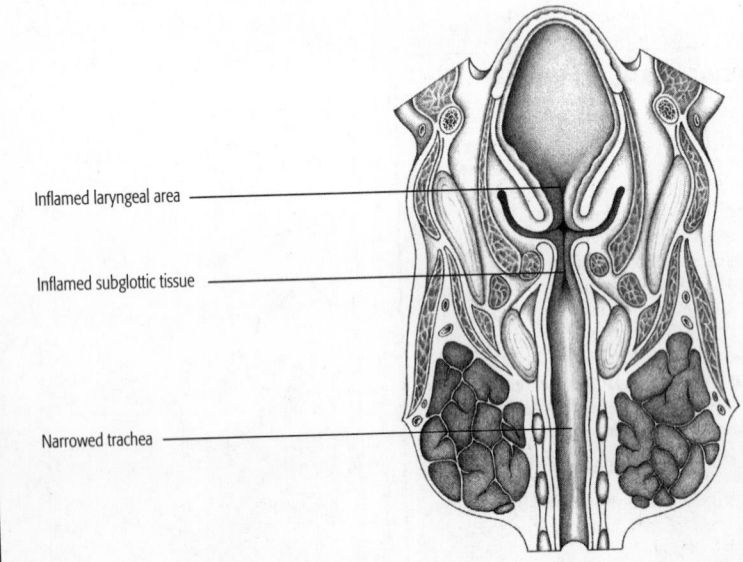

Inflamed laryngeal area

Inflamed subglottic tissue

Narrowed trachea

Test results

LABORATORY
- Throat cultures show bacteria and sensitivity to antibiotic.

IMAGING
- X-ray of the neck may show upper airway narrowing and edema in subglottic folds; helps to differentiate croup from bacterial epiglottitis
- Computed tomography scan helps differentiate between croup, epiglottitis, and noninfection.

DIAGNOSTIC PROCEDURES
- Laryngoscopy may reveal inflammation and obstruction in epiglottal and laryngeal areas.

TREATMENT

General
- Home or hospitalized care
- Humidification during sleep
- Intubation if other means of preventing respiratory failure are unsuccessful

Diet
- As tolerated
- Parenteral fluids (possibly)

Activity
- Rest

Medication
- Oxygen therapy as needed
- Antipyretics
- Antibiotics, if cause is bacterial
- Aerosolized racemic epinephrine for moderately severe croup
- Corticosteroids for acute laryngotracheobronchitis (controversial)

Surgery
- Rarely, tracheostomy

❖ NURSING CONSIDERATIONS

Nursing diagnoses
- Anxiety
- Compromised family coping
- Deficient knowledge (croup)
- Fear
- Hyperthermia
- Impaired gas exchange
- Ineffective airway clearance

Key outcomes
The patient will:
- report feeling less anxious
- use effective coping strategies and available support systems
- verbalize understanding of the disorder
- express feelings of fear related to the diagnosis
- maintain normal temperature
- maintain adequate ventilation and oxygenation
- maintain a patent airway.

Nursing interventions
- Administer medications as ordered.
- Keep the child as quiet as possible, but avoid sedation.
- Provide quiet diversional activities.
- Engage parents in the care of the infant or child.
- Position an infant in an infant seat or prop him up with a pillow.
- Position an older child in Fowler's position.
- Provide humidification.
- Offer water-based ices for sore throat.
- Avoid mild-based fluids if the patient has thick mucus or swallowing difficulties.
- Provide frequent mouth care.
- Isolate patients for respiratory syncytial virus and parainfluenza infections.
- Use sponge baths and hypothermia blanket, as ordered, for temperatures above 102° F (38.9° C).

Monitoring
- Vital signs
- Intake and output
- Respiratory status
- Signs and symptoms of dehydration

▶ PATIENT TEACHING

Be sure to cover:
- disorder, diagnostic tests, and treatment
- medication administration, dosage, and possible adverse effects
- when to notify the physician
- humidification
- hydration
- signs and symptoms of ear infection
- signs and symptoms of pneumonia.

✺ RESOURCES

Organizations
American Academy of Pediatrics: *www.aap.org*

Selected references
Bjornson, C.L., and Johnson, D.W. "Croup—Treatment Update," *Pediatric Emergency Care* 21(12):863-70, December 2005.

Diseases, 4th ed., Philadelphia: Lippincott Williams & Wilkins, 2006.

Pilliteri, A. *Maternal and Child Health Nursing: Core of the Childbearing and Childrearing Family,* 5th ed. Philadelphia: Lippincott Williams & Wilkins, 2006.

Savoy, N.B. "Differentiating Stridor in Children in Triage: It's Not Always Croup," *Journal of Emergency Nursing* 31(5):503-505, October 2005.

Cryptococcosis

● OVERVIEW

Description
- Usually begins as asymptomatic pulmonary infection in patient who presents with meningoencephalitis on diagnosis
- Also known as *torulosis* and *European blastomycosis*

Pathophysiology
- Small granulomas and cysts in the cerebral cortex and later in deep cerebral tissues produce a minimal inflammatory response.
- In chronic cases, dense basilar arachnoiditis occurs.
- Lung lesions with intense granulomatous inflammation occur.

Causes
- Airborne fungus *Cryptococcus neoformans* found in dust particles contaminated by pigeon stool
- Transmission by inhalation of cryptococci

Incidence
- Prevalent in immunocompromised patients (such as those with acquired immunodeficiency syndrome) and those taking immunosuppressant drugs

Common characteristics
- Disseminates to extrapulmonary sites, including the central nervous system (CNS), skin, bones, prostate gland, liver, and kidneys
- Without treatment, leads to CNS infection and death
- Mortality dramatically reduced with treatment; neurologic deficits, such as paralysis and hydrocephalus, not necessarily reduced with treatment

Complications
- Optic atrophy
- Ataxia
- Hydrocephalus
- Deafness
- Paralysis
- Organic mental syndrome
- Personality changes
- Coma
- Death

✳ ASSESSMENT

History
- Human immunodeficiency virus infection or other immunosuppressive disorder
- Usually asymptomatic, but patient may complain of dull chest pain and cough producing slight amount of white, blood-streaked sputum

Physical findings
- Progressively severe frontal and temporal headache
- Diplopia, blurred vision, papilledema
- Tinnitus, dizziness, ataxia, and aphasia
- Vomiting
- Memory changes, inappropriate behavior, irritability, and psychosis
- Facial weakness
- Hyperactive reflexes and seizures in the late stage
- Pain in the long bones, skull, spine, and joints
- Red facial papules and other skin abscesses, with or without ulceration
- Rarely, pleural friction rub or crackles

Test results
LABORATORY
- Analysis or cultures of the sputum, urine, prostatic secretions, or bone marrow aspirate show *C. neoformans.*
- Tissue or neural biopsy shows myriad cryptococci.
- India ink preparation of cerebrospinal fluid (CSF) diagnoses CNS infection when *C. neoformans* is detected.
- Blood cultures are positive only in severe infection.
- Antigen titers are elevated in serum and CSF in disseminated infection.
- Protein levels are elevated and white blood cell count is increased in CNS infection.
- CSF glucose levels are moderately decreased (in about 50% of patients).

IMAGING
- Chest X-ray or computed tomography scan of the chest shows lesions in pulmonary cryptococcosis.

OTHER
- Lumbar puncture shows increased CSF pressure.

◆ TREATMENT

General
- Early treatment for cryptococcal disease

Diet
- No restriction

Activity
- No restriction

Medication
- Combination of antifungal antibiotics amphotericin B and flucytosine, or amphotericin B alone

✤ NURSING CONSIDERATIONS

Nursing diagnoses
- Acute pain
- Impaired gas exchange
- Impaired physical mobility
- Ineffective breathing pattern
- Ineffective tissue perfusion: Cardiopulmonary, cerebral
- Risk for injury

Key outcomes
The patient will:
- express feelings of increased comfort and decreased pain
- maintain adequate ventilation and oxygenation
- attain the highest degree of mobility possible within the confines of the disorder
- maintain normal arterial blood gas levels
- maintain patent airway
- maintain hemodynamic stability
- remain free from injury.

Nursing interventions
- Administer medication as ordered.
- Before therapy, draw serum for testing to determine electrolyte levels and baseline renal status.
- Observe for adverse effects such as diarrhea.
- Evaluate the need for long-term venous access for administering amphotericin B.
- Provide psychological support to help cope with long-term treatment.
- If vision loss occurs, provide a safe environment.
- Encourage verbalization and provide support.

Monitoring
- Vital signs
- Neurologic checks
- Headache, vomiting, and nuchal rigidity
- Urine output
- Blood urea nitrogen, creatinine levels, and complete blood count results
- Urinalysis results
- Magnesium and potassium levels and hepatic function test results
- Blood levels of flucytosine

▶ PATIENT TEACHING

Be sure to cover:
- medication administration, dosage, possible adverse effects, and need for long-term treatment.

Discharge planning
- Urge the patient to return for follow-up care and evaluation every few months for 1 year.
- Refer the patient for resource and support services, as needed.

✱ RESOURCES

Organizations
Centers for Disease Control and Prevention: *www.cdc.gov*
Harvard University Consumer Health Information: *www.intelihealth.com*
National Health Information Center: *www.health.gov/nhic/*
National Library of Medicine: *www.nlm.nih.gov*

Selected references
Kasper., D.L., et al., eds. *Harrison's Principles of Internal Medicine*, 16th ed. New York: Mc-Graw-Hill Book Co., 2005.
Kiertiburanakul, S., et al. "Cryptococcosis in Human Immunodeficiency Virus-Negative Patients," *International Journal of Infectious Diseases* 10(1):72-76, January 2006.
Mandell, G.L., et al. *Principles and Practice of Infectious Diseases*, 6th ed. New York: Churchill Livingstone Inc., 2005.

Cushing's syndrome

● OVERVIEW

Description
- Clinical manifestations of glucocorticoid excess, particularly cortisol
- May also reflect excess secretion of mineralocorticoids and androgens
- Classified as primary, secondary, or iatrogenic, depending on etiology
- Prognosis dependent on early diagnosis, identification of underlying cause, and effective treatment

Pathophysiology
- A loss of normal feedback inhibition by cortisol occurs.
- Elevated levels of cortisol don't suppress hypothalamic and anterior pituitary secretion of corticotropin-releasing hormone and adrenocorticotropic hormone (ACTH).
- The result is excessive levels of circulating cortisol.

Causes
- Pituitary microadenoma
- Excess production of corticotropin
- Corticotropin-producing tumor in another organ
- Administration of synthetic glucocorticoids or corticotropin
- Cortisol-secreting adrenal tumor

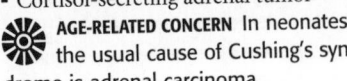 **AGE-RELATED CONCERN** In neonates, the usual cause of Cushing's syndrome is adrenal carcinoma.

Incidence
- More common in females
- Can strike at any age

Common characteristics
- Adiposity of the face, neck, and trunk
- Purple striae on the skin
- Truncal weight gain
- Glucose intolerance

Complications
- Osteoporosis and pathologic fractures
- Peptic ulcer
- Dyslipidemia
- Impaired glucose tolerance
- Diabetes mellitus
- Frequent infections
- Slow wound healing
- Suppressed inflammatory response
- Hypertension
- Ischemic heart disease; heart failure
- Menstrual disturbances
- Sexual dysfunction
- Psychiatric problems, ranging from mood swings to frank psychosis

✳ ASSESSMENT

History
- Use of synthetic steroids
- Fatigue
- Muscle weakness
- Sleep disturbances
- Water retention
- Amenorrhea
- Decreased libido, impotence
- Irritability; emotional instability
- Symptoms resembling those of hyperglycemia, such as polyuria and thirst

Physical findings
- Thin hair
- Moon-shaped face
- Hirsutism
- A buffalo-humplike back
- Thin extremities
- Muscle wasting
- Petechiae, ecchymoses, and purplish striae
- Delayed wound healing
- Swollen ankles
- Hypertension
- Central obesity
- Acne

Test results
LABORATORY
- Salivary free cortisol levels are elevated.
- ACTH levels are decreased in adrenal disease and increased in excess pituitary or ectopic secretion of ACTH.
- Blood chemistry may show hypernatremia, hypokalemia, hypocalcemia, and elevated blood glucose.
- Urinary free cortisol levels are elevated.
- Serum cortisol levels are elevated.

IMAGING
- Ultrasonography, computed tomography scan, and magnetic resonance imaging may show the location of a pituitary or adrenal tumor.

DIAGNOSTIC PROCEDURES
- A low-dose dexamethasone suppression test shows failure of plasma cortisol levels to be suppressed.

◆ TREATMENT

General
- Management to restore hormone balance and reverse Cushing's syndrome, including radiation, drug therapy, or surgery

Diet
- High-protein, high-potassium
- Low-calorie, low-sodium

Activity
- As tolerated

Medication
- Aminoglutethimide
- Antifungal agents
- Antihypertensives
- Diuretics
- Glucocorticoids
- Potassium supplements
- Antineoplastic, antihormone agents

◆ **NURSING ALERT** Glucocorticoid administration on the morning of surgery can help prevent acute adrenal insufficiency during surgery. Cortisol therapy is essential during and after surgery to help the patient tolerate the physiologic stress caused by removal of the pituitary or adrenal glands.

Surgery
- Possible hypophysectomy or pituitary irradiation
- Bilateral adrenalectomy
- Excision of nonendocrine, corticotropin-producing tumor, followed by drug therapy

NURSING CONSIDERATIONS

Nursing diagnoses
- Activity intolerance
- Deficient knowledge (Cushing's syndrome)
- Disturbed body image
- Excess fluid volume
- Impaired skin integrity
- Ineffective coping
- Risk for infection
- Risk for injury
- Sexual dysfunction

Key outcomes
The patient will:
- perform activities of daily living as tolerated within the confines of the disorder
- verbalize understanding of the disorder
- express positive feelings about self
- maintain balanced fluid volume
- maintain skin integrity
- demonstrate appropriate coping strategies
- remain free from infection
- remain free of injury
- verbalize feelings related to sexual functioning.

Nursing interventions
- Administer medications as ordered.
- Consult a dietitian.
- Use protective measures to reduce the risk of infection.
- Use meticulous hand-washing technique.
- Schedule adequate rest periods.
- Institute safety precautions.
- Provide meticulous skin care.
- Encourage verbalization of feelings.
- Offer emotional support.
- Help to develop effective coping strategies.

WITH TRANSSPHENOIDAL APPROACH TO HYPOPHYSECTOMY
- Keep the head of the bed elevated at least 30 degrees.
- Maintain nasal packing.
- Provide frequent mouth care.
- Avoid activities that increase intracranial pressure (ICP).

Monitoring
- Vital signs
- Intake and output
- Daily weights
- Serum electrolyte results

AFTER BILATERAL ADRENALECTOMY AND HYPOPHYSECTOMY
- Neurologic and behavioral status
- Severe nausea, vomiting, and diarrhea
- Bowel sounds
- Adrenal hypofunction
- Increased ICP
- Hypopituitarism
- Transient diabetes insipidus
- Hemorrhage and shock

AFTER TRANSSPHENOIDAL APPROACH TO HYPOPHYSECTOMY
- Cerebrospinal fluid leak

PATIENT TEACHING

Be sure to cover:
- disorder, diagnostic tests, and treatment
- medication administration, dosage, and possible adverse effects
- when to notify the physician
- lifelong steroid replacement
- signs and symptoms of adrenal crisis
- medical identification bracelet
- prevention of infection
- stress reduction strategies.

Discharge planning
- Refer the patient to a mental health professional for additional counseling, if necessary.

RESOURCES

Organizations
Addison and Cushing International Foundation: *www.nvacp.nl/page.php?main=5*
Cushing's Support and Research Foundation, Inc.: *www.world.std.com/~CSRF*
Endocrine Society: *www.endosociety.org/*
National Adrenal Diseases Foundation: *www.medhelp.org/www/nadf.htm*

Selected references
Holcomb, S.S. "Confronting Cushing's Syndrome," *Nursing2005* 35(9):32hn1-32hn6, September 2005.
Maddox, T., and Parker, D.M. "Going Up? Rapid ACTH Screening," *Nursing Made Incredibly Easy!* 4(3):62-63, May-June 2006.
Nettina, S.M. *Lippincott Manual of Nursing Practice,* 8th ed. Philadelphia: Lippincott Williams & Wilkins, 2006.

Cystic fibrosis

● OVERVIEW

Description
- Chronic, progressive, inherited, fatal disease affecting exocrine (mucus-secreting) glands
- Most common genetic disease of white children
- Transmitted as an autosomal recessive trait
- Genetic mutation that involves chloride transport across epithelial membranes (more than 100 specific mutations of the gene identified)
- Characterized by major aberrations in sweat gland, respiratory, and GI functions
- Accounts for almost all cases of pancreatic enzyme deficiency in children
- Clinical effects apparent soon after birth or take years to develop
- Death typically from pneumonia, emphysema, or atelectasis

Pathophysiology
- The viscosity of bronchial, pancreatic, and other mucous gland secretions increases, obstructing glandular ducts.
- The accumulation of thick, tenacious secretions in the bronchioles and alveoli causes respiratory changes, eventually leading to severe atelectasis and emphysema.
- The disease also causes characteristic GI effects in the intestines, pancreas, and liver.
- Obstruction of the pancreatic ducts results in a deficiency of trypsin, amylase, and lipase. This prevents the conversion and absorption of fat and protein in the intestinal tract and interferes with the digestion of food and absorption of fat-soluble vitamins.
- In the pancreas, fibrotic tissue, multiple cysts, thick mucus, and fat replace the acini, producing signs of pancreatic insufficiency.

Causes
- Autosomal recessive mutation of gene on chromosome 7

Incidence
- When both parents are carriers of the recessive gene, 25% chance of transmission with each pregnancy
- Highest in people of northern European ancestry
- Less common in Blacks, Native Americans, and people of Asian ancestry
- Equally common in both sexes

Common characteristics
- Wheezy respirations
- Dry, nonproductive, paroxysmal cough
- Dyspnea
- Poor weight gain

Complications
- Bronchiectasis
- Pneumonia
- Atelectasis
- Dehydration
- Distal intestinal obstructive syndrome
- Malnutrition
- Gastroesophageal reflux
- Cor pulmonale
- Hepatic disease
- Diabetes
- Arthritis
- Biliary disease
- Clotting problems
- Retarded bone growth
- Delayed sexual development
- Azoospermia in males
- Secondary amenorrhea in females
- Electrolyte imbalances
- Cardiac arrhythmias
- Potentially fatal shock
- Death

✳ ASSESSMENT

History
- Recurring bronchitis and pneumonia
- Nasal polyps and sinusitis
- Wheezing
- Dry, nonproductive cough
- Shortness of breath
- Abdominal distention, vomiting, constipation
- Frequent, bulky, foul-smelling, and pale stool with a high fat content
- Poor weight gain
- Poor growth
- Ravenous appetite
- Hematemesis

✸ **AGE-RELATED CONCERN** Neonates may exhibit meconium ileus and develop symptoms of intestinal obstruction: abdominal distention, vomiting, constipation, dehydration, and electrolyte imbalance.

Physical findings
- Wheezy respirations
- Dry, nonproductive, paroxysmal cough
- Dyspnea
- Tachypnea
- Barrel chest
- Cyanosis, and clubbing of the fingers and toes
- Distended abdomen
- Thin extremities
- Sallow skin with poor turgor
- Delayed sexual development
- Neonatal jaundice
- Hepatomegaly
- Rectal prolapse
- Failure to thrive

Test results
LABORATORY
- Stool specimen analysis shows absence of trypsin.
- Deoxyribonucleic acid testing shows presence of the delta F 508 deletion.
- Liver enzyme tests may show hepatic insufficiency.
- Sputum culture may show organisms such as *Pseudomonas* and *Staphylococcus*.
- Serum albumin levels are decreased.
- Serum electrolytes may show hypochloremia and hyponatremia.

IMAGING
- Chest X-rays may show early signs of lung obstruction.

DIAGNOSTIC PROCEDURES
- Sweat tests using pilocarpine solution show positive results.
- Pulmonary function tests show decreased vital capacity, elevated residual volume, and decreased forced expiratory volume in 1 second.

 TREATMENT

General
- To help patient lead as normal a life as possible
- Dependent on organ systems involved
- Chest physiotherapy, nebulization and breathing exercises several times per day
- Gene therapy (experimental)
- Annual influenza vaccine

Diet
- Salt supplements
- High-fat, high-protein, and high in calories
- Nutritional supplementation

Activity
- As tolerated

Medication
- Dornase alfa, a pulmonary enzyme given by aerosol nebulizer
- Antibiotics
- Oxygen therapy, as needed
- Oral pancreatic enzymes
- Bronchodilators
- Prednisone

Surgery
- Heart-lung transplantation

☘ NURSING CONSIDERATIONS

Nursing diagnoses
- Anxiety
- Compromised family coping
- Deficient knowledge (cystic fibrosis)
- Delayed growth and development
- Fear
- Imbalanced nutrition: Less than body requirements
- Impaired gas exchange
- Ineffective airway clearance
- Ineffective breathing pattern
- Ineffective tissue perfusion: Cardiopulmonary

Key outcomes
The patient will:
- identify strategies to reduce anxiety and fear
- use a support system to assist with coping
- express an understanding of the illness
- achieve age-appropriate growth and development milestones to fullest extent possible
- express concerns about coping with the illness
- consume adequate calories daily
- maintain adequate ventilation and oxygenation and a patent airway
- maintain adequate cardiopulmonary tissue perfusion.

Nursing interventions
- Administer medications, as ordered.
- Administer pancreatic enzymes with meals and snacks.
- Perform chest physiotherapy, as ordered.
- Administer oxygen therapy, as needed.
- Provide a well-balanced, high-calorie, high-protein diet; include adequate fats.
- Provide vitamin A, D, E, and K supplements, if indicated.
- Ensure adequate oral fluid intake.
- Provide exercise and activity periods.
- Encourage breathing exercises.
- Provide the young child with play periods.
- Enlist the help of the physical therapy department and play therapists, if available.
- Provide emotional support to the parents of children with cystic fibrosis.
- Encourage discussion of fears and concerns.
- Be flexible with care and visiting hours during hospitalization.
- Allow the child to continue schoolwork and friendships.
- Include family members in all phases of the child's care.

Monitoring
- Vital signs
- Intake and output
- Daily weight
- Hydration
- Pulse oximetry
- Respiratory status

▶ PATIENT TEACHING

Be sure to cover:
- disorder, diagnostic tests, and treatment
- medication administration, dosage, and possible adverse effects
- when to notify the physician
- aerosol therapy
- chest physiotherapy
- aerobic exercise, if prescribed
- signs and symptoms of infection
- complications.

Discharge planning
- Refer family members for genetic counseling, as appropriate.
- Refer the patient and family members to a local support group such as the Cystic Fibrosis Foundation.

✳ RESOURCES

Organizations
American Academy of Pediatrics: *www.aap.org*
Cystic Fibrosis Foundation: *www.cff.org*
National Institute of Diabetes and Digestive and Kidney Diseases: *www.niddk.nih.gov*

Selected references
Diseases, 4th ed. Philadelphia: Lippincott Williams & Wilkins, 2006.
Flume, P. et al. "Emergency Preparedness for the Chronically Ill: Hurricanes and Cystic Fibrosis: Preparing the Patient," *AJN* 104(3):68-72, March 2005.
Grossman, S., and Grossman, L.C. "Pathophysiology of Cystic Fibrosis: Implications for Critical Care Nurses," *Critical Care Nurse* 25(4):46-51, August 2005.

Cytomegalovirus infection

● OVERVIEW

Description
- Also called *generalized salivary gland disease* and *cytomegalic inclusion disease*

Pathophysiology
- Cytomegalovirus (CMV) is found in the saliva, urine, semen, breast milk, feces, blood, and vaginal and cervical secretions of infected people. It can be detected in body fluids for weeks or months after infection.
- CMV usually remains latent, but reactivation occurs when T-lymphocyte-mediated immunity is compromised, as in organ transplantation, lymphoid neoplasms, and certain acquired immunodeficiencies.
- CMV spreads through the body in lymphocytes or mononuclear cells to the lungs, liver, GI tract, eyes, and central nervous system (CNS), typically producing inflammatory reactions.

Causes
- Results from a deoxyribonucleic acid virus belonging to the herpes family
- Transmitted by human contact; once infected, a person carries CMV for life
- Transmission through direct contact with secretions and excretions, through blood transfusions, transplacentally, and through transplanted organs
- May be transmitted in semen during homosexual activity (such transmission not yet proved in heterosexual men)

Incidence
- Occurs worldwide
- Occurs in approximately 30% to 50% of acquired immunodeficiency syndrome patients
- One of the most opportunistic pathogens in patients infected with human immunodeficiency virus

Common characteristics
- Mild fatigue, myalgia, and headache or no clinical symptoms

Complications
- Pneumonia
- Hepatitis
- Ulceration of the GI tract and esophagus
- Retinitis
- Encephalopathy

NEONATAL COMPLICATIONS
- Stillbirth
- Neonatal retinitis
- Microcephaly
- Mental retardation
- Seizures
- Hearing loss
- Thrombocytopenia
- Hemolytic anemia

✱ ASSESSMENT

History
- Immunosuppressive condition

Physical findings
- Fever (common)
- In immunocompromised patient with CMV mononucleosis, 3 or more weeks of irregular high (fever may be only finding)
- Tachypnea, dyspnea, cyanosis, cough
- Jaundice, spider angiomas, hepatomegaly
- Splenomegaly
- In infants, CNS damage (mental retardation, hearing loss, seizures), jaundice, petechial rash, respiratory distress

Test results
LABORATORY
- Isolating the virus or demonstrating increasing serologic titers by complement fixation studies, hemagglutination inhibition antibody tests and, in congenital infections, indirect immunofluorescent tests for CMV immunoglobulin M antibody allows diagnosis.

IMAGING
- Chest X-ray reveals bilateral, diffuse, white infiltrates.
- Computed tomography scan or magnetic resonance imaging shows CNS involvement.

◆ TREATMENT

General
- No current treatment for CMV infection in the healthy individual
- Antiviral therapy being evaluated in neonates
- Vaccines still in the research and development stage

Diet
- No restriction

Activity
- Rest, as needed

Medication
- Antiviral agents
- Immune serums

♣ NURSING CONSIDERATIONS

Nursing diagnoses
- Activity intolerance
- Acute pain
- Diarrhea
- Fatigue
- Hyperthermia
- Impaired gas exchange
- Ineffective breathing pattern
- Risk for infection
- Risk for injury

Key outcomes
The patient will:
- demonstrate skill in conserving energy while carrying out daily activities to tolerance level
- articulate factors that intensify pain and modify behavior accordingly
- return to a normal elimination pattern
- report having an increased energy level
- remain afebrile
- maintain adequate ventilation and oxygenation
- maintain an effective breathing pattern
- remain free from signs of infection and avoid injury.

Nursing interventions
- Institute standard precautions.
- Administer medications, as ordered.
- If vision becomes impaired, provide a safe environment and encourage optimal independence.

Monitoring
- Intake and output
- Ventilation and oxygenation, if the respiratory system is involved

▶ PATIENT TEACHING

Be sure to cover:
- good hand-washing technique
- need for parents to wear gloves when in contact with secretions or changing diapers and to dispose of diapers or soiled articles properly and wash hands thoroughly
- need for female health care workers trying to get pregnant to have CMV titers drawn to identify their risk of contracting the infection
- need for an immunosuppressed or pregnant patient to avoid contact with any person who has confirmed or suspected CMV infection
- need for an immunosuppressed patient who is CMV-seronegative to carry this information with him so he won't be given CMV-positive blood.

Discharge planning
- Provide emotional support and counseling to the parents of a child with severe CMV infection. Help them find support systems, and coordinate referrals to other health care professionals.
- For information and support, refer the patient and family members to a local chapter of the National Center for Infectious Diseases.

✳ RESOURCES

Organizations
Centers for Disease Control and Prevention: www.cdc.gov
Harvard University Consumer Health Information: www.intelihealth.com
National Health Information Center: www.health.gov/nhic
National Library of Medicine: www.nlm.nih.gov

Selected references
Diseases, 4th ed. Philadelphia: Lippincott Williams & Wilkins, 2006.
Kasper, D.L. et al., eds. *Harrison's Principles of Internal Medicine,* 16th ed. New York: McGraw-Hill Book Co., 2005.
Lawson, C.A. "Cytomegalovirus After Kidney Transplantation: A Case Review," *Progress in Transplantation* 15(2):157-60, June 2005.
Mandell, G.L., et al. *Principles and Practice of Infectious Diseases,* 6th ed. New York: Churchill Livingstone Inc., 2005.

Dermatitis

● OVERVIEW

Description
- Characterized by inflammation of the skin
- Can be acute or chronic
- Occurs in several forms, including contact, seborrheic, nummular, exfoliative, and stasis dermatitis (see *Types of dermatitis*, pages 162 and 163)
- Typically associated with other atopic diseases

Pathophysiology
- The allergic mechanism of hypersensitivity results in a release of inflammatory mediators through sensitized antibodies of immunoglobulin (Ig) E.
- Histamine and other cytokines induce an inflammatory response resulting in edema, skin breakdown, and pruritus.

Causes
- Exact cause unknown
- Possible underlying metabolic or biochemical causes
- Possible genetic link to elevated serum IgE levels
- Possible defective T-cell function
- Precipitating factors:
  - infections
  - allergens
  - temperature extremes
  - humidity
  - sweating
  - stress

Incidence
- Common in infants and toddlers between ages 6 months and 2 years
- Common in those with strong family histories of atopic disease
- Affects about 9 of every 1,000 persons

Common characteristics
- Pruritus
- Skin lesions

Complications
- Permanent skin damage
- Lichenification
- Altered pigmentation
- Scarring
- Bacterial, fungal, and viral infections
- Kaposi's varicelliform eruption

✳ ASSESSMENT

History
- Dependent on type of dermatitis
- Family history of atopic dermatitis
- Exposure to an allergen or irritant
- Intense itching

Physical findings
- Dependent on type of dermatitis
- Erythematous patches in excessively dry areas

✸ **AGE-RELATED CONCERN** In children, look for lesions on the forehead, cheeks, and extensor surfaces of the arms and legs.

- Lesions usually at flexion points in adults
- During a flare-up: edema, scaling, and vesiculation; pus-filled vesicles
- In chronic disease: multiple areas of dry, scaly skin, with white dermatographism, blanching, and lichenification

Test results
- Dependent on type of dermatitis

LABORATORY
- Serum analysis shows elevated IgE levels.
- Tissue cultures may rule out bacterial, viral, or fungal superinfections.
- Allergy testing may disclose allergic rhinitis or asthma.

DIAGNOSTIC PROCEDURES
- Patch testing and distribution of lesions are used to pinpoint the provoking allergen.

OTHER
- Firm stroking of the patient's skin with a blunt instrument causes a white — not reddened — hive to appear on the skin of 70% of patients with atopic dermatitis.
- Food elimination diet may help to identify at least one allergen.

◆ TREATMENT

General
- Dependent on type of dermatitis
- Elimination of allergens
- Avoidance of precipitating factors
- Ultraviolet B light therapy to increase the thickness of the stratum corneum

Diet
- Avoidance of food allergens

Activity
- Avoidance of overheating

Medication
- Antihistamines
- Corticosteroids
- Bland emollients
- Antibiotics
- Antifungals
- Antivirals

Surgery
- Vein stripping, sclerotherapy, or skin grafts in stasis dermatitis

Nursing diagnoses
- Acute pain
- Deficient knowledge (dermatitis)
- Disturbed body image
- Impaired oral mucous membrane
- Impaired skin integrity
- Risk for infection

Key outcomes
The patient will:
- report feelings of increased comfort and decreased pain
- demonstrate understanding of skin care regimen
- verbalize feelings about changes in body image
- exhibit improved or healed lesions or wounds
- remain free of infection.

Nursing interventions
- Nursing interventions are guided by the type of dermatitis.
- Assist the patient in daily skin care.
- Trim fingernails short.
- Apply intermittent occlusive dressings to lichenified skin.
- Apply cool, moist compresses.
- Encourage verbalization of feelings.
- Offer emotional support and reassurance.

Monitoring
- Adverse reactions
- Response to treatment
- Complications

Be sure to cover:
- disorder, diagnostic tests, and treatment
- skin care
- medication administration, dosage, and possible adverse effects
- signs and symptoms of corticosteroid overdose and notifying the physician immediately if they occur
- control of pruritus
- meticulous hand washing and good personal hygiene
- use of plain, tepid water (96° F [35.6° C]) and nonfatty, nonperfumed soaps
- application of occlusive dressings
- application of wet-to-dry dressings
- identification and avoidance of aggravating factors.

Discharge planning
- Refer the patient to the American Academy of Dermatology.

Organizations
American Academy of Dermatology: *www.aad.org*
Dermatology Foundation: *www.dermfnd.org*

Selected references
Bliss, D.Z., et al. "Prevalence and Correlates of Perineal Dialysis in Nursing Home Residents," *Nursing Research* 55(4):243-51, July-August 2006.
Borgers, M., et al. "Fungal Infections of the Skin: Infection Process and Antimycotic Therapy," *Current Drug Targets* 6(8):849-62, December 2005.
Wjst, M. "Reducing the Burden of Atopic Dermatitis," *Archives of Disease in Childhood* 92(3):279, March 2007.

Dermatitis

TYPES OF DERMATITIS

Type	Causes	Assessment findings	Diagnosis	Treatment and intervention
CHRONIC DERMATITIS Characterized by inflammatory eruptions of the hands and feet	• Usually unknown but may result from progressive contact dermatitis • Secondary factors: trauma, infections, redistribution of normal flora, photosensitivity, and food sensitivity, which may perpetuate this condition	• Thick, lichenified, single or multiple lesions on any part of the body (commonly on the hands) • Inflammation and scaling • Recurrence after long remissions	• No characteristic pattern or course; diagnosis based on detailed history and physical findings	• Elimination of known allergens and decreased exposure to irritants, wearing protective clothing such as gloves, and washing immediately after contact with irritants or allergens • Antibiotics for secondary infection • Avoidance of excessive washing and drying of hands and accumulation of soaps and detergents under rings • Use of emollients with topical steroids
CONTACT DERMATITIS Commonly, sharply demarcated skin inflammation and irritation due to contact with concentrated substances to which the skin is sensitive, such as perfumes or chemicals	• Mild irritants: chronic exposure to detergents or solvents • Strong irritants: damage on contact with acids or alkalis • Allergens: sensitization after repeated exposure	• Mild irritants and allergens: erythema and small vesicles that ooze, scale, and itch • Strong irritants: blisters and ulcerations • Classic allergic response: clearly defined lesions, with straight lines following points of contact • Severe allergic reaction: marked edema of affected areas	• Patient history • Patch testing to identify allergens • Shape and distribution of lesions	• Same as for chronic dermatitis • Topical anti-inflammatory agents (such as steroids), systemic steroids for edema and bullae, antihistamines, and local applications of Burow's solution (for blisters) • Other nursing interventions similar to those for atopic dermatitis
EXFOLIATIVE DERMATITIS Severe, chronic skin inflammation characterized by redness and widespread erythema and scaling	• Progression of preexisting skin lesions to exfoliative stage, as in contact dermatitis, drug reaction, lymphoma, or leukemia	• Generalized dermatitis, with acute loss of stratum corneum, and erythema and scaling • Sensation of tight skin • Hair loss • Possibly fever, sensitivity to cold, shivering, gynecomastia, and lymphadenopathy	• Identification of the underlying cause	• Hospitalization, with protective isolation and hygienic measures to prevent secondary bacterial infection • Open wet dressings, with colloidal baths • Bland lotions over topical steroids • Maintenance of constant environmental temperature to prevent chilling or overheating • Careful monitoring of renal and cardiac status • Systemic antibiotics and steroids • Other nursing interventions similar to those for atopic dermatitis
LOCALIZED NEURODERMATITIS (LICHEN SIMPLEX CHRONICUS, ESSENTIAL PRURITUS) Superficial skin inflammation characterized by itching and papular eruptions that appear on thickened, hyperpigmented skin	• Chronic scratching or rubbing of a primary lesion or insect bite, or other skin irritation	• Intense, sometimes continual scratching • Thick, sharp-bordered, possibly dry, scaly lesions, with raised papules • Usually affects easily reached areas, such as ankles, lower legs, anogenital area, back of neck, and ears	• Physical findings	• Scratching cessation; then erosions disappear in 2 weeks • Fixed dressing or Unna's boot to cover affected area • Topical steroids (occlusive dressings or intralesional injections) • Antihistamines and open wet dressings • Emollients

TYPES OF DERMATITIS *(continued)*

Type	Causes	Assessment findings	Diagnosis	Treatment and intervention
NUMMULAR DERMATITIS Chronic form of dermatitis characterized by coin-shaped, vesicular, crusted scales and, possibly, pruritic lesions	• Possibly precipitated by stress; or dryness, irritants, or scratching	• Round, nummular (coin-shaped) lesions, usually on arms and legs, with distinct borders of crusts and scales • Possibly oozing and severe itching • Summertime remissions common, with wintertime recurrence	• Physical findings and patient history; history of atopic dermatitis in middle-aged or older patient • Exclusion of fungal infections, atopic or contact dermatitis, and psoriasis	• Elimination of known irritants • Measures to relieve dry skin: increased humidification, limited frequency of baths and use of bland soap and bath oils, and application of emollients • Wet dressings in acute phase • Topical steroids (occlusive dressings or intralesional injections) for persistent lesions • Tar preparations and antihistamines for itching and antibiotics for secondary infection • Other interventions similar to those for atopic dermatitis
SEBORRHEIC DERMATITIS An acute or subacute disease that affects the scalp, face and, occasionally, other areas and is characterized by lesions covered with yellow or brownish gray scales	• Unknown; stress and neurologic conditions may be predisposing factors	• Eruptions in areas with many sebaceous glands (usually scalp, face, and trunk) and in skin folds • Itching, redness, and inflammation of affected areas; lesions that may appear greasy; possibly fissures • Indistinct, occasionally yellowish scaly patches from excess stratum corneum (dandruff may be mild seborrheic dermatitis)	• Patient history and physical findings, especially distribution of lesions in sebaceous gland areas • Exclusion of psoriasis	• Removal of scales by frequent washing and shampooing with selenium sulfide suspension, zinc pyrithione, tar and salicylic acid shampoo or ketoconazole shampoo • Application of topical steroids and antifungal agents to nonhairy areas
STASIS DERMATITIS Condition usually caused by impaired circulation and characterized by eczema of the legs with edema, hyperpigmentation, and persistent inflammation	• Secondary to peripheral vascular diseases affecting legs, such as recurrent thrombophlebitis and resultant chronic venous insufficiency	• Varicosities and edema common, but obvious vascular insufficiency not always present • Usually affects the lower leg, just above internal malleolus, or sites of trauma or irritation • Early signs: dusky red deposits of hemosiderin in skin, with itching and dimpling of subcutaneous tissue; later signs: edema, redness, and scaling of large area of legs • Possibly fissures, crusts, and ulcers	• Positive history of venous insufficiency and physical findings such as varicosities	• Measures to prevent venous stasis: avoidance of prolonged sitting or standing, use of support stockings, and weight reduction for obese patients • Corrective surgery for underlying cause • After ulcer develops, rest periods with legs elevated; open wet dressings; Unna's boot (provides continuous pressure to areas); and antibiotics for secondary infection after wound culture

Diabetes insipidus

● OVERVIEW

Description
- Disorder of water balance regulation
- Characterized by excessive fluid intake and hypotonic polyuria
- Two types of diabetes insipidus: primary and secondary
- Transient form possibly occurring during pregnancy, usually after the fifth or sixth month of gestation
- Impaired or absent thirst mechanism increasing risk of complications
- If uncomplicated, good prognosis
- If complicated by underlying disorder, such as cancer, variable prognosis
- Also referred to as *DI*

Pathophysiology
- Vasopressin (antidiuretic hormone) is synthesized in the hypothalamus and stored by the posterior pituitary gland.
- Once released into the general circulation, vasopressin acts on the distal and collecting tubules of the kidneys.
- Vasopressin increases the water permeability of the tubules and causes water reabsorption.
- The absence of vasopressin allows filtered water to be excreted in the urine instead of being reabsorbed.

Causes
- Failure of vasopressin secretion in response to normal physiologic stimuli
- Failure of the kidneys to respond to vasopressin, called *nephrogenic DI*
- Medications such as lithium
- Damage to hypothalamus or pituitary gland
- Familial
- Idiopathic
- Congenital malformation of the central nervous system (CNS)
- Infection
- Trauma
- Tumors
- Neurosurgery, skull fracture, or head trauma
- Granulomatous disease
- Vascular lesions
- Psychogenic
- Pregnancy (gestational DI)

Incidence
- More common in men than in women
- Slightly higher today than in the past
- Primary DI in 50% of patients

Common characteristics
- Polyuria with low specific gravity and osmolality
- Nocturia
- Dehydration
- Polydipsia

Complications
- Hypovolemia
- Hyperosmolality
- Circulatory collapse
- Loss of consciousness
- CNS changes
- Bladder distention
- Hydroureter
- Hydronephrosis

✱ ASSESSMENT

History
- Abrupt onset of extreme polyuria
- Extreme thirst, resulting in markedly increased oral fluid intake
- Weight loss
- Dizziness, weakness, fatigue
- Constipation
- Nocturia

❂ **AGE-RELATED CONCERN** In children, reports of enuresis, sleep disturbances, irritability, anorexia, thirst, and decreased weight gain and linear growth are common.

Physical findings
- Signs of dehydration
- Fever
- Dyspnea
- Pale, voluminous urine
- Poor skin turgor
- Tachycardia
- Decreased muscle strength
- Hypotension

Test results
LABORATORY
- Urinalysis shows colorless urine with low osmolality and specific gravity.
- Serum sodium is increased.
- Serum osmolality is increased.
- Serum vasopressin is decreased.
- 24-hour urine shows decreased specific gravity and increased volume.
- Blood urea nitrogen (BUN) and creatinine levels are elevated.

DIAGNOSTIC PROCEDURES
- Dehydration test or water deprivation test shows an increase in urine osmolality after vasopressin administration exceeding 9%.

General

- Identification and treatment of underlying cause

Diet

- Control of fluid balance
- Dehydration prevention
- Free access to oral fluids
- With nephrogenic DI, low-sodium diet

Activity

- No restrictions

Medication

- Vasopressin
- Synthetic vasopressin analogue
- Vasopressin stimulant
- Thiazide diuretics in nephrogenic DI
- I.V. fluids
  - If serum sodium level greater than 150, 5% dextrose in water
  - If serum sodium level less than 150, normal saline solution

Surgery

- Not indicated, unless required to treat underlying cause such as a tumor

Nursing diagnoses

- Anxiety
- Deficient fluid volume
- Deficient knowledge (diabetes insipidus)
- Delayed growth and development
- Impaired oral mucous membrane
- Impaired urinary elimination
- Ineffective coping

Key outcomes

The patient will:
- identify strategies to reduce anxiety
- demonstrate balanced fluid volume
- verbalize understanding of the disorder
- demonstrate age-appropriate skills and behavior to the extent possible
- maintain intact oral mucous membranes
- have balanced intake and output
- display adaptive coping behaviors.

Nursing interventions

- Administer medications as ordered.
- Institute safety precautions.
- Provide meticulous skin and mouth care.
- Avoid trauma to the oral mucosa.

NURSING ALERT Use caution when administering vasopressin to a patient with coronary artery disease because the drug can cause coronary artery constriction.

- Encourage verbalization of feelings.
- Offer encouragement while providing a realistic assessment of the situation.
- Help the patient develop effective coping strategies.

Monitoring

- Intake and output
- Vital signs
- Daily weight
- Urine specific gravity
- Serum electrolytes and blood urea nitrogen
- Signs and symptoms of hypovolemic shock
- Changes in mental or neurologic status
- Cardiac rhythm
- Anginal symptoms

Be sure to cover:
- disorder, diagnostic tests, and treatment
- medication administration, dosage, and possible adverse effects
- when to notify the physician
- signs and symptoms of dehydration
- daily weights
- intake and output
- use of a hydrometer to measure urine specific gravity
- need for medical identification bracelet
- maintenance of fluid intake during the day
- limitation of fluid intake in the evening
- alterations in normal growth and development
- need for ongoing medical care.

Discharge planning

- Refer the patient to a mental health professional for additional counseling, as indicated.

Organizations

American Association of Clinical Endocrinologists: *www.aace.com*
Diabetes Insipidus Foundation, Inc.: *www.diabetesinsipidus.maxinter.net*
Endocrine Society: *www.endosociety.org*

Selected references

Brewster, U.C., and Hayslett, J.P. "Diabetes Insipidus in the Third Trimester of Pregnancy," *Obstetrics & Gynecology* 105(5 part 2) Supplement; 1173-176, May 2005.

Davies, J.H., et al. "Clinical Features, Diagnosis and Molecular Studies of Familial Central Diabetes Insipidius," *Hormone Research* 64(5):231-37, Epub October 2005.

Jani, R., et al. "Heparin-induced Thrombocytopenia Presenting as Central Diabetes Insipidus," *Endocrinologist* 15(6):374-76, November-December 2005.

Diabetes mellitus

⬤ OVERVIEW

Description
- Chronic disease of absolute or relative insulin deficiency or resistance
- Characterized by disturbances in carbohydrate, protein, and fat metabolism
- Two primary forms:
  - Type 1, characterized by absolute insufficiency
  - Type 2, characterized by insulin resistance with varying degrees of insulin secretory defects

Pathophysiology
- The effects of diabetes mellitus (DM) result from insulin deficiency or resistance to endogenous insulin.
- Insulin allows glucose transport into the cells for use as energy or storage as glycogen.
- Insulin also stimulates protein synthesis and free fatty acid storage in the adipose tissues.
- Insulin deficiency compromises the body tissues' access to essential nutrients for fuel and storage.

Causes
- Genetic factors
- Autoimmune disease (type 1)

Risk factors
- Viral infections (type 1)
- Obesity (type 2)
- Physiologic or emotional stress
- Sedentary lifestyle (type 2)
- Pregnancy
- Medication, such as thiazide diuretics, adrenal corticosteroids, and oral contraceptives

Incidence
- Type 1 — usually occurs before age 30, although it may occur at any age
- Type 2 — usually occurs in obese adults after age 30, although it may be seen in obese North American youths of African-American, Native American, or Hispanic descent
- Affects about 8% of the population of the United States
- About one-third of patients undiagnosed
- Increases with age (type 2)

Common characteristics
- Polyuria
- Polydipsia
- Polyphagia
- Weight loss
- Fatigue

Complications
- Ketoacidosis
- Hyperosmolar, hyperglycemic syndrome
- Cardiovascular disease
- Peripheral vascular disease
- Retinopathy, blindness
- Nephropathy, renal failure
- Diabetic dermopathy
- Peripheral neuropathy
- Autonomic neuropathy
- Amputations
- Impaired resistance to infection
- Cognitive depression

✴ **AGE-RELATED CONCERN** Neonates of diabetic mothers have a two- to three-times-greater incidence of congenital malformations and fetal distress unless the mothers' blood glucose levels are well-controlled before conception and during pregnancy.

✳ ASSESSMENT

History
- Polyuria, nocturia
- Dehydration
- Polydipsia
- Dry mucous membranes
- Poor skin turgor
- Weight loss and hunger
- Weakness; fatigue
- Vision changes
- Frequent skin and urinary tract infections
- Dry, itchy skin
- Sexual problems
- Numbness or pain in the hands or feet
- Postprandial feeling of nausea or fullness
- Nocturnal diarrhea

TYPE 1
- Rapidly developing symptoms

TYPE 2
- Vague, long-standing symptoms that develop gradually
- Family history of DM
- History of gestational diabetes

- Delivery of a neonate weighing more than 9 lb (4.1 kg)
- Severe viral infection
- Other endocrine diseases
- Recent stress or trauma
- Use of drugs that increase blood glucose levels

Physical findings
- Retinopathy or cataract formation
- Skin changes, especially on the legs and feet
- Muscle wasting and loss of subcutaneous fat (type 1)
- Obesity, particularly in the abdominal area (type 2)
- Poor skin turgor
- Dry mucous membranes
- Decreased peripheral pulses
- Cool skin temperature
- Diminished deep tendon reflexes
- Orthostatic hypotension
- Characteristic "fruity" breath odor in ketoacidosis
- Possible hypovolemia and shock in ketoacidosis and hyperosmolar hyperglycemic state

Test results
LABORATORY
- Fasting plasma glucose level is greater than or equal to 126 mg/dl on at least two occasions.
- Random blood glucose level is greater than or equal to 200 mg/dl.
- Two-hour postprandial blood glucose level is greater than or equal to 200 mg/dl.
- Glycosylated hemoglobin (Hb) is increased.
- Urinalysis may show acetone or glucose.

DIAGNOSTIC PROCEDURES
- Ophthalmologic examination may show diabetic retinopathy.

◆ TREATMENT

General
- Exercise and diet for type 2 diabetes
- Tight glycemic control for prevention of complications in type 1 and type 2
- American Diabetes Association recommendations to reach target glucose, Hb A_{1c} lipid, and blood pressure levels

Diet

- Modest caloric restriction for weight loss or maintenance

Activity

- Regular aerobic exercise

Medication

- Exogenous insulin (type 1)
- Oral antihyperglycemic drugs (type 2); insulin (possible)

Surgery

- Pancreas transplantation

❖ NURSING CONSIDERATIONS

Nursing diagnoses

- Deficient fluid volume
- Disabled family coping
- Disturbed sensory perception: Tactile, visual
- Imbalanced nutrition: Less than body requirements
- Imbalanced nutrition: More than body rquirements
- Impaired skin integrity
- Impaired urinary elimnation
- Ineffective coping
- Ineffective tissue perfusion: Cardiopulmonary, peripheral, renal
- Risk for infection
- Risk for injury
- Sexual dysfunction

Key outcomes

The patient will:

- maintain adequate fluid balance
- develop adequate coping mechanisms and support systems
- maintain optimal functioning within the confines of the tactile and visual impairment
- maintain daily calorie requirements
- maintain weight within an acceptable range
- maintain skin integrity
- have balanced intake and output
- demonstrate adaptive coping behaviors
- exhibit signs of adequate cardiopulmonary, peripheral, and renal perfusion
- remain free from signs and symptoms of infection
- avoid injury and complications

- discuss feelings about sexual impairment.

Nursing interventions

- Administer medications as ordered.
- Give rapidly absorbed carbohydrates for hypoglycemia or, if the patient is unconscious, glucagon or I.V. dextrose, as ordered.
- Administer I.V. fluids and insulin replacement for hyperglycemic crisis as ordered.
- Provide meticulous skin care, especially to the feet and legs.
- Treat all injuries, cuts, and blisters immediately.
- Avoid constricting hose, slippers, or bed linens.
- Encourage adequate fluid intake.
- Consult a dietitian.
- Encourage verbalization of feelings.
- Offer emotional support.
- Help to develop effective coping strategies.

Monitoring

- Vital signs
- Intake and output
- Daily weights
- Serum glucose
- Urine acetone
- Renal status
- Cardiovascular status
- Signs and symptoms of:
  - hypoglycemia
  - hyperglycemia
  - hyperosmolar coma
  - urinary tract and vaginal infections
  - diabetic neuropathy

▶ PATIENT TEACHING

Be sure to cover:

- disorder, diagnostic tests, and treatment
- medication administration, dosage, and possible adverse effects
- when to notify the physician
- prescribed meal plan
- prescribed exercise program
- signs and symptoms of:
  - infection
  - hypoglycemia
  - hyperglycemia
  - diabetic neuropathy
- self-monitoring of blood glucose

- complications of hyperglycemia
- foot care
- annual regular ophthalmologic examinations
- safety precautions
- management of diabetes during illness.

Discharge planning

- Refer the patient to a podiatrist if indicated.
- Refer the patient to an ophthalmologist.
- Refer the adult diabetic patients who are trying to conceive for preconception counseling.
- Refer the patient to the Juvenile Diabetes Research Foundation, the American Association of Diabetes Educators, and the American Diabetes Association to obtain additional information.

✳ RESOURCES

Organizations

American Diabetes Association: *www.diabetes.org*
Juvenile Diabetes Foundation International: *www.jdf.org*
National Institute of Diabetes, Digestive, and Kidney Diseases: *www.niddk.nih.gov*

Selected references

"Ask an Expert: How Should I Administer An Insulin Injection?" *Nursing Made Incredibly Easy* 2(2):64, March-April 2004.

"Drug News: Inhaled Insulin Earns FDA Approval," *Nursing* 36(3):30, March 2006.

Moshang, J. "Ask an Expert: Is Splitting an Insulin Glargine Dose OK?" *Nursing Made Incredibly Easy* 3(3):64, May-June 2005.

Sieggreen, M.Y. "Stepping up Care for Diabetic Food Ulcers," *Nursing* 35(10):36-41, October 2005.

Sperling, M.A. "Neonatal Diabetes Mellitus: From Understudy to Center Stage," *Current Opinion in Pediatrics* 17(4):512-18, August 2005.

Stuebe, A.M., et al. "Duration of Lactation and Incidence of Type 2 Diabetes," *JAMA* 294(20)2601-610, November 2005.

Watkinson, S., and Chetram, N. "A Nurse-led Approach to Diabetic Retinal Screening," *Nursing Times* 101(36):32-34, September 2005.

Dislocations and subluxations

● OVERVIEW

Description
- Dislocation: displacement of joint bones so that articulating surfaces totally lose contact (see *Common dislocation*)
- Subluxation: partial displacement of articulating surfaces
- May accompany joint fractures

Pathophysiology
- Trauma causes displacement of the joint, leading to damage of oint structures (blood vessels, ligaments, tendons and nerves).
- Injuries may result in deposition of fracture fragments between joint surfaces, damaging surrounding structures.
- Joint function is impaired.

Causes
- Congenital
- Trauma
- Paget's disease of surrounding joint tissues

Risk factors
- Participation in contact sports

Incidence
- Shoulder dislocations—account for more than half of dislocations seen in emergency rooms
- Hip dislocations—from trauma, more common in those under 35 years old; from falls, more common in those over age 65

Common characteristics
- Visible deformity of affected extremity
- Shortening of affected extremity
- Local pain
- Swelling
- Limitation of function
- Numbness of affected extremity

Complications
- Avascular necrosis
- Bone necrosis

✳ ASSESSMENT

History
- Trauma or fall
- Extreme pain at injury site

Physical findings
- Joint surface fractures
- Deformity around the joint
- Change in the length of the involved extremity
- Impaired joint mobility
- Point tenderness

Test results
IMAGING
- X-rays are used to confirm the diagnosis and show any associated fractures.

◆ TREATMENT

General
- Immediate reduction and immobilization that can prevent additional tissue damage and vascular impairment
- Closed reduction

Diet
- Nothing by mouth if surgery scheduled
- No restriction

Activity
- Limitations based on injury
- Active range-of-motion (ROM) exercises for adjacent joints that aren't immobilized

Medications
- Sedation
- Analgesics
- Muscle relaxants

Surgery
- Open reduction
- Skeletal traction
- Ligament repair

Nursing diagnoses
- Acute pain
- Disturbed body image
- Dressing or grooming self-care deficit
- Impaired physical mobility
- Ineffective tissue perfusion: Peripheral
- Risk for disuse syndrome

Key outcomes
The patient will:
- articulate factors that intensify pain and will modify behavior accordingly
- express positive feelings about self
- perform self-care activities at the highest level possible
- attain the highest degree of mobility possible within the confines of the injury
- show signs of adequate peripheral perfusion
- maintain joint ROM and muscle strength.

Nursing interventions
- Administer medications as ordered.
- Provide proper positioning of the affected area.
- Apply ice as ordered.
- Encourage ROM exercises, as ordered, for adjacent nonmobilized joints.
- Provide meticulous skin care.

◈ **NURSING ALERT** Immediately report signs and symptoms of severe vascular compromise, such as pallor, pain, loss of pulse, paralysis, and paresthesia; the patient needs an immediate orthopedic examination and emergency reduction.

Monitoring
- Respiratory status when I.V. sedatives used
- Neurovascular status of extremity involved
- Integrity of skin

Be sure to cover:
- need to report numbness, pain, cyanosis, and coldness of the extremity below the cast or splint
- how to evaluate skin integrity
- how to assess neurovascular status
- use of assistive devices
- importance of follow-up visits
- medication administration, dosage, and possible adverse effects.

Discharge planning
- Refer the patient to a rehabilitation program if appropriate.
- Refer the patient for home health care if appropriate.

COMMON DISLOCATION

Normal elbow joint

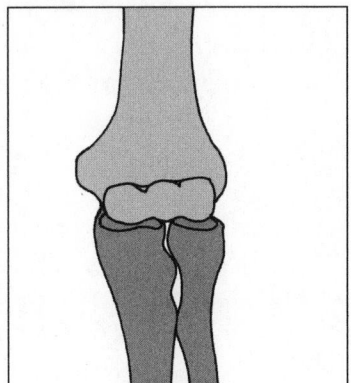

Elbow joint with lateral dislocation

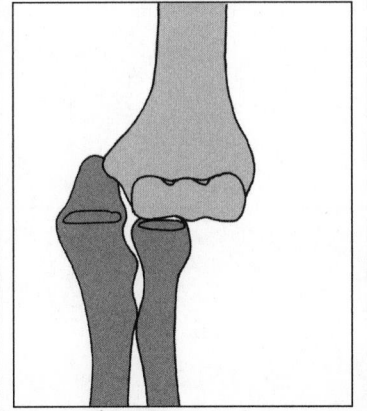

Organizations
American Academy of Neurology: *www.aan.com*
American Academy of Orthopedic Surgeons: *www.aaos.org*
American Academy of Pediatric Sports Medicine: *www.aapsm.org*
Southern California Orthopedic Institute: *www.scoi.com*
Totally Hip Support Group: www.*members.tripod.com/totallyhip1/index1.htm*

Selected references
Flanigan, D.C., and Kaplan, L.D. "Elbow Dislocations and Instability," *Current Opinion in Orthopedics* 15(4):280-85, August 2004.

Shinoda-Tagawa, T., et al. "Resident-to-Resident Violent Incidents in Nursing Homes," *JAMA* 291(17):2074-2075, May 2005.

Yasukawa, A., et al. "Shoulder Support for Children with Subluxation: A Case Study," *JPO: Journal of Prosthetics & Orthotics* 17(3):74-79, July 2005.

Disseminated intravascular coagulation

● OVERVIEW

Description
- Complicates diseases and conditions that accelerate clotting, causing occlusion of small blood vessels, organ necrosis, depletion of circulating clotting factors and platelets, and activation of the fibrinolytic system
- Also known as *DIC, consumption coagulopathy,* and *defibrination syndrome*

Pathophysiology
- Typical accelerated clotting results in generalized activation of prothrombin and a consequent excess of thrombin.
- Excess thrombin converts fibrinogen to fibrin, producing fibrin clots in the microcirculation.
- This process consumes exorbitant amounts of coagulation factors (especially platelets, factor V, prothrombin, fibrinogen, and factor VIII), causing thrombocytopenia, deficiencies in factors V and VIII, hypoprothrombinemia, and hypofibrinogenemia.
- Circulating thrombin activates the fibrinolytic system, which lyses fibrin clots into fibrinogen degradation products (FDPs).
- The hemorrhage that occurs may be due largely to the anticoagulant activity of FDPs and depletion of plasma coagulation factors.

Causes
- Infection, sepsis
- Obstetric complications
- Neoplastic disease
- Disorders that produce necrosis, such as extensive burns and trauma
- Other disorders, such as heatstroke, shock, incompatible blood transfusion, drug reactions, cardiac arrest, surgery necessitating cardiopulmonary bypass, adult respiratory distress syndrome, diabetic ketoacidosis, pulmonary embolism, and sickle cell anemia

Incidence
- Dependent on the cause

Common characteristics
- Abnormal bleeding
- Hemorrhage

Complications
- Renal failure
- Hepatic damage
- Stroke
- Ischemic bowel
- Respiratory distress
- Death (mortality is greater than 50%)

✳ ASSESSMENT

History
- Abnormal bleeding *without* a history of a serious hemorrhagic disorder; bleeding possibly occurring at all bodily orifices
- Possible presence of one of the causes of DIC
- Possible signs of bleeding into the skin, such as cutaneous oozing, petechiae, ecchymoses, and hematomas
- Possible bleeding from surgical or invasive procedure sites, such as incisions or venipuncture sites
- Possible nausea and vomiting; severe muscle, back, and abdominal pain; chest pain; hemoptysis; epistaxis; seizures; and oliguria
- Possible GI bleeding, hematuria

Physical findings
- Petechiae
- Acrocyanosis
- Dyspnea, tachypnea
- Mental status changes, including confusion

Test results
LABORATORY
- Serum platelet count is decreased (less than 100,00/mm³).
- Serum fibrinogen level is decreased (less than 150 mg/dl).
- Prothrombin time is prolonged (more than 15 seconds).
- Partial thromboplastin time is prolonged (more than 80 seconds).
- FDPs are increased (commonly greater than 45 mcg/ml, or positive at less than 1:100 dilution).
- D-dimer test is positive (specific fibrinogen test for DIC) at less than 1:8 dilution.
- Thrombin time is prolonged.
- Blood clotting factors V and VIII are diminished.
- Complete blood count shows decreased hemoglobin levels (less than 10 g/dl).
- Blood urea nitrogen (greater than 25 mg/dl) and serum creatinine levels (greater than 1.3 mg/dl) are elevated.

◆ TREATMENT

General
- Possibly supportive care alone if the patient isn't actively bleeding

Diet
- No restrictions

Activity
- As tolerated

Medication
IF THE PATIENT IS ACTIVELY BLEEDING
- Administration of blood, fresh frozen plasma, platelets, or packed red blood cells
- Heparin therapy
- Antithrombin III and gabexate
- Fluid replacement

♣ NURSING CONSIDERATIONS

Nursing diagnoses
- Acute pain
- Anxiety
- Fatigue
- Fear
- Impaired gas exchange
- Impaired physical mobility
- Impaired tissue integrity
- Ineffective tissue perfusion: GI, cerebral, renal
- Risk for deficient fluid volume
- Risk for injury

Key outcomes
The patient will:
- express feelings of increased comfort and decreased pain
- report feeling less anxious
- demonstrate increased energy and less fatigue
- use available support systems to assist in coping with fears
- maintain adequate ventilation and oxygenation
- perform activities of daily living with the maximum level of mobility and independence
- maintain adequate tissue integrity
- demonstrate blood pressure that remains high enough to maintain cerebral perfusion pressure, but low enough to prevent intracranial bleeding and cerebral swelling
- maintain balanced intake and output
- remain free of injury.

Nursing interventions
◉ **NURSING ALERT** Focus on early recognition of signs of abnormal bleeding, prompt treatment of the underlying disorders, and prevention of further bleeding.
- Keep family members informed of the patient's progress. Provide emotional support. Listen to the patient's and family members' concerns.
- If the patient can't tolerate activities because of blood loss, provide rest periods.
- Administer prescribed analgesics for pain, as necessary.
- Reposition the patient every 2 hours and provide meticulous skin care.
- Administer oxygen therapy, as ordered.

◉ **NURSING ALERT** To prevent clots from dislodging and causing fresh bleeding, don't vigorously rub affected areas when bathing.
- Protect the patient from injury. Enforce complete bed rest during bleeding episodes. If the patient is agitated, pad the side rails.
- If bleeding occurs, use pressure and topical hemostatic agents to control bleeding.
- After injection or removal of I.V. catheters or needles, apply pressure to injection sites for at least 10 minutes. Alert other personnel to the patient's tendency to hemorrhage.
- Limit venipunctures whenever possible.
- Watch for transfusion reactions and signs of fluid overload.
- To measure the amount of blood lost, weigh dressings and linen and record drainage.
- Weigh the patient daily, particularly in renal involvement.
- Watch for bleeding from the GI and genitourinary (GU) tracts.
- Perform bladder irrigations, as ordered, for GU bleeding.

Monitoring
- Vital signs
- Results of serial blood studies
- Venipuncture sites
- Abdominal girth
- Signs of shock
- Intake and output, especially when administering blood products
- Stool and urine for occult blood

▶ PATIENT TEACHING

Be sure to cover (with the patient and family):
- disorder, diagnostic tests, and treatment.

✱ RESOURCES

Organizations
American Heart Association: *www.americanheart.org*
Mayo Health Clinic: *www.mayohealth.org*

Selected references
Backhouse, R. "Understanding Disseminated Intravascular Coagulation," *Nursing Times* 100(36):38-42, September 2004.

Dressler, D.K. "DIC: Coping with a Coagulation Crisis," *Nursing* 34(5):58-62, May 2004.

Kasper, D.L., et al., eds. *Harrison's Principles of Internal Medicine,* 16th ed. New York: McGraw-Hill Book Co., 2005.

Toh, C., and Towney, C. "Back to the Future: Testing in Disseminated Intravascular Coagulation," *Blood Coagulation & Fibrinolysis* 16(8):535-42, November 2005.

Diverticular disease

OVERVIEW

Description
- Bulging pouches (diverticula) in GI wall that push mucosal lining through surrounding muscle
- Sigmoid colon: most common site, but may develop anywhere, from proximal end of the pharynx to the anus
- Other typical sites: the duodenum, near the pancreatic border or the ampulla of Vater; the jejunum
- Diverticular disease of the ileum (Meckel's diverticulum): most common congenital anomaly of the GI tract
- Two clinical forms:
  - Diverticulosis (diverticula are present but don't cause symptoms)
  - Diverticulitis (diverticula become inflamed and can cause complications)

Pathophysiology
- Pressure in the intestinal lumen is exerted on weak areas, such as points where blood vessels enter the intestine, causing a break in the muscular continuity of the GI wall, creating a diverticulum.
- Diverticulitis occurs when retained undigested food mixed with bacteria accumulates in the diverticulum, forming a hard mass (fecalith). This substance cuts off the blood supply to the diverticulum's thin walls, increasing its susceptibility to attack by colonic bacteria.
- Inflammation follows bacterial infection, causing abdominal pain.

Causes
- Diminished colonic motility and increased intraluminal pressure
- Defects in colon wall strength

Risk factors
- Age
- Low-fiber diet

Incidence
- Most common in adults ages 45 and older
- Affects 30% of adults over age 60
- More common in women than men

Common characteristics
- Abdominal pain
- Diarrhea or constipation
- Palpable mass

Complications
- Ruptured diverticula that cause abdominal abscesses or peritonitis
- Intestinal obstruction
- Rectal hemorrhage
- Portal pyemia
- Fistula

ASSESSMENT

History
DIVERTICULOSIS
- May be asymptomatic
- Occasional intermittent pain in the left lower abdominal quadrant, which may be relieved by defecation or the passage of flatus
- Alternating bouts of constipation and diarrhea

DIVERTICULITIS
- History of diverticulosis
- Low fiber consumption
- Recent consumption of foods containing seeds or kernels or indigestible roughage, such as celery and corn
- Complaints of moderate dull or steady pain in the left lower abdominal quadrant, aggravated by straining, lifting, or coughing
- Mild nausea, gas, diarrhea, or intermittent bouts of constipation, sometimes accompanied by rectal bleeding

Physical findings
DIVERTICULITIS
- Distressed appearance
- Left lower quadrant abdominal tenderness
- Low-grade fever
- Palpabable mass
ACUTE DIVERTICULITIS
- Muscle spasms
- Signs of peritoneal irritation
- Guarding and rebound tenderness

Test results
LABORATORY
- Complete blood count reveals leukocytosis.
- Erythrocyte sedimentation rate is elevated in diverticulitis.
- Stool test is positive for occult blood in 20% of patients with diverticulitis.

IMAGING
- Barium studies reveal barium-filled diverticula or outlines, but barium doesn't fill diverticula blocked by impacted stools. This procedure isn't performed for acute diverticulitis because of potential rupture.
- Radiography may reveal colonic spasm if irritable bowel syndrome accompanies diverticular disease.
- Abdominal X-rays rule out perforation.
- Computed tomography of abdomen identifies possible abscesses.

DIAGNOSTIC PROCEDURES
- Colonoscopy or flexible sigmoidoscopy shows diverticula. It isn't usually performed in the acute phase.
- Biopsy results may rule out cancer.

◆ TREATMENT

General
- Generally, no treatment for asymptomatic diverticulosis
- Nasogastric (NG) decompression for severe diverticulitis

Diet
FOR DIVERTICULOSIS
- Liquid or low-residue diet (if experiencing pain)
- Increased water consumption, if appropriate
- High-residue diet
FOR SEVERE DIVERTICULITIS
- Nothing by mouth

Activity
- Bed rest

Medication
FOR DIVERTICULOSIS
- Stool softeners
- Bulk medication
FOR DIVERTICULITIS
- Antibiotics
- Analgesics
- Antispasmodics
- I.V. therapy for severe diverticulitis

Surgery
- Colon resection
- May require temporary colostomy to drain abscesses or to rest the colon for 6 to 8 weeks
- Needed for rupture or to correct cases refractory to medical treatment

❖ NURSING CONSIDERATIONS

Nursing diagnoses
- Acute pain
- Anxiety
- Constipation
- Diarrhea
- Deficient fluid volume
- Deficient knowledge (diverticular disease)
- Ineffective tissue perfusion: GI

Key outcomes
The patient will:
- express feelings of increased comfort and decreased pain
- identify measures to reduce anxiety
- have bowel movements that return to normal
- maintain fluid volume balance
- verbalize understanding of the disease process and treatment regimen
- exhibit signs of adequate GI perfusion.

Nursing interventions
◆ **NURSING ALERT** Remember that diverticulitis produces more serious signs and symptoms, as well as complications, and requires more interventions than diverticulosis.
- If the patient is anxious, provide psychological support.
- Administer medications, as ordered.
- Maintain bed rest for acute diverticulitis.
- Maintain the diet as ordered.
- If surgery is scheduled, provide routine preoperative care.
AFTER COLON RESECTION
- Provide meticulous wound care.
- Encourage coughing and deep breathing to prevent atelectasis.
- Administer I.V. fluids and medications as ordered.
- Provide colostomy care, if appropriate.

Monitoring
- Pain control
- Stools for color, consistency, and frequency
- NG drainage if appropriate
- Signs and symptoms of complications

AFTER COLON RESECTION
- Signs of infection and postoperative bleeding
- Intake and output
- Vital signs

▶ PATIENT TEACHING

Be sure to cover:
- bowel and dietary habits (in uncomplicated diverticulosis)
- disorder, diagnostic tests, and treatment
- preoperative teaching (for a patient needing surgery)
- postoperative teaching (for a patient who must care for his colostomy, as needed)
- medication administration, dosage, and possible adverse effects
- recommended dietary changes.

Discharge planning
- Refer the patient to an enterostomal therapist, if appropriate.
- Refer the patient to a dietitian, if needed.

✹ RESOURCES

Organizations
Digestive Disease National Coalition: *www.ddnc.org*
National Digestive Diseases Information Clearinghouse: *www.niddk.nih.gov/health/digest/nddic.htm*
National Institute of Diabetes and Digestive and Kidney Disorders: *www.niddk.nih.gov*

Selected references
Burch, J. "Exploring the Conditions Leading to Stoma-forming Surgery," *British Journal of Nursing* 14(2):94-98, January-February 2005.
Diseases, 4th ed. Philadelphia: Lippincott Williams & Wilkins, 2006.
Yamada, T., et al. *Handbook of Gastroenterology,* 2nd ed. Philadelphia: Lippincott Williams & Wilkins, 2005.

Down syndrome

● OVERVIEW

Description
- Chromosomal aberration that results in mental retardation, abnormal facial features, and other distinctive physical abnormalities
- Commonly associated with heart defects and other congenital disorders
- Average IQ between 30 and 50 (some higher)
- Also known as *trisomy 21 syndrome*

Pathophysiology
- Down syndrome is an aberration in which chromosome 21 has three copies instead of the normal two because of faulty meiosis (nondisjunction) of the ovum or, sometimes, the sperm.
- There's unbalanced translocation, in which the long arm of chromosome 21 breaks and attaches to another chromosome.
- The result is a karyotype of 47 chromosomes instead of the normal 46.

Causes
- Trisomy 21
- Deterioration of the oocyte resulting from age or cumulative effects of radiation and viruses

Risk factors
- Maternal age, especially over age 35

Incidence
- Occurs in 1 per 800 to 1,000 live births
- Increases with maternal age, especially after age 35

Common characteristics
- Characteristic craniofacial appearance

Complications
- Death
- Congenital heart defects
- Premature senile dementia
- Leukemia
- Acute and chronic infections
- Diabetes mellitus
- Thyroid disorders

✳ ASSESSMENT

History
- Neonate lethargic and a poor feeder

Physical findings
- Slanting, almond-shaped eyes
- Small, open mouth, protruding tongue
- Single transverse palmar crease
- Brushfield's spots on the iris
- Small skull
- Flat bridge across the nose
- Flattened face
- Small external ears
- Short neck with excess skin
- Dry, sensitive skin with decreased elasticity
- Umbilical hernia
- Short stature
- Short extremities with broad, flat, and squarish hands and feet
- Dysplastic middle phalanx of the fifth finger
- Wide space between the first and second toes
- Abnormal fingerprints and footprints
- Impaired reflex development
- Absent Moro's reflex and hyperextensible joints
- Impaired posture, coordination, and balance
- Clubfoot
- Imperforate anus
- Cleft lip and palate
- Pelvic bone abnormalities

Test results
LABORATORY
- Karyotype analysis or chromosome mapping shows the chromosomal abnormality and confirms the diagnosis.
- Serum alpha-fetoprotein reveals reduced levels of alpha-fetoprotein prenatally.

IMAGING
- Prenatal ultrasonography may suggest Down syndrome if a duodenal obstruction or an atrioventricular canal defect is present.

OTHER
- Developmental screening tests show severity and progress of retardation.
- Amniocentesis allows prenatal diagnosis.

◆ TREATMENT

General
- Early intervention
- Special education programs
- Special athletic programs

Diet
- No restriction

Activity
- Maximal environmental simulation for infants
- Safety precautions for children and adults in a controlled environment

Medication
- Antibiotic therapy for recurrent infections
- Thyroid hormone replacement for hypothyroidism

Surgery
- Open-heart surgery to correct cardiac defects, such as ventricular septal defects or atrial septal defects
- Plastic surgery to correct congenital abnormalities, such as protruding tongue, cleft lip, and cleft palate

❖ NURSING CONSIDERATIONS

Nursing diagnoses
- Bathing or hygiene self-care deficit
- Compromised family coping
- Delayed growth and development
- Ineffective health maintenance
- Risk for impaired parenting

Key outcomes
The patient will:
- demonstrate age-appropriate skills and behaviors to the extent possible
- perform health maintenance activities according to level of ability
- participate in developmental stimulation programs to increase skill levels
- express understanding of norms for growth and development.

Nursing interventions
- Establish a trusting relationship with the child's parents.
- Encourage verbalization and provide support.
- Encourage the parents to hold and nurture their child.

Monitoring
- Response to treatment
- Signs and symptoms of infection
- Complications
- Nutritional status
- Growth and development
- Thyroid function test results
- Heart sounds

▶ PATIENT TEACHING

Be sure to cover:
- need for adequate exercise and maximal environmental stimulation
- realistic goals for the parents and child
- information about a balanced diet
- importance of remembering the emotional needs of other children in the family.

Discharge planning
- Refer the parents to infant stimulation classes.
- Refer the parents and older siblings for genetic and psychological counseling, as appropriate.
- Refer the patient to support services.

✴ RESOURCES

Organizations
National Association for Down Syndrome: *www.nads.org*
National Down Syndrome Congress: *www.ndsccenter.org*
National Down Syndrome Society: *www.ndss.org*

Selected references
Diagnostic and Statistical Manual of Mental Disorders, 4th ed., Text Revision. Washington, D.C.: American Psychiatric Association, 2000.

Kasper, D.L., et al., eds. *Harrison's Principles of Internal Medicine,* 16th ed. New York: McGraw-Hill Book Co., 2005.

Melville, C., et al. "Obesity in Adults with Down Syndrome: A Case Control Study," *Journal of Intellectual Disability Research* 49(2):125-33, February 2005.

Zindler, I. "Ethical Decision Making in First Trimester Pregnancy Screening," *Journal of Perinatal & Neonatal Nursing* 19(2):122-31, April-June 2005.

Ectopic pregnancy

● OVERVIEW

Description
- Implantation of a fertilized ovum outside the uterine cavity, most commonly in the fallopian tube (see *Implantation sites of ectopic pregnancy*)
- Good prognosis with prompt diagnosis, appropriate surgical intervention, and control of bleeding
- Very few carried to term; rarely, with abdominal implantation, fetus survives to term
- About 1 in 3 women with ectopic pregnancy giving birth to live neonate in subsequent pregnancy

Pathophysiology
- Transport of a blastocyst to the uterus is delayed.
- The blastocyst implants at another available vascularized site, usually the fallopian tube lining.
- Normal signs of pregnancy are initially present.
- Uterine enlargement occurs in about 25% of cases.
- Human chorionic gonadotropin (HCG) levels are lower than in uterine pregnancies.
- If not interrupted, internal hemorrhage occurs with rupture of the fallopian tube.

Causes
- Endosalpingitis
- Diverticula
- Tumors pressing against the tube
- Previous surgery, such as tubal ligation or resection
- Transmigration of the ovum
- Congenital defects in reproductive tract
- Ectopic endometrial implants in the tubal mucosa
- Sexually transmitted tubal infection
- Intrauterine device

Incidence
- In whites, about 1 of 200 pregnancies
- In nonwhites, about 1 of 120 pregnancies

Risk factors
- Increasing age
- Cigarette smoking
- Use of fertility drugs
- Exposure to DES

Common characteristics
- Abdominal tenderness
- Abdominal discomfort
- Minimal vaginal bleeding
- Amenorrhea

Complications
- Rupture of fallopian tube
- Hemorrhage
- Shock
- Peritonitis
- Infertility
- Disseminated intravascular coagulation
- Death

✳ ASSESSMENT

History
- Amenorrhea
- Abnormal menses (after fallopian tube implantation)
- Slight vaginal bleeding
- Unilateral pelvic pain over the mass
- If fallopian tube ruptures, sharp lower abdominal pain, possibly radiating to the shoulders and neck

◆ **NURSING ALERT** Ectopic pregnancy sometimes produces symptoms of normal pregnancy or no symptoms other than mild abdominal pain (especially in abdominal pregnancy), making diagnosis difficult.

Physical findings
- Possible extreme pain when cervix is moved and adnexa palpated
- Boggy and tender uterus
- Adnexa possibly enlarged

Test results
LABORATORY
- Serum HCG is abnormally low; when repeated in 48 hours, level remains lower than levels found in a normal intrauterine pregnancy.
IMAGING
- Real-time ultrasonography shows intrauterine pregnancy or ovarian cyst.
DIAGNOSTIC PROCEDURES
- Culdocentesis shows free blood in the peritoneum.
- Laparoscopy may reveal pregnancy outside the uterus.

IMPLANTATION SITES OF ECTOPIC PREGNANCY

In about 95% of patients with ectopic pregnancy, the ovum implants in part of the fallopian tube: the fimbria, ampulla, or isthmus. Other possible abnormal sites of implantation include the interstitium, ovarian ligament, ovary, abdominal viscera, and internal cervical os.

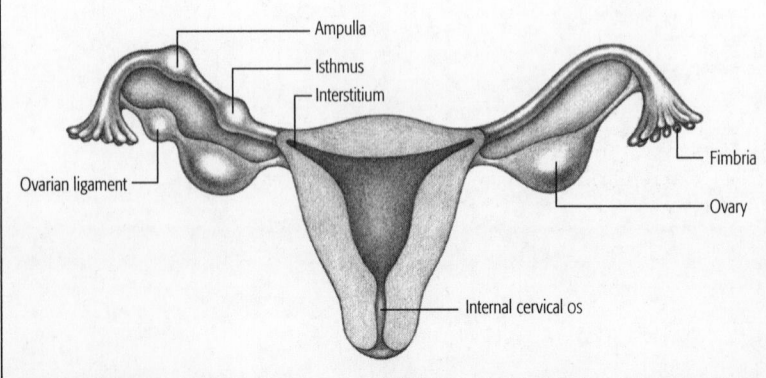

◆ TREATMENT

General
- Initially, in the event of pelvic-organ rupture, management of shock

Diet
- Determined by clinical status

Activity
- Determined by clinical status

Medication
- Transfusion with whole blood or packed red blood cells
- Broad-spectrum I.V. antibiotics
- Supplemental iron
- Methotrexate

Surgery
- Laparotomy and salpingectomy if culdocentesis shows blood in the peritoneum; possibly after laparoscopy to remove affected fallopian tube and control bleeding
- Microsurgical repair of the fallopian tube for patients who wish to have children
- Oophorectomy for ovarian pregnancy
- Hysterectomy for interstitial pregnancy
- Laparotomy to remove the fetus for abdominal pregnancy

✿ NURSING CONSIDERATIONS

Nursing diagnoses
- Acute pain
- Anxiety
- Anticipatory grieving
- Deficient fluid volume
- Deficient knowledge (ectopic pregnancy)
- Fear
- Ineffective coping

Key outcomes
The patient will:
- verbalize feelings of increased comfort and decreased pain
- express feelings of anxiety and grief about the current situation
- maintain adequate fluid volume
- verbalize understanding of the disorder
- discuss fears and concerns of loss
- use available support systems to aid in coping.

Nursing interventions
- Prepare the patient with excessive blood loss for emergency surgery.
- Administer blood transfusions, as ordered.
- Provide emotional support.
- Administer analgesics, as ordered.
- Administer $Rh_o(D)$ immune globulin (RhoGAM), as ordered, if the patient is Rh-negative.
- Determine the date and description of her last menstrual period.
- Provide a quiet, relaxing environment.
- Encourage the patient to express her feelings of fear, loss, and grief.
- Help the patient to develop effective coping strategies.

Monitoring
- Vital signs
- Vaginal bleeding
- Pain
- Intake and output
- Signs of hypovolemia
- Signs of impending shock

▶ PATIENT TEACHING

Be sure to cover:
- disorder, diagnostic tests, and treatment
- surgery
- postoperative care
- prevention of recurrent ectopic pregnancy
- prompt treatment of pelvic infections
- risk factors for ectopic pregnancy, including surgery involving the fallopian tubes and pelvic inflammatory disease.

Discharge planning
- Refer the patient to a mental health professional for additional counseling, if necessary.

✷ RESOURCES

Organizations
American College of Obstetricians and Gynecologists: *www.acog.org*
American Society for Reproductive Medicine: *www.asrm.org*

Selected references
Kirk, E., et al. "The Non-Surgical Management of Ectopic Pregnancy," *Ultrasound in Obstetrics & Gynecology* 27(1):91-100, January 2006.
Latchaw, G., et al. "Risk Factors Associated with the Rupture of Tubal Ectopic Pregnancy," *Gynecologic and Obstetric Investigation* 60(3):177-80, 2005.
Lozeau, A.M., and Poter, B. "Dianogis and Management of Ectopic Pregnancy," *American Family Practitioner* 72(9):1707-714, November 2005.
"Myths and Facts...About Ectopic Pregnancy," *Nursing* 36(8):70, August 2006.

Electric shock

OVERVIEW

Description
- Electric current that passes through body
- Damage dependent on intensity of current, resistance of the tissues it passes through, kind of current, and frequency and duration of current flow
- Classified as lightning, low voltage (less than 600 V), and high voltage (greater than 600 V)

Pathophysiology
- Electrical energy results in altered cell membrane resting potential, causing depolarization in muscles and nerves.
- Electric shock alters normal electrical activity of the heart and brain.
- Electric shock resulting from a high-frequency current generates more heat in tissues than a low-frequency current, resulting in burns and local tissue coagulation and necrosis.
- Muscle tetany is elicited.
- Tissue destruction and coagulative necrosis occurs.

Causes
- Accidental contact with an exposed part of an electrical appliance or wiring
- Lightning
- Flash of electric arcs from high-voltage power lines or machines

Incidence
- Causes more than 500 deaths annually
- More common in men ages 20 to 40

Common characteristics
- Cutaneous burn
- Variable deep tissue damage

Complications
- Sepsis
- Neurologic dysfunction
- Cardiac dysfunction
- Psychiatric dysfunction
- Renal failure
- Electrolyte abnormalities
- Peripheral nerve injuries
- Vascular disruption
- Thrombi

ASSESSMENT

History
- Exposure to electricity or lightening
- Loss of consciousness
- Muscle pain
- Fatigue
- Headache
- Nervous irritability

Physical findings
- Determined by voltage exposure
- Burns
- Local tissue coagulation
- Entrance and exit injuries
- Cyanosis
- Apnea
- Markedly decreased blood pressure
- Cold skin
- Unconsciousness
- Numbness or tingling or sensorimotor deficits

Test results
LABORATORY
- Urinalysis shows evidence of myoglobin.

IMAGING
- Computed tomography or magnetic resonance imaging aids in ruling out intracranial bleeding or brain contusion if patient is unresponsive or unconscious.
- Chest X-rays reveal internal damage, such as fractures.

OTHER
- Electrocardiogram (ECG) reveals cardiac arrhythmias.

TREATMENT

General
- Separation of victim from current source
- Stabilization of cervical spine
- Emergency measures
- Treatment of acid-base imbalance
- Vigorous fluid replacement

Diet
- No restrictions if swallowing ability intact

Activity
- Based on outcome of interventions

Medication
- Osmotic diuretic
- Tetanus prophylaxis

❖ NURSING CONSIDERATIONS

Nursing diagnoses

- Acute pain
- Anxiety
- Decreased cardiac output
- Impaired skin integrity
- Impaired spontaneous ventilation
- Ineffective tissue perfusion: Cardio-pulmonary
- Risk for injury
- Risk for posttrauma syndrome

Key outcomes

The patient will:

- report pain relief with analgesic or other measures
- express feelings of decreased anxiety
- maintain cardiac output
- regain skin integrity
- maintain adequate ventilation either spontaneously or with assisted ventilation
- exhibit signs of adequate cardiopulmonary perfusion
- verbalize methods to prevent future injury from electric shock
- express feelings and fears about the traumatic event.

Nursing interventions

- Separate the victim from the current source.
- Provide emergency treatment.
- Give rapid I.V. fluid infusion.
- Obtain a 12-lead ECG.
- Administer medications, as ordered.

Monitoring

- Cardiac rhythm (continuously)
- Intake and output (hourly)
- Neurologic status
- Sensorimotor deficits
- Peripheral neurovascular status

▶ PATIENT TEACHING

Be sure to cover:

- information about the injury, diagnosis, and treatment
- how to avoid electrical hazards at home and at work
- electrical safety regarding children.

✳ RESOURCES

Organizations

Harborview Injury Prevention and Research Center:
www.depts.washington.edu/hiprc/
National Center for Injury Prevention and Control: *www.cdc.ncipc*

Selected references

Diseases, 4th ed. Philadelphia: Lippincott Williams & Wilkins, 2006.
Hendler, N. "Overlooked Diagnoses in Chronic Pain: Analysis of Survivors of Electric Shock and Lightning Strike," *Journal of Occupational & Environmental Medicine* 47(8):796-805, August 2005.

Emphysema

● OVERVIEW

Description
- Characterized by exertional dyspnea
- One of several diseases usually labeled collectively as chronic obstructive pulmonary disease or chronic obstructive lung disease

Pathophysiology
- Recurrent inflammation associated with the release of proteolytic enzymes from lung cells causes abnormal, irreversible enlargement of the air spaces distal to the terminal bronchioles.
- This enlargement leads to the destruction of alveolar walls, which results in a breakdown of elasticity. (See *What happens in emphysema.*)

Causes
- Genetic deficiency of alpha$_1$-antitrypsin (AAT)
- Cigarette smoking

Incidence
- Most common cause of death from respiratory disease in the United States
- Appears to be more prevalent in men than in women
- Approximately 2 million Americans affected
- Affects 1 in 3,000 neonates

Common characteristics
- Exertional dyspnea
- Chronic cough
- Shortness of breath
- Anorexia and weight loss
- Malaise

Complications
- Recurrent respiratory tract infections
- Cor pulmonale
- Respiratory failure
- Peptic ulcer disease
- Spontaneous pneumothorax
- Pneumomediastinum

✳ ASSESSMENT

History
- Long-time smoking
- Shortness of breath
- Chronic cough
- Anorexia and weight loss
- Malaise

Physical findings
- Barrel chest
- Pursed-lip breathing
- Use of accessory muscles
- Cyanosis
- Clubbed fingers and toes
- Tachypnea
- Decreased tactile fremitus
- Decreased chest expansion
- Hyperresonance
- Decreased breath sounds
- Crackles
- Inspiratory wheeze
- Prolonged expiratory phase with grunting respirations
- Distant heart sounds

Test results
LABORATORY
- Arterial blood gas analysis shows decreased partial pressure of oxygen; partial pressure of carbon dioxide is normal until late in the disease.
- Red blood cell count shows an increased hemoglobin level late in the disease.

IMAGING
- Chest X-ray may show:
  - flattened diaphragm
  - reduced vascular markings at the lung periphery
  - overaeration of the lungs
  - vertical heart
  - enlarged anteroposterior chest diameter
  - large retrosternal air space.

DIAGNOSTIC PROCEDURES
- Pulmonary function tests typically show:
  - increased residual volume and total lung capacity
  - reduced diffusing capacity
  - increased inspiratory flow.
- Electrocardiography may show tall, symmetrical P waves in leads II, III, and aV$_F$; a vertical QRS axis; and signs of right ventricular hypertrophy late in the disease.

◆ TREATMENT

General
- Chest physiotherapy
- Possible transtracheal catheterization and home oxygen therapy
- Mechanical ventilation (for acute exacerbations)

Diet
- Adequate hydration
- High-protein, high-calorie

Activity
- As tolerated

WHAT HAPPENS IN EMPHYSEMA

In normal, healthy breathing, air moves in and out of the lungs to meet metabolic needs. A change in airway size compromises the lungs' ability to circulate sufficient air.

In a patient with emphysema, recurrent pulmonary inflammation damages and eventually destroys the alveolar walls, creating large air spaces. This breakdown leaves the alveoli unable to recoil normally after expanding and results in bronchiolar collapse on expiration. This traps air within the lungs.

Associated pulmonary capillary destruction usually allows a patient with severe emphysema to match ventilation to perfusion and thus avoid cyanosis.

NORMAL ALVEOLI

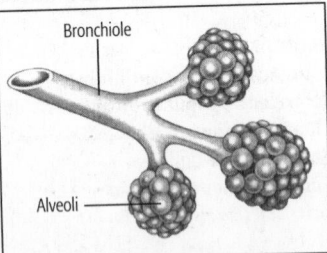

ABNORMAL ALVEOLI

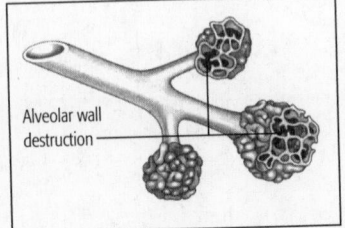

Medication

- Bronchodilators
- Anticholinergics
- Mucolytics
- Corticosteroids
- Antibiotics
- Oxygen

Surgery

- Chest tube insertion for pneumothorax

♣ NURSING CONSIDERATIONS

Nursing diagnoses

- Activity intolerance
- Anxiety
- Deficient knowledge (emphysema)
- Fatigue
- Fear
- Imbalanced nutrition: Less than body requirements
- Impaired gas exchange
- Ineffective airway clearance
- Ineffective breathing pattern
- Interrupted family processes
- Rick of infection

Key outcomes

The patient will:

- perform daily activities to tolerance level
- demonstrate effective coping strategies
- express understanding of the illness
- demonstrate energy conservation techniques
- verbalize feelings of fear related to the diagnosis
- consume adequate calories daily
- maintain adequate ventilation and oxygenation
- maintain a patent airway
- identify appropriate support systems (family)
- remain free from signs and symptoms of infection.

Nursing interventions

- Administer medications, as ordered.
- Provide supportive care.
- Help the patient adjust to lifestyle changes necessitated by a chronic illness.
- Encourage him to express his fears and concerns.
- Include the patient and family members in care-related decisions.
- Perform chest physiotherapy.
- Provide a high-calorie, protein-rich diet.
- Give small, frequent meals.
- Provide frequent mouth care.
- Ensure adequate hydration.
- Encourage daily activity and diversional activities.
- Provide frequent rest periods.

Monitoring

- Vital signs
- Intake and output
- Daily weight
- Complications
- Respiratory status
- Activity tolerance

▶ PATIENT TEACHING

Be sure to cover:

- disorder, diagnostic tests, and treatment
- medication administration, dosage, and possible adverse effects
- when to notify the physician
- avoidance of smoking and areas where smoking is permitted
- avoidance of crowds and people with known infections
- home oxygen therapy, if indicated
- transtracheal catheter care, if needed
- postural drainage and chest percussion
- coughing and deep-breathing exercises
- proper use of handheld inhalers
- high-calorie, protein-rich diet
- adequate oral fluid intake
- avoidance of respiratory irritants
- prevention of bronchospasm
- signs and symptoms of peptic ulcer disease
- signs and symptoms that suggest ruptured alveolar blebs and bullae
- spontaneous pneumothorax.

◈ **NURSING ALERT** Urge the patient to notify the physician if he experiences a sudden onset of worsening dyspnea or sharp pleuritic chest pain exacerbated by chest movement, breathing, or coughing.

Discharge planning

- Refer the patient to a smoking-cessation program, if indicated.
- Refer the patient for influenza and pneumococcal pneumonia immunizations, as needed.
- Refer family members of patients with familial emphysema for AAT deficiency screening.

✸ RESOURCES

Organizations

National Emphysema Foundation: *www.emphysemafoundation.org*
National Institute on Drug Abuse: *www.nida.nih.gov*
Office on Smoking and Health: *www.cdc.gov/tobacco*

Selected references

Nettina, S.M. *Lippincott Manual of Nursing Practice,* 8th ed. Philadelphia: Lippincott Williams & Wilkins, 2006.

Richmond, R.J., and Zellner, K.M. "Al-Antitrypsin Deficiency Incidence and Implications," *Dimensions of Critical Care Nursing* 24(6):255-260, November-December 2005.

Wright, J.L. and Churg, A. "Current Concepts in Mechanisms of Emphysema," *Toxocologic Pathology* 35(1):111-15, 2007.

Encephalitis

● OVERVIEW

Description
- Severe inflammation of the brain

Pathophysiology
- Intense lymphocytic infiltration of brain tissues and the leptomeninges results in:
  - cerebral edema
  - degeneration of the brain's ganglion cells
  - diffuse nerve cell destruction (gray matter more than white).

Causes
- Mosquito- or tick-borne arboviruses specific to rural areas
- Enteroviruses in urban areas (coxsackievirus, poliovirus, and echovirus)
- Herpesvirus
- Mumps virus
- Adenoviruses
- Demyelinating diseases after measles, varicella, rubella, or vaccination
- Human immunodeficiency virus
- Swimming in fresh water (amebic)
- Sytemic viral infection

Incidence
- Determining true incidence nearly impossible because reporting policies differ

Common characteristics
- Dysuria; pyuria
- Fever
- Nausea and vomiting
- Myalgia
- Photophobia
- Stiff neck; headache
- Localized seizures
- Acute confusion or amnesic state

Complications
- Bronchial pneumonia
- Urinary retention and urinary tract infection
- Pressure ulcers
- Coma
- Parkinsonism
- Mental deterioration
- Seizures
- Stroke

✳ ASSESSMENT

History
- Systemic symptoms including:
  - headache
  - muscle stiffness and malaise
  - sore throat and upper respiratory tract symptoms
  - sudden onset of altered levels of consciousness
  - seizures

Physical findings
- Confusion, disorientation, or hallucinations
- Tremors
- Cranial nerve palsies
- Exaggerated deep tendon reflexes and absent superficial reflexes
- Paresis or paralysis of the extremities
- Stiff neck when the head is bent forward
- Fever
- Nausea and vomiting
- Cerebral hemispheres
- Aphasia
- Involuntary movements
- Ataxia
- Sensory defects

Test results
- Diagnosis is readily made from the clinical findings and patient history.

LABORATORY
- Blood analysis identifys the virus.
- Serologic studies in herpes encephalitis show rising titers of complement-fixing antibodies.

IMAGING
- Computed tomography scan rules out cerebral hematoma.

DIAGNOSTIC PROCEDURES
- Cerebrospinal fluid (CSF) analysis identifies the virus.
- Lumbar puncture discloses CSF pressure.

OTHER
- EEG shows slowing of waveforms.

◆ TREATMENT

General
- Supportive measures
- Airway maintenance
- Oxygen administration

Diet
- Adequate fluid and electrolyte intake
- As tolerated

Activity
- As tolerated

Medication
- Osmotic diuretics
- Corticosteroids
- Anticonvulsants
- Aspirin or acetaminophen
- Antibiotics
- Antiviral agent. vidarabine

❖ NURSING CONSIDERATIONS

Nursing diagnoses
- Acute pain
- Anxiety
- Deficient knowledge (encephalitis)
- Disturbed thought processes
- Hyperthermia
- Imbalanced nutrition: Less than body requirements
- Impaired gas exchange
- Impaired physical mobility
- Risk for deficient fluid volume
- Risk for impaired skin integrity

Key outcomes
The patient will:
- verbalize feelings of increased comfort and and decreased pain
- report feeling less anxious
- verbalize understanding of the disorder
- exhibit temperature within normal limits
- consume adequate calorie requirements daily
- maintain adequate ventilation and oxygenation
- maintain joint mobility and muscle strength
- exhibit fluid balance within normal limits
- maintain skin integrity.

Nursing interventions
- Assure adequate fluid intake.
- Administer medications, as ordered.
- Position and turn the patient often.
- Assist with range-of-motion exercises.
- Maintain adequate nutrition.
- Administer laxatives or stool softeners.
- Administer mouth care.
- Maintain a quiet environment.
- Start seizure precautions, if necessary.
- Reorient the patient often, if necessary.

Monitoring
- Neurologic function (continuous) for cranial nerve involvement
- Intake and output
- Response to medications
- Intracranial pressure (severe cases)

▶ PATIENT TEACHING

Be sure to cover:
- disorder, diagnosis, and treatment
- transient behavior changes
- medication administration, dosage, and possible adverse effects
- follow-up care.

Discharge planning
- Refer the patient to an outpatient rehabilitation program, as indicated.

✳ RESOURCES

Organizations
American Academy of Neurology: *www.aan.com*
National Institutes of Health: *www.nih.gov*
WebMD: *www.webmd.com*

Selected references
De Tiege, X., et al. "Herpes Simplex Encephalitis: Diagnostic Probems and Late Relapse," *Developmental Medicine and Child Neurology* 48(1):60-63, January 2006.

Diseases, 4th ed. Philadelphia: Lippincott Williams & Wilkins, 2006.

Handbook of Pathophysiology, 2nd ed. Philadelphia: Lippincott Williams & Wilkins, 2005.

Mandell, G.L., et al. *Principles and Practice of Infectious Diseases,* 6th ed. New York: Churchill-Livingstone, Inc., 2005.

Endocarditis

Description
- Infection of the endocardium, heart valves, or cardiac prosthesis
- Includes three types: native valve (acute and subacute) endocarditis, prosthetic valve (early and late) endocarditis, and endocarditis related to I.V. drug abuse (usually involving the tricuspid valve)

Pathophysiology
- Fibrin and platelets cluster on valve tissue and engulf circulating bacteria or fungi. (See *Degenerative changes in endocarditis*.)
- This produces vegetation, which in turn may cover the valve surfaces, causing deformities and destruction of valvular tissue and may extend to the chordae tendineae, causing them to rupture, leading to valvular insufficiency.
- Vegetative growth on the heart valves, endocardial lining of the heart chamber, or the endothelium of a blood vessel may embolize to the spleen, kidneys, central nervous system, and lungs.

Causes
NATIVE VALVE ENDOCARDITIS
- Alpha-hemolytic *Streptococcus* or enterococci (subacute form)
- Group B hemolytic *Streptococcus*
- *Staphylococcus aureus*
PROSTHETIC VALVE
- Alpha-hemolytic *Streptococcus*, enterococci, and *Staphylococcus* (late; 60 days or more after implant)
- *Staphylococcus*, gram-negative bacilli, and *Candida* (early; within 60 days after implant)
RELATED TO I.V. DRUG ABUSE
- *S. aureus*

Incidence
- No underlying heart disease in up to 40% of affected patients
- More common in males (especially drug abusers) than in females
- Most patients over age 50
- Uncommon in children
- Rheumatic valvular disease accounts for about 25% of all cases

- Mitral valve most common valve involved

Common characteristics
- Heart murmur

Complications
- Left-sided heart failure
- Valve stenosis or regurgitation
- Myocardial erosion
- Embolic debris lodged in the small vasculature of the visceral tissue

History
- Predisposing condition
- Complaints of nonspecific symptoms, such as weakness, fatigue, weight loss, anorexia, arthralgia, night sweats, and intermittent fever that may recur for weeks
- Dyspnea and chest pain common with I.V. drug abusers

Physical findings
- Petechiae on the skin (especially common on the upper anterior trunk) and on the buccal, pharyngeal, or conjunctival mucosa
- Splinter hemorrhages under the nails
- Clubbing of the fingers in patients with long-standing disease
- Heart murmur in all patients except those with early acute endocarditis and I.V. drug users with tricuspid valve infection
- Osler's nodes
- Roth's spots
- Janeway lesions
- A murmur that changes suddenly or a new murmur that develops in the presence of fever—a classic finding
- Splenomegaly in long-standing disease
- Dyspnea, tachycardia, and bibasilar crackles possible with left-sided heart failure
- Splenic infarction causing pain in the upper left quadrant, radiating to the left shoulder, and abdominal rigidity
- Renal infarction causing hematuria, pyuria, flank pain, and decreased urine output

- Cerebral infarction causing hemiparesis, aphasia, and other neurologic deficits
- Pulmonary infarction causing cough, pleuritic pain, pleural friction rub, dyspnea, and hemoptysis
- Peripheral vascular occlusion causing numbness and tingling in arm, leg, finger, or toe or signs of impending peripheral gangrene

Test results
LABORATORY
- Three or more blood cultures during a 24- to 48-hour period identify the causative organism (in up to 90% of patients).
- White blood cell count and differential are normal or elevated.
- Complete blood count and anemia panel show normocytic, normochromic anemia in subacute infective endocarditis.
- Erythrocyte sedimentation rate and serum creatinine levels are elevated.
- Serum rheumatoid factor is positive in about half of all patients with endocarditis after the disease is present for 6 weeks.
- Urinalysis shows proteinuria and microscopic hematuria.
IMAGING
- Echocardiography may identify valvular damage in up to 80% of patients with native valve disease.

DEGENERATIVE CHANGES IN ENDOCARDITIS

This illustration shows typical vegetations on the endocardium produced by fibrin and platelet deposits on infection sites.

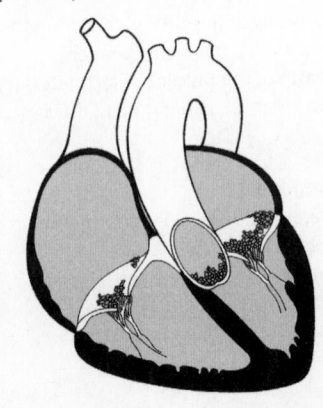

DIAGNOSTIC PROCEDURES
- An electrocardiogram reading may show atrial fibrillation and other arrhythmias that accompany valvular disease.

◆ TREATMENT

General
- Prompt therapy that continues for several weeks
- Selection of anti-infective drug based on type of infecting organism and sensitivity studies
- For negative blood cultures (10% to 20% of subacute cases), possible I.V. antibiotic therapy (usually for 4 to 6 weeks) against probable infecting organism

Diet
- Sufficient fluid intake

Activity
- Bed rest

Medication
- Aspirin
- Antibiotics

Surgery
- For severe valvular damage, especially aortic insufficiency or infection of a cardiac prosthesis, possible corrective surgery if refractory heart failure develops or if an infected prosthetic valve must be replaced

❖ NURSING CONSIDERATIONS

Nursing diagnoses
- Activity intolerance
- Decreased cardiac output
- Deficient diversional activity
- Impaired gas exchange
- Ineffective role performance

Key outcomes
The patient will:
- carry out activities of daily living without weakness or fatigue
- maintain hemodynamic stability with adequate cardiac output
- exhibit no arrhythmias
- express interest in using leisure time meaningfully
- maintain adequate ventilation and oxygenation
- express feelings about diminished capacity to perform usual roles.

Nursing interventions
- Stress the importance of bed rest.
- Provide a bedside commode.
- Allow the patient to express his concerns.
- Obtain a history of allergies.
- Administer antibiotics on time.
- Administer oxygen.

Monitoring
 NURSING ALERT Watch for signs of embolization, a common occurrence during the first 3 months of treatment. Tell the patient to watch for and report these signs.
- Renal status
- Frequent cardiovascular status assessment
- Arterial blood gas evaluation, as needed

▶ PATIENT TEACHING

Be sure to cover:
- disorder, diagnosis, and treatment
- anti-infectives the patient needs to continue taking
- need to watch closely for fever, anorexia, and other signs of relapse about 2 weeks after treatment stops
- need for prophylactic antibiotics before dental work and some surgical procedures
- proper dental hygiene and to avoid flossing the teeth
- how to recognize symptoms of endocarditis, and to notify the physician immediately if such symptoms occur.

✳ RESOURCES

Organizations
Mayo Health Clinic: *www.mayohealth.org*
National Heart, Lung and Blood Institute: *www.nhlbi.nih.gov/nhlbi/cardio*

Selected references
Eftychiou, C., et al. "Factors Associated with Non-bacterial Thrombotic Endocarditis: Case Report and Literature Review," *Journal of Heart Valve Disease* 14(6):859-62, November 2005.

Habib, G. "Management of Infective Endocarditis," *Heart* 92(1):124-30, January 2006.

Kasper, D.L., et al., eds. *Harrison's Principles of Internal Medicine,* 16th ed. New York: McGraw-Hill Book Co., 2005.

The Merck Manual, 18th ed. Whitehouse Station, N.J.: Merck and Co., Inc., 2006.

Endometriosis

● OVERVIEW

Description
- Poorly understood gynecological condition characterized by pain occurring with menstruation
- Endometrial tissue appearring outside uterine cavity lining
- Ectopic tissue generally confined to the pelvic area, but can appear anywhere in the body

Pathophysiology
- Endometrial cells respond to estrogen and progesterone with proliferation and secretion.
- During menstruation, ectopic tissue bleeds and causes inflammation of the surrounding tissues.
- Inflammation leads to fibrosis.
- Fibrosis leads to adhesions that produce pain and infertility.

Causes
- Exact cause unknown
- Familial susceptibility
- Direct implantation
- Transportation (retrograde menstruation)
- Formation in situ
- Induction
- Immune system defects
- Lymphatic spread theory
- Inflammatory influence
- Environmental contaminants

Incidence
- Usually occurs between ages 20 and 40
- More common in women who postpone childbearing
- Uncommon before age 20

Common characteristics
- Early menarche
- Menstrual flow lasting more than 7 days
- Cycles lasting more than 27 days
- Family history of endometriosis
- Multiparity
- Cyclic pelvic pain
- Severe dysmenorrhea

Complications
- Infertility
- Spontaneous abortion
- Anemia secondary to excessive bleeding
- Emotional problems secondary to infertility
- Pelvic adhesions
- Severe dysmenorrhea
- Ovarian cyst

✳ ASSESSMENT

History
- Cyclic pelvic pain that peaks 5 to 7 days before menses and lasts 2 to 3 days
- Infertility
- Acquired dysmenorrhea
- Pain in lower abdomen, vagina, posterior pelvis and back; often radiates down legs
- Additional symptoms dependent on site of involvement include:
  - Hypermenorrhea (oviducts and ovaries)
  - Deep-thrust dyspareunia (ovaries and cul-de-sac)
  - Suprapubic pain, dysuria, and hematuria (bladder)
  - Dyschezia, rectal bleeding with menses, and pain in the coccyx or sacrum (rectovaginal septum and colon)
  - Nausea and vomiting that worsen before menses (small bowel and appendix)
  - Abdominal cramps (small bowel and appendix)

Physical findings
- Multiple tender nodules on uterosacral ligaments or rectovaginal septum that enlarge and become more tender during menses
- Ovarian enlargement with endometrial cysts on the ovaries
- Thickened, nodular adnexa

Test results
DIAGNOSTIC PROCEDURES
- A scoring and staging system created by the American Fertility Society quantifies endometrial implants according to size, character, and location:
  - Stage I is minimal disease (1 to 5 points).
  - Stage II signifies mild disease (6 to 15 points).
  - Stage III indicates moderate disease (16 to 40 points).
  - Stage IV indicates severe disease (more than 40 points).
- Laparoscopy results confirm the diagnosis and identify the disease stage.

◆ TREATMENT

General
- Stage of disease, patient's age, and desire to have children determining course of treatment
- Pregnancy, if possible, is temporary treatment

Diet
- No restrictions

Activity
- As tolerated

Medication
- Progestins
- Hormonal contraceptives
- Gonadotropin-releasing analogues
- Androgens
- Analgesics

Surgery
- Laparoscopy to lyse adhesions, remove small implants, and cauterize implants and for laser vaporization of implants; usually followed by hormonal therapy to suppress return of endometrial implants
- Total abdominal hysterectomy with bilateral salpingo-oophorectomy in stages III and IV

❖ NURSING CONSIDERATIONS

Nursing diagnoses
- Anxiety
- Chronic pain
- Deficient knowledge (endometriosis)
- Disturbed body image
- Fear
- Ineffective coping
- Risk for infection
- Sexual dysfunction

Key outcomes
The patient will:
- report feeling less anxious
- express feelings of increased comfort and decreased pain
- express understanding of the disorder and treatment
- express positive feelings about self and decreased feelings of fear
- develop adequate coping behaviors
- remain free from infection
- verbalize feelings related to changes in sexual functioning.

Nursing interventions
- Encourage the patient to express her feelings about the disorder.
- Offer the patient emotional support.
- Encourage using open communication before and during intercourse.
- Help the patient to develop effective coping strategies.

Monitoring
- Response to treatment
- Complications
- Adverse drug reactions
- Coping ability

▶ PATIENT TEACHING

Be sure to cover:
- disorder, diagnosis, and treatment
- misconceptions about the disorder
- associated complications
- infertility
- using sanitary napkins instead of tampons in adolescents
- avoiding minor gynecologic procedures immediately before and during menstruation
- not postponing childbearing due to potential for infertility
- importance of annual pelvic examination and Papanicolaou test.

Discharge planning
- Refer the patient and her partner to a mental health professional for additional counseling, if necessary.
- Refer the patient to a support group, such as the Endometriosis Association.

✷ RESOURCES

Organizations
American College of Obstetricians and Gynecologists: *www.acog.org*
American Society for Reproductive Medicine: *www.asrm.org*
Endometriosis Association: *www.endometriosisassn.org*

Selected references
Huntington, A., and Gilmour, J.A. "A Life Shaped by Pain: Women and Endometriosis," *Journal of Clinical Nursing* 14(9):1124-132, October 2005.
Jackson, L.W., et al. "Oxidative Stress and Endometriosis," *Human Reproduction* 29(7):2014-2020, July 2005.
"Myths and Facts...About Endometriosis," *Nursing* 35(4):28, April 2005.
Pilliterri, A. *Maternal and Child Health Nursing: Care for the Childbearing and Childrearing Family,* 5th ed. Philadelphia: Lippincott Williams & Wilkins, 2006.

Enterobacteriaceae infections

● OVERVIEW

Description
- Family of mostly aerobic, gram-negative bacilli
- Cause local and systemic infections, including invasive diarrhea resembling shigellosis and noninvasive, toxin-mediated diarrhea resembling cholera
- *Escherichia coli* most common cause of nosocomial infections

Pathophysiology
- When infected, incubation takes 12 to 72 hours.
- Noninvasive diarrhea results from two toxins produced by enterotoxigenic or enteropathogenic strains of *E. coli*.
- Toxins interact with intestinal juices and promote excessive loss of chloride and water.
- The invasive form directly attacks the intestinal mucosa without producing enterotoxins, causing local irritation, inflammation, and diarrhea. This form produces sporadic and outbreak-associated bloody diarrhea due to hemorrhagic colitis, which can be life threatening at age extremes.

Causes
- Some strains of *E. coli* that are part of normal GI flora but cause infection in immunocompromised patients
- Infection usually from nonindigenous strains
- Transmission directly from an infected person
- Ingestion of contaminated food or water or contact with contaminated utensils (ground beef most common food source)
- Enterotoxigenic *E. coli* (major cause of diarrhea among those who travel from industrialized to developing regions)

Incidence
- May be major cause of diarrheal illness in children in United States
- Incidence highest among travelers returning from other countries, especially Mexico (noninvasive form), Southeast Asia (noninvasive form), and South America (invasive form)

Common characteristics
- Diarrhea (cardinal symptom)

Complications
- Bacteremia
- Severe dehydration and life-threatening electrolyte disturbances
- Acidosis
- Shock

✳ ASSESSMENT

History
- Recent travel to another country
- Ingestion of contaminated food or water
- Recent close contact with a person who has diarrhea
- Abrupt onset of watery diarrhea

Physical findings
- Cramping abdominal pain with hyperactive bowel sounds
- Blood and pus in infected stools
- Vomiting and anorexia
- Low-grade fever
- Signs of dehydration, especially in children
- Signs and symptoms of hyponatremia, hypokalemia, hypomagnesemia, and hypocalcemia from electrolyte losses
- Orthostatic hypotension
- Rapid, thready pulse
- Initially in infants, loose, watery stools that change from yellow to green and contain little mucus or blood
- Listlessness and irritability in infants

Test results
LABORATORY
- Cultures—any growth of *E. coli* in a normally sterile location, including the bloodstream, cerebrospinal fluid, biliary tract, pleural fluid, or peritoneal cavity—suggest *E. coli* infection at that site.

◆ TREATMENT

General
- Contact precautions if patient is incontinent
- Correction of fluid and electrolyte imbalances

Diet
- Initially, nothing by mouth
- Increased fluid intake (if appropriate)
- Avoidance of foods that cause diarrhea
- Small frequent meals until bowel function returns to normal

Medication
- I.V. antibiotics
- Bismuth subsalicylate or tincture of opium

NURSING CONSIDERATIONS

Nursing diagnoses
- Acute pain
- Deficient fluid volume
- Diarrhea
- Imbalanced nutrition: Less than body requirements
- Ineffective tissue perfusion: Cardio-pulmonary, GI
- Risk for infection

Key outcomes
The patient will:
- express feelings of increased comfort and decreased pain
- regain or maintain normal fluid and electrolyte balance
- exhibit an elimination pattern that returns to normal
- show no further evidence of weight loss
- maintain normal cardiac output and GI perfusion
- remain free from signs and symptoms of infection.

Nursing interventions
- Institute contact precautions and use proper hand-washing technique.
- Replace fluids and electrolytes as needed.
- Clean the perianal area and lubricate it after each episode of diarrhea.
- Administer antibiotics, as ordered.
- During epidemics, screen all facility personnel and visitors for diarrhea, and prevent people with the disorder from having direct patient contact.

Monitoring
- Intake and output
- Stool volume measurement and presence of blood and pus
- Serum electrolyte results
- Signs and symptoms of gram-negative septic shock
- Signs and symptoms of dehydration
- Vital signs (to detect early indications of circulatory collapse)
- Routine surveillance cultures and evaluation of culture and sensitivity tests to find resistant strains of *E. coli* in patients on antibiotic therapy

PATIENT TEACHING

Be sure to cover:
- disorder, diagnostic tests, and treatment
- proper hand-washing technique for facility personnel, patients, and their families
- importance of washing hands before eating or preparing food and after defecating, changing diapers, or having contact with stool
- need for travelers to other countries to avoid unbottled water, ice, unpeeled fruit, and uncooked vegetables
- signs of dehydration and seeking prompt medical attention if these occur (if the patient is to be cared for at home).

RESOURCES

Organizations
Centers for Disease Control and Prevention: *www.cdc.gov*
Harvard University Consumer Health Information: *www.intelihealth.com*
National Health Information Center: *www.health.gov/nhic/*
National Library of Medicine: *www.nlm.nih.gov*

Selected references
Kasper, D.L., et al., eds. *Harrison's Principles of Internal Medicine,* 16th ed. New York: McGraw-Hill Book Co., 2005.
Mandell, G.L., et al. *Principles and Practice of Infectious Diseases,* 6th ed. New York: Churchill-Livingstone, Inc., 2005.

Epididymitis

● OVERVIEW

Description
- Infection of the epididymis (cordlike excretory duct of the testis)
- One of most common infections of the male reproductive tract

Pathophysiology
- Organisms enter the epididymis by the vas deferens or lymphatics, resulting in inflammation.
- Other organs, such as the testes and prostate, may be affected.

Causes
- Brucellosis
- Certain drugs (such as amiodarone [Cordarone])
- Leprosy
- Obstruction
- Pyogenic organisms, such as staphylococci, *Escherichia coli,* streptococci, chlamydia, *Neisseria gonorrhoeae,* and *Treponema pallidum*
- Sarcoidosis
- Trauma
- Tuberculosis

Risk factors
- Urinary tract infection
- Unprotected sex
- Prostatitis
- Trauma

Incidence
- Usually affects boys and men ages 15 to 30 or older than 60
- Rare before puberty
- Affects 1 in 1,000 men annually

Common characteristics
- Dull, aching groin pain
- Fever

Complications
- Orchitis (see *Understanding orchitis*)
- Infertility
- Abscess
- Atrophy
- Pyocele
- Infarction

✳ ASSESSMENT

History
- Unilateral, dull, aching pain
- Pain that radiates to spermatic cord, lower abdomen, and flank
- Extremely heavy feeling in scrotum
- Dysuria, frequency, urgency

Physical findings
- Erythema
- High fever
- Characteristic waddle (attempt to protect groin and scrotum while walking)
- Mild scrotal cellulitis
- Urethral discharge
- Prehn's sign
- Tenderness and induration in epididymal tail

Test results
LABORATORY
- Urinalysis shows an increased white blood cell (WBC) count, indicating infection.
- Urine culture and sensitivity tests may show the causative organism.
- Serum WBC count is greater than 10,000/μl, indicating infection.
IMAGING
- Ultrasonography shows enlarged epididymis (greater than 17 mm); can rule out testicular torsion.

◆ TREATMENT

General
- Scrotal elevation
- Ice bag to groin

Diet
- Increased oral fluids

Activity
- Bed rest until condition improves
- Use of an athletic supporter until recovered

Medication
- Broad-spectrum antibiotics
- Analgesics
- Antipyretics
- Anti-inflammatory agents

Surgery
- Serotal exploration for complications of epididymitis
- Epididymectomy under local anesthesia when disease is refractory to antibiotic therapy

---

UNDERSTANDING ORCHITIS

Orchitis, an infection of the testes, is a serious complication of epididymitis. It also may result from mumps, which can lead to sterility or, less commonly, another systemic infection.

Signs and symptoms
Typical effects of orchitis include unilateral or bilateral tenderness and redness, sudden onset of pain, and swelling of the scrotum and testes. Nausea and vomiting also occur. Sudden cessation of pain indicates testicular ischemia, which can cause permanent damage to one or both testes. Hydrocele also may be present.

Treatment
Appropriate treatment consists of immediate antibiotic therapy in bacterial infection or, in mumps orchitis, injection of 20 ml of lidocaine near the spermatic cord of the affected testis, which may relieve swelling and pain. Severe orchitis may require surgery to incise and drain the hydrocele and to improve testicular circulation. Other treatments are similar to those for epididymitis.

To prevent mumps orchitis, suggest that prepubertal males receive the mumps vaccine (or gamma globulin injection after contracting mumps).

Nursing diagnoses

- Acute pain
- Disturbed body image
- Hyperthermia
- Impaired urinary elimination
- Ineffective sexuality patterns
- Risk for infection
- Risk for injury
- Sexual dysfunction

Key outcomes

The patient will:

- express feelings of increased comfort and decreased pain
- express positive feelings about self-concept and body image
- maintain a normal body temperature
- demonstrate skill in managing urinary elimination problem
- express feelings about potential or actual changes in sexual activity
- remain free from signs or symptoms of infection
- avoid or minimize injury
- resume sexual activity to the fullest extent possible.

Nursing interventions

- Administer medications as ordered.
- Apply ice packs for comfort.

Monitoring

- Signs of abscess formation
- Vital signs
- Pain control
- Intake and output

Be sure to cover:

- disorder, diagnostic tests, and treatment
- medication administration, dosage, and possible adverse effects
- use of a scrotal support while sitting, standing, or walking
- safer sex practices.

Organizations

American Association of Kidney Patients: *www.aakp.org*

National Institute of Diabetes & Digestive & Kidney Diseases: *www.niddk.nih.gov*

Selected references

Brissom, P., et al. "Torsion of the Epididymis," *Journal of Pediatric Surgery* 40(1):1795-797, November 2005.

Diseases, 4th ed. Philadelphia: Lippincott Williams & Wilkins, 2006.

Ringdahl, E. and Teague, L. "Testicular Tortion," *American Family Physician* 74(10):1739-43, November 15, 2006.

Wilson, S.R. and Katz, D.S. "Computed Tomography Demonstration of Epididymitis with Extension to Vas Deferens," *Urology* 68(6):1339-40, December 2006.

Epiglottiditis

● OVERVIEW

Description
- Acute inflammation of the epiglottis and surrounding area
- Life-threatening emergency that rapidly causes edema and induration
- If untreated, results in complete airway obstruction
- Mortality 8% to 12%, typically in children ages 2 to 8

Pathophysiology
- An infection of the epiglottis and surrounding area leads to intense inflammation of the supraglottic region.
- Swelling of the epiglottis, aryepiglottic folds, arytenoid cartilage, and ventricular bands leads to acute airway obstruction.

Causes
- Bacterial infection, usually *Haemophilus influenzae* type B
- Pneumococci or group A streptococci
- Thermal injuries

Incidence
- Occurs from infancy to adulthood
- Occurs in any season
- Males accounting for 60% of cases

Common characteristics
- Sore throat
- Dysphagia
- Apprehension
- Irritability

Complications
- Airway obstruction
- Death

✳ ASSESSMENT

History
- Recent upper respiratory tract infection
- Sore throat
- Dysphagia
- Sudden onset of high fever

Physical findings
- Red and inflamed throat
- Fever
- Drooling
- Pale or cyanotic skin
- Restlessness and irritability
- Nasal flaring
- Patient may sit in tripod position
- Thick and muffled voice sounds

Test results
LABORATORY
- Arterial blood gas analysis may show hypoxia.

IMAGING
- Lateral neck X-rays show an enlarged epiglottis and distended hypopharynx.

DIAGNOSTIC PROCEDURES
- Direct laryngoscopy shows a swollen, beefy-red epiglottis.

OTHER
- Pulse oximetry may show decreased oxygen saturation.

◆ TREATMENT

General
- Emergency hospitalization
- Humidification
- Parenteral fluids

Diet
- As tolerated

Activity
- As tolerated

Medication
- Parenteral antibiotics
- Corticosteroids
- Oxygen therapy

Surgery
- Possible tracheotomy

✤ NURSING CONSIDERATIONS

Nursing diagnoses
- Anxiety
- Deficient fluid volume
- Fear
- Imbalanced nutrition: Less than body requirements
- Impaired gas exchange
- Impaired verbal communication
- Ineffective airway clearance

Key outcomes
The patient will:
- use effective coping strategies
- maintain adequate fluid volume
- verbalize feelings and concerns
- maintain adequate caloric intake
- maintain adequate ventilation and oxygenation
- use alternate means of communication
- maintain a patent airway. (See *Airway crisis.*)

Nursing interventions
- Administer medications, as ordered.
- Place the patient in a sitting position.
- Place the patient in a cool-mist tent.
- Encourage the parents to remain with their child.
- Offer reassurance and support.
- Ensure adequate fluid intake.
- Minimize external stimuli.

Monitoring
- Vital signs
- Intake and output
- Respiratory status
- ABG results
- Pulse oximetry
- Signs and symptoms of secondary infection
- Signs and symptoms of dehydration

▶ PATIENT TEACHING

Be sure to cover:
- disorder, diagnostic tests, and treatment
- medication administration, dosage, and possible adverse effects
- when to call the physician
- humidification
- signs and symptoms of respiratory distress
- signs and symptoms of dehydration.

Discharge planning
- Refer the patient for *H. influenzae* b conjugate vaccine, preferably at age 2 months, if indicated.

AIRWAY CRISIS

Epiglottiditis can progress to complete airway obstruction within minutes. To prepare for this medical emergency, keep the following tips in mind:

- Watch for the inability to speak; weak, ineffective cough; high-pitched sounds or no sounds while inhaling; increased difficulty breathing; and possible cyanosis. These are warning signs of total airway obstruction and the need for an emergency tracheotomy.
- Keep the following equipment available at the patient's bedside in case of sudden, complete airway obstruction: a tracheotomy tray, endotracheal tubes, a manual resuscitation bag, oxygen equipment, and a laryngoscope with blades of various sizes.
- Remember that using a tongue blade or throat culture swab can initiate sudden, complete airway obstruction.
- Before examining the patient's throat, request trained personnel, such as an anesthesiologist, to stand by if emergency airway insertion is needed.

✻ RESOURCES

Organizations
American Academy of Pediatrics: *www.aap.org*

Selected references
Diseases, 4th ed. Philadelphia: Lippincott Williams & Wilkins, 2006.

Katori, H., and Tsukuda, M. "Acute Epiglottitis: Analysis of Factors Associated with Airway Interventions," *Journal of Laryngology and Otology* 119(12):967-72, December 2006.

Pillitterri, A. *Maternal and Child Health Nursing: Care for the Childbearing and Childrearing Family,* 5th ed. Philadelphia: Lippincott Williams & Wilkins, 2006.

Epilepsy

● OVERVIEW

Description
- Susceptibility to recurrent seizures
- Doesn't affect intelligence
- In 80% of patients, good seizure control with strict adherence to prescribed treatment
- Also known as *seizure disorder*

Pathophysiology
- Seizures are paroxysmal events involving abnormal electrical discharges of neurons in the brain and cell membrane potential that's less negative than usual.
- On stimulation, the neuron fires, the discharge spreads to surrounding cells, and stimulation continues to one side or both sides of the brain.

Causes
- Half of cases idiopathic

NONIDIOPATHIC EPILEPSY
- Birth trauma
- Anoxia
- Perinatal infection
- Genetic abnormalities (tuberous sclerosis and phenylketonuria)
- Perinatal injuries
- Metabolic abnormalities (hypoglycemia, pyridoxine deficiency, hypoparathyroidism)
- Brain tumors or other space-occupying lesions
- Meningitis, encephalitis, or brain abscess
- Traumatic injury
- Ingestion of toxins, such as mercury, lead, or carbon monoxide
- Cerebrovascular accident
- Apparent familial incidence in some seizure disorders

Incidence
- First seizure usually occurring in childhood or after age 50
- Affects 1% to 2% of population

Common characteristics
- Recurring seizures

Complications
- Anoxia
- Traumatic injury

✳ ASSESSMENT

History
- Seizure occurrence unpredictable and unrelated to activities
- Precipitating factors or events possibly reported
- Headache
- Mood changes
- Lethargy
- Myoclonic jerking
- Description of an aura
- Pungent smell
- GI distress
- Rising or sinking feeling in the stomach
- Dreamy feeling
- Unusual taste in the mouth
- Visual disturbance
- Family history of epilepsy

Physical findings
- Findings possibly normal while patient isn't having a seizure and when the cause is idiopathic
- Findings related to underlying cause of the seizure

Test results
LABORATORY
- Serum glucose and calcium study results rule out other diagnoses.

IMAGING
- Computed tomography scan and magnetic resonance imaging may indicate abnormalities in internal structures.
- Skull radiography may show certain neoplasms within the brain substance or skull fractures.
- Brain scan may show malignant lesions when X-ray findings are normal or questionable.
- Cerebral angiography may show cerebrovascular abnormalities, such as aneurysm or tumor.

OTHER
- EEG shows paroxysmal abnormalities. A negative EEG doesn't rule out epilepsy because paroxysmal abnormalities occur intermittently.

◆ TREATMENT

General
- Vagal nerve stimulation by pacemaker (see *Vagal nerve stimulation*)
- Detailed presurgical evaluation to characterize seizure type, frequency, site of onset, psychological functioning, and degree of disability to select candidates for surgery in medically intractable patients
- Safety measures; seizure precautions

Diet
- No restrictions
- Regular meals

Activity
- As tolerated

Medication
- Anticonvulsants

Surgery
- Removal of a demonstrated focal lesion
- Correction of the underlying problem

VAGAL NERVE STIMULATION

The vagal nerve stimulator is a Food and Drug Administration–approved method to treat medically refractory epilepsy. The stimulator device is about the size of a pacemaker and is surgically placed in a pocket under the skin in the upper chest. Lead wires from the stimulator are tunneled under the skin to a neck incision where the vagal nerve has been exposed. The electrode coils are then placed around the nerve. The treating physician has a computer that can be used to alter the stimulation parameters, thereby optimizing the treatment of seizures.

The device stimulates the vagus nerve for 30 seconds every 5 minutes to prevent seizure occurrence. A magnet over the area can activate the device to give extra, on-demand stimulation if the patient feels a seizure coming on. Adverse effects include voice change, throat discomfort, shortness of breath, and coughing and are usually only felt when the device is "on."

✣ NURSING CONSIDERATIONS

Nursing diagnoses
- Anxiety
- Deficient knowledge (epilepsy)
- Fear
- Ineffective coping
- Risk for injury
- Social isolation

Key outcomes
The patient will:
- express feelings of decreased anxiety
- communicate understanding of the condition and treatment regimen
- express feelings of decreased fear
- use support systems and develop adequate coping
- remain free from injury
- resume active participation in social situations and activities.

Nursing interventions
- Institute seizure precautions.
- Prepare the patient for surgery, if indicated.
- Administer anticonvulsants, as ordered.

Monitoring
- Response to anticonvulsants
- Vital signs
- Seizure activity
- Respiratory status
- Adverse drug reactions
- Associated injuries

▶ PATIENT TEACHING

Be sure to cover:
- disorder, diagnostic tests, and treatment
- maintaining a normal lifestyle
- medication administration, dosage, and possible adverse effects
- care during a seizure
- importance of regular meals and checking with the doctor before dieting
- importance of carrying a medical identification card.

Discharge planning
- Refer the patient to the Epilepsy Foundation of America.
- Refer the patient to his state's motor vehicle department for information about a driver's license.

✴ RESOURCES

Organizations
American Academy of Pediatrics: *www.aap.org*
Epilepsy Foundation of America: *www.efa.org*
National Institutes of Health: *www.nih.gov*

Selected references
Crawford, P. "Best Practice Guidelines for the Management of Women with Epilepsy," *Epilepsia* 46:117-24, 2005.

Diseases, 4th ed. Philadelphia: Lippincott Williams & Wilkins, 2006.

Handbook of Pathophysiology, 2nd ed. Philadelphia: Lippincott Williams & Wilkins, 2005.

Leppik, I.E. Epilepsy Foundation of America. "Choosing an Antiepileptic: Selecting Drugs for Older Patients with Epilepsy," *Geriatrics* 60(11):42-47, November 2005.

Marin, S. "The Impact of Epilepsy on the Adolescent," *MCN, The American Journal of Maternal/Child Nursing* 30(5):321-26, September-October 2005.

Smy, J. "Improving the Lives of Epilepsy Patients," *Nursing Times* 101(27):44-45, July 2005.

Erectile dysfunction

● OVERVIEW

Description
- Inability to attain or maintain penile erection long enough to complete intercourse
- Classified as primary or secondary:
  - primary impotence—never achieving sufficient erection
  - secondary impotence—patient has achieved erection and completed intercourse in the past
- Also called *impotence*

Pathophysiology
- A lack of autonomic signal or impairment of perfusion may interfere with arteriolar dilation due to inappropriate adrenergic stimulation, causing premature collapse of the sacs of the corpus cavernosum.
- Pelvic steal syndrome can cause loss of erection before ejaculation due to increased blood flow to pelvic muscles.

Causes
- 80% of cases believed to have an organic cause, such as vascular insufficiency and veno-occlusive dysfunction
- 20% of cases believed to be psychogenic in origin

Risk factors
- Medication
- Pelvic injury or surgery
- Alcohol use
- Increasing age
- Smoking
- Obesity
- Hypertension
- Cardiovascular disease
- Diabetes
- Stroke
- Performance anxiety

Incidence
- Affects men of all age-groups but incidence increasing with age

Common characteristics
- Depression
- Inability to obtain or maintain an erection

Complications
- Serious disruption of marital or other sexual relationships

✳ ASSESSMENT

History
- Long-standing inability to achieve erection
- Sudden loss of erectile function
- Gradual decline in function
- Medical disorders, drug therapy, or psychological trauma
- Achievement of erection through masturbation but not with a partner

Physical findings
- Anxious appearance
- Signs of depression

DSM-IV-TR criteria
- Diagnosis confirmed when patient meets either of two criteria:
  - persistent or recurrent partial or complete failure to attain or maintain erection until completion of sexual activity
  - marked distress or interpersonal difficulty occurring as a result of erectile dysfunction
- In addition, this disorder doesn't occur only during course of other Axis I disorder such as major depression.

Test results
LABORATORY
- Serum testosterone levels may be decreased.
- Glycosylated hemoglobin level may be elevated, indicating uncontrolled diabetes mellitus.
- Urinalysis results may be abnormal, indicating kidney damage or diabetes mellitus.
- Lipid profiles may be increased, indicating atherosclerosis.
- Blood glucose levels may be increased, indicating diabetes mellitus.
- Serum creatinine levels may be elevated, indicating kidney damage.
- Prostate-specific antigen results help rule out prostate cancer.

IMAGING
- Ultrasonography evaluates vascular function.
- Angiography evaluates vaso-occlusive disease.

OTHER
- Direct injection of alprostadil (Caverject) into the corpora evaluates the quality of erection.
- Nocturnal penile tumescence testing helps distinguish psychogenic potence from organic potence.

◆ TREATMENT

General
- Sex therapy for psychogenic impotence
- Elimination of cause for organic impotence
- Psychological counseling

Diet
- Avoidance of alcohol

Activity
- No restrictions

Medication
- Sildenafil
- Vardenfil
- Tadalafil
- Alprostadil
- Intracavernosal injection therapy
- Medication Urethral System for Erections
- Intraurethral suppository

Surgery
- Surgically inserted inflatable or semirigid penile prosthesis

NURSING CONSIDERATIONS

Nursing diagnoses
- Anxiety
- Ineffective sexuality patterns
- Interrupted family processes
- Situational low self-esteem
- Sexual dysfunction

Key outcomes
The patient will:
- acknowledge a problem in sexual function
- voluntarily discuss condition
- agree to obtain sexual evaluation and therapy if needed.
- discuss with his partner feelings and perceptions about changes in sexual performance
- develop and maintain a positive attitude toward sexuality and sexual performance.

Nursing interventions
- Encourage verbalization and provide support.
- As needed, refer the patient to a physician, nurse, psychologist, social worker, or counselor trained in sex therapy.

AFTER PENILE PROSTHESIS SURGERY
- Apply ice packs to the penis for 24 hours.
- Empty the drainage device when it's full.
- If the patient has an inflatable prosthesis, provide instructions for use.

Monitoring
- Response to treatment
- Adverse effects of medication
- Complications
- Postoperative bleeding
- Postoperative infection

PATIENT TEACHING

Be sure to cover:
- disorder, diagnostic tests, and treatment
- anatomy and physiology of the reproductive system and the human sexual response cycle
- need to avoid intercourse until the incision heals, usually 6 weeks after penile implant surgery
- signs of infection.

Discharge planning
- Refer the patient to support services.

RESOURCES

Organizations
American Association of Sex Educators, Counselors, and Therapists: *www.aasect.org*
American Psychiatric Association: *www.helping.apa.org*
American Urological Association: *www.auanet.org*
National Cancer Institute: *www.nci.nih.gov*

Selected references
Diagnostic and Statistical Manual of Mental Disorders, 4th Edition, Text Revision. Washington, D.C.: American Psychiatric Association, 2000.
Ferrer, E., Mural, M.A., and Bozzo, J. "The Role of Statins in Erectile Dysfunction," *Drugs Today* 43(1):55-9, January 2007.
Reffelmann, T., and Keoner, R.A. "Sexual Function in Hypertensive Patients Receiving Treatment," *Vascular Health and Risk Management* 2(4):447-55, 2006.
Weeks, B., and Ficorelli, C.T. "Health Matters: How New Drugs Treat Erectile Dysfunction," *Nursing* 36(1):18-19, January 2006.

Esophageal cancer

Description
- Esophageal tumors usually fungating and infiltrating and nearly always fatal
- Liver and lungs common sites of metastasis
- Includes two types of malignant tumors: squamous cell carcinoma and adenocarcinoma
- Grim prognosis for esophageal cancer: 5-year survival rates occurring in fewer than 5% of cases; most patients dying within 6 months of diagnosis

Pathophysiology
- Most esophageal cancers are poorly differentiated squamous cell carcinomas (50% occur in the lower portion of the esophagus; 40%, in the middle portion; 10%, in the upper or cervical esophagus).
- Adenocarcinomas occur less frequently and are contained to the lower third of the esophagus.
- The tumor partially constricts the lumen of the esophagus.
- Regional metastasis occurs early by way of submucosal lymphatics, often fatally invading adjacent vital intrathoracic organs. (If the patient survives primary extension, the liver and lungs are the usual sites of distant metastases; unusual metastasis sites include the bone, kidneys, and adrenal glands.)

Causes
- Exact cause unknown

Risk factors
- Chronic irritation from heavy smoking
- Excessive use of alcohol
- Stasis-induced inflammation, as in achalasia or stricture
- Previous head and neck tumors
- Nutritional deficiency, such as in untreated sprue and Plummer-Vinson syndrome

Incidence
- Most common in men over age 60
- Occurs worldwide; most common in Japan, Russia, China, Middle East, and Transkei region of South Africa

Common characteristics
- Dysphagia
- Weight loss
- Esophageal obstruction
- Acute pain
- Hoarseness, coughing
- Cachexia

Complications
- Direct invasion of adjoining structures
- Inability to control secretions
- Obstruction of the esophagus
- Loss of lower esophageal sphincter control (may result in aspiration pneumonia)

History
- Feeling of fullness, pressure, indigestion, or substernal burning
- Dysphagia and weight loss; degree of dysphagia varies, depending on the extent of disease
- Hoarseness
- Pain on swallowing or pain that radiates to the back
- Anorexia, vomiting, and regurgitation of food

Physical findings
- Chronic cough (possibly from aspiration)
- Cachexia and dehydration

Test results
IMAGING
- X-rays of the esophagus, with barium swallow and motility studies, delineate structural and filling defects and reduced peristalsis.
- Computed tomography scan may help to diagnose and monitor esophageal lesions.
- Magnetic resonance imaging permits evaluation of the esophagus and adjacent structures.

DIAGNOSTIC PROCEDURES
- Esophagoscopy, punch and brush biopsies, and exfoliative cytologic tests confirm esophageal tumors.
- Bronchoscopy (usually performed after an esophagoscopy) may reveal tumor growth in the tracheobronchial tree.
- Endoscopic ultrasonography of the esophagus combines endoscopy and ultrasound technology to measure the depth of penetration of the tumor.

General
- Surgery and other treatments to relieve disease effects because esophageal cancer usually advanced when diagnosed
- Palliative therapy used to keep esophagus open:
  - Dilatation of the esophagus
  - Laser therapy
  - Radiation therapy
  - Installation of prosthetic tubes (such as Celestin's tube)

Diet
- Liquid to soft, as tolerated
- High-calorie supplements

Activity
- No restrictions

Medication
- Chemotherapy
- Analgesics

Surgery
- Radical surgery to excise tumor and resect esophagus or stomach and esophagus
- Gastrostomy or jejunostomy

Other
- Endoscopic laser treatment and bipolar electrocoagulation
- Radiation therapy

Nursing diagnoses
- Acute pain
- Anxiety
- Deficient fluid volume
- Fatigue
- Fear
- Imbalanced nutrition: Less than body requirements
- Impaired swallowing
- Risk for aspiration
- Risk for infection

Key outcomes
The patient will:
- express feelings of increased comfort and decreased pain
- express feelings of decreased anxiety
- maintain fluid volume within the normal range
- express feelings of energy and decreased fatigue
- express concerns and fears related to his diagnosis and condition
- maintain weight within an acceptable range
- swallow without coughing or choking
- not aspirate
- remain free from signs and symptoms of infection.

Nursing interventions
- Provide support and encourage verbalization.
- Position the patient properly to prevent food aspiration.
- Provide tube feedings as ordered.
- Administer medications as ordered.

Monitoring
POSTOPERATIVELY
- Vital signs
- Hydration and nutritional status
- Electrolyte levels
- Intake and output
- Postoperative complications
- Swallowing ability
- Pain control

Be sure to cover:
- the disease process, treatment, and postoperative course
- dietary needs
- the need for rest between activities.

Discharge planning
- Arrange for home care follow-up after discharge.
- Refer the patient to the American Cancer Society.

Organizations
American Cancer Society: *www.cancer.org*
Guide to Internet Resources for Cancer: *www.cancerindex.org*
National Cancer Institute: *www.nci.org*

Selected references
Atlas of Pathophysiology, 2nd ed. Philadelphia: Lippincott Williams & Wilkins, 2005.
Odelli, C., et al. "Nutrition Support Improves Patient Outcomes, Treatment Tolerance and Admission Characteristics in Oesophageal Cancer," *Clinical Oncology* 17(8):639-45, December 2005.

Fibromyalgia syndrome

● OVERVIEW

Description
- Diffuse pain syndrome
- Referred to as *FMS*
- Previously called *fibrositis*

Pathophysiology
- There are several theories describing FMS:
  - Blood flow to the muscle is decreased (due to poor muscle aerobic conditioning, rather than other physiologic abnormalities).
  - Blood flow in the thalamus and caudate nucleus is decreased, leading to a lowered pain threshold.
  - Endocrine dysfunction—such as abnormal pituitary-adrenal axis responses or abnormal levels of the neurotransmitter serotonin in brain centers—affect pain and sleep.
  - The functioning of other pain-processing pathways is abnormal.

Causes
- Unknown
- May be primary disorder or associated with underlying disease, such as infection
- May be multifactorial and influenced by stress, physical conditioning, abnormal-quality sleep, neuroendocrine factors, psychiatric factors and, possibly, hormonal factors (due to predominance in women)

Incidence
- Observed in up to 15% of patients seen in general rheumatology practice and 5% of general medicine clinic patients
- More common in women than in men
- May occur at almost any age; peak incidence among those ages 20 to 60

Common characteristics
- Widespread pain and fatigue

Complications
- Pain
- Depression
- Sleep deprivation

✱ ASSESSMENT

History
- Diffuse, dull, aching pain across neck and shoulders and in lower back and proximal limbs
- Pain typically worse in morning, sometimes with stiffness; can be exacerbated by stress, lack of sleep, weather changes, and inactivity
- Sleep disturbances with frequent arousal and fragmented sleep or frequently waking throughout night (patient unaware of arousals)
- Possible report of irritable bowel syndrome, tension headaches, puffy hands, and paresthesia

Physical findings
- Tender points elicited by applying a moderate amount of pressure to specific location (see *Tender points of fibromyalgia*)

Test results
- Diagnostic testing in FMS not associated with an underlying disease is generally negative for significant abnormalities.

TENDER POINTS OF FIBROMYALGIA

The patient with fibromyalgia syndrome may complain of specific areas of tenderness, which are shown in the illustrations below.

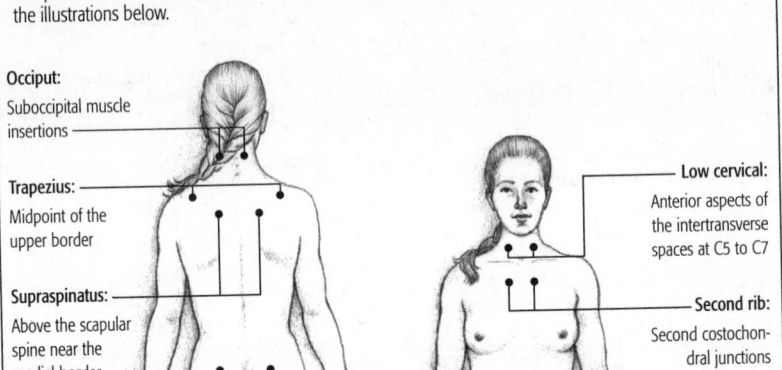

Occiput: Suboccipital muscle insertions

Trapezius: Midpoint of the upper border

Supraspinatus: Above the scapular spine near the medial border

Gluteal: Upper outer quadrants of buttocks

Greater trochanter: Posterior to the trochanteric prominence

Low cervical: Anterior aspects of the intertransverse spaces at C5 to C7

Second rib: Second costochondral junctions

Lateral epicondyle: 2 cm distal to the epicondyles

Knee: Medial fat pad proximal to the joint line

◆ TREATMENT

General
- Massage therapy
- Ultrasound treatments

Diet
- No restrictions

Activity
- Regular, low-impact aerobic exercise program such as water aerobics
- Preexercise and postexercise stretching to minimize injury

Medication
- Amitriptyline, nortriptyline (Pamelor), or cyclobenzaprine (Amrix)
- Tricyclic antidepressant and serotonin uptake inhibitor
- Nonsteroidal anti-inflammatory drugs
- Magnesium supplements
- Pramipexole (Mirapex), adopamine agonist (possibly helpful in some patients)
- Steroid or lidocaine injections

❖ NURSING CONSIDERATIONS

Nursing diagnoses
- Activity intolerance
- Chronic pain
- Disturbed energy field
- Fatigue
- Hopelessness
- Impaired physical mobility
- Ineffective health maintenance
- Ineffective role performance
- Powerlessness
- Risk for infection

Key outcomes
The patient will:
- verbalize importance of balancing rest and activity
- express feelings of increased comfort and decreased pain
- express an increased sense of well-being
- report an increase in energy
- state positive aspects about life and condition

- attain the highest degree of mobility possible within the confines of the disease
- demonstrate participation in treatments and follow-up care
- state her feelings about limitations
- remain free from signs and symptoms of infection.

Nursing interventions
- Administer analgesics, as ordered.
- Provide emotional support.
- Encourage the patient to regularly perform stretching exercises safely and effectively.
- Reassure her that FMS is common and can be treated.

Monitoring
- Sensory disturbances
- Level of pain
- Response to treatment
- Fatigue
- Depression

▶ PATIENT TEACHING

Be sure to cover:
- disorder, diagnostic tests, and treatment
- explanation that exercise (low-impact, aerobic) can be helpful in maintaining muscle conditioning, improving energy and, possibly, improving sleep quality
- reassurance that if increased muscle pain occurs with a new exercise program, the patient may reduce the duration or intensity of the exercise without stopping exercising altogether (unless specifically told to do so)
- importance of taking the tricyclic antidepressant dose 1 to 2 hours before bedtime, which can improve sleep benefits while reducing the morning-after effect
- avoidance of decongestants and caffeine before bedtime
- need for a low-fat diet, high in complex carbohydrates, to decrease symptoms.

Discharge planning
- Refer the patient to appropriate counseling, as needed.

✴ RESOURCES

Organizations
American Fibromyalgia Syndrome Association, Inc.: *www.afsafund.org*
Arthritis Foundation: *www.arthritis.org*

Selected references
D'Arcy, Y. "Following New Guidelines to Treat Fibromyalgia Pain," *Nursing* 35(10):17-18, October 2005.
Schultz, M.A., et al. "Help Patients Cope with Fibromyalgia," *RN* 67(9):46-48, 50, September 2004.

Gas gangrene

● OVERVIEW

Description
- Rare condition caused by local infection with an anaerobic, spore-forming, gram-positive, rod-shaped bacillus *Clostridium perfringens* or another clostridial species
- Occurs in devitalized tissues and results from compromised arterial circulation after trauma or surgery

Pathophysiology
- Incubation is 1 to 4 days but can vary from 3 hours to 6 weeks or longer.
- *C. perfringens* invades soft tissues, producing thrombosis of regional blood vessels, tissue necrosis, and localized edema. (See *Effects of* Clostridium perfringens.)
- Necrosis releases carbon dioxide and hydrogen subcutaneously, producing interstitial gas bubbles.

Causes
- *C. perfringens*
- Transmission when organism enters the body during trauma or surgery

Incidence
- Rare, although more than 30% of deep wounds infected with clostridia
- Most common in deep wounds, especially when tissue necrosis further reduces oxygen supply
- Most common in extremities and abdominal wounds; less common in uterus

Common characteristics
- Sudden, severe pain at wound site

Complications
- Renal failure
- Hypotension and shock
- Hemolytic anemia
- Tissue death requiring amputation of the affected body part

✳ ASSESSMENT

History
- Recent surgery (within 72 hours)
- Traumatic injury
- Septic abortion
- Delivery

Physical findings
- Normothermia, followed by a moderate increase, usually not above 101° F (38.3° C)
- Toxemia (hypotension, tachycardia, tachypnea)
- Localized swelling and discoloration (often dusky brown or reddish)
- Bullae and tissue necrosis
- Dark red or black necrotic muscle
- Foul-smelling, watery or frothy discharge
- Subcutaneous emphysema (hallmark of gas gangrene)
- In later stages, altered level of consciousness that may deteriorate to delirium and coma

Test results
LABORATORY
- Anaerobic cultures of wound drainage show *C. perfringens.*
- Gram stain of wound drainage shows large, gram-positive, rod-shaped bacteria.
- Blood studies show leukocytosis and, later, hemolysis.
IMAGING
- X-rays reveal gas in tissues.

◆ TREATMENT

General
- Hyperbaric oxygenation

Diet
- Adequate hydration
- Nothing by mouth if surgery planned

Activity
- Bed rest until recovery begins

Medication
- I.V. antibiotics
- Analgesics

Surgery
- Immediate wide surgical excision of all affected tissues and necrotic muscle in myositis
- Amputation of the affected part

EFFECTS OF *CLOSTRIDIUM PERFRINGENS*

As *C. perfringens* grows in a closed wound, it destroys cell walls and causes hemolysis, local tissue death, and increasing edema.

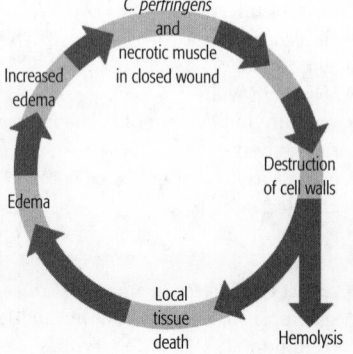

Nursing diagnoses

- Acute pain
- Anxiety
- Fear
- Impaired skin integrity
- Impaired tissue integrity
- Ineffective tissue perfusion: Cardio-pulmonary, peripheral
- Risk for infection

Key outcomes

The patient will:

- express feelings of increased comfort and decreased pain
- report a decrease in level of anxiety
- verbalize areas of concern and fear
- have skin that remains warm, dry, and intact
- exhibit signs of wound healing
- maintain adequate hemodynamic stability and collateral circulation
- exhibit no further signs and symptoms of infection.

Nursing interventions

- Provide adequate fluid replacement.
- Maintain the airway and ventilation.
- Provide good skin and meticulous wound care; place the patient on an air mattress or an air-fluidized bed.
- Prepare the patient emotionally for a large wound after surgical excision and for possible daily debridement.
- Dispose of drainage material properly (double-bag dressings in plastic bags for incineration), and wear sterile gloves when changing dressings.
- Encourage verbalization and provide support.

Monitoring

- Intake and output
- Pulmonary and cardiac function
- Wound site

Be sure to cover:

- disorder, diagnostic tests, and treatment
- need to report severe pain at the wound site immediately
- the need to report foul odor or drainage.

Discharge planning

- After recovery, refer the patient for physical rehabilitation, as necessary.
- After extensive surgery, such as amputation, refer the patient for psychological support, as necessary.

Organizations

Centers for Disease Control and Prevention: *www.cdc.gov*
Harvard University Consumer Health Information: *www.intelihealth.com*
National Health Information Center: *www.health.gov/nhic*
National Library of Medicine: *www.nlm.nih.gov*

Selected references

Titball, R.W. "Gas Gangrene: An Open and Closed Case," *Microbiology* 151(Pt 9):2821-828, September 2005.

Yildiz, T., et al. "Spontaneous Nontraumatic Gas Gangrene Due to Clostridium Perfringens," *International Journal of Infectious Diseases* 10(1):83-85, January 2006.

Gastric cancer

● OVERVIEW

Description
- Classified according to gross appearance (polyploid, ulcerating, ulcerating and infiltrating, or diffuse)
- Prognosis dependent on stage of disease at time of diagnosis (5-year survival rate about 15%)

Pathophysiology
- The most commonly affected areas of the stomach are the pylorus and antrum.
- The remaining areas affected in order of descending frequency are the lesser curvature of the stomach, the cardia, the body of the stomach, and the greater curvature of the stomach.
- Rapid metastasis occurs to the regional lymph nodes, omentum, liver, and lungs.

Causes
- Exact cause unknown

Risk factors
- Gastritis with gastric atrophy
- People with type A blood (10% increased risk)
- Family history of gastric cancer
- Smoked foods, pickled vegetables, and salted fish and meat
- High alcohol consumption
- Smoking

Incidence
- Second most common cancer-related death in the world
- Seventeenth most common cancer and seventh leading cause of cancer death in the United States
- Slightly more common in men than women; usually occurs between ages 40 and 70

Common characteristics
- Feeling of fullness, abdominal distention
- Back, epigastric, or retrosternal pain

Complications
- Malnutrition
- GI obstruction
- Iron deficiency anemia
- Metastasis

✱ ASSESSMENT

History
- Back, epigastric, or retrosternal pain not relieved with nonprescription medications
- Vague feeling of fullness, heaviness, and moderate abdominal distention after meals
- Weight loss, nausea, vomiting
- Weakness and fatigue
- Dysphagia

Physical findings
- Palpable mass
- Palpable lymph nodes, especially the supraclavicular and axillary nodes
- Other assessment findings dependent on extent of disease and location of metastasis

Test results
LABORATORY
- Complete blood count may show iron deficiency anemia.
- Liver function studies may be elevated with metastatic spread of tumor to liver.
- Carcinoembryonic antigen radioimmunoassay may be elevated.

IMAGING
- Barium X-rays of the GI tract with fluoroscopy shows changes that suggest gastric cancer, including a tumor or filling defect in the outline of the stomach, loss of flexibility and distensibility, and abnormal gastric mucosa with or without ulceration.

DIAGNOSTIC PROCEDURES
- Gastroscopy with fiber-optic endoscope is used to help to rule out other diffuse gastric mucosal abnormalities by allowing direct visualization.
- Gastroscopic biopsy permits evaluation of gastric mucosal lesions.

OTHER
- Gastric acid stimulation test discloses whether the stomach secretes acid properly.

◆ TREATMENT

General
- Radiation therapy combined with chemotherapy (not indicated preoperatively because it may damage viscera and impede healing)

Diet
- Based on extent of disorder
- Parenteral feeding (with inability to consume adequate calories)

Activity
- No restrictions

Medication
- Chemotherapy
- Antiemetics
- Sedatives and tranquilizers
- Opioid analgesics

Surgery
- Excision of lesion with appropriate margins (in more than one-third of patients)
- Gastroduodenostomy
- Gastrojejunostomy
- Partial gastric resection
- Total gastrectomy (with metastasis, possible removal of omentum and spleen)

NURSING CONSIDERATIONS

Nursing diagnoses
- Acute pain
- Anxiety
- Diarrhea
- Fatigue
- Fear
- Imbalanced nutrition: Less than body requirements
- Impaired gas exchange
- Impaired oral mucous membrane
- Impaired skin integrity
- Impaired swallowing
- Risk for aspiration

Key outcomes
The patient will:
- report feelings of pain relief
- express feelings of decreased anxiety
- return to a normal elimination pattern
- express feelings of increased energy
- verbalize feelings and concerns about his diagnosis and condition
- maintain weight within an acceptable range
- maintain adequate ventilation
- maintain intact oral mucous membranes
- maintain skin integrity
- be able to swallow without coughing or choking
- not aspirate.

Nursing interventions
- Provide a high-protein, high-calorie diet with dietary supplements.
- Administer medications, as ordered.
- Provide parenteral nutrition, as appropriate.
- After surgery, provide supportive care.

Monitoring
- Pain control
- Vital signs
- Hydration and nutritional status
- Nasogastric tube function and drainage
- Wound site
- Postoperative complications
- Effects of medication

PATIENT TEACHING

Be sure to cover (with the patient or family):
- disorder, diagnostic tests, and treatment
- dietary plan
- effective pulmonary toileting
- avoidance of crowds and people with known infection
- relaxation techniques
- medication administration, dosage, and possible adverse effects.

Discharge planning
- Direct the patient and family members to support services.
- Refer for home care services, as necessary.
- Refer to hospice, if indicated.

RESOURCES

Organizations
American Cancer Society: *www.cancer.org*
Guide to Internet Resources for Cancer: *www.cancerindex.org*
National Cancer Institute: *www.nci.org*
National Institute of Diabetes, Digestive, and Kidney: *www.niddk.nih.gov*

Selected references
Atlas of Pathophysiology, 2nd ed. Philadelphia: Lippincott Williams & Wilkins, 2005.
Leung, T. "Chemotherapy and Radiotherapy in the Management of Gastric Cancer," *Current Opinion in Gastroenterology* 21(6): 673-78, November 2005.

Gastritis

● OVERVIEW

Description
- Inflammation of the gastric mucosa
- May be acute or chronic
- Most common stomach disorder (acute)

Pathophysiology

ACUTE GASTRITIS
- The protective mucosal layer is altered.
- Acid secretion produces mucosal reddening, edema, and superficial surface erosion.

CHRONIC GASTRITIS
- Progressive thinning and degeneration of gastric mucosa occur.

Causes

ACUTE GASTRITIS
- Chronic ingestion of irritating foods and alcohol
- Such drugs as aspirin and other nonsteroidal anti-inflammatory drugs (in large doses), cytotoxic agents, caffeine, corticosteroids, antimetabolites, phenylbutazone, and indomethacin
- Ingested poisons, especially DDT, ammonia, mercury, carbon tetrachloride, or corrosive substances
- Endotoxins released from infecting bacteria, such as staphylococci, *Escherichia coli*, and salmonella
- Complication of acute illness

CHRONIC GASTRITIS
- Recurring exposure to irritating substances, such as drugs, alcohol, cigarette smoke, and environmental agents
- Pernicious anemia, renal disease, or diabetes mellitus
- *Helicobacter pylori* infection (common cause of nonerosive gastritis)

Risk factors
- Older than age 60
- Exposure to toxic substances
- Hemodynamic disorder

Incidence
- May occur at any age; increased incidence of *H. pylori* older than age 60
- Occurs equally in men and women
- Acute gastritis in 8 of 1,000 people; chronic gastritis in 2 of 10,000 people

Common characteristics
- Abdominal pain
- Indigestion

Complications
- Hemorrhage
- Obstruction
- Perforation
- Peritonitis
- Gastric cancer

✳ ASSESSMENT

History
- Evidence of one or more causative agents
- Rapid onset of symptoms (acute gastritis)
- Epigastric discomfort
- Indigestion
- Cramping
- Anorexia
- Nausea, hematemesis, and vomiting
- Coffee-ground emesis or melena if GI bleeding present

Physical findings
- Possible normal appearance
- Grimacing
- Restlessness
- Pallor
- Tachycardia
- Hypotension
- Abdominal distention, tenderness, and guarding
- Normoactive to hyperactive bowel sounds

Test results

LABORATORY
- Occult blood appears in vomitus or stools (or both) if the patient has gastric bleeding.
- Hemoglobin level and hematocrit are decreased.
- Urea breath test shows *H. pylori*.

DIAGNOSTIC PROCEDURES
- Upper GI endoscopy reveals gastritis when it's performed within 24 hours of bleeding.
- Biopsy reveals inflammatory process.

◆ TREATMENT

General
- Elimination of cause
- For massive bleeding:
  – Blood transfusion
  – Iced saline lavage
  – Angiography with vasopressin

Diet
- Nothing by mouth, if bleeding occurs
- Elimination of irritating foods

Activity
- As tolerated, bed rest during acute phase

Medication
- Histamine antagonists
- Antacids
- Proton pump inhibitors
- Prostaglandins
- Vitamin B_{12}
- Triple therapy—two antibiotics and bismuth subsalicylate
- Dual therapy—antibiotic and proton pump inhibitor

Surgery
- Indicated when conservative treatment fails
- Vagotomy, pyloroplasty
- Rarely, partial or total gastrectomy

❖ NURSING CONSIDERATIONS

Nursing diagnoses
- Acute pain
- Deficient knowledge (gastritis)
- Imbalanced nutrition: Less than body requirements
- Ineffective coping
- Risk for deficient fluid volume

Key outcomes
The patient will:
- express feelings of increased comfort and decreased pain
- verbalize understanding of the disorder and treatment regimen
- maintain weight
- express concerns about his current condition
- maintain normal fluid volume.

Nursing interventions
- Provide physical and emotional support.
- Administer medications and I.V. fluids.
- Assist the patient with diet modification.
- If surgery is necessary, prepare the patient preoperatively and provide appropriate postoperative care.

Monitoring
- Vital signs
- Fluid intake and output
- Electrolyte and hemoglobin levels
- Returning symptoms as food is reintroduced
- Response to medication
- Pain control

▶ PATIENT TEACHING

Be sure to cover:
- disorder, diagnostic tests, and treatment
- lifestyle and diet modifications
- preoperative teaching if surgery is necessary
- stress-reduction techniques
- medication administration, dosage, and possible adverse effects.

Discharge planning
- Refer the patient to a smoking-cessation program, if indicated.

✷ RESOURCES

Organizations
The National Digestive Diseases Information Clearinghouse: *www.niddk.nih.gov/health/digest/nddic.htm*

Selected references
Handbook of Diseases, 3rd ed. Philadelphia: Lippincott Williams & wilkins, 2004.

Krumberger, J.M. "How to Manage an Acute Upper GI Bleed," *RN* 68(3):34-39, March 2005.

Rugge, M., and Genta, R.M. "Staging Gastritis: An International Proposal," *Gastroenterology* 129(5):1807-808, November 2005.

Yamada, T., et al. *Atlas of Gastroenterology,* 3rd ed. Philadelphia: Lippincott Williams & Wilkins, 2003.

Gastroenteritis

● OVERVIEW

Description
- Self-limiting inflammation of the stomach and small intestine
- Also known as *intestinal flu, traveler's diarrhea, viral enteritis,* and *food poisoning*

Pathophysiology
- The bowel reacts to the various causes of gastroenteritis with increased luminal fluid that can't be absorbed.
- This results in abdominal pain, vomiting, severe diarrhea (primarily), and secondary depletion of intracellular fluid.
- Dehydration and electrolyte loss occurs.

Causes
- Bacteria, such as *Staphylococcus aureus, Salmonella, Shigella, Clostridium botulinum, Clostridium perfringens,* and *Escherichia coli*
- Amoebae, especially *Entamoeba histolytica*
- Parasites, such as *Ascaris, Enterobius,* and *Trichinella spiralis*
- Viruses, such as adenoviruses, echoviruses, and coxsackieviruses
- Ingestion of toxins, such as poisonous plants and toadstools
- Drug reactions from antibiotics
- Food allergens
- Enzyme deficiencies

Incidence
- Occurs at any age
- Major cause of morbidity and mortality in underdeveloped nations
- Ranks second to common cold as cause of lost work time in the United States
- Fifth most common cause of death among young children
- Can be life-threatening in elderly and debilitated patients

Common characteristics
- Diarrhea
- Nausea and vomiting

Complications
- Severe dehydration
- Electrolyte imbalance

✳ ASSESSMENT

History
- Acute onset of diarrhea
- Abdominal pain and discomfort
- Nausea, vomiting
- Malaise and fatigue
- Exposure to contaminated food
- Recent travel (see *Preventing traveler's diarrhea*)

Physical findings
- Slight abdominal distention
- Poor skin turgor (with dehydration)
- Hyperactive bowel sounds
- Decreased blood pressure

Test results
LABORATORY
- Gram stain, stool culture (by direct rectal swab), or blood culture shows the causative bacteria.

PREVENTING TRAVELER'S DIARRHEA

If the patient travels, especially to developing nations, discuss precautions that he can take to reduce his chances of getting traveler's diarrhea. Explain that traveler's diarrhea is caused by inadequate sanitation and occurs after bacteria-contaminated food or water is ingested. These organisms attach to the lining of the small intestine, where they release a toxin that causes diarrhea and cramps. To minimize this risk, advise him to:

- Drink water (or brush his teeth with water) only if it's chlorinated. Chlorination protects the water supply from bacterial contaminants such as *Escherichia coli*.
- Avoid beverages in glasses that may have been washed in contaminated water.
- Refuse ice cubes that may have been made from contaminated water.
- Drink only beverages made with boiled water, such as coffee and tea, or those in bottles or cans.
- Sanitize impure water by adding 2% tincture of iodine (5 drops/L of clear water, 10 drops/L of cloudy water) or by adding liquid laundry bleach (about 2 drops/L of clear water; 4 drops/L of cloudy water).
- Avoid uncooked vegetables, unpeeled fresh fruits, salads, unpasteurized milk, and other dairy products.
- Beware of foods offered by street vendors.

If traveler's diarrhea occurs despite precautions, bismuth subsalicylate, diphenoxylate with atropine, or loperamide can be used to relieve symptoms.

◆ TREATMENT

General
- Supportive treatment for nausea, vomiting, and diarrhea

Diet
- Rehydration
- Initially, clear liquids, as tolerated
- Electrolyte solutions
- Avoidance of milk products

Activity
- Bed rest

Medication
- Antidiarrheal therapy
- Antiemetics
- Antibiotics
- I.V. fluids

NURSING CONSIDERATIONS

Nursing diagnoses
- Acute pain
- Diarrhea
- Imbalanced nutrition: Less than body requirements
- Risk for deficient fluid volume

Key outcomes
The patient will:
- express feelings of increased comfort and decreased pain
- return to normal elimination pattern
- maintain weight without further loss
- maintain adequate fluid volume.

Nursing interventions
- Allow uninterrupted rest periods.
- Replace lost fluids and electrolytes through diet or I.V. fluids.
- Administer medication, as ordered.

Monitoring
- Intake and output
- Vital signs
- Signs of dehydration
- Electrolytes

PATIENT TEACHING

Be sure to cover:
- disorder, diagnostic tests, and treatment
- dietary modifications
- medication administration, dosage, and possible adverse effects
- preventive measures
- how to perform warm sitz baths three times per day to relieve anal irritation.

RESOURCES

Organizations
The National Digestive Diseases Information Clearinghouse: *www.niddk.nih.gov/health/digest/nddic.htm*

Selected references
Handbook of Diseases, 3rd ed. Philadelphia: Lippincott Williams & Wilkins, 2004.

Krumberger, J.M. "How to Manage an Acute Upper GI Bleed," *RN* 68(3):34-39, March 2005.

Rugge, M., and Genta, R.M. "Staging Gastritis: An International Proposal," *Gastroenterology* 129(5):1807-808, November 2005.

Yamada, T., et al. *Atlas of Gastroenterology,* 3rd ed. Philadelphia: Lippincott Williams & Wilkins, 2003.

Gastroesophageal reflux disease

● OVERVIEW

Description
- Backflow of gastric or duodenal contents, or both, into the esophagus and past the lower esophageal sphincter (LES), without associated belching or vomiting
- Reflux of gastric acid, causing acute epigastric pain, usually after a meal
- Popularly called *heartburn*
- Also called *GERD*

Pathophysiology
- Reflux occurs when LES pressure is deficient or pressure in the stomach exceeds LES pressure. The LES relaxes and gastric contents regurgitate into the esophagus.
- The degree of mucosal injury is based on the amount and concentration of refluxed gastric acid, proteolytic enzymes, and bile acids.

Causes
- Pyloric surgery (alteration or removal of the pylorus), which allows reflux of bile or pancreatic juice
- Hiatal hernia with incompetent sphincter
- Any condition or position that increases intra-abdominal pressure

Risk factors
- Any agent that lowers LES pressure: acidic and fatty food, alcohol, cigarettes, anticholinergics (atropine, belladonna, propantheline) or other drugs (morphine, diazepam, calcium channel blockers, meperidine)
- Nasogastric (NG) intubation for more than 4 days

Incidence
- Affects approximately 7 million Americans
- Affects all ethnic groups and socioeconomic classes
- Most common in people ages 45 to 64

Common characteristics
- Epigastric pain, usually after a meal or when lying down

Complications
- Reflux esophagitis
- Esophageal stricture
- Esophageal ulcer
- Barrett's esophagus (metaplasia and possible increased risk of neoplasm)
- Anemia from esophageal bleeding
- Reflux aspiration leading to chronic pulmonary disease

✳ ASSESSMENT

History
- Minimal or no symptoms in one-third of patients
- Heartburn that typically occurs 30 minutes to 2 hours after eating
- Heartburn that worsens with vigorous exercise, bending, lying down, wearing tight clothing, coughing, constipation, and obesity
- Reported relief by using antacids or sitting upright
- Regurgitation without associated nausea or belching
- Feeling of fluid accumulation in the throat without a sour or bitter taste.
- Chronic pain radiating to the neck, jaws, and arms that may mimic angina pectoris
- Nocturnal hypersalivation and wheezing

Physical findings
- Odynophagia (sharp substernal pain on swallowing), possibly followed by a dull substernal ache
- Bright red or dark brown blood in vomitus
- Laryngitis and morning hoarseness
- Chronic cough

Test results
IMAGING
- Barium swallow with fluoroscopy shows evidence of recurrent reflux.
DIAGNOSTIC PROCEDURES
- Gastroesophageal scintillation testing shows reflux.
- Esophageal manometry reveals abnormal LES pressure and sphincter incompetence.
- Acid perfusion (Bernstein) test result confirms esophagitis.
- Esophagoscopy and biopsy results confirm pathologic changes in the mucosa.
- 24-hour intraesophageal monitoring shows frequent acidic spikes that correlate with patient's complaints in symptom/activity diary.

◆ TREATMENT

General
- Modification of lifestyle
- Positional therapy
- Removal of cause
- Parenteral nutrition or tube feeding
- Weight reduction

Diet
- Avoidance of dietary causes
- Avoidance of eating 2 hours before sleep (see *Factors affecting LES pressure*)
- Parenteral nutrition or tube feedings

Activity
- No restrictions
- Lifting restrictions for surgical treatment

Medication
- Antacids
- Cholinergics
- Histamine-2 receptor antagonists
- Proton pump inhibitors

FACTORS AFFECTING LES PRESSURE

Various dietary and lifestyle elements can increase or decrease lower esophageal sphincter (LES) pressure. Consider these as you plan the patient's treatment program.

What increases LES pressure
- Protein
- Carbohydrates
- Nonfat milk
- Low-dose ethanol

What decreases LES pressure
- Fat
- Whole milk
- Orange juice
- Tomatoes
- Antiflatulent (simethicone)
- Chocolate
- High-dose ethanol
- Cigarette smoking
- Lying on right or left side
- Sitting

Surgery

- Hiatal hernia repair
- Vagotomy or pyloroplasty
- Nissen fundoplication (open or laproscopic)
- Esophagectomy

❖ NURSING CONSIDERATIONS

Nursing diagnoses

- Acute pain
- Anxiety
- Deficient knowledge (gastroesophageal reflux)
- Imbalanced nutrition: Less than body requirements
- Risk for aspiration

Key outcomes

The patient will:

- express feelings of increased comfort and decreased pain
- verbalize methods to reduce anxiety
- demonstrate understanding of gastroesphageal reflux disease
- achieve adequate calorie and nutritional intake
- show no signs of aspiration.

Nursing interventions

- Offer the patient emotional and psychological support.
- Assist the patient with diet modification.
- Perform chest physiotherapy.
- Use semi-Fowler's position for the patient with an NG tube.

Monitoring
AFTER SURGERY

- Respiratory status
- Pain
- Intake and output
- Vital signs
- Chest tube drainage

▶ PATIENT TEACHING

Be sure to cover:

- disorder, diagnostic tests, and treatment
- causes of gastroesophageal reflux
- prescribed antireflux regimen of medication, diet, and positional therapy such as sleeping with the head of the bed elevated
- developing a dietary plan
- need to sit upright after meals and snacks and to eat small, frequent meals
- need to identify situations or activities that increase intra-abdominal pressure
- need to refrain from using substances that reduce sphincter control
- signs and symptoms to watch for and report.

✳ RESOURCES

Organizations

American Gastroenterological Association: www.gastro.org
National Digestive Diseases Information Clearinghouse: www.niddk.nih.gov/health/digest/nddic.htm
Pediatric/Adolescent Gastroesophageal Reflux Association, Inc.: www.reflux.org
The Society of American Gastrointestinal and Endoscopic Surgeons: www.sages.org

Selected references

Chen, Y.K. "Endoscopic Approaches to the Treatment of Gastroesophageal Reflux Disease," *Current Opinion in Internal Medicine* 4(6):643-48, December 2005.
Handbook of Diseases, 3rd ed. Philadelphia: Lippincott Williams & Wilkins, 2004.
Henry, S.M. "Discerning Differences: Gastroespoahgeal Reflux and Gastroesophageal Reflux Disease in Infants," *Advances in Neonatal Care* 4(4):234-47, August 2004.
Simpson, T., and Ivey, J. "Pediatric Management Problems. GERD," *Pediatric Nursing* 31(3):214-15, May-June 2005.
The Society of American Gastrointestinal and Endoscopic Surgeons (2001). Guidelines for Surgical Treatment of Gastroesophageal Reflux Disease (GERD). Available at: *www.sages.org* Accessed 9/1/2006.
Yamada, T., et al. *Atlas of Gastroenterology,* 3rd ed. Philadelphia: Lippincott Williams & Wilkins, 2003.

Genital warts

Description
- Papillomas that consist of fibrous tissue overgrowth from the dermis and thickened epithelial coverings
- Also known as *venereal warts* and *condylomata acuminata*

Pathophysiology
- It's transmitted by sexual contact and incubates for 1 to 6 months (2 months, average) before warts erupt.
- Infection of the basal cells occurs, with proliferation of all epidermal layers, producing acanthosis, parakeratosis, and hyperkeratosis.

Causes
- Infection with one of more than 60 known strains of human papillomavirus
- Receptive anal intercourse is suggested cause of perianal warts in men

Incidence
- One of the most common sexually transmitted diseases (STDs) in the United States

Common characteristics
- Appearance of small pink to red, moist warts with irregular surfaces
- Usually located around the external genitalia and possibly inside the urethra or vagina or on the cervix
- No symptoms in most patients

Complications
- During pregnancy, genital warts in the vaginal and cervical walls that grow large enough to impede vaginal delivery
- Genital tract dysplasia
- Cervical and vulvar cancer in women, penile cancer in men, and some rectal carcinomas in both genders

History
- Unprotected sexual contact with a partner with a known infection, a new partner, or many partners

Physical findings
- Warts on moist genital surfaces (subpreputial sac, urethral meatus, penile shaft, scrotum, vulva, vaginal and cervical walls)
- In women, anogenital warts appearing first at the posterior introitus and adjacent labia, then spreading to other parts of the vulva, commonly involving the vagina and cervix
- Tiny red or pink swellings that may grow as large as 4″ (10 cm) and that may be pedunculated
- Infected lesions that become malodorous

Test results
LABORATORY
- Dark-field microscopy of wart-cell scrapings show marked epidermal cell vascularization.
- Application of 5% acetic acid (white vinegar) turns warts white if they're papillomas.

General
- Chronic treatment because relapse is frequent
- Circumcision (may prevent recurrence)

Diet
- No restrictions

Activity
- No restrictions

Medication
- Topical antimetabolites
- Topical podophyllum resin
- Topical interferon
- Vaccine preparations

Surgery
- Cryosurgery
- Electrodesiccation
- Surgical excision
- Laser ablation

✤ NURSING CONSIDERATIONS

Nursing diagnoses
- Acute pain
- Disturbed body image
- Impaired skin integrity
- Ineffective sexuality patterns
- Risk for infection
- Risk for injury

Key outcomes
The patient will:
- express feelings of increased comfort and decreased pain
- acknowledge the change in body image
- exhibit improved or healed lesions or wounds
- voice feelings about potential or actual changes in sexuality
- remain free from signs and symptoms of infection and injury.

Nursing interventions
- Use standard precautions.
- Provide a nonthreatening, nonjudgmental atmosphere that encourages verbalization, and provide support.
- Remove podophyllum resin with soap and water 4 to 6 hours after applying it to warts.

Monitoring
- Response to treatment
- Adverse effects of medication
- Signs and symptoms of infection (postoperative)
- Concomitant STDs or infections
- Papanicolaou (Pap) test results

▶ PATIENT TEACHING

Be sure to cover:
- disorder, diagnostic tests, and treatment
- need for sexual abstinence or condom use during intercourse until healing is complete
- evaluation of the patient's sexual partners
- importance of testing for human immunodeficiency virus infection and other STDs
- emphasis that genital warts can recur and that the virus can mutate, causing infection with warts of a different strain
- recommendation that female patients have a Pap test every 6 months.

✵ RESOURCES

Organizations
Centers for Disease Control and Prevention: *www.cdc.gov*
Harvard University Consumer Health Information: *www.intelihealth.com*
National Health Information Center: *www.health.gov/nhic/*
National Library of Medicine: *www.nlm.nih.gov*

Selected references
Kahn, J.A., and Bernstein, D.J. "Human Papillomavirus Vaccines and Adolescents," *Current Opinion in Obstetrics & Gynecology* 17(5):476-82, October 2005.

Kasper, D.L., et al., eds. *Harrison's Principles of Internal Medicine,* 16th ed. New York: McGraw-Hill Book Co., 2005.

O'Mahony, C. "Genital Warts: Current and Future Management Options," *American Journal of Clinical Dermatology* 6(4):239-43, 2005.

Gestational hypertension

● OVERVIEW

Description
- High blood pressure, most often occurring after the 20th week of gestation in a nulliparous woman
- Carries a high risk for fetal mortality because of the increased incidence of premature delivery
- Among the most common causes of maternal death in developed countries (especially when complications occur)
- Nonconvulsive form (also called *preeclampsia*): occurs after the 20th week of gestation; may be mild or severe
- Convulsive form (also called *eclampsia*): occurs between the 24th week of gestation and the end of the first postpartum week

Pathophysiology
- Generalized arteriolar vasoconstriction is thought to cause decreased blood flow through the placenta and maternal organs, leading to intrauterine growth retardation or restriction, placental infarcts, and abruptio placentae.

Causes
- Exact cause unknown
- Contributing factors:
  – Autointoxication
  – Autolysis of placental infarcts
  – Diabetes
  – Geographic, ethnic, racial, nutritional, immunologic, and familial factors
  – Maternal age
  – Maternal sensitization to total proteins
  – Preexisting vascular disease
  – Pyelonephritis
  – Uremia

☀ **AGE-RELATED CONCERN** Adolescents and primiparas older than age 35 are at higher risk for preeclampsia.

Risk factors
- First-time pregnancy
- Multiple fetuses
- History of vascular disease

Incidence
- Occurs in about 7% of pregnancies and is more common in women from lower socioeconomic groups

- Roughly a 5% incidence of preeclampsia progressing to eclampsia.

Common characteristics
- Hypertension
- Sudden weight gain
- Irritability

Complications
- Abruptio placentae
- HELLP syndrome: hemolysis, elevated liver enzyme levels, low platelet count
- Coagulopathy
- Stillbirth
- Seizures
- Coma
- Preterm labor
- Renal failure
- Maternal hepatic damage

✳ ASSESSMENT

History
- Sudden weight gain
- Irritability
- Emotional tension
- Severe frontal headache
- Blurred vision
- Epigastric pain or heartburn

Physical findings
- Preeclampsia: blood pressure of 160/110 mm Hg or higher
- Eclampsia: systolic blood pressure of 180 or 200 mm Hg or higher
- Generalized edema, especially of the face
- Pitting edema of the legs and feet
- Hyperreflexia
- Oliguria
- Vascular spasm, papilledema, retinal edema or detachment, and arteriovenous nicking or hemorrhage (seen on ophthalmoscopy)
- Seizures

Test results
LABORATORY
- In preeclampsia, proteinuria exceeds 300 mg/24 hours [1+].
- In severe eclampsia, proteinuria is 5 g/24 hours [5+] or more.
- In HELLP syndrome, hemolysis, elevated liver enzymes, and decreased platelet count are present.

IMAGING
- Ultrasonography aids evaluation of fetal well-being.
DIAGNOSTIC PROCEDURES
- Stress and nonstress tests and biophysical profiles help evaluate fetal well-being.

◆ TREATMENT

General
- Measures to halt progression of the disorder and ensure fetal survival
- Prompt labor induction, especially if the patient is near term (advocated by some clinicians)

Diet
- Adequate nutrition
- Low-sodium, if indicated
- Limited caffeine

Activity
- Complete bed rest
- Left lateral lying position

Medications
- Antihypertensives
- Magnesium sulfate
- Oxytocin
- Oxygen

Surgery
- Possible cesarean delivery

❖ NURSING CONSIDERATIONS

Nursing diagnoses
- Activity intolerance
- Anxiety
- Disturbed sensory perception: Visual
- Excess fluid volume
- Fear
- Impaired urinary elimination
- Ineffective coping
- Ineffective tissue perfusion: Cerebral, peripheral
- Risk for injury

Key outcomes
The patient will:
- perform activities of daily living within limits of condition
- identify strategies to reduce anxiety

- maintain optimal functioning within the confines of the visual impairment
- maintain adequate fluid volume
- verbalize fears and concerns
- maintain urine output within normal limits
- demonstrate adaptive coping behaviors
- exhibit signs of adequate cerebral and peripheral perfusion
- remain free from injury.

Nursing interventions
- Give prescribed drugs.
- Elevate edematous arms or legs.
- Eliminate constricting hose, slippers, and bed linens.
- Assist with or insert an indwelling urinary catheter, if necessary.
- Provide a quiet, darkened room.
- Enforce absolute bed rest.
- Provide emotional support.
- Encourage the patient to express her feelings.
- Help the patient develop effective coping strategies. (See *Emergency interventions for gestational hypertension.*)

EMERGENCY INTERVENTIONS FOR GESTATIONAL HYPERTENSION

When caring for a patient with gestational hypertension, be prepared to perform the following interventions:

- Observe for signs of fetal distress by closely monitoring results of stress and nonstress tests.
- Keep emergency resuscitative equipment and anticonvulsants at hand in case of seizures and cardiac or respiratory arrest.
- Carefully monitor magnesium sulfate administration. Signs of drug toxicity include absence of patellar reflexes, flushing, muscle flaccidity, decreased urinary output, significant blood pressure drop (> 15 mm Hg), and a respiratory rate less than 12 per minute. Keep calcium gluconate at the bedside to counteract the toxic effects of magnesium sulfate.
- Prepare for emergency cesarean delivery, if indicated. Alert the anesthesiologist and pediatrician.
- To protect the patient from injury, maintain seizure precautions. Don't leave an unstable patient unattended. Maintain a patent airway, and have supplemental oxygen readily available.

Monitoring
- Vital signs
- Fetal heart rate
- Vision
- Edema
- Daily weight
- Intake and output; urine protein levels
- Level of consciousness
- Deep tendon reflexes
- Headache unrelieved by medication
- Complications

▶ PATIENT TEACHING

Be sure to cover:
- disorder, diagnostic tests, and treatment
- signs and symptoms of preeclampsia and eclampsia
- importance of bed rest in the left lateral position, as ordered
- adequate nutrition and a low-sodium diet
- good prenatal care
- control of preexisting hypertension
- early recognition and prompt treatment of preeclampsia
- likelihood that the neonate will be small for gestational age, with the probability that he'll do better than other preterm neonates of the same weight.

Discharge planning
- Refer the patient for professional counseling, as indicated.

✱ RESOURCES

Organizations
American College of Obstetricians and Gynecologists: *www.acog.org*
American Heart Association: *www.americanheart.org*
American Society for Reproductive Medicine: *www.asrm.org*

Selected references
Alexander, J.M., et.al. "Selective Magnesium Sulfate Prophylaxis for the Prevention of Eclampsia in Women with Gestational Hypertension," *Obstetrics & Gynecology* 108(4): 826-832, October 2006.

Arafeh, J.M. "Preeclampsia: Pieces of the Puzzle Revealed," *Journal of Perinatal and Neonatal Nursing* 20(1):85-87, March 2006.

Ehrenberg, H.M., and Mercer, B.M. "Abbreviated Postpartum Magnesium Sulfate Therapy for Women with Mild Preeclampsia: A Randomized Controlled Trial," *Obstetrics & Gynecology* 108(4):833-38, October 2006.

Kisters, K., et al. "Preventing Pregnancy-Induced Hypertension: The Role of Calcium and Magnesium," *Journal of Hypertension* 24(1):201, January 2006.

Nabukera, S., et.al. "First-Time Births Among Women 30 Years and Older in the United States: Patterns and Risk of Adverse Outcomes," *Journal of Reproductive Medicine* 51(9):676-682, September 2006.

Roberts, J.M., and Gammill, H.S. "Preeclampsia: Recent Insights," *Hypertension* 46(6):1243-249, December 2005.

Sibai, B.M. "Diagnosis and Management of Gestational Hypertension and Preeclampsia," *Obstetrics & Gynecology* 102(1):181-92, July 2003.

Giardiasis

● OVERVIEW

Description
- Infection of the small bowel by *Giardia lamblia*, a symmetrical flagellate protozoan
- Reinfection possible because infection doesn't confer immunity
- Also called *G. enteritis* and *lambliasis*

Pathophysiology
- Cysts enter the small bowel and release trophozoites, which attach to the bowel's epithelial surface.
- Attachment causes superficial mucosal invasion and destruction, inflammation, and irritation.
- Trophozoites become encysted again, travel down the colon, and are excreted. (Unformed stool may contain trophozoites as well as cysts.)

Causes
- Ingestion of *G. lamblia* cysts in stool-contaminated water
- Fecal-oral transfer of cysts from an infected person

Incidence
- Occurs worldwide but is most common in developing countries and other areas where sanitation and hygiene are poor (*G. lamblia* has been found in municipal water sources, nursing homes, and day care centers.)
- Children more likely to develop giardiasis than adults
- In the United States, most common in travelers who recently returned from endemic areas, campers who drink water from contaminated streams, male homosexuals, patients with congenital immunoglobulin A deficiency, and children in day care centers

Common characteristics
- Prominent early symptoms:
  - Diarrhea
  - Abdominal pain
  - Bloating
  - Belching
  - Flatus
  - Nausea and vomiting

Complications
- Malabsorption
- Dehydration
- Lactose intolerance
- Possible death, in hypogammaglobulinemia

✳ ASSESSMENT

History
- Recent travel to an area with poor sanitation
- Sexual practices that involve oral-anal contact
- Ingestion of suspect water
- Institutionalization

Physical findings
- Possibly, no intestinal symptoms in mild infection
- Abdominal cramps, bloating
- Belching, flatus
- Nausea, vomiting
- Explosive pale, loose, greasy, malodorous, frequent stools (occurring 2 to 10 times daily)
- Fatigue, weight loss
- Hyperactive bowel sounds in the right upper and left lower quadrants just before bowel movements
- General upper and right lower quadrant discomfort and guarding

Test results
LABORATORY
- Examination of a fresh stool specimen shows cysts; examination of duodenal aspirate or biopsy shows trophozoites.

◆ TREATMENT

General
- Possible testing and treatment for people living with an infected person or those who have had sexual contact with an infected person

Diet
- Parenteral fluid replacement to prevent dehydration

Activity
- No restrictions

Medication
- Metronidazole

✤ NURSING CONSIDERATIONS

Nursing diagnoses
- Acute pain
- Deficient fluid volume
- Diarrhea
- Fatigue
- Imbalanced nutrition: Less than body requirements
- Impaired skin integrity
- Risk for infection

Key outcomes
The patient will:
- express feelings of increased comfort and decreased pain
- maintain normal electrolyte levels
- have an elimination pattern that returns to normal
- verbalize an increase in energy levels
- experience no further weight loss
- remain free from skin breakdown or infection
- maintain stable vital signs.

Nursing interventions
- Institute enteric precautions, and quickly dispose of all fecal material.
- Place a child or an incontinent adult in a private room.
- Keep the perianal area clean, especially after each bowel movement.
- Administer I.V. fluid therapy, as needed.
- Provide nutritionally adequate foods.
- Administer medication, as ordered.
- Report epidemic situations to public health authorities.

Monitoring
- Frequency and characteristics of bowel movements
- Nutritional intake (to prevent malnutrition)
- Adverse drug effects
- Skin integrity
- Signs and symptoms of dehydration

▶ PATIENT TEACHING

Be sure to cover:
- medication administration, dosage, and possible adverse effects.
- need for the patient who is taking metronidazole or furazolidone to avoid alcohol while taking the drug and for 3 days afterward
- need for family members and others in contact with the patient to have their stools tested for *G. lamblia* cysts
- need for good personal hygiene, especially proper hand washing as well as correct handling of infectious material by the patient and family members
- importance of safer sex practices
- need for campers to purify all stream and lake water before drinking it
- need for travelers to endemic areas to avoid drinking tap or suspect water and to avoid eating uncooked and unpeeled fruits or vegetables.

Discharge planning
- Encourage the patient to return for follow-up appointments because relapses can occur.

✴ RESOURCES

Organizations
Centers for Disease Control and Prevention: *www.cdc.gov*
Harvard University Consumer Health Information: *www.intelihealth.com*
National Health Information Center: *www.health.gov/nhic/*
National Library of Medicine: *www.nlm.nih.gov*

Selected references
Dawson, D. "Foodborne Protozoan Parasites," *International Journal of Food Microbiology* 103(2):207-27, August 2005.
Diseases, 4th ed. Philadelphia: Lippincott Williams & Wilkins, 2006.
Kasper, D.L., et al., eds. *Harrison's Principles of Internal Medicine,* 16th ed. New York: McGraw-Hill Book Co., 2005.

Glaucoma

● OVERVIEW

Description

- Group of disorders characterized by high intraocular pressure (IOP) and optic nerve damage
- Leading cause of blindness
- Two forms:
  - Open-angle (also known as *chronic, simple,* or *wide-angle*) glaucoma: begins insidiously and progresses slowly
  - Angle-closure (also known as *acute* or *narrow-angle*) glaucoma: occurs suddenly and can cause permanent vision loss in 48 to 72 hours

Pathophysiology
OPEN-ANGLE GLAUCOMA
- Degenerative changes in the trabecular meshwork block the flow of aqueous humor from the eye, increasing IOP and resulting in optic nerve damage.

ANGLE-CLOSURE GLAUCOMA
- Obstruction to the outflow of aqueous humor is caused by an anatomically narrow angle between the iris and the cornea.
- IOP increases suddenly.

Causes
OPEN-ANGLE GLAUCOMA
- Degenerative changes
ANGLE-CLOSURE GLAUCOMA
- Anatomically narrow angle between the iris and the cornea
- Attacks triggered by trauma, pupillary dilation, stress, or ocular changes that push the iris forward

Risk factors
OPEN-ANGLE GLAUCOMA
- Family history
- Myopia
- Ethnic origin
ANGLE-CLOSURE GLAUCOMA
- Family history
- Cataracts
- Hyperopia

Incidence
- Affects about 2% of Americans older than age 40
- Accounts for about 12% of newly diagnosed blindness in the United States
- Highest incidence among males and African-American and Asian populations

Common characteristics
- Decreased visual acuity
- Nausea and vomiting

Complications
- Varying degrees of vision loss
- Total blindness

OPTIC DISK CHANGES

Ophthalmoscopy and slit-lamp examination show cupping of the optic disk, characteristic of glaucoma.

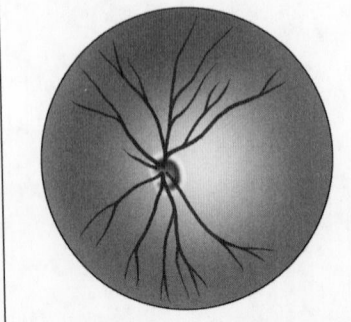

✳ ASSESSMENT

History
OPEN-ANGLE GLAUCOMA
- Possibly no symptoms
- Dull, morning headache
- Mild aching in the eyes
- Loss of peripheral vision
- Halos around lights
- Reduced visual acuity (especially at night) not corrected by glasses

ANGLE-CLOSURE GLAUCOMA

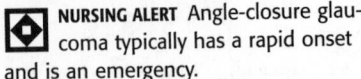 **NURSING ALERT** Angle-closure glaucoma typically has a rapid onset and is an emergency.

- Pain and pressure over the eye
- Blurred vision
- Decreased visual acuity
- Halos around lights
- Nausea and vomiting (from increased IOP)

Physical findings
- Unilateral eye inflammation
- Cloudy cornea
- Moderately dilated pupil, nonreactive to light
- With gentle fingertip pressure to the closed eyelids, one eye feels harder than the other (in angle-closure glaucoma)

Test results
DIAGNOSTIC PROCEDURES
- Tonometry measurement shows increased IOP.
- Slit-lamp examination shows effects of glaucoma on the anterior eye structures.
- Gonioscopy shows angle of the eye's anterior chamber.
- Ophthalmoscopy aids visualization of the fundus. (See *Optic disk changes.*)
- Perimetry or visual field tests show extent of peripheral vision loss.
- Fundus photography shows optic disk changes.

◆ TREATMENT

General
- Reduction of IOP by decreasing aqueous humor production with medications

Diet
- No restrictions

Activity
- Bed rest (with acute angle-closure glaucoma)

Medication
- Topical adrenergic agonists
- Cholinergic agonists
- Beta-adrenergic blockers
- Topical or oral carbonic anhydrase inhibitors

◈ **NURSING ALERT** Occasionally, systemic absorption of a beta-adrenergic blocker from eyedrops can be sufficient to cause bradycardia, hypotension, heart block, bronchospasm, impotence, or depression.

Surgery
- For patients who don't respond to drug therapy:
  - Argon laser trabeculoplasty
  - Trabeculectomy

ANGLE-CLOSURE GLAUCOMA
- Laser iridectomy
- Surgical peripheral iridectomy
- In end-stage glaucoma, tube shunt or valve

❖ NURSING CONSIDERATIONS

Nursing diagnoses
- Acute pain
- Anxiety
- Disturbed sensory perception: Visual
- Fear
- Risk for injury

Key outcomes
The patient will:
- express areas of fear and concern openly
- express feelings of increased comfort and decreased pain
- express feelings and concerns
- regain visual function
- sustain no harm or injury.

Nursing interventions
- Give medication, as ordered.
- Prepare for surgery, if indicated.
- Administer cycloplegic eyedrops in affected eye only (may precipitate attack of angle-closure glaucoma and threaten residual vision).
- After trabeculectomy, give medications, as ordered, to dilate the pupil.
- Apply topical corticosteroids, as ordered, to rest the pupil.
- After surgery, protect the affected eye.
- Administer pain medication, as ordered.
- Encourage ambulation immediately after surgery.
- Encourage the patient to express his concerns related to the chronic condition.

Monitoring
- Vital signs
- Response to treatment
- Visual acuity

▶ PATIENT TEACHING

Be sure to cover:
- disorder, diagnostic tests, and treatment
- need for meticulous compliance with prescribed drug therapy
- how lost vision can't be restored but treatment can usually prevent further loss
- modification of the patient's environment for safety
- signs and symptoms that require immediate medical attention, such as sudden vision change or eye pain
- importance of glaucoma screening for early detection and prevention.

Discharge planning
- Refer the patient for home care follow-up, if indicated.

✴ RESOURCES

Organizations
Glaucoma Research Foundation:
www.glaucoma.org
Prevent Blindness America:
www.preventblindness.org

Selected references
Grieshaber, M.C., and Flammer, J. "Blood Flow in Glaucoma," *Current Opinion in Ophthalmology* 16(2):79-83, April 2005.

Jonas, J.B., et al. "Central Corneal Thickness and Development of Glaucomatous Optic Disk Hemorrhages," *American Journal of Ophthalmology* 140(6):1139-141, December 2005.

Marquis, R.E., and Whitson, J.T. "Management of Glaucoma: Focus on Pharmacological Therapy," *Drugs & Aging* 22(1):1-21, 2005.

Gonorrhea

Description
- Common venereal disease that usually starts as infection of the genitourinary tract; can also begin in rectum, pharynx, or eyes
- Left untreated, spreads through the blood to the joints, tendons, meninges, and endocardium
- May lead to chronic pelvic inflammatory disease (PID) and sterility (in women)

Pathophysiology
- Gonococci infect mucus-secreting epithelial surfaces and penetrate through or between the cells to the connective tissue.
- Inflammation and spread of the infection results.

Causes
- Transmission of *Neisseria gonorrhoeae*, the causative organism, through sexual contact with an infected person
- For child born to infected mother, acquisition of gonococcal ophthalmia neonatorum during passage through the birth canal
- Acquisition of gonococcal conjunctivitis by touching the eyes with a contaminated hand

Incidence
- Among sexually active individuals, incidence highest in those with multiple partners, teenagers, nonwhites, the poor, the poorly educated, city dwellers, and unmarried people who live alone
- Reinfection common

Common characteristics
- Possible dysuria in males
- Possible absence of symptoms (in both sexes) or symptoms related to the area infected
- Most common infection site in female children older than age 1 is vagina

Complications
- PID
- Acute epididymitis
- Proctitis
- Salpingitis
- Septic arthritis
- Dermatitis
- Perihepatitis
- Corneal ulceration
- Blindness
- Meningitis
- Osteomyelitis
- Pneumonia
- Acute respiratory distress syndrome

✳ ASSESSMENT

History
- Unprotected sexual contact (vaginal, oral, or anal) with an infected person, an unknown partner, or multiple sex partners
- History of sexually transmitted disease

Physical findings
- Fever
- Purulent discharge from urethral meatus
- Female urethral meatus possibly red and edematous
- Friable cervix and a greenish yellow discharge
- Engorged, red, swollen vagina with profuse purulent discharge
- Rectal infection
- Ocular infection
- Pharyngeal infection
- Papillary skin lesions on hands and feet
- PID
- Perihepatitis
- Pain and a cracking noise when moving an involved joint

Test results
LABORATORY
- Culture from the infection site of the urethra, cervix, rectum, or pharynx, grown on a Thayer-Martin agar, usually establishes the diagnosis.
- Culture of conjunctival scrapings confirms gonococcal conjunctivitis.
- In males, a Gram stain shows gram-negative diplococci, possibly confirming gonorrhea.
- Gonococcal arthritis requires identification of gram-negative diplococci on smear from joint fluid and skin lesions.
- Complement fixation and immunofluorescent assays of serum reveals antibody titers four times the normal rate.
- Venereal Disease Research Laboratory test may be reactive in a patient with syphilis.
- Rapid plasma reagin test may be reactive in a patient with syphilis.

◆ TREATMENT

General
- Follow-up cultures 4 to 7 days after treatment and again in 6 months
- For a pregnant patient, final follow-up before delivery
- Effective therapy (ends communicability within hours)

Diet
- No restrictions

Activity
- Abstinence from sexual activity until infection is treated

Medication
- Cephalosporins
- 1% silver nitrate drops or erythromycin ointment in neonates to prevent gonococcal ophthalmia neonatorum

Nursing diagnoses
- Acute pain
- Ineffective sexuality patterns
- Risk for infection
- Situational low self-esteem

Key outcomes
The patient will:
- express feelings of increased comfort and decreased pain
- voice feelings about potential or actual changes in sexual activity
- identify signs and symptoms of infection, and experience no further signs and symptoms of infection
- express concerns and feelings about self-concept, esteem, and body image.

Nursing interventions
- Practice standard precautions.
- Isolate the patient if his eyes are infected.
- With gonococcal arthritis, apply moist heat to ease pain in affected joints.
- Administer medications, as ordered.
- Report all cases of gonorrhea to the local public health authorities as required.
- Report all cases of gonorrhea in children to child abuse authorities.
- Routinely instill prophylactic medications, according to facility protocol, in the eyes of all neonates on admission to the nursery.
- Check the neonate of an infected mother for signs of infection, and obtain specimens for culture from the neonate's eyes, pharynx, and rectum.

Monitoring
- Response to treatment
- Adverse effects of medication
- Complications
- Follow-up culture results

Be sure to cover:
- disorder, diagnostic tests, and treatment
- need to inform all sexual partners of the infection so that they can seek treatment
- need to avoid sexual contact until cultures are negative and infection is eradicated
- need for the patient and all sexual partners to be tested for human immunodeficiency virus and hepatitis B infection
- need to be careful when coming into contact with any bodily discharge to avoid contaminating the eyes
- safer sex practices
- need to take anti-infective drugs for the time prescribed
- importance of returning for follow-up testing. (See *Preventing gonorrhea.*)

Discharge planning
- Refer to community health agency for follow-up testing as necessary.

PREVENTING GONORRHEA

To prevent gonorrhea, provide the following patient teaching:

- Tell the patient to avoid sexual contact until cultures prove negative and infection is eradicated.
- Advise the partner of an infected person to receive treatment even if the partner doesn't have a positive culture. Recommend that the partner avoid sexual contact with anyone until treatment is complete because reinfection is extremely common.
- Counsel the patient and all sexual partners to be tested for the human immunodeficiency virus and hepatitis B infection.
- Instruct the patient to be careful when coming into contact with any bodily discharges to avoid contaminating the eyes.
- Tell the patient to take anti-infective drugs for the time prescribed.
- To prevent reinfection, tell the patient to avoid sexual contact with anyone *suspected* of being infected, to use condoms during intercourse, to wash genitalia with soap and water before and after intercourse, and to avoid sharing washcloths or douche equipment.
- Advise returning for follow-up testing.

Organizations
Centers for Disease Control and Prevention: *www.cdc.gov*
Harvard University Consumer Health Information: *www.intelihealth.com*
National Health Information Center: *www.health.gov/nhic/*
National Library of Medicine: *www.nlm.nih.gov*

Selected references
Feroli, K.L., and Burstein, G.R. "Adolescent Sexually Transmitted Diseases: New Recommendations for Diagnosis, Treatment, and Prevention," *MCN The American Journal of Maternal/Child Nursing* 28(2):113-18, March-April 2003.

Kasper, D.L., et al., eds. *Harrison's Principles of Internal Medicine,* 16th ed. New York: McGraw-Hill Book Co., 2005.

Nsuami, M., et al. "Chlamydia and Gonorrhea Co-occurrence in a High School Population," *Sexually Transmitted Diseases* 31(7):424-27, July 2004.

Warner, L., et al. "Condom Use and Risk of Gonorrhea and Chlamydia: A Systemic Review of Design and Measurement Factors Assessed in Epidemiologic Studies," *Sexually Transmitted Diseases* 33(1):36-41, January 2006.

Goodpasture's syndrome

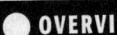

OVERVIEW

Description
- Pulmonary renal syndrome
- Characterized by hemoptysis and rapidly progressive glomerulonephritis

Pathophysiology
- Abnormal production and deposition of antibodies against glomerular basement membrane (GBM) and alveolar basement membrane activate the complement and inflammatory responses, resulting in glomerular and alveolar tissue damage.

Causes
- Exact cause unknown
- May be associated with exposure to hydrocarbons or with type II hypersensitivity reaction
- Possible genetic predisposition

Incidence
- Occurs at any age; most commonly in men between ages 20 and 30

Common characteristics
- Hemoptysis
- Rapidly progressive glomerulonephritis

Complications
- Renal failure
- Pulmonary edema and hemorrhage

ASSESSMENT

History
- Possible complaints of malaise, fatigue, and pallor
- Possible pulmonary bleeding for months or years before developing overt hemorrhage and signs of renal disease

Physical findings
- Hematuria
- Decreased urine output
- Dyspnea, tachypnea, orthopnea
- Restlessness
- Hemoptysis, ranging from a cough with blood-tinged sputum to frank pulmonary hemorrhage
- Pulmonary crackles and rhonchi

Test results
LABORATORY
- Immunofluorescence of alveolar basement membrane shows linear deposition of immunoglobulins as well as C3 and fibrinogen.
- Immunofluorescence of GBM also shows linear deposition of immunoglobulins.
- Serum anti-GBM antibody reveals the presence of circulating anti-GBM antibodies that distinguishes Goodpasture's syndrome from other pulmonary-renal syndromes, such as Wegener's granulomatosis, polyarteritis, and systemic lupus erythematosus.
- Serum creatinine and blood urea nitrogen (BUN) levels are typically increased to two to three times their normal level.
- Urinalysis may reveal red blood cells and cellular casts, which typify glomerular inflammation; may also show granular casts and proteinuria.

IMAGING
- Chest X-rays reveal pulmonary infiltrates in a diffuse, nodular pattern.

DIAGNOSTIC PROCEDURES
- Lung biopsy shows interstitial and intra-alveolar hemorrhage with hemosiderin-laden macrophages.
- Renal biopsy usually shows focal necrotic lesions and cellular crescents.

TREATMENT

General
- Plasmapheresis
- Dialysis

Diet
- Low-protein, low-sodium

Activity
- As tolerated

Medication
- High-dose I.V. corticosteroids
- Cyclophosphamide (Cytoxan)

Surgery
- Kidney transplantation

❖ NURSING CONSIDERATIONS

Nursing diagnoses
- Activity intolerance
- Anxiety
- Excess fluid volume
- Fatigue
- Impaired gas exchange
- Impaired urinary elimination
- Ineffective airway clearance
- Ineffective breathing pattern
- Risk for injury

Key outcomes
The patient will:
- demonstrate measures to balance rest and activity
- verbalize feelings and concerns
- exhibit fluid balance that remains within range; intake will equal output
- express feelings of increased energy
- maintain adequate ventilation and oxygenation
- maintain a patent airway
- maintain effective breathing pattern
- remain free from complications or injury.

Nursing interventions
- Elevate the head of the bed and administer humidified oxygen, as ordered.
- Encourage the patient to conserve his energy.
- Provide range-of-motion exercises.
- Assist with activities of daily living, and provide frequent rest periods.
- Transfuse blood and administer corticosteroids, as ordered. Watch closely for signs of adverse reactions.

Monitoring
- Respiratory rate and breath sounds
- Quantity and quality of sputum
- Vital signs and arterial blood gas levels
- Intake and output and daily weight
- Creatinine clearance, BUN, and serum creatinine levels
- Hematocrit and coagulation studies

▶ PATIENT TEACHING

Be sure to cover:
- disorder, diagnostic tests, and treatment
- information about the disease process
- importance of conserving energy
- explanation that fluid intake may be restricted
- name, dosage, purpose, and adverse effects of all medications
- how to effectively deep breathe and cough
- need to obtain regular follow-up care
- use of sugarless hard candy if the patient has a sore, dry mouth
- how to recognize the signs of respiratory or genitourinary bleeding and the need to report such signs to the physician at once.

Discharge planning
- If dialysis or kidney transplantation is required, refer the patient to a renal support group.

✳ RESOURCES

Organizations
National Kidney and Urologic Diseases Information Clearinghouse: *www.niddk.nih.gov*
National Kidney Foundation: www.*kidney.org*

Selected references
Bergs, L. "Goodpasture Syndrome," *Critical Care Nurse* 25(5):50-54, 56, 57-58, October 2005.
Kasper, D.L., et al., eds. *Harrison's Principles of Internal Medicine,* 16th ed. New York: McGraw-Hill Book Co., 2005.
The Merck Manual of Diagnosis and Therapy, 18th ed. Whitehouse Station, N.J.: Merck and Co., Inc., 2006.

Gout

● OVERVIEW

Description
- Inflammatory arthritis caused by uric acid and cyrstal deposits
- Red, swollen, and acutely painful joints
- Mostly affects feet, great toe, ankle, and midfoot
- Primary gout patient symptom-free for years between attacks
- First acute attack: strikes suddenly and peaks quickly
- Delayed attacks: associated with olecranon bursitis
- Chronic polyarticular gout: final, unremitting stage of the disease marked by persistent painful polyarthritis

Pathophysiology
- Uric acid crystallizes in blood or body fluids and the precipitate accumulates in connective tissue (tophi).
- Crystals trigger an immune response.
- Neutrophils secrete lysosomes for phagocytosis.
- Lysosomes damage tissue and exacerbate the immune response.

Causes
- Decreased renal excretion of uric acid
- Genetic defect in purine metabolism (hyperuricemia)
- Hereditary factors
- Oversecretion of uric acid
- Radical dieting practices involving starvation
- Secondary gout that develops with other diseases:
  - Obesity
  - Diabetes mellitus
  - Hypertension
  - Polycythemia
  - Leukemia
  - Myeloma
  - Sickle cell anemia
  - Renal disease
- Secondary gout that follows treatment with drugs (hydrochlorothiazide or pyrazinamide)

Incidence
- Primary gout typical in men older than age 30 and postmenopausal women who take diuretics

Common characteristics
- Extreme pain
- Redness and swelling in joints
- Tophi in great toe, ankle, or pinna of ear
- Elevated skin temperature

Complications
- Renal calculi
- Atherosclerotic disease
- Cardiovascular lesions
- Stroke
- Coronary thrombosis
- Hypertension
- Infection (when tophi rupture)

✳ ASSESSMENT

History
- Sedentary lifestyle
- Hypertension
- Renal calculi
- Waking during the night with pain in great toe
- Initial moderate pain that grows intense
- Chills; mild fever

Physical findings
- Swollen, dusky red or purple joint
- Limited movement of joint
- Tophi, especially in the outer ears, hands, and feet (see *Recognizing gouty tophi*)
- Skin over tophi that may ulcerate and release chalky white exudate or pus
- Secondary joint degeneration
- Erosions, deformity, and disability
- Warmth over joint
- Extreme tenderness
- Fever
- Hypertension

Test results
LABORATORY
- Serum uric acid levels are elevated with a gout attack.
- White blood cell count is elevated in acute attack.
- Urine uric acid level is elevated in 20% of patients.
IMAGING
- X-ray of the articular cartilage and subchondral bone shows evidence of chronic gout.

DIAGNOSTIC PROCEDURES
- Needle aspiration of synovial fluid shows needlelike intracellular crystals.

◆ TREATMENT

General
- Termination of acute attack
- Protection of inflamed, painful joints
- Treatment for hyperuricemia
- Local application of cold
- Prevention of recurrent gout
- Prevention of renal calculi
- Weight loss program, if indicated

Diet
- Avoidance of alcohol
- Sparing use of purine-rich foods (such as anchovies, liver, and sardines)

Activity
- Bed rest (in acute attack)
- Immobilization of joint

Medication
- Analgesics
- Nonsteroidal anti-inflammatory drugs
- Colchicine
- Allopurinol
- Probenecid or sulfinpyrazone
- Corticosteroids

Nursing diagnoses

- Acute pain
- Anxiety
- Deficient knowledge (gout)
- Disturbed sleep pattern
- Impaired physical mobility
- Ineffective coping
- Risk for injury

Key outcomes

The patient will:

- express feelings of increased comfort and decreased pain
- exhibit decreased anxiety
- demonstrate knowledge of the condition and treatment regimen.
- verbalize feelings of being well rested
- maintain joint mobility and range of motion
- perform activities of daily living within confines of the disease
- demonstrate adequate coping skills.

Nursing interventions

- Allow adequate time for self-care.
- Institute bed rest.
- Use a bed cradle if appropriate.
- Give pain medication, as needed.
- Apply cold packs.
- Identify techniques and activities that promote rest and relaxation.
- Administer anti-inflammatory medication.
- Provide a purine-poor diet.

Monitoring

- Intake and output
- Serum uric acid levels
- Acute gout attacks 24 to 96 hours after surgery

Be sure to cover:

- disorder, diagnostic tests, and treatment
- need to drink plenty of fluids (up to 2 L per day)
- relaxation techniques
- need to avoid purine-rich foods because these substances raise the urate level
- need to report adverse drug reactions immediately
- importance of compliance with the medication regimen
- need to control hypertension.

Discharge planning

- Refer the patient to a weight-reduction program, if appropriate.

RECOGNIZING GOUTY TOPHI

In advanced gout, urate crystal deposits develop into hard, irregular, yellow-white nodules called *tophi*. These bumps commonly protrude from the great toe and ear.

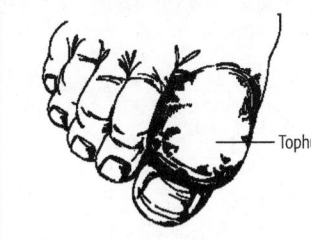
Tophus

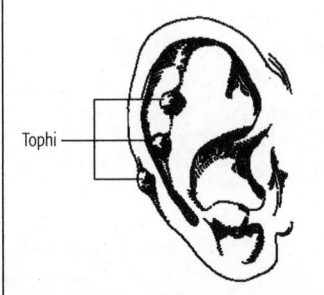
Tophi

Organizations

National Institutes of Health: *www.nih.gov*
WebMD: *www.webmd.com*

Selected references

Diseases, 4th ed. Philadelphia: Lippincott Williams & Wilkins, 2006.

Handbook of Pathophysiology, 2nd ed. Philadelphia: Lippincott Williams & Wilkins, 2005.

Masseoud, D., et al. "Overview of Hyperuricaemia and Gout," *Current Pharmaceutical Design* 11(32):4117-124, 2005.

Moreland, L.W. "Febuxostat—Treatment for Hyperuricemia and Gout?" *New England Journal of Medicine* 353(23):2505-507, December 2005.

Graft rejection syndrome

● OVERVIEW

Description
- Rejection of a donated organ that occurs when the host's immune responses are directed against the graft
- Three subtypes based on time of onset and mechanisms involved:
  - Hyperacute rejection
  - Acute rejection
  - Chronic rejection

Pathophysiology
- Hyperacute rejection occurs within minutes to hours after graft transplantation. Circulating host antibodies recognize and bind to graft antigens. Binding of these antibodies leads to initiation of the complement cascade, recruitment of neutrophils, platelet activation, damage to graft endothelial cells, and stimulation of coagulation reactions.
- Acute rejection may occur several hours to days (even weeks) after transplantation. Alloantigen-reactive T cells from the host infiltrate the graft and are activated by contact with foreign, graft-related proteins that are presented to them by antigen-presenting cells. These T cells may cause graft tissue damage.
- Chronic rejection is characterized by the development of blood vessel luminal occlusion due to progressive thickening of the intimal layers of medium and large arterial walls. Large amounts of intimal matrix are produced, leading to increasingly occlusive vessel wall thickening. A slowly progressing reduction in blood flow results in regional tissue ischemia, cell death, and tissue fibrosis.

Causes
- Immune system response to the graft

Incidence
- Hyperacute rejection rare; affects less than 1% of transplant recipients
- Acute rejection in 50% of transplant patients (only 10% progress to graft loss)
- Chronic rejection in 50% of transplant patients within 10 years after transplantation

Common characteristics
- Rapid or gradual progression of organ dysfunction

Complications
- Rapid thrombosis
- Loss of graft function

✳ ASSESSMENT

History
- Signs and symptoms variable; dependent on type of rejection, underlying illnesses, and type of organ transplanted

Physical findings
- Oliguria and increasing serum creatinine and blood urea nitrogen levels with kidney transplant
- Elevated transaminase levels, decreased albumin levels, and hypocoagulability with liver transplant
- Hypotension, heart failure, and edema with heart transplant

Test results
DIAGNOSTIC PROCEDURES
- Graft rejection can be confirmed with a biopsy of the transplanted tissue.
- Hyperacute rejection is characterized by large numbers of polymorphonuclear leukocytes in the graft blood vessels, widespread microthrombi, platelet accumulation, and interstitial hemorrhage. There's little or no interstitial inflammation.

◆ TREATMENT

General
- Close monitoring of function of grafted organ
- Surveillance, with prophylactic measures against opportunistic infections

Diet
- Restrictions based on organ system affected

Activity
- As tolerated

Medication
- Immunosuppressants
- Antirejection therapies
- Antibiotics

NURSING CONSIDERATIONS

Nursing diagnoses
- Activity intolerance
- Disturbed body image
- Fatigue
- Hopelessness
- Hyperthermia
- Imbalanced nutrition: Less than body requirements
- Impaired skin integrity
- Ineffective coping
- Ineffective health maintenance
- Ineffective tissue perfusion: Renal, cardiopulmonary
- Interrupted family processes
- Risk for deficient fluid volume
- Risk for infection
- Social isolation

Key outcomes
The patient will:
- verbalize the importance of balancing activity, as tolerated, with rest
- express feelings related to a changed body image
- make decisions on his own behalf
- maintain a normal body temperature
- exhibit no signs of malnutrition
- exhibit normal healing of wounds and lesions
- experience decreased areas of redness, swelling, and inflammation
- use support systems to assist with coping
- perform health maintenance activities according to the level of his ability
- maintain adequate renal and cardiopulmonary perfusion
- voice feelings about the condition
- express feelings of control over his well-being
- maintain a normal fluid balance
- experience no fever, chills, or other signs or symptoms of illness
- maintain social interaction to the extent possible.

Nursing interventions
- Administer immunosuppressants, as ordered.
- Administer antirejection therapies, as ordered.
- Administer antibiotics for infection, as ordered.

Monitoring
- Vital signs
- Function of the transplanted organ
- Signs and symptoms of infection
- Signs and symptoms of rejection

PATIENT TEACHING

Be sure to cover:
- disorder, diagnostic tests, and treatment
- how to recognize signs and symptoms of organ dysfunction
- need to immediately report fever, chills, and other symptoms of infection
- why long-term or lifelong medication compliance is vital to successful immunosuppressive therapy for the prevention of acute graft rejection.

Discharge planning
- Refer the patient and his family to social support, including psychological support services, as indicated.

RESOURCES

Organizations
Centers for Disease Control and Prevention: *www.cdc.gov*
National Institutes of Health: *www.nih.gov*

Selected references
Diseases, 4th ed. Philadelphia: Lippincott Williams & Wilkins, 2006.
Kasper, D.L., et al., eds. *Harrison's Principles of Internal Medicine,* 16th ed. New York: McGraw-Hill Book Co., 2005.
Storm, T.B. "Rejection—More than the Eye Can See," *New England Journal of Medicine* 353(22):2394-396, December 2005.

Guillain-Barré syndrome

● OVERVIEW

Description
- Form of polyneuritis
- Acute, rapidly progressive, and potentially fatal
- Three phases:
  - Acute: lasting from first symptom, ending in 1 to 3 weeks
  - Plateau: lasting several days to 2 weeks
  - Recovery: coincides with remyelination and axonal process regrowth; extends over 4 to 6 months and may take up to 2 to 3 years; recovery possibly not complete

Pathophysiology
- Segmented demyelination of peripheral nerves occurs, preventing normal transmission of electrical impulses.
- Sensorimotor nerve roots are affected; autonomic nerve transmission may also be affected. (See *Understanding sensorimotor nerve degeneration.*)

Causes
- Exact cause unknown
- Virus that causes cell-mediated immunologic attack on peripheral nerves

---

UNDERSTANDING SENSORIMOTOR NERVE DEGENERATION

Guillain-Barré syndrome attacks the peripheral nerves so that they can't transmit messages to the brain correctly. Here's what goes wrong:

The myelin sheath degenerates for unknown reasons. This sheath covers the nerve axons and conducts electrical impulses along the nerve pathways. With degeneration comes inflammation, swelling, and patchy demyelination. As this disorder destroys myelin, the nodes of Ranvier (at the junctures of the myelin sheaths) widen. This delays and impairs impulse transmission along the dorsal and ventral nerve roots.

Because the dorsal nerve roots handle sensory function, the patient may experience sensations, such as tingling and numbness, when the nerve root is impaired. Similarly, because the ventral roots are responsible for motor function, impairment causes varying weakness, immobility, and paralysis.

Risk factors
- Surgery
- Rabies or swine influenza vaccination
- Viral illness
- Hodgkin's or some other malignant disease
- Lupus erythematosus

Incidence
- Occurs equally in both sexes
- Occurs between ages 30 and 50

Common characteristics
- Symmetrical muscle weakness initially in lower extremities and progressing to upper extremities
- Paresthesia
- Diplegia
- Dysphagia
- Hypotonia
- Areflexia

Complications
- Thrombophlebitis
- Pressure ulcers
- Contractures
- Muscle wasting
- Aspiration
- Respiratory tract infections
- Life-threatening respiratory and cardiac compromise

✳ ASSESSMENT

History
- Minor febrile illness 1 to 4 weeks before current symptoms
- Tingling and numbness in the legs
- Progression of symptoms to arms, trunk and, finally, the face
- Stiffness and pain in the calves

Physical findings
- Muscle weakness (major neurologic sign)
- Sensory loss, usually in the legs (spreads to arms)
- Difficulty talking, chewing, and swallowing
- Paralysis of the ocular, facial, and oropharyngeal muscles
- Loss of position sense
- Diminished or absent deep tendon reflexes

Test results
DIAGNOSTIC PROCEDURES
- Cerebrospinal fluid (CSF) analysis may show a normal white blood cell count, an elevated protein count and, in severe disease, increased CSF pressure.

OTHER
- Electromyography may demonstrate repeated firing of the same motor unit instead of widespread sectional stimulation.
- Nerve conduction studies show marked slowing of nerve conduction velocities.

TREATMENT

General
- Primarily supportive
- Possible endotracheal intubation or tracheotomy
- Volume replacement
- Plasmapheresis

Diet
- Possible tube feedings with endotracheal intubation
- Adequate caloric intake

Activity
- Exercise program to prevent contractures

Medication
- I.V. beta-adrenergic blockers
- Parasympatholytics
- I.V. immune globulin

Surgery
- Possible tracheostomy
- Possible gastrostomy or jejunotomy feeding tube insertion

NURSING CONSIDERATIONS

Nursing diagnoses
- Anxiety
- Fear
- Imbalanced nutrition: Less than body requirements
- Impaired gas exchange
- Impaired physical mobility
- Impaired urinary elimination
- Impaired verbal communication
- Ineffective breathing pattern

Key outcomes
The patient will:
- identify strategies to decrease anxiety
- express fears and concerns
- maintain required daily caloric intake
- maintain a patent airway and adequate ventilation and oxygenation
- maintain joint mobility and range of motion (ROM)
- establish routine urinary elimination patterns
- develop alternate means of expressing self
- maintain effective breathing pattern.

Nursing interventions
- Establish a means of communication before intubation is required.
- Turn and reposition the patient.
- Encourage coughing and deep breathing.
- Begin respiratory support at the first sign of dyspnea.
- Provide meticulous skin care.
- Administer passive ROM exercises.
- In case of facial paralysis, provide eye and mouth care.
- Prevent constipation.
- Provide emotional support.
- Administer medications, as ordered.

Monitoring
- Vital signs
- Breath sounds
- Arterial blood gas measurements
- Level of consciousness
- Continual respiratory function
- Pulse oximetry
- Signs of thrombophlebitis
- Signs of urine retention
- Response to medications

PATIENT TEACHING

Be sure to cover:
- disorder, diagnostic tests, and treatment
- effective means of communication
- appropriate home care plan
- instructions about medications
- adverse drug reactions.

Discharge planning
Refer the patient to:
- physical rehabilitation sources, as indicated
- occupational and speech rehabilitation resources, as indicated
- Guillain-Barré Syndrome Foundation.

RESOURCES

Organizations
Guillain-Barré Syndrome Foundation, International: *www.webmast.com*
National Institutes of Health: *www.nih.gov*

Selected references
Diseases, 4th ed. Philadelphia: Lippincott Williams & Wilkins, 2006.

Gregory, M.A., et al. "Understanding Guillian-Barré Syndrome and Central Nervous System Involvement," *Rehabilitative Nursing* 30(5):207-12, September-October 2005.

Halderman, D., and Zulkosky, K. "Treatment and Nursing Care for a Patient with Guillain-Barré Syndrome," *Dimensions of Critical Care Nursing* 24(6):267-72, November-December 2005.

Handbook of Pathophysiology, 2nd ed. Philadelphia: Lippincott Williams & Wilkins, 2005.

Kuwabara, S. "Guillain-Barré Syndrome: Epidemiology, Pathophysiology and Management," *Drugs* 64(6):597-610, 2004.

Haemophilus influenzae infection

● OVERVIEW

Description
- Most commonly attacks respiratory system
- Common cause of epiglottiditis, laryngotracheobronchitis, pneumonia, bronchiolitis, otitis media, and meningitis
- Infrequent cause of bacterial endocarditis, conjunctivitis, facial cellulitis, septic arthritis, and osteomyelitis

Pathophysiology
- Antigenic response occurs with invasion of bacteria.
- Systemic disease results from invasion and hematogenous spread to distant sites (meninges, bones, and joints).
- Local invasion occurs on the mucosal surfaces.
- Otitis media occurs when bacteria reach the middle ear through the eustachian tube.

Causes
- *H. influenzae*, a gram-negative, pleomorphic aerobic bacillus
- Transmission by direct contact with secretions or airborne droplets

Incidence
- *H. influenzae* type B (Hib) infection predominantly affecting children at a rate of 3% to 5%; incidence lower when vaccine is administered at ages 2, 4, 6, and 15 months
- *H. influenza* epiglottiditis most common in children between ages 3 and 7 but can occur at any age
- Higher incidence of meningitis due to Hib in black children
- Ten times higher incidence in Native Americans, possibly due to exposure, socioeconomic conditions, and genetic differences in immune response

Common characteristics
- Generalized malaise
- High fever

Complications
- Permanent neurologic sequelae from meningitis
- Complete upper airway obstruction from epiglottiditis
- Cellulitis
- Pericarditis, pleural effusion
- Respiratory failure from pneumonia

✳ ASSESSMENT

History
- Possible report of recent viral infection

Physical findings
EPIGLOTTIDITIS
- Restlessness and irritability
- Use of accessory muscles, inspiratory retractions, stridor
- Sitting up, leaning forward with mouth open, tongue protruding, and nostrils flaring
- Expiratory rhonchi; diminishing breath sounds as the condition worsens
- Pharyngeal mucosa that may look reddened (rarely, with soft yellow exudate)
- Epiglottis that appears cherry red with considerable edema
- Severe pain that makes swallowing difficult or impossible

PNEUMONIA
- Shaking chills
- Tachypnea
- Productive cough
- Impaired or asymmetrical chest movement caused by pleuritic pain
- Dullness over areas of lung consolidation

MENINGITIS
- Altered level of consciousness
- Seizures and coma as disease progresses
- Positive Brudzinski's and Kernig's signs
- Exaggerated and symmetrical deep tendon reflexes
- Nuchal rigidity
- Opisthotonos

Test results
LABORATORY
- Isolation of the organism in blood culture confirms infection.
- Hib meningitis is detected in cerebrospinal fluid cultures.

◆ TREATMENT

General
- Airway maintenance (critical in epiglottiditis)

Diet
- Based on respiratory status (possible need for small frequent meals)
- Nothing by mouth with inability to swallow adequately

Activity
- Rest periods, as needed

Medication
- Cephalosporin
- Chloramphenicol and ampicillin (alternate regimen)
- Glucocorticoids

Nursing diagnoses

- Acute pain
- Anxiety
- Deficient fluid volume
- Imbalanced nutrition: Less than body requirements
- Impaired gas exchange
- Ineffective airway clearance
- Ineffective breathing pattern
- Risk for aspiration
- Risk for infection

Key outcomes

The patient will:

- express feelings of increased comfort and decreased pain
- report a decrease in anxiety
- attain and maintain normal fluid and electrolyte balance
- achieve adequate nutritional intake
- maintain adequate gas exchange
- maintain a patent airway
- maintain effective breathing pattern without adventitious breath sounds
- exhibit no signs of aspiration
- remain free from signs and symptoms of infection.

Nursing interventions

- Maintain infection control precautions.
- Maintain adequate respiratory function through cool humidification; oxygen, as needed; and croup or face tents.
- Keep emergency resuscitation equipment readily available.
- Suction, as needed.
- Administer medication, as ordered.
- Maintain adequate nutrition and elimination.

Monitoring

- Pulse oximetry
- Arterial blood gas results
- Complete blood count for signs of bone marrow depression when therapy includes ampicillin or chloramphenicol
- Intake and output
- Respiratory status
- Neurologic status

Be sure to cover:

- disorder, diagnostic tests, and treatment
- importance of continuing the prescribed antibiotic until entire prescription is finished
- using a room humidifier or breathing moist air from a shower or bath, as necessary, for home treatment of a respiratory infection
- coughing and deep-breathing exercises to clear secretions
- the disposal of secretions and use of proper hand-washing technique.

Discharge planning

- Refer the patient to an infectious disease specialist if necessary.
- Encourage the patient to receive vaccinations to prevent future infections.

Organizations

Centers for Disease Control and Prevention: *www.cdc.gov*
Harvard University Consumer Health Information: *www.intelihealth.com*
National Health Information Center: *www.health.gov/nhic*
National Library of Medicine: *www.nlm.nih.gov*

Selected references

Heininger, U., and Zuberbuhler, M. "Immunization Rates and Timely Adminisrtaion in Pre-school and School-aged Children," *European Journal of Pediatrics* 165(2):124-29, February 2006.

Kasper, D.L., et al., eds. *Harrison's Principles of Internal Medicine,* 16th ed. New York: McGraw-Hill Book Co., 2005.

Sheff, B. "Haemophilus Infleunzae Type B (Hib)," *Nursing* 36(1):31, January 2006.

Hantavirus pulmonary syndrome

● OVERVIEW

Description
- Viral disease that causes flulike symptoms
- Rapidly progresses to respiratory failure

Pathophysiology
- Rodents shed virus in stool, urine, and saliva.
- Human infection occurs from inhalation, ingestion (of contaminated food or water, for example), contact with rodent excrement, or rodent bites. (See *Sin Nombre virus.*)

Causes
- Hantaviruses
- Transmission with exposure to infected rodents (deer mice, pinion mice, brush mice, and western chipmunks)
- Farming, hiking, or camping in rodent-infested areas and occupying rodent-infested dwellings

Incidence
- Occurs mainly in southwestern United States

Common characteristics
- Noncardiogenic pulmonary edema
- Myalgia, fever, headache, nausea, vomiting, and cough

Complications
- Respiratory failure
- Death (in 80% of cases)

✳ ASSESSMENT

History
- Vague prodromal symptoms that may become severe enough to seek medical attention

Physical findings
- Fever, cough
- Myalgia
- Hypotension
- Tachycardia, tachypnea
- Severe hypoxemia and respiratory failure

Test results
- The Centers for Disease Control and Prevention and state health departments can perform definitive testing for hantavirus exposure and antibody formation.

LABORATORY
- White blood cell count is elevated, with a predominance of neutrophils, myeloid precursors, and atypical lymphocytes.
- Hematocrit is elevated.
- Platelet count is decreased.
- Partial thromboplastin time is elevated.
- Fibrinogen level is normal.
- Serum creatinine levels are no greater than 2.5 mg/dl.

IMAGING
- Chest X-rays eventually show bilateral diffuse infiltrates in almost all patients (findings consistent with acute respiratory distress syndrome).

◆ TREATMENT

General
- Intubation and aggressive respiratory management
- Adequate oxygenation
- Stabilization of heart rate and blood pressure
- Cautious fluid volume replacement

Diet
- Nothing by mouth until recovery begins

Activity
- Bed rest

Medication
- Vasopressors
- Ribavirin (Virazole)

SIN NOMBRE VIRUS

This illustration shows the Sin Nombre virus, the most common cause of hantavirus pulmonary syndrome in the United States and Canada. It exists primarily in western states and provinces.

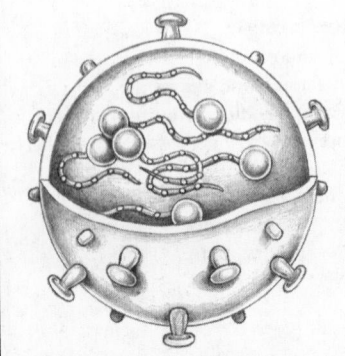

❖ NURSING CONSIDERATIONS

Nursing diagnoses
- Acute pain
- Fatigue
- Hyperthermia
- Impaired gas exchange
- Ineffective airway clearance
- Ineffective breathing pattern
- Ineffective health maintenance
- Risk for deficient fluid volume
- Risk for infection

Key outcomes
The patient will:
- verbalize increased comfort and decreased pain
- verbally report having an increased energy level
- exhibit a temperature within an acceptable range
- maintain adequate gas exchange
- maintain a patent airway with a respiratory rate within 5 breaths/minute of baseline
- express feelings of comfort while maintaining adequate air exchange
- maintain an adequate fluid volume
- remain free from signs and symptoms of infection.

Nursing interventions
- Maintain a patent airway by suctioning. Ensure adequate humidification and check mechanical ventilator settings frequently.
- Administer medication, as ordered.
- Provide I.V. fluid therapy based on results of hemodynamic monitoring.
- Provide emotional support.
- Report cases of hantavirus pulmonary syndrome to your state health department.

Monitoring
- Serum electrolyte levels
- Respiratory status
- Neurologic status

▶ PATIENT TEACHING

Be sure to cover:
- disorder, diagnostic tests, and treatment
- need to immediately report signs or symptoms of respiratory distress
- prevention guidelines, with a focus on rodent control.

Discharge planning
- Refer the patient for follow up with a pulmonologist, if indicated.

✳ RESOURCES

Organizations
Centers for Disease Control and Prevention: *www.cdc.gov*
Harvard University Consumer Health Information: *www.intelihealth.com*
National Health Information Center: *www.health.gov/nhic*
National Library of Medicine: *www.nlm.nih.gov*

Selected references
Dara, S.J., et al. "Acute Sin Nombre Hantavirus Infection Complicated by Renal Failure Requiring Hemodialysis," *Mayo Clinic Proceedings* 80(5):703-704, May 2005.

Kasper, D.L., et al., eds. *Harrison's Principles of Internal Medicine.* 16th ed. New York: McGraw-Hill Book Co., 2005.

Miedzinski, I. "Community-Acquired Pneumonia: New Facets of an Old Disease—Hantavirus Pulmonary Syndrome," *Respiratory Care Clinics of North America* 11(1):45-58, March 2005.

Overtruf, G.D. "Clinical Sin Nombre Hantaviral Infections in Children," *The Pediatric Infectious Disease Journal* 24(4):373-74, April 2005.

Headache

● OVERVIEW

Description

- Head pain that may or may not be a symptom of an underlying disorder
- Classified as vascular or muscle contraction, or a combination, in 90% of all headaches
- Migraine headaches: throbbing, vascular headaches

Pathophysiology

HEADACHE

- Sustained muscle contractions directly deform pain receptors.
- Inflammation or direct pressure affects the cranial nerves.
- Pain-sensitive structures respond, including the skin, scalp, muscles, arteries, and veins; cranial nerves V, VII, IX, and X; and cervical nerves 1, 2, and 3.

MIGRAINE

- Biochemical abnormalities occur, including local leakage of a vasodilator polypeptide through the dilated arteries and a decreased plasma level of serotonin.

Causes

HEADACHE

- Underlying intracranial disorder
- Systemic disorder
- Psychological disorders
- Tension (muscle contraction)
- Emotional stress
- Fatigue
- Menstruation
- Environmental stimuli
- Glaucoma
- Inflammation of the eyes or mucosa of the nasal or paranasal sinuses
- Diseases of the scalp, teeth, extracranial arteries, or external or middle ear
- Muscle spasms of the face, neck, or shoulders
- Vasodilators
- Systemic disease
- Hypoxia
- Hypertension
- Head trauma and tumors
- Intracranial bleeding, abscess, or aneurysm

MIGRAINE

- Constriction and dilation of intracranial and extracranial arteries

Incidence

HEADACHE

- Affects 60% to 80% of people in the United States at any given time

MIGRAINE

- Affects up to 10% of Americans
- First appears in childhood or adolescence, recurring throughout adulthood
- More common in females than in males
- Strong familial incidence

Common characteristics

- Pain that's aching or tight
- Hatband like pattern around head
- Nausea
- Photophobia
- Phonophobia

Complications

- Worsening of already existing hypertension
- Photophobia
- Emotional lability
- Motor weakness

✳ ASSESSMENT

History

HEADACHE

- Location (bilateral or unilateral), characteristics (frequency and intensity), onset and duration (continuous or intermittent)
- Precipitating factors that may include tension, menstruation, loud noises, menopause, and alcohol consumption
- Aggravating factors that may include coughing, sneezing, sunlight, and interference with daily activities
- Associated symptoms that may include nausea or vomiting, weakness, facial pain, scotomas, and allergies
- Use of headache-inducing medications
- Family history of headaches

MIGRAINE

- Unilateral, pulsating pain that gradually becomes more generalized
- May be preceded by scintillating scotoma, hemianopsia, unilateral paresthesia, or speech disorders
- May be accompanied by irritability, anorexia, nausea or vomiting, and photophobia

Physical findings

HEADACHE

- Possible signs of infection
- Possible bruits
- If no underlying problem, normal physical findings
- Possible crepitus or tender spots of the head and neck

MIGRAINE

- Pallor
- Possible extraocular muscle palsies
- Possible ptosis
- Possible neurologic deficits

Test results

IMAGING

- Skull X-rays may show skull fracture or sinusitis.
- Computed tomography scan may show tumor or subarachnoid hemorrhage or other intracranial pathology; may show pathology of sinuses.
- Magnetic resonance imaging may show tumor.

DIAGNOSTIC PROCEDURES

- Lumbar puncture may show increased intracranial pressure suggesting tumor, edema, or hemorrhage.
- EEG may show alterations in the brain's electrical activity, suggesting intracranial lesion, head injury, meningitis, or encephalitis.

General

- Yoga, mediation, or other relaxation-type therapy
- Identification and elimination of causative factors
- Psychotherapy, if emotional stress involved

Diet

- For migraine patient, adequate oral fluid intake; avoidance of dietary triggers

Activity

- For migraine patient, bed rest in a darkened room

Medication

HEADACHE

- Analgesics
- Tranquilizers
- Muscle relaxants

MIGRAINE

- Ergotamine preparations
- Preventive drugs
- Triptan agents
- Serotonin receptor agonists

Nursing diagnoses

- Acute pain
- Anxiety
- Energy field disturbance
- Fatigue
- Hopelessness
- Ineffective health maintenance
- Interrupted family processes

Key outcomes

The patient will:
- express feelings of increased comfort and decreased pain
- feel increasingly relaxed
- express an increased sense of well-being
- verbalize feeling well rested
- participate in self-care and make decisions regarding care
- demonstrate methods of promoting relaxation and inner well-being
- use support systems to assist with coping.

Nursing interventions

- Encourage the use of relaxation techniques.
- Keep the patient's room dark and quiet.
- Place ice packs on the patient's forehead or a cold cloth over her eyes.
- Administer pain medications, as ordered.

Monitoring

- Headaches
- Response to analgesics and other treatment
- Vital signs, especially blood pressure
- Neurologic status

Be sure to cover:
- disorder, diagnostic tests, and treatment
- migraine prevention
- avoidance of migraine triggers
- lifestyle changes
- nonpharmacologic strategies
- monitoring of headaches with headache diary
- appropriate use of preventive medications
- possible adverse effects of medications.

Discharge planning

- Refer the patient who experiences migraine headaches to the National Headache Foundation.

Organizations

National Headache Foundation: *www.headaches.org*
National Institutes of Health: *www.nih.gov*

Selected references

Davis, G.C., and Grassley, J.S. "Measurement of the Experience of Living with Primary Recurrent Headache," *Pain Management Nursing* 6(1):37-44, March 2005.

Diseases, 4th ed. Philadelphia: Lippincott Williams & Wilkins, 2006.

Gurney, D. "Patients with Chief Complaint of Headache: High-Risk Decision-Making at Triage," *Journal of Emergency Nursing* 31(1):115-16, February 2006.

Handbook of Pathophysiology, 2nd ed. Philadelphia: Lippincott Williams & Wilkins, 2005.

Linde, K., et al. "Acupuncture for Patients with Migraine: A Randomized Controlled Trial," *JAMA* 293(17):2118-125, May 2005.

Hearing loss

● OVERVIEW

Description
- Mechanical or nervous impediment to the transmission of sound waves to the brain
- Classified as conductive, sensorineural, or mixed
- Presbycusis: most common type of sensorineural hearing loss
- Congenital hearing loss: may be conductive or sensorineural
- Sudden hearing loss: may be conductive, sensorineural, or mixed; usually affects only one ear
- Noise-induced hearing loss: may be transient or permanent
- Depending on the cause, with prompt treatment (within 48 hours), hearing possibly restored

Pathophysiology
- In conductive hearing loss, sound wave transmission is interrupted between the external canal and inner ear (junction of the stapes and oval window).
- In sensorineural hearing loss, sound wave transmission is interrupted between the inner ear and brain, with accompanying cochlea or acoustic nerve dysfunction.
- Mixed hearing loss involves a combination of conduction and sensorineural transmission dysfunction.

Causes
CONDUCTIVE HEARING LOSS
- Cerumen (wax) impaction
- Blockage of the external ear
- Tympanic membrane thickening, retraction, scarring, or perforation
- Otitis media; otitis externa
- Otosclerosis
- Cholesteatoma
- Trauma
- Tumor
SENSORINEURAL HEARING LOSS
- Impairment of the cochlea, eighth cranial or acoustic nerve
- Loss of hair cells and nerve fibers in the cochlea
- Drug toxicity
- Infectious diseases
- Arteriosclerosis
- Otospongiosis
- Head or ear injury
- Organ of Corti degeneration
- Prolonged exposure to loud noise (85 to 90 dB)
- Brief exposure to extremely loud noise (greater than 90 dB)
- Acoustic neuroma
CONGENITAL HEARING LOSS
- Sensorineural or conductive
- May be transmitted as a dominant, autosomal dominant, autosomal recessive, or sex-linked recessive trait
HEARING LOSS IN NEONATES
- Trauma during delivery
- Toxicity
- Infection during pregnancy or delivery
- Known hereditary disorders
- Maternal exposure to rubella or syphilis during pregnancy
- Use of ototoxic drugs during pregnancy
- Prolonged fetal anoxia during delivery
- Congenital abnormalities of the ears, nose, or throat
SUDDEN HEARING LOSS
- Occlusion of internal auditory artery by spasm or thrombosis
- Subclinical mumps
- Bacterial and viral infections
- Acoustic neuroma
- Ménière's disease
- Metabolic, vascular, or neurologic disorders
- Blood dyscrasias
- Ototoxic drugs

Risk factors
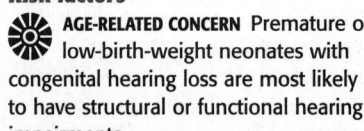 AGE-RELATED CONCERN Premature or low-birth-weight neonates with congenital hearing loss are most likely to have structural or functional hearing impairments.
- Neonates with serum bilirubin levels greater than 20 mg/dl (toxic effects on the brain)

Incidence
- Most common disability in the United States
- Third most prevalent disorder in adults older than age 65
- Presbycusis prevalent in adults older than age 50

Common characteristics
- Hearing loss
- Tinnitus

Complications
- Tympanic membrane perforation
- Cholesteatoma
- Permanent hearing loss

✳ ASSESSMENT

History
- Deficient response to auditory stimuli within 2 to 3 days after birth
- Older child with hearing loss that impairs speech development
- Recent upper respiratory tract infection
- Use of ototoxic substances
SUDDEN DEAFNESS
- Recent exposure to loud noise
- Brief exposure to an extremely loud noise
- Persistent tinnitus
- Transient vertigo

Physical findings
- Obvious hearing difficulty

Test results
IMAGING
- Computed tomography scan shows vestibular and auditory pathways.
- Magnetic resonance imaging shows acoustic tumors and brain lesions.
DIAGNOSTIC PROCEDURES
- Auditory brain response shows activity in auditory nerve and brain stem.
- Pure tone audiometry shows presence and degree of hearing loss.
- Electronystagmography shows vestibular function.
- Otoscopic or microscopic examination shows middle ear disorders; removes debris.
- Rinne and Weber's tests show whether hearing loss is conductive or sensorineural.

◆ TREATMENT

General
- Varies with the type and cause of impairment
- Hearing aids or other effective means of aiding communication

Diet
- Low-fat, low-cholesterol

Activity
- Avoiding activities that allow water to enter ear, with perforated eardrum

Medication
- Antibiotics
- Agents to dissolve cerumen
- Decongestants
- Analgesics
- Antipyretics
- Sedatives

Surgery
- Correction of tympanic membrane perforation

❖ NURSING CONSIDERATIONS

Nursing diagnoses
- Acute pain
- Anxiety
- Deficient knowledge (hearing loss)
- Disturbed sensory perception: Auditory
- Fear
- Impaired verbal communication
- Ineffective coping
- Risk for infection
- Risk for injury
- Situational low self-esteem

Key outcomes
The patient will:
- express feelings of increased comfort and decreased pain
- identify methods to relieve anxiety
- express understanding of the condition and treatment
- express feelings and concerns about the disorder
- regain hearing or develop alternate means of communication
- develop methods for communicating feelings and needs

- exhibit adequate coping mechanisms
- reman free from signs and symptoms of infection or injury
- express positive feelings related to self-esteem.

Nursing interventions
- Encourage discussion of concerns about hearing loss.
- Offer the patient reassurance when appropriate.
- Give clear, concise explanations.
- Face the patient when speaking.
- Enunciate words clearly, slowly, and in a normal tone.
- Allow adequate time for the patient to process what you said.
- Provide a pencil and paper to aid communication.
- Alert staff to communication problem.
- When speaking to a patient who can read lips:
  - approach within his visual range and attract his attention by raising your arm or waving
  - stand directly in front of him, with the light on your face
  - speak slowly and distinctly.

Monitoring
- Response to medication
- Progression of hearing loss
- Adaptation to hearing aid

▶ PATIENT TEACHING

Be sure to cover:
- disorder, diagnostic tests, and treatment
- preoperative and postoperative instructions
- danger of exposure to drugs, chemicals, and infection
- proper technique for ear cleaning or irrigation
- how to instill otic medications
- operation and maintenance of hearing aids
- danger of excessive noise exposure and need for protective devices in a noisy environment
- prescribed antibiotics and decongestants and their possible adverse effects
- need to report significant earache.

Discharge planning
- If hearing deteriorates, refer the patient for speech and hearing rehabilitation.
- Refer a child to an audiologist or otolaryngologist for further evaluation, as indicated.
- Refer the patient to special augmentation services for telephone use.
- Refer the patient to community resources, as appropriate.

✷ RESOURCES

Organizations
Alexander Graham Bell Association for the Deaf, Inc.:
www.agbell.org/index.html
National Institute on Deafness and Other Communication Disorders:
www.nidcd.nik.gov

Selected references
Folmer, R.I. "Noise-induced Hearing Loss in Young People," *Pediatrics* 117(1):248-49, January 2006.

Mamak, A., et al. "A Study of Prognostic Factors in Sudden Hearing Loss," *Ear, Nose & Throat Journal* 84(1):641-44, October 2005.

Williams, D. "Does Irrigation of the Ear to Remove Impacted Wax Improve Hearing?" *British Journal of Community Nursing* 19(5):228-32, May 2005.

Wills, T. "Learning How to Communicate Better with Deafened Patients," *Nursing Times* 101(3):44, January 2005.

Heart failure

● OVERVIEW

Description
- Myocardium: can't pump effectively enough to meet the body's metabolic needs
- Usually occurs in a damaged left ventricle, but it may happen in right ventricle primarily, or secondary to left-sided heart failure

Pathophysiology
LEFT-SIDED HEART FAILURE
- Pumping ability of the left ventricle fails and cardiac output falls.
- Blood backs up into the left atrium and lungs, causing pulmonary congestion.

RIGHT-SIDED HEART FAILURE
- Ineffective contractile function of the right ventricle leads to blood backing up into the right atrium and the peripheral circulation, which results in peripheral edema and engorgement of the kidneys and other organs.

Causes
- Mitral stenosis secondary to rheumatic heart disease, constrictive pericarditis, or atrial fibrillation
- Mitral or aortic insufficiency
- Arrhythmias
- Pregnancy
- Thyrotoxicosis
- Pulmonary embolism
- Hypertension
- Infections
- Anemia
- Emotional stress
- Increased salt or water intake

Incidence
- Affects 1% of people older than age 50
- Affects 10% of people older than age 80

Common characteristics
- Reduced cardiac output

Complications
- Pulmonary edema
- Organ failure, especially the brain and kidneys
- Myocardial infarction

✱ ASSESSMENT

History
- Disorder or condition that can precipitate heart failure
- Dyspnea or paroxysmal nocturnal dyspnea
- Peripheral edema
- Fatigue
- Weakness
- Insomnia
- Anorexia
- Nausea
- Sense of abdominal fullness (particularly in right-sided heart failure)

Physical findings
- Cough that produces pink, frothy sputum
- Cyanosis of the lips and nail beds
- Pale, cool, clammy skin
- Diaphoresis
- Jugular vein distention
- Ascites
- Tachycardia
- Pulsus alternans
- Hepatomegaly and, possibly, splenomegaly
- Decreased pulse pressure
- S_3 and S_4 heart sounds
- Moist, bibasilar crackles, rhonchi, and expiratory wheezing
- Decreased urinary output

Test results
LABORATORY
- B-type natriuretic peptide immunoassay is elevated.

IMAGING
- Chest X-rays show increased pulmonary vascular markings, interstitial edema, or pleural effusion and cardiomegaly.

DIAGNOSTIC PROCEDURES
- Electrocardiography reflects heart strain or enlargement or ischemia. It may also reveal atrial enlargement, tachycardia, and extrasystole.
- Pulmonary artery pressure monitoring typically shows elevated pulmonary artery and pulmonary artery wedge pressures, left ventricular end-diastolic pressure in left-sided heart failure, and elevated right atrial or central venous pressure in right-sided heart failure.

◆ TREATMENT

General
- Antiembolism stockings
- Elevation of lower extremities

Diet
- Sodium restriction
- Fluid restriction
- Calorie restriction, if indicated
- Low-fat, if indicated

Activity
- As tolerated
- Walking program

Medication
- Diuretics
- Oxygen
- Inotropic drugs
- Vasodilators
- Angiotensin-converting enzyme inhibitors
- Angiotensin-receptor blockers
- Cardiac glycosides
- Diuretics
- Potassium supplements
- Beta-adrenergic blockers
- Anticoagulants

Surgery
- For valvular dysfunction with recurrent acute heart failure, surgical replacement
- Heart transplantation
- Ventricular assist device
- Stent placement

❖ NURSING CONSIDERATIONS

Nursing diagnoses

- Activity intolerance
- Decreased cardiac output
- Deficient knowledge (heart failure)
- Excess fluid volume
- Fatigue
- Imbalanced nutrition: Less than body requirements
- Ineffective airway clearance
- Ineffective breathing pattern
- Ineffective tissue perfusion: Cardio-pulmonary

Key outcomes

The patient will:
- demonstrate methods to balance activity and rest
- maintain adequate cardiac output
- develop no complications from excess fluid volume
- carry out activities of daily living without excess fatigue or decreased energy
- maintain adequate hemodynamic stability
- maintain a patent airway
- maintain adequate nutritional intake
- maintain adequate ventilation and oxygenation.

Nursing interventions

- Place the patient in Fowler's position and give supplemental oxygen.
- Provide continuous cardiac monitoring during acute and advanced stages.
- Assist the patient with range-of-motion exercises. Enforce bed rest, and apply antiembolism stockings. Check for calf pain and tenderness.

Monitoring

- Daily weight for peripheral edema and other signs and symptoms of fluid overload
- Intake and output
- Vital signs
- Mental status
- Abnormal heart and breath sounds
- Peripheral edema

◈ **NURSING ALERT** Auscultate for abnormal heart and breath sounds and report changes immediately.

- Blood urea nitrogen and serum creatinine, potassium, sodium, chloride, and magnesium levels

▶ PATIENT TEACHING

Be sure to cover:
- disorder, diagnostic testing, and treatment
- signs and symptoms of worsening heart failure
- when to notify the physician
- importance of follow-up care
- need to avoid high-sodium foods
- need to avoid fatigue
- instructions about fluid restrictions
- need to weigh himself every morning, at the same time, before eating, and after urinating; keeping a record of his weight; and reporting a weight gain of 3 to 5 lb in 1 week.

Discharge planning

- Refer the patient to a smoking-cessation program, if appropriate.
- Arrange for follow-up home care, if indicated.

✳ RESOURCES

Organizations

American Heart Association: *www.americanheart.org*
Heart Failure Online: *www.heartfailure.org*

Selected references

D'Amico, C.I. "Cardiac Transplantation: Patient Selection in the Current Era," *Journal of Cardiovascular Nursing* 20(5 Suppl):S4-13, September-October 2005.

Jarcho, J.A. "Resynchronizing Ventricular Contraction in Heart Failure," *New England Journal of Medicine* 352(15):1594-597, April 2005.

Tsukui, H., et al. "Biventricular Assist Device Utilization for Patients with Morbid Congestive Heart Failure: A Justifiable Strategy," *Circulation* 112(Suppl):S65-72, August 2005.

Heat syndrome

● OVERVIEW

Description
- Heat exhaustion: acute heat injury with hyperthermia due to dehydration
- Heat stroke: extreme hyperthermia with thermoregulatory failure

Pathophysiology
- Normal regulation of temperature is through evaporation (30% of body's heat loss) or vasodilation. When heat is generated or gained by the body faster than it can dissipate, the thermoregulatory mechanism is stressed and eventually fails.
- Hyperthermia accelerates.
- Cerebral edema and cerebrovascular congestion occurs.
- Cerebral perfusion pressure increases and cerebral perfusion decreases.
- Tissue damage occurs when temperature exceeds 107.6° F (42° C), resulting in tissue necrosis, organ dysfunction, and failure.

Causes
- Illness
- Heart disease
- Endocrine disorders
- Neurologic disorder
- Infection (fever)
- Dehydration
- Excessive physical activity
- Excessive clothing
- Lack of acclimatization
- Hot environment without ventilation
- Inadequate fluid intake
- Drugs, such as phenothiazines, anticholinergics, and amphetamines

Risk factors
- Obesity
- Salt and water depletion
- Alcohol use
- Age

Incidence
- Affects men and women equally
- Increased incidence among elderly patients and neonates during excessively hot summer days

Common characteristics
- Temperature elevation
- Tachycardia greater than 130 beats/minute
- Widened pulse pressure
- Changes in level of consciousness
- Tonic-dystonic contractions of the muscles
- Coma
- Tachypnea
- Hypoxia

Complications
- Hypovolemic shock
- Cardiogenic shock
- Cardiac arrhythmias
- Renal failure
- Disseminated intravascular coagulation
- Hepatic failure

✳ ASSESSMENT

History
HEAT EXHAUSTION
- Prolonged activity in a very warm or hot environment
- Muscle cramps
- Nausea and vomiting
- Thirst
- Weakness
- Headache
- Fatigue
HEAT STROKE
- Same signs as heat exhaustion
- Exposure to high temperature and humidity without air circulation
- Blurred vision
- Confusion
- Hallucinations
- Decreased muscle coordination

Physical findings
HEAT EXHAUSTION
- Rectal temperature over 100° F (37.8° C)
- Pale skin
- Thready, rapid pulse
- Cool, moist skin
- Decreased blood pressure
- Irritability
- Syncope
- Impaired judgment
- Hyperventilation

HEAT STROKE
- Rectal temperature of at least 104° F (40° C)
- Red, diaphoretic, and hot skin in early stages
- Gray, dry, and hot skin in later stages
- Tachycardia
- Slightly elevated blood pressure in early stages
- Decreased blood pressure in later stages
- Signs of central nervous system dysfunction
- Altered mental status
- Hyperpnea
- Cheyne-Stokes respirations
- Anhydrosis (late sign)

Test results
LABORATORY
- Elevated serum electrolytes may show hyponatremia and hypokalemia.
- Arterial blood gas levels may show respiratory alkalosis.
- Complete blood count may show leukocytosis and thrombocytopenia.
- Coagulation studies may show increased bleeding and clotting times.
- Urinalysis may show concentrated urine and proteinuria with tubular casts and myoglobinuria.
- Blood urea nitrogen may be elevated.
- Serum calcium may be decreased.
- Serum phosphorus may be decreased.
- Possibly myoglobinuria indicating rhabdomyolysis.

♦ TREATMENT

General
HEAT EXHAUSTION
- Cool environment
- Oral or I.V. fluid administration

HEAT STROKE
- Lowering the body temperature as rapidly as possible
- Evaporation, hypothermia blankets, and ice packs to the groin and axillae
- Supportive respiratory and cardiovascular measures

Diet
- Increased hydration; cool liquids only
- Avoidance of caffeine

Activity
- Rest

♣ NURSING CONSIDERATIONS

Nursing diagnoses
- Decreased cardiac output
- Deficient fluid volume
- Deficient knowledge (heat injury)
- Hyperthermia
- Impaired gas exchange

Key outcomes
The patient will:
- exhibit signs of adequate cardiac output
- express understanding of the need to maintain adequate fluid intake
- verbalize understanding of how to prevent recurrent episodes of hyperthermia
- maintain a normal body temperature
- maintain adequate ventilation and oxygenation.

Nursing interventions
- Perform rapid cooling procedures.
- Provide supportive measures.
- Provide adequate fluid intake.
- Administer medication, as ordered.

Monitoring
- Vital signs
- Pulse oximetry readings
- Complications
- Level of consciousness
- Cardiac rhythm
- Intake and output
- Myoglobin test results

▶ PATIENT TEACHING

Be sure to cover:
- disorder, diagnostic tests, and treatment
- how to avoid reexposure to high temperatures
- maintaining adequate fluid intake
- need to wear loose clothing
- limiting activity in hot weather.

Discharge planning
- Refer the patient to social services, if appropriate.

✱ RESOURCES

Organizations
National Center for Injury Prevention and Control: *www.cdc.ncipc*
National Institutes of Health: *www.nih.gov*

Selected references
Auber, G. "Taking the Heat Off: How to Manage Heat Injuries," *Nursing* 34(7):50-52, July 2004.
Deleu, D., et al. "Downbeat Nystagmus Following Classical Heat Stroke," *Clinical Neurology and Neurosurgery* 108(1):102-104, December 2005.
Glazer, J.L. "Management of Heatstroke and Heat Exhaustion," *American Family Physician* 71(11):2133-140, June 2005.
Sucholeiki, R. "Heatstroke," *Seminars in Neurology: Tropical Neurology* 25(3):307-14, September 2005.
Wolfson, A.B., et al. *Harwood-Nuss' Clinical Practice of Emergency Medicine*, 4th ed. Philadelphia: Lippincott Williams & Wilkins, 2005.

Hemophilia

● OVERVIEW

Description
- Hereditary bleeding disorder that's incurable
- Characterized by greatly prolonged coagulation time
- Results from deficiency of specific clotting factors
- Hemophilia A (classic hemophilia): affects more than 80% of hemophiliacs; results from deficiency of factor VIII
- Hemophilia B (Christmas disease): affects 15% of hemophiliacs; results from deficiency of factor IX
- Incurable

Pathophysiology
- Hemophilia is a disruption in the normal intrinsic clotting cascade due to a low level or absence of blood protein necessary for clotting.
- It produces abnormal bleeding, which may be mild, moderate, or severe, depending on the degree of factor deficiency.
- After a platelet plug at a bleeding site, the lack of clotting factors impairs formation of a stable fibrin clot.
- Immediate hemorrhage isn't prevalent; delayed bleeding is common.

Causes
- Hemophilia A and B inherited as X-linked recessive traits
- Spontaneous mutation
- Acquired immunologic process

Incidence
- Most common X-linked genetic disease
- Occurs in about 1.25 of 10,000 live male births

Common characteristics
- Painful and swollen joints
- Abnormal tendency to bleed

Complications
- Pain, swelling, extreme tenderness, and permanent deformity of joints and muscles
- Peripheral neuropathies, pain, paresthesia, and muscle atrophy
- Ischemia and gangrene
- Shock and death

✳ ASSESSMENT

History
- Pain and swelling in a weight-bearing joint, such as the hip, knee, and ankle
- With mild hemophilia or after minor trauma, lack of spontaneous bleeding, but prolonged bleeding with major trauma or surgery
- Moderate hemophilia producing only occasional spontaneous bleeding episodes
- Severe hemophilia causing spontaneous bleeding
- Prolonged bleeding after surgery or trauma or joint pain in spontaneous bleeding into muscles or joints
- Signs of internal bleeding, such as abdominal, chest, or flank pain; episodes of hematuria or hematemesis; and tarry stools
- Activity or movement limitations and need for assistive devices, such as splints, canes, or crutches

Physical findings
- Hematomas on extremities, torso, or both
- Joint swelling in episodes of bleeding into joints
- Limited and painful joint range of motion (ROM) in episodes of bleeding into joints

Test results
LABORATORY
HEMOPHILIA A
- Factor VIII assay is 0% to 25% of normal.
- Partial thromboplastin time (PTT) is prolonged.
- Platelet count and function, bleeding time, and prothrombin time are normal.
HEMOPHILIA B
- Factor IX assay is deficient.
- Baseline coagulation results are similar to those of hemophilia A, with normal factor VIII.
HEMOPHILIA A OR B
- The degree of factor deficiency defines severity:
  - mild hemophilia—factor levels are 5% to 25% of normal
  - moderate hemophilia—factor levels are 1% to 5% of normal
  - severe hemophilia—factor levels are less than 1% of normal.

◆ TREATMENT

General
- Correct treatment to quickly stop bleeding by increasing plasma levels of deficient clotting factors

Diet
- Food high in vitamin K

Activity
- Limitations guided by degree of factor deficiency

Medication
- Aminocaproic acid
HEMOPHILIA A
- Cryoprecipitated antihemophilic factor (AHF), lyophilized AHF, or both
- Desmopressin
HEMOPHILIA B
- Factor IX concentrate

♣ NURSING CONSIDERATIONS

Nursing diagnoses
- Activity intolerance
- Anxiety
- Deficient knowledge (hemophilia)
- Impaired physical mobility
- Ineffective coping
- Ineffective tissue perfusion: Cardiopulmonary
- Powerlessness
- Risk for deficient fluid volume
- Risk for injury
- Social isolation

Key outcomes
The patient will:
- verbalize methods to balance activity and rest
- express feelings of comfort
- maintain ROM and joint mobility
- demonstrate adequate coping skills
- show evidence of hemodynamic stability
- maintain fluid volume within normal range
- maintain existing social relationships.

Nursing interventions

- Provide emotional support, and listen to the patient's fears and concerns. Offer reassurance when indicated.
- If the newly diagnosed patient has difficulty adjusting to diagnosis, reassure him that feelings of fear and anxiety are normal. Arrange for others with the same problem to speak with the patient and family.
- Allow the patient private time with family and friends to help overcome feelings of social isolation.

DURING BLEEDING EPISODES

- If the patient has surface cuts or epistaxis, apply pressure, which is often the only treatment needed.
- With deeper cuts, pressure may stop the bleeding temporarily. Cuts deep enough to require suturing may also require factor infusions to prevent further bleeding.
- Give the deficient clotting factor or plasma, as ordered. The body uses up AHF in 48 to 72 hours; therefore, repeat infusions, as ordered, until the bleeding stops.
- Apply cold compresses or ice bags, and elevate the injured part.
- To prevent recurrence of bleeding, restrict activity for 48 hours after bleeding is under control.
- Control pain with analgesics, as ordered.
- Avoid I.M. injections because of possible hematoma formation at the injection site.
- Avoid aspirin and aspirin-containing medications, which are contraindicated because they decrease platelet adherence and may increase bleeding.
- If the patient can't tolerate activities because of blood loss, provide frequent rest periods.

DURING BLEEDING IN A JOINT

- Immediately elevate the joint.
- To restore joint mobility, begin ROM exercises at least 48 hours after the bleeding is controlled.
- Restrict weight bearing until bleeding stops and swelling subsides.
- Administer analgesics for the pain associated with hemarthrosis.
- Apply ice packs and elastic bandages to alleviate pain.

Monitoring

- PTT
- Adverse reactions to blood products
- Signs and symptoms of decreased tissue perfusion
- Vital signs
- Bleeding from the skin, mucous membranes, and wounds

▶ PATIENT TEACHING

Be sure to cover:
- benefits of regular isometric exercises
- how parents can protect their child from injury while avoiding unnecessary restrictions that impair normal development
- avoidance of contact sports, which increase the risk of injury and can cause serious bleeding problems
- if an injury occurs, directions for parents to apply cold compresses or ice bags and to elevate the injured part or apply light pressure to bleeding
- need for parents to restrict the child's activity for 48 hours after bleeding is under control
- need to notify the physician immediately after even a minor injury
- need for parents to watch for signs of internal bleeding
- importance of avoiding aspirin, combination medications that contain aspirin, and over-the-counter anti-inflammatory agents; tell parents to use acetaminophen instead
- importance of good dental care and the need to check with the physician before dental extractions or surgery
- importance of protecting the patient's veins to facilitate lifelong therapy
- need for the child to wear a medical identification bracelet at all times.

WHEN RECEIVING BLOOD COMPONENTS

Be sure to cover:
- how to administer blood factor components at home
- proper venipuncture and infusion techniques; urge parents not to delay treatment during bleeding episodes
- need to keep blood factor concentrate and infusion equipment available at all times, even on vacation
- adverse reactions that can result from replacement factor procedures

- signs and symptoms of anaphylaxis; teach the patient to administer epinephrine and that he must contact the physician immediately
- need for the patient or parents to watch for early signs of hepatitis
- information that all donated blood and plasma are screened for antibodies to human immunodeficiency virus (HIV) and that all freeze-dried products are heat-treated to kill HIV.

Discharge planning

- Refer the new patient to a hemophilia treatment center for evaluation.
- Refer the patient's family to the National Hemophilia Foundation.

✳ RESOURCES

Organizations

Centers for Disease Control and Prevention: *www.cdc.gov*
National Hemophilia Foundation: *www.hemophilia.org*

Selected references

Dunn, A.L. "Management and Prevention of Recurrent Hemarthrosis in Patients with Hemophilia," *Current Opinion in Hematology* 12(95):390-94, September 2005.

Kasper, D.L., et al., eds. *Harrison's Principles of Internal Medicine,* 16th ed. New York: McGraw-Hill Book Co., 2005.

Millier, K.L. "Factor Products in the Treatment of Hemophilia." *Journal of Pediatric Health Care* 18(3):156-57, May-June 2004.

Tierney, L., et al. *Current Medical Diagnosis and Treatment 2006.* New York: McGraw-Hill Book Co., 2006.

Hemothorax

● OVERVIEW

Description
- Blood in the pleural cavity
- May result in lung collapse

Pathophysiology
- Damaged intercostal, pleural, mediastinal, and sometimes lung parenchymal vessels cause blood to enter the pleural cavity.
- The amount of bleeding and the cause is associated with varying degrees of lung collapse and mediastinal shift.

Causes
- Damaged intercostal, pleural, or mediastinal vessels
- Damaged parenchymal vessels
- Blunt or penetrating chest trauma
- Thoracic surgery
- Pulmonary infarction
- Neoplasm
- Dissecting thoracic aneurysm
- Anticoagulant therapy
- Thoracic endometriosis
- Central venous catheter insertion
- Tuberculosis

Incidence
- Occurs in about 25% of patients with chest trauma

Common characteristics
- Chest pain
- Sudden shortness of breath

Complications
- Mediastinal shift
- Ventilatory compromise
- Lung collapse
- Cardiopulmonary arrest
- Pneumothorax
- Empyema

✳ ASSESSMENT

History
- Recent trauma
- Recent thoracic surgery

Physical findings
- Tachypnea
- Dusky skin color
- Diaphoresis
- Hemoptysis
- Restlessness
- Anxiety
- Cyanosis
- Stupor
- Affected side possibly expanding and stiffening
- Unaffected side possibly rising with gasping respirations
- Dullness over affected side
- Decreased or absent breath sounds over affected side
- Tachycardia
- Hypotension

Test results
LABORATORY
- Pleural fluid analysis shows hematocrit greater than 50% of serum hematocrit.
- Arterial blood gas (ABG) analysis may show increased partial pressure of carbon dioxide and decreased partial pressure of oxygen.
- Serum hemoglobin level may be decreased, depending on blood loss.

IMAGING
- Chest X-ray and computed tomography scan of the thorax shows the presence and extent of hemothorax.

USING AUTOTRANSFUSION FOR CHEST WOUNDS

Autotransfusion is used most often in patients with chest wounds, especially those that involve hemothorax. Through autotransfusion, a patient's own blood is collected, filtered, and reinfused. The procedure may also be used when two or three units of pooled blood can be recovered, such as in cardiac or orthopedic surgery.

Autotransfusion eliminates the patient's risk of transfusion reaction or blood-borne disease, such as cytomegalovirus, hepatitis, and human immunodeficiency virus. It's contraindicated in patients with sepsis or cancer.

How autotransfusion works
A large-bore chest tube connected to a closed drainage system is used to collect the patient's blood from a wound or chest cavity. This blood passes through a filter, which catches most potential thrombi, including clumps of fibrin and damaged red blood cells (RBCs). The filtered blood passes into a collection bag. From the bag, the blood is reinfused immediately, or it may be processed in a commercial cell washer that reduces anticoagulated whole blood to washed RBCs for later infusion.

Assisting with autotransfusion
Set up the blood collection system as you would any closed chest drainage system. Attach the collection bag according to the manufacturer's instructions.

If ordered, inject an anticoagulant, such as heparin or acid-citrate-dextrose solution, into the self-sealing port on the connector of the patient's drainage tubing.

During reinfusion, monitor the patient for complications, such as blood clotting, hemolysis, coagulopathies, thrombocytopenia, particulate and air emboli, sepsis, and citrate toxicity (from the acid-citrate-dextrose solution).

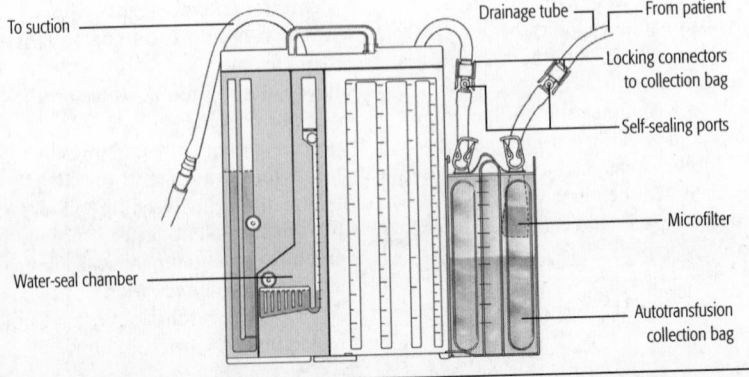

DIAGNOSTIC PROCEDURES
- Thoracentesis may yield blood or serosanguineous fluid.

 TREATMENT

General
- Stabilization of the patient's clinical condition
- Stoppage of bleeding
- Evacuation of blood from the pleural cavity
- Reexpansion of the affected lung
- Thoracentesis
- Insertion of chest tube
- Suction
- Autotransfusion, if blood loss approaches or exceeds 1 L (see *Using autotransfusion for chest wounds*)

Diet
- As tolerated
- I.V. therapy

Activity
- As tolerated

Medication
- Oxygen
- Analgesics

Surgery
- Thoracotomy if chest tube doesn't improve condition

✥ NURSING CONSIDERATIONS

Nursing diagnoses
- Acute pain
- Anxiety
- Deficient fluid volume
- Impaired gas exchange
- Ineffective breathing pattern
- Ineffective tissue perfusion: Cardiopulmonary
- Risk for infection

Key outcomes
The patient will:
- express feelings of increased comfort and decreased pain and anxiety
- maintain adequate fluid volume
- maintain adequate ventilation and oxygenation
- maintain effective breathing pattern
- maintain adequate cardiopulmonary perfusion
- verbalize understanding of the illness
- remain free from signs and symptoms of infection.

Nursing interventions
- Administer medications, as ordered.
- Listen to the patient's fears and concerns, and offer reassurance.
- Promote comfort and relaxation.
- Include family members in care-related decisions whenever possible.
- Give oxygen, as ordered.
- Administer I.V. fluids and blood transfusions, as ordered.
- Assist with thoracentesis.
- Prepare the patient for surgery, if needed.
- Don't clamp the chest tube.
- Change the chest tube dressing, as needed.
- Avoid tubing kinks.
- Tape all chest tube connections.

◈ **NURSING ALERT** Immediately report a chest tube drainage system that's warm and full of blood as well as a rapidly rising bloody fluid level.

Monitoring
- Vital signs
- Intake and output
- Chest tube drainage
- Central venous pressure
- ABG results
- Chest X-ray results
- Complete blood count results
- Respiratory status
- Complications
- Signs and symptoms of infection

▶ PATIENT TEACHING

Be sure to cover:
- disorder, diagnostic tests, and treatment
- medication administration, dosage, and possible adverse effects
- when to notify the physician
- preoperative and postoperative care, if needed
- mechanical ventilation, if needed
- deep-breathing exercises
- thoracentesis
- chest tube and drainage system.

✳ RESOURCES

Organizations
American Thoracic Society: *www.thoracic.org*

Selected references
Mason, R.J., et al. *Murray and Nadel's Textbook of Respiratory Medicine,* 4th ed. Philadelphia: W.B. Saunders Co., 2005.

Wiklund, C.U., et al. "Misplacement of Central Vein Catheters in Patients with Hemothorax: A New Approach to Resolve the Problem," *Journal of Trauma-Injury Infection & Critical Care* 59(4):1029-1031, October 2005.

Yamamoto, I., et al. "Thoracic Trauma: The Deadly Dozen," *Critical Care Nursing Quarterly* 28(1):22-40, January-March 2005.

Hepatic encephalopathy

● OVERVIEW

Description
- Neurologic syndrome that develops as a complication of aggressive fulminant hepatitis or chronic hepatic disease
- Most common in patients with cirrhosis
- May be acute and self-limiting or chronic and progressive
- In advanced stages, poor prognosis despite vigorous treatment

Pathophysiology
- Normally, the ammonia produced by protein breakdown in the bowel is metabolized to urea in the liver. When portal blood shunts past the liver, ammonia directly enters the systemic circulation and is carried to the brain.
- Such shunting may result from the collateral venous circulation that develops in portal hypertension or from surgically created portal-systemic shunts.
- Cirrhosis further compounds this problem because impaired hepatocellular function prevents conversion of ammonia that reaches the liver.

Causes
- Exact cause unknown
- Ammonia intoxication of the brain

Risk factors
- Excessive protein intake
- Sepsis
- Excessive accumulation of nitrogenous body wastes (from constipation or GI hemorrhage)
- Bacterial action on protein and urea to form ammonia
- Fluid and electrolyte imbalance (especially metabolic alkalosis)
- Hypoxia
- Azotemia
- Impaired glucose metabolism
- Infection
- Use of sedatives, opioids, and general anesthetics

Incidence
- Occurs in approximately 4 of 100,000 people
- Seen in 70% of patients with cirrhosis

Common characteristics
- Changes in mental status
- Jaundice
- Muscle tremors

Complications
- Irreversible coma
- Death

● ASSESSMENT

History
PRODROMAL STAGE
- Slight personality changes, such as agitation, belligerence, disorientation, and forgetfulness
- Trouble concentrating or thinking clearly
- Fatigue
- Mental changes, such as confusion and disorientation
- Sleep-wake reversal
IMPENDING STAGE
- Mental changes (confusion and disorientation)
STUPOROUS STAGE
- Marked mental confusion
COMATOSE STAGE
- Unable to arouse

Physical findings
PRODROMAL STAGE
- Slurred or slowed speech
- Slight tremor
IMPENDING STAGE
- Tremors that have progressed to asterixis
- Lethargy
- Aberrant behavior
- Apraxia
- Possible incontinence
STUPOROUS STAGE
- Drowsy and stuporous
- Noisy and abusive when aroused
- Hyperventilation
- Muscle twitching
- Asterixis

COMATOSE STAGE
- Obtunded
- Seizures
- Hyperactive reflexes
- Positive Babinski's sign
- Fetor hepaticus (musty, sweet breath odor)

Test results
LABORATORY
- Serum ammonia levels are elevated and, together with characteristic clinical features, strongly suggest hepatic encephalopathy.
- Serum bilirubin is elevated.
- Prothrombin time is prolonged.
DIAGNOSTIC PROCEDURES
- EEG shows slowing waves as the disease progresses.

TREATMENT

General
- Elimination of underlying cause
- I.V. fluid administration
- Control of GI bleeding
- Life-support measures (if appropriate)
- Bowel cleansing

Diet
- Limited protein
- Nothing by mouth with decreased responsiveness
- Parenteral or enteral feedings (if appropriate)

Activity
- Bed rest until condition improves

Medication
- Lactulose
- Neomycin
- Potassium supplements
- Salt-poor albumin

Surgery
- Possible liver transplant

NURSING CONSIDERATIONS

Nursing diagnoses
- Acute pain
- Anxiety
- Deficient fluid volume
- Diarrhea
- Disturbed sensory perception: All
- Fear
- Imbalanced nutrition: Less than body requirements
- Ineffective tissue perfusion: Cerebral, GI
- Risk for injury

Key outcomes
The patient will:
- express feelings of increased comfort and decreased pain and anxiety
- maintain normal fluid volume
- regain normal bowel function
- maintain orientation to environment
- discuss feelings and concerns
- ingest adequate nutrition
- maintain adequate cerebral and GI perfusion
- remain free from injury.

Nursing interventions
- Promote rest, comfort, and a quiet atmosphere.
- Administer medications, as ordered.
- Use appropriate safety measures to protect the patient from injury
- Inspect skin regularly.
- Perform passive range-of-motion exercises.
- Provide emotional support.

Monitoring
- Level of consciousness
- Intake and output
- Fluid and electrolyte balance
- Weight and abdominal girth
- Signs of anemia, alkalosis, GI bleeding, and infection
- Serum ammonia level
- Changes in handwriting for progression of neurologic involvement

PATIENT TEACHING

Be sure to cover:
- disorder, diagnostic tests, and treatment
- signs of complications or worsening symptoms
- dietary modifications
- medication administration, dosage, and possible adverse effects.

Discharge planning
- Refer the patient to social services, as indicated.

RESOURCES

Organizations
American Liver Foundation:
www.liverfoundation.org
Digestive Disease National Coalition:
www.ddnc.org
National Digestive Diseases Information:
www.niddk.nih.gov/health/digest/nddic.htm

Selected references
Amodio, P., and Gatta, A. "Neurophysiological Investigation of Hepatic Encephalopathy," *Metabolic Brain Diseases* 20(4):369-79, December 2005.
Blei, A.T. "Albumin Dialysis for the Treatment of Hepatic Encephalopahty," *Journal of Gastroenterology & Hepatology* 19(Suppl 7):S224-228, December 2005.
Handbook of Diseases, 3rd ed. Philadelphia: Lippincott Williams & Wilkins, 2004.

Hepatitis, viral

● OVERVIEW

Description

- Six types recognized—A, B, C, D, E, and G—and a seventh suspected
- Marked by hepatic cell destruction, necrosis, and autolysis, leading to anorexia, jaundice, and hepatomegaly
- In most patients, hepatic cells eventually regenerating with little or no residual damage, allowing recovery
- Complications more likely with advanced age and serious underlying disorders
- Prognosis poor if edema and hepatic encephalopathy develop

Pathophysiology

- Hepatic inflammation caused by virus leads to diffuse injury and necrosis of hepatocytes.
- Hypertrophy and hyperplasia of Kupffer cells and sinusoidal lining cells occurs.
- Bile obstruction may occur.

Causes

- Infection with the causative viruses for each of six major forms of viral hepatitis

TYPE A
- Transmittal by the fecal-oral or parenteral route
- Ingestion of contaminated food, milk, or water

TYPE B
- Transmittal by contact with contaminated human blood, secretions, and stool

TYPE C
- Transmittal primarily through sharing of needles by I.V. drug users, blood transfusions, tattoo needles, or sharing nasal paraphenalia used for sniffing cocaine

TYPE D
- Found only in patients with an acute or a chronic episode of hepatitis B

TYPE E
- Transmittal by parenteral route and commonly water-borne

TYPE G
- Thought to be blood-borne, with transmission similar to that of hepatitis B and C

Incidence

- Hepatitis A virus (HAV): occurs in nationwide epidemics
- Chronic hepatitis B virus (HBV): affects 1.25 million Americans
- Chronic hepatitis C virus (HCV): affects 3.9 million Americans

Common characteristics

- Malaise, fatigue
- Dark-colored urine
- Clay-colored stools
- Abdominal tenderness
- Fever
- Jaundice
- Nausea

Complications

- Life-threatening fulminant hepatitis
- Death
- Chronic active hepatitis (in hepatitis B)
- Syndrome resembling serum sickness, characterized by arthralgia or arthritis, rash, and angioedema; can lead to misdiagnosis of hepatitis B as rheumatoid arthritis or lupus erythematosus (in hepatitis B)
- Primary liver cancer (in hepatitis B or C)
- Mild or asymptomatic form of hepatitis B that flares into severe, progressive chronic active hepatitis and cirrhosis (in hepatitis D)

✳ ASSESSMENT

History

- Revelation of a source of transmission

PRODROMAL STAGE
- Patient easily fatigued, with generalized malaise
- Anorexia, mild weight loss
- Depression
- Headache, photophobia
- Weakness
- Arthralgia, myalgia
- Nausea or vomiting
- Changes in the senses of taste and smell

CLINICAL JAUNDICE STAGE
- Pruritus
- Abdominal pain or tenderness
- Indigestion
- Anorexia

- Possible jaundice of sclerae, mucous membranes, and skin

POSTICTERIC STAGE
- Most symptoms decreasing or subsiding

Physical findings

PRODROMAL STAGE
- Fever (100° to 102° F [37.8° to 38.9° C])
- Dark-colored urine
- Clay-colored stools

CLINICAL JAUNDICE STAGE
- Rashes, erythematous patches, or hives
- Abdominal tenderness in the right upper quadrant
- Enlarged and tender liver
- Splenomegaly
- Cervical adenopathy

POSTICTERIC STAGE
- Decrease in liver enlargement

Test results

LABORATORY
- In suspected viral hepatitis, hepatitis profile is routinely performed; result identifies antibodies specific to the causative virus and establishes the type of hepatitis:
  - Type A—Detection of an antibody to hepatitis A (anti-HAV) confirms the diagnosis.
  - Type B—The presence of hepatitis B surface antigens (HBsAg) and hepatitis B antibodies (anti-HBs) confirms the diagnosis.
  - Type C—Diagnosis depends on serologic testing for the specific antibody one or more months after the onset of acute illness; until then, diagnosis is principally established by obtaining negative test results for hepatitis A, B, and D.
  - Type D—Detection of intrahepatic delta antigens or immunoglobulin (Ig) M antidelta antigens in acute disease (or IgM and IgG in chronic disease) establishes the diagnosis.
  - Type E—Detection of hepatitis E antigens support the diagnosis; however, diagnosis may also rule out hepatitis C.
  - Type G—Detection of hepatitis G ribonucleic acid supports the diagnosis; serologic assays are being developed.

- Additional findings from liver function studies support the diagnosis:
  - Serum aspartate aminotransferase and serum alanine aminotransferase levels are increased in the prodromal stage of acute viral hepatitis.
  - Serum alkaline phosphatase levels are slightly increased.
  - Serum bilirubin levels are elevated; levels may remain elevated late in the disease, especially with severe disease.
  - Prothrombin time (PT) is prolonged; PT more than 3 seconds longer than normal indicates severe liver damage.
  - White blood cell count commonly reveals transient neutropenia and lymphopenia followed by lymphocytosis.

DIAGNOSTIC PROCEDURES
- Liver biopsy shows chronic hepatitis.

◆ TREATMENT

General
FOR HCV
- Aimed at clearing HCV from the body, stopping or slowing of hepatic damage, and symptom relief

Diet
- Small, high-calorie, high-protein meals (reduced protein intake if signs of precoma—lethargy, confusion, mental changes—develop)
- Parenteral feeding (if appropriate)
- Avoidance of alcohol

Activity
- Frequent rest periods as needed
- Avoidance of contact sports and strenuous activity

Medication
- Standard Ig
- Vaccine
- Alfa-2b interferon (HBV, HCV)
- Antiemetics
- Cholestyramine
- Lamivudine (HBV)
- Ribavirin (HCV)

Surgery
- Possible liver transplant (HCV)

❁ NURSING CONSIDERATIONS

Nursing diagnoses
- Activity intolerance
- Anxiety
- Deficient knowledge (viral hepatitis)
- Fear
- Imbalanced nutrition: Less than body requirements
- Risk for infection
- Risk for injury

Key outcomes
The patient will:
- perform activities of daily living within the confines of the disease process
- verbalize a decrease in anxiety
- verbalize understanding of the disorder and treatment regimen
- express feelings and concerns
- demonstrate adequate nutritional intake
- remain free from signs and symptoms of infection or injury.

Nursing interventions
- Observe standard precautions to prevent transmission of the disease.
- Provide rest periods throughout the day.
- Administer medications, as ordered.
- Encourage oral fluid intake.

PREVENTING THE SPREAD OF VIRAL HEPATITIS

In your teaching, review the following measures to prevent the spread of viral hepatitis:

- Stress the importance of thorough and frequent hand washing.
- Tell the patient not to share food, eating utensils, or toothbrushes.
- If the patient has hepatitis A or E, warn him not to contaminate food or water with fecal matter because the disease is transmitted by the fecal-oral route.
- If the patient has hepatitis B, C, D, or G, explain that transmission occurs through exchange of blood or body fluids that contain blood. While infected, he shouldn't donate blood or have sexual relations.
- Advise the patient to take extra care to avoid cutting himself.

Monitoring
- Hydration and nutritional status
- Daily weight
- Intake and output
- Stool for color, consistency, amount, and frequency
- Signs of complications

▶ PATIENT TEACHING

Be sure to cover:
- disorder, diagnostic tests, and treatment
- measures to prevent the spread of disease (see *Preventing the spread of viral hepatitis*)
- importance of rest and a proper diet
- need to abstain from alcohol
- medication administration, dosage, and possible adverse effects
- need to avoid over-the-counter medication unless approved by the physician
- need for follow-up care.

Discharge planning
- Refer the patient to Alcoholics Anonymous, if indicated.

✳ RESOURCES

Organizations
American Liver Foundation:
www.liverfoundation.org
Digestive Disease National Coalition:
www.ddnc.org
National Digestive Diseases Information:
www.niddk.nih.gov/health/digest/nddic.htm

Selected references
Diseases, 4th ed. Philadelphia: Lippincott Williams & Wilkins, 2006.
Durston, S. "What You Need To Know About Viral Hepatitis," *Nursing* 35(8):36-41, August 2005.
Leone, N., and Bean, K.B. "The ABCs of Hepatitis," *Gastroenterology Nursing* 28(2):171, March-April 2005.
McPhee, S.J., et al. *Current Medical Diagnosis and Treatment 2007.* New York: McGraw-Hill Book Co., 2007.
Strategies for Managing Multisystem Disorders. Philadelphia: Lippincott Williams & Wilkins, 2005.

Hereditary hemorrhagic telangiectasia

● OVERVIEW

Description
- Inherited vascular disorder
- Also called *Osler-Weber-Rendu disease*

Pathophysiology
- Venules and capillaries dilate to form fragile masses of thin convoluted vessels (telangiectases), resulting in an abnormal tendency to hemorrhage.

Causes
- Transmitted by autosomal dominant inheritance

Incidence
- Affects both sexes but may cause less severe bleeding in females
- Occurs in 1 in 50,000 births

Common characteristics
- Recurrent epistaxis

Complications
- Secondary iron deficiency anemia
- Vascular malformation causing pulmonary arteriovenous fistulas (rare)
- Recurring cerebral embolism and brain abscess
- Hemorrhagic shock
- Intracranial hemorrhage

✳ ASSESSMENT

History
- Established familial pattern of bleeding disorders
- Epistaxis, hemoptysis, or tarry stools

Physical findings
- Localized aggregations of dilated capillaries on the skin of the face, ears, scalp, hands, arms, and feet, and under the nails
- Characteristic telangiectases that are violet, bleed spontaneously, flat or raised, blanch on pressure, and are nonpulsatile
- Signs of capillary fragility (may exist without overt telangiectasia): Spontaneous bleeding, petechiae, ecchymoses, and spider hemangiomas of varying size (see *Typical lesions of hereditary hemorrhagic telangiectasia*)
- Clubbing of the digits

Test results
LABORATORY
- Platelet count may be abnormal.
- Complete blood count and anemia panel may show hypochromic, microcytic anemia.

IMAGING
- Chest X-rays may show arteriovenous malformation.
- Echocardiography may show "high-output" cardiac failure.

DIAGNOSTIC PROCEDURES
- Bone marrow aspiration shows depleted iron stores and confirms secondary iron deficiency anemia.

◆ TREATMENT

General
- Supportive therapy, including blood transfusions and supplemental iron administration
- Ancillary treatment consisting of applying pressure and topical hemostatic agents to bleeding sites, cauterizing bleeding sites not readily accessible, and protecting the patient from trauma and unnecessary bleeding

Diet
- No restrictions

Activity
- Avoidance of activities that have the potential for trauma

Medication
- Parenteral iron
- Antipyretics or antihistamines

TYPICAL LESIONS OF HEREDITARY HEMORRHAGIC TELANGIECTASIA

The illustrations below show the commonly encountered lesions of hereditary hemorrhagic telangiectasia.

Dilated capillaries, either flat or raised, appear in localized aggregations, as on the fingers.

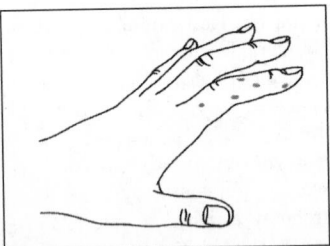

On the face, spider hemangiomas reflect capillary fragility.

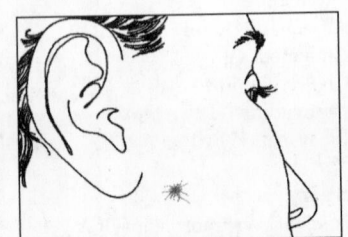

Nursing diagnoses

- Activity intolerance
- Anxiety
- Deficient knowledge (hereditary hemorrhagic telangiectasia)
- Disturbed body image
- Impaired skin integrity
- Ineffective tissue perfusion: Cardiopulmonary
- Risk for deficient fluid volume
- Risk for infection

Key outcomes

The patient will:
- demonstrate measures to balance activity and rest
- verbalize a decrease in anxiety
- demonstrate positive signs of coping and decreased anxiety
- verbalize positive feelings about self and body image
- demonstrate improvement in lesion
- maintain hemodynamic stability
- maintain adequate fluid balance
- remain free from signs and symptoms of infection.

Nursing interventions

- Provide emotional and psychological support.
- Administer ordered blood transfusions.
- Encourage fluid intake if the patient is bleeding or hypovolemic.
- Provide meticulous skin care and hygiene.
- Use aseptic technique when caring for the patient.

Monitoring

- Vital signs
- Intake and output
- Signs of febrile or allergic transfusion reaction
- Indications of GI bleeding
- Organ function through physical examination
- Laboratory values to detect possible renal, hepatic, or respiratory failure

Be sure to cover:
- disorder, diagnostic tests, and treatment
- iron supplements and the importance of following dosage instructions and of taking oral iron with meals to minimize GI irritation
- warning that iron turns stools dark green or black and may cause constipation
- management of minor bleeding episodes, especially recurrent epistaxis
- how to recognize major bleeding episodes that require emergency intervention.

Discharge planning

- Refer the patient for genetic counseling, as appropriate.

Organizations

Mayo Clinic: *www.mayohealth.org*
National Heart, Lung and Blood Institute: *www.nhlbi.nih.gov*

Selected references

Gallitelli, M., et al. "Emergencies in Hereditary Haemorrhagic Telangiectasia," *QIM* 99(1):15-22, January 2006.

Kasper, D.L., et al., eds. *Harrison's Principles of Internal Medicine,* 16th ed. New York: McGraw-Hill Book Co., 2005.

McPhee, S.J., et al. *Current Medical Diagnosis and Treatment 2007.* New York: McGraw-Hill Book Co., 2007.

Nguyen, N.Q., "Herediatry Hemorrhagic Telangiectasia," *Dermatology Online Journal* 11(4):19, December 2005.

Post, M.C., et al. "A Pulmonary Right-to-Left Shunt in Patients with Hereditary Hemorrhagic Telangiectasia is Associated with an Increased Prevalence of Migraine," *Chest* 128(4):2485-489, October 2005.

Hernia, hiatal

● OVERVIEW

Description
- Defect in the diaphragm that permits a portion of the stomach to pass through the diaphragmatic opening into the chest
- Three types: sliding, rolling (paraesophageal), and mixed (see "Hernia, paraesophageal," pages 256 and 257)

Pathophysiology
SLIDING HERNIA
- The muscular collar around the esophageal and diaphragmatic junction loosens.
- Increased intra-abdominal pressure causes the lower portion of the esophagus and the upper portion of the stomach to rise into the chest.

Causes
SLIDING HERNIA
- Normal aging
- Secondary to esophageal carcinoma, kyphoscoliosis, trauma, or surgery
- Diaphragmatic malformations that can cause congenital weakness

Risk factors
- Obesity
- Smoking

Incidence
- Sliding hernia: 3 to 10 times more common than rolling and mixed hernias combined
- Increases with age
- By age 60, 60% of people affected by hiatal hernias
- Higher prevalence in women than in men

Common characteristics
- May produce no symptoms
- Heartburn

Complications
- Esophageal stricture
- Incarceration
- In association with gastroesophageal reflux disease:
  - Esophagitis
  - Esophageal ulceration and perforation
  - Hemorrhage
  - Peritonitis
  - Mediastinitis
  - Aspiration
  - Strangulation and gangrene of herniated portion of stomach

✳ ASSESSMENT

History
- Heartburn 1 to 4 hours after eating; aggravated by reclining, belching, or conditions that increase intra-abdominal pressure
- Regurgitation or vomiting
- Retrosternal or substernal chest pain (typically after meals or at bedtime)
- Feeling of fullness after eating
- Feeling of breathlessness or suffocation
- Chest pain resembling angina pectoris
- Chronic cough

Physical findings
- Possibly none
- Dysphagia

Test results
LABORATORY
- Fecal occult blood test may be positive.
- Analysis of gastric contents may reveal blood.

IMAGING
- Chest X-ray reveals an air shadow behind the heart in a large hernia; lower lobe infiltrates with aspiration.
- Barium swallow with fluoroscopy detects a hiatal hernia and diaphragmatic abnormalities.

DIAGNOSTIC PROCEDURES
- Endoscopy and biopsy results identify the mucosal junction and the edge of the diaphragm indenting the esophagus; differentiate hiatal hernia, varices, and other small gastroesophageal lesions; and rule out malignant tumors.
- Esophageal motility studies reveal esophageal motor or lower esophageal pressure abnormalities before surgical repair of the hernia.
- pH studies identify reflux of gastric contents.
- Acid perfusion (Bernstein) test identifies esophageal reflux.

◆ TREATMENT

General
- Smoking cessation (smoking stimulates gastric acid production)
- Weight reduction

Diet
- Six small meals per day
- Elimination of spicy or irritating foods, alcohol, and coffee
- No food or fluids 1 to 2 hours before bedtime

Activity
- Restriction of activity that increases intra-abdominal pressure
- Upright posture for 2 to 3 hours after eating

Medication
- Antacids
- Histamine-2 receptor antagonists
- Cholinergics
- Motility agents
- Antiemetics
- Cough suppressants

Surgery
- Hernia repair

Nursing diagnoses
- Acute pain
- Deficient knowledge (hiatal hernia)
- Imbalanced nutrition: Less than body requirements
- Impaired swallowing
- Risk for aspiration

Key outcomes
The patient will:
- express feelings of increased comfort and decreased pain
- verbalize understanding of the disorder and treatment regimen
- achieve adequate caloric and nutritional intake
- experience no choking or coughing when swallowing
- maintain a patent airway
- show no evidence of aspiration.

Nursing interventions
- Prepare the patient for diagnostic tests.
- Teach positional therapy.
- If surgery is necessary, provide appropriate preoperative and postoperative care.

Monitoring
NURSING ALERT After endoscopy, watch for signs of perforation, including decreasing blood pressure, rapid pulse, shock, and sudden pain.
- Response to prescribed antacids and other medications

Be sure to cover:
- disorder, diagnostic tests, and treatment
- development of a dietary plan
- need to sit upright after meals and snacks
- situations or activities that increase intra-abdominal pressure
- medication administration, dosage, and possible adverse effects
- need to sleep with the head of the bed elevated about 6″.

Discharge planning
- Refer the patient to a smoking-cessation program, if appropriate.
- Refer the patient to a weight-reduction program, if appropriate.

Organizations
American Gastroenterological Association: *www.gastro.org*
International Foundation for Functional Gastrointestinal Disorders: *www.iffgd.org*
National Digestive Diseases Information Clearinghouse: *www.niddk.nih.gov/health/digest/nddic.htm*

Selected references
Agrawal, A., et al. "Identification of Hiatal Hernia by Esophageal Manometry: Is it Reliable?" *Diseases of the Esophagus* 18(5):316-19, October 2005.
Handbook of Diseases, 3rd ed. Philadelphia: Lippincott Williams & Wilkins, 2004.
Stylopoulos, N., and Rattner, D.W. "The History of Hiatal Hernia Surgery: From Bowditch to Laparascopy," *Annals of Surgery* 41(1):185-93, January 2005.
Yamada, T., et al. *Atlas of Gastroenterology,* 3rd ed. Philadelphia: Lippincott Williams & Wilkins, 2003.

Hernia, inguinal

● OVERVIEW

Description
- Part of an internal organ that protrudes through an abnormal opening in the wall of the cavity that surrounds it
- Most common type of hernia (see *Common sites of hernia*)
- May be direct or indirect
- Also called *ruptures*

Pathophysiology
- In an inguinal hernia, the large or small intestine, omentum, or bladder protrudes into the inguinal canal.
- In an indirect hernia, abdominal viscera leave the abdomen through the inguinal ring and follow the spermatic cord (in males) or round ligament (in females); they emerge at the external ring and extend down into the inguinal canal, usually into the scrotum or labia.
- In a direct inguinal hernia, instead of entering the canal through the internal ring, the hernia passes through the posterior inguinal wall, protrudes directly through the transverse fascia of the canal (in an area known as *Hesselbach's triangle*), and comes out at the external ring.

Causes
- Weak abdominal muscles or increased intra-abdominal pressure
- Direct hernia: weakness in fascial floor of inguinal canal
- Indirect hernia: weakness in fascial margin of internal inguinal ring

Risk factors
- Congenital malformation
- Trauma
- Aging
- Heavy lifting
- Pregnancy
- Obesity
- Straining

Incidence
- Indirect hernias: may develop at any age, are three times more common in males, and are especially prevalent in infants
- Direct hernias: occur more commonly in middle-age and older people

Common characteristics
- Pain

Complications
- Strangulation
- Intestinal obstruction
- Infection (after surgery)

✳ ASSESSMENT

History
- Sharp or "catching" pain when lifting or straining

Physical findings
- Obvious swelling or lump in the inguinal area (large hernia) (see *Identifying a hernia*)

Test results
LABORATORY
- White blood cell count is elevated, with intestinal obstruction.

OTHER
- Physical examination helps confirm the diagnosis.

COMMON SITES OF HERNIA

There are four common sites of hernia: umbilical, incisional, inguinal, and femoral. Here are descriptions of each type with an illustration demonstrating where each type is located.

Umbilical
Umbilical hernia results from abnormal muscular structures around the umbilical cord. This hernia is quite common in neonates but also occurs in women who are obese or who have had several pregnancies. Because most umbilical hernias in infants close spontaneously, surgery is warranted only if the hernia persists for more than 4 or 5 years. Taping or binding the affected area or supporting it with a truss may relieve symptoms until the hernia closes. A severe congenital umbilical hernia, which allows the abdominal viscera to protrude outside the body, must be repaired immediately.

Incisional
Incisional (ventral) hernia develops at the site of previous surgery, usually along vertical incisions. This hernia may result from a weakness in the abdominal wall, caused by an infection, impaired wound healing, inadequate nutrition, extreme abdominal distention, or obesity. Palpation of an incisional hernia may reveal several defects in the surgical scar. Effective repair requires pulling the layers of the abdominal wall together without creating tension or, if this isn't possible, the use of Teflon, Marlex mesh, or tantalum mesh to close the opening.

Inguinal
Inguinal hernia can be direct or indirect. An indirect inguinal hernia causes the abdominal viscera to

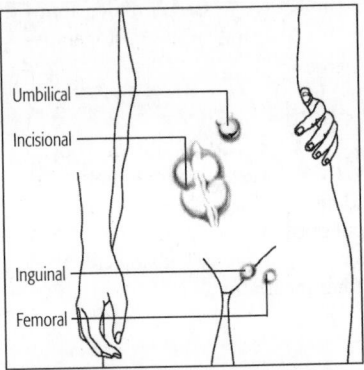

protrude through the inguinal ring and follow the spermatic cord (in males) or round ligament (in females). A direct inguinal hernia results from a weakness in the fascial floor of the inguinal canal.

Femoral
Femoral hernia occurs where the femoral artery passes into the femoral canal. Typically, a fatty deposit within the femoral canal enlarges and eventually creates a hole big enough to accommodate part of the peritoneum and bladder. A femoral hernia appears as a swelling or bulge at the pulse point of the large femoral artery. It's usually a soft, pliable, reducible, nontender mass but commonly becomes incarcerated or strangulated.

◆ TREATMENT

General
- Manual reduction
- Truss

Diet
- Nothing by mouth (if surgery necessary)

Activity
- As tolerated

Medications
- Analgesics
- Antibiotics
- Electrolyte replacement

Surgery
- Herniorrhaphy
- Hernioplasty
- Bowel resection (with strangulation or necrosis)

❖ NURSING CONSIDERATIONS

Nursing diagnoses
- Activity intolerance
- Acute pain
- Ineffective tissue perfusion: GI
- Risk for infection
- Risk for injury

Key outcomes
The patient will:
- perform activities of daily living within the confines of the disease process
- express feelings of increased comfort and decreased pain
- exhibit adequate GI perfusion
- remain free from signs and symptoms of infection and injury.

Nursing interventions
- Apply a truss after a hernia has been reduced.
- Give prescribed drugs for pain.
- Encourage coughing and deep breathing.

Monitoring
- Vital signs
- Pain control
- Signs of strangulation or incarceration

IDENTIFYING A HERNIA

Palpation of the inguinal area while the patient is performing Valsalva's maneuver confirms the diagnosis of inguinal hernia. To detect a hernia in a male patient, ask the patient to stand with his ipsilateral leg slightly flexed and his weight resting on the other leg. Insert an index finger into the lower part of the scrotum and invaginate the scrotal skin so the finger advances through the external inguinal ring to the internal ring (about ½″ to 2″ [1 to 5 cm] through the inguinal canal). Tell the patient to cough. If pressure is felt against the fingertip, an indirect hernia exists; if pressure is felt against the side of the finger, a direct hernia exists.

▶ PATIENT TEACHING

Be sure to cover:
- avoidance of lifting heavy objects or straining during bowel movements
- signs and symptoms of infection (oozing, tenderness, warmth, and redness) at the incision site
- wound care
- after surgery, not returning to normal activity or work without the surgeon's permission.

Discharge planning
- Encourage the patient to schedule follow-up appointments, as recommended by the surgeon.

✱ RESOURCES

Organizations
Mayo Clinic: *www.mayoclinic.com*
The Merck Manuals Online Medical Library: *www.merck.com/mmhe*
National Digestive Diseases Information Clearinghouse: *www.niddk.nih.gov/health/digest/nddic.htm*

Selected references
Kasper, D.L., et al., eds. *Harrison's Principles of Internal Medicine,* 16th ed. New York: McGraw-Hill Book Co., 2005.

Twu, C.M., et al. "Predicting Risk Factors for Inguinal Hernia after Radical Retropubic Prostatectomy," *Urology* 66(4):814-18, October 2005.

Zisholtz, B. "Laparoscopic Inguinal Hernia Repair," *Journal of the American College of Surgeons* 201(3):488-89, September 2005.

Hernia, paraesophageal

● OVERVIEW

Description
- Defect in the diaphragm allowing a portion of the stomach to protrude into the thoracic cavity
- Rolling type of hiatal hernia
- Potentially life-threatening condition
- May be congenital or acquired

Pathophysiology
- A defect occurs in the diaphragm.
- A portion of the stomach herniates into the thoracic cavity and remains there regardless of the patient's position.
- The gastroesophageal junction remains below the diaphragm; it may rise above the diaphragm but it's below the level of the herniated portion of the stomach.

CONGENITAL PARAESOPHAGEAL HERNIA
- The esophagus is congenitally short and straight and a portion of the stomach is malpositioned or displaced in the thoracic cavity.

ACQUIRED PARAESOPHAGEAL HERNIA
- Increased intra-abdominal pressure causes a portion of the stomach to herniate into the thoracic cavity through the defect in the diaphragm.
- The portion of the stomach that herniates is typically anterior to the esophagus.

◈ **NURSING ALERT** Paraesophageal hernias tend to enlarge over time, such that entire portions of the stomach may herniated into the thoracic cavity.

Causes
- Exact cause unknown

Risk factors
- Obesity
- Ascites
- Pregnancy

Incidence
- Accounts for about 3% to 5% of all hiatal hernias

✹ **AGE-RELATED CONCERN** The incidence of acquired paraesophageal hernias increases with age, with most occurring in elderly patients.

Common characteristics
- Epigastric discomfort
- Bloating
- Dysphagia

Complications
- Herniation of intestines into thoracic cavity
- Volvulus
- Incarceration
- Strangulation
- Death

✳ ASSESSMENT

History
- Possibly asymptomatic
- Vague abdominal pain, which increases after eating
- Bloating
- Heartburn (reflux; rare)
- Feelings of breathlessness
- Severe pain (indicative of incarceration)

Physical findings
- Unremarkable
- Shock, suggesting incarceration
- Blood in stool or vomitus, suggesting ulceration

Test results
LABORATORY
- Serum hemoglobin level and hematocrit are decreased with bleeding from esophageal or gastric ulceration.

IMAGING
- Chest X-ray reveals air-filled structure above the diaphragm.
- Barium swallow with fluoroscopy identifies hernia and evidence of esophageal and diaphragmatic abnormalities; double contrast study may show an ulceration on the lesser curvature of the stomach.
- Computed tomography scanning may depict presence of a totally intrathoracic stomach especially if volvulus is suspected.
- Magentic resonance imaging may detect a retrocardiac mass.
- Ultrasound provides information about the location of the gastroesophageal junction position.

DIAGNOSTIC PROCEDURES
- pH studies aid in identifying possible reflux.
- Endoscopy and biopsy help reveal the mucosal junction and edge of diaphragm indenting the esophagus and also aids in diagnosing complications.

◆ TREATMENT

General
- Supportive
- Weight reduction

Diet
- Food and fluid restriction before surgery
- As tolerated after surgery

Activity
- Restriction of activity that increases intra-abdominal pressure

Medications
- Antacids, histamine-2 receptor antagonists, or proton pump inhibitors if reflux present
- Antiemetics

Surgery
- Emergency laparoscopic or open repair of diaphragmatic defect and removal of the herniated sac
- Possible tacking down of stomach or temporary gastrostomy to help decompress the stomach and anchor it in place in abdominal cavity

❖ NURSING CONSIDERATIONS

Nursing diagnoses
- Acute pain
- Anxiety
- Deficient knowledge (paraesophageal hernia, surgery)
- Imbalanced nutrition: Less than body requirements
- Impaired swallowing
- Risk for injury

Key outcomes
The patient will:
- express feelings of increased comfort and and decreased pain
- identify strategies to reduce anxiety
- demonstrate an understanding of condition and treatment plan
- achieve adequate caloric and nutritional intake
- demonstrate ability to swallow without aspiration
- remain free from injury.

Nursing interventions
- Prepare the patient for surgery.
- Complete preoperative and postoperative teaching.
- Offer emotional support.
- Assist with diet.
- Provide postoperative care, including gastrostomy care, if performed.

Monitoring
- Respiratory status
- Pain
- Intake and output
- Vital signs
- Bowel function
- Appetite
- Gastrostomy site (if applicable)

▶ PATIENT TEACHING

Be sure to cover:
- disorder, diagnostic tests, and treatment
- lifestyle changes, including diet plan, if indicated
- preoperative and postoperative care measures
- signs and symptoms of complications
- need to seek medical attention if symptoms increase or new symptoms develop
- gastrostomy site care (if applicable).

Discharge planning
- Refer the patient to community support services, as necessary.
- Arrange for follow-up home health care for assistance with temporary gastrostomy care.

✳ RESOURCES

Organizations
American Gastroenterological Association: *www.gastro.org*
International Foundation for Functional Gastrointestinal Disorders: *www.iffgd.org*
National Digerstive Diseases Information Clearinghouse: *www.niddk.nih.gov/heatlh/digest/nddic.htm*

Selected references
Handbook of Diseases, 3rd ed. Philadelphia: Lippincott Williams & Wilkins, 2004.
Imamo, I.M., et al. "Congenital Paraesophageal Hiatal Hernia: Pitfalls in the Diagnosis and Treatment," *Journal of Pediatric Surgery* 40(7):1128-133, 2005. Available at: *www.medscape.com/medline/abstract/16034757.* Accessed 11/15/06.
Khan, A.N., et al. "Hiatal Hernia," Available at *www.emedicine.com/radio/topic337.htm.* Accessed 11/15/06.
Yamada, T., et al. *Atlas of Gastroenterology,* 3rd ed. Philadelphia: Lippincott Williams & Wilkins, 2003.

Herniated intervertebral disk

● OVERVIEW

Description
- Protrusion of part of the nucleus pulposus—disk's gelatinous center, through a tear in the posterior rim of the outer ring or annulus fibrosus
- Results in pressure on spinal nerve roots or spinal cord that causes back pain and other symptoms of nerve root irritation
- Most common site for herniation L4-L5 disk space; other sites, L5-S1, L2-L3, L3-L4, C6-C7, and C5-C6
- Clinical manifestations determined by:
  - Location and size of the herniation into the spinal canal
  - Amount of space that exists inside the spinal canal
- Also known as *herniated nucleus pulposus* or *slipped disk*

Pathophysiology
- The ligament and posterior capsule of the disk are usually torn, allowing the nucleus pulposus to extrude, compressing the nerve root.
- Occasionally, the injury tears the entire disk loose, causing protrusion onto the nerve root or compression of the spinal cord.
- Large amounts of extruded nucleus pulposus or complete disk herniation of the capsule and nucleus pulposus may compress the spinal cord.

Causes
- Trauma or strain
- Degenerative disk disease

Risk factors
- Advanced age
- Congenitally small lumbar spinal canal
- Osteophytes along the vertebrae

Incidence
- About 90% affect lumbar (L) and lumbosacral spine; 8% in cervical (C) spine; 1% to 2% in thoracic (T) spine
- Lumbar herniation more common in people ages 20 to 45
- Cervical herniation more common in people age 45 or older
- Herniated disks more common in men than in women

Common characteristics
- Pain
- Limited range of motion (ROM)
- Paresthesia
- Motor weakness

Complications
- Neurologic deficits
- Bowel and bladder dysfunction
- Sexual dysfunction

✱ ASSESSMENT

History
- Previous traumatic injury or back strain
- Unilateral, lower back pain
- Pain that may radiate to the buttocks, legs, and feet
- Pain that may begin suddenly, subside in a few days, and then recur at shorter intervals with progressive intensity
- Sciatic pain beginning as a dull ache in the buttocks, worsening with Valsalva's maneuver, coughing, sneezing, or bending
- Pain that may subside with rest
- Muscle spasms

Physical findings
- Limited ability to bend forward
- Posture that favors the affected side
- Muscle atrophy, in later stages
- Tenderness over the affected region
- Radicular pain with straight leg raising, in lumbar herniation
- Increased pain with neck movement in cervical herniation (see *Two tests for a herniated disk*)

Test results
IMAGING
- X-ray studies of the spine show degenerative changes.
- Myelography shows the level of the herniation.
- Computed tomography scan shows bone and soft-tissue abnormalities; can also show spinal canal compression.
- Magnetic resonance imaging shows soft-tissue abnormalities.
DIAGNOSTIC PROCEDURES
- Nerve conduction studies show sensory and motor loss.

- Electromyography measures muscle response to nerve stimulation.

◆ TREATMENT

General
- Initial treament conservative, unless neurologic impairment progresses rapidly
- Possible traction
- Supportive devices such as a brace
- Heat or ice applications
- Transcutaneous electrical nerve stimulation
- Chemonucleolysis

Diet
- As tolerated

Activity
- Bed rest, initially
- Prescribed physical therapy program
- Avoidance of repetitive activity

Medication
- Nonsteroidal anti-inflammatory drugs
- Steroids
- Muscle relaxants
- Analgesics

Surgery
- Laminectomy
- Spinal fusion
- Microdiskectomy

TWO TESTS FOR A HERNIATED DISK

The straight-leg-raising test and its variant, Lasègue's sign, are perhaps the best tests to perform when a herniated disk is suspected.

Straight-leg-raising test
Have the patient lie in a supine position. Place one hand on the patient's ilium to stabilize the pelvis and the other hand under the patient's ankle. Slowly raise the patient's leg. If the patient complains of posterior leg (sciatic) pain—*not back pain*—suspect a herniated disk.

Lasègue's sign
To do this test, have the patient lie in a supine position with his hip and knee flexed (to a 90-degree angle). Resistance and pain as well as loss of ankle or knee-jerk reflex indicates spinal root compression.

♣ NURSING CONSIDERATIONS

Nursing diagnoses
- Activity intolerance
- Acute pain
- Anxiety
- Dressing or grooming self-care deficit
- Fear
- Impaired physical mobility
- Risk for injury

Key outcomes
The patient will:
- perform activities of daily living within the confines of the disorder
- express feelings of increased comfort and decreased pain
- verbalize a decrease in anxiety
- participate in self-care to maximum degree possible
- verbalize concerns and feelings
- demonstrate adequate joint mobility and ROM
- achieve the highest level of mobility possible within the confines of the disease
- remain free from injury.

Nursing interventions
- Administer medications, as ordered.
- Plan a pain-control regimen.
- Offer supportive care.
- Provide encouragement.
- Help the patient cope with chronic pain and impaired mobility.
- Include the patient and his family in all phases of his care.
- Encourage the patient to express his concerns.
- Encourage performance of self-care.
- Help the patient identify activities that promote rest and relaxation.
- Prepare the patient for myelography, if indicated.
- Periodically remove traction to inspect skin.
- Institute measures to prevent deep vein thrombosis and footdrop.
- Ensure a consistent regimen of leg- and back-strengthening exercises.
- Encourage adequate oral fluid intake.
- Encourage coughing and deep-breathing exercises.
- Provide meticulous skin care.
- Provide a fracture bedpan for the patient on complete bed rest.

◈ **NURSING ALERT** During conservative treatment, watch for a deterioration in neurologic status, especially during the first 24 hours after admission, which may indicate an urgent need for surgery.

AFTER SURGERY
- Enforce bed rest as ordered.
- Use the logrolling technique to turn the patient.
- Assist the patient during his first attempt to walk.
- Provide a straight-backed chair for the patient to sit in briefly.

Monitoring
- Vital signs
- Intake and output
- Pain
- ROM
- Mobility
- Motor strength
- Deep vein thrombosis
- Bowel and bladder function

AFTER SURGERY
- Blood drainage system
- Drainage
- Incisions
- Dressings
- Neurovascular status
- Bowel sounds and abdominal distention

▶ PATIENT TEACHING

Be sure to cover:
- disorder, diagnostic tests, and treatment
- medication administration, dosage, and possible adverse effects
- when to notify the physician
- bed rest
- traction
- heat application
- exercise program
- myelography, if indicated
- preoperative and postoperative care, if indicated
- relaxation techniques
- proper body mechanics
- skin care.

Discharge planning
- Refer the patient to physical therapy, if indicated.
- Refer the patient to occupational therapy, if indicated.
- Refer the patient to a weight-reduction program, if appropriate.

✴ RESOURCES

Organizations
American Academy of Orthopaedic Surgeons: *www.aaos.org*
American College of Sports Medicine: *www.acsm.org*
American Physical Therapy Association: *www.apta.org*

Selected references
Jansson, K.A., et al. "Health-related Quality of Life in Patients Before and After Surgery for a Herniated Lumbar Disc," *Journal of Bone and Joint Surgery* (British volume) 87(7):959-64, July 2005.

Puschak, T.J., and Sasso, R.C. "Use of Artificial Disc Replacement in Degenerative Conditions of the Cervical Spine," *Current Opinion in Orthopedics* 15(3):175-79, June 2004.

Strayer, A. "Lumbar Spine: Common Pathology and Interventions," *Journal of Neuroscience Nursing* 37(4):181-93, August 2005.

Herpes simplex virus

● OVERVIEW

Description
- Common infection that may be latent in patient (carrier) for years
- After initial herpes simplex virus (HSV) infection, patient susceptible to recurrent attacks
- Recurrent infections possibly provoked by fever, menses, stress, heat, cold, lack of sleep, sun exposure, and contact with reactivated disease (kissing, sharing cosmetics)

Pathophysiology
- Virus enters mucosal surfaces or abraded skin sites and initiates replication in cells of the epidermis and dermis.
- Replication continues to permit infection of sensory or autonomic nerve endings.
- Virus enters the neuronal cell and is transported intra-axonally to nerve cell bodies in ganglia (where the virus establishes latency) and spreads by the peripheral sensory nerves. (See *Understanding the genital herpes cycle.*)

Causes
- Type 1 (HSV-1)—*Herpesvirus hominis* transmitted primarily by contact with oral secretions; mainly affects oral, labial, ocular, or skin tissues
- Type 2 (HSV-2)—*Herpesvirus hominis* transmitted primarily by contact with genital secretions; mainly affects genital structures

Incidence
- Occurs worldwide and equally in males and females
- Affects lower socioeconomic groups more commonly, probably because of crowded living conditions
- HSV-1 infection more common and occurs earlier in life than HSV-2 infection

Common characteristics
- Fever, malaise, and headache
- Tender inguinal adenopathy
- Typical primary lesions that erupt following prodromal tingling and itching
- Ruptured vesicles that produce painful ulcers, followed by yellow crusting

Complications
- Primary (or initial) HSV infection during pregnancy leading to abortion, premature labor, microcephaly, and uterine growth retardation
- Congenital herpes transmitted during vaginal birth, producing a subclinical neonatal infection or severe infection with seizures, chorioretinitis, skin vesicles, and hepatosplenomegaly
- HSV-1 causing life-threatening nonepidemic encephalitis in infants
- Gingivostomatitis in children ages 1 to 3
- Blindness from ocular infection
- Increased risk for cervical cancer
- Urethral stricture from recurrent genital herpes
- Perianal ulcers
- Colitis
- Esophagitis (more common in the impaired host)
- Pneumonitis
- Neurologic disorders
- Viremia with multiple-organ involvement

UNDERSTANDING THE GENITAL HERPES CYCLE

After a patient is infected with genital herpes, a latency period follows. The virus takes up permanent residence in the nerve cells surrounding the lesions, and intermittent viral shedding may take place.

Repeated outbreaks may develop at any time, again followed by a latent stage during which the lesions heal completely. Outbreaks may recur as often as three to eight times yearly. Although the cycle continues indefinitely, some people remain symptom-free for years.

```
┌─────────────────────────────────┐
│        INITIAL INFECTION         │
│ Highly infectious period marked  │
│ by fever, aches, adenopathy,     │
│ pain, and ulcerated skin and     │
│ mucous membranes                 │
└─────────────────────────────────┘
                │
                ▼
┌─────────────────────────────────┐
│            LATENCY               │
│ Intermittently infectious period │
│ marked by viral dormancy or      │
│ viral shedding and no disease    │
│ symptoms                         │
└─────────────────────────────────┘
                │
                ▼
┌─────────────────────────────────┐
│       RECURRENT INFECTION        │
│ Highly infectious period similar │
│ to initial infection with milder │
│ symptoms that resolve faster     │
└─────────────────────────────────┘
```

✱ ASSESSMENT

History
- Oral, vaginal, or anal sexual contact with an infected person or other direct contact with lesions
- With recurrent infection, various precipitating factors identified

Physical findings
PRIMARY PERIORAL HSV
- Sore throat, fever, anorexia, adenopathy
- Increased salivation
- Severe mouth pain, halitosis
- Small vesicles on an erythematous base possibly present on pharyngeal and oral mucosa

PRIMARY GENITAL HSV
- Malaise, tender inguinal adenopathy
- Dysuria, leukorrhea
- Dyspareunia
- Fluid-filled vesicles on the cervix, labia, perianal skin, vulva, and vagina; and on glans penis, foreskin, and penile shaft
- Extragenital lesions possibly seen on the mouth or anus

PRIMARY OCULAR INFECTION
- Photophobia, excessive tearing
- Follicular conjunctivitis, chemosis
- Blepharitis, vesicles on eyelids
- Lethargy and fever
- Regional adenopathy

Test results
LABORATORY
- Staining of scrapings from the base of the lesion demonstrates characteristic giant cells or intranuclear inclusions of herpes virus infection.
- Tissue culture shows isolation of virus.
- Tissue analysis shows HSV antigens or deoxyribonucleic acid in scrapings from lesions.

◆ TREATMENT

General
- Symptomatic and supportive therapy
- Ophthalmologist treatment for eye infections: drops, ointments, or surgery to drain the eye

Diet
- Avoidance of acidic foods (with stomatitis)

Activity
- No restrictions
- Abstinence from sexual activity during active phase (with genital lesions)

Medication
- Antipyretics and analgesics
- Anesthetic mouthwashes
- Bicarbonate-based mouth rinse
- Drying agents
- Ophthalmic medications
- Antivirals
- Docosanol (Abreva)

♣ NURSING CONSIDERATIONS

Nursing diagnoses
- Acute pain
- Impaired oral mucous membrane
- Impaired skin integrity
- Impaired social interaction
- Ineffective sexuality patterns
- Powerlessness
- Risk for infection
- Risk for injury
- Social isolation

Key outcomes
The patient will:
- express feelings of increased comfort and decreased pain
- remain free from complications related to trauma to oral mucous membranes
- exhibit improved or healed lesions or wounds
- resume effective communication patterns with spouse or partner
- voice feelings about potential or actual changes in sexuality
- verbalize feelings of control of situation
- experience no further signs and symptoms of infection
- remain free from injury
- maintain relationships with family and friends.

Nursing interventions
- Observe standard precautions.
- Administer medications, as ordered.
- Encourage the patient to express his feelings, and provide support.

Monitoring
- Response to treatment
- Adverse reactions to medication
- Complications
- Lesions

▶ PATIENT TEACHING

Be sure to cover:
- disorder, diagnostic tests, and treatment
- good hand-washing techniques
- recommended use of lip balm with sunscreen (with oral lesions)
- instructions to keep lesions dry, except for applying prescribed medications
- medication administration, dosage, and possible adverse effects
- recommendation that sexual partners be screened for sexually transmitted diseases (with genital herpes)
- recommendation to use warm compresses or take sitz baths several times per day and avoid all sexual contact during outbreaks of active infection (with genital herpes).

Discharge planning
- Referral to an ophthalmologist may be necessary for a patient with an eye infection.
- Refer the patient to a support group, such as the Herpes Resource Center, as appropriate.

✴ RESOURCES

Organizations
Centers for Disease Control and Prevention: *www.cdc.gov*
Harvard University Consumer Health Information: *www.intelihealth.com*
The Herpes Resource Center: *www.metalab.unc.edu/ASHA/herpes/hrc.html*
National Health Information Center: *www.health.gov/nhic*
National Library of Medicine: *www.nlm.nih.gov*

Selected references
Ensor, D. "The Significance of Herpes Simplex for School Nurses," *Journal of School Nursing* 21(1):10-16, February 2005.
Novak, N., and Peng, W.M. "Dancing with the Enemy: The Interplay of Herpes Simplex Virus with Dentrite Cells," *Clinical & Experimental Immunology* 142(3):405-10, December 2005.
Rodrigues, F., et al. "Herpes Simplex Virus Esophagitis in Immunocompetent Children," *Journal of Pediatric Gastrenterology & Nutrition* 39(5):560-63, November 2004.

Herpes zoster virus

● OVERVIEW

Description
- Acute unilateral and segmental inflammation of dorsal root ganglia
- Also called *shingles*

Pathophysiology
- Herpes zoster erupts when the virus reactivates after dormancy in the cerebral ganglia (extramedullary ganglia of the cranial nerves) or the ganglia of posterior nerve roots.
- The virus may multiply as it reactivates, and antibodies remaining from the initial infection may neutralize it.
- Without opposition from effective antibodies, the virus continues to multiply in the ganglia, destroys neurons, and spreads down the sensory nerves to the skin.

Causes
- Varicella-zoster virus (herpesvirus that also causes chickenpox)

Incidence
- Most common in adults between ages 50 and 70
- Bone marrow transplant patients especially at risk
- Possibly more prevalent in people who had chickenpox at a young age

Common characteristics
- Localized vesicular skin lesions, confined to a dermatome; thoracic, cervical and ophthalmic dermatomes most commonly involved
- Severe neuralgic pain in peripheral areas innervated by the nerves arising in the inflamed root ganglia
- Pain that generally precedes rash by 2 to 3 days
- Lesions that pustulate, crust, and heal in 3 to 4 weeks

Complications
- Deafness
- Secondary skin infection
- Postherpetic neuralgia
- Meningoencephalitis
- Cutaneous dissemination
- Ocular involvement with facial zoster
- Hepatitis
- Pneumonitis
- Peripheral motor weakness
- Guillain-Barré syndrome
- Cranial nerve syndrome

✳ ASSESSMENT

History
- Typical patient reports no history of exposure to others with varicella-zoster virus
- Complaints of fever, malaise, pain that mimics appendicitis, pleurisy, musculoskeletal pain, or other conditions
- In 2 to 4 days, possible severe, deep pain; pruritus; and paresthesia or hyperesthesia (usually affecting the trunk and occasionally the arms and legs)

Physical findings
- Small, red, nodular skin lesions that spread unilaterally around the thorax or vertically over the arms or legs
- Vesicles that may be filled with clear fluid or pus
- Vesicles that dry, forming scabs or even becoming gangrenous (see *A look at herpes zoster*)
- Enlarged regional lymph nodes

GENICULATE INVOLVEMENT
- Vesicle formation in the external auditory canal and ipsilateral facial palsy
- Hearing loss, dizziness, and loss of taste

TRIGEMINAL INVOLVEMENT
- Eye pain
- Corneal and scleral damage and impaired vision
- Conjunctivitis, extraocular weakness, ptosis, and paralytic mydriasis
- Secondary glaucoma

Test results
LABORATORY
- Vesicular fluid and infected tissue analyses show eosinophilic intranuclear inclusions and varicella virus.
- Staining antibodies from vesicular fluid and identification under fluorescent light aid differentiation of herpes zoster from herpes simplex virus.
- Cerebrospinal fluid analysis demonstrates increased protein levels and, possibly, pleocytosis.
- Specific antibody immune globulin measurement of varicella antibodies is elevated.

DIAGNOSTIC PROCEDURES
- Lumbar puncture indicates increased pressure.

◆ TREATMENT

General
- Transcutaneous peripheral nerve stimulation for postherpetic neuralgia
- Sooth baths
- Cold compresses

Diet
- No restrictions

Activity
- No restrictions

Medication
- Antivirals
- Antipruritics
- Analgesics
- Tricyclic antidepressants
- Demulcent and skin protectant
- Systemic antibiotics
- Corticosteroids
- Tranquilizers and sedatives
- Patient-controlled analgesia

Nursing diagnoses

- Acute pain
- Disturbed body image
- Impaired skin integrity
- Impaired social interaction
- Risk for infection

Key outcomes

The patient will:

- express feelings of increased comfort and decreased pain
- acknowledge change in body image
- exhibit improved or healed lesions or wounds
- participate in decision-making about his care
- demonstrate effective social interaction skills in one-on-one and group settings
- remain free from further signs and symptoms of infection.

Nursing interventions

- Administer medications, as ordered.
- Maintain meticulous hygiene to prevent spreading the infection to other parts of the patient's body.
- With open lesions, follow contact isolation precautions to prevent the spread of infection.

Monitoring

- Response to treatment
- Adverse reaction to medication
- Signs and symptoms of infection
- Lesions

Be sure to cover:

- use of a soft toothbrush, eating soft foods, and using a saline- or bicarbonate-based mouthwash and oral anesthetics to decrease discomfort from oral lesions
- need for meticulous hygiene to prevent spreading infection to other parts of the body
- need to avoid scratching lesions
- need to apply a cold compress if vesicles rupture.

Discharge planning

- Refer the patient to an ophthalmologist for ocular involvement.
- Refer the patient to a pain management specialist for postherpetic neuralgia.

Organizations

Centers for Disease Control and Prevention: *www.cdc.gov*
Harvard University Consumer Health Information: *www.intelihealth.com*
National Health Information Center: *www.health.gov/nhic*
National Library of Medicine: *www.nlm.nih.gov*

Selected references

Bielan, B. "What's Your Assessment? Herpes Zoster," *Dermatology Nursing* 16(5):431-32, October 2004.
Crider, E.F. "Herpes Zoster," *New England Journal of Medicine* 348(20):2044-2045, May 2003.
Kasper, D.L., et al., eds. *Harrison's Principles of Internal Medicine,* 16th ed. New York: McGraw-Hill Book Co., 2005.
Sandy, M.C. "Herpes Zoster: Medical and Nursing Management," *Clinical Journal of Oncology Nursing* 9(4):443-46, August 2005.
Wung, P.K., et al. "Herpes Zoster in Immunocompromised Patients: Incidence, Timing, and Risk Factors," *American Journal of Medicine* 118(12):1416, December 2005.

A LOOK AT HERPES ZOSTER

These characteristic herpes zoster lesions are fluid-filled vesicles that dry and form scabs after about 10 days. Unilateral vesicular lesions in a dermatomal pattern should rapidly lead to a diagnosis of herpes zoster.

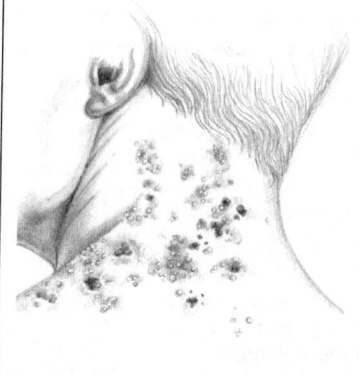

Hip fracture

● OVERVIEW

Description
- Break in the head (most common site) or neck of the femur
- Most common fall-related injury resulting in hospitalization
- Leading cause of disability among older adults
- May permanently change level of functioning and independence
- Within 1 year following hip fracture, fatal in one-fourth of patients

Pathophysiology
- With bone fracture, the periosteum and blood vessels in the marrow, cortex, and surrounding soft tissues are disrupted.
- This results in bleeding from the damaged ends of the bone and from the neighboring soft tissue.
- Clot formation occurs within the medullary canal, between the fractured bone ends, and beneath the periosteum.
- Bone tissue immediately adjacent to the fracture dies, and the necrotic tissue causes an intense inflammatory response.
- Vascular tissue invades the fracture area from surrounding soft tissue and marrow cavity within 48 hours, increasing blood flow to the entire bone.
- Bone-forming cells in the periosteum, endosteum, and marrow are activated to produce subperiosteal procallus along the outer surface of the shaft and over the broken ends of the bone.
- Collagen and matrix, which become mineralized to form callus, are synthesized by osteoblasts within the procallus.
- During the repair process, remodeling occurs; unnecessary callus is resorbed and trabeculae are formed along stress lines.
- New bone, not scar tissue, is formed over the healed fracture.

Causes
- Falls
- Trauma
- Cancer metastasis
- Osteoporosis
- Skeletal disease

Incidence
- Affects more than 200,000 people annually
- Occurs in one of five women by age 80
- More common in females than in males

Common characteristics
- Impaired function
- Deformity
- Edema
- Muscle spasm
- Pain and tenderness
- Impaired sensation

Complications
- Pneumonia
- Venous thrombosis
- Pressure ulcers
- Social isolation
- Depression
- Bladder dysfunction
- Deep vein thrombosis
- Pulmonary embolus
- Hip dislocation
- Death

✳ ASSESSMENT

History
- Falls or trauma to the bones
- Pain in the affected hip and leg
- Pain exacerbated by movement

Physical findings
- Outward rotation of affected extremity, which may appear shorter
- Limited or abnormal range of motion (ROM)
- Edema and discoloration of the surrounding tissue
- In an open fracture, bone protruding through the skin

Test results
IMAGING
- X-rays show the location of the fracture.
- Computed tomography scan shows abnormalities in complicated fractures.

◆ TREATMENT

General
- Dependent on age, comorbidities, cognitive functioning, support systems, and functional ability
- Possible skin traction
- Physical therapy
- Non–weight-bearing transfers

Diet
- Well-balanced
- Foods rich in vitamin C and A, calcium, and protein
- Adequate vitamin D

Activity
- Bed rest initially
- Ambulation as soon as possible after surgery
- Physical therapy

Medication
- Analgesics

Surgery
- Total hip arthroplasty
- Hemiarthroplasty
- Percutaneous pinning
- Internal fixation using a compression screw and plate

✤ NURSING CONSIDERATIONS

Nursing diagnoses
- Acute pain
- Anxiety
- Dressing or grooming self-care deficit
- Impaired physical mobility
- Impaired skin integrity
- Ineffective role performance
- Ineffective tissue perfusion: Peripheral
- Risk for infection
- Risk for injury

Key outcomes
The patient will:
- express feelings of increased comfort and decreased pain and anxiety
- verbalize feelings about present condition
- perform self-care activities to the fullest extent possible
- maintain muscle strength and tone and joint ROM
- maintain skin integrity
- carry out previous roles within the limitations of the condition
- demonstrate signs of adequate peripheral perfusion
- remain free from signs and symptoms of infection or injury.

Nursing interventions
- Administer medications, as ordered.
- Cover exposed bone and open wound with sterile dressings.
- Administer prophylactic anticoagulation after surgery, as ordered.
- If the patient has skin traction, remove it daily to check skin integrity.
- Maintain traction, as ordered.
- Maintain proper body alignment.
- Use an abductor splint or trochanter roll between the legs.
- Use logrolling techniques to turn the patient in bed.
- Maintain non–weight-bearing status, as ordered.
- Increase the patient's activity level, as prescribed.
- Consult physical therapy as early as possible.
- Assist with active ROM exercises to unaffected limbs.
- Encourage coughing and deep-breathing exercises.
- Keep the patient's skin clean and dry.
- Prevent skin breakdown.

- Encourage good nutrition; offer high-protein, high-calorie snacks.
- Perform daily wound care, as ordered.

> **⊙ NURSING ALERT** Don't massage the patient's extremities to promote circulation. Massage could increase the risk of thromboembolism.

Monitoring
- Vital signs
- Intake and output
- Pain
- Mobility and ROM
- Incision and dressings
- Complications
- Coagulation study results
- Signs of bleeding
- Neurovascular status
- Skin integrity
- Signs and symptoms of infection

> **⊙ NURSING ALERT** Following surgery, assess the patient for complications, such as deep vein thrombosis, pulmonary embolus, and hip dislocation.

▶ PATIENT TEACHING

Be sure to cover:
- disorder, diagnostic tests, and treatment
- medication administration, dosage, and possible adverse effects
- ROM exercises
- meticulous skin care
- proper body alignment
- wound care
- signs of infection
- coughing and deep-breathing exercises and incentive spirometry
- assistive devices
- activity restrictions and lifestyle changes
- safe ambulation practices
- nutritious diet and adequate fluid intake.

Discharge planning
- Refer the patient to physical and occupational therapy programs, as indicated.
- Refer the patient to home health or rehabilitation care as necessary.

✱ RESOURCES

Organizations
American Academy of Orthopaedic Surgeons: *www.aaos.org*
American Fracture Association: (309) 663-6272
The Merck Manual Online Medical Library: *www.merck.com/mmhe*
National Osteoporosis Foundation: *www.nof.org*

Selected references
Cole, A. "Nurse-adminstered Femoral Nerve Block after Hip Fracture," *Nursing Times* 101(37):34-36, September 2005.

Latham, N.K., et al. "Pattern of Functional Change During Rehabilitation of Patients with Hip Fracture," *Archives of Physical Medicine and Rehabilitation* 87(1):111-16, January 2006.

Wald, H., et al. "Extended Use of Indwelling Urinary Catheters in Postoperative Hip Fracture Patients," *Medical Care* 43(10):1009-1017, October 2005.

Williams, A., and Jester, R. "Delayed Surgical Fixation of Fractured Hips in Older People: Impact on Mortality," *Journal of Advanced Nursing* 52(1):63-69, October 2005.

Histoplasmosis

● OVERVIEW

Description
- Fungal infection
- Three forms in the United States:
  - Primary acute histoplasmosis
  - Progressive disseminated histoplasmosis (acute disseminated or chronic disseminated disease)
  - Chronic pulmonary (cavitary) histoplasmosis
- Also known as *Ohio Valley disease*, *Central Mississippi Valley disease*, *Appalachian Mountain disease*, and *Darling's disease*

Pathophysiology
- Spores reach alveoli and are transformed into budding forms.
- Intense granulomatous reaction occurs and caseation necrosis or calcification (resembling tuberculosis) occurs.
- Transient dissemination can leave granulomas in the spleen.

Causes
- Caused by *Histoplasma capsulatum*, which is found in the stool of birds and bats and in soil contaminated by their stool (near roosts, chicken coops, barns, caves, and underneath bridges)
- Transmitted to humans by inhalation of *H. capsulatum* or *H. capsulatum* var. *duboisii* spores or invasion of spores after minor skin trauma

Incidence
- Occurs worldwide, especially in temperate areas of Asia, Africa, Europe, and North and South America
- In the United States, most prevalent in southeastern, mid-Atlantic, and central states
- Primary acute histoplasmosis most common in infants, young children, and immunocompromised patients

Common characteristics
- Incubation period that ranges from 5 to 18 days, although chronic pulmonary histoplasmosis possibly progressing slowly for many years
- Chronic pulmonary infections that occurs more commonly in males older than age 40, particularly with a history of cigarette smoking or emphysema

Complications
- Vascular or bronchial obstruction
- Acute pericarditis
- Pleural effusion
- Mediastinal fibrosis or granuloma
- Intestinal ulceration
- Addison's disease
- Endocarditis
- Meningitis

✳ ASSESSMENT

History
- Possible history of an immunocompromised condition
- Exposure to contaminated soil in an endemic area

Physical findings
- Fever, which may rise as high as 105° F (40.6° C)

PRIMARY ACUTE HISTOPLASMOSIS
- Usually no characteristic signs
- Mild respiratory illness, cough
- Malaise, headache, myalgia, anorexia
- Chest pain

PROGRESSIVE DISSEMINATED HISTOPLASMOSIS
- Anorexia and weight loss
- Pain
- Hoarseness, tachypnea in later stages
- Ulceration of the oropharynx, dysphagia
- Pallor from anemia
- Jaundice and ascites
- Hepatosplenomegaly
- Lymphadenopathy

CHRONIC PULMONARY HISTOPLASMOSIS
- Productive cough, dyspnea, hemoptysis
- Shortness of breath, cyanosis
- Extreme weakness, weight loss
- Upper lobe fibrocavitary pneumonia

Test results
LABORATORY
- Blood cultures done by lysis-centrifugation technique shows presence of the etiologic organism.
- In disseminated forms, culture of bone marrow, mucosal lesions, liver, and bronchoalveolar lavage is helpful in showing organisms.
- Sputum cultures (preferred in chronic pulmonary histoplasmosis), which may take 2 to 4 weeks to culture, show growth of the organism.
- Radioactive assay for histoplasma antigen in blood or urine shows presence of the antigen.

IMAGING
- Chest X-ray shows lung damage.

◆ TREATMENT

General
- Oxygen for respiratory distress
- Parenteral fluids for dysphagia caused by oral or laryngeal ulcerations
- Cool mist humdifier
- Smoking cessation

Diet
- Soft, bland foods (with oropharyngeal ulceration)
- Small, frequent meals

Activity
- Frequent rest periods

Medication
- Antifungal therapy
- Glucocorticoids

Surgery
- Lung resection to remove pulmonary nodules
- Shunt for increased intracranial pressure
- Cardiac repair for constrictive pericarditis

❖ NURSING CONSIDERATIONS

Nursing diagnoses
- Activity intolerance
- Acute pain
- Decreased cardiac output
- Imbalanced nutrition: Less than body requirements
- Impaired gas exchange
- Ineffective airway clearance
- Ineffective breathing pattern
- Risk for injury

Key outcomes
The patient will:
- express feelings of increased comfort and decreased pain
- demonstrate measures to balance activity and rest
- maintain adequate cardiac output
- experience no further weight loss
- maintain adequate gas exchange with arterial blood gas levels that return to baseline
- maintain patent airway
- express feelings of comfort in maintaining air exchange
- maintain hemodynamic stability
- remain free from injury.

Nursing interventions
- Administer medications, as ordered.
- Provide oxygen therapy if needed.
- Plan rest periods.
- Consult with the dietitian and patient concerning food preferences.

Monitoring
- Hypoglycemia and hyperglycemia, which indicate adrenal dysfunction
- Respiratory status
- Neurologic status

▶ PATIENT TEACHING

Be sure to cover:
- disorder, diagnostic tests, and treatment
- medication administration, dosage, and possible adverse effects
- cardiac and pulmonary signs that could indicate effusions
- need to watch for early signs of this infection and to seek treatment promptly to help prevent the spread of histoplasmosis for people in endemic areas
- need for people who risk occupational exposure to contaminated soil to wear face masks.

Discharge planning
- Stress the need for follow-up care on a regular basis for at least 1 year.
- Refer the patient with chronic pulmonary or disseminated histoplasmosis for psychological support to cope with long-term treatment, as appropriate.
- Refer the patient to a social worker or an occupational therapist, as needed.
- Help parents of a child with the disease arrange for a visiting teacher.

✹ RESOURCES

Organizations
Centers for Disease Control and Prevention: *www.cdc.gov*
Harvard University Consumer Health Information: *www.intelihealth.com*
National Health Information Center: *www.health.gov/nhic*
National Library of Medicine: *www.nlm.nih.gov*

Selected references
Adderson, F. "Histoplasmosis," *Pediatric Infectious Disease Journal* 25(1):73-74, January 2006.
Adderson, F. "Histoplasmosis in a Pediatric Oncology Center," *Journal of Pediatrics* 144(1):100-106, January 2004.
Kasper, D.L., et al., eds. *Harrison's Principles of Internal Medicine,* 16th ed. New York: McGraw-Hill Book Co., 2005.
Tropin, J., and Mutlu, G.M. "Images in Clinical Medicine. Splenic and Mediastinal Calcification in Histoplasmosis," *New England Journal of Medicine* 354(2):179, January 2006.

Hodgkin's disease

● OVERVIEW

Description
- Neoplastic disorder characterized by painless, progressive enlargement of lymph nodes, spleen, and other lymphoid tissue
- With appropriate treatment, 5-year survival rate about 90%

Pathophysiology
- Enlarged lymphoid tissue results from proliferation of lymphocytes, histiocytes, eosinophils, and Reed-Sternberg cells.
- Untreated Hodgkin's disease follows a variable but relentlessly progressive and ultimately fatal course.

Causes
- Exact cause unknown

Risk factors
- Genetic
- Viral
- Environmental

Common characteristics
- Painless swelling of lymph nodes
- Fever, night sweats

Incidence
- Peaks in two age-groups: ages 15 to 38 and after age 50
- Occurs in all races; slightly more common in whites
- Most common in young adults, except in Japan (exclusively in people older than age 50)
- Greater incidence in men than in women

Complications
- Multiple organ failure

✻ ASSESSMENT

History
- Painless swelling of one of the cervical, axillary, or inguinal lymph nodes
- Persistent fever and night sweats
- Weight loss despite an adequate diet, with resulting fatigue and malaise
- Increasing susceptibility to infection

Physical findings
- Edema of the face and neck and jaundice
- Enlarged, rubbery lymph nodes in the neck (these nodes enlarge during periods of fever and then revert to normal size)

Test results
LABORATORY
- Hematologic tests show mild to severe normocytic anemia, normochromic anemia in 50% of patients, and elevated, normal, or reduced white blood cell count and differential, showing any combination of neutrophilia, lymphocytopenia, monocytosis, and eosinophilia.
- Serum alkaline phosphatase levels are elevated, indicating liver or bone involvement.

DIAGNOSTIC PROCEDURES
- Tests must first rule out other disorders that cause lymph node enlargement.
- Lymph node biopsy confirms the presence of Reed-Sternberg cells, abnormal histiocyte proliferation, and nodular fibrosis and necrosis. Lymph node biopsy is also used to determine lymph node and organ involvement.
- A staging laparotomy is necessary for patients younger than age 55 and for those without obvious stage III or stage IV disease, lymphocyte predominance subtype histology, or medical contraindications.

◆ TREATMENT

General
- For patient with stage I or II disease, radiation therapy alone
- For patient with stage III disease, radiation therapy and chemotherapy
- For patient with stage IV disease, chemotherapy alone (or chemotherapy and radiation therapy to involved sites), sometimes inducing complete remission
- Autologous bone marrow transplantation or autologous peripheral blood sternal transfusions and immunotherapy

Diet
- Well-balanced; no restrictions

Activity
- Frequent rest periods
- No restrictions

Medication
- Chemotherapy
- Antiemetics
- Sedatives
- Antidiarrheals

✿ NURSING CONSIDERATIONS

Nursing diagnoses

- Acute pain
- Anxiety
- Disabled family coping
- Fatigue
- Fear
- Imbalanced nutrition: Less than body requirements
- Impaired oral mucous membrane
- Impaired skin integrity
- Ineffective coping
- Risk for infection

Key outcomes

The patient will:

- express feelings of increased comfort and decreased pain and anxiety
- express feelings of increased energy
- exhibit no further weight loss
- exhibit intact mucous membranes
- verbalize feelings and concerns
- maintain adequate skin integrity
- demonstrate effective coping mechanisms
- remain free from signs and symptoms of infection.

Nursing interventions

- Provide a well-balanced, high-calorie, high-protein diet.
- Provide for periods of rest.
- Administer medications, as ordered.
- Provide emotional support

Monitoring

- Complications of treatment
- Pain control
- Lymph node enlargement
- Body temperature
- Fatigue
- Daily weight
- Signs and symptoms of infection
- Response to treatment
- Signs and symptoms of dehydration

▶ PATIENT TEACHING

Be sure to cover:

- disorder, diagnostic tests, and treatment
- signs and symptoms of infection
- importance of maintaining good nutrition
- pacing of activities to counteract therapy-induced fatigue
- importance of good oral hygiene
- avoidance of crowds and people with known infection
- importance of checking the lymph nodes
- medication administration, dosage, and possible adverse effects.

Discharge planning

- Refer the patient to resource and support services.

✳ RESOURCES

Organizations

American Cancer Society: *www.cancer.org*
Guide to Internet Resources for Cancer: *www.cancerindex.org*
National Cancer Institute: *www.nci.org*

Selected references

Atlas of Pathophysiology, 2nd ed. Philadelphia: Lippincott Williams & Wilkins, 2005.

Casciato, D.A. *Manual of Clinical Oncology,* 5th ed. Philadelphia: Lippincott Williams & Wilkins, 2004.

Cole, S., and Dunne, K. "Hodgkin's Lymphoma," *Nursing Standard* 18(19):46-52, January 2004.

Krasin, M.J., et al. "Patterns of Treatment Failure in Pediatric and Young Adult Patients with Hodgkin's Disease: Local Disease Control with Combined Modality Therapy," *Journal of Clinical Oncology* 23(33):8406-413, November 2005.

Kupers, R., et al. "Advances in Biology, Diagnostics, and Treatment of Hodgkin's Disease," *Biology of Blood and Marrow Transplantation* 12(1 Suppl 1):66-76, January 2006.

Huntington's disease

● OVERVIEW

Description
- Degenerative brain disease that causes dementia
- Usually fatal 10 to 15 years after onset
- Also called *Huntington's chorea, hereditary chorea, chronic progressive chorea,* or *adult chorea*

Pathophysiology
- Degeneration in the cerebral cortex and basal ganglia leads to chronic progressive chorea (dancelike movements).
- The final stage is mental deterioration, which ends in dementia.

Causes
- Genetic link
- Transmitted as autosomal dominant trait (either sex can transmit and inherit it)

Incidence
- Most common between ages 25 and 55 (average age 35)
- 2% of cases in children
- 5% of cases as late as age 60
- 50% chance of inheritance in each child of a parent with disease
- In child who doesn't inherit disease, can't pass it on
- Affects men and women equally

Common characteristics
- Emotional changes, irritability
- Clumsiness, bradykinesia
- Bouts of anger
- Purposeless movements
- Grimacing
- Dysarthria
- Writhing and twitching
- Loss of motor control; rigidity
- Dysphagia
- Oral apraxia, aprosody

Complications
- Choking and aspiration
- Pneumonia
- Heart failure
- Infections

✳ ASSESSMENT

History
- Findings dependent on disease progression
- Family history of the disorder
- Emotional and mental changes
- Insidious onset
- Total dependency through:
  - Intellectual decline
  - Emotional disturbances
  - Loss of musculoskeletal control
- Reports of feeling clumsy, irritable, or impatient
- Subject to fits of anger
- Periods of suicidal depression, apathy, or elation
- Ravenous appetite, especially for sweets
- Loss of bladder and bowel control in later stages

Physical findings
- Choreic movements
- Rapid, usually violent, and purposeless movements
- Unilateral
- More prominent in the face and arms than in the legs

EARLY STAGES
- Mild fidgeting
- Grimacing, tongue smacking
- Dysarthria
- Athetoid movements related to emotional state
- Torticollis

LATER STAGES
- Constant writhing and twitching
- Unintelligible speech
- Difficulty chewing and swallowing
- Ambulation impossible
- Appears emaciated and exhausted

Test results
LABORATORY
- Deoxyribonucleic acid analysis may show disease.

IMAGING
- Positron emission tomography may show disease.
- Magnetic resonance imaging shows characteristic butterfly dilation of the brain's lateral ventricles.
- Computed tomography scan shows brain atrophy.

◆ TREATMENT

General
- No known cure
- Supportive and protective treatment, based on symptoms
- Psychotherapy
- Safety measures

Diet
- No restrictions; may need soft diet

Activity
- No restrictions

Medication
- Tranquilizers
- Dopamine agonists
- Neuroleptics
- Selective serotonin reuptake inhibitors
- Antidepressants

❖ NURSING CONSIDERATIONS

Nursing diagnoses
- Anxiety
- Chronic low self-esteem
- Dressing or grooming self-care deficit
- Feeding self-care deficit
- Impaired physical mobility
- Impaired verbal communication
- Ineffective health maintenance
- Risk for aspiration
- Risk for infection
- Risk for injury
- Toileting self-care deficit
- Total urinary incontinence

Key outcomes
The patient will:
- exhibit a decrease in anxiety
- express positive feelings about self
- perform activities of daily living within the limitations of the disorder
- maintain joint mobility and range of motion
- develop alternative means of communication to express self
- demonstrate measures to maintain good health
- maintain a patent airway without evidence of aspiration
- remain free from signs and symptoms of infection and injury
- identify strategies to reduce incontinent episodes.

Nursing interventions
- Provide psychological support.
- Identify self-care deficits.
- Encourage the patient to be independent.
- Provide communication aids.
- Help the patient with difficulty walking.
- Maintain a turning schedule.
- Elevate the head of the bed during eating.
- Administer medications, as ordered.
- Protect the patient from infections.

Monitoring
- Response to medications
- Possible suicide attempts
- Temperature
- White blood cell count

▶ PATIENT TEACHING

Be sure to cover:
- disorder, diagnostic tests, and treatment
- medication administration, dosage, and possible adverse effects
- aspiration precautions
- signs and symptoms of infection
- communication strategies.

Discharge planning
- Refer the patient to the Huntington's Disease Society of America.
- Refer the patient to appropriate community organizations.
- Refer affected families for genetic counseling.
- Refer the patient for psychotherapy, as appropriate.

✳ RESOURCES

Organizations
Huntington's Disease Society of America: *www.hdsa.org*
National Institutes of Health: *www.nih.gov*

Selected references
Diseases, 4th ed. Philadelphia: Lippincott Williams & Wilkins, 2006.
Handbook of Pathophysiology, 2nd ed. Philadelphia: Lippincott Williams & Wilkins, 2005.
King, N. "Palliatve Care Management of a Child with Juvenile Onset Huntington's Disease," *International Journal of Palliative Nursing* 11(6):278-83, June 2005.
Skirton, J. "Huntington's Disease: A Nursing Perspective," *Medsurg Nursing* 14(3):167-72, June 2005.

Hydrocephalus

● OVERVIEW

Description
- Refers to a variety of conditions characterized by an excess of fluid within the cranial vault, subarachnoid space, or both
- Occurs because of interference with cerebrospinal fluid (CSF) flow caused by increased fluid production, obstruction within the ventricular system, or defective reabsorption of CSF
- Types:
  - Noncommunicating hydrocephalus: obstruction within the ventricular system
  - Communicating hydrocephalus: impaired absorption of CSF

Pathophysiology
- The obstruction of CSF flow associated with hydrocephalus produces dilation of the ventricles proximal to the obstruction.
- The obstructed CSF is under pressure, causing atrophy of the cerebral cortex and degeneration of the white matter tracts. There's selective preservation of gray matter.
- When excess CSF fills a defect caused by atrophy, a degenerative disorder, or a surgical excision, the fluid isn't under pressure and atrophy and degenerative changes aren't induced.

Causes
NONCOMMUNICATING HYDROCEPHALUS
- Aqueduct stenosis
- Arnold-Chiari malformation
- Congenital abnormalities in the ventricular system
- Mass lesions such as a tumor that compresses one of the structures of the ventricular system

COMMUNICATING HYDROCEPHALUS
- Adhesions from inflammation, such as with meningitis or subarachnoid hemorrhage
- Compression of the subarachnoid space by a mass such as a tumor
- Congenital abnormalities of the subarachnoid space
- High venous pressure within the sagittal sinus
- Head injury
- Cerebral atrophy

Incidence
- Congenital hydrocephalus rare
- Noncommunicating hydrocephalus more common in children
- Communicating hydrocephalus more common in adults

Common characteristics
- Enlargement of head clearly disproportionate to growth
- Distended scalp veins
- Thin, shiny, fragile-looking scalp skin
- Underdeveloped neck muscles
- Depressed orbital roof
- Downward displacement of eyes
- High-pitched, shrill cry; irritability
- Projectile vomiting
- Skull widening

Complications
- Mental retardation
- Impaired motor function
- Vision loss
- Death (increased intracranial pressure [ICP])
- Infection and malnutrition (more common in infants)

✳ ASSESSMENT

History
INFANTS
- History that may disclose cause
- High-pitched, shrill cry; irritability
- Anorexia
- Episodes of projectile vomiting
ADULTS AND OLDER CHILDREN
- Frontal headaches
- Nausea and vomiting (may be projectile)
- Symptoms cause wakening or occur on awakening
- Diplopia
- Restlessness

Physical findings
INFANTS
- Enlarged head that's clearly disproportionate to the infant's growth
- Head that may appear normal in size, but with bulging fontanels
- Distended scalp veins
- Thin, fragile, and shiny scalp skin
- Underdeveloped neck muscles
- Depression of the roof of the eye orbit
- Displacement of the eyes downward
- Prominent sclera (sunset sign)
- Abnormal muscle tone of the legs
ADULTS AND OLDER CHILDREN
- Decreased level of consciousness
- Ataxia
- Impaired intellect
- Incontinence
- Signs of increased ICP

Test results
IMAGING
- Skull X-rays show thinning of the skull with separation of sutures and widening of the fontanels in infants.
- Angiography, computed tomography scan, and magnetic resonance imaging show differentiation between hydrocephalus and intracranial lesions and Arnold-Chiari deformity.

◆ TREATMENT

General
- Shunting of CSF directly from the ventricular system to some point beyond the obstruction

Diet
- Small, frequent feedings

Activity
- Decreased movement during and immediately after meals

Medication
- Possible preoperative and postoperative antibiotics

Surgery
- Surgical correction (the only treatment for hydrocephalus) including:
  - removal of obstruction to CSF flow
  - implantation of a ventriculoperitoneal shunt to divert CSF flow from the brain's lateral ventricle into the peritoneal cavity
  - with concurrent abdominal problem, ventriculoatrial shunt to divert CSF flow from the brain's lateral ventricle into the right atrium of the heart

Nursing diagnoses

- Acute pain
- Anxiety
- Decreased intracranial capacity
- Delayed growth and development
- Disturbed body image
- Imbalanced nutrition: Less than body requirements
- Impaired skin integrity
- Ineffective airway clearance
- Ineffective tissue perfusion: Cerebral
- Interrupted family processes
- Risk for disorganized infant behavior
- Risk for infection

Key outcomes

The patient (or family) will:
- express feelings of increased comfort and decreased pain and anxiety
- remain free from signs and symptoms of increased ICP
- achieve age-appropriate growth , behaviors, and skills to fullest extent possible
- maintain skin integrity
- maintain a patent airway
- maintain adequate ventilation and oxygenation
- maintain and improve current level of consciousness
- remain free from signs and symptoms of infection
- verbalize effect of patient's condition on daily life
- remain free from seizure activity.

Nursing interventions

- Promote maternal-infant bonding.
- Elevate the head of the bed to 30 degrees.
- Administer oxygen, as needed.
- Provide small, frequent feedings.
- Decrease the patient's movement during and immediately after meals.
- Feed the infant slowly.
- After feeding, place the infant on his side.
- Reposition the infant every 2 hours, or prop him up in an infant seat.
- Provide skin care.

AFTER SHUNT SURGERY
- Place the infant on the side opposite the operative site.
- Administer I.V. fluids.
- Administer analgesics, as ordered.

Monitoring

- Fontanels for tension or fullness
- Head circumference
- Signs and symptoms of increased ICP
- Complications
- Growth and development
- Neurologic status
- Intake and output

AFTER SHUNT SURGERY

◆ **NURSING ALERT** Monitor for vomiting, which may be an early sign of shunt malfunction.

- Signs and symptoms of meningitis
- Redness, swelling, and other signs and symptoms of local infection
- Dressing for drainage
- Response to analgesics

▶ PATIENT TEACHING

Be sure to cover:
- disorder, diagnostic tests, and treatment
- shunt surgery, including hair loss and the visibility of a mechanical device
- need to focus on the child's strengths, not weaknesses
- postoperative shunt care
- signs and symptoms of increased ICP or shunt malfunction
- infant's needs for sensory stimulation
- signs and symptoms of infection
- signs and symptoms of paralytic ileus
- need for periodic shunt surgery to lengthen the shunt as the child grows older.

Discharge planning

- Refer the patient to special education programs, as appropriate.

✴ RESOURCES

Organizations

The American Academy of Pediatrics: *www.aap.org*
National Institutes of Health: *www.nih.gov*

Selected references

Diseases, 4th ed. Philadelphia: Lippincott Williams & Wilkins, 2006.

Handbook of Pathophysiology, 2nd ed. Philadelphia: Lippincott Williams & Wilkins, 2005.

Mangano, E.T., et al. "Early Programmable Valve Malfunctions in Pedatric Hydrocephalus," *Journal of Neurosurgery* 103(6 Suppl): 501-507, December 2005.

McGirt, M.J., et al. "Diagnosis, Treatment, and Analysis of Long-Term Outcomes in Idiopathic Normal-Pressure Hydrocephalus," *Neurosurgery* 57(4):699-705, October 2005.

Rudy, C. "Hydrocephalus," *Journal of Pediatric Health Care* 19(2):111, 127-28, March-April 2005.

Hydronephrosis

● OVERVIEW

Description
- Abnormal dilation of the renal pelvis and calyces of one or both kidneys
- Caused by obstruction of urine flow in the genitourinary tract
- May be acute or chronic

Pathophysiology
- With obstruction in the urethra or bladder, hydronephrosis is usually bilateral.
- With obstruction in a ureter, hydronephrosis is usually unilateral.
- Obstructions distal to the bladder cause the bladder to dilate, acting as a buffer zone, delaying hydronephrosis.
- Total obstruction of urine flow with dilation of the collecting system ultimately causes complete cortical atrophy and glomerular filtration ceases.

Causes
- Benign prostatic hyperplasia (BPH)
- Urethral strictures
- Renal calculi
- Strictures or stenosis of the ureter or bladder outlet
- Congenital abnormalities
- Bladder, ureteral, or pelvic tumors
- Blood clots
- Neurogenic bladder
- Gram-negative infection
- Ureterocele

Incidence
- Approximately 1 of 100 people affected by unilateral hydronephrosis
- Approximately 1 of 200 people affected by bilateral hydronephrosis

Common characteristics
- Decreased urine output
- Flank pain

Complications
- Pyelonephritis
- Paralytic ileus
- Renal failure
- Infection
- Sepsis
- Renovascular hypertension

✳ ASSESSMENT

History
- Varies depending on cause of obstruction
- With partial obstruction and hydronephrosis, may initially be asymptomatic, however increasing pressure behind the obstruction eventually resulting in renal dysfunction
- Mild pain and slightly decreased urine flow
- Severe, colicky renal pain or dull flank pain that radiates to the groin
- Hematuria, pyuria, dysuria
- Alternating oliguria and polyuria, anuria
- Nausea, vomiting, and abdominal fullness
- Pain on urination, dribbling, and urinary hesitancy
- Change in voiding pattern

Physical findings
- Hematuria, pyuria
- Urinary tract infection
- Palpable kidney
- Distended bladder

Test results
LABORATORY
- Renal function studies are abnormal.
- Urine studies confirm inability to concentrate urine, decreased glomerular filtration rate, and pyuria if infection is present.

IMAGING
- Excretory urography, retrograde pyelography, and renal ultrasonography confirm diagnosis.
- I.V. urogram may show site of obstruction.
- Nephrogram may show delayed appearance time.
- Radionuclide scan may show site of obstruction.

◆ TREATMENT

General
- For inoperable obstructions, decompression and drainage of the kidney, using a nephrostomy tube placed temporarily or permanently in the renal pelvis

Diet
- If renal function affected, low-protein, low-sodium, and low-potassium

Activity
- No restrictions

Medication
- Antibiotics
- Analgesics
- Oral alkalinization therapy (for uric acid calculi)
- Steroid therapy (for retroperitoneal fibrosis)

Surgery
- Dilatation for urethral stricture
- Prostatectomy for BPH
- Percutaneous nephrostomy tube placement

❖ NURSING CONSIDERATIONS

Nursing diagnoses
- Acute pain
- Anxiety
- Deficient fluid volume
- Imbalanced nutrition: Less than body requirements
- Impaired urinary elimination
- Risk for infection

Key outcomes
The patient will:
- express feelings of increased comfort and decreased pain and anxiety
- maintain fluid balance
- maintain hemodynamic stability
- demonstrate adequate nutritional intake
- maintain adequate urinary function
- remain free from signs and symptoms of infection.

Nursing interventions
- Administer medications, as ordered.
- Administer I.V. fluids, as ordered.
- Allow the patient to express his fears and anxieties.

Monitoring
- Renal function studies
- Intake and output
- Vital signs
- Fluid and electrolyte status
- Nephrostomy tube function and drainage (if appropriate)
- Wound site (postoperatively)

▶ PATIENT TEACHING

Be sure to cover:
- disorder, diagnostic tests, and treatment
- (if surgery is scheduled) the procedure and postoperative care
- nephrostomy tube care, if appropriate
- medication administration, dosage, and possible adverse effects
- dietary changes
- hydronephrosis symptom recognition and reporting.

Discharge planning
- Arrange for follow-up to evaluate recovery and monitor urinary function.

✷ RESOURCES

Organizations
American Association of Kidney Patients: *www.aakp.org*
National Institute of Diabetes & Digestive & Kidney Diseases: *www.niddk.nih.gov*

Selected references
Diseases, 4th ed. Philadelphia: Lippincott Williams & Wilkins, 2006.
Esklid-Jensen, A., et al. "Interpretation of the Renogram: Problems and Pitfalls in Hydronephrosis in Children," *BJU International* 94(6):887-92, October 2004.
Pates, J.A., and Dashe, J.S. "Prenatal Diagnosis and Management of Hydronephrosis," *Early Human Development* 82(1):3-8, January 2006.
Tsai, J.D., et al. "Intermittent Hydronephrosis Secondary to Ureteropelvic Junction Obstruction: Clinical and Imaging Features," *Pediatrics* 117(1):139-46, January 2006.

Hyperlipoproteinemia

● OVERVIEW

Description
- Increased plasma concentrations of one or more lipoproteins
- Primary form: includes at least five distinct and inherited metabolic disorders
- May occur secondary to other conditions such as diabetes mellitus
- Clinical changes ranging from relatively mild symptoms, managed by diet, to potentially fatal pancreatitis

Pathophysiology
- Increased low-density lipoprotein (LDL) and decreased high-density lipoprotein (HDL) levels lead to accelerated development of atherosclerosis.

Causes
- Primary hyperlipoproteinemia
  - Types I and III transmitted as autosomal recessive traits
  - Types II, IV, and V transmitted as autosomal dominant traits
- Secondary hyperlipoproteinemia
  - Diabetes mellitus
  - Pancreatitis
  - Hypothyroidism
  - Renal disease

Incidence
TYPE I
- Present at birth (relatively rare)

TYPE II
- Occurs between ages 10 and 30

TYPE III
- Usually occurs after age 20 (although uncommon)

TYPE IV
- Relatively common, especially in middle-age men

TYPE V
- Usually occurs in late adolescence or early adulthood (although uncommon)

Common characteristics
- Increased plasma concentrations of one or more lipoproteins

Complications
- Coronary artery disease (CAD)
- Pancreatitis

✱ ASSESSMENT

History
TYPE I
- Recurrent attacks of severe abdominal pain
- Abdominal pain usually preceded by fat intake
- Malaise and anorexia

TYPE II
- History of premature and accelerated coronary atherosclerosis

TYPE III
- Aggravating factors, such as obesity, hypothyroidism, and diabetes mellitus

TYPE IV
- Atherosclerosis
- Early CAD
- Excessive alcohol consumption
- Poorly controlled diabetes mellitus
- Birth control pills containing estrogen (can precipitate severe hypertriglyceridemia)
- Hypertension
- Hyperuricemia

TYPE V
- Abdominal pain associated with pancreatitis
- Complaints related to peripheral neuropathy

Physical findings
TYPE I
- Papular or eruptive xanthomas over pressure points and extensor surfaces
- Ophthalmoscopic examination: lipemia retinalis (reddish white retinal vessels)
- Abdominal spasm, rigidity, or rebound tenderness
- Hepatosplenomegaly, with liver or spleen tenderness
- Fever possible

TYPE II
- Tendinous xanthomas on the Achilles tendons and tendons of the hands and feet
- Tuberous xanthomas, xanthelasma
- Juvenile corneal arcus

TYPE III
- Tuberoeruptive xanthomas over elbows and knees
- Palmar xanthomas on the hands, particularly the fingertips

TYPE IV
- Obesity

- Xanthomas may be noted during exacerbations

TYPE V
- Eruptive xanthomas on extensor surface of arms and legs
- Ophthalmoscopic examination: lipemia retinalis
- Hepatosplenomegaly

Test results
LABORATORY
- Serum lipid profiles show elevated levels of total cholesterol, triglycerides, very-low-density lipoproteins, LDLs, or HDLs.

◆ TREATMENT

General
- Weight reduction
- Elimination or treatment of aggravating factors, such as diabetes mellitus, alcoholism, and hypothyroidism
- Reduction of risk factors for atherosclerosis
- Smoking cessation
- Treatment of hypertension
- Avoidance of oral and estrogen-containing contraceptive drugs

Diet
- Avoidance of alcoholic beverages to decrease plasma triglyceride levels
- Inclusion of polyunsaturated vegetable oils to reduce plasma LDLs

TYPE I
- Restricted fat intake (less than 20 g/day); 20- to 40-g/day, medium-chain triglyceride diet to supplement calorie intake

TYPE II
- Restriction of cholesterol intake to less than 300 mg/day for adults and less than 150 mg/day for children; restricted triglyceride intake to less than 100 mg/day for children and adults; increased polyunsaturated fats

TYPE III
- Restricted cholesterol intake (to less than 300 mg/day) and carbohydrates; increased polyunsaturated fats

TYPE IV
- Restricted cholesterol intake; increased polyunsaturated fats

TYPE V

- Long-term maintenance of a low-fat diet; 20- to 40-g/day medium-chain triglyceride diet

Activity

- Maintenance of exercise and physical fitness program

Medication

- Nicotinic acid
- Clofibrate and niacin
- Niacin, clofibrate, gemfibrozil
- HMG-CoA reductase inhibitors such as atorvastatin (Lipitor), simvastatin (Zocor), and lovosatin (Mevacor)

Surgery

- If unable to tolerate drug therapy, surgical creation of an ileal bypass
- For severely affected homozygote children, portacaval shunt as a last resort to reduce plasma cholesterol levels

❖ NURSING CONSIDERATIONS

Nursing diagnoses

- Anxiety
- Deficient knowledge (hyperlipoproteinemia)
- Fear
- Ineffective tissue perfusion: Cardiopulmonary
- Risk for injury

Key outcomes

The patient will:

- report decreased anxiety
- verbalize understanding of the disorder and treatment regimen
- verbalize feelings and concerns
- maintain adequate cardiopulmonary perfusion
- remain free from complications and injury.

Nursing interventions

- Administer antilipemics, as ordered.
- Prevent or minimize adverse reactions.
- Urge the patient to adhere to the prescribed diet.
- Assist the patient with additional lifestyle changes.
- Encourage verbalization of fears related to premature CAD.

Monitoring

- Vital signs
- Adverse reactions
- Serum lipoproteins
- Response to treatment
- Signs and symptoms related to CAD or its sequelae

▶ PATIENT TEACHING

Be sure to cover:

- disorder, diagnostic tests, and treatment
- (for the 2 weeks preceding serum cholesterol and serum triglyceride tests) need to maintain a steady weight and strictly adhere to the prescribed diet, and to fast for 12 hours before the test
- need to avoid excessive sugar intake and alcoholic beverages
- minimized intake of saturated fats (higher in meats and coconut oil)
- increased intake of polyunsaturated fats (vegetable oils)
- avoiding hormonal contraceptives or drugs that contain estrogen
- foods high in cholesterol and saturated fats
- medication administration, dosage, and possible adverse effects
- signs and symptoms requiring medical evaluation.

Discharge planning

- Refer the patient for a medically supervised exercise program.
- Refer the patient to a smoking-cessation program, if indicated.
- Refer the patient to a dietitian, if necessary.

✷ RESOURCES

Organizations

American Heart Association: *www.americanheart.org*
Food and Nutrition Information Center: *www.na1.usda.gov*

Selected references

Burnside, N.J., et al. "Type III Hyperlipoproteinemia with Xanthomas and Mutiple Myeloma," *Journal of the American Acdemy of Dermatology* 53(5 Suppl I):S281-84, November 2005.

Carroll, M.D., et al. "Trends in Serum Lipids and Lipoproteins of Adults, 1960-2002," *JAMA* 294(14):1773-781, October 2005.

Diseases, 4th ed. Philadelphia: Lippincott Williams & Wilkins, 2006.

Hollman, G., et al. "Meaning of Quality of Life among Patients with Familiar Hypercholesterolemia," *Journal of Cardiovascular Nursing* 19(4):243-50, July-August 2004.

Thompson, G.R., "Additive Effects of Plant Sterol and Stanol Esters to Statin Therapy," *American Journal of Cardiology* 96(1A):37D-39D, July 2005.

Hyperparathyroidism

● OVERVIEW

Description
- Characterized by a greater than normal secretion of parathyroid hormone (PTH)
- Classified as either primary or secondary

Pathophysiology
- In primary hyperparathyroidism, one or more of the parathyroid glands enlarges, increasing PTH secretion and elevating serum calcium levels or an adenoma secretes PTH, unresponsive to negative feedback of serum calcium.
- In secondary hyperparathyroidism, excessive compensatory production of PTH stems from a hypocalcemia-producing abnormality outside the parathyroid gland, which isn't responsive to PTH such as decreased intestinal absorption of calcium or vitamin D.
- Increased PTH levels act directly on the bone and the kidney tubules, resulting in an increase in extracellular calcium.
- Renal excretion and uptake into the soft tissues or skeleton can't compensate for increased calcium.

Causes
- Adenoma
- Genetic disorders
- Multiple endocrine neoplasia
- Dietary vitamin D or calcium deficiency
- Decreased intestinal absorption of vitamin D or calcium
- Chronic renal failure
- Osteomalacia
- Ingestion of drugs such as phenytoin
- Laxative ingestion
- Idiopathic

Incidence
- Most common in women
- Increased incidence in posmenopausal women
- Onset usually between ages 35 and 65

Common characteristics
- Bone pain and tenderness
- Renal calculi
- Abdominal distress
- Anxiety and depression

Complications
- Chondrocalcinosis
- Osteoporosis
- Bone cysts and brown tumors
- Subperiosteal resorption
- Severe osteopenia
- Juxta-articular surface erosions
- Subchondral fractures
- Traumatic synovitis
- Pseudogout
- Nephrolithiasis
- Hypercalciuria
- Renal calculi and colic
- Renal insufficiency and failure
- Peptic ulcers
- Cholelithiasis
- Cardiac arrhythmias
- Vascular damage
- Heart failure
- Muscle atrophy
- Depression

◈ **NURSING ALERT** Severe hypercalcemia can cause parathyroid poisoning, which includes central nervous system changes, renal failure, rapid precipitation of calcium throughout the soft tissues and, possibly, coma.

✱ ASSESSMENT

History
- Recurring nephrolithiasis
- Polyuria
- Hematuria
- Chronic lower back pain
- Easy fracturing
- Osteoporosis
- Constant, severe epigastric pain that radiates to the back
- Abdominal pain
- Anorexia, nausea, and vomiting
- Constipation
- Polydipsia
- Muscle weakness, particularly in the legs
- Lethargy
- Personality disturbances
- Depression
- Overt psychosis
- Cataracts
- Anemia

Physical findings
- Muscle weakness and atrophy
- Psychomotor disturbances
- Stupor and, possibly, coma

- Skin necrosis
- Subcutaneous calcification

Test results
LABORATORY
PRIMARY DISEASE
- Alkaline phosphatase levels are increased.
- Osteocalcin levels are increased.
- Tartrate-resistant acid phosphatase levels are increased.
- Serum PTH levels are increased.
- Serum calcium levels are increased.
- Serum phosphorus levels are decreased.
- Urine and serum calcium and serum chloride levels are increased.
- Creatinine levels may be increased.
- Basal acid secretion may be increased.
- Serum amylase may be increased.

SECONDARY DISEASE
- Serum calcium levels are normal or slightly decreased.
- Serum phosphorus levels are variable.
- Serum PTH levels are increased.

IMAGING
- X-rays show diffuse bone demineralization, bone cysts, outer cortical bone absorption, and subperiosteal erosion of the phalanges and distal clavicles in primary disease.
- X-ray spectrophotometry shows increased bone turnover in primary disease.
- Esophagography, thyroid scan, parathyroid thermography, ultrasonography, thyroid angiography, computed tomography scan, and magnetic resonance imaging may show location of parathyroid lesions.

◆ TREATMENT

General
- In primary disease, treatment to decrease calcium levels
- In renal failure, dialysis
- In secondary disease, treatment to correct underlying cause of parathyroid hypertrophy

Diet
- Increased oral fluid intake

Activity
- As tolerated

Medication

PRIMARY DISEASE

- Biphosphonates
- Oral sodium or potassium phosphate
- Calcitonin
- Plicamycin, if primary disease is metastatic

SECONDARY DISEASE

- Vitamin D therapy
- Aluminum hydroxide
- Glucocorticoids

POSTOPERATIVELY

- I.V. magnesium and phosphate
- Sodium phosphate
- Supplemental calcium
- Vitamin D or calcitriol

Surgery

- With primary hyperparathyroidism, removal of adenoma or all but half of one gland (see *Surgery for patients with primary hyperparathyroidism*)

❖ NURSING CONSIDERATIONS

Nursing diagnoses

- Activity intolerance
- Chronic pain
- Decreased cardiac output
- Deficient knowledge (hyperparathyroidism)
- Disturbed body image
- Disturbed thought processes
- Excess fluid volume
- Fear
- Imbalanced nutrition: Less than body requirements
- Ineffective coping

Key outcomes

The patient will:

- perform activities of daily living without excessive fatigue
- verbalize increased comfort and decreased pain
- maintain adequate cardiac output
- express positive feelings about self
- maintain balanced fluid volume status
- express feelings and concerns
- maintain current weight
- demonstrate positive coping methods.

Nursing interventions

- Obtain baseline serum potassium, calcium, phosphate, and magnesium levels before treatment.

- Provide at least 3 L of fluid per day.
- Institute safety precautions.
- Schedule frequent rest periods.
- Provide comfort measures.
- Administer medications, as ordered.
- Help the patient turn and reposition every 2 hours.
- Support affected extremities with pillows.
- Consult a dietitian.
- Encourage the patient to express her feelings.
- Offer emotional support.
- Help the patient to develop effective coping strategies.

AFTER PARATHYROIDECTOMY

- Keep a tracheotomy tray and endotracheal tube setup at the bedside.
- Maintain seizure precautions.
- Place the patient in semi-Fowler's position.
- Support her head and neck with sandbags.
- Have the patient ambulate as soon as possible.

◈ **NURSING ALERT** Watch for complaints of tingling in the hands and around the mouth. If these symptoms don't subside quickly, they may be prodromal signs of tetany, so keep I.V. calcium gluconate or calcium chloride available for emergency administration.

Monitoring

- Vital signs
- Intake and output
- Serum calcium levels
- Urine for calculi
- Signs and symptoms of pulmonary edema
- Respiratory status
- Cardiovascular status

SURGERY FOR PATIENTS WITH PRIMARY HYPERPARATHYROIDISM

Patients with primary hyperparathyroidism should be considered for surgery when:

- calcium levels are 1 mg/dl or more above normal
- osteoporosis or hypercalcemia is present
- recurrent peptic ulcer disease is present
- nephrolithiasis is present
- impaired kidney function is noted
- the patient is young or consistent follow-up values are unavailable.

AFTER PARATHYROIDECTOMY

- Increased neuromuscular irritability
- Complications
- Neck edema
- Chvostek's sign
- Trousseau's sign

▶ PATIENT TEACHING

Be sure to cover:

- disorder, diagnostic tests, and treatment
- medication administration, dosage, and possible adverse effects
- when to notify the physician
- signs and symptoms of tetany, respiratory distress, and renal dysfunction
- need for periodic blood tests
- avoidance of calcium-containing antacids and thiazide diuretics
- need to wear a medical identification bracelet.

Discharge planning

- Refer the patient to a mental health professional for additional counseling, if necessary.

✸ RESOURCES

Organizations

American Association of Clinical Endocrinologists: *www.aace.com*
Endocrine Society: *www.endo-society.org/index.htm*

Selected references

Donovan, P.I. "Outpatient Parathyroidectomy: A New Paradigm from a Nursing Perspective," *Current Opinion in Oncology* 17(1):28-32, January 2005.

Levine, M.A., "Primary Hyperparathyroidism: 7,000 Years of Progress," *Cleveland Clinic Journal of Medicine* 72(12): 1084-1085, 1088, 1091-1092 passim., December 2005.

Peregrin, T. "Early Assessment of Secondary Hyperparathyroidism," *Journal of the American Dietetic Association* 106(1):22-23, January 2006.

Strategies for Managing Multisystem Disorders. Philadelphia: Lippincott Williams & Wilkins, 2006.

Hyperpituitarism

● OVERVIEW

Description
- Chronic, progressive disease marked by hormonal dysfunction and startling skeletal overgrowth
- Prognosis dependent on cause
- Life expectancy usually reduced
- Appears in two forms: acromegaly and gigantism
- Also referred to as *growth hormone (GH) excess*

Pathophysiology
- Progressive excessive secretion of pituitary GH occurs.
- Acromegaly occurs after epiphyseal closure, causing bone thickening and transverse growth and visceromegaly.
- Gigantism occurs before epiphyseal closure with excess GH, causing proportional overgrowth of all body tissues.
- A large tumor may cause loss of other trophic hormones, such as thyroid-stimulating hormone, luteinizing hormone, follicle-stimulating hormone, and corticotropin, which may cause dysfunction of target organs.

Causes
- GH-producing adenoma of the anterior pituitary gland
- Excessive GH secretion
- Excessive GH releasing hormone
- Possible genetic cause

Incidence
ACROMEGALY
- Occurs equally among men and women
- Usually occurs between ages 30 and 50
GIGANTISM
- Affects infants and children

Common characteristics
- Progressive enlargement of the face, hands and feet, thorax, and soft tissue
- Coarsening of features
- Headache
- Menstrual disturbances

Complications
- Arthritis
- Carpal tunnel syndrome
- Osteoporosis
- Kyphosis
- Hypertension
- Arteriosclerosis
- Cardiomegaly and heart failure
- Blindness
- Severe neurologic disturbances
- Glucose intolerance
- Diabetes mellitus
- Severe psychological stress

✱ ASSESSMENT

History
- Gradual onset of acromegaly
- Relatively abrupt onset of gigantism
- Soft-tissue swelling
- Hypertrophy of the face and extremities
- Diaphoresis, oily skin
- Fatigue, sleep disturbances
- Weight gain
- Headaches, decreased vision
- Decreased libido, impotence
- Oligomenorrhea, infertility
- Joint pain
- Hypertrichosis
- Irritability, hostility, and other psychological disturbances

Physical findings
- Enlarged jaw, thickened tongue
- Enlarged and weakened hands
- Coarsened facial features
- Oily or leathery skin
- Prominent supraorbital ridge
- Deep, hollow-sounding voice
- Cartilaginous and connective tissue overgrowth
- Skeletal abnormalities

✿ **AGE-RELATED CONCERN** In infants, inspection reveals a highly arched palate, muscular hypotonia, slanting eyes, and exophthalmos.

Test results
LABORATORY
- GH radioimmunoassay shows increased plasma GH levels and levels of insulin-like growth factor I.
- Glucose suppression test fails to suppress the hormone level to below the accepted norm of 2 ng/ml.
IMAGING
- Skull X-ray, computed tomography scan, or magnetic resonance imaging shows location of pituitary tumor.
- Bone X-rays show a thickening of the cranium and long bones and osteoarthritis in the spine.

◆ TREATMENT

General
- Treatment to curb overproduction of GH
- Pituitary radiation therapy

Diet
- No restrictions

Activity
- No restrictions

Medication
- Replacement of thyroid, cortisone, and gonadal hormones postoperatively if entire pituitary removed
- GH synthesis inhibitor
- Long-acting analogue of somatostatin

Surgery
- Transsphenoidal hypophysectomy

❖ NURSING CONSIDERATIONS

Nursing diagnoses
- Activity intolerance
- Deficient knowledge (excess GH)
- Delayed growth and development
- Disturbed body image
- Disturbed sensory perception: Visual
- Impaired oral mucous membrane
- Impaired physical mobility
- Ineffective coping
- Sexual dysfunction

Key outcomes
The patient will:
- perform activities of daily living within the confines of the disease process
- demonstrate age-appropriate skills and behaviors to the extent possible
- express positive feelings about self
- maintain optimal functioning within the limits of visual disturbance
- maintain intact oral mucous membranes
- maintain joint mobility and range of motion (ROM)
- demonstrate positive coping skills
- verbalize feelings about actual or perceived sexual impairment.

Nursing interventions
- Provide emotional support.
- Provide reassurance that mood changes result from hormonal imbalances and can be reduced with treatment.
- Administer medications, as ordered.
- Provide comfort measures.
- Perform or assist with ROM exercises.
- Evaluate muscle weakness.
- Institute safety precautions.
- Provide meticulous skin care.
- Assist with early postoperative ambulation.

◈ **NURSING ALERT** Report large increases in urine output after surgery, which may indicate diabetes insipidus.

Monitoring
- Vital signs
- Intake and output
- Serum glucose levels
- Signs and symptoms of hyperglycemia

AFTER SURGERY
- Signs and symptoms of increased intracranial pressure (ICP) and intracranial bleeding
- Respiratory status
- Surgical incisions and dressings
- Complications
- Signs and symptoms of infection
- Signs and symptoms of hormonal deficiency

▶ PATIENT TEACHING

Be sure to cover:
- disorder, diagnostic tests, and treatment
- medication administration, dosage, and possible adverse effects
- when to notify the physician
- avoidance of activities that increase ICP
- deep breathing through the mouth if nasal packing is in place postoperatively
- hormone replacement therapy, if ordered
- need to wear a medical identification bracelet
- follow-up examinations
- possible tumor recurrence.

Discharge planning
- Refer the patient for psychological counseling to help cope with body image changes and sexual dysfunction, as needed.

✹ RESOURCES

Organizations
Endocrine Society: *www.endo-society.org/index.htm*
Pituitary Tumor Network Association: *www.pituitary.com*

Selected references
Ezzat, S. "Pharmacological Options in the Treatment of Acromegaly," *Current Opinion in Investigational Drugs* 6(10):1023-1027, October 2005.

Hanberg, A. "Common Disorders of the Pituitary Gland: Hyposecretion versus Hypersecretion," *Journal of Infusion Nursing* 28(1):46-44, January-February 2005.

Strategies for Managing Multisystem Disorders. Philadelphia: Lippincott Williams & Wilkins, 2006.

Hypertension

Description

- Intermittent or sustained elevation of diastolic or systolic blood pressure
- Usually begins as benign disease, slowly progressing to accelerated or malignant state
- Two major types: essential (also called *primary* or *idiopathic*) hypertension and secondary hypertension, which results from renal disease or another identifiable cause
- Malignant hypertension: severe, fulminant form commonly arising from both types; a medical emergency

Pathophysiology

SEVERAL THEORIES

- Changes in arteriolar bed causes increased peripheral vascular resistance.
- Abnormally increased tone in the sympathetic nervous system originates in the vasomotor system centers, causing increased peripheral vascular resistance.
- Increased blood volume results from renal or hormonal dysfunction.
- An increase in arteriolar thickening caused by genetic factors, leads to increased peripheral vascular resistance.
- Abnormal renin release results in the formation of angiotensin II, which constricts the arterioles and increases blood volume.

Causes

- Exact cause unknown

Risk factors

- Family history
- Black race in United States
- Stress
- Obesity
- Diet high in sodium or saturated fat
- Use of tobacco or hormonal contraceptives
- Excess alcohol intake
- Sedentary lifestyle
- Aging

Incidence

- Affects 15% to 20% of adults in the United States
- Essential hypertension accounting for 90% to 95% of cases

Common characteristics

- Serial blood pressure measurements greater than 140/90 mm Hg in people younger than age 50 or greater than 150/95 mm Hg in those older than age 50

Complications

- Stroke
- Cardiac disease
- Renal failure
- Blindness

History

- In many cases, no symptoms; may be revealed incidentally during evaluation for another disorder or during a routine blood pressure screening program
- Symptoms that reflect the effect of hypertension on the organ systems
- Awakening with a headache in the occipital region, which subsides spontaneously after a few hours
- Dizziness, fatigue, and confusion
- Palpitations, chest pain, dyspnea
- Epistaxis
- Hematuria
- Blurred vision

Physical findings

- Peripheral edema in late stages
- Hemorrhages, exudates, and papilledema of the eye in late stages (if hypertensive retinopathy present)
- Pulsating abdominal mass, suggesting an abdominal aneurysm
- Elevated blood pressure on at least two consecutive occasions after initial screenings
- Bruits over the abdominal aorta and femoral arteries or the carotids

Test results

LABORATORY

- Urinalysis may show protein, red blood cells, or white blood cells, suggesting renal disease; or glucose, suggesting diabetes mellitus.
- Serum potassium levels less than 3.5 mEq/L may indicate adrenal dysfunction (primary hyperaldosteronism).
- Blood urea nitrogen levels are normal or elevated to more than 20 mg/dl and serum creatinine levels are normal or elevated to more than 1.5 mg/dl, suggesting renal disease.

IMAGING

- Excretory urography may reveal renal atrophy, indicating chronic renal disease; one kidney more than ⅝″ (1.6 cm) shorter than the other suggests unilateral renal disease.
- Chest X-rays may demonstrate cardiomegaly.
- Renal arteriography may show renal artery stenosis.

DIAGNOSTIC PROCEDURES

- Electrocardiography may show left ventricular hypertrophy or ischemia.
- An oral captopril challenge may be done to test for renovascular hypertension.
- Ophthalmoscopy reveals arteriovenous nicking and, in hypertensive encephalopathy, edema.

General

- Lifestyle modification, such as weight control, limiting alcohol, regular exercise, and smoking cessation
- For a patient with secondary hypertension, correction of the underlying cause and control of hypertensive effects

Diet

- Low in saturated fats and sodium
- Adequate calcium, magnesium, and potassium

Activity

- Regular exercise program

Medication

- Diuretics
- Beta-adrenergic blockers
- Calcium channel blockers
- Angiotensin-converting enzyme inhibitors
- Alpha-receptor antagonists
- Vasodilators
- Angiotensin receptor blockers
- Aldosterone antagonists

❖ NURSING CONSIDERATIONS

Nursing diagnoses
- Deficient knowledge (hypertension)
- Fatigue
- Ineffective tissue perfusion: Cardio-pulmonary
- Ineffective coping
- Noncompliance (risk factor modification)
- Risk for injury

Key outcomes
The patient will:
- express feelings of increased energy
- maintain adequate cardiac output and hemodynamic stability
- demonstrate positive coping methods
- develop no arrhythmias
- comply with the therapy regimen
- remain free from injury.

Nursing interventions
- Find out if the patient was taking prescribed antihypertensive medication.
- When routine blood pressure screening reveals elevated pressure, make sure the sphygmomanometer cuff size is appropriate for the patient's upper arm circumference.
- Take the pressure in both arms in lying, sitting, and standing positions. Ask the patient if he smoked, drank a beverage containing caffeine, or was emotionally upset before the test.
- Encourage public participation in blood pressure screening programs.
- Routinely screen all patients, especially those at risk.
- Administer medications, as ordered.
- Encourage dietary and lifestyle changes.
- Help the patient identify risk factors and make dietary and lifestyle changes, as necessary.

Monitoring
- Vital signs, especially blood pressure
- Signs and symptoms of target end-organ damage
- Complications
- Response to treatment
- Risk factor modification
- Adverse effects of antihypertensive agents

▶ PATIENT TEACHING

Be sure to cover:
- disorder, diagnostic tests, and treatment
- how to use a self-monitoring blood pressure cuff and to record the reading in a journal for review by the physician
- need to keep a record of drugs used in the past, noting especially which ones are or aren't effective
- importance of compliance with antihypertensive therapy and establishing a daily routine for taking medication
- need to report adverse effects of drugs
- need to avoid high-sodium antacids and over-the-counter cold and sinus medications containing harmful vasoconstrictors
- examining and modifying lifestyle, including diet
- need for a routine exercise program, particularly aerobic walking
- need to avoid high-sodium foods, table salt, and foods high in cholesterol and saturated fat
- the importance of follow-up care.

Discharge planning
- Refer the patient to stress-reduction therapies or support groups, as needed.
- Refer the patient to weight-reduction or smoking-cessation groups, as indicated.

✴ RESOURCES

Organizations
American Heart Association:
www.americanheart.org
American Medical Association:
www.ama-assn.org

Selected references
Cheng, S.L. "Treating HTN Crisis. How Low? How Fast?" *RN* 68(6):37-41, June 2005.

Coy, V. "Genetics of Essential Hypertension," *Journal of the American Academy of Nurse Practitioners* 17(6):219-24, June 2005.

Jacobs, T.F., and Ramsey, L.A. "Angiotensin Receptor Blockers. Applications Beyond Hypertension," *Advanced Nurse Practitioner* 13(1):27-30, January 2005.

Lloyd-Jones, D.M., et al. "Hypertension in Adults Across the Age Spectrum: Current Outcomes and Control in the Community," *JAMA* 294(4):466-72, July 2005.

Nettina, S.M. *Lippincott Manual of Nursing Practice,* 8th ed. Philadelphia: Lippincott Williams & Willkins, 2006.

Hypoparathyroidism

Description
- Deficiency in parathyroid hormone (PTH) secretion by the parathyroid glands or the decreased action of PTH in the periphery
- Because parathyroid glands primarily regulate calcium balance, neuromuscular symptoms ranging from paresthesia to tetany
- May be acute or chronic
- Classified as idiopathic, acquired, or reversible

Pathophysiology
- PTH normally maintains serum calcium levels by increasing bone resorption and by stimulating renal conversion of vitamin D to its active form, which enhances GI absorption of calcium and bone resorption.
- PTH also maintains the inverse relationship between serum calcium and phosphate levels by inhibiting phosphate reabsorption in the renal tubules and enhancing calcium reabsorption.
- Abnormal PTH production in hypoparathyroidism disrupts this delicate balance.

Causes
- Autoimmune genetic disorder
- Congenital absence or malformation of the parathyroid glands
- Accidental removal of or injury to one or more parathyroid glands during surgery
- Ischemia or infarction of the parathyroid glands during surgery
- Hemochromatosis
- Sarcoidosis
- Amyloidosis
- Tuberculosis
- Neoplasms
- Trauma
- Massive thyroid irradiation
- Hypomagnesemia-induced impairment of hormone secretion
- Suppression of normal gland function due to hypercalcemia
- Delayed maturation of parathyroid function
- Abnormalities of the calcium-sensor receptor

Incidence
- Idiopathic and reversible forms most common in children
- Acquired form most common in older patients who have undergone thyroid gland surgery

Common characteristics
- Muscle spasms
- Hyperreflexia
- Neuromuscular excitability

Complications
- Heart failure
- Cataracts
- Tetany
- Increased intracranial pressure
- Irreversible calcification of basal ganglia
- Bone deformities
- Laryngospasm, respiratory stridor, anoxia
- Paralysis of the vocal cords
- Seizures
- Death

⚙ **AGE-RELATED CONCERN** Hypoparathyroidism that develops during childhood results in malformed teeth.

History
- Neck surgery or irradiation
- Malabsorption disorders
- Alcoholism
- Tingling in the fingertips, around the mouth and, occasionally, in the feet
- Muscle tension and spasms
- Feeling like throat is constricted
- Dysphagia
- Difficulty walking and a tendency to fall
- Nausea, vomiting, abdominal pain
- Constipation or diarrhea
- Personality changes
- Fatigue

Physical findings
- Brittle nails
- Dry skin
- Coarse hair, alopecia
- Transverse and longitudinal ridges in the fingernails
- Loss of eyelashes and fingernails
- Stained, cracked, and decayed teeth
- Tetany

- Positive Chvostek's and Trousseau's signs (see *Eliciting signs of hypocalcemia*)
- Increased deep tendon reflexes
- Irregular, slow or rapid pulse

ELICITING SIGNS OF HYPOCALCEMIA

When the patient complains of muscle spasms and paresthesia in his limbs, try eliciting Chvostek's and Trousseau's signs — indications of tetany associated with calcium deficiency.

Follow the procedures described below, keeping in mind the discomfort they typically cause. If you detect these signs, notify the physician immediately. During these tests, watch the patient for laryngospasm, monitor his cardiac status, and have resuscitation equipment nearby.

Chvostek's sign
To elicit this sign, tap the patient's facial nerve just in front of the earlobe and below the zygomatic arch or between the zygomatic arch and the corner of the mouth, as shown below.

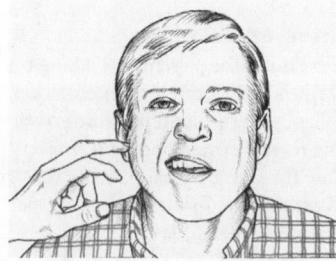

A positive response (indicating latent tetany) ranges from simple mouth-corner twitching to twitching of all facial muscles on the side tested. Simple twitching may be normal in some patients. However, a more pronounced response usually confirms Chvostek's sign.

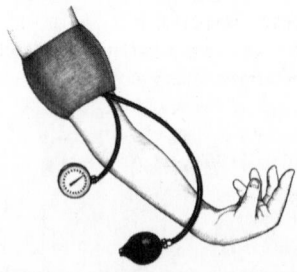

Trousseau's sign
In this test, occlude the brachial artery by inflating a blood pressure cuff on the patient's upper arm to a level between diastolic and systolic blood pressure. Maintain this inflation for 3 minutes while observing the patient for carpal spasm (shown above), which is Trousseau's sign.

Test results

LABORATORY

- Radioimmunoassay for PTH is decreased.
- Serum and urine calcium levels are decreased.
- Serum phosphate levels are increased.
- Urine creatinine levels are decreased.

IMAGING

- Computed tomography scan may show frontal lobe and basal ganglia calcifications.
- X-rays may show increased bone density and bone malformation.

DIAGNOSTIC PROCEDURES

- Electrocardiography shows a prolonged QT interval.

◆ TREATMENT

General

- To restore the calcium and associated mineral balance within the body
- For an acute life-threatening attack or hypoparathyroid tetany, supportive care

Diet

- High-calcium, low-phosphorus

Activity

- As tolerated

Medication

- Vitamin D
- Supplemental calcium
- Calcitriol

ACUTE, LIFE-THREATENING TETANY

- I.V. administration of 10% calcium gluconate, 10% calcium glucepate, or 10% calcium chloride
- Sedatives
- Anticonvulsants

Surgery

- To treat underlying cause such as tumor

❖ NURSING CONSIDERATIONS

Nursing diagnoses

- Anxiety
- Decreased cardiac output
- Deficient knowledge (hypoparathyroidism)
- Disturbed body image
- Disturbed thought processes
- Impaired skin integrity
- Ineffective breathing pattern
- Ineffective coping

Key outcomes

The patient will:

- identify strategies to reduce anxiety
- maintain normal cardiac output
- verbalize an understanding of the disorder and treatment regimen
- express positive feelings about self
- maintain intact skin integrity
- maintain adequate ventilation and oyxgenation
- demonstrate positive coping methods.

Nursing interventions

- Administer medications, as ordered.
- Maintain a patent I.V. line.
- Keep emergency equipment readily available.
- Maintain seizure precautions.
- Provide meticulous skin care.
- Institute safety precautions.
- Encourage the patient to express his feelings.
- Offer emotional support.
- Help the patient to develop effective coping strategies.

Monitoring

- Vital signs
- Intake and output
- Serum calcium and phosphorus levels
- Electrocardiogram for QT interval changes and arrhythmias
- Signs and symptoms of decreased cardiac output
- Chvostek's sign
- Trousseau's sign

> **NURSING ALERT** Closely monitor the patient receiving digoxin and calcium because calcium potentiates the effect of digoxin. Stay alert for signs of digoxin toxicity.

▶ PATIENT TEACHING

Be sure to cover:

- disorder, diagnostis tests, and treatment
- medication administration, dosage, and possible adverse effects
- when to notify the physician
- follow-up care
- complications
- periodic checks of serum calcium levels. (See *Living with hypoparathyroidism.*)

Discharge planning

- Refer the patient to a mental health professional for additional counseling, if necessary.

✶ RESOURCES

Organizations

American Association of Clinical Endocrinologists: *www.aace.com*

Endocrine Society: *www.endo-society.org/index.htm*

Selected references

Adorni, A., et al. "Extensive Brain Calcification and Dementia in Postsurgical Hypoparathyrodism," *Neurology* 65(9):1501, November 2005

Diseases, 4th ed. Philadelphia: Lippincott Williams & Wilkins, 2006.

Heymann, R.S., et al. "Anaplastic Thyroid Carcinoma with Thyrotoxicosis and Hypoparathyroidism," *Endocrine Practice* 11(4):281-84, July-August 2005.

LIVING WITH HYPOPARATHYROIDISM

To help the patient learn to live with hypoparathyroidism, follow these guidelines:

- Tell the patient to take calcium supplements with or after meals and to chew the tablets well. Instruct him to always wear a medical identification bracelet and carry his medication with him at all times.
- Teach the patient and his family to identify and report signs and symptoms of hypercalcemia, tetany, and respiratory distress.
- Teach the patient techniques for decreasing stress and avoiding fatigue.
- Advise the patient to follow a high-calcium, low-phosphorus diet. Discuss high-calcium foods, including dairy products, salmon, egg yolks, shrimp, and green, leafy vegetables. Caution him to avoid high-phosphate foods, such as spinach, rhubarb, and asparagus.

Hypopituitarism

Description

- Partial or complete failure of the anterior pituitary gland to produce its vital hormones: corticotropin, thyroid-stimulating hormone (TSH), luteinizing hormone (LH), follicle-stimulating hormone (FSH), growth hormone (GH), and prolactin
- May be primary or secondary, resulting from dysfunction of the hypothalamus
- Clinical features typically developing slowly and don't become apparent until 75% of the pituitary gland is destroyed
- Total loss of all hormones is fatal without treatment
- Prognosis good with adequate replacement therapy and correction of the underlying causes
- Absence of all hormones called *panhypopituitarism*

Pathophysiology

- The pituitary gland is extremely vulnerable to ischemia and infarction because it's highly vascular.
- Any event that leads to circulatory collapse and compensatory vasospasm may result in gland ischemia, tissue necrosis, or edema.
- Expansion of the pituitary within the fixed compartment of the sella turcica further impedes blood supply to the pituitary.

Causes

- Tumor
- Congenital defects
- Pituitary gland hypoplasia or aplasia
- Pituitary infarction
- Partial or total hypophysectomy by surgery, irradiation, or chemical agents
- Granulomatous disease
- Deficiency of hypothalamus releasing hormones
- Idiopathic
- Infection
- Trauma

Incidence

- Relatively rare
- Occurs in adults and children
- Affects males and females equally

Common characteristics

- Metabolic dysfunction
- Sexual immaturity
- Growth retardation
- Fatigue

Complications

- Any combination of deficits in the production of the six major hormones
- GH deficiency
- TSH deficiency
- Corticotropin deficiency
- Gonadotropin and prolactin deficiency
- Pituitary apoplexy (a medical emergency) (see *What happens in pituitary apoplexy*)
- High fever, shock, coma, and death
- Diabetes insipidus

WHAT HAPPENS IN PITUITARY APOPLEXY

Five percent to 10% of patients with pituitary tumors develop pituitary apoplexy, a potentially life-threatening condition caused by hemorrhage into the tumor. Pituitary apoplexy usually occurs suddenly when rapid adenoma growth causes infarction or rupture of the tumor's thin-walled vessels. Patients with acromegaly, Cushing's disease, or large nonfunctioning tumors have a higher-than-average incidence of pituitary apoplexy.

Signs and symptoms

Assessment findings for pituitary apoplexy include:
- sudden, severe headache
- blurred vision
- diplopia
- blindness (from optic chiasma compression)
- eye deviation and pupil dilation (from oculomotor nerve paralysis)
- altered level of consciousness (possibly progressing to unconsciousness)
- nausea and vomiting
- hyperpyrexia
- nuchal rigidity.

Diagnosis and treatment

Diagnosis is based on the patient's history and test results, which may include leukocytosis, xanthochromic or frankly bloody cerebrospinal fluid (CSF), elevated CSF pressure and protein concentration, or suprasellar extension (as shown by a computed tomography scan).

Treatment is controversial, but it may involve corticosteroid administration. If visual deterioration continues, surgical evacuation of the hematoma may be performed to preserve vision.

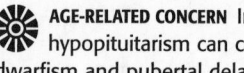 **AGE-RELATED CONCERN** In children, hypopituitarism can cause dwarfism and pubertal delay.

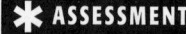 **ASSESSMENT**

History

- Signs and symptoms dependent on which pituitary hormones are deficient, patient's age, and severity of disorder

FSH AND LH DEFICIENCY (WOMEN)
- Amenorrhea
- Dyspareunia
- Infertility
- Reduced libido

FSH AND LH DEFICIENCY (MEN)
- Impotence
- Reduced libido

TSH DEFICIENCY
- Cold intolerance
- Constipation
- Menstrual irregularity
- Lethargy
- Severe growth retardation in children despite treatment

CORTICOTROPIN DEFICIENCY
- Fatigue
- Nausea, vomiting, anorexia
- Weight loss

PROLACTIN DEFICIENCY
- Absent postpartum lactation
- Amenorrhea

Physical findings

GH DEFICIENCY
- Physical signs possibly not apparent in neonate
- Growth retardation usually apparent at age 6 months
  In children:
- Chubbiness from fat deposits in the lower trunk
- Short stature
- Delayed secondary tooth eruption
- Delayed puberty
- Average height of 4′ (1.2 m), with normal proportions

FSH AND LH DEFICIENCY (WOMEN)
- Breast atrophy
- Sparse or absent axillary and pubic hair
- Dry skin

FSH AND LH DEFICIENCY (MEN)
- Decreased muscle strength
- Testicular softening and shrinkage

- Retarded secondary sexual hair growth

TSH DEFICIENCY
- Dry, pale, puffy skin
- Slow thought processes
- Bradycardia

CORTICOTROPIN DEFICIENCY
- Depigmentation of skin and nipples
- Hypothermia and hypotension during periods of stress

PROLACTIN DEFICIENCY
- Sparse or absent growth of pubic and axillary hair

PANHYPOPITUITARISM
- Mental abnormalities, including lethargy and psychosis
- Physical abnormalities, including orthostatic hypotension and bradycardia

Test results

LABORATORY
- Serum thyroxin levels are decreased in diminished thyroid gland function due to lack of TSH.
- Radioimmunoassay shows decreased plasma levels of some or all of the pituitary hormones.
- Increased prolactin levels may indicate a lesion in the hypothalamus or pituitary stalk.

IMAGING
- Computed tomography scan, magnetic resonance imaging, or cerebral angiography may show the presence of intrasellar or extrasellar tumors.

DIAGNOSTIC PROCEDURES
- Oral administration of metyrapone may show the source of low hydroxycorticosteroid levels.
- Insulin administration shows low levels of corticotropin, indicating pituitary or hypothalamic failure.
- Dopamine antagonist administration evaluates prolactin secretory reserve.
- I.V. administration of gonadotropin-releasing hormone may distinguish pituitary and hypothalamic causes of gonadotropin deficiency.
- Provocative testing shows persistently low GH and insulin-like growth factor-1 levels confirming GH deficiency.

◆ TREATMENT

General
- If caused by a lesion or tumor, removal or radiation or both, followed

by possible life long hormone replacement therapy
- Endocrine substitution therapy for affected organs

Diet
- High-calorie, high-protein

Activity
- Regular exercise program
- Rest, for fatigue

Medication
- Hormone replacement

✳ **AGE-RELATED CONCERN** Children with hypopituitarism may also need adrenal and thyroid hormone replacement and, as they approach puberty, sex hormones.

Surgery
- For pituitary tumor

❖ NURSING CONSIDERATIONS

Nursing diagnoses
- Deficient knowledge (hypopituitarism)
- Delayed growth and development
- Disturbed body image
- Hypothermia
- Risk of infection
- Situational low self-esteem
- Sexual dysfunction

Key outcomes
The patient will:
- demonstrate age-appropriate skills and behavior to the extent possible
- maintain body weight
- express positive feelings about self
- maintain normal body temperature
- remain free from signs and symptoms of infection
- verbalize feelings about impaired sexual function
- verbalize feelings of positive self-esteem

Nursing interventions
- Administer medications, as ordered.
- Encourage adequate caloric intake.
- Offer frequent small meals.
- Keep the patient warm.
- Institute safety precautions.
- Provide emotional support.

- Encourage the patient to express his feelings.

Monitoring
- Laboratory tests for hormonal deficiencies
- Caloric intake
- Daily weight
- Vital signs
- Intake and output
- Signs and symptoms of anemia
- Neurologic status

▶ PATIENT TEACHING

Be sure to cover:
- disorder, diagnostic tests, and treatment
- long-term hormonal replacement therapy and adverse reactions
- when to notify the physician
- regular follow-up appointments
- energy-conservation techniques
- need for adequate rest
- need for a balanced diet.

Discharge planning
- Refer parents for psychological counseling or to community resources.

✷ RESOURCES

Organizations
American Association of Clinical Endocrinologists: www.aace.com
National Organization for Rare Diseases: www.rarediseases.org

Selected references
Agha, A., et al. "The Natural History of Post-Traumatic Hypopituitarism: Implications for Assessment and Treatment," American Journal of Medicine 118(12):1416, December 2005.

Hanberg, A. "Common Disorders of the Pituitary Gland: Hyposecretion versus Hypersecretion," Journal of Infusion Nursing 28(1):36-44, January-February 2005.

Mondok, A., et al. "Treatment of Pituitary Tumors: Radiation," Endocrine 28(1):77-85, October 2005.

Hypothyroidism

Description

- Clinical condition characterized by either decreased circulating levels of or resistance to free thyroid hormone (TH)
- Classified as primary or secondary
- Severe hypothyroidism known as *myxedema*

Pathophysiology

- In primary hypothyroidism, a decrease in TH production is a result of the loss of thyroid tissue.
- This results in an increased secretion of thyroid-stimulating hormone (TSH) that leads to a goiter.
- In secondary hypothyroidism, the pituitary typically fails to synthesize or secrete adequate amounts of TSH, or target tissues fail to respond to normal blood levels of TH.
- Either type may progress to myxedema, which is clinically more severe and considered a medical emergency. (See *Managing myxedema coma.*)

Causes

- Thyroid gland surgery
- Radioactive iodine therapy
- Inflammatory conditions
- Autoimmune thyroiditis
- Endemic iodine deficiency
- Antithyroid drugs
- Congenital defects
- Amyloidosis
- Sarcoidosis
- External radiation to the neck
- Drugs, such as iodides and lithium
- Pituitary failure to produce TSH
- Hypothalamic failure to produce thyrotropin-releasing hormone
- Postpartum pituitary necrosis
- Pituitary tumor
- Idiopathic

Incidence

- Most prevalent in women
- In United States, increased incidence in people older than age 40

Common characteristics

- Decreased energy metabolism
- Decreased heat production

Complications

CARDIOVASCULAR

- Hypercholesterolemia
- Arteriosclerosis
- Ischemic heart disease
- Peripheral vascular disease
- Cardiomegaly
- Heart failure
- Pleural and pericardial effusion

GI

- Achlorhydria
- Anemia
- Dynamic colon
- Megacolon
- Intestinal obstruction
- Bleeding tendencies

OTHER

- Conductive or sensorineural deafness
- Psychiatric disturbances
- Carpal tunnel syndrome
- Benign intracranial hypertension
- Impaired fertility
- Myxedema coma

History

- Vague and varied symptoms that have developed slowly over time
- Energy loss, fatigue
- Forgetfulness
- Sensitivity to cold
- Unexplained weight gain
- Constipation
- Anorexia
- Decreased libido
- Menorrhagia
- Paresthesia
- Joint stiffness
- Muscle cramping

Physical findings

- Slight mental slowing to severe obtundation
- Thick, dry tongue
- Hoarseness; slow, slurred speech
- Dry, flaky, inelastic skin
- Puffy face, hands, and feet
- Periorbital edema; drooping upper eyelids
- Dry, sparse hair with patchy hair loss
- Loss of the outer third of the eyebrow
- Thick and brittle nails with transverse and longitudinal grooves
- Ataxia, intention tremor; nystagmus
- Doughy skin that feels cool
- Weak pulse and bradycardia
- Muscle weakness
- Sacral or peripheral edema
- Delayed reflex relaxation time
- Possible goiter
- Absent or decreased bowel sounds

MANAGING MYXEDEMA COMA

Myxedema coma is a medical emergency that usually has a fatal outcome. Progression is typically gradual, but when stress aggravates severe or prolonged hypothyroidism, coma may develop abruptly. Examples of severe stress are infection, exposure to cold, and trauma. Other precipitating factors include thyroid medication withdrawal and the use of sedatives, opioids, or anesthetics.

Patients in myxedema coma have significantly depressed respirations, so their partial pressure of arterial carbon dioxide may increase. Decreased cardiac output and worsening cerebral hypoxia may also occur. The patient is stuporous and hypothermic, and her vital signs reflect bradycardia and hypotension.

Lifesaving interventions

If the patient becomes comatose, begin these interventions as soon as possible:

- Maintain airway patency with ventilatory support, if necessary.
- Maintain circulation through I.V. fluid replacement.
- Provide continuous electrocardiogram monitoring.
- Monitor arterial blood gas measurements to detect hypoxia and metabolic acidosis.
- Warm the patient by wrapping her in blankets. Don't use a warming blanket because it might increase peripheral vasodilation, causing shock.
- Monitor the patient's body temperature with a low-reading thermometer, until stable.
- Replace thyroid hormone by administering large I.V. levothyroxine doses, as ordered. Monitor vital signs because rapid correction of hypothyroidism can cause adverse cardiac effects.
- Monitor intake and output and daily weight. With treatment, urine output should increase and body weight should decrease; if not, report this to the physician.
- Replace fluids and other substances such as glucose. Monitor serum electrolyte levels.
- Administer corticosteroids, as ordered.
- Check for possible sources of infection, such as blood, sputum, or urine, which may have precipitated coma. Treat infections or other underlying illnesses.

- Hypotension
- A gallop or distant heart sounds
- Adventitious breath sounds
- Abdominal distention or ascites

Test results
LABORATORY
- Radioimmunoassay shows decreased serum levels of T_3 and T_4.
- Serum TSH level is increased with thyroid insufficiency; decreased with hypothalamic or pituitary insufficiency.
- Serum cholesterol, alkaline phosphatase, and triglycerides levels are elevated.
- Serum electrolytes show low serum sodium levels in myxedema coma.
- Arterial blood gas analysis shows decreased pH and increased partial pressure of carbon dioxide in myxedema coma.

IMAGING
- Skull X-ray, computed tomography scan, and magnetic resonance imaging may show pituitary or hypothalamic lesions.

◆ TREATMENT

General
- To restore and maintain a normal thyroid state
- Need for long-term thyroid replacement

Diet
- Low-fat, low-cholesterol
- High-fiber
- Low-sodium
- Possible fluid restriction

Activity
- As tolerated

Medication
- Synthetic hormone levothyroxine
- Synthetic liothyronine

Surgery
- For underlying cause such as pituitary tumor

❖ NURSING CONSIDERATIONS

Nursing diagnoses
- Chronic low self-esteem
- Constipation
- Decreased cardiac output
- Deficient knowledge (hypothyroidism)
- Disturbed body image
- Excess fluid volume
- Imbalanced nutrition: More than body requirements
- Ineffective coping
- Ineffective tissue perfusion: Cardiopulmonary
- Risk for impaired skin integrity

Key outcomes
The patient will:
- express positive feelings about self
- resume normal bowel elimination
- maintain adequate cardiac output
- demonstrate understanding of condition and treatment
- express positive feelings about self
- maintain adequate fluid volume
- consume adequate daily calorie requirements
- demonstrate positive coping strategies
- exhibit hemodynamic stability
- maintain skin integrity.

Nursing interventions
- Administer medications, as ordered.
- Provide adequate rest periods.
- Apply antiembolism stockings.
- Encourage coughing and deep-breathing exercises.
- Maintain fluid restrictions and a low-sodium diet.
- Provide a high-bulk, low-calorie diet.
- Reorient the patient, as needed.
- Offer support and encouragement.
- Provide meticulous skin care.
- Keep the patient warm, as needed.
- Encourage the patient to express her feelings.
- Help the patient to develop effective coping strategies.

Monitoring
- Vital signs
- Intake and output
- Daily weight
- Cardiovascular status
- Pulmonary status
- Edema

- Bowel sounds, abdominal distention, frequency of bowel movements
- Mental and neurologic status
- Signs and symptoms of hyperthyroidism

▶ PATIENT TEACHING

Be sure to cover:
- disorder, diagnostic tests, and treatment
- medication administration, dosage, and possible adverse effects
- when to notify the physician
- physical and mental changes
- signs and symptoms of myxedema
- need for lifelong hormone replacement therapy
- need to wear a medical identification bracelet
- importance of accurate records of daily weight
- need for a well-balanced, high-fiber, low-sodium diet
- energy-conservation techniques.

Discharge planning
- Refer the patient and her family to a mental health professional for additional counseling, if needed.

✷ RESOURCES

Organizations
American Foundation of Thyroid Patients: *www.thyroidfoundation.org*
American Thyroid Association: *www.thyroid.org*
Thyroid Foundation of America, Inc.: *www.clark.net/puB/tfa*

Selected references
Col, N.F., et al. "Subclinical Thyroid Disease: Clinical Applications," *JAMA* 291(2):239-43, January 2004.
Holcomb, S.S. "Detecting Thyroid Disease," *Nursing* 35(10 Suppl):4-8, October 2005.
Strategies for Managing Multisystem Disorders. Philadelphia: Lippincott Williams & Wilkins, 2006.

Impetigo

Description
- Contagious, superficial bacterial skin infection
- Nonbullous and bullous forms
- May complicate chickenpox, eczema, and other skin disorders marked by open lesions
- Most commonly appears on face and extremities

Pathophysiology
NONBULLOUS IMPETIGO
- Eruption occurs when bacteria inoculate traumatized skin cells.
- Lesions begin as small vesicles, which rapidly erode.
- Honey-colored crusts surrounded by erythema are formed.
BULLOUS IMPETIGO
- Eruption occurs in nontraumatized skin via bacterial toxin or exotoxin.
- Lesions begin as thin-walled bullae and vesicles.
- Lesions contain clear to turbid yellow fluid; some crusting exists.

Causes
NONBULLOUS IMPETIGO
- Beta-hemolytic streptoccci
BULLOUS IMPETIGO
- Coagulase-positive *Staphylococcus aureus*

COMPARING ECTHYMA AND IMPETIGO

Ecthyma is a superficial skin infection that usually causes scarring. It generally results from infection by group A beta-hemolytic streptococci.

Ecthyma differs from impetigo in that its characteristic ulcer results from deeper penetration of the skin by the infecting organism (involving the lower epidermis and dermis) and the overlying crust tends to be raised (3/8" to 1 1/4" [1 to 3 cm]).

These lesions usually are found on the legs after a scratch or an insect bite. Autoinoculation can transmit ecthyma to other parts of the body, especially to sites that have been scratched open.

Therapy is basically the same as for impetigo, beginning with removal of the crust, but the patient's response may be slower. Parenteral antibiotics also are used.

Risk factors
- Poor hygiene
- Untreated minor trauma
- Overcrowded living conditions
- Lesions of preexisting eczema, chickenpox, scabies
- Other skin rashes
- Anemia
- Malnutrition

Incidence
- Most common among infants, children, and young adults
- More common in warm ambient temperatures
- Predominant during late summer and early fall

Common characteristics
- Painlessness
- Tender red macule or papule
- Pustules

Complications
- Acute glomerulonephritis
- Ecthyma (see *Comparing ecthyma and impetigo*)
- Exfoliative eruption (staphylococcal scalded-skin syndrome)

History
- Presence of risk factors
- Absence of pain
- Possible pruritus

Physical findings
NONBULLOUS IMPETIGO
- Small, red macule or vesicle that becomes pustular within a few hours
- Characteristic thick, honey-colored crust formed from the exudate
- Satellite lesions caused by autoinoculation
BULLOUS IMPETIGO
- Thin-walled vesicle
- Thin, clear crust formed from exudate (see *Recognizing impetigo*)
- Lesion that appears as a central clearing circumscribed by an outer rim

Test results
LABORATORY
- Gram stain of vesicular fluid shows infecting organism.
- Culture and sensitivity testing of exudate or denuded crust shows infecting organism.
- White blood cell count is elevated.

◆ TREATMENT

General
- Removal of exudate by washing lesions two to three times per day with soap and water
- Warm soaks or compresses of normal saline solution or a diluted soap solution for stubborn crusts
- Prevention by benzoyl peroxide soap

Diet
- No restrictions

Activity
- No restrictions

Medication
- Antibiotics
- Antihistamines

❖ NURSING CONSIDERATIONS

Nursing diagnoses
- Disturbed body image
- Impaired skin integrity
- Impaired tissue integrity
- Risk for infection

Key outcomes
The patient will:
- verbalize feelings about changed body image
- exhibit improved or healed wounds or lesions
- remain free from complications or infection.

Nursing interventions
- Use meticulous hand-washing technique.
- Follow standard precautions.
- Trim fingernails short.
- Remove crusts by gently washing with bactericidal soap and water.
- Administer medications, as ordered.
- Encourage verbalization of feelings about body image.
- Comply with local public health standards and guidelines.

Monitoring
- Response to treatment
- Adverse drug reactions
- Complications

▶ PATIENT TEACHING

Be sure to cover:
- disorder, diagnostic tests, and treatment
- meticulous hand-washing technique
- trimming fingernails short
- regular bathing with bactericidal soap
- avoiding sharing clothes and linens
- identification of characteristic lesions
- medication administration, dosage, and possible adverse effects
- lesion care.

✳ RESOURCES

Organizations
American Academy of Dermatology: *www.aad.org*
Dermatology Foundation: *www.dermfnd.org*

Selected references
Kuniyuki, S., et al. "Topical Antibiotic Treatment of Impetigo with Tetracycline," *Journal of Dermatology* 32(10):788-92, October 2005.
Sandhu, K., and Kanwar, A.J. "Generalized Bullous Impetigo in a Neonate," *Pediatric Dermatology* 21(6):667-69, November-December 2004.
Watkins, P. "Impetigo: Aetiology, Complications and Treatment Options," *Nursing Standard* 19(36):50-54, May 2005.

RECOGNIZING IMPETIGO

In impetigo, when the vesicles break, crust forms from the exudate. This infection is especially contagious among young children.

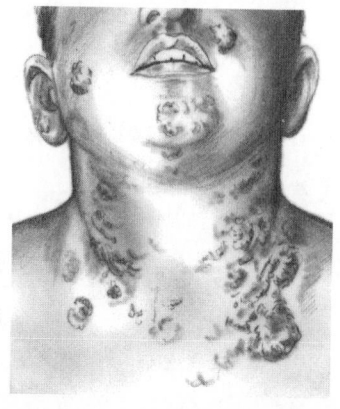

Infectious mononucleosis

● OVERVIEW

Description
- Acute infectious disease that causes fever, sore throat, and cervical lymphadenopathy

Pathophysiology
- Virus enters and replicates in epithelial cells of the oropharynx and B cells of tonsillar tissue, causing alteration of shape and function of the infected cells.
- Infected B cells activate cell-mediated immunity with proliferation of abnormal cytotoxic T cells in lymphoid tissues.
- Lymphoproliferation stops when cytotoxic T cells are able to destroy infected B cells.

Causes
- Epstein-Barr virus (EBV), a member of the herpes group
- Spread by contact with oral secretions (kissing)
- Also transmitted during bone marrow transplantation and blood transfusion

Incidence
- Primarily affects young adults and children
- Common and widespread in early childhood in developing countries and socioeconomically depressed populations

Common characteristics
- Incubation period of about 4 to 6 weeks in young adults
- Prodromal symptoms, including headache, malaise, and profound fatigue
- After 3 to 5 days, triad of symptoms, including sore throat, cervical lymphadenopathy, and temperature fluctuations, with an evening peak of 101° to 102° F (38.3° to 38.9° C)

Complications
- Splenic rupture
- Aseptic meningitis
- Encephalitis
- Hemolytic anemia
- Pericarditis
- Guillain-Barré syndrome

✳ ASSESSMENT

History
- Contact with a person who has infectious mononucleosis

Physical findings
- Exudative tonsillitis, pharyngitis
- Palatal petechiae
- Periorbital edema
- Maculopapular rash that resembles rubella
- Cervical adenopathy; possible inguinal and axillary adenopathy
- Splenomegaly, hepatomegaly, jaundice

Test results
LABORATORY
- White blood cell (WBC) count is 10,000 to 20,000/µl during the second and third weeks of illness; lymphocytes and monocytes account for 50% to 70% of the total WBC count; 10% of the lymphocytes are atypical.
- Fourfold increase in heterophil antibodies (agglutinins for sheep red blood cells) during the acute phase and at 3- to 4-week intervals.
- Antibodies to EBV and cellular antigens are shown by indirect immunofluorescence.
- Liver function studies are abnormal.

◆ TREATMENT

General
- Essentially supportive

Diet
- Nutritious foods
- Soft food (with throat soreness)

Activity
- Frequent rest periods
- Avoidance of strenuous activity or contact sports until fully recovered

Medication
- Aspirin or another salicylate
- Steroids
- Antibiotics

Surgery
- Splenectomy for splenic rupture

✣ NURSING CONSIDERATIONS

Nursing diagnoses
- Activity intolerance
- Acute pain
- Imbalanced nutrition: Less than body requirements
- Fatigue
- Hyperthermia
- Impaired skin integrity
- Impaired social interaction
- Risk for deficient fluid volume

Key outcomes
The patient will:
- express feelings of increased comfort and decreased pain
- demonstrate measures to balance activity and rest
- conserve energy while performing daily activities to tolerance level
- maintain temperature within normal limits
- maintain adequate nutritional intake
- demonstrate intact skin
- engage in appropriate social interactions
- maintain adequate fluid volume.

Nursing interventions
- Administer medications, as ordered.
- Provide warm saline gargles for symptomatic relief of sore throat.
- Provide adequate fluids and nutrition.
- Plan care to provide frequent rest periods.

Monitoring
- Response to treatment
- Fatigue
- Nutritional status
- Liver function tests
- Complications

▶ PATIENT TEACHING

Be sure to cover:
- disorder, diagnostic tests, and treatment
- explanation that convalescence may take several weeks
- need for bed rest during the acute illness
- explanation that there's a period of prolonged communicability (stress good hand washing and avoidance of salivary contamination)
- benefits of bland foods, milk shakes, fruit juices, and broths to minimize throat discomfort.

Discharge planning
- Refer the patient to an otolaryngologist for marked tonsillar swelling or a neurologist for central nervous system complications.

✳ RESOURCES

Organizations
Centers for Disease Control and Prevention: *www.cdc.gov*
Harvard University Consumer Health Information: *www.intelihealth.com*
National Health Information Center: *www.health.gov/nhic/*
National Institute of Allergy and Infectious Diseases: *www.niaid.nih.gov*
National Library of Medicine: *www.nlm.nih.gov*

Selected references
Diseases, 4th ed. Philadelphia: Lippincott Williams & Wilkins, 2006.
Foreman, B.H., et al. "Clinical Inquiries. Can We Prevent Splenic Rupture for Patients with Infectious Monoucleosis?" *Journal of Family Practice* 54(6):547-48, June 2005.
Kasper, D.L., et al., eds. *Harrison's Principles of Internal Medicine,* 16th ed. New York: McGraw-Hill Book Co., 2005.
Statter, M.B., and Liu, D.C. "Nonoperative Management of Blunt Splenic Injury in Infectious Mononucleosis," *The American Surgeon* 71(5):376-78, May 2005.

Inflammatory bowel disease

● OVERVIEW

Description
- Chronic inflammation of intestines
- Two major forms: Crohn's disease and ulcerative colitis

CROHN'S DISEASE
- Inflammatory bowel disease that may affect any part of GI tract but commonly involves terminal ileum
- Fifty percent of cases involving colon and small bowel; 33%, terminal ileum; 10% to 20%, only colon
- Extends through all layers of the intestinal wall; may involve regional lymph nodes and mesentery

ULCERATIVE COLITIS
- Episodic inflammatory chronic disease that causes ulcerations of the mucosa in the colon
- Begins in the rectum and sigmoid colon and may extend upward into the entire colon
- Rarely affects the small intestine, except for the terminal ileum
- Produces congestion, edema (leading to mucosal friability), and ulcerations
- Range in severity from mild, localized disorder to fulminant disease that causes many complications

Pathophysiology

CROHN'S DISEASE
- Crohn's disease involves slow, progressive inflammation of the bowel.
- Lymphatic obstruction is caused by enlarged lymph nodes.
- Edema, mucosal ulceration, fissures, and abscesses occur.
- Elevated patches of closely packed lymph follicles (Peyer's patches) develop in the small intestinal lining.
- Fibrosis occurs, thickening the bowel wall and causing stenosis.
- Inflamed bowel loops adhere to other diseased or normal loops.
- The diseased bowel becomes thicker, shorter, and narrower.

ULCERATIVE COLITIS
- The disorder primarily involves the bowel mucosa and submucosa.
- Crypt abscesses and mucosal ulceration may occur.
- The mucosa typically appears granular and friable.
- The colon becomes a rigid, foreshortened tube.

- In severe ulcerative colitis, areas of hyperplastic growth occur, with swollen mucosa surrounded by inflamed mucosa with shallow ulcers.
- Submucosa and the circular and longitudinal muscles may be involved.

Causes
- Exact cause unknown

Risk factors

CROHN'S DISEASE
- History of allergies
- Immune disorders
- Genetic predisposition: 10% to 20% of patients having one or more affected relatives; sometimes occurring in monozygotic twins

ULCERATIVE COLITIS
- Stress
- Family history
- Jewish ancestry

Incidence

CROHN'S DISEASE
- Occurs equally in males and females
- Occurs more commonly in Jewish people
- Usually begins before age 30

ULCERATIVE COLITIS
- Occurs primarily in young adults, especially women
- More prevalent among Jewish people and higher socioeconomic groups
- Affects about 1 in 1,000 people
- Commonly peaks between ages 15 and 30; again between ages 50 and 70

Common characteristics
- Bloody diarrhea
- Fatigue
- Weakness
- Anorexia
- Abdominal cramping

Complications
- Nutritional deficiencies due to malabsorption and maldigestion
- Anal fistula
- Perineal abscess
- Strictures, intestinal obstruction
- Toxic megacolon
- Perforation
- Peritonitis

CROHN'S DISEASE
- Fistulas of the bladder or vagina or to the skin in an old scar area

ULCERATIVE COLITIS
- Cancer
- Cirrhosis
- Pyoderma gangrenosum on legs and ankles
- Uveitis
- Cholangiocarcinoma
- Arthritis

✳ ASSESSMENT

History
- Gradual onset of signs and symptoms, marked by periods of remission and exacerbation
- Fatigue and weakness
- Fever, flatulence, nausea
- Steady, colicky, or cramping abdominal pain that usually occurs in the right lower abdominal quadrant
- Bloody diarrhea; may worsen after emotional upset or ingestion of poorly tolerated foods, such as milk, fatty foods, and spices (Crohn's); recurrent episodes as often as 10 to 25 times daily (ulcerative colitis)
- Anorexia, weight loss

Physical findings
- Abdominal tenderness or distention

CROHN'S DISEASE
- Possible soft or semiliquid stool, usually without gross blood
- Possible abdominal mass, indicating adherent loops of bowel
- Hyperactive bowel sounds
- Bloody diarrhea
- Perianal and rectal abscesses

ULCERATIVE COLITIS
- Liquid stools with visible pus, mucus, and blood
- Perianal irritation, hemorrhoids, and fissures
- Jaundice
- Joint pain

Test results

LABORATORY
- Stool specimen analysis reveals blood, pus, and mucus but no pathogenic organisms.
- Other supportive laboratory tests show decreased serum potassium, magnesium, hemoglobin, and albumin as well as leukocytosis and increased prothrombin time; an ele-

vated erythrocyte sedimentation rate correlates with the severity of the attack.

IMAGING

CROHN'S DISEASE

- Small bowel X-rays may show irregular mucosa, ulceration, and stiffening.
- Barium enema reveals the string sign (segments of stricture separated by normal bowel) and may also show fissures and narrowing of the lumen in Crohn's disease; may disclose extent of ulcerative colitis and possible complications such as carcinoma.

◈ **NURSING ALERT** Barium enema shouldn't be performed in a patient with active signs and symptoms.

DIAGNOSTIC PROCEDURES

- Sigmoidoscopy and colonoscopy show areas of inflammation; cobblestone appearance of mucosa in Crohn's disease; and inflammatory exudates and mucosal friability in ulcerative colitis erosions.
- Biopsy performed during colonoscopy helps to confirm the diagnosis.

◆ TREATMENT

General

- Stress reduction
- I.V. fluid replacement
- Blood transfusion (if needed)

Diet

- Nothing by mouth (if severe)
- Parenteral nutrition (if severe)
- Supplemental feeding
- Avoidance of foods that worsen diarrhea

Activity

- Rest periods during exacerbation

Medication

- Corticosteroids
- Immunosuppressants
- Sulfonamides
- Anti-inflammatories
- Antispasmodics and antidiarrheals

Surgery

- For acute intestinal obstruction

CROHN'S DISEASE

- Colectomy with ileostomy

ULCERATIVE COLITIS

- Treatment of last resort
- Proctocolectomy with ileostomy
- Pouch ileostomy
- Ileoanal reservoir with loop ileostomy
- Colectomy (after 10 years of disease)

❖ NURSING CONSIDERATIONS

Nursing diagnoses

- Acute pain
- Diarrhea
- Disturbed body image
- Imbalanced nutrition: Less than body requirements
- Ineffective coping
- Ineffective tissue perfusion: GI
- Risk for deficient fluid volume
- Risk for impaired skin integrity
- Risk for injury

Key outcomes

The patient will:

- express feelings of increased comfort and decreased pain
- regain normal intestinal function
- express positive feelings about self
- maintain adequate caloric intake
- exhibit adequate coping mechanisms and seek sources of support
- exhibit signs of adequate GI perfusion
- maintain normal fluid volume
- maintain skin integrity
- remain free from injury.

Nursing interventions

- Provide emotional support to the patient and his family.
- Provide meticulous skin care after each bowel movement.
- Schedule patient care to include rest periods throughout the day.
- Assist with dietary changes and intake.
- Give prescribed medications, supplements, and blood transfusions.

Monitoring

- Abdominal pain and distention
- Vital signs
- Intake and output, including amount of stool
- Daily weight
- Serum electrolytes and glucose, hemoglobin, and stools for occult blood
- Signs of infection or obstruction

- Bleeding

AFTER SURGERY

- Wound site
- Pain level
- Bowel function

▶ PATIENT TEACHING

Be sure to cover:

- disorder, diagnostic tests, and treatment
- dietary instructions
- importance of rest
- medication administration, dosage, and possible adverse effects
- ostomy care, if appropriate
- importance of regular physical examination due to increased risk for cancer (with ulcerative colitis).

Discharge planning

- Refer the patient to a smoking-cessation program, if appropriate.
- Refer the patient to an enterostomal therapist, if indicated.

☀ RESOURCES

Organizations

Digestive Disease National Coalition: *www.ddnc.org*

National Digestive Diseases Information Clearinghouse: *www.niddk.nih.gov/health/digest/nddic.htm*

Selected references

Ghosh, S., et al. "Is Thiopurine Therapy in Ulcerative Colitis as Effective as in Crohn's Disease?" *Gut* 55(1):6-8, January 2006.

Influenza

Description
- An acute, highly contagious infection of the respiratory tract
- Has capacity for antigenic variation (ability to mutate into different strains so that no immunologic resistance is present in those at risk)
- Antigenic variation characterized as antigenic drift (minor changes that occur yearly or every few years) and antigenic shift (major changes that lead to pandemics)
- Also called *the grippe* or *the flu*

Pathophysiology
- Virus invades the epithelium of the respiratory tract, causing inflammation and desquamation.
- After attaching to the host cell, viral ribonucleic acid enters the cell and uses host components to replicate its genetic material and protein, which are then assembled into new virus particles.
- Newly produced viruses burst forth to invade other healthy cells.
- Viral invasion destroys host cells, impairing respiratory defenses (especially mucociliary transport system) and predisposing the patient to secondary bacterial infection.

Causes
- Infection transmitted by inhaling a respiratory droplet from an infected person or by indirect contact (drinking from a contaminated glass)
- Type A: most prevalent and strikes every year with new serotypes causing epidemics every 3 years
- Type B: strikes annually but causes epidemics only every 4 to 6 years
- Type C: endemic and causes only sporadic cases

Incidence
- Affects all age-groups; highest incidence occurring school-age children
- Greatest severity (may lead to death) in young children, elderly people, and those with chronic diseases

- Occurs sporadically or in epidemics (usually during colder months) with peak within 2 to 3 weeks after initial cases and lasting 2 to 3 months

Common characteristics
- After an incubation period of 24 to 48 hours, flu symptoms appearing
- Sudden onset of chills, fever (101° to 104° F [38.3° to 40° C]), headache, malaise, myalgia (particularly in the back and limbs), photophobia, a nonproductive cough and, occasionally, laryngitis, hoarseness, rhinitis, and rhinorrhea

Complications
- Pneumonia
- Myositis
- Exacerbation of chronic obstructive pulmonary disease
- Reye's syndrome
- Myocarditis
- Pericarditis
- Transverse myelitis
- Encephalitis

History
- Usually, recent exposure (typically within 48 hours) to a person with influenza
- No influenza vaccine during the past season
- Headache, malaise, myalgia

Physical findings
- Fever (usually higher in children)
- Signs of croup, dry cough
- Tired and listless feeling, weakness
- Red, watery eyes; clear nasal discharge
- Erythema of the nose and throat without exudate
- Tachypnea, shortness of breath, cyanosis
- With bacterial pneumonia, purulent or bloody sputum
- Cervical adenopathy and tenderness
- Diminished breath sounds in areas of consolidation

Test results
- After an epidemic is confirmed, diagnosis requires only observation of clinical signs and symptoms.

LABORATORY
- Inoculation of chicken embryos with nasal secretions from infected patients shows influenza virus.
- Throat swabs, nasopharyngeal washes, or sputum culture shows isolation of the influenza virus.
- Immunodiagnostic techniques show viral antigens in tissue culture or in exfoliated nasopharyngeal cells obtained by washings.
- Leukocyte counts are elevated in secondary bacterial infection.
- Leukocyte counts are decreased in overwhelming viral or bacterial infection.

◆ TREATMENT

General
- Fluid and electrolyte replacements
- Oxygen and assisted ventilation if indicated

Diet
- Increased fluid intake

Activity
- Rest periods, as needed

Medication
- Acetaminophen or aspirin
- Guaifenesin or expectorant
- Antivirals such as amantadine
- Antibiotics

❖ NURSING CONSIDERATIONS

Nursing diagnoses
- Acute pain
- Fatigue
- Hyperthermia
- Ineffective breathing pattern
- Ineffective health maintenance
- Risk for deficient fluid volume
- Risk for infection

Key outcomes
The patient will:
- express a feeling of increased comfort and decreased pain
- report an increased energy level
- maintain a normal temperature
- maintain respiratory rate within 5 breaths/minute of baseline
- maintain his current health status
- maintain adequate fluid volume
- remain free from further signs and symptoms of infection.

Nursing interventions
- Administer medications, as ordered.
- Follow standard precautions.
- Administer oxygen therapy, if warranted.

Monitoring
- Temperature
- Signs and symptoms of dehydration
- Respiratory status
- Response to treatment
- Complications

▶ PATIENT TEACHING

Be sure to cover:
- disorder, diagnostic tests, and treatment
- mouthwash or warm saline gargles to ease sore throat
- importance of increased fluids to prevent dehydration
- warm bath or a heating pad to relieve myalgia
- proper hand-washing technique and tissue disposal to prevent the virus from spreading
- influenza immunization.

✺ RESOURCES

Organizations
Centers for Disease Control and Prevention: www.cdc.gov
Harvard University Consumer Health Information: www.intelihealth.com
National Health Information Center: www.health.gov/nhic/
National Institute of Allergy and Infectious Diseases: www.niaid.nih.gov
National Library of Medicine: www.nlm.nih.gov
World Health Organization: www.who.int

Selected references
Hara, M., et al. "Immune Response to Influenza Vaccine in Healthy Adults and the Elderly: Association with Nutritional Status," *Vaccine* 23(12):1457-463, February 2005.

Kasper, D.L., et al., eds. *Harrison's Principles of Internal Medicine,* 16th ed. New York: McGraw-Hill Book Co., 2005.

Munoz, E.M., et al. "Safety of Influenza Vaccination During Pregnancy," *American Journal of Obstetrics & Gynecology* 192(4):1098-106, April 2005.

Nelson, R. "Health Care Workers: Few Feel the Flu Shot," *AJN* 104(10):24-25, October 2004.

Insect bites and stings

● OVERVIEW

Description
- Bite or sting from an insect or other arthropod, such as a tick, brown recluse spider, black widow spider, bee, wasp, yellow jacket, or fire ant

Pathophysiology
- A bite or sting can injure the skin, and secretions released from a bite or sting can cause a physiologic response specific to the insect or arthropod.
- Exposure to secretions ranges from barely noticeable to life-threatening.
- Transmission of disease may result from a bite or sting.
- Mouthparts of an insect or arthropod are classified as piercing-sucking, sponging, or biting-chewing.

Causes
- Toxic effects of venom
- Hypersensitivity response

Incidence
- Not known

Common characteristics
LOCAL REACTION
- Mild discomfort to moderate or severe pain
- Erythema and warmth
- Tenderness
- Edema of surrounding tissues
- Severe local reaction
- Generalized erythema
- Urticaria
- Pruritic edema

SYSTEMIC RESPONSE
- All of the above symptoms
- Anxiety, disorientation
- Weakness
- GI disturbances
- Dizziness
- Hypotension
- Stridor
- Dyspnea and cough
- Cardiovascular collapse

Complications
- Anaphylaxis
- Thrombocytopenia (rare complication of brown recluse spider bite)
- Hemolytic anemia

✳ ASSESSMENT

History
TICK BITE
- Itching at the affected site
- Tick exposure lesion

BROWN RECLUSE SPIDER BITE
- Minimal initial pain that increases over time
- Fever, chills, malaise, weakness
- Nausea, vomiting
- Joint pain

BLACK WIDOW SPIDER BITE
- Pinprick sensation, followed by dull, numbing pain
- Severe pain and large-muscle cramping (if leg bite)
- Vertigo
- Chills and sweats

BEE, WASP, OR YELLOW JACKET STING
- Pain and pruritus
- Generalized weakness
- Chest tightness
- Dizziness
- Nausea and vomiting
- Abdominal cramps
- Throat constriction

FIRE ANT STING
- Immediate pain, itching, and burning

Physical findings
TICK BITE
- Tick paralysis
- Expanding skin lesion, erythema migrans

BROWN RECLUSE SPIDER BITE
- Petechiae

BLACK WIDOW SPIDER BITE
- Rigid, painful abdomen
- Rigidity and pain in the chest, shoulders, and back (if arm bite)
- Extreme restlessness (systemic)
- Pallor
- Seizures, especially in children
- Hyperactive reflexes
- Hypertension
- Tachycardia with thready pulse
- Circulatory collapse

BEE, WASP, OR YELLOW JACKET STING
- Raised, reddened wheal, possibly with a protruding stinger from the bee
- Wheezing
- Hypotension

FIRE ANT STING
- Clear vesicles with surrounding erythema
- Pustule

Test results
LABORATORY
- Urinalysis shows hematuria (black widow spider bite).
- White blood cell count is increased (black widow spider bite).
- Anemia panel shows hemolytic anemia (brown recluse spider bite).
- Platelet count shows thrombocytopenia (brown recluse spider bite).

OTHER
- Identification of the insect is difficult unless stung by a honeybee or bumblebee, which commonly leave a stinger with a venom sac in the lesion.

◆ TREATMENT

General
TICK BITE
- Tick removal
- Symptomatic therapy for severe symptoms

BROWN RECLUSE SPIDER BITE
- No known specific treatment
- I.V. fluids

BLACK WIDOW SPIDER BITE
- Ice packs)

BEE, WASP, YELLOW JACKET, OR FIRE ANT STING
- Ice application
- Elevation of affected extremity
- Supportive treatment

Diet
- No restrictions
- Nothing by mouth if severe, systemic reaction

Activity
- Rest to limit toxic effects of venom

Medication
TICK BITE
- Antipruritics
- Antibiotics (Lyme disease treatment or Rocky Mountain spotted fever treatment)

BROWN RECLUSE SPIDER BITE
- Corticosteroids
- Antibiotics
- Antihistamines
- Tranquilizers
- Tetanus prophylaxis

BLACK WIDOW SPIDER BITE
- Antivenin I.V.

- Calcium gluconate I.V.
- Muscle relaxants
- Adrenaline or antihistamines
- Tetanus immunization
- Antibiotics
- Oxygen for respiratory difficulty

BEE, WASP, YELLOW JACKET, OR FIRE ANT STING
- Antihistamines
- Steroids for severe reactions

Surgery
- Lesion excision for brown recluse spider bite

❖ NURSING CONSIDERATIONS

Nursing diagnoses
- Acute pain
- Deficient fluid volume
- Impaired skin integrity
- Ineffective airway clearance
- Ineffective breathing pattern
- Ineffective tissue perfusion: Cardiopulmonary, peripheral
- Risk for poisoning

Key outcomes
The patient will:
- express feelings of increased comfort and decreased pain
- maintain normal fluid volume
- regain skin integrity
- maintain adequate ventilation and oxygenation and a patent airway
- exhibit signs of adequate cardiopulmonary perfusion
- remain free from signs and symptoms of poisoning.

Nursing interventions
- Keep the affected part immobile.
- Clean the bite or sting site with antiseptic.
- Apply ice.
- Administer medication, as ordered.
- Provide emergency resuscitation.

TICK BITE
- Remove the tick promptly and carefully.
- Use tweezers to grasp the tick near its head or mouth and gently pull to remove the whole tick without crushing it.
- If possible, seal the tick in a plastic bag and keep it in case the patient needs to see a physician. Otherwise, flush the tick down the toilet.

BROWN RECLUSE SPIDER BITE
- Clean the lesion with a 1:20 Burow's aluminum acetate solution.
- Apply antibiotic ointment as ordered.

BLACK WIDOW SPIDER BITE
- Remove all jewelry.
- Apply cool compresses.
- Avoid cutting into the wound or applying suction.

BEE, WASP, OR YELLOW JACKET STING
- Scrape stinger off; don't pull or squeeze it, which releases more toxin.

FIRE ANT STING
- Apply cool compresses.
- Gently wash the bite area, leaving the blister intact.
- Be prepared to intervene for an acute severe allergic reaction (rare).

Monitoring
- Vital signs
- Respiratory status
- General appearance
- Changes at the bite or sting site

▶ PATIENT TEACHING

Be sure to cover:
- avoidance of insect bites and stings
- examination of the body for ticks after being outdoors
- removal of ticks
- medical identification bracelet or card
- anaphylaxis kit use
- insect repellent use.

✳ RESOURCES

Organizations
American Academy of Allergy, Asthma, and Immunology: *www.aaaai.org*
National Center for Injury Prevention and Control: *www.cdc.gov/ncipc/ncipchm.htm*
National Institutes of Health: *www.nih.gov*

Selected references
McIntyre, C.L., et al. "Administration of Epinephrine for Life-Threatening Allergic Reactions in School Settings," *Pediatrics* 116(5):1134-140, November 2005.
Nunnelee, J.D. "Summer Injuries. Bites & Stings," *RN* 68(4):56-58, 60-61, April 2005.
Rash, E.M., "Arthropod Bites and Stings. Recognition and Treatment," *Advance for Nurse Practitioners* 11(9):87-90, 92, 102, September 2003.
Wolfson, A.B., et al. *Harwood-Nuss' Clinical Practice of Emergency Medicine*, 4th ed. Philadelphia: Lippincott Williams & Wilkins 2005.

Intestinal obstruction

● OVERVIEW

Description
- Partial or complete blockage of the lumen of the small or large bowel
- Commonly a medical emergency
- Most likely after abdominal surgery or with congenital bowel deformities
- Without treatment, complete obstruction in any part of bowel possibly causing death within hours from shock and vascular collapse

Pathophysiology
- Mechanical or nonmechanical (neurogenic) blockage of the lumen occurs.
- Fluid, air, or gas collects near the site.
- Peristalsis increases temporarily in an attempt to break through the blockage.
- Intestinal mucosa is injured, and distention at and above the site of obstruction occurs.
- Venous blood flow is impaired and normal absorptive processes cease.
- Water, sodium, and potassium are secreted by the bowel into the fluid pooled in the lumen.

Causes
MECHANICAL OBSTRUCTION
- Adhesions
- Strangulated hernias
- Carcinomas
- Foreign bodies
- Compression of the bowel wall from stenosis, intussusception, volvulus of the sigmoid or cecum, tumors, and atresia

NONMECHANICAL OBSTRUCTION
- Paralytic ileus
- Electrolyte imbalances
- Toxicity, such as that associated with uremia or generalized infection
- Neurogenic abnormalities
- Thrombosis or embolism of mesenteric vessels

Risk factors
- Abdominal surgery
- Radiation therapy
- Gallstones
- Inflammatory bowel disease

Incidence
- Diagnosed in approximately 20% of hospital admissions for abdominal illness
- Occurs equally in men and women

Common characteristics
- Abdominal pain
- Change in bowel habits

Complications
- Perforation
- Peritonitis
- Septicemia
- Secondary infection
- Metabolic alkalosis or acidosis
- Death

✻ ASSESSMENT

History
- Recent change in bowel habits
- Hiccups
MECHANICAL OBSTRUCTION
- Colicky pain
- Nausea, vomiting
- Constipation
NONMECHANICAL OBSTRUCTION
- Diffuse abdominal discomfort
- Frequent vomiting
- Severe abdominal pain (if obstruction results from vascular insufficiency or infarction)

Physical findings
MECHANICAL OBSTRUCTION
- Distended abdomen
- Borborygmi and rushes (occasionally loud enough to be heard without a stethoscope)
- Abdominal tenderness
- Rebound tenderness
NONMECHANICAL OBSTRUCTION
- Abdominal distention
- Decreased bowel sounds (early), then absent bowel sounds

Test results
LABORATORY
- Serum sodium, chloride, and potassium levels are decreased.
- White blood cell count is elevated.
- Serum amylase level is increased if pancreas is irritated by a bowel loop.
IMAGING
- Abdominal X-rays reveal the presence and location of intestinal gas or fluid. In small-bowel obstruction, a typical "stepladder" pattern emerges, with alternating fluid and gas levels apparent in 3 to 4 hours.
- Barium enema reveals a distended, air-filled colon or a closed loop of sigmoid with extreme distention (in sigmoid volvulus).
- Abdominal computed tomography scan, ultrasound, or magnetic resonance imaging may show specific nature and characteristics of the obstruction.

◆ TREATMENT

General
- Correction of fluid and electrolyte imbalances
- Decompression of the bowel to relieve vomiting and distention
- Treatment of shock and peritonitis

Diet
- Nothing by mouth (NPO)
- Parenteral nutrition until bowel is functioning
- High-fiber diet when obstruction is relieved

Activity
- Bed rest during acute phase
- Postoperatively, avoidance of lifting and contact sports

Medication
- Broad-spectrum antibiotics
- Analgesics
- Blood replacement

Surgery
- Usually the treatment of choice (exception is paralytic ileus in which nonoperative therapy is usually attempted first)
- Type of surgery dependent on cause of blockage

❖ NURSING CONSIDERATIONS

Nursing diagnoses
- Acute pain
- Deficient fluid volume
- Imbalanced nutrition: Less than body requirements
- Ineffective tissue perfusion: GI

Key outcomes
The patient will:
- express feelings of increased comfort and decreased pain
- maintain normal fluid volume
- maintain adequate nutritional status
- have normal bowel function
- exhibit signs of adequate GI perfusion.

Nursing interventions
- Keep the patient on NPO status.
- Insert a nasogastric (NG) tube and attach to low-pressure, intermittent suction.
- Maintain the patient in semi-Fowler's position.
- Provide mouth and nose care.
- Begin and maintain I.V. therapy, as ordered.
- Administer medications, as ordered.

Monitoring
- Vital signs
- Signs and symptoms of shock
- Bowel sounds and signs of returning peristalsis
- NG tube function and drainage
- Pain control
- Abdominal girth measurement to detect progressive distention
- Hydration and nutritional status
- Electrolytes and signs and symptoms of metabolic derangements
- Wound site (postoperatively)

▶ PATIENT TEACHING

Be sure to cover:
- disorder, focusing on the patient's type of intestinal obstruction; diagnostic tests; and treatment
- techniques for coughing and deep breathing, and use of incentive spirometry
- how to care for a colostomy or ileostomy
- incision care
- postoperative activity limitations and why these restrictions are necessary
- proper use of prescribed medications, focusing on their correct administration, dosage, and adverse effects
- importance of following a structured bowel regimen, particularly if the patient had a mechanical obstruction from fecal impaction.

Discharge planning
- Refer the patient to an enterostomal therapist, if indicated.

✸ RESOURCES

Organizations
Digestive Disease National Coalition: *www.ddnc.org*
National Digestive Diseases Information Clearinghouse: *www.niddk.nih.gov/health/digest/nddic.htm*

Selected references
Ben-Sassi, A., et al. "Distal Intestinal Obstruction Syndrome: A Childhood Illness Now Seen in Adults," *Colorectal Disease Supplement* 6(Suppl 1):83, July 2004.
Fisichella, P., and Helton, W. "(2004). Section 5 Gastrointestinal Tract and Abdomen: Assessment of Intestinal Obstruction. Available at: *www.acssurgery.com.* Accessed 9/1/2006.
Handbook of Diseases, 3rd ed. Philadelphia: Lippincott Williams & Wilkins, 2004.
Hughes, E. "Caring for a Patient with an Intestinal Obstruction," *Nursing Standard* 19(47):56-64, August 2005
Saddler, D. "A Literature Review of Fecal Impaction," *Gastroenterology Nursing* 28(1):49-50, January-February 2005.

Intussusception

Description
- Can be fatal if treatment delayed more than 24 hours
- Pediatric emergency

Pathophysiology
- Intussusception occurs when a portion of the bowel telescopes or invaginates into an adjacent bowel portion. (See *Understanding intussusception*.)
- It may be linked to viral infections because of seasonal peaks.

Causes
INFANTS
- Exact cause unknown
OLDER CHILDREN
- Polyps
- Hemangioma
- Lymphosarcoma
- Lymphoid hyperplasia
- Meckel's diverticulum
- Alterations in intestinal motility
ADULTS
- Benign or malignant tumors (65% of patients)
- Polyps
- Meckel's diverticulum
- Gastroenterostomy with herniation
- Appendiceal stump

Incidence
- Most common in infants
- Three times more common in males than in females
- About 87% of children with intussusception under age 2; about 70% of these children between 4 and 11 months old
- Seasonal peaks in late spring and early summer

Common characteristics
- Intermittent attacks of colicky pain
- Vomiting
- Abdominal guarding

Complications
- Strangulation of the intestine
- Gangrene of the bowel
- Shock
- Bowel perforation
- Peritonitis
- Death

History
- Intermittent attacks of colicky pain
- Pain that causes the child to scream, draw his legs up to his abdomen, turn pale and diaphoretic and, possibly, grunt
- Vomiting, initially stomach contents; later, bile-stained or fecal material
- "Currant jelly" stools, which contain mixture of blood and mucus

Physical findings
- Distended, tender abdomen
- Guarding over the intussusception site
- Palpable sausage-shaped abdominal mass in the right upper quadrant or in the midepigastric area if transverse colon is involved
- Bloody mucus found on rectal examination
- In adults, abdominal pain localized in right lower quadrant, radiating to the back, and increasing with eating

Test results
LABORATORY
- White blood cell count up to 15,000/µl indicates obstruction; more than 15,000/µl, strangulation; and more than 20,000/µl, bowel infarction.
IMAGING
- Barium enema confirms colonic intussusception when it shows the characteristic coiled-spring sign; it also delineates the extent of intussusception.
- Upright abdominal X-rays may show a soft-tissue mass and signs of complete or partial obstruction, with dilated loops of bowel.

UNDERSTANDING INTUSSUSCEPTION

In intussusception, a bowel section invaginates and is propelled along by peristalsis, pulling in more bowel. This illustration shows intussusception of a portion of the transverse colon. Intussusception typically produces edema, hemorrhage from venous engorgement, incarceration, and obstruction.

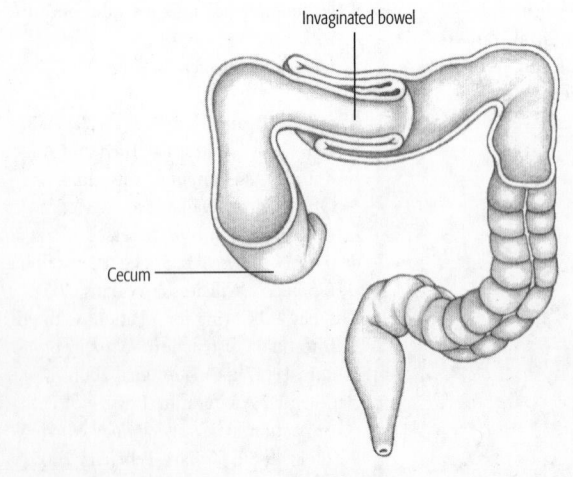

Invaginated bowel

Cecum

◆ TREATMENT

General
- Hydrostatic reduction
- Bowel decompression

Diet
- Nothing by mouth until bowel functioning properly

Activity
- Bed rest until condition is resolved

Medication
- Analgesics
- Antibiotics

Surgery
- Indicated for children with recurrent intussusception, those who show signs of shock or peritonitis, and those in whom symptoms present longer than 24 hours
- In adults, surgery always treatment of choice

❖ NURSING CONSIDERATIONS

Nursing diagnoses
- Acute pain
- Anxiety
- Deficient fluid volume
- Fear
- Ineffective tissue perfusion: GI
- Risk for infection

Key outcomes
The patient will:
- express feelings of increased comfort and decreased pain
- identify measures to decrease anxiety
- maintain normal fluid volume
- verbalize feelings and concerns
- exhibit signs of adequate GI perfusion
- remain free from signs and symptoms of infection.

Nursing interventions
- Offer reassurance and emotional support to the patient and, if the patient is a child, to his parents.
- Administer I.V. fluids, as ordered.
- Encourage coughing and deep breathing.
- Administer antibiotics, as ordered.

Monitoring
- Vital signs
- Intake and output
- Hydration status
- Nasogastric tube function and drainage
- Bowel sounds, stools, abdominal distention
- Wound site (after surgery)
- For recurrence in the first 36 to 48 hours after reduction

▶ PATIENT TEACHING

Be sure to cover:
- disorder, diagnostic tests, and treatment
- parental participation in their child's care to minimize the stress of hospitalization (be flexible about visiting hours)
- medication administration, dosage, and possible adverse effects
- wound care
- signs and symptoms of infection.

Discharge planning
- Refer the patient for follow-up with home care or support services, as necessary.

✴ RESOURCES

Organizations
Digestive Disease National: *www.ddnc.org*
National Digestive Diseases Information Clearinghouse: *www.niddk.nih.gov/health/digest/nddic.htm*

Selected references
Grosfeld, J.I., "Intussusception Then and Now: A Historical Vignette," *Journal of the American College of Surgeons* 291(6):830-33, December 2005.
Handbook of Diseases, 3rd ed. Philadelphia: Lippincott Williams & Wilkins 2004.
Kim, K.H., et al. "Intussusception after Gastric Surgery," *Endoscopy* 37(12):1237-243, December 2005.
McNally, P. *GI/Liver Secrets,* 3rd ed. Philadelphia: Hanley & Belfus, Inc., 2006.

Irritable bowel syndrome

● OVERVIEW

Description
- Common condition marked by chronic or periodic diarrhea alternating with constipation
- Accompanied by straining and abdominal cramps
- Initial episodes early in life and late teens to twenties
- Good prognosis
- Also known as *spastic colon, spastic colitis,* and *mucous colitis*

Pathophysiology
- It involves a change in bowel motility, reflecting an abnormality in the neuromuscular control of intestinal smooth muscle.

Causes
- Exact cause unknown
- Anxiety and stress
- Dietary factors, such as fiber, raw fruits, coffee, alcohol, and foods that are cold, highly seasoned, or laxative in nature

OTHER POSSIBLE TRIGGERS
- Hormones
- Laxative abuse
- Allergy to certain foods or drugs
- Lactose intolerance

Incidence
- Occurs mostly in women, with symptoms first emerging before age 40

Common characteristics
- Chronic constipation or diarrhea
- Lower abdominal pain

Complications
- Diverticulitis and colon cancer
- Chronic inflammatory bowel disease

✳ ASSESSMENT

History
- Chronic constipation, diarrhea, or both
- Lower abdominal pain (typically in the left lower quadrant) usually relieved by defecation or passage of gas
- Stools are small with visible mucus or small, pasty, and pencil-like stools instead of diarrhea
- Dyspepsia
- Abdominal bloating
- Heartburn
- Faintness and weakness
- Contributing psychological factors, such as a recent stressful life change, that may have triggered or aggravated symptoms
- Anxiety and fatigue

Physical findings
- Normal bowel sounds
- Tympany over a gas-filled bowel

Test results
- Assessment involves studies to rule out other, more serious disorders.

LABORATORY
- Stool examination is negative for occult blood, parasites, and pathogenic bacteria.
- Complete blood count, serologic tests, serum albumin, and erythrocyte sedimentation rate are normal.

IMAGING
- Barium enema may reveal colonic spasm and a tubular appearance of the descending colon. It's also used to rule out certain other disorders, such as diverticula, tumors, and polyps.

DIAGNOSTIC PROCEDURES
- Sigmoidoscopy may disclose spastic contractions.

◆ TREATMENT

General
- Stress management
- Lifestyle modifications

Diet
- Based on the patient's symptoms
- Initially, an elimination diet
- Avoidance of sorbitol, nonabsorbable carbohydrates, and lactose-containing foods
- Increased dietary bulk
- Increased fluid intake

Activity
- Regular exercise

Medication
- Anticholinergic, antispasmodic drugs
- Antidiarrheals
- Laxatives
- Antiemetics
- Simethicone
- Mild tranquilizers
- Tricyclic antidepressants

☘ NURSING CONSIDERATIONS

Nursing diagnoses
- Acute pain
- Constipation
- Deficient knowledge (irritable bowel syndrome)
- Diarrhea
- Disturbed body image
- Ineffective coping

Key outcomes
The patient will:
- express feelings of increased comfort and decreased pain
- achieve normal bowel function
- demonstrate understanding of the disease process and treatment regimen
- maintain adequate caloric intake
- express positive feelings about self
- exhibit effective coping behaviors.

Nursing interventions
- Because the patient with irritable bowel syndrome isn't hospitalized, nursing interventions almost always focus on patient teaching.

Monitoring
- Weight
- Diet
- Bowel movements

▶ PATIENT TEACHING

Be sure to cover:
- disorder, diagnostic tests, and treatment
- dietary plans and implementation
- need to drink 8 to 10 glasses of water or other compatible fluids daily
- medication administration, dosage, and possible adverse effects
- need to implement lifestyle changes that reduce stress
- smoking cessation
- need for regular physical examinations. (For patients older than age 40, emphasize the need for colorectal cancer screening, including annual proctosigmoidoscopy and rectal examinations.)

✸ RESOURCES

Organizations
Digestive Disease National Coalition: *www.ddnc.org*
National Digestive Diseases Information Clearinghouse: *www.niddk.nih.gov/health/digest/nddic.htm*

Selected references
Bruno, M. "Irritable Bowel Syndrome and Inflammatory Bowel Disease in Pregnancy," *Journal of Perinatal & Neonatal Nursing* 18(4):341-50, October-December 2004.

Handbook of Diseases, 3rd ed. Philadelphia: Lippincott Williams & Wilkins 2004.

McNally, P. *GI/Liver Secrets,* 3rd ed. Philadelphia: Hanley & Belfus, Inc., 2006.

Tierney, L., et al. *Current Medical Diagnosis and Treatment 2006.* New York: McGraw-Hill Book Co., 2006.

Watson, A.R., and Bowling, T.E. "Irritable Bowel Syndrome: Diagnosis and Bowel Management," *British Journal of Community Nursing* 10(3):118-22, March 2005.

Juvenile rheumatoid arthritis

Description
- Several conditions characterized by chronic synovitis and joint swelling, pain, and tenderness
- Major types: systemic (Still's disease or acute febrile type), polyarticular, and pauciarticular

Pathophysiology
- If juvenile rheumatoid arthritis (JRA) isn't arrested, the inflammatory process in the joints occurs in four stages:
  - Synovitis develops from congestion and edema of the synovial membrane and joint capsule.
  - Pannus covers and invades cartilage and eventually destroys the joint capsule and bone.
  - Fibrous tissue and ankylosis occludes the joint space.
  - Fibrous tissue calcifies, resulting in bony ankylosis and total immobility.

Causes
- Suggested link to genetic factors or an abnormal immune response
- Viral or bacterial (streptococcal) infection, trauma, and emotional stress

Incidence
- May occur as early as age 6 weeks but seldom before age 6 months; peak onset between ages 1 and 3 and 8 and 12
- Occurs in estimated 150,000 to 250,000 children in United States; affects twice as many girls as boys

Common characteristics
- Joint stiffness in the morning

Complications
- Flexion contractures
- Ocular damage and loss of vision

History
- Common complaint of joint stiffness in morning or after periods of inactivity
- Young children with JRA typically irritable and listless

Physical findings
SYSTEMIC JRA
- Mild, transient arthritis or frank polyarthritis with fever and rash
- Behavior that may clearly suggest joint pain and fatigue
- Painful breathing and nonspecific abdominal pain
- Fatigue, shortness of breath, palpitations, and fever
- Resting or exertional tachycardia; arrhythmias; neck vein distention; heart murmurs
- Hepatic, splenic, and lymph node enlargement
- Friction rub associated with pericarditis

POLYARTICULAR JRA
- Pain in the wrists, elbows, knees, ankles, and small joints of the hands and feet
- Pain in larger joints, including the temporomandibular, cervical spine, hips, and shoulders
- Tenderness, stiffness, and swelling of joints
- Possible low-grade fever with daily peaks
- Weight loss
- Noticeable developmental retardation
- Hepatic, splenic, and lymph node enlargement
- Subcutaneous nodules on the elbows or heels

PAUCIARTICULAR JRA
- Pain in the hips, knees, heels, feet, ankles, and elbows
- Eye redness, blurred vision, and photophobia
- Lower back pain

Test results
LABORATORY
- Serum hemoglobin levels are decreased and neutrophil (neutrophilia) and platelet (thrombocytosis) levels are increased; other results include an elevated erythrocyte sedimentation rate and elevated C-reactive protein, serum haptoglobin, immunoglobulin, and C3 complement levels.
- Antinuclear antibody test is positive in patients with polyarticular JRA and in those with pauciarticular JRA with chronic iridocyclitis.
- Rheumatoid factor (RF) appears in about 15% of patients with JRA; in contrast, about 85% of patients with RA test positive for RF; patients with polyarticular JRA may test positive for RF.
- Human leukocyte antigen-B27 forecasts later development of ankylosing spondylitis.

IMAGING
- X-ray studies demonstrate early structural changes associated with JRA. These include soft-tissue swelling, effusion, and periostitis in affected joints. Later evidence includes osteoporosis and accelerated bone growth followed by subchondral erosions, joint-space narrowing, bone destruction, and fusion.

◆ TREATMENT

General
- Physical therapy
- Splints
- Heat application during passive exercises

Diet
- No restrictions
- Adequate iron, protein, calcium, and caloric intake

Activity
- As tolerated

Medication
- Aspirin
- Nonsteroidal anti-inflammatory drugs (NSAIDs)
- Gold salts
- Hydroxychloroquine
- Penicillamine
- Low-dose cytotoxic agents
- Monoclonal antibodies

Surgery
- Soft-tissue releases to improve mobility
- Joint replacement (delayed until child matures physically and can tolerate vigorous rehabilitation)

❖ NURSING CONSIDERATIONS

Nursing diagnoses
- Activity intolerance
- Chronic pain
- Compromised family coping
- Delayed growth and development
- Dressing or grooming self-care deficit
- Fatigue
- Impaired physical mobility
- Ineffective coping
- Ineffective role performance
- Powerlessness
- Risk for injury

Key outcomes
The patient and family will:
- demonstrate measures to balance activity and rest
- express feelings of increased comfort and decreased pain
- use age-appropriate skills and behaviors as much as possible
- participate in self-care activities to the fullest extent possible
- express feelings of increased energy
- attain optimal mobility
- demonstrate effective coping behaviors
- verbalize feelings related to changes in roles and functions
- recognize and express feelings about limitations due to illness
- remain free from injury.

Nursing interventions
- Focus nursing care on reducing pain and promoting mobility.
- During inflammatory exacerbations, administer NSAIDs or prescribed medication on a regular schedule.
- Allow the patient to rest frequently throughout the day to conserve energy for times when she must be mobile.
- Arrange the patient's environment for participation in activities of daily living so that she feels capable of accomplishing tasks.

Monitoring
- Pain level
- Response to treatment
- Signs and symptoms of bleeding
- Nutritional status
- Joint mobility
- Adverse drug reactions

▶ PATIENT TEACHING

Be sure to cover:
- disorder, diagnostic tests, and treatment
- need to encourage the child to be as independent as possible
- need for regular slit-lamp examinations to enable early diagnosis and treatment of iridocyclitis
- signs and symptoms of bleeding caused by aspirin or NSAID therapy; and instructions to take with meals or milk to reduce adverse GI reactions
- signs and symptoms of exacerbation, and the need to notify the pediatrician about these symptoms
- need for proper nutrition and caloric consumption
- child's special needs (teachers and the school principal should be notified).

Discharge planning
- Consult an occupational therapist to assess the patient's home care needs.

✷ RESOURCES

Organizations
American Academy of Pediatrics: *www.aap.org*
Arthritis Foundation: *www.arthritis.org*

Selective references
Kasper, D.L., et al., eds. *Harrison's Principles of Internal Medicine*, 16th ed. New York: McGraw-Hill Book Co., 2005.

Mason, T.G., and Reed, A.M. "Update in Juvenile Rheumatoid Arthritis," *Arthritis and Rheumatism* 53(5):795-99, October 2005.

The Merck Manual of Diagnosis & Therapy, 18th ed. Whitehouse Station, N.J.: Merck & Co., Inc., 2006.

Phelan, J.D., et al. "Susceptibility to JRA/JHA: Complementing General Autoimmune and Arthritis Traits," *Genes and Immunity* 7(1):1-10, January 2006.

Schikler, K.N. "Growth Hormone Therapy in Juvenile Arthritis: Importance of Classification," *Journal of Pediatrics* 145(3):423-24, September 2004.

Kaposi's sarcoma

● OVERVIEW

Description
- Most common acquired immunodeficiency syndrome (AIDS)-related cancer
- Characterized by obvious, colorful lesions
- Most common internal sites: lungs and GI tract (esophagus, oropharynx, and epiglottis)

Pathophysiology
- Kaposi's sarcoma causes structural and functional damage.
- When associated with AIDS, it progresses aggressively, involving the lymph nodes, the viscera, and, possibly, GI structures.

Causes
- Exact cause unknown

Risk factors
- Immunosuppression
- Genetic or hereditary predisposition

Incidence
- Originally affected 35% of AIDS patients; now declining with earlier detection of AIDS
- Possibly more common in middle-aged and older Mediterranean, Eastern European, and Jewish men

Common characteristics
- History of AIDS
- Lesions of various shapes, sizes, and colors

Complications
- Severe pulmonary involvement, resulting in respiratory distress
- GI involvement, leading to digestive problems

✳ ASSESSMENT

History
- Possible history of AIDS
- Pain (in advanced cases)

Physical findings
- Several lesions of various shapes, sizes, and colors (ranging from red-brown to dark purple) on the skin, buccal mucosa, hard and soft palates, lips, gums, tongue, tonsils, conjunctiva, and sclera (the most common sites)
- In advanced disease, lesions that may merge, becoming one large plaque
- Untreated lesions that may appear as large, ulcerative masses
- Dyspnea
- Edema from lymphatic obstruction
- Wheezing and hypoventilation

Test results
DIAGNOSTIC PROCEDURES
- Tissue biopsy shows the type and stage of the lesion. (See *Laubenstein's stages in Kaposi's sarcoma*.)

LAUBENSTEIN'S STAGES IN KAPOSI'S SARCOMA

L.J. Laubenstein proposed this staging system to evaluate and treat patients with acquired immunodeficiency syndrome and Kaposi's sarcoma:
- Stage I—locally indolent cutaneous lesions
- Stage II—locally aggressive cutaneous lesions
- Stage III—mucocutaneous lesions and lymph node involvement
- Stage IV—visceral involvement.

  Within each stage, a patient may have different symptoms further classified as stage subtype A or B, which are:
- Subtype A—no systemic signs or symptoms
- Subtype B—one or more systemic signs and symptoms, including 10% weight loss, fever of unknown origin that exceeds 100° F (37.8° C) for longer than 2 weeks, chills, lethargy, night sweats, anorexia, and diarrhea.

◆ TREATMENT

General
- Radiation therapy for palliation of symptoms (pain from obstructing lesions in the oral cavity or extremities and edema caused by lymphatic blockage); also for cosmetic improvement

Diet
- High-calorie, high-protein
- Small meals

Activity
- Limited activity
- Frequent rest periods

Medication
- Chemotherapy
- Biological response modifier

Surgery
- Removal of lesion from skin (especially if lesion is small), using local excision, electrodesiccation and curettage, or cryotherapy

Nursing diagnoses
- Acute pain
- Anxiety
- Disturbed body image
- Fatigue
- Fear
- Grieving
- Imbalanced nutrition: Less than body requirements
- Impaired gas exchange
- Impaired skin integrity
- Ineffective breathing pattern
- Ineffective coping
- Risk for infection

Key outcomes
The patient will:
- report feelings of increased comfort and decreased pain
- express feelings and concerns about condition and potential loss
- express positive feelings about self
- verbalize an increase in energy
- verbalize fears and concerns
- maintain weight
- maintain adequate ventilation and oxygenation
- remain free from skin breakdown
- maintain an effective breathing pattern
- demonstrate effective coping mechanisms
- remain free from signs and symptoms of further infection.

Nursing interventions
- Encourage verbalization and offer support.
- Inspect the skin for new lesions and skin breakdown.
- Administer medications, as ordered.
- Provide rest periods.

Monitoring
- Adverse effects of treatment
- Vital signs
- Pain control
- Nutritional status
- Respiratory status

Be sure to cover:
- disorder, diagnostic tests, and treatment
- medication administration, dosage, and possible adverse effects
- infection prevention techniques and, if necessary, basic hygiene measures to prevent infection (especially if the patient also has AIDS)
- need for ongoing treatment and care.

Discharge planning
- Refer the patient to resource and support services.
- Arrange for referral for home-health care or hospice care, as indicated.

Organizations
American Cancer Society: *www.cancer.org*
Guide to Internet Resources for Cancer: *www.cancerindex.org*
National Cancer Institute: *www.nci.nih.gov*

Selected references
Casciato, D.A. *Manual of Clinical Oncology,* 5th ed. Philadelphia: Lippincott Williams & Wilkins, 2004.
Gutmann-Yassky, E., et al. "Classic Kaposi Sarcoma," *Cancer* 106(2):413-19, January 2006.

Keratitis

Description
- Infection of the cornea
- Usually affects only one eye
- May be acute or chronic

Pathophysiology
- Inflammation of the cornea results from corneal infection.
- Inflammation may be deep or superficial.

Causes
- Viral, bacterial, or fungal infection
- Tear deficiency
- Denervation
- Immune reactions
- Ischemia
- Trauma
- Congenital syphilis

Incidence
- Fairly common
- May develop at any age

Common characteristics
- Photophobia
- Pain
- Lacrimation

Complications
- Blindness
- Corneal scarring or perforation

History
- Recent upper respiratory tract infection, accompanied by cold sores
- Eye pain
- Central vision loss
- Sensitivity to light
- Sensation of a foreign body in eye
- Blurred vision

Physical findings
- Cornea that lacks normal luster
- Characteristic branched lesion of the cornea with herpes simplex virus type 1

Test results
DIAGNOSTIC PROCEDURES
- Slit-lamp examination with sodium fluorescein staining may show corneal inflammation or abrasion; small branchlike (dendritic) lesions indicate possible herpes simplex virus infection.

General
- Eye shield or patch

Diet
- No restrictions

Activity
- No restrictions

Medication
ACUTE DENDRITIC KERATITIS
- Trifluridine eyedrops
- Vidarabine therapy
- Broad-spectrum antibiotic
CHRONIC DENDRITIC KERATITIS
- Vidarabine therapy
- Possible long-term topical therapy
FUNGAL KERATITIS
- Natamycin

Surgery
- Corneal transplantation for severe ulcerations with residual scarring

Nursing diagnoses
- Acute pain
- Disturbed sensory perception: Visual
- Ineffective health maintenance
- Risk for infection
- Risk for injury

Key outcomes
The patient will:
- express feelings of increased comfort and decreased pain
- regain visual function
- maintain current health status
- remain free from signs and symptoms of infection or injury.

Nursing interventions
◈ **NURSING ALERT** Watch for keratitis in patients predisposed to cold sores. Corneal infection is commonly caused by a virus, such as adenovirus or herpes simplex—the same viruses that cause cold sores. Be sure to tell patients never to put their fingers to their eyes after touching their mouths.
- Wear gloves when in contact with eyes or ocular drainage with herpes simplex virus.
- Apply warm compresses.
- Dim the lights in case of photophobia.
- Administer medications, as ordered.

Monitoring
- Response to treatment
- Visual acuity

Be sure to cover:
- disorder, diagnostic tests, and treatment
- medication administration, dosage, and possible adverse effects
- how stress, traumatic injury, fever, colds, and sun overexposure can trigger flare-up of keratitis
- wearing sunglasses for photophobia
- meticulous hand washing
- preventing spread of infection.

Discharge planning
- Refer the patient to an ophthalmologist, as indicated.

Organizations
American Academy of Ophthalmology: *www.eyenet.org*
National Eye Institute: *www.nei.nih.gov*

Selected references
Gagnon, M.R., and Walter, K.A. "A Case of Acanthamoeba Keratitis as a Result of a Cosmetic Contact Lens," *Eye & Contact Lens* 32(1):37-38, January 2006.

Parmar, P., et al. "Microbial Keratitis at Extremes of Age," *Cornea* 25(2):153-58, February 2006.

Sun, X., et al. "Acanthamoeba Keratitis Clinical Characteristics and Management," *Ophthalmology* 113(3):412-16, March 2006.

Kidney cancer

● OVERVIEW

Description
- Proliferation of cancer cells in the kidney
- 85% originating in kidneys; 15% metastasizing from various primary-site carcinomas
- Also called *nephrocarcinoma, renal carcinoma, hypernephroma,* and *Grawitz's tumor*
- Kidney cancer may affect either kidney; occasionally tumors are bilateral or multifocal.
- The prognosis is better for patients with the clear cell type than for the other types; in general, however, the prognosis depends more on the cancer's stage than on its type. The overall prognosis has improved considerably, with the 5-year survival rate about 50%.

Pathophysiology
- Most kidney tumors are large, firm, nodular, encapsulated, unilateral, and solitary, arising from the tubular epithelium.
- Tumor margins are usually clearly defined.
- Tumors can include areas of ischemia, necrosis, and focal hemorrhage.
- Tumor cells may be well differentiated to anaplastic.
- Kidney cancer can be separated histologically into clear cell, granular cell, and spindle cell types.

Causes
- Exact cause unknown

Risk factors
- Heavy cigarette smoking
- Regular hemodialysis treatments
- Obesity
- Occupational exposure to petroleum products, asbestos, or heavy metals

Incidence
- Twice as common in men as in women
- More common after age 40
- Renal pelvic tumors and Wilms' tumor most common in children

Common characteristics
- Hematuria
- Flank pain

Complications
- Hemorrhage
- Metastasis

✳ ASSESSMENT

History
- Hematuria
- Dull, aching flank pain
- Weight loss (rare)
- Fever
- Night sweats

Physical findings
- Palpable smooth, firm, nontender abdominal mass
- Gross hematuria
- Hypertension
- Supraclavicular adenopathy

Test results
LABORATORY
- Alkaline phosphatase, bilirubin, and transaminase levels are increased.
- Prothrombin time is prolonged.
IMAGING
- Renal ultrasonography and computed tomography scan can be used to verify renal cancer.
- Excretory urography, nephrotomography, and kidney-ureter-bladder radiography are used to aid diagnosis and help in staging.

◆ TREATMENT

General
- Because of radiation resistance, radiation used only when cancer has spread into perinephric region or lymph nodes or when primary tumor or metastatic sites can't be completely excised

Diet
- Low-protein

Activity
- Postoperatively, no heavy lifting or contact sports for 6 to 8 weeks

Medication
- Chemotherapy
- Biotherapy with lymphokine-activated killer cells plus recombinant interleukin-2
- Interferon

Surgery
- Radical nephrectomy, with or without regional lymph node dissection

❖ NURSING CONSIDERATIONS

Nursing diagnoses
- Acute pain
- Anxiety
- Deficient knowledge (cancer and treatment)
- Fear
- Impaired physical mobility
- Ineffective breathing pattern
- Ineffective tissue perfusion: Renal
- Risk for imbalanced fluid volume
- Risk for injury

Key outcomes
The patient will:
- express feelings of increased comfort and decreased pain and anxiety
- demonstrate a decrease in anxiety
- communicate understanding of medical regimen, medications, diet, and activity restrictions
- verbalize fears and concerns openly
- maintain joint mobility and range of motion
- maintain adequate ventilation and oxygenation
- exhibit signs of adequate renal perfusion
- maintain adequate fluid balance
- remain free from injury.

Nursing interventions
- Administer medications, as ordered.
- Encourage verbalization and provide support.

Monitoring
- Wound site
- Intake and output
- Complete blood count; serum chemistry results
- Pain control

▶ PATIENT TEACHING

Be sure to cover:
- disorder, diagnostic tests, and treatment
- medication administration, dosage, and possible adverse effects
- need for a healthy, well-balanced diet and regular exercise
- importance of checking with the physician before taking vitamins or other dietary supplements
- importance of follow-up care.

Discharge planning
Refer the patient to:
- support services
- weight reduction program, if indicated
- smoking-cessation program, if indicated.

✳ RESOURCES

Organizations
American Cancer Society: *www.cancer.org*
Guide to Internet Resources for Cancer: *www.cancerindex.org*
National Cancer Institute: *www.nci.nih.gov*
National Institute of Diabetes and Digestive and Kidney Diseases: *www.niddk.nih.gov*

Selected references
Atlas of Pathophysiology, 2nd ed. Philadelphia: Lippincott Williams & Wilkins, 2005.
Galli, B., et al. "Laparoscopic Radical Nephrectomy in Renal Cell Carcinoma," *Urologic Nursing* 25(2):83-86, April 2005.
Weiss, R.H., and Lin, P.Y. "Kidney Cancer: Identification of Novel Targets for Therapy," *Kidney International* 69(2):224-32, January 2005.
Weizer, A.Z., et al. "Complications after Percutaneous Radiofrequency Ablation of Renal Tumors," *Urology* 66(6):1176-180, December 2005.

Labyrinthitis

● OVERVIEW

Description
- Inflammation of the labyrinth of the inner ear
- Typically produces severe vertigo with head movement and sensorineural hearing loss
- Viral labyrinthitis most prevalent form

Pathophysiology
- Lesion within vestibular pathways (inner ear to cerebral cortex) results in an imbalance in the vestibular system.

Causes
- Viral or bacterial infections
- Cholesteatoma
- Drug toxicity
- Head injury
- Tumor
- Vasculitis

Incidence
- Affects all ages beyond infancy
- Affects males and females equally

Common characteristics
- Severe vertigo with head movement
- Nausea and vomiting
- Sensorineural hearing loss

Complications
- Meningitis
- Permanent balance disability
- Permanent hearing loss

✳ ASSESSMENT

History
- Severe vertigo from any movement of the head
- Nausea and vomiting
- Unilateral or bilateral hearing loss
- Recent upper respiratory tract infection
- Loss of balance and falling in the direction of the affected ear

Physical findings
- Spontaneous nystagmus
- Jerking movements of eyes toward unaffected ear
- Purulent drainage

Test results
LABORATORY
- Culture and sensitivity tests show the infecting organism.
IMAGING
- Computed tomography scan rules out brain lesion.
DIAGNOSTIC PROCEDURES
- Audiometric testing reveals sensorineural hearing loss.
- A flat tympanogram may suggest fluid in the middle ear, a perforated tympanic membrane, or impacted cerumen. Fluctuations on the tympanogram, synchronous with the patient's pulse, suggest a glomangioma in the middle ear.
- Electronystagmography may show decreased velocity from one side that indicates hypofunction or canal paresis. An inability to induce nystagmus with ice water denotes a dead labyrinth.

◆ TREATMENT

General
- Based on relieving symptoms

Diet
- Increased oral fluids

Activity
- During acute attacks, bed rest in darkened room with head immobilized between pillows

Medication
- Meclizine to relieve vertigo
- Antiemetics
- Antibiotics
- I.V. fluids for severe dehydration

Surgery
- Surgical excision of cholesteatoma
- Drainage of middle and inner ear infected areas
- Labyrinthectomy

❖ NURSING CONSIDERATIONS

Nursing diagnoses
- Activity intolerance
- Anxiety
- Deficient knowledge (labyrinthitis)
- Disturbed sensory perception: Auditory
- Fear
- Risk for deficient fluid volume
- Risk for infection
- Risk for injury

Key outcomes
The patient will:
- perform activities of daily living to the fullest extent possible
- express feelings of increased comfort and decreaed anxiety
- verbalize understanding of the condition and treatment
- regain hearing or develop other means of communication
- verbalize fears and concerns openly
- maintain normal fluid volume
- remain free from signs and symptoms of infection
- remain free from injury or harm.

Nursing interventions
- Encourage expression of concerns about hearing loss.
- Offer the patient reassurance when appropriate.
- Maintain bed rest in a darkened room with his head immobilized during acute attacks.
- Administer medications, as ordered.
- Encourage oral fluid intake.

PATIENT WITH HEARING LOSS
- Give clear, concise explanations.
- Face him when speaking.
- Enunciate words clearly, slowly, and in a normal tone.
- Allow adequate time to grasp what's said.
- Provide a pencil and paper to aid communication.
- Alert staff to communication problem.
- Assist with ambulation, as needed.

Monitoring
- Response to medication
- Vital signs
- Signs of dehydration
- Intake and output
- Auditory acuity
- Complications

▶ PATIENT TEACHING

Be sure to cover:
- disorder, diagnostic tests, and treatment
- limitation of activities to avoid danger from vertigo
- recovery time (up to 6 weeks)
- prompt treatment of upper respiratory tract and systemic infections
- controlling use of salicylates and other potentially toxic substances
- medication administration, dosage, and possible adverse effects
- preoperative and postoperative instructions, as indicated
- management of labyrinthitis. (See *Managing labyrinthitis.*)

Discharge planning
- Refer the patient to support services and community assistance

✴ RESOURCES

Organizations
American Academy of Otolaryngology-Head and Neck Surgery: *www.sinuscarecenter.com/AAOHNS.htm*
The Vestibular Disorders Association: *www.vestibular.org*

Selected references
Barreire, S.O. "Spin Cycle: Evaluation and Management of Dizziness and Vertigo," *Advance for Nurse Practitioners* 13(3):22-27, March 2005.
Trinidad, A., et al. "Labyrinthitis Secondary to Experimental Otitis Media," *American Journal of Otolaryngology* 26(4):226-29, July-August 2005.
Westerlaan, H.E., et al. "Labyrinthitis Ossificans Associated with Sensorineural Deafness," *Ear, Nose & Throat Journal* 84(1):14-15, January 2005.

MANAGING LABYRINTHITIS

- Tell the patient to avoid sudden position changes.
- Help the patient assess how much this disability will affect his daily life.
- Work with the patient to identify hazards in the home, such as throw rugs and dark stairways.
- Discuss the patient's anxieties and concerns about vertigo attacks and decreased hearing.
- Stress the importance of maintaining and resuming normal diversions or social activities when balance disturbance is absent.

Laryngeal cancer

● OVERVIEW

Description
- Cancer of the larynx or voice box
- Squamous cell carcinoma most common form (95% of cases)
- Adenocarcinoma and sarcoma rare (5% of cases)
- May be intrinsic (located on the true vocal cords; tends not to spread because underlying connective tissues lack lymph nodes) or extrinsic (located on another part of the larynx; tends to spread easily)

Pathophysiology
- Laryngeal cancer is classified by its location:
  - supraglottic (on the false vocal cords)
  - glottic (on the true vocal cords)
  - subglottic (rare downward extension from the vocal cords).
- Malignant cells that proliferate can cause swallowing and breathing impairment.
- A tumor can decrease mobility of the vocal cords.

Causes
- Exact cause unknown

Risk factors
- Smoking
- Alcoholism
- Chronic inhalation of noxious fumes
- Familial disposition
- History of gastroesophageal reflux disease

Incidence
- About nine times more common in men than women
- Most victims between ages 50 and 65

Common characteristics
INTRINSIC LARYNGEAL CANCER
- Hoarseness lasting longer than 3 weeks
EXTRINSIC LARYNGEAL CANCER
- Lump in the throat
- Pain or burning of the throat when drinking hot liquid or citrus drinks
WITH METASTASIS
- Dysphagia
- Dyspnea
- Cough
- Pain, most often radiating to the ear
- Enlarged cervical lymph nodes

Complications
- Increased swallowing difficulty and pain
- Metastasis

✳ ASSESSMENT

History
STAGE I
- Complaints of local throat irritation
- 2-week history of hoarseness
STAGES II AND III
- Hoarseness
- Sore throat
- Voice volume reduced to whisper
STAGE IV
- Pain radiating to ears
- Dysphagia
- Dyspnea

Physical findings
STAGE I
- None
STAGE II
- Possible abnormal movement of vocal cords
STAGE III
- Abnormal movement of vocal cords; possible lymphadenopathy
STAGE IV
- Neck mass or enlarged cervical nodes

Test results
IMAGING
- Xeroradiography, laryngeal tomography, computed tomography scan, and laryngography confirm the presence of a mass.
- Chest X-ray rules out metastasis.
DIAGNOSTIC PROCEDURES
- Laryngoscopy allows definitive staging by obtaining multiple biopsy specimens to establish a primary diagnosis, to determine the extent of the disease, and to identify additional premalignant lesions or second primaries.
- Biopsy identifies cancer cells.

◆ TREATMENT

General
- Precancerous lesions—laser surgery
- Early lesions—laser surgery or radiation therapy
- Advanced lesions—radiation therapy and chemotherapy
- Speech preservation
- Speech rehabilitation (when speech preservation impossible)—esophageal speech, prosthetic devices, or experimental surgical reconstruction of the voice box

Diet
- Based on treatment options
- May require enteral feeding

Activity
- No restrictions
- Frequent rest periods

Medication
- Chemotherapeutic agents
- Analgesics

Surgery
- Cordectomy
- Partial or total laryngectomy
- Supraglottic laryngectomy or total laryngectomy with laryngoplasty

❖ NURSING CONSIDERATIONS

Nursing diagnoses
- Acute pain
- Disturbed body image
- Fear
- Impaired gas exchange
- Impaired swallowing
- Impaired verbal communication
- Ineffective airway clearance
- Ineffective coping
- Risk for infection

Key outcomes
The patient will:
- report feeling less tension or pain
- express positive feelings about body image
- recognize and express feelings about limitations due to illness
- maintain adequate ventilation and oxygenation
- demonstrate ability to swallow without coughing or choking
- use an appropriate method to communicate effectively
- maintain a patent airway
- demonstrate appropriate coping mechanisms
- remain free from signs and symptoms of infection.

Nursing interventions
- Provide supportive psychological, preoperative, and postoperative care.
- Encourage verbalization and provide support.
- Assist with establishing a method of communication.
- Prepare patient for functional losses (inability to smell, blow his nose, whistle, gargle, sip, or suck on a straw).
- Provide frequent mouth care.
- Suction when needed.
- After total laryngectomy, elevate the head of the bed 30 to 45 degrees and support the back of the neck to prevent tension on sutures and, possibly, wound dehiscence.

Monitoring
AFTER PARTIAL LARYNGECTOMY
- Hydration and nutritional status
- Tracheostomy tube care
- Use of voice

AFTER TOTAL LARYNGECTOMY
- Laryngectomy tube care
- Vital signs
- Postoperative complications
- Pain control
- Nasogastric (NG) tube placement and function

▶ PATIENT TEACHING

Be sure to cover:
- disorder, diagnostic tests, and treatment
- appropriate oral hygiene practices (before partial or total laryngectomy)
- postoperative procedures, such as suctioning, NG tube feeding, and laryngectomy tube care
- preparation for any functional losses.

Discharge planning
- Arrange for rehabilitation measures (including laryngeal speech, esophageal speech, an artificial larynx, and various mechanical devices).
- Refer the patient to resource and support services.

✵ RESOURCES

Organizations
American Cancer Society: *www.cancer.org*
Guide to Internet Resources for Cancer: *www.cancerindex.org*
International Association of Laryngectomees: *www.larynxlink.com*
National Cancer Institute: *www.nci.nih.gov*

Selected references
Atlas of Pathophysiology, 2nd ed. Philadelphia: Lippincott Williams & Wilkins, 2005.

Bianco, A.J., and Chao, C. "Management of Radiation-Induced Head and Neck Injury," *Cancer Treatment and Research* 128:23-41, 2006.

Dias, F.L. "Therapeutic Options in Advanced Laryngeal Cancer: An Overview," *ORT Journal* 67(6):311-18, December 2005.

Garavello, W., et al. "Type of Alcoholic Beverage and the Risk for Laryngeal Cancer," *European Journal of Cancer Prevention* 15(1):69-73, February 2006.

Nishike, S., et al. "Laryngeal Tuberculosis Following Laryngeal Carcinoma," *Journal of Laryngology and Otology* 120(2):151-53, February 2006.

Laryngitis

Description
- Common acute or chronic inflammation of vocal cords
- Isolated infection or part of a generalized bacterial or viral upper respiratory tract infection
- Typical viral infection mild, with limited duration
- Inflammatory changes caused by repeated attacks (associated with chronic laryngitis)

Pathophysiology
- Inflammatory response to cell damage by viruses results in hyperemia and fluid exudation.
- Irritant receptors are triggered.
- Kinins and other inflammatory mediators may induce spasm of upper airway smooth muscle.

  ✳ **AGE-RELATED CONCERN** Developmental differences in the upper airway structures of young children may result in severe narrowing of the upper airways with inflammation, to the degree that respiratory failure may result from hypoventilation.

Causes
- Infection
- Overuse of the voice
- Inhalation of smoke or fumes
- Aspiration of caustic chemicals
- Chronic laryngitis
- Chronic upper respiratory tract disorders
- Mouth breathing
- Smoking
- Constant exposure to dust or other irritants
- Alcohol abuse
- Gastroesophageal reflux
- Reflux esophagitis

Incidence
- Affects all ages
- Affects males and females equally

Common characteristics
- Hoarseness
- Dry cough

Complications
- Chronic hoarseness
- Permanent laryngeal tissue changes
- Airway obstruction

✱ ASSESSMENT

History
- Hoarseness ranging from mild to complete loss of voice
- Feeling of throat rawness
- Throat pain
- Dry cough
- Malaise
- Difficulty swallowing

Physical findings
- Cough
- Fever
- Regional lymphadenopathy
- Stridor (in children)

Test results
LABORATORY
- White blood cell count is elevated (in bacterial infection).

DIAGNOSTIC PROCEDURES
- Indirect laryngoscopy reveals red, inflamed and, occasionally, hemorrhagic vocal cords exudate.

◆ TREATMENT

General
- Symptom-based
- Elimination of underlying cause
- Resting the voice (primary treatment)
- Humidification
- Avoidance of smoking
- Avoidance of whispering

Diet
- No restrictions
- Cold fluids

Activity
- Rest during febrile period, with head of bed elevated

Medication
- Analgesics
- Throat lozenges
- Antibiotics (bacterial infection)
- Systemic corticosteroids

Surgery
- Tracheotomy with chronic laryngitis

✤ NURSING CONSIDERATIONS

Nursing diagnoses
- Acute pain
- Anxiety
- Deficient knowledge (laryngitis)
- Fatigue
- Fear
- Impaired verbal communication
- Ineffective airway clearance
- Ineffective breathing pattern
- Risk for aspiration
- Risk for infection

Key outcomes
The patient will:
- express feelings of increased comfort and decreased pain
- demonstrate a decrease in anxiety
- express understanding of the condition and treatment
- demonstrate measures to balance activity and rest
- verbalize fears and concerns openly
- exhibit appropriate means for effective communication
- maintain a patent airway
- exhibit an adequate breathing pattern
- remain free from signs of infection
- remain free of signs and symptoms of aspiration.

Nursing interventions
- Encourage discussion of concerns.
- Keep tracheotomy tray at bedside.
- Encourage modification of predisposing factors.
- Restrict verbal communication.
- Provide alternative communication means.
- Anticipate needs.
- Administer medications, as ordered.

Monitoring
- Response to treatment
- Respiratory status

◈ **NURSING ALERT** With severe, acute laryngitis, monitor the patient for signs and symptoms of airway obstruction.

▶ PATIENT TEACHING

Be sure to cover:
- disorder, diagnostic tests, and treatment
- why the patient shouldn't talk
- alternate methods of communication
- speaking softly rather than whispering
- maintenance of adequate humidification
- smoking cessation
- medication administration, dosage, and possible adverse effects
- importance of completing prescribed antibiotics
- avoidance of occupational hazards.

Discharge planning
- Refer the patient to a smoking cessation program, if indicated.
- Refer the patient to voice retraining, as needed.

✱ RESOURCES

Organizations
Johns Hopkins Center for Laryngeal and Voice Disorders-Laryngitis: *www.med.jhu.edu/voice/laryngitis.html*
National Institute of Allergy and Infectious Diseases: *www.niaid.nih.gov*

Selected references
Beaver, M.E., et al. "Acute Ulcerative Laryngitis," *Ear, Nose & Throat Journal* 84(5):268, May 2005.
Ebell, M.H. "Antibiotics for Acute Laryngitis in Adults," *American Family Physician* 72(1):76-77, July 2005.
Savoy, N.B. "Differentiating Stridor in Children at Triage: It's Not Always Croup," *Journal of Emergency Nursing* 31(5):503-505, October 2005.

Latex allergy

● OVERVIEW

Description
- An immunoglobulin (Ig) E-mediated immediate hypersensitivity reaction to products that contain natural latex
- Can range from local dermatitis to life-threatening anaphylactic reaction

Pathophysiology
- Mast cells release histamine and other secretory products in response to contact with latex-containing products.
- Vascular permeability increases, and vasodilation and bronchoconstriction occur.
- Chemical sensitivity dermatitis is a type IV delayed hypersensitivity reaction to the chemicals used in the processing rather than to the latex itself.
- In a cell-mediated allergic reaction, sensitized T lymphocytes are triggered, stimulating the proliferation of other lymphocytes and mononuclear cells, resulting in tissue inflammation and contact dermatitis.

Causes
- Frequent contact with products containing latex (see *Products that contain latex*)

Risk factors
- Medical and dental professionals
- Workers in latex manufacturing or supply companies
- Patients with spina bifida or other conditions that require multiple surgeries involving latex material
- History of:
  - asthma or allergies, especially to bananas, avocados, tropical fruits, or chestnuts
  - multiple intra-abdominal or genitourinary surgeries
  - frequent intermittent urinary catheterization

Incidence
- Present in 1% to 5% of the U.S. population
- Affects 10% to 30% of health care workers
- Most prevalent (20% to 68%) in patients with spina bifida and urogenital abnormalities
- Affects men and women equally

Common characteristics
- Respiratory difficulties
- Rash

Complications
- Respiratory obstruction
- Systemic vascular collapse
- Death

PRODUCTS THAT CONTAIN LATEX

Medical products
- Adhesive bandages
- Airways, Levin tube
- Blood pressure cuff, tubing, and bladder
- Catheter leg straps
- Catheters
- Dental dams
- Elastic bandages
- Electrode pads
- Fluid-circulating hypothermia blankets
- Handheld resuscitation bags
- Hemodialysis equipment
- I.V. catheters
- Latex or rubber gloves
- Medication vials
- Pads for crutches
- Protective sheets
- Reservoir breathing bags
- Rubber airways and endotracheal tubes
- Tape
- Tourniquets

Nonmedical products
- Adhesive tape
- Balloons (excluding Mylar)
- Cervical diaphragms
- Condoms
- Disposable diapers
- Elastic stockings
- Glue
- Latex paint
- Nipples and pacifiers
- Rubber bands
- Tires

✳ ASSESSMENT

History
- Exposure to latex

Physical findings
- Signs of anaphylaxis
- Rash
- Angioedema
- Conjunctivitis
- Wheezing, stridor

Test results
- Diagnosis of latex allergy is based mainly on history and physical assessment

LABORATORY
- Radioallergosorbent test results show specific IgE antibodies to latex (safest for use in patients with a history of type I hypersensitivity).

DIAGNOSTIC PROCEDURES
- Patch test reaction is positive, as indicated by hives with itching or redness.

◆ TREATMENT

General
- Prevention of exposure, including use of latex-free products, to decrease possible exacerbation of hypersensitivity
- Maintenance of patent airway

Diet
- No restrictions

Activity
- As tolerated

Medications
Before and after possible exposure to latex:
- Corticosteroids
- Antihistamines
- Histamine-2 receptor blockers

ACUTE TREATMENT
- Epinephrine (1:1,000)
- Oxygen therapy
- Volume expanders
- I. V. vasopressors
- Aminophylline and albuterol

Nursing diagnoses
- Impaired gas exchange
- Impaired skin integrity
- Ineffective airway clearance
- Ineffective breathing pattern
- Latex allergy response
- Risk for injury

Key outcomes
The patient will:
- maintain adequate ventilation and oxygenation
- maintain skin integrity
- maintain a patent airway
- maintain effective breathing pattern
- exhibit no signs or symptoms of latex allergy response
- remain free from signs and symptoms of injury.

Nursing interventions
- Maintain airway, breathing, and circulation.
- Give prescribed drugs.
- ◈ **NURSING ALERT** When adding medication to an I.V. bag, inject the drug through the spike port, not the rubber latex port.
- Monitor the patient for sensitivity to tropical nuts or bananas.
- Keep the patient's environment latex-free.

Monitoring
- Vital signs
- Respiratory status

Be sure to cover:
- disorder, diagnostic tests, and treatment
- potential for life-threatening reaction
- importance of wearing medical identification jewelry that identifies allergy
- how to use an epinephrine autoinjector.

Discharge planning
- Refer the patient to support services and community resources, as necessary.

Organizations
American Academy of Allergy Asthma & Immunology: *www.aaaai.org*
American Latex Allergy Association: *www.latexallergyresources.org*
U.S. Department of Labor Occupational Safety & Health Administration: *www.osha-slc.gov*

Selected references
Filon, E.L., and Radman, G. "Latex Allergy: A Follow-Up Study of 1,040 Healthcare Workers," *Occupational and Environmental Medicine* 63(2):121-25, February 2006.

Reines, R.D., and Seifert, P.C. "Patient Safety: Latex Allergy," *Surgical Clinics of North America* 85(6):1329-340, December 2005.

Rolland, I.M., et al. "Advances in Development of Hypoallergenic Latex Immunotherapy," *Current Opinion in Allergy and Clinical Immunology* 5(6):544-51, December 2005.

Legionnaires' disease

Description

- Acute bronchopneumonia produced by a gram-negative bacillus
- Illness ranging from mild (with or without pneumonitis) to serious multilobed pneumonia with mortality as high as 15%
- Outbreaks (usually in late summer and early fall) epidemic or confined to a few cases

Pathophysiology

- The legionella enter the lungs after aspiration or inhalation.
- Although alveolar macrophages phagocytize the legionella, the organisms aren't killed and proliferate intracellularly.
- The cells rupture, releasing the legionella, and the cycle starts again.
- Lesions develop a nodular appearance, and alveoli become filled with fibrin, neutrophils, and alveolar macrophages.

Causes

- *Legionella pneumophila,* an aerobic, gram-negative bacillus that's probably transmitted by air
- Water distribution systems (such as whirlpool spas and decorative fountains) primary reservoir for the organism

Incidence

- Most likely to affect men (more than women) and others, including:
  - elderly patients
  - immunocompromised patients
  - patients with chronic underlying disease such as diabetes
  - alcoholics
  - cigarette smokers

Common characteristics

- Nonspecific prodromal symptoms
- Initial nonproductive cough that then becomes productive

Complications

- Hypoxia and acute respiratory failure
- Hypotension
- Delirium
- Seizures
- Heart failure
- Arrhythmias
- Renal failure
- Shock

History

- Presence at a suspected source of infection
- Prodromal symptoms including anorexia, malaise, myalgia, and headache

Physical findings

- Rapidly rising fever with chills
- Grayish or rust-colored, nonpurulent, occasionally blood-streaked sputum
- Tachypnea
- Bradycardia (in about 50% of patients)
- Neurologic signs (altered level of consciousness [LOC])
- Dullness over areas of secretions and consolidation or pleural effusions
- Fine crackles that develop into coarse crackles as the disease progresses

Test results

LABORATORY

- Gram staining reveals numerous neutrophils but no organism.
- Definitive method of diagnosis involves isolation of the organisms from respiratory secretions or bronchial washings or through thoracentesis.
- Definitive tests include direct immunofluorescence of *L. pneumophila* and indirect fluorescent serum antibody testing.
- Leukocytosis is present, and erythrocyte sedimentation rate is increased.
- Partial pressure of oxygen is decreased; partial pressure of carbon dioxide is initially decreased.
- Serum sodium level isless than 131 mg/L, indicating hyponatremia.

IMAGING

- Chest X-ray typically shows patchy, localized infiltration, which progresses to multilobed consolidation (usually involving the lower lobes) and pleural effusion.
- In fulminant disease, chest X-ray reveals opacification of the entire lung.

General

- Fluid replacement
- Oxygen administration
- Mechanical ventilation, as necessary

Diet

- No restrictions

Activity

- No restrictions

Medication

- Antibiotics
- Antipyretics
- Vasopressors

✤ NURSING CONSIDERATIONS

Nursing diagnoses
- Acute pain
- Deficient fluid volume
- Hyperthermia
- Impaired gas exchange
- Ineffective airway clearance
- Ineffective breathing pattern
- Ineffective tissue perfusion: Cardiopulmonary

Key outcomes
The patient will:
- express feelings of increased comfort and decreased pain
- regain and maintain normal fluid and electrolyte balance
- remain normothermic
- maintain adequate ventilation and oxygenation
- cough effectively and expectorate sputum effectively
- have normal breath sounds
- exhibit signs and symptoms of adequate cardiopulmonary perfusion.

Nursing interventions
- Give tepid sponge baths or use hypothermia blankets to lower fever.
- Provide frequent mouth care. If necessary, apply soothing cream to irritated nostrils.
- Replace fluids and electrolytes, as needed.
- Institute seizure precautions.
- Administer medications, as ordered.

Monitoring
- Vital signs
- Respiratory status and arterial blood gases
- LOC

▶ PATIENT TEACHING

Be sure to cover:
- disorder, diagnostic tests, and treatment
- prevention of infection
- importance of disinfection of water supply
- purpose of postural drainage, and how to perform coughing and deep-breathing exercises
- proper hand washing and disposal of soiled tissues to prevent disease transmission.

Discharge planning
- Refer the patient to a pulmonologist, if necessary.

✱ RESOURCES

Organizations
Centers for Disease Control and Prevention: *www.cdc.gov*
Harvard University Consumer Health Information: *www.intelihealth.com*
National Health Information Center: *www.health.gov/nhic/*
National Institute of Allergy and Infectious Diseases: *www.niaid.nih.gov*
National Library of Medicine: *www.nlm.nih.gov*

Selected references
Kasper, D.L., et al., eds. *Harrison's Principles of Internal Medicine*, 16th ed. New York: McGraw-Hill Book Co., 2005.
Makin, T. "Legionella Bacteria and Water Systems in Health Care Premises," *Nursing Times* 101(3):48-49, September-October 2005.
Murray., S. "Legionella Infection," *Canadian Medical Association Journal* 173(11):1322, November 2005.
Todd, B. "Legionella Pneumonia: Many Cases of Legionnaire Disease Go Unreported or Unrecognized," *AJN* 105(11):35-36, 38, November 2005.

Leukemia, acute

● OVERVIEW

Description
- Malignant proliferation of white blood cell (WBC) precursors, or blasts, in bone marrow or lymph tissue; blasts accumulating in peripheral blood, bone marrow, and body tissues
- Most common form of cancer among children
- Common forms:
  - Acute lymphoblastic (lymphocytic) leukemia (ALL): characterized by abnormal growth of lymphocyte precursors (lymphoblasts)
  - Acute myeloblastic (myelogenous) leukemia (AML): causes rapid accumulation of myeloid precursors (myeloblasts)
  - Acute monoblastic (monocytic) leukemia, or Schilling's type: results in marked increase in monocyte precursors (monoblasts)
- In ALL, treatment inducing remissions in 90% of children (average survival time: 5 years) and 65% of adults (average survival time: 1 to 2 years); children ages 2 to 8 having best survival rate—about 50%—with intensive therapy
- In AML, average survival time only 1 year after diagnosis, even with aggressive treatment (remissions lasting 2 to 10 months occurring in 50% of children; adults surviving only about 1 year after diagnosis, even with treatment)
- Without treatment, invariably fatal

Pathophysiology
- Immature, nonfunctioning WBCs appear to accumulate first in the tissue where they originate, such as lymphocytes in lymph tissue and granulocytes in bone marrow.
- The immature, nonfunctioning WBCs spill into the bloodstream and overwhelm red blood cells (RBCs) and platelets; from there, they infiltrate other tissues.

Causes
- Exact cause unknown

Risk factors
- Radiation (especially prolonged exposure)
- Certain chemicals and drugs
- Viruses
- Genetic abnormalities
- Chronic exposure to benzene

IN CHILDREN
- Down syndrome
- Ataxia
- Telangiectasia
- Congenital disorders, such as albinism and congenital immunodeficiency syndrome

Incidence
- More common in males than females
- More common in whites (especially of Jewish ancestry)
- More common in children between ages 2 and 5 (80% of leukemias in this age group are ALL), and those who live in urban and industrialized areas

Common characteristics
- Sudden onset of high fevers
- Bleeding
- Night sweats
- Malaise

Complications
- Infection
- Organ malfunction through encroachment or hemorrhage

✳ ASSESSMENT

History
- Sudden onset of high fever
- Abnormal bleeding
- Fatigue and night sweats
- Weakness, lassitude, recurrent infections, and chills
- Abdominal or bone pain in patient with ALL, AML, or acute monoblastic leukemia

Physical findings
- Tachycardia, palpitations, and a systolic ejection murmur
- Decreased ventilation
- Pallor
- Lymph node enlargement
- Liver or spleen enlargement

Test results
LABORATORY
- Blood counts show thrombocytopenia and neutropenia and a WBC differential shows the cell type.

IMAGING
- Computed tomography scan shows the affected organs, and cerebrospinal fluid analysis shows abnormal WBC invasion of the central nervous system.

DIAGNOSTIC PROCEDURES
- Bone marrow aspiration that shows a proliferation of immature WBCs confirms acute leukemia; if the aspirate is dry or free from leukemic cells but the patient has other typical signs of leukemia, a bone marrow biopsy, usually of the posterior superior iliac spine, must be performed.
- Lumbar puncture is used to detect meningeal involvement.

◆ TREATMENT

General
- Transfusions of platelets to prevent bleeding
- Transfusions of RBCs to prevent anemia
- Bone marrow transplantation in some patients
- Radiation therapy in case of brain or testicular infiltration
- Chemotherapeutic and radiation treatment, depending on diagnosis

Diet
- Well-balanced; no restrictions

Activity
- Frequent rest periods

Medication
MENINGEAL INFILTRATION
- Intrathecal instillation of methotrexate or cytarabine with cranial radiation

ALL
- Vincristine, prednisone, high-dose cytarabine, and daunorubicin
- Intrathecal methotrexate or cytarabine because ALL carries 40% risk of meningeal infiltration

AML
- Combination of I.V. daunorubicin and cytarabine or some or all of the following drugs: a combination of cyclophosphamide, vincristine, prednisone, or methotrexate; high-dose cytarabine alone or with other drugs; amsacrine; etoposide; and 5-azacytidine and mitoxantrone.

ACUTE MONOBLASTIC LEUKEMIA
- Cytarabine and thioguanine with daunorubicin or doxorubicin
- Anti-infectives, such as antibiotics, antifungals, and antivirals and granulocyte injections

❖ NURSING CONSIDERATIONS

Nursing diagnoses
- Acute pain
- Anticipatory grieving
- Anxiety
- Disabled family coping
- Fatigue
- Fear
- Imbalanced nutrition: Less than body requirements
- Impaired oral mucous membrane
- Impaired tissue integrity
- Ineffective coping
- Ineffective protection
- Risk for imbalanced body temperature
- Risk for infection
- Risk for injury

Key outcomes
The patient (or family) will:
- express feelings of increased comfort and decreased pain
- express feelings about condition and potential loss
- verbalize a decrease in anxiety
- report feelings of increased energy
- verbalize fears and concerns
- exhibit no further weight loss
- exhibit intact mucous membranes
- exhibit intact tissue integrity
- demonstrate positive coping behaviors (self and family)
- demonstrate use of protective measures, including conserving energy, maintaining a balanced diet, and getting adequate rest
- remain free from infection and injury.

Nursing interventions
- Encourage verbalization and provide comfort.
- Provide adequate hydration.
- After bone marrow transplantation, keep the patient in protective isolation, administer antibiotics, and transfuse packed RBCs, as necessary.
- Administer medications, as ordered.
- Control mouth ulceration by checking often for obvious ulcers and gum swelling and by providing frequent mouth care and saline rinses.

Monitoring
- Complications from treatment
- Hydration and nutritional status
- Urine pH (should be above 7.5)
- Vital signs
- Signs and symptoms of bleeding

▶ PATIENT TEACHING

Be sure to cover:
- disorder, diagnostic tests, and treatment
- medication administration, dosage, and possible adverse effects
- use of a soft toothbrush and avoidance of hot, spicy foods and commercial mouthwashes
- signs and symptoms of infection
- signs and symptoms of abnormal bleeding
- planned rest periods during the day.

Discharge planning
- Refer the patient to resource and support services.

✹ RESOURCES

Organizations
American Cancer Society: *www.cancer.org*
Guide to Internet Resources for Cancer: *www.cancerindex.org*
The Leukemia and Lymphoma Society: *www.leukemia.org*
National Cancer Institute: *www.nci.nih.gov*

Selected references
Atlas of Pathophysiology, 2nd ed. Philadelphia: Lippincott Williams & Wilkins, 2005.
Dick, J.F,. and Lapidot, T. "Biology of Normal and Acute Myeloid Leukemia Stem Cells," *International Journal of Hematology* 82(5):389-96, December 2005.
Mohren, M., et al. "Increased Risk for Thromboembolism in Patients with Acute Leukaemia," *British Journal of Cancer* 94(2):200-202, January 2006.

Leukemia, chronic granulocytic

● OVERVIEW

Description
- Characterized by abnormal over-growth of granulocytic precursors (myeloblasts, promyelocytes, meta-myelocytes, and myelocytes) in bone marrow, peripheral blood, and body tissues
- Always fatal (average survival time is 3 to 4 years after onset of chronic phase and 3 to 6 months after onset of acute phase)
- Proceeds in two distinct phases:
  - Insidious chronic phase (characterized by anemia and bleeding abnormalities)
  - Acute phase (blast crisis; or myeloblasts, the most primitive granulocytic precursors, proliferate rapidly)
- During acute phase: either lymphoblastic or myeloblastic disease may develop (despite vigorous treatment, chronic granulocytic leukemia rapidly advancing after onset of acute phase)
- Also called chronic myelogenous (or myelocytic) leukemia (CML)

Pathophysiology
- CML is a myeloproliferative disorder, originating in a progenitor stem cell.
- Malignant transformation is identified in erythroid, megakaryocytic, and macrophage cell lines.
- Malignant transformation arises from pluripotetial stem cells or lymphoid stem cells.

Causes
- Exact cause unknown

Risk factors
- Presence of the Philadelphia chromosome (found in almost 90% of patients)
- Myeloproliferative diseases

Incidence
- Most common in young and middle-aged adults
- Slightly more common in men than women; rare in children
- In United States, 3,000 to 4,000 cases of chronic granulocytic leukemia annually (about 20% of all leukemias)

Common characteristics
- Fatigue
- Weakness
- Weight loss
- History of gouty arthritis or renal calculi

Complications
- Infection
- Hemorrhage
- Pain

✳ ASSESSMENT

History
- Renal calculi or gouty arthritis
- Fatigue, weakness, dyspnea, decreased exercise tolerance, and headache
- Recent weight loss and anorexia

Physical findings
- Evidence of bleeding and clotting disorders
- Low-grade fever and tachycardia
- Pallor
- Difficulty breathing
- Retinal hemorrhage
- Hepatosplenomegaly with abdominal discomfort and pain
- Sternal and rib tenderness

Test results
LABORATORY
- Chromosomal studies of peripheral blood or bone marrow show the Philadelphia chromosome.
- Low leukocyte alkaline phosphatase levels confirm chronic granulocytic leukemia.
- White blood cell (WBC) abnormalities are present, including:
  - leukocytosis (WBC count over 50,000/mcg, rising as high as 250,000/mcg)
  - occasionally leukopenia (WBC count under 5,000/mcg)
  - neutropenia (neutrophil count under 1,500/mcg) despite high WBC count.
- Circulating myeloblasts are increased.
- Hemoglobin level is decreased (below 10 g/dl) and hematocrit is low (less than 30%).
- Thrombocytosis is present (more than 1 million thrombocytes/mcg).

- Serum uric acid levels may exceed 8 mg/dl.
IMAGING
- Computed tomography scan may show the affected organs.
DIAGNOSTIC PROCEDURES
- Bone marrow aspirate or biopsy (performed only if the aspirate is dry) may be hypercellular, characteristically showing bone marrow infiltration by a significantly increased number of myeloid elements; in the acute phase, myeloblasts predominate.

◆ TREATMENT

General
- Bone marrow transplantation (during chronic phase, more than 60% of patients who receive transplant achieving remission)
- Local splenic radiation
- Leukapheresis (selective leukocyte removal) to reduce the WBC count

Diet
- Well-balanced; no restrictions

Activity
- Frequent rest periods

Medication
- Busulfan and hydroxyurea
- Aspirin
- Allopurinol
- Antibiotics

Surgery
- Splenectomy

Nursing diagnoses

- Acute pain
- Anxiety
- Constipation
- Disabled family coping
- Fatigue
- Fear
- Grieving
- Imbalanced nutrition: Less than body requirements
- Impaired oral mucous membrane
- Impaired tissue integrity
- Ineffective coping
- Ineffective protection
- Risk for imbalanced body temperature
- Risk for infection
- Risk for injury

Key outcomes

The patient (or family) will:

- express feelings of increased comfort and decreased pain
- express their feelings about condition and potential loss
- demonstrate a decrease in anxiety
- regain a regular bowel elimination pattern
- report increased energy
- verbalize fears and concerns openly
- have no further weight loss
- have intact mucous membranes
- maintain tissue integrity
- demonstrate positive coping methods (self and family)
- demonstrate use of protective measures, including conserving energy, maintaining a balanced diet, and getting adequate rest
- maintain normothermia
- remain free from infection and injury.

Nursing interventions

- Plan your care to minimize fatigue.
- Regularly check skin and mucous membranes for pallor, petechiae, and bruising.
- Encourage deep-breathing and coughing exercises.
- Encourage verbalization and provide comfort.
- Administer medications, as ordered.
- After bone marrow transplantation, keep the patient in protective isolation, and administer antibiotics and packed red blood cells, as ordered.

Monitoring

- Adverse effects of treatment
- Signs and symptoms of bleeding
- Signs and symptoms of infection
- Complete blood count
- Vital signs
- Hydration and nutritional status

▶ PATIENT TEACHING

Be sure to cover:

- disorder, diagnostic tests, and treatment
- how to minimize bleeding and infection risks (such as by using a soft-bristled toothbrush, an electric razor, and other safety devices)
- diet high in calories and protein
- if the patient is to undergo bone marrow transplantation, reinforcement of the explanation of the procedure, possible outcome, and potential adverse effects
- medication administration, dosage, and possible adverse effects
- signs and symptoms of infection and thrombocytopenia.

Discharge planning

- Refer the patient to resource and support services.

✺ RESOURCES

Organizations

American Cancer Society: *www.cancer.org*
Guide to Internet Resources for Cancer: *www.cancerindex.org*
The Leukemia and Lymphoma Society: *www.leukemia.org*
National Cancer Institute: *www.nci.nih.gov*

Selected references

Atlas of Pathophysiology, 2nd ed. Philadelphia: Lippincott Williams & Wilkins, 2005.

D'Antonio, J. "Chronic Myelogenous Leukemia," *Clinical Journal of Oncology Nursing* 9(5):535-38, October 2005.

Goldman, J. "Is Imatinib a Cost-Effective Treatment for Newly Diagnosed Chronic Myeloid Leukemia Patients?" *Nature Clinical Practice Oncology* 2(3):126-27, March 2005.

Morris, E.L, and Dutcher, J.P. "Blastic Phase of Chronic Myelogenous Leukemia," *Clinical Advances in Hematology and Oncology* 3(7):547-52, July 2005.

Leukemia, chronic lymphocytic

● OVERVIEW

Description
- Most benign and slowly progressive form of leukemia
- Prognosis poor if anemia, thrombocytopenia, neutropenia, bulky lymphadenopathy, and severe lymphocytosis develop

Pathophysiology
- Chronic lymphocytic leukemia is a generalized, progressive disease marked by an uncontrollable spread of abnormal, small lymphocytes in lymphoid tissue, blood, and bone marrow.
- Once these cells infiltrate bone marrow, lymphoid tissue, and organ systems, clinical signs begin to appear.
- Gross bone marrow replacement by abnormal lymphocytes is the most common cause of death, usually within 4 to 5 years of diagnosis.

Causes
- Exact cause unknown

Risk factors
- Hereditary factors
- Undefined chromosomal abnormalities
- Certain immunologic defects, such as ataxia-telangiectasia or acquired agammaglobulinemia

Common characteristics
- Fever, malaise, weakness
- Enlarged lymph nodes

Incidence
- Most common in elderly people; nearly all afflicted are men over age 50
- Chronic lymphocytic leukemia accounting for almost one-third of new leukemia cases annually
- Higher incidence recorded within families

Complications
- Infection
- In end-stage disease: anemia, progressive splenomegaly, leukemic cell replacement of the bone marrow, and profound hypogammaglobulinemia, which usually terminates with fatal septicemia

✳ ASSESSMENT

History
- Fatigue, malaise, fever, weight loss, and frequent infections
- Weakness, palpitations

Physical findings
- Macular or nodular eruptions and evidence of skin infiltration
- Enlarged lymph nodes, liver, and spleen
- Bone tenderness and edema from lymph node obstruction
- Pallor, dyspnea, tachycardia, bleeding, and infection from bone marrow involvement
- Signs of opportunistic fungal, viral, or bacterial infections

Test results
LABORATORY
- Miscellaneous blood tests reveal the disease. (Typically, chronic lymphocytic leukemia is an incidental finding during a routine complete blood count that reveals numerous abnormal lymphocytes.)
  - In the early stages, the patient has a mildly but persistently elevated white blood cell (WBC) count; granulocytopenia is the rule, although the WBC count climbs as the disease progresses.
  - Hemoglobin level is under 11g/dl.
  - WBC differential shows neutropenia (less than 1,500/mcg) and lymphocytosis (more than 10,000/mcg).
  - Platelet count shows thrombocytopenia (less than 150,000/mcg).
  - Serum protein electrophoresis shows hypogammaglobulinemia.
IMAGING
- Computed tomography scan shows affected organs.
DIAGNOSTIC PROCEDURES
- Bone marrow aspiration and biopsy show lymphocytic invasion.

◆ TREATMENT

General
- Radiation therapy to relieve symptoms (generally for patient with enlarged lymph nodes, painful bony lesions, or massive splenomegaly)

Diet
- High-calorie, high-protein
- Avoidance of hot and spicy foods for patient with impaired oral membranes

Activity
- Frequent rest periods

Medication
- Systemic chemotherapy

❖ NURSING CONSIDERATIONS

Nursing diagnoses
- Acute pain
- Anxiety
- Disabled family coping
- Fatigue
- Fear
- Grieving
- Imbalanced nutrition: Less than body requirements
- Impaired tissue integrity
- Ineffective coping
- Ineffective protection
- Risk for infection
- Risk for injury

Key outcomes
The patient (or family) will:
- express feelings of increased comfort and decreased pain
- express feelings about condition and potential loss
- demonstrate a decrease in anxiety
- report feelings of increased energy
- verbalize fears and concerns openly
- experience no further weight loss
- exhibit intact tissue integrity
- demonstrate positive coping methods (self and family)
- demonstrate use of protective measures, including conserving energy, maintaining a balanced diet, and getting adequate rest
- remain free from infection and injury.

Nursing interventions
- Help establish an appropriate rehabilitation program during remission.
- Place in protective isolation, if necessary.
- Administer medications, as ordered.
- Encourage verbalization and provide support.
- Administer blood component therapy, as necessary.

Monitoring
- Signs and symptoms of bleeding and thrombocytopenia
- Adverse effects of treatment
- In rectal area, induration, swelling, erythema, skin discoloration, and drainage
- Pain control
- Vital signs

▶ PATIENT TEACHING

Be sure to cover:
- disorder, diagnostic tests, and treatment
- use of a soft toothbrush and avoidance of commercial mouthwashes to prevent irritating the mouth ulcers that result from chemotherapy
- medication administration, dosage, and possible adverse effects
- signs and symptoms of infection, bleeding, and recurrence
- avoidance of anyone with an infection
- importance of follow-up care
- signs and symptoms of recurrence.

Discharge planning
- Refer the patient to resource and support services.

✳ RESOURCES

Organizations
American Cancer Society: *www.cancer.org*
Guide to Internet Resources for Cancer: *www.cancerindex.org*
The Leukemia and Lymphoma Society: *www.leukemia.org*
National Cancer Institute: *www.nci.nih.gov*

Selected references
Abbott, B.L. "Chronic Lymphocytic Leukemia: Recent Advances in Diagnosis and Treatment," *Oncologist* 11(1):21-30, January 2006.

Atlas of Pathophysiology, 2nd ed. Philadelphia: Lippincott Williams & Wilkins, 2005.

Hamblin, T.J. "Autoimmune Complications of Chronic Lymphocytic Leukemia," *Seminars in Oncology* 33(2):230-39, April 2006.

Liver cancer

● OVERVIEW

Description
- Growth of malignant cells in the tissues of the liver
- Rapidly fatal, usually within 6 months
- After cirrhosis, leading cause of fatal hepatic disease
- Liver metastasis occurring as solitary lesion (the first sign of recurrence after a remission)

Pathophysiology
- Most (90%) of primary liver tumors originate in the parenchymal cells and are hepatomas. Others originate in the intrahepatic bile ducts (cholangiomas).
- Approximately 30% to 70% of patients with hepatomas also have cirrhosis.
- Rare tumors include a mixed-cell type, Kupffer cell sarcoma, and hepatoblastoma.
- The liver is one of the most common sites of metastasis from other primary cancers.

Causes
- Exact cause unknown
- Environmental exposure to carcinogens
- Possibly androgens and oral estrogens
- Hepatitis B, C, D viruses

Risk factors
- Cirrhosis
- Excessive alcohol intake
- Malnutrition

Incidence
- Most prevalent in men over age 60
- Primary liver cancer roughly 2% of all cancers in North America and 10% to 50% of cancers in Africa and parts of Asia

Common characteristics
- Right upper quadrant pain
- Fatigue

Complications
- GI hemorrhage
- Progressive cachexia
- Liver failure

✱ ASSESSMENT

History
- Weight loss
- Weakness, fatigue, and fever
- Severe pain in the epigastrium or right upper quadrant

Physical findings
- Jaundice
- Dependent edema
- Abdominal bruit, hum, or rubbing sound
- Tender, nodular, enlarged liver
- Ascites
- Palpable mass in the right upper quadrant

Test results
LABORATORY
- Liver function studies are abnormal.
- Alpha-fetoprotein levels are greater than 500 mcg/ml.
- Electrolyte levels are abnormal.
IMAGING
- Liver scan may show filling defects.
- Arteriography may define large tumors.
- Ultrasonography and computed tomography may reveal hepatic lesions.
DIAGNOSTIC PROCEDURES
- Liver biopsy by needle or open biopsy reveals cancerous cells.

◆ TREATMENT

General
- Radiation therapy (alone or with chemotherapy)

Diet
- High-calorie, low-protein

Activity
- Frequent rest periods
- Postoperative avoidance of heavy lifting and contact sports

Medication
- Chemotherapeutic drugs

Surgery
- Liver resection (lobectomy or partial hepatectomy)
- Liver transplantation

♣ NURSING CONSIDERATIONS

Nursing diagnoses
- Acute pain
- Anxiety
- Excess fluid volume
- Fatigue
- Fear
- Hyperthermia
- Imbalanced nutrition: Less than body requirements
- Impaired gas exchange
- Impaired skin integrity
- Ineffective coping
- Ineffective tissue perfusion: Cardiopulmonary

Key outcomes
The patient will:
- express feelings of increased comfort and decreased pain and anxiety
- maintain normal fluid volume
- demonstrate measures to balance activity and rest
- express fears and concerns openly
- exhibit a body temperature within acceptable parameters
- exhibit adequate nutritional status
- maintain adequate ventilation and oxygenation
- maintain skin integrity
- exhibit adequate coping behaviors
- maintain hemodynamic stability and cardiac output

Nursing interventions
- Administer medications, as ordered.
- Provide meticulous skin care.
- Encourage verbalization and provide support.

Monitoring
- Vital signs
- Hydration and nutritional status
- Weight
- Pain control
- Neurologic status
- Complete blood count; liver function tests
- Postoperative complications
- Wound site

▶ PATIENT TEACHING

Be sure to cover:
- disorder, diagnostic tests, and treatment
- dietary restrictions
- relaxation techniques
- medication administration, dosage, and possible adverse effects.

Discharge planning
- Refer the patient and family members to support services.

✳ RESOURCES

Organizations
American Cancer Society: *www.cancer.org*
Guide to Internet Resources for Cancer: *www.cancerindex.org*
National Cancer Institute: *www.nci.nih.gov*

Selected references
Atlas of Pathophysiology, 2nd ed. Philadelphia: Lippincott Williams & Wilkins, 2005.

Weber, S.M., and Lee, F.T., Jr. "Expanded Treatment of Hepatic Tumors with Radiofrequency Ablation and Cryoablation," *Oncology* (Williston Park) 19(11 Suppl 4):27-32, October 2005.

Yoshida, H., et al. "Early Liver Cancer: Concepts, Diagnosis, and Management," *International Journal of Clinical Oncology* 10(6):384-90, December 2005.

Zavaglia, C., et al. "Predictors of Long-Term Survival after Liver Transplantation for Hepatocellular Carcinoma," *American Journal of Gastroenterology* 100(12):2708-716, December 2005.

Lung cancer

● OVERVIEW

Description
- Tumors arising from the respiratory epithelium
- Most common types: epidermoid (squamous cell), adenocarcinoma, small-cell (oat cell), and large-cell (anaplastic)
- Most common site: wall or epithelium of bronchial tree
- Prognosis poor for most patients; dependent on extent of cancer when diagnosed and cells' growth rate (only about 13% of patients with lung cancer surviving 5 years after diagnosis)

Pathophysiology
- Individuals with lung cancer demonstrate bronchial epithelial changes progressing from squamous cell alteration or metaplasia to carcinoma in situ.
- Tumors originating in the bronchi are thought to be more mucus producing.
- Partial or complete obstruction of the airway occurs with tumor growth, resulting in lobar collapse distal to the tumor.
- Early metastasis occurs to other thoracic structures, such as hilar lymph nodes or the mediastinum.
- Distant metastasis occurs to the brain, liver, bone, and adrenal glands.

Causes
- Exact cause unknown

Risk factors
- Tobacco smoking
- Exposure to carcinogenic and industrial air pollutants (asbestos, arsenic, chromium, coal dust, iron oxides, nickel, radioactive dust, and uranium)
- Genetic predisposition

Incidence
- Family susceptibility

✳ **AGE-RELATED CONCERN** Lung cancer is the most common cause of death from cancer in men and women ages 50 to 75.

Common characteristics
EPIDERMOID AND SMALL-CELL
- Smoker's cough
- Hoarseness
- Wheezing
- Dyspnea
- Hemoptysis
- Chest pain
- Cushing's and carcinoid syndromes
- Hypercalcemia

ADENOCARCINOMA AND LARGE-CELL
- Fever
- Weakness
- Weight loss
- Anorexia
- Shoulder pain
- Gynecomastia
- Hypertrophic pulmonary osteoarthropathy

Complications
- Spread of primary tumor to intrathoracic structures
- Tracheal obstruction
- Esophageal compression with dysphagia
- Phrenic nerve paralysis with hemidiaphragm elevation and dyspnea
- Sympathetic nerve paralysis with Horner's syndrome
- Spinal cord compression
- Lymphatic obstruction with pleural effusion
- Hypoxemia
- Anorexia and weight loss, sometimes leading to cachexia, digital clubbing, and hypertrophic osteoarthropathy
- Neoplastic and paraneoplastic syndromes, including Pancoast's syndrome and syndrome of inappropriate secretion of antidiuretic hormone

✳ ASSESSMENT

History
- Possibly asymptomatic
- Exposure to carcinogens
- Coughing
- Hemoptysis
- Shortness of breath
- Hoarseness
- Fatigue

Physical findings
- Dyspnea on exertion
- Finger clubbing
- Edema of the face, neck, and upper torso
- Dilated chest and abdominal veins (superior vena cava syndrome)
- Weight loss
- Enlarged lymph nodes
- Enlarged liver
- Decreased breath sounds
- Wheezing
- Pleural friction rub

Test results
LABORATORY
- Cytologic sputum analysis shows diagnostic evidence of pulmonary malignancy.
- Liver function tests are abnormal, especially with metastasis.

IMAGING
- Chest X-rays show advanced lesions and can show a lesion up to 2 years before signs and symptoms appear; findings may indicate tumor size and location.
- Contrast studies of the bronchial tree (chest tomography, bronchography) demonstrate size and location as well as spread of lesion.
- Bone scan is used to detect metastasis.
- Computed tomography is used to detect metastasis.
- Positron emission tomography aids in diagnosis of primary and metastatic site.
- Magnetic resonance imaging may reveal tumor invasion.
- Gallium scans of liver and spleen help to detect metastasis.

DIAGNOSTIC PROCEDURES
- Bronchoscopy can be used to identify the tumor site. Bronchoscopic washings provide material for cytologic and histologic study.

- Needle biopsy of the lungs (relies on biplanar fluoroscopic visual control to locate peripheral tumors before withdrawing a tissue specimen for analysis) allows firm diagnosis in 80% of patients.
- Tissue biopsy of metastatic sites (including supraclavicular and mediastinal nodes and pleura) is used to assess disease extent. Based on histologic findings, staging describes the disease's extent and prognosis and is used to direct treatment.
- Thoracentesis allows chemical and cytologic examination of pleural fluid.

◆ TREATMENT

General
- Various combinations of surgery, radiation therapy, and chemotherapy to improve prognosis
- Palliative (most treatments)
- Preoperative and postoperative radiation therapy
- Laser therapy (investigational)

Diet
- Well-balanced

Activity
- As tolerated per breathing capacity

Medication
- Chemotherapy drug combinations
- Immunotherapy (investigational)

Surgery
- Partial removal of lung (wedge resection, segmental resection, lobectomy, radical lobectomy)
- Total removal of lung (pneumonectomy, radical pneumonectomy)

⁘ NURSING CONSIDERATIONS

Nursing diagnoses
- Acute pain
- Anxiety
- Deficient fluid volume
- Fatigue
- Imbalanced nutrition: Less than body requirements
- Impaired gas exchange
- Impaired physical mobility
- Impaired skin integrity
- Ineffective airway clearance
- Ineffective breathing pattern
- Risk for infection
- Risk for injury

Key outcomes
The patient will:
- express feelings of increased comfort and decreased pain and anxiety
- maintain normal fluid volume
- carry out activities of daily living without weakness or fatigue
- maintain adequate nutritional intake
- maintain adequate ventilation and oxygenation
- maintain muscle strength and joint range of motion
- maintain intact skin
- maintain a patent airway
- exhibit signs of adequate breathing pattern
- remain free from infection and injury.

Nursing interventions
- Provide supportive care.
- Encourage verbalization.
- Give medications, as ordered.

Monitoring
- Chest tube function and drainage
- Postoperative complications
- Wound site
- Vital signs
- Sputum production
- Hydration and nutrition
- Oxygenation
- Pain control

▶ PATIENT TEACHING

Be sure to cover:
- disorder, diagnostic tests, and treatment
- postoperative procedures and equipment
- chest physiotherapy
- exercises to prevent shoulder stiffness
- medication administration, dosage, and possible adverse effects
- risk factors for recurrent cancer.

Discharge planning
- Refer smokers to local branches of the American Cancer Society or Smokenders.
- Provide information about group therapy, individual counseling, and hypnosis.
- Refer the patient to resource and support services.

✸ RESOURCES

Organizations
American Cancer Society: *www.cancer.org*
Guide to Internet Resources for Cancer: *www.cancerindex.org*
National Cancer Institute: *www.nci.nih.gov*
Smokenders: *www.smokenders.com*

Selected references
Godtfresen, N.S., et al. "Effect of Smoking Reduction on Lung Cancer Risk," *JAMA* 294(12):1505-510, September 2005.

Haiman, C.A., et al. "Ethnic and Racial Differences in the Smoking-Related Risk for Lung Cancer," *New England Journal of Medicine* 354(4):333-42, January 2006.

Thompson, E., et al. "Non-Invasive Interventions for Improving Well-Being and Quality of Life in Patients with Lung Cancer—a Systematic Review of the Evidence," *Lung Cancer* 50(2):163-76, November 2005.

Tishelman, C., et al. "Symptoms in Patients with Lung Carcinoma: Distinguishing Distress from Intensity," *Cancer* 104(9):2013-2021, November 2005.

Lyme disease

OVERVIEW

Description
- Multisystem disorder caused by a spirochete
- Also known as *chronic lyme neuroborreliosis*

Pathophysiology
- A tick injects spirochete-laden saliva into the bloodstream or deposits fecal matter on the skin.
- After incubating for 3 to 32 days, the spirochetes migrate outward on the skin, causing a rash, and disseminate to other skin sites or organs through the bloodstream or lymph system.
- Spirochetes may survive for years in the joints, or die after triggering an inflammatory response in the host.

Causes
- The spirochete *Borrelia burgdorferi*, carried by the minute tick *Ixodes dammini* (also called *I. scapularis*) or another tick in the Ixodidae family

Incidence
- Affects all ages and both sexes
- Onset during the summer months
- Occurs in geographic ranges of ixodid ticks

Common characteristics
- Typically begins with classic skin lesion, erythema migrans (EM)
- Skin lesions with bright red outer rims and white centers appearing on axilla, thigh, and groin
- Initial reported symptoms include fatigue, malaise, migratory myalgia, and arthralgia

Complications
- Myocarditis
- Pericarditis
- Arrhythmias
- Meningitis
- Encephalitis
- Cranial or peripheral neuropathies
- Arthritis

ASSESSMENT

History
- Recent exposure to ticks
- Onset of symptoms in warmer months
- Severe headache and stiff neck with rash eruption
- Fever (up to 104° F [40° C]) and chills
- Myalgia
- Arthralgia

Physical findings
- Regional lymphadenopathy
- Tenderness in the skin lesion site or the posterior cervical area

EARLY STAGE
- Tachycardia or irregular heartbeat
- Mild dyspnea
- EM

LATER STAGE
- Neurologic signs such as memory impairment
- Bell's palsy
- Intermittent arthritis (see *Differentiating Lyme disease*)
- Ocular signs such as conjunctivitis
- Cardiac signs such as heart failure and pericarditis

Test results

LABORATORY
- Assays for anti-*B. burgdorferi* (anti-B) show evidence of previous or current infection.
- Enzyme-linked immunosorbent technology (ELISA or EIA) or indirect immunofluorescence microscopy (IFA) show immunoglobulin (Ig) M levels that peak 3 to 6 weeks after infection; IgG antibodies detected several weeks after infection may continue to develop for several months and generally persist for years.
- Positive Western blot assay shows serologic evidence of past or current infection with *B. burgdorferi*.
- Polymerase chain reaction test is used when joint and cerebrospinal fluid involvement is present; detects genetic material found in Lyme disease bacteria.

> **NURSING ALERT** Serologic testing isn't useful early in the course of Lyme disease because of the low sensitivity of tests. Serologic testing may be more useful later in the disease process, at which time sensitivity and specificity of the test is improved.

DIAGNOSTIC PROCEDURES
- Lumbar puncture with analysis of cerebrospinal fluid may show antibodies to *B. burgdorferi*.
- Biopsy of skin specimen may be done to detect *B. burgdorferi*.

TREATMENT

General
- Prompt tick removal using proper technique

Diet
- No restrictions

Activity
- Rest periods when needed

Medication
- I.V. or oral antibiotics (initiated as soon as possible after infection)

❖ NURSING CONSIDERATIONS

Nursing diagnoses
- Acute pain
- Decreased cardiac output
- Fatigue
- Hyperthermia
- Impaired physical mobility
- Impaired skin integrity
- Ineffective tissue perfusion: Cardiopulmonary, cerebral, peripheral
- Risk for infection

Key outcomes
The patient will:
- express feelings of increased comfort and decreased pain
- maintain adequate cardiac output without evidence of arrhythmias
- return to pre-illness energy level
- remain afebrile
- attain the highest degree of mobility possible
- exhibit a decrease in extent of rash
- demonstrate effective tissue perfusion
- remain free from further signs and symptoms of infection.

Nursing interventions
- Plan care to provide adequate rest.
- Administer medications, as ordered.
- Assist with range-of-motion and strengthening exercises (with arthritis).
- Encourage verbalization and provide support.

Monitoring
- Skin lesions
- Response to treatment
- Adverse drug reactions
- Complications

▶ PATIENT TEACHING

Be sure to cover:
- disorder, diagnostic tests, and treatment
- medication administration, dosage, and possible adverse effects
- importance of follow-up care and reporting recurrent or new symptoms to the physician
- prevention of Lyme disease, such as avoiding tick-infested areas, covering the skin with clothing, using insect repellants, inspecting exposed skin for attached ticks at least every 4 hours, and removing ticks
- proper tick removal
- information about the vaccine for persons at risk for contracting Lyme disease.

Discharge planning
- If the patient is in the late stages of the disease, refer to a dermatologist, neurologist, cardiologist, or infectious disease specialist, as indicated.

✱ RESOURCES

Organizations
Centers for Disease Control and Prevention: *www.cdc.gov*
Harvard University Consumer Health Information: *www.intelihealth.com*
National Health Information Center: *www.health.gov/nhic/*
National Institute of Allergy and Infectious Diseases: *www.niaid.nih.gov*
National Library of Medicine: *www.nlm.nih.gov*

Selected references
Bratton, R.I., and Corey, R. "Tick-borne Disease," *American Family Physician* 71(12):2323-330, June 2005.

Kasper, D.L., et al., eds. *Harrison's Principles of Internal Medicine,* 16th ed. New York: McGraw-Hill Book Co., 2005.

Phillips, S.E., et al. "Rash Decisions about Southern Tick-Associated Rash Illness and Lyme Disease," *Clinical Infectious Diseases* 42(2):306-307, January 2006.

Rudd-Arieta, M.P. "Lyme Disease in Children. An Overview," *Advance for Nurse Practitioners* 11(6):77-78, June 2003.

DIFFERENTIATING LYME DISEASE

Lyme disease needs to be differentiated from chronic fatigue syndrome or fibromyalgia, which is difficult late in the disease because of chronic pain and fatigue. The other diseases produce more generalized and disabling symptoms; also, patients lack evidence of joint inflammation, have normal neurologic tests, and have a greater degree of anxiety and depression than patients with Lyme disease.

Lymphoma, non-Hodgkin's

● OVERVIEW

Description
- Heterogeneous group of malignant diseases that originate in lymph glands and other lymphoid tissue
- Usually classified according to histologic, anatomic, and immunomorphic characteristics developed by the National Cancer Institute (Rappaport histologic and Lukes and Collins classifications also used in some facilities)
- Newly identified categories of non-Hodgkin's lymphoma: mantle zone lymphoma and marginal zone lymphoma
- Uses the Hodgkin's disease staging system
- Also called *malignant lymphoma* and *lymphosarcoma*

Pathophysiology
- Non-Hodgkin's lymphoma is similar to Hodgkin's disease, but Reed-Sternberg cells aren't present and the lymph node destruction is different.
- Lymphoid tissue is defined by the pattern of infiltration as diffuse or nodular. Nodular lymphomas yield a better prognosis than the diffuse form, but in both, the prognosis is less hopeful than in Hodgkin's disease.

Causes
- Exact cause unknown

Risk factors
- History of autoimmune disease

Incidence
- Non-Hodgkin's lymphoma three times more common than Hodgkin's disease
- Incidence increasing, especially in patients with autoimmune disorders and those receiving immunosuppressant treatment

  ✳ AGE-RELATED CONCERN Men older than age 60 have the highest incidence of non-Hodgkin's lymphoma.

Common characteristics
- Enlarged lymph nodes
- Fever, malaise
- Weight loss

Complications
- Hypercalcemia
- Hyperuricemia
- Lymphomatosis
- Meningitis
- Anemia
- Liver, kidney, and lung problems (with tumor growth)
- Central nervous system involvement that leads to increased intracranial pressure

✳ ASSESSMENT

History
- Symptoms that mimic those of Hodgkin's disease
- Painless, swollen lymph glands (swelling may have appeared and disappeared over several months)
- Complaints of fatigue, malaise, weight loss, and night sweats
- Trouble breathing, cough (usually children)

Physical findings
- Enlarged tonsils and adenoids
- Rubbery nodes in the cervical and supraclavicular areas

Test results
LABORATORY
- Complete blood count shows anemia.
- Uric acid levels may be normal or elevated.
- Calcium levels are elevated, resulting from bone lesions.
IMAGING
- Miscellaneous scans (chest X-rays; lymphangiography; liver, bone, and spleen scans; computed tomography scan of the abdomen; and excretory urography) show disease progression.
DIAGNOSTIC PROCEDURES
- Biopsies of lymph nodes; of tonsils, bone marrow, liver, bowel, or skin; or, as needed, of tissue removed during exploratory laparotomy help to differentiate a malignant lymphoma from Hodgkin's disease.

◆ TREATMENT

General
- Radiation therapy used mainly during the localized stage of the disease
- Total nodal irradiation often effective in nodular and diffuse lymphomas

Diet
- Well-balanced, high-calorie, high-protein
- Increased fluid intake
- Small, frequent meals

Activity
- Limited activity
- Frequent rest periods

Medication
- Chemotherapy in combinations (cyclophosphamide, vincristine, and prednisone or cycloshosphamide, hydroxydaunomycin, vincristine, and prednisone)

Surgery
- Debulking procedure (such as subtotal or, in some cases, total gastrectomy) before chemotherapy for perforation (common in patients with gastric lymphomas)

✤ NURSING CONSIDERATIONS

Nursing diagnoses
- Acute pain
- Anxiety
- Fatigue
- Fear
- Imbalanced nutrition: Less than body requirements
- Ineffective coping
- Ineffective protection
- Risk for infection

Key outcomes
The patient will:
- express feelings of increased comfort and decreased pain and anxiety
- express feelings of increased energy
- verbalize fears and concerns openly
- experience no further weight loss
- demonstrate effective coping mechanisms
- demonstrate use of protective measures, including conserving energy, maintaining a balanced diet, and getting adequate rest
- remain free from signs and symptoms of infection.

Nursing interventions
- Administer medication, as ordered.
- Provide for rest periods.
- Encourage verbalization and provide support.

Monitoring
- Adverse effects of treatment
- Vital signs
- Pain control
- Hydration and nutritional status

▶ PATIENT TEACHING

Be sure to cover:
- disorder, diagnostic tests, and treatment
- preoperative and postoperative procedures
- dietary plan
- mouth care using a soft-bristled toothbrush and avoidance of commercial mouthwashes
- relaxation and comfort measures
- medication administration, dosage, and possible adverse effects.

Discharge planning
- Refer the patient to resource and support services.

✵ RESOURCES

Organizations
American Cancer Society: *www.cancer.org*
Guide to Internet Resources for Cancer: *www.cancerindex.org*
The Leukemia and Lymphoma Society: *www.leukemia.org*
National Cancer Institute: *www.nci.nih.gov*

Selected references

Atlas of Pathophysiology, 2nd ed. Philadelphia: Lippincott Williams & Wilkins, 2005.

Casciato, D.A. *Manual of Clinical Oncology* 5th ed. Philadelphia: Lippincott Williams & Wilkins, 2004.

Grulich, A.E. , and Vajdic, C.M. "The Epidemiology of Non-Hodgkin's Lymphoma," *Pathology* 37(6):409-19, December 2005.

Hohenstein, M., et al. "Patient-Specific Vaccine Therapy for Non-Hodgkin's Lymphoma, " *Clinical Journal of Oncology Nursing* 9(1):85-90, February 2005.

Lee, W.J., et al. "Asthma History, Occupational Exposure to Pesticides and the Risk for Non-Hodgkin's Lymphoma," *International Journal of Cancer* 118(12):3174-176, June 2006.

Major depression

● OVERVIEW

Description
- Persistent sad, dysphoric mood; may be life-threatening
- Unipolar depressive disorder with onset in early adulthood and recurrences throughout life (at least two more episodes in 50% to 60% of patients)
- Recurrences possible after protracted symptom-free period or occurring sporadically, increasing in frequency, or occurring in clusters

Pathophysiology
- Changes occur in the receptor-neurotransmitter relationships in the limbic system.
- Changes in the hypothalamic-pituitary-adrenal regulation system may be an adaptive deregulation of the stress response.
- There's a possible defect on chromosome II or X.

Causes
- Psychological stress
- Genetic, familial, biochemical, physical, and social
- Many physical causes resulting in secondary depression
- Seasonal depression

Risk factors
- Female gender
- Family history of major depression or bipolar disorder
- Chronic illness
- Chronic pain
- Substance abuse
- Adverse reaction to medication such as beta-adrenergic blockers

Incidence
- Affects approximately 17.6 million Americans each year
- Affects 5% to 20% of general population at some time in their lives
- 6% to 8% of patients in care settings meeting diagnostic criteria
- Incidence increasing with age
- Twice as common in women as men, regardless of age

Common characteristics
- Depressed mood daily for 2 weeks or longer
- History of personal loss or severe stress
- Expression of doubts about self-worth or ability to cope
- Appearance of being unhappy and apathetic

Complications
- Profound alteration of social, family, and occupational functioning
- Suicide

✳ ASSESSMENT

History
- Profound loss of pleasure in all enjoyable activities for a full month to 1 or more years
- Life problems or losses
- Physical disorder
- Use of prescription, nonprescription, or illegal drugs
- Change in eating and sleeping patterns
- Lack of interest in sex
- Constipation or diarrhea

Physical findings
- Difficulty concentrating or thinking clearly
- Easily distracted
- Indecisiveness
- Delusions of persecution or guilt
- Agitation
- Psychomotor retardation
- Somatic delusions

DSM-IV-TR criteria
A diagnosis is confirmed when five or more of the following symptoms present during the same 2-week period and represent a change from previous functioning:
- Depressed mood (irritable mood in children and adolescents) most of the day, nearly every day, as indicated by either subjective account or observation by others
- Markedly diminished interest or pleasure in all, or almost all, activities most of the day, nearly every day
- Significant weight loss or weight gain (greater than 5% of the patient's body weight in a month) when not dieting or a change in appetite nearly every day
- Insomnia or hypersomnia nearly every day
- Psychomotor agitation or retardation
- Fatigue or loss of energy
- Feelings of worthlessness and excessive or inappropriate guilt
- Diminished ability to think or concentrate, or indecisiveness
- Recurrent thoughts of death, recurrent suicidal ideation without a specific plan, or suicide attempt or a specific plan for committing suicide (see *Suicide prevention guidelines*)
- Symptoms that aren't due to a mixed episode, a medical condition, the effects of a medication or other substance, or bereavement

Test results
LABORATORY
- Toxicology screening suggests a drug-induced depression.
DIAGNOSTIC PROCEDURES
- Dexamethasone suppression test may show a failure to suppress cortisol secretion.
- Beck Depression Inventory shows the onset, severity, duration, and progression of depressive symptoms.

◆ TREATMENT

General
- Electroconvulsive therapy
- Short-term psychotherapy (a combination of individual, family, or group psychotherapy)

Diet
- Well-balanced

Activity
- Scheduled activities of daily living

Medication
- Selective serotonin-reuptake inhibitors
- Maprotiline
- Tricyclic antidepressants
- Monoamine oxidase inhibitors

✿ NURSING CONSIDERATIONS

Nursing diagnoses
- Chronic or situational low self-esteem
- Impaired social interaction
- Ineffective coping
- Ineffective role performance
- Insomnia
- Risk for self-directed violence or other-directed violence
- Social isolation

Key outcomes
The patient will:
- voice feelings related to positive self-esteem
- engage in social interactions with others
- develop effective coping behaviors
- achieve a regular sleep pattern
- maintain roles and responsibilities to fullest extent possible
- make a verbal contract not to harm self or others.

Nursing interventions
- Encourage participation in individual and group therapy.
- Encourage verbalization and expression of feelings.
- Listen attentively and respectfully.
- Provide a structured routine and distraction from self-absorption.
- Encourage interaction with others.
- Document observations and significant conversations.
- Assume an active role in initiating communication.
- Plan activities for when the patient's energy levels are highest.

Monitoring
- Adverse effects of medication
- Suicidal ideations
- Self-care
- Social interaction
- Functioning level
- Response to treatment

▶ PATIENT TEACHING

Be sure to cover:
- disorder, diagnostic tests, and treatment
- depression and its effects on daily living
- medication administration, dosage, and possible adverse effects and interactions with other substances
- need for adherence to medication regimen.

Discharge planning
- Refer the patient to support services and community assistance.

✱ RESOURCES

Organizations
American Association of Suicidology:
www.suicidology.org
American Psychiatric Association:
www.psych.org
American Psychological Association:
www.helping.apa.org

Selected references
Diagnostic and Statistical Manual of Mental Disorders, Fourth Edition, Text revision, Washington, D.C.: American Psychiatric Association, 2000.

Ebmeier, K.P,. et al. "Recent Developments and Current Controversies in Depression," *Lancet* 367(9505):153-67, January 2006.

Gunderson, A., and Tomkowiak, J. "Major Depression in Rehabilitation Care," *Rehabilitation Nursing* 30(6):219-20, November-December 2005.

Kendler, K.S., et al. "Toward a Comprehensive Developmental Model for Major Depression in Men," *American Journal of Psychiatry* 163(1):114-24, January 2006.

Montgomery, S.A. "Why Do We Need New and Better Antidepressants?" *International Clinical Psychopharmacology* 21(Suppl 1):S1-10, February 2006.

SUICIDE PREVENTION GUIDELINES

To help deter potential suicide in the patient with major depression, keep in mind these guidelines.

Assess for clues to suicide
Watch for such clues as communicating suicidal thoughts, threats, and messages; hoarding medication; talking about death and feelings of futility; giving away prized possessions; describing a suicide plan; and changing behavior, especially as depression begins to lift.

Provide a safe environment
Check patient areas and correct dangerous conditions, such as exposed pipes, windows without safety glass, and access to the roof or open balconies.

Remove dangerous objects
Remove such objects as belts, razors, suspenders, light cords, glass, knives, nail files, and clippers from the patient's environment.

Consult with staff
Recognize and document verbal and nonverbal suicidal behaviors, keep the physician informed, share data with all staff, clarify the patient's specific restrictions, assess risk and plan for observation, and clarify day and night staff responsibilities and frequency of consultation.

Observe the suicidal patient
Be alert when the patient is using a sharp object (shaving), taking medication, or using the bathroom (to prevent hanging or other injury). Assign the patient to a room near the nurses' station and with another patient. Continuously observe the acutely suicidal patient.

Maintain personal contact
Help the suicidal patient feel that he isn't alone or without resources or hope. Encourage continuity of care and consistency of primary nurses. Building emotional ties to others is the ultimate technique for preventing suicide.

Mastitis

OVERVIEW

Description
- Inflammation of the breast
- Lactating breast infection
- Good prognosis

Pathophysiology
- A pathogen (typically originating in nursing infant's nose or pharynx) invades the breast tissue, entering through a fissured or abraded nipple.
- The result is parenchymatous inflammation of the mammary glands, which disrupts normal lactation.
- Systemic manifestations of inflammation may also result.

Causes
- Most common pathogen is *Staphylococcus aureus;* less frequently, *S. epidermidis* or *beta-hemolytic streptococci*
- Disseminated tuberculosis (rare)
- Mumps virus (rare)

Risk factors
- Fissure or abrasion of the nipple
- Blocked milk ducts
- Incomplete letdown reflex
- Tight fitting bra
- Prolonged intervals between breast-feedings

Incidence
- Occurs in about 1% of lactating women
- More common in breast-feeding primiparas
- Occurs occasionally in nonlactating women
- Rare in men

Common characteristics
- Red, swollen, warm, and tender breasts
- Nipple cracks or fissures
- Enlarged axillary lymph nodes

Complications
- Abscess

ASSESSMENT

History
- Fever
- Malaise
- Flulike symptoms
- Tenderness

Physical findings
- Nipple abrasion or fissure
- Enlarged axillary lymph nodes
- Involved breast is red, edematous, warm, and hard

Test results
LABORATORY
- Cultures of expressed milk confirm generalized mastitis.
- Cultures of breast skin confirm localized mastitis.

TREATMENT

General
- Warm soaks
- Avoidance of tight fitting bras and other clothing
- Continuation of breast-feeding from both breasts to prevent engorgement, with proper infant sucking and changing of feeding positions to drain the milk

Diet
- No restrictions

Activity
- No restrictions

Medication
- Broad-spectrum antibiotics
- Analgesics

Surgery
- Breast abscess incision and drainage

✤ NURSING CONSIDERATIONS

Nursing diagnoses
- Acute pain
- Deficient knowledge (mastitis)
- Ineffective breast-feeding
- Risk for impaired skin integrity
- Risk for infection

Key outcomes
The patient will:
- express feelings of increased comfort and decreased pain
- express understanding of the condition and treatment
- resume breast-feeding without further complications
- maintain skin integrity
- remain free from further signs or symptoms of infection.

Nursing interventions
- Give medications, as ordered.
- Provide warm soaks.
- Use meticulous hand-washing technique.
- Provide meticulous skin care.

Monitoring
- Signs and symptoms of infection
- Abscess development
- Breast engorgement
- Skin integrity
- Breast-feeding process

▶ PATIENT TEACHING

Be sure to cover:
- disorder, diagnostic tests, and treatment
- prescribed antibiotic therapy and potential adverse reactions
- reassurance that breast-feeding won't harm the infant because he's the source of the infection
- offering the infant the unaffected breast first to promote complete emptying and prevent clogged ducts
- need to stop breast-feeding with abscessed breast
- use of a breast pump until abscess heals
- continuation of breast-feeding on the unaffected side
- prevention of mastitis. (See *Preventing mastitis.*)

Discharge planning
- Refer the patient to a lactation specialist, if indicated.

✵ RESOURCES

Organizations
American College of Obstetricians and Gynecologists: *www.acog.org*
La Leche League International: *www.lalecheleague.org*

Selected references
Mass, S. "Breast Pain: Engorgement, Nipple Pain and Mastitis," *Clinical Obstetrics and Gynecology* 47(3):676-82, September 2004.
Potter, B. "A Multi-Method Approach to Measuring Mastitis Incidence," *Community Practitioner* 78(5):169-73, May 2005.
Potter, B. "Women's Experiences of Managing Mastitis," *Community Practitioner* 78(6):209-12, June 2005.

PREVENTING MASTITIS

To help your patient prevent mastitis from recurring, follow these guidelines while breastfeeding:
- Stress the importance of emptying the breasts completely because milk stasis can cause infection and mastitis.
- Teach the patient to alternate feeding positions and to rotate pressure areas on the nipples.
- Remind the patient to position the infant properly on the breast with the entire areola in his mouth.
- Advise her to expose sore nipples to the air as often as possible.
- Teach the patient proper hand-washing technique and personal hygiene.
- Instruct her to get plenty of rest and consume sufficient fluids and a balanced diet to enhance breast-feeding.
- Suggest applying a warm, wet towel to the affected breast or taking a warm shower to relax and improve breast-feeding.

Meconium aspiration syndrome

● OVERVIEW

Description
- Inhalation of meconium that's mixed with amniotic fluid
- Typically occurs while fetus is in utero or with neonate's first breath

Pathophysiology
- Meconium is the thick, sticky, greenish black substance that constitutes the neonate's first feces and is present in the bowel of the fetus as early as 10 weeks' gestation.
- When hypoxia occurs in the fetus, peristalsis increases and the anal sphincter relaxes, allowing meconium to be passed
- The neonate gasps or inhales the meconium while in utero or with the first breath, partially or completely blocking the neonate's airways so that air becomes trapped during exhalation.
- Meconium irritates the neonate's airways, making breathing difficult.
- The severity of meconium aspiration syndrome depends on the amount of meconium aspirated and the consistency of the meconium.
- Neonates with meconium aspiration syndrome increase their respiratory efforts to create greater negative intrathoracic pressures and improve air flow to the lungs.
- Hyperinflation, hypoxemia, and acidemia cause increased peripheral vascular resistance.
- Right-to-left shunting often follows.

Causes
- Exact cause unknown

Risk factors
- Maternal diabetes
- Maternal hypertension
- Difficult delivery
- Fetal distress
- Intrauterine hypoxia
- Advanced gestational age (greater than 40 weeks)
- Poor intrauterine growth

Incidence
- Occurs in approximately 20% of pregnancies at term

Common characteristics
- Greened stained amniotic fluid or skin
- Respiratory distress

Complications
- Bronchopulmonary dysplasia
- Pneumothorax
- Aspiration pneumonia

✳ ASSESSMENT

History
- Maternal evidence of risk factors

Physical findings
- Dark, greenish staining or streaking of the amniotic fluid
- Obvious presence of meconium in the amniotic fluid
- Skin with a greenish stain (if the meconium was passed long before delivery)
- Staining of vocal cords
- Limp appearance at birth
- Cyanosis
- Rapid, labored breathing
- Apnea
- Signs of postmaturity, such as peeling skin and long nails
- Low heart rate before birth
- Low Apgar score
- Hypothermia
- Hypoglycemia
- Hypocalcemia

Test results
LABORATORY
- Arterial blood gases reveal low blood pH and hypoxemia.
IMAGING
- Chest X-ray reveals patches or streaks of meconium in the lungs if air is trapped or if hyperinflation has occurred.

◆ TREATMENT

General
- Suctioning of neonate's nose and mouth as soon as the head is delivered
- Tracheal suctioning, if necessary, to remove all of the meconium before the first breath is taken
- Chest physiotherapy
- Chest tube insertion (for pneumothorax)
- Radiant warmer
- Maternal amnioinfusion before delivery
- Extracorporeal membrane oxygenation (last resort)

Diet
- Gavage feeding or parenteral nutrition

Activity
- As tolerated; clustering care to minimize energy expenditure

Medications
- I.V. fluids
- Antibiotics
- Vasopressors and pulmonary vasodilators
- Supplemental oxygen
- Surfactant therapy if neonate is preterm
- Nitric oxide

Surgery
None

✣ NURSING CONSIDERATIONS

Nursing diagnoses
- Compromised family coping
- Delayed growth and development
- Impaired gas exchange
- Ineffective airway clearance
- Risk for infection
- Risk for injury

Key outcomes
The patient (or family) will
- demonstrate effective coping behaviors
- demonstrate age-appropriate skills and behaviors
- achieve and maintain adequate ventilation and oxygenation
- maintain a patent airway
- remain free from signs and symptoms of infection and injury.

Nursing interventions
- Give prescribed drugs.
- Suction, as necessary.
- Change the transcutaneous PaO_2 monitor lead placement site every 2 to 4 hours.
- Implement measures to prevent infection.
- Encourage parents to participate in neonate's care.
- Encourage parents to ask questions and to express their fears and concerns.
- Offer emotional support.

⬥ **NURSING ALERT** If the neonate requires mechanical ventilation, watch carefully for signs of barotrauma and accidental disconnection from the ventilator. Check ventilator settings and alarms frequently.

Monitoring
- Vital signs
- ABG values
- Intake and output
- Signs and symptoms of infection
- Pulse oximetry
- Daily weight
- Skin color
- Respiratory status
- Skin integrity
- Mechanical ventilation settings

⬥ **NURSING ALERT** Watch for evidence of complications from oxygen therapy: lung capillary damage, decreased mucus flow, impaired ciliary functioning, and widespread atelectasis. Also be alert for signs of patent ductus arteriosus, heart failure, retinopathy, pulmonary hypertension, necrotizing enterocolitis, and neurologic abnormalities.

▶ PATIENT TEACHING

Be sure to cover (with the parents):
- disorder, diagnostic tests, and treatment
- medication administration, dosage, possible adverse effects
- explanations of respiratory equipment, alarm sounds, and mechanical noise
- potential complications
- signs and symptoms of when to notify the physician.

Discharge planning
- Refer the parents to pastoral counselors and social worker, as indicated.
- Refer the patient for follow-up care with a developmental specialist and neonatal ophthalmologist, as indicated.

✳ RESOURCES

Organizations
American Academy of Pediatrics: *www.aap.org*
American Association for Respiratory Care: *www.aarc.org*
American Lung Association: *www.lungusa.org*
National Heart, Lung, and Blood Institute: *www.nhlbi.nih.gov*

Selected references
Fraser, W.D., et. al. "Amnioinfusion for the Prevention of the Meconium Aspiration Syndrome," *New England Journal of Medicine* 353(9):909-17, September 2005.

Jobe, A.H. "Surfactant in Meconium Aspiration Syndrome," *Journal of Pediatrics* 49(5):A3, November 2006.

Pillitteri, A. *Maternal and Child Health Nursing,* 5th ed. Philadelphia: Lippincott Williams and Wilkins, 2007.

Ross, M.G. "Meconium Aspiration Syndrome — More Than Intrapartum Meconium," *New England Journal of Medicine* 353(9):946-48, September 2005.

Melanoma, malignant

● OVERVIEW

Description
- Neoplasm that arises from melanocytes
- Potentially the most lethal of the skin cancers
- Common sites: head and neck in men, legs in women, and backs of people exposed to excessive sunlight
- Four types:
  - Superficial spreading melanoma: most common type; usually develops between ages 40 and 50
  - Nodular melanoma: grows vertically, invades the dermis, and metastasizes early; usually develops between ages 40 and 50
  - Acral-lentiginous melanoma: occurs on the palms and soles and in sublingual locations; most common melanoma among Hispanics, Asians, and Blacks
  - Lentigo maligna melanoma: relatively rare; most benign, slowest growing, and least aggressive of the four types; most commonly occurs in areas heavily exposed to the sun; arises from a lentigo maligna on an exposed skin surface; usually occurs between ages 60 and 70

Pathophysiology
- Malignant melanoma arises as a result of malignant degeneration of melanocytes located either along the basal layer of the epidermis or in a benign melanocytic nevus.
- Up to 70% of malignant melanomas arise from a preexisting nevus.
- Malignant melanoma spreads through the lymphatic and vascular systems and metastasizes to the regional lymph nodes, skin, liver, lungs, and central nervous system.
- Malignant melanoma follows an unpredictable course; recurrence and metastasis may not appear for more than 5 years after resection of the primary lesion.

Causes
- Ultraviolet rays from the sun that damage the skin and can cause malignant melanoma

Risk factors
- Excessive exposure to sunlight
- Skin type (blond or red hair, fair skin, and blue eyes; prone to sunburn; and Celtic or Scandinavian ancestry)
- Hormonal factors (pregnancy)
- Family history
- Past history of melanoma
- Preexisting pigmented mole or nevus

Incidence
- Account for 1% to 2% of all malignant tumors
- Slightly more common in women than in men
- Unusual in children
- Peak incidence between ages 50 and 70, but incidence in younger age groups increasing

Common characteristics
- Sore that doesn't heal
- Preexisting lesion or nevus that changes in appearance

Complications
- Metastasis to the lungs, liver, or brain

✳ ASSESSMENT

History
- A sore that doesn't heal, a persistent lump or swelling, and changes in preexisting skin markings, such as moles, birthmarks, scars, freckles, or warts
- Preexisting skin lesion or nevus that enlarges, changes color, becomes inflamed or sore, itches, ulcerates, bleeds, changes texture, or shows signs of surrounding pigment regression

Physical findings
- Lesions on the ankles or the inside surfaces of the knees
- Uniformly discolored nodule on knee or ankle
- Small, elevated tumor nodules that may ulcerate and bleed
- Palpable polypoid nodules that resemble the surface of a blackberry
- Pigmented lesions on the palms and soles or under the nails
- Long-standing lesion that has ulcerated
- Flat nodule with smaller nodules scattered over the surface

Test results
LABORATORY
- Complete blood count with differential shows anemia.
- Erythrocyte sedimentation rate is elevated.
- Platelet count is abnormal (if metastasis).
- Liver function studies are abnormal (if metastasis).
IMAGING
- Chest X-ray assists in staging.
DIAGNOSTIC PROCEDURES
- Excisional biopsy and full-depth punch biopsy with histologic examination can show tumor thickness and disease stage.

◆ TREATMENT

General
- Close long-term follow-up care to detect metastasis and recurrences
- Radiation therapy (usually for metastatic disease)

Diet
- Well-balanced; no restrictions

Activity
- Avoidance of sun exposure

Medication
- Chemotherapy
- Biotherapy
- Immunotherapy
- Immunostimulants

Surgery
- Surgical resection to remove lesion and 3- to 5-cm margin
- Regional lymphadenectomy

Nursing diagnoses

- Acute pain
- Anxiety
- Disturbed body image
- Fear
- Grieving
- Imbalanced nutrition: Less than body requirements
- Impaired skin integrity
- Ineffective coping
- Risk for infection

Key outcomes

The patient (or family) will:

- express feelings of increased comfort and decreased pain
- express feelings about condition and potential loss
- exhibit signs of a decrease in anxiety
- express positive feelings about self
- verbalize fears and concerns about diagnosis and condition
- maintain weight within acceptable range
- experience healing of wound
- demonstrate effective coping mechanisms
- remain free from signs and symptoms of infection.

Nursing interventions

- Encourage verbalization and provide support.
- Provide appropriate wound care.
- Administer medications as ordered.
- Provide a high-protein, high-calorie diet.

Monitoring

- Complications of treatment
- Pain control
- Wound site
- Postoperative complications

Be sure to cover:

- disorder, diagnostic tests, and treatment
- preoperative and postoperative care
- need for close follow-up care to detect recurrences early
- signs and symptoms of recurrence
- detrimental effects of overexposure to solar radiation and benefits of regular use of a sunblock or a sunscreen.

Discharge planning

- Refer the patient to resource and support services.

Organizations

American Cancer Society: *www.cancer.org*
Guide to Internet Resources for Cancer: *www.cancerindex.org*
National Cancer Institute: *www.nci.nih.gov*

Selected references

Atlas of Pathophysiology, 2nd ed. Philadelphia: Lippincott Williams & Wilkins, 2005.

Casciato, D.A. *Manual of Clinical Oncology,* 5th ed. Philadelphia: Lippincott Williams & Wilkins, 2004.

Christopoulou, A., et al. "Integration of Gamma Knife Surgery in the Management of Cerebral Metastases from Melanoma," *Melanoma Research* 16(1):51-57, February 2006.

Demierre, M.F., et al. "New Treatments for Melanoma," *Dermatology Nursing* 17(14):287-95, August 2005.

Lee, D.A., et al. "Are All Melanomas the Same? Spitzoid Melanoma is a Distinct Subtype of Melanoma," *Cancer* 106(4):907-13, February 2006.

Niendorf, K.B., and Tsao, H. "Cutaneous Melanoma: Family Screening and Genetic Testing," *Dermatologic Therapy* 18(1):1-8, January-February 2006.

Meningitis

● OVERVIEW

Description
- Inflammation of brain and spinal cord meninges
- May affect all three meningeal membranes (dura mater, arachnoid membrane, and pia mater)
- Usually follows onset of respiratory symptoms
- Sudden onset, causing serious illness within 24 hours
- Bacterial meningitis: acute infection in the subarachnoid space
- Good prognosis; complications rare
- ❋ AGE-RELATED CONCERN Prognosis is poorer for infants and elderly people.

Pathophysiology
- Inflammation of pia-arachnoid progresses to congestion of adjacent tissues.
- Nerve cells are destroyed.
- Intracranial pressure (ICP) increases because of exudates.
- Results can include:
  - engorged blood vessels
  - disrupted blood supply
  - edema of brain tissue
  - thrombosis
  - rupture
  - acute hydrocephalus.

Causes
- Bacterial infection, usually from *Neisseria meningitidis* and *Streptococcus pneumoniae* (Before the 1990s, *Haemophilus influenzae* type b [Hib] was the leading cause of bacterial meningitis. However, new vaccines have reduced its occurrence in children.)
- Viruses
- Protozoa
- Fungi
- Secondary to another bacterial infection such as pneumonia
- May follow skull fracture, penetrating head wound, lumbar puncture, or ventricular shunting procedures

Incidence
- ❋ AGE-RELATED CONCERN Infants, children, and elderly people have highest risk. It's also an increasing risk with college students.

Common characteristics
- Headache
- Fever
- Meningismus, typically with signs of cerebral dysfunction

Complications
- Visual impairment, optic neuritis
- Cranial nerve palsies, deafness
- Paresis or paralysis
- Endocarditis
- Coma
- Vasculitis
- Cerebral infarction
- Seizures

✳ ASSESSMENT

History
- Headache
- Fever
- Nausea, vomiting
- Weakness
- Myalgia
- Photophobia
- Confusion, delirium
- Seizures

Physical findings
- Meningismus
- Rigors
- Profuse sweating
- Kernig's and Brudzinski's signs elicited in only 50% of adults
- Decreasing level of consciousness (LOC)
- Cranial nerve palsies
- Focal neurologic deficits such as visual field defects
- Signs of increased ICP (in later stages)
- ❋ AGE-RELATED CONCERN Meningismus and fever are commonly absent in neonates, and the only clinical clues may be nonspecific, such as refusal to feed, high-pitched cry, and irritability.
- ❋ AGE-RELATED CONCERN Elderly patients may have an insidious onset, exhibiting lethargy and variable signs of meningismus and no fever.

Test results
LABORATORY
- White blood cell count shows leukocytosis.
- Blood cultures are positive in bacterial meningitis, depending on the pathogen.
- Coagglutination tests reveal causative agent.

IMAGING
- Chest X-rays may reveal pneumonia.
- Neuroimaging techniques, such as computed tomography and magnetic resonance imaging, may detect complications and a parameningeal source of infection.

DIAGNOSTIC PROCEDURES
- Lumbar puncture with cerebrospinal fluid analysis shows:
  - increased opening pressure
  - neutrophilic pleocytosis
  - elevated protein, decreased glucose level

– hypoglycorrhachia
– positive Gram stain
– positive culture
– enterovirus via Xpert EV test (distinguishes viral meningitis from bacterial meningitis).

◆ TREATMENT

General
- Fever reduction
- Fluid therapy
- Pain management

Diet
- Generally no restrictions

Activity
- Bed rest (in acute phase)

Medication
- I.V. antibiotics
- Oral antibiotics
- Antiarrhythmics
- Osmotic diuretics
- Anticonvulsants
- Aspirin or acetaminophen

❖ NURSING CONSIDERATIONS

Nursing diagnoses
- Acute pain
- Anxiety
- Hyperthermia
- Impaired gas exchange
- Risk for deficient fluid volume
- Risk for impaired skin integrity

Key outcomes
The patient will:
- express feelings of increased comfort and decreased pain
- demonstrate a decrease in anxiety
- have normal temperature
- maintain adequate ventilation and oxygenation
- maintain normal fluid volume
- maintain skin integrity.

Nursing interventions
- Administer oxygen, as ordered.
- Position the patient in proper body alignment.
- Maintain droplet precautions for first 24 hours (with *H. influenzae* or meningococcus infection)
- Encourage active range-of-motion (ROM) exercises when appropriate.
- Provide passive ROM exercises when appropriate.
- Maintain adequate nutrition.
- Administer laxatives or stool softeners, as ordered.
- Provide meticulous skin and mouth care.
- Administer prescribed medications, as ordered.

Monitoring
- Neurologic status
- Vital signs
- Signs and symptoms of cranial nerve involvement
- Signs and symptoms of increased ICP
- Seizures
- Respiratory status
- Arterial blood gas results
- Fluid balance
- Response to medications
- Complications

▶ PATIENT TEACHING

Be sure to cover:
- disorder, diagnostic tests, and treatment
- contagion risks for close contacts
- medication administration, dosage, and possible adverse effects
- signs and symptoms of meningitis
- polysaccharide meningococcal vaccine, pneumococcal vaccine, and Hib vaccine.

✺ RESOURCES

Organizations
National Institutes of Health: *www.nih.gov*
Web MD: *www.webmd.com*

Selected references
Diseases, 4th ed. Philadelphia: Lippincott Williams & Wilkins, 2006.

Estep, M. "Meningococcal Meningitis in Critical Care: An Overview, New Treatments/Preventions, and a Case Study," *Critical Care Nursing Quarterly* 28(2):111-21, April-June 2005.

Handbook of Pathophysiology, 2nd ed. Philadelphia: Lippincott Williams & Wilkins, 2004.

Harrison, L.H., "Prospects for Vaccine Prevention of Meningococcal Infection," *Clinical Microbiology Reviews* 19(1):142-64, January 2006.

Snyder, C.H. "Coccidioidal Meningitis Presenting as Memory Loss," *Journal of the American Academy of Nurse Practitioners* 17(5):18-16, May 2005.

Metabolic syndrome

Description

- Cluster of symptoms triggered by insulin resistance: abdominal fat; obesity; high blood pressure; and high levels of blood glucose, triglycerides, and cholesterol
- Associated with increased risk of diabetes, heart disease, and stroke
- Often unrecognized
- Also known as *syndrome X, insulin resistance syndrome, dysmetabolic syndrome,* and *multiple metabolic syndrome*

Pathophysiology

- The body breaks down food into basic components; one of these components is glucose, which provides energy for cellular activity.
- Insulin, which is secreted by the pancreas, stores excess glucose in cells for future use.
- In those with metabolic syndrome, glucose doesn't respond to insulin's attempt to guide it into storage cells—called insulin resistance.
- To overcome this resistance, the pancreas produces excess insulin, which causes damage to arterial lining, promotes fat storage deposits, and prevents fat breakdown.
- This series of events can lead to diabetes, blood clots, and coronary events.

Causes

- Acquired factors (see "Risk factors")
- Genetic predisposition

Risk factors

- Obesity
- High-fat, high-carbohydrate diet
- Insufficient physical activity
- Aging
- Hyperinsulinemia/impaired glucose tolerance
- Previous heart attack

Incidence

- Affects an estimated 47 million people in the United States
- Most common in Mexican Americans (highest rate at 32%)
- In Black and Mexican-American populations, women more susceptible

than men; otherwise, men and women equally affected

Common characteristics

- Abdominal obesity
- Hypertension
- Altered lipoprotein levels

Complications

- Coronary artery disease
- Diabetes
- Hyperlipidemia
- Premature death

History

- Familial history
- Hypertension
- High low-density lipoprotein (LDL) and triglyceride levels
- Low high-density lipoprotein (HDL) levels
- Abdominal obesity
- Sedentary lifestyle
- Poor diet

Physical findings

- Abdominal obesity (see *Why abdominal obesity is dangerous*)

Test results

LABORATORY

- Glucose level is elevated.
- LDL and triglyceride levels are increased.
- HDL level is decreased.
- Blood tests show hyperinsulinemia.
- Serum uric acid level is elevated.

OTHER

- Blood pressure is greater than 130/85 mm Hg.

WHY ABDOMINAL OBESITY IS DANGEROUS

People with excess weight around the waist have a greater risk of developing metabolic syndrome than people with excess weight around the hips. That's because intra-abdominal fat tends to be more resistant to insulin than fat in other areas of the body. Insulin resistance increases the release of free fatty acid into the portal system, leading to increased apolipoprotein B, increased low-density lipoprotein, decreased high-density lipoprotein, and increased triglyceride levels. As a result, the risk of cardiovascular disease increases.

◆ TREATMENT

General
- Supportive

Diet
- Low alcohol intake
- Low-cholesterol
- High in complex carbohydrates (grains, beans, vegetables, fruit) and low in refined carbohydrates (soda, table sugar, high-fructose corn syrup)

Activity
- Daily physical activity of at least 20 minutes
- Weight reduction program

Medications
- Oral antidiabetic agents
- Antihypertensives
- Statins

❖ NURSING CONSIDERATIONS

Nursing diagnoses
- Fatigue
- Imbalanced nutrition: More than body requirements
- Risk for injury

Key outcomes
The patient will:
- express feelings of increased energy
- identify appropriate food choices according to a prescribed diet and maintain a healthy weight
- remain free from injury.

Nursing Interventions
- Promote lifestyle changes and give appropriate support.

Monitoring
- Blood pressure
- Ordered laboratory tests

▶ PATIENT TEACHING

Be sure to cover:
- disorder, diagnostic tests, and treatment
- principles of a healthy diet
- relationship of diet, inactivity, and obesity to metabolic syndrome
- benefits of increased physical activity
- medication administration, dosage, and possible adverse effects.

Discharge planning
- Assist with referrals to weight reduction programs or support services.

✹ RESOURCES

Organizations
American Diabetes Association: *www.diabetes.org*
American Heart Association: *www.americanheart.org*
Cleveland Clinic Health Information Center: *www.clevelandclinic.org/health*

Selected references
Appel, S.J. "Sizing Up Patients for Metabolic Syndrome," *Nursing* 35(12):20-21, December 2005.

Bell-Anderson, K., and Sarnman, S. "Nutrition and Metabolism: Race, Sex and the Metabolic Syndrome," *Current Opinion in Lipidology* 17(1):82-84, February 2006.

Fowler, S.B., et al. "Metabolic Syndrome: Contributing Factors and Treatment Strategies," *Journal of Neuroscience Nursing* 37(4):220-23, August 2003.

Venkatapuram, S., and Shannon, R.P. "Managing Atherosclerosis in Patients with Type 2 Diabetes and Metabolic Syndrome," *American Journal of Therapeutics* 13(1):64-71, January-February 2006.

Methicillin-resistant *Staphylococcus aureus*

● OVERVIEW

Description
- Mutation of a very common bacterium easily spread by direct person-to-person contact
- Also known as *MRSA*

Pathophysiology
- 90% of *Staphylococcus aureus* isolates or strains are penicillin-resistant, and about 27% of all *S. aureus* isolates are resistant to methicillin, a penicillin derivative. These strains may also resist cephalosporins, aminoglycosides, erythromycin, tetracycline, and clindamycin.
- When natural defense systems break down (after invasive procedures, trauma, or chemotherapy), the usually benign bacteria can invade tissue, proliferate, and cause infection.
- The most frequent colonization site is the anterior nares (40% of adults and most children become transient nasal carriers). The groin, axilla, and gut are less common colonization sites.

Causes
- MRSA that enters a health care facility through an infected or colonized patient (symptom-free carrier of the bacteria) or colonized health care worker
- Transmitted mainly by health care workers' hands

Risk factors
- Immunosuppression
- Prolonged facility stays
- Extended therapy with multiple or broad-spectrum antibiotics
- Close proximity to others colonized or infected with MRSA

Incidence
- Endemic in nursing homes, long-term care facilities, and community facilities

Common characteristics
- Dependent upon body system affected

Complications
- Sepsis
- Death

✳ ASSESSMENT

History
- Possible risk factors for MRSA
- Carrier patient often asymptomatic

Physical findings
- In symptomatic patients, signs and symptoms related to the primary diagnosis (respiratory, cardiac, or other major system symptoms)

Test results
LABORATORY
- Cultures from suspicious wounds, skin, urine, or blood show MRSA.

◆ TREATMENT

General
- Infection control precautions: contact precautions for wound, skin, and urine infections; droplet precautions for respiratory/sputum infections
- Isolation of patient with MRSA infection
- No treatment needed for patient with colonization only

Diet
- High-protein

Activity
- Rest periods, as needed

Medication
- Linezolid

❖ NURSING CONSIDERATIONS

Nursing diagnoses
- Acute pain
- Decreased cardiac output
- Deficient fluid volume
- Hyperthermia
- Impaired gas exchange
- Impaired tissue integrity
- Ineffective tissue perfusion: Cardiopulmonary

Key outcomes
The patient will:
- express feelings of increased comfort and decreased pain
- maintain adequate cardiac output
- have an adequate fluid volume
- remain afebrile
- maintain adequate ventilation and oxygenation
- have wounds that remain free from infection
- attain hemodynamic stability and maintain collateral circulation.

Nursing interventions
- Provide emotional support to the patient and family members.
- Consider grouping infected patients together and having the same nursing staff care for them.
- Use proper hand-washing technique.
- Use appropriate infection control precautions.

Monitoring
- Vital signs
- Culture results
- Response to treatment
- Adverse drug reactions
- Complications

▶ PATIENT TEACHING

Be sure to cover:
- disorder, diagnostic tests, and treatment
- difference between MRSA infection and colonization
- prevention of MRSA spread
- proper hand-washing technique
- need for family and friends to wear protective garb when they visit the patient and proper disposal
- medication administration, dosage, and possible adverse effects
- need to take antibiotics for the full prescription period, even as the patient begins to feel better.

Discharge planning
- Refer the patient to an infectious disease specialist, if indicated.

✱ RESOURCES

Organizations
Centers for Disease Control and Prevention: *www.cdc.gov*
Harvard University Consumer Health Information: *www.intelihealth.com*
National Health Information Center: *www.health.gov/nhic/*
National Library of Medicine: *www.nlm.nih.gov*

Selected references
Cowan, T. "A Victory Against MRSA," *Journal of Wound Care* 14(8):372, September 2005.

Kasper, D.L., et al., eds. *Harrison's Principles of Internal Medicine,* 16th ed. New York: McGraw-Hill Book Co., 2005.

Mylotte, J.M. "Nursing Home-Acquired Bloodstream Infection," *Infection Control and Hospital Epidemiology* 26(10):833-37, October 2005.

Ott, M., et al. "Evidence-Based Practice for Control of Methicillin-Resistant *Staphylococcus Aureus*," *AORN Journal* 81(2):361-64, 367-72, February 2005.

Mitral insufficiency

● OVERVIEW

Description
- Valvular disease of the mitral valve that allows the backflow of blood from the left ventricle to the left atrium
- May be acute (sudden volume overload of the left ventricle), chronic compensated (left ventricle compensates and left ventricular enlargement occurs), or chronic decompensated (left ventricle unable to sustain forward cardiac output)
- Also known as *mitral regurgitation*

Pathophysiology
- Blood from the left ventricle flows back into the left atrium during systole, causing the atrium to enlarge to accommodate the backflow.
- As a result, the left ventricle dilates to accommodate the increased volume of blood from the atrium and to compensate for diminishing cardiac output.
- Ventricular hypertrophy and increased end-diastolic pressure result in increased pulmonary artery pressure, eventually leading to left- and right-sided heart failure.

Causes
- Hypertrophic cardiomyopathy
- Infective endocarditis
- Mitral valve prolapse
- Myocardial infarction
- Rheumatic fever
- Ruptured chordae tendineae
- Scleroderma
- Severe left-sided heart failure
- Systemic lupus erythematosus
- Trauma

Risk factors
- Congenital anomalies such as transposition of the great arteries

Incidence
- Can occur at any age
- Affects both sexes equally

Common characteristics
- Pansystolic murmur
- Orthopnea
- Dyspnea
- Palpitation

Complications
- Heart failure
- Pulmonary edema
- Thromboembolism
- Endocarditis
- Arrhythmias

✳ ASSESSMENT

History
- Causal occurrence
- Orthopnea
- Dyspnea
- Fatigue
- Angina
- Palpitations

Physical findings
- Tachycardia
- Crackles in the lungs
- Hepatomegaly (right-sided failure)
- Holosystolic murmur at the apex (see *Identifying the murmur of mitral valve insufficiency*)
- Possible split S_2
- S_3

Test results
IMAGING
- Chest X-ray reveals left atrial and ventricular enlargement and pulmonary congestion.
- Echocardiogram shows abnormal valve leaflet motion and left atrial enlargement.

DIAGNOSTIC PROCEDURES
- Cardiac catheterization reveals mitral insufficiency with increased left ventricular end-diastolic volume and pressure, increased atrial pressure and pulmonary artery wedge pressure, and decreased cardiac output.

- Electrocardiography may show left atrial and ventricular hypertrophy, sinus tachycardia. or atrial fibrillation.

◆ TREATMENT

General
- Appropriate treatment of underlying cause

Diet
- Low-sodium

Activity
- As tolerated

Medications
- Diuretics
- Inotropic agents
- Angiotensin-converting enzyme inhibitors
- Oxygen
- Anticoagulants
- Prophylactic antibiotics before and after surgery or dental care to prevent endocarditis
- Beta-adrenergic blockers or digoxin to slow the ventricular rate in atrial fibrillation or atrial flutter

Surgery
- Annuloplasty or valvuloplasty to reconstruct or repair the valve
- Valve replacement with a prosthetic valve

IDENTIFYING THE MURMUR OF MITRAL INSUFFICIENCY

A high-pitched, rumbling pansystolic murmur that radiates from the mitral area to the left axillary line characterizes mitral insufficiency.

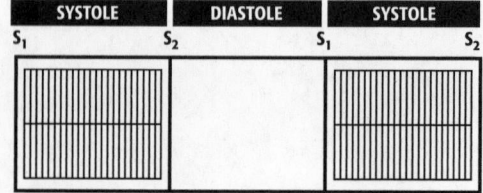

SYSTOLE		DIASTOLE	SYSTOLE	
S_1		S_2	S_1	S_2

NURSING CONSIDERATIONS

Nursing diagnoses
- Activity intolerance
- Decreased cardiac output
- Excess fluid volume
- Fatigue
- Impaired gas exchange
- Impaired physical mobility
- Ineffective coping
- Ineffective tissue perfusion: Cardiopulmonary
- Risk for infection

Key outcomes
The patient will:
- carry out activities of daily living without weakness or fatigue
- maintain hemodynamic stability and adequate cardiac output, with no arrhythmias
- experience no complications from fluid excess
- verbalize the importance of balancing activity with adequate rest periods
- maintain adequate ventilation and oxygenation
- maintain joint mobility and muscle strength
- exhibit adequate coping mechanisms
- maintain adequate cardiopulmonary perfusion
- remain free from signs and symptoms of infection.

Nursing interventions
- Give prescribed oxygen.
- Watch for signs of heart failure or pulmonary edema.

Monitoring
- Vital signs and pulse oximetry
- Cardiac rhythm
- Pulmonary artery catheter readings
- Intake and output
- Adverse effects of drug therapy

PATIENT TEACHING

Be sure to cover:
- disorder, diagnostic tests, and treatment
- dietary restrictions
- medications administration, dosage, and possible adverse effects.

RESOURCES

Organizations
American Heart Association: *www.americanheart.org*
Cleveland Clinic Health Information Center: *www.clevelandclinic.org/health*
HeartCenterOnline: *www.heart.healthcentersonline.com*
Mayo Foundation for Medical Education and Research: *www.mayoclinic.com*
National Institutes of Health: *www.nih.gov*

Selected references
Sanchez, P.L., et al. "The Impact of Age in the Immediate and Long-Term Outcomes of Percutaneous Mitral Balloon Valvuloplasty," *Journal of Interventional Cardiology* 18(4):217-25, August 2005.

Todd, B.A., and Higgins, K. "Recognizing Aortic and Mitral Valve Disease," *Nursing* 35(6):58-63, June 2005.

Ziegler, K., and Quillen, T.E "Mitral Valve Regurgitation after Myocardial Infarction," *Nursing* 35(11):88, November 2005.

Mitral stenosis

● OVERVIEW

Description
- Narrowing of the mitral valve orifice, which is normally 3 to 6 cm
- Mild mitral stenosis: valve orifice of 2 cm
- Moderate mitral stenosis: valve orifice between 1 and 2 cm
- Severe mitral stenosis: valve orifice of 1 cm

Pathophysiology
- Valve leaflets become diffusely thickened by fibrosis and calcification.
- The mitral commissures and the chordae tendineae fuse and shorten, the valvular cusps become rigid, and the valve's apex becomes narrowed. This obstructs blood flow from the left atrium to the left ventricle.
- Left atrial volume and pressure increase, and the atrial chamber dilates.
- Increased resistance to blood flow causes pulmonary hypertension, right ventricular hypertrophy and, eventually, right-sided heart failure and reduced cardiac output.

Causes
- Rheumatic fever
- Congenital anomalies
- Atrial myxoma
- Endocarditis
- Adverse effects of fenfluramine and phentermine (Fen-phen) diet drug combination

Incidence
- Females accounting for two-thirds of all mitral stenosis patients
- Occurs in approximately 40% of patients with rheumatic heart disease

Common characteristics
- Gradual decline in exercise tolerance
- Dyspnea on exertion
- Shortness of breath

Complications
- Cardiac arrhythmias, especially atrial fibrillation
- Thromboembolism

✻ ASSESSMENT

History
MILD MITRAL STENOSIS
- Asymptomatic
MODERATE TO SEVERE MITRAL STENOSIS
- Gradual decline in exercise tolerance
- Dyspnea on exertion, shortness of breath
- Paroxysmal nocturnal dyspnea
- Orthopnea
- Weakness
- Fatigue
- Palpitations
- Cough

Physical findings
- Hemoptysis
- Peripheral and facial cyanosis
- Malar rash
- Jugular vein distention
- Ascites
- Peripheral edema
- Hepatomegaly
- A loud S_1 or opening snap
- A diastolic murmur at the apex (see *Identifying the murmur of mitral stenosis*)
- Crackles over lung fields
- Right ventricular lift
- Resting tachycardia; irregularly irregular heart rhythm

Test results
IMAGING
- Chest X-rays show left atrial and ventricular enlargement (in severe mitral stenosis), straightening of the left border of the cardiac silhouette, enlarged pulmonary arteries, dilation of the upper lobe pulmonary veins, and mitral valve calcification.
- Echocardiography discloses thickened mitral valve leaflets and left atrial enlargement.
DIAGNOSTIC PROCEDURES
- Cardiac catheterization shows a diastolic pressure gradient across the valve, elevated pulmonary artery wedge pressure (greater than 15 mm Hg), and pulmonary artery pressure in the left atrium with severe pulmonary hypertension.
- Electrocardiography reveals left atrial enlargement, right ventricular hypertrophy, right axis deviation, and (in 40% to 50% of cases) atrial fibrillation.

◆ TREATMENT

General
- Synchronized electrical cardioversion to correct atrial fibrillation

Diet
- Sodium-restricted

Activity
- As tolerated

Medication
- Digoxin
- Diuretics
- Oxygen
- Beta-adrenergic blockers
- Calcium-channel blockers
- Anticoagulants
- Infective endocarditis antibiotic prophylaxis
- Nitrates

Surgery
- Commissurotomy or valve replacement
- Percutaneous balloon valvuloplasty

❖ NURSING CONSIDERATIONS

Nursing diagnoses
- Activity intolerance
- Decreased cardiac output
- Excess fluid volume
- Fatigue
- Impaired gas exchange
- Impaired physical mobility
- Ineffective coping
- Ineffective role performance
- Ineffective tissue perfusion: Cardio-pulmonary
- Risk for infection

Key outcomes
The patient will:
- carry out activities of daily living without weakness or fatigue
- maintain adequate cardiac output
- maintain adequate fluid volume
- report an increase in energy level
- maintain adequate ventilation and oxygenation
- maintain joint mobillity and muscle strength
- cope with condition without demonstrating severe signs of anxiety
- express feelings about diminished capacity to perform usual roles
- maintain adequate cardiopulmony perfusion
- remain free from signs and symptoms of infection.

Nursing interventions
- Check for hypersensitivity reaction to antibiotics.
- Stress the importance of bed rest, if needed. Provide a bedside commode.
- Allow the patient to express concerns over her inability to meet responsibilities because of activity restrictions.
- Place the patient in an upright position to relieve dyspnea, if needed.
- Provide a low-sodium diet.

Monitoring
- Vital signs and hemodynamics
- Intake and output
- Signs and symptoms of heart failure and pulmonary edema
- Signs and symptoms of thromboembolism
- Adverse drug reactions
- Cardiac arrhythmias

- Postoperatively: hypotension, arrhythmias, and thrombus formation

▶ PATIENT TEACHING

Be sure to cover:
- disorder, diagnostic tests, and treatment
- need to plan for periodic rest in daily routine
- how to take the pulse
- dietary restrictions
- medication administration, dosage, and possible adverse effects
- signs and symptoms to report
- importance of consistent follow-up care
- when to notify the physician.

✱ RESOURCES

Organizations
American Heart Association: *www.americanheart.org*
Cleveland Clinic Health Information Center: *www.clevelandclinic.org/health*
HeartCenterOnline: *www.heart.healthcentersonline.com*
Mayo Foundation for Medical Education and Research: *www.mayoclinic.com*
National Institutes of Health: *www.nih.gov*

Selected references
Kasper, D.L., et al., eds. *Harrison's Principles of Internal Medicine*, 16th ed. New York: McGraw-Hill Book Co., 2005.
The Merck Manual of Diagnosis & Therapy, 18th ed. Whitehouse Station N.J.: Merck & Co., Inc., 2006.
Sebag, I.A., et al. "Usefulness of Three-Dimensionally Guided Assessment of Mitral Stenosis Using Matrix-Array Ultrasound," *American Journal of Cardiology* 96(8):1151-156, October 2005.
Todd, B.A., and Higgins, K. "Recognizing Aortic and Mitral Valve Disease," *Nursing* 35(6):58-63, June 2005.

IDENTIFYING THE MURMUR OF MITRAL STENOSIS

A low, rumbling crescendo-decrescendo murmur in the mitral valve area characterizes mitral stenosis.

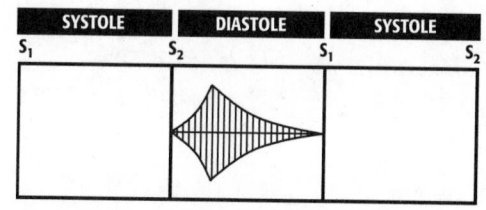

Mitral valve prolapse

● OVERVIEW

Description
- Portion of the mitral valve (MV) that prolapses into the left atrium during ventricular contraction (systole)
- Also known as *MVP*

Pathophysiology
- Myxomatous degeneration of MV leaflets with redundant tissue leads to prolapse of the MV into the left atrium during systole.
- In some patients, this results in leakage of blood into the left atrium from the left ventricle.

Causes
- Connective tissue disorders, such as systemic lupus erythematosus and Marfan syndrome
- Congenital heart disease
- Acquired heart disease, such as coronary artery disease and rheumatic heart disease

Incidence
- More prevalent in females than males
- Usually detected in young adulthood
- Affects 2.5% to 5% of the general population

 AGE-RELATED CONCERN MVP is most common in women ages 20 to 40.

Common characteristics
- Palpitations
- Atypical chest pain

Complications
- Arrhythmias
- Infective endocarditis
- Mitral insufficiency from chordal rupture

✳ ASSESSMENT

History
- Usually asymptomatic
- Possible fatigue, syncope, palpitations, chest pain, or dyspnea on exertion

Physical findings
- Orthostatic hypotension
- Mid-to-late systolic click and late systolic murmur

Test results
IMAGING
- Echocardiography may reveal MVP with or without mitral insufficiency.

DIAGNOSTIC PROCEDURES
- Electrocardiography (ECG) is usually normal but may reveal atrial or ventricular arrhythmia.
- Signal-averaged ECG may show ventricular and supraventricular arrhythmias.
- Holter monitor worn for 24 hours may show an arrhythmia.

◆ TREATMENT

General
- Usually requires no treatment; regular monitoring necessary, however

Diet
- Decreased caffeine intake
- Increased fluid intake to maintain hydration

Activity
- No restrictions

Medication
- Antibiotic prophylaxis
- Beta-adrenergic blockers
- Anticoagulants
- Antiarrhythmics

❖ NURSING CONSIDERATIONS

Nursing diagnoses
- Activity intolerance
- Anxiety
- Decreased cardiac output
- Fatigue
- Impaired gas exchange
- Ineffective coping
- Ineffective tissue perfusion: Cardio-pulmonary
- Risk for infection

Key outcomes
The patient will:
- carry out activities of daily living without fatigue or anxiety
- maintain adequate cardiac output, without arrhythmias
- report increased energy
- demonstrate adequate ventilation and oxygenation
- exhibit positive coping methods for current medical condition
- maintain adequate cardiopulmonary perfusion
- remain free from signs and symptoms of infection.

Nursing interventions
- Provide reassurance and comfort if the patient experiences anxiety.
- Plan rest periods, as needed.

Monitoring
- Vital signs
- Blood pressure while lying, sitting, and standing
- Heart sounds
- Signs and symptoms of mitral insufficiency
- Serial echocardiograms
- ECG for arrhythmias

▶ PATIENT TEACHING

Be sure to cover:
- disorder, diagnostic tests, and treatment
- need to perform the most important activities of the day when energy levels are highest
- need for antibiotic prophylaxis therapy before dental or surgical procedures, as indicated (Not all patients with MVP require antibiotic prophylaxis.)
- medication administration, dosage, and possible adverse effects
- importance of adequate hydration
- avoidance of foods and beverages high in caffeine.

Discharge planning
- If being discharged with a Holter monitor, make sure the patient understands the importance of documenting her activities throughout the monitoring process.
- Refer the patient to an MVP support group.

✳ RESOURCES

Organizations
American Heart Association: *www.americanheart.org*
Cleveland Clinic Health Information Center: *www.clevelandclinic.org/health*
Mayo Foundation for Medical Education and Research: *www.mayoclinic.com*
National Heart, Lung, and Blood Institute: *www.nhlbi.nih.gov*
National Institutes of Health: *www.nih.gov*

Selected references
Kasper, D.L., et al., eds. *Harrison's Principles of Internal Medicine*, 16th ed. New York: McGraw-Hill Book Co., 2005.
The Merck Manual of Diagnosis & Therapy, 18th ed. Whitehouse Station, N.J.: Merck & Co., Inc., 2006.
Scordo, K.A. "Mitral Valve Prolapse Syndrome Health Concerns, Symptoms, and Treatments," *Western Journal of Nursing Research* 27(4):390-405, June 2005.
Weyman, A.F., and Scherrer-Crosbie, M. "Marfan Syndrome and Mitral Valve Prolapse," *Journal of Clinical Investigation* 114(11):1543-546, December 2004.

Monkeypox

● OVERVIEW

Description
- Rare, viral disease that occurs primarily in the rainforest countries of central and West Africa
- Originally discovered in laboratory monkeys in 1958, then later recovered from an African squirrel (thought to be the natural host)
- May also infect other rodents (rats and mice) and rabbits
- First human cases of monkeypox reported in remote African locations in 1970
- Twelve day incubation period; lasts approximately 2 to 4 weeks

Pathophysiology
- The monkeypox virus (related to variola virus [smallpox] and cowpox), belonging to the Orthopoxvirus group of viruses, causes monkeypox.
- The virus is less infectious than smallpox.

Causes
- Direct contact with an infected person's body fluids or with virus-contaminated objects, such as bedding or clothing
- Person-to-person spread via respiratory droplets during direct and prolonged face-to-face contact
- Transmission to humans by an infected animal through a bite or direct contact with the animal's blood, body fluids, or lesions

Incidence
- In June 2003, outbreak occurred in the United States that involved individuals who became infected following contact with infected prairie dogs

Common characteristics
- Papular rash
- Fever
- Malaise

Complications
- May include encephalitis and death (rare)
- Fatal in 10% of those who contract the disease in Africa

✳ ASSESSMENT

History
- Signs and symptoms similar to those of smallpox but milder
- Fever, headache, myalgia, backache, swollen lymph nodes, and a general feeling of discomfort and exhaustion

Physical findings
- Papular rash that begins on the face or other area of the body within 1 to 3 days of the onset of fever
- Lesions that go through several stages before crusting and falling off

Test results
LABORATORY
- The virus may be isolated from vesicular fluid to aid in diagnosis and differentiation from other rash-producing viruses.
OTHER
- Diagnosis is based on the patient's history and his presenting signs and symptoms.

◆ TREATMENT

General
- No specific treatment; supportive

Diet
- As tolerated

Activity
- As tolerated

Medications
- Smallpox vaccine (recommended by the CDC for people who are investigating monkeypox outbreaks, people caring for infected individuals or animals, and those exposed to individuals or animals confirmed to have monkeypox [up to 14 days after exposure])
- Immune globulin vaccination for severely immunocompromised patients
- Cidofovir (Vistide) for human monkeypox cases (no effectiveness data available)

♣ NURSING CONSIDERATIONS

Nursing diagnoses
- Acute pain
- Fatigue
- Impaired skin integrity

Key outcomes
The patient will:
- express feelings of increased comfort and decreased pain
- report increased levels of energy
- maintain warm, dry, and intact skin with healed or improved lesions or wounds.

Nursing interventions
- Notify the local health department immediately if you suspect monkeypox in a patient.
- Adhere to a combination of standard, contact, and droplet precautions in all health care settings.

◈ **NURSING ALERT** Because of the risk of airborne transmission, droplet precautions should be applied whenever possible using a NIOSH-certified N95 (or comparable) filtering disposable respirator that has been fit-tested. Surgical masks may be worn if a respirator is not available. Isolation should continue until all lesions are crusted over or until the local or state health department advises that isolation is no longer necessary.

- Perform strict hand washing after contact with an infected patient or contaminated objects.
- Eye protection should be used if splash or spray of body fluids is possible.
- Place the patient in a private room. Use a negative pressure room, if available.
- When transporting the patient, place a mask over his nose and mouth, and cover the exposed skin lesions with a sheet or gown. If the patient is to remain at home, he should maintain the same precautions.

▶ PATIENT TEACHING

Be sure to cover:
- disorder, diagnostic tests, and treatment
- need to wear a mask over his nose and mouth and to cover exposed lesions with a sheet or gown when he's in contact with others
- proper hand-washing practices.

Discharge planning
- Assist with referrals to community services and resources.

✳ RESOURCES

Organizations
Centers for Disease Control and Prevention: *www.cdc.gov*
U.S. Food and Drug Administration: *wwwfda.gov*
World Health Organization: *www.who.int*

Selected references
Fishman, M., et al.. "Patient Safety Tools: SARS, Smallpox, Monkeypox, and Avian Flu," *Disaster Management & Response* 3(3):86-90, July-September 2005.

Heeney, J., "Zoonotic Viral Diseases and the Frontier of Early Diagnosis, Control, and Prevention," *Journal of Internal Medicine* 260(5):399-408, November 2006.

Nalca, A, et al. "Re-Emergence of Monkeypox: Prevalence, Diagnostics, and Countermeasures," *Clinical Infectious Diseases* 41(12):1765-771, December 2005.

Multiple myeloma

● OVERVIEW

Description
- Disseminated neoplasm of marrow plasma cells
- Usually not diagnosed until it has infiltrated the vertebrae, pelvis, skull, ribs, clavicles, and sternum (by then, skeletal destruction is widespread and, without treatment, leads to vertebral collapse; within 3 months of diagnosis, 52% of patients die; within 2 years, 90% die)
- With early diagnosis and treatment, life often prolonged by 3 to 5 years
- Also called *malignant plasmacytoma, plasma cell myeloma,* and *myelomatosis*

Pathophysiology
- Infiltration of the bone produces osteolytic lesions throughout the skeleton.
- In late stages, multiple myeloma infiltrates the body organs.

Causes
- Exact cause unknown

Risk factors
- Genetic factors
- Occupational exposure to radiation

Incidence
- Most commonly affects men over age 40

Common characteristics
- History of neoplastic fractures
- Joint and back pain

Complications
- Infections (such as pneumonia)
- Pyelonephritis, renal calculi, and renal failure
- Hematologic imbalance
- Fractures
- Hypercalcemia
- Hyperuricemia
- Dehydration

✳ ASSESSMENT

History
- History of neoplastic fractures
- Severe, constant back pain, which may increase with exercise
- Arthritic symptoms
- Peripheral paresthesia
- Progressive weakness
- History of pneumonia
- Pain on movement or weight bearing, especially in the thoracic and lumbar vertebrae

Physical findings
- Noticeable thoracic deformities and reduction in body height of 5″ (12.7 cm)

Test results
LABORATORY
- Complete blood count shows moderate or severe anemia; the differential may show 40% to 50% lymphocytes but seldom more than 3% plasma cells; Rouleau formation, often the first clue, is seen on differential smear and results from elevation of the erythrocyte sedimentation rate.
- Urine studies may show protein urea, Bence Jones protein, and hypercalciuria; absence of Bence Jones protein doesn't rule out multiple myeloma, but its presence almost invariably confirms the disease.
- Serum electrophoresis shows an elevated globulin spike that's electrophoretically and immunologically abnormal.

IMAGING
- X-rays during the early stages may reveal only diffuse osteoporosis. Eventually, they show the characteristic lesions of multiple myeloma: multiple, sharply circumscribed osteolytic, or punched out lesions, particularly on the skull, pelvis, and spine.

DIAGNOSTIC PROCEDURES
- Bone marrow aspiration reveals myelomatous cells and abnormal number of immature plasma cells (10% to 95% instead of the normal 3% to 5%).

◆ TREATMENT

General
- Adjuvant local radiation
- Dialysis (if renal complications develop)
- Plasmapheresis to remove the M protein from the blood and return the cells to the patient (temporary effect)
- Peripheral blood stem cell transplantation

Diet
- Well-balanced; no restrictions

Activity
- May be limited by symptoms

Medication
- Bisphosphonates
- Analgesics
- Chemotherapeutic agents
- Possible use of thalidomide
- Immunotherapy

Surgery
- Laminectomy if the patient develops vertebral compression

Nursing diagnoses

- Acute pain
- Anxiety
- Fear
- Hopelessness
- Imbalanced nutrition: Less than body requirements
- Impaired physical mobility
- Ineffective breathing pattern
- Ineffective coping
- Ineffective protection

Key outcomes

The patient (or family) will:
- express feelings of increased comfort and decreased pain and anxiety
- verbalize an improvement in feelings of well-being
- recognize and express fears and concerns about illness and limitations
- maintain adequate nutritional intake
- maintain muscle strength and joint mobility
- maintain adequate ventilation and oxygenation
- demonstrate effective coping skills
- demonstrate use of protective measures, including conserving energy, maintaining a balanced diet, and getting adequate rest.

Nursing interventions

- Encourage fluid intake (3 to 4 qt [3,000 to 4,000 ml] daily).
- Administer medications, as ordered.

AFTER SURGERY
- Encourage mobilization.

Monitoring

- Complications of treatment
- Signs and symptoms of severe anemia and fractures
- Proper positioning (alignment)
- Pain control

Be sure to cover:
- disease process, diagnostic tests, and treatment
- importance of deep breathing and changing position every 2 hours after surgery
- appropriate dress for weather conditions (the patient may be sensitive to cold)
- avoidance of crowds and people with known infections
- medication administration, dosage, and possible adverse effects.

Discharge planning

- Refer the patient to resource and support services.

Organizations

American Cancer Society: *www.cancer.org*
Guide to Internet Resources for Cancer: *www.cancerindex.org*
International Myeloma Foundation: *www.myeloma.org*
National Cancer Institute: *www.nci.nih.gov*

Selected references

Atlas of Pathophysiology, 2nd ed. Philadelphia: Lippincott Williams & Wilkins, 2005.

Collins, C.D. "Problems Monitoring Response in Multiple Myeloma," *Cancer Imaging* 5 (Suppl):S119-126, November 2005.

Govindan, R., *The Washington Manual of Oncology,* 2nd ed. Philadelphia: Lippincott Williams & Wilkins, 2007.

Hideshima, T., et al. "Current Therapeutic Uses of Lenalidomide in Multiple Myeloma," *Expert Opinion on Investigational Drugs* 15(2):171-79, February 2006.

Richardson, P., and Anderson, K. "Thalidomide and Dexamethasone: A New Standard of Care for Initial Therapy in Multiple Myeloma," *Journal of Clinical Oncology* 24(3):334-36, January 2006.

Multiple organ dysfunction syndrome

● OVERVIEW

Description
- Condition that occurs when two or more organs or organ systems are unable to function in their role of maintaining homeostasis
- Not considered an illness itself; rather, a manifestation of another progressive underlying condition
- Classified as primary or secondary
- Also called *MODS*

Pathophysiology
PRIMARY
- Organ or organ system failure is caused by a direct injury (such as trauma, aspiration, or near drowning) or a primary disorder (such as pneumonia or pulmonary embolism).
- The syndrome commonly involves the lungs.
- Acute respiratory distress syndrome (ARDS) develops, which progresses to encephalopathy and coagulopathy.
- Eventually, other organ systems are affected.
SECONDARY
- Organ or organ system fails due to sepsis.
- Typically, the infection source isn't associated with the lungs.
- The most common infection sources include intra-abdominal sepsis, extensive blood loss, pancreatitis, or major vascular injuries.
- The development of ARDS is more rapid (than in the primary form), with progressive involvement of other organs and organ systems.

Causes
- Widespread systemic inflammation triggered by infection, ischemia, trauma, reperfusion injury, or multisystem injury that overtaxes a patient's compensatory mechanisms

Risk factors
- Use of chemotherapeutic drugs
- Malignancy
- Severe trauma
- Burns
- Immunocompromised patients

Incidence
- Increased in patients with sepsis
- High mortality, possibly as high as 90%

Common characteristics
- Acute illness
- Fever
- Tachycardia
- Tachypnea
- Decreased urine output

Complications
- Progressive organ involvement
- Disseminated intravascular coagulation
- Renal failure
- Respiratory failure
- Cardiac failure
- Death

✳ ASSESSMENT

History
- Acute illness
- Fever
- Chills
- Malaise

Physical findings
EARLY FINDINGS
- Fever, usually greater than 101° F (38.3° C)
- Tachycardia
- Narrowed pulse pressure
- Tachypnea
- Decreased pulmonary artery pressure (PAP), pulmonary artery wedge pressure (PAWP), and central venous pressure and increased cardiac output
PROGRESSIVE FINDINGS
- Decreased level of consciousness
- Respiratory depression
- Diminished bowel sounds
- Jaundice
- Oliguria or anuria
- Increased PAP and PAWP and decreased cardiac output
- Poor distal perfusion, cool skin, cool extremities, and delayed capillary refill

Test results
No single test confirms MODS; test results depend on the cause and which organs are affected.
LABORATORY
- Arterial blood gas (ABG) analysis may reveal hypoxemia with respiratory acidosis or metabolic acidosis.
- Complete blood count may reveal decreased hemoglobin level and hematocrit as well as leukocytosis.
- Platelet count may be decreased at the onset of serious stress and fall with continued progression of infection.
- Serum creatinine and blood urea nitrogen may be elevated if renal system is involved.
- Alkaline phosphate and alanine aminotransferase may be altered if liver is involved.
- Altered prothrombin time and partial thromboplastin time may suggest coagulopathy.
- Urinalysis and urine culture may indicate infectious organism with urinary tract infection.
- Blood or specimen cultures may reveal source or presence of bacterial infection or bacteremia.
IMAGING
- X-rays may reveal fractures, cervical spine injury, pulmonary infiltrates, or abnormal air or fluid in the chest or abdominal organs.
- Computed tomography and magnetic resonance imaging may help identify source of infection or underlying causative condition.
DIAGNOSTIC PROCEDURES
- Lumbar puncture may reveal meningitis as the causative infection.
- Pulmonary artery catheterization may show evidence of altered cardiac output and tissue hypoxia.

◆ TREATMENT

General
- Supportive
- Endotracheal intubation; mechanical ventilation
- Hemodynamic monitoring
- Serial laboratory testing
- Dialysis (for renal involvement)

Diet
- Enteral or parenteral nutritional support

Activity
- As tolerated; energy conservation measures
- Bedrest, until condition stabilizes

Medications
- Crystalloid and colloid I.V. fluids
- Vasopressors
- Analgesics
- Sedation
- Drotrecogin alpha (Xigris) for sepsis
- Oxygen
- Antimicrobials

Surgery
- Drainage of abscess or lesion if cause of the infection

❖ NURSING CONSIDERATIONS

Nursing diagnoses
- Anxiety
- Decreased cardiac output
- Deficient fluid volume
- Disabled family coping
- Fatigue
- Impaired gas exchange
- Ineffective tissue perfusion: Cardiopulmonary, renal
- Risk for imbalanced body temperature
- Risk for infection
- Risk for injury

Key outcomes
The patient (family) will
- verbalize strategies to reduce anxiety
- maintain adequate cardiac output and achieve hemodynamic stability
- maintain adequate fluid volume

- express feelings and develop adequate coping mechanisms
- report increased energy and decreased fatigue
- maintain adequate ventilation and oxygenation
- maintain adequate cardiopulmonary and renal perfusion
- maintain a normal body temperature
- remain free from further signs and symptoms of infection
- remain free from complications or injury.

Nursing interventions
- Maintain the patient's airway and breathing with the use of mechanical ventilation and supplemental oxygen.
- Provide endotracheal tube care as per facility policy.
- Remove or replace invasive catheters, and send them to the laboratory to culture for the presence of the causative organism.
- Give prescribed I.V. fluids.
- Administer prescribed antimicrobials.
- Notify the physician if urine output is less than 30 ml/hour.
- Provide emotional support to the patient and his family.

Monitoring
- ABG levels and pulse oximetry
- Intake and output (hourly for urine output)
- Vital signs and peripheral pulses
- Oxygen saturation levels
- Hemodynamics
- Cardiac rhythm
- Heart and breath sounds

NURSING ALERT Watch for a progressive drop in blood pressure accompanied by a thready pulse. This usually signals inadequate cardiac output from reduced intravascular volume. Notify the physician immediately.

▶ PATIENT TEACHING

Be sure to cover:
- disorder, diagnostic tests, and treatment
- all procedures, equipment, and their purpose
- risks associated with condition
- medication administration, dosage, and possible adverse effects
- possible complications
- infection control measures.

Discharge planning
- Refer the patient to appropriate rehabilitation program, as necessary.
- Arrange for follow-up home care, if indicated.

✴ RESOURCES

Organizations
National Heart, Lung, and Blood Institute: *www.nhlbi.nih.gov*

Selected references
Kasper, D., et.al., eds. *Harrison's Principles of Internal Medicine,* 16th ed. New York: McGraw-Hill Book Co., 2005.

Marshall, J.C. "Multiple Organ Dysfunction Syndrome: Approach to Multiple Organ Dysfunction Syndrome," *American College of Surgeons Surgery Online.* Available at: *http://www.medscape.vom/viewarticle/525763*

Nettina, S.M. *Lippincott Manual of Nursing Practice,* 8th ed. Philadelphia: Lippincott Williams & Wilkins, 2006.

Rivers, E.P. "Early Goal-Directed Therapy in Severe Sepsis and Septic Shock: Converting Science to Reality," *Chest* 129(2):217-18, February 2006.

Tantalean, J.A. "Multiple Organ Dysfunction Syndrome in Children," *Pediatric Critical Care Medicine* 4(2):2003. Available at: *http://www.medscape.com/viewarticle/452721.* Accessed 11/18/2006.

Walsh, C.R. "Multiple Organ Dysfunction Syndrome after Multiple Trauma," *Orthopaedic Nursing* 24(5):324-33, September-October 2005.

Multiple sclerosis

● OVERVIEW

Description
- Progressive demyelination of white matter of brain and spinal cord
- Characterized by exacerbations and remissions
- May progress rapidly, causing death within months
- Prognosis variable (70% leading active lives with prolonged remissions)

Pathophysiology
- Sporadic patches of demyelination occur in the central nervous system, resulting in widespread and varied neurologic dysfunction. (See *Describing multiple sclerosis.*)

Causes
- Exact cause unknown
- Slowly acting viral infection
- Autoimmune response of the nervous system
- Allergic response
- Events that precede the onset:
  - Emotional stress
  - Overwork
  - Fatigue
  - Pregnancy
  - Acute respiratory tract infections
- Possible genetic factors

Risk factors
- Trauma
- Anoxia
- Toxins
- Nutritional deficiencies
- Vascular lesions
- Anorexia nervosa

Incidence
- Highest in women
- Highest among people in northern urban areas
- Highest in higher socioeconomic groups
- Low incidence in Japan
- Family history increasing incidence
- Increased incidence in cold, damp climates

⚙ **AGE-RELATED CONCERN** Multiple sclerosis is a major cause of chronic disability in young adults ages 20 to 40.

Common characteristics
- Dependent on the extent and site of myelin destruction
- Sensory impairment
- Muscle dysfunction
- Bladder and bowel disturbances
- Speech problems
- Fatigue

Complications
- Injuries from falls
- Urinary tract infections
- Constipation
- Contractures
- Pressure ulcers
- Pneumonia
- Depression

DESCRIBING MULTIPLE SCLEROSIS

Multiple sclerosis (MS) may be described using various terms:

- *Elapsing-remitting:* clear relapses (or acute attacks or exacerbations) with full recovery and lasting disability. Between attacks, the disease doesn't worsen.
- *Primary progressive:* steady progression or worsening of the disease from the onset with minor recovery or plateaus. This form is uncommon and may involve different brain and spinal cord damage than other forms.
- *Secondary progressive:* begins as a pattern of clear-cut relapses and recovery but becomes steadily progressive and worsens between acute attacks.
- *Progressive-relapsing:* steadily progressive from the onset but also has clear, acute attacks. This form is rare.

In addition, differential diagnosis must rule out spinal cord compression, foramen magnum tumor (which may mimic the exacerbations and remission of MS), multiple small strokes, syphilis or another infection, thyroid disease, and chronic fatigue syndrome.

✳ ASSESSMENT

History
- Symptoms related to extent and site of myelin destruction, extent of remyelination, and adequacy of subsequent restored synaptic transmission
- Symptoms possibly transient or lasting for hours or weeks
- Symptoms unpredictable and difficult to describe
- Visual problems and sensory impairment (the first signs)
- Blurred vision or diplopia
- Urinary problems
- Emotional lability
- Dysphagia
- Bowel disturbances (involuntary evacuation or constipation)
- Fatigue (typically the most disabling symptom)

Physical findings
- Poor articulation
- Muscle weakness of the involved area
- Spasticity; hyperreflexia
- Intention tremor
- Gait ataxia
- Paralysis, ranging from monoplegia to quadriplegia
- Nystagmus; scotoma
- Optic neuritis
- Ophthalmoplegia

Test results
LABORATORY
- Cerebrospinal fluid analysis shows mononuclear cell pleocytosis, an elevation in the level of total immunoglobulin (Ig) G, and presence of oligoclonal Ig.

IMAGING
- Magnetic resonance imaging is the most sensitive method of detecting multiple sclerosis focal lesions.

DIAGNOSTIC PROCEDURES
- EEG abnormalities occur in one-third of patients.
- Evoked potential studies show slowed conduction of nerve impulses.
- Years of testing and observation may be required for diagnosis.

◆ TREATMENT

General
- Symptomatic for acute exacerbations and related signs and symptoms

Diet
- High fluid and fiber intake (for constipation)

Activity
- Frequent rest periods

Medication
- I.V. steroids followed by oral steroids
- Immunosuppressants
- Antimetabolites
- Alkylating drugs
- Biological response modifiers
- Antidepressants
- Glatiromer acetate

✿ NURSING CONSIDERATIONS

Nursing diagnoses
- Activity intolerance
- Chronic low self-esteem
- Chronic pain
- Constipation
- Fatigue
- Imbalanced nutrition: Less than body requirements
- Impaired physical mobility
- Impaired urinary elimination
- Ineffective coping
- Ineffective role performance
- Interrupted family processes
- Risk for infection
- Risk for injury

Key outcomes
The patient (or family) will:
- perform activities of daily living within the confines of the disorder
- voice feelings of increased self-esteem
- express feelings of increased comfort and decreased pain
- maintain a normal bowel elimination pattern
- express feelings of increased energy and decreased fatigue
- show no signs of malnutrition
- maintain joint mobility and range of motion
- develop regular bowel and bladder habits
- demonstrate effective coping skills
- resume regular roles and responsibilities to the fullest extent possible
- discuss the impact of the patient's condition on the family unit
- remain free from signs and symptoms of infection
- remain free from injury.

Nursing interventions
- Provide emotional and psychological support.
- Assist with physical therapy program.
- Provide adequate rest periods.
- Promote emotional stability.
- Keep the bedpan or urinal readily available because the need to void is immediate.
- Provide bowel and bladder training, if indicated.
- Administer medications.
- Schedule activities of daily living in the morning to conserve patient's energy.

Monitoring
- Response to medications
- Adverse drug reactions
- Sensory impairment
- Muscle dysfunction
- Energy level
- Signs and symptoms of infection
- Speech
- Elimination patterns
- Vision changes
- Laboratory results

▶ PATIENT TEACHING

Be sure to cover:
- disorder, diagnostic tests, and treatment
- medication administration, dosage, and possible adverse effects
- avoidance of stress, infections, and fatigue
- maintaining independence
- avoiding exposure to bacterial and viral infections
- nutritional management
- adequate fluid intake and regular urination.

Discharge planning
- Refer the patient to the National Multiple Sclerosis Society.
- Refer the patient to physical and occupational rehabilitation programs, as indicated.

✴ RESOURCES

Organizations
Multiple Sclerosis Association of America: *www.msaa.com*
National Institutes of Health: *www.nih.gov*
National Multiple Sclerosis Society: *www.nmss.org*

Selected references
Coyle, P.K., et al. "Multiple Sclerosis Gender Issues: Clinical Practices of Women Neurologists," *Multiple Sclerosis* 10(5):582-88, October 2004.

Diseases, 4th ed. Philadelphia: Lippincott Williams & Wilkins, 2005.

Handbook of Pathophysiology, 2nd ed. Philadelphia: Lippincott Williams & Wilkins, 2005.

Higginson, I., et al. "Symptom Prevalence and Severity in People Severely Affected By Multiple Sclerosis," *Journal of Palliative Care* 22(3):158-65 Autumn 2006.

Traboulsee, A.L., and Li, D.K. "The Role of MRI in the Diagnosis of Multiple Sclerosis," *Advances in Neurology* 98:125-46, 2006.

Mumps

● OVERVIEW

Description
- Acute inflammation of one or both parotid glands, and sometimes the sublingual or submaxillary glands
- Transmitted by droplets or by direct contact with the saliva of an infected person
- Also called *infectious* or *epidemic parotitis*

Pathophysiology
- Replication of the virus occurs in the epithelium of the upper respiratory tract, leading to viremia.
- Infection of the central nervous system (CNS) or glandular tissues (or both) occurs, resulting in perivascular and interstitial mononuclear cell infiltrates with edema.
- Necrosis of acinar and epithelial duct cells occurs in the salivary glands and germinal epithelium of the seminiferous tubules.

Causes
- Paramyxovirus found in the saliva of an infected person

Incidence
- Seldom occurs in infants under age 1 because of passive immunity from maternal antibodies
- Young adults accounting for about 50% of cases; remainder in young children or immunocompromised adults
- Peak incidence during late winter and early spring

Common characteristics
- Initially, prodromal symptoms that last for 24 hours
- Myalgia, anorexia, malaise, headache, an earache aggravated by chewing, and pain when drinking sour or acidic liquids; may have a fever of 101° to 104° F (38.3° to 40° C)

Complications
- Epididymo-orchitis
- Meningoencephalitis
- Sterility
- Pancreatitis
- Transient sensorineural hearing loss
- Arthritis
- Nephritis
- Spontaneous abortion (with contact during the first trimester)

✱ ASSESSMENT

History
- Inadequate immunization and exposure to someone with mumps within the preceding 2 to 3 weeks
- Myalgia, headache
- Malaise, fever
- Earache aggravated by chewing

Physical findings
- Swelling and tenderness of the parotid glands
- Simultaneous or subsequent swelling of one or more other salivary glands (see *Parotid inflammation in mumps*)

Test results
LABORATORY
- Serologic testing shows mumps antibodies.

◆ TREATMENT

General
- Rest
- Cold compresses for swollen glands
- Use of athletic supporter if testicles are tender

Diet
- Liquid to mechanical soft until able to swallow
- Increased fluid intake

Activity
- Bed rest until fever resolves
- Periods of rest when fatigued

Medication
- Analgesics
- Antipyretics

PAROTID INFLAMMATION IN MUMPS

The mumps virus (paramyxovirus) attacks the parotid glands — the main salivary glands. Inflammation causes characteristic swelling and discomfort associated with eating, drinking, swallowing, and talking.

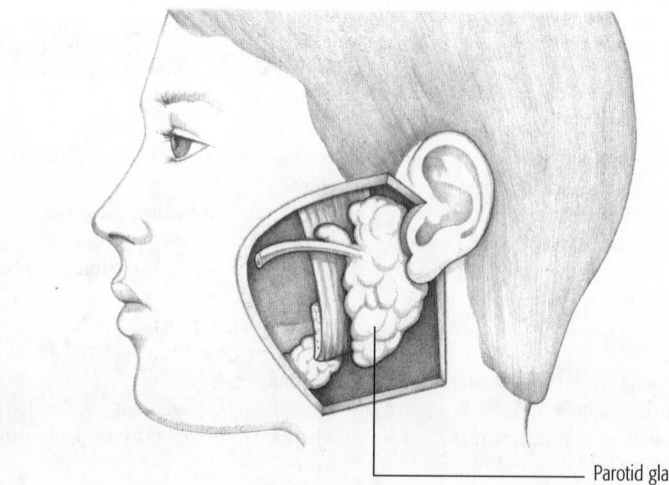

Parotid gland

✿ NURSING CONSIDERATIONS

Nursing diagnoses
- Acute pain
- Anxiety
- Deficient fluid volume
- Disturbed body image
- Hyperthermia
- Imbalanced nutrition: Less than body requirements
- Impaired swallowing
- Risk for infection

Key outcomes
The patient will:
- express feelings of increased comfort and decreased pain and anxiety
- maintain adequate fluid volume
- express feelings about changed body image
- remain afebrile
- achieve adequate nutritional intake
- swallow without pain or aspiration
- remain free from signs and symptoms of infection.

Nursing interventions
- Apply warm or cool compresses to the neck area to relieve pain.
- Administer medications, as ordered.
- Provide scrotal support, if needed.
- Report all cases of mumps to local public health authorities.
- Disinfect articles soiled with nose and throat secretions.

Monitoring
- Response to treatment
- Signs of CNS involvement
- Auditory acuity
- Complications

▶ PATIENT TEACHING

Be sure to cover:
- disorder, diagnostic tests, and treatment
- need to stay away from school or work from days 12 through 25 after exposure
- importance of having children immunized with live attenuated mumps vaccine at age 15 months or older, if applicable
- if epididymoorchitis occurs, reassurance that it won't cause impotence and sterility (occurs only with bilateral orchitis)
- need for bed rest during febrile period
- need to avoid spicy, irritating foods, and those that require much chewing; advise a soft, bland, diet
- need for family members to follow droplet isolation precautions until symptoms subside.

Discharge planning
- Refer the patient to a urologist for orchitis, if indicated.

✳ RESOURCES

Organizations
Centers for Disease Control and Prevention: *www.cdc.gov*
Harvard University Consumer Health Information: *www.intelihealth.com*
National Health Information Center: *www.health.gov/nhic/*
National Institute of Allergy and Infectious Diseases: *www.niaid.nih.gov*
National Library of Medicine: *www.nlm.nih.gov*

Selected references
Bedford, H. "Mumps: Current Outbreaks and Vaccination Recommendations," *Nursing Times* 101(39):53-54, 56, September-October 2005.
Francois, G., et al. "Vaccine Safety Controversies and the Future of Vaccination Programs," *Pediatric Infectious Disease Journal* 24(11):953-61, November 2005.
Hviid, A., et al. "Childhood Vaccination and Nontargeted Infectious Disease Hospitalization," *JAMA* 294(6):699-705, August 2005.

Muscular dystrophy

● OVERVIEW

Description
- Hereditary disorders characterized by progressive symmetrical wasting of skeletal muscles
- No neural or sensory defects
- Four main types: Duchenne's (pseudohypertrophic), Becker's (benign pseudohypertrophic), Landouzy-Dejerine (facioscapulohumeral), and Erb's (limb-girdle) dystrophy
- Duchenne's beginning during early childhood with death occurring within 10 to 15 years

Pathophysiology
- Muscle fibers necrotize and regenerate in various states.
- Regeneration slows and degeneration dominates.
- Fat and connective tissue replace muscle fibers, resulting in weakness.

Causes
- Various genetic mechanisms (band Xp 21)
- Duchenne's and Becker's: X-linked recessive
- Landouzy-Dejerine: autosomal dominant
- Erb's: usually autosomal recessive

Incidence
- Duchenne's and Becker's affecting males almost exclusively
- Landouzy-Dejerine and Erb's affecting both sexes equally

Common characteristics
- Waddling gait
- Toe walking
- Lumbar lordosis
- Frequent falls
- Dyspnea

Complications
- Crippling disability
- Contractures, fractures
- Pneumonia
- Arrhythmias
- Cardiac hypertrophy
- Dysphagia
- Speech impairment

✱ ASSESSMENT

History
- Evidence of genetic transmission
- Progressive muscle weakness

DUCHENNE'S
- Onset insidious
- Onset between ages 3 and 5
- Pelvic muscle weakness
- Interferes with child's ability to run, climb, and walk

BECKER'S
- Onset after age 5
- Symptoms the same as Duchenne's, but slower progression

LANDOUZY-DEJERINE
- Onset before age 10
- Weakness of eye, face, and shoulder muscles
- Inability to raise arms over head
- Inability to close eyes
- Inability to pucker lips or whistle
- Abnormal facial movements
- Absence of facial movements when laughing or crying
- Pelvic muscle weakness as the disease progresses

ERB'S
- Symptoms the same as in Landouzy-Dejerine but slower in progression
- Less disability than in Landouzy-Dejerine
- Onset between ages 6 and 10
- Muscle weakness of upper arm and pelvic muscles

Physical findings

DUCHENNE'S AND BECKER'S
- Wide stance and waddling gait
- Gowers' sign when rising from a sitting or supine position
- Muscle hypertrophy and atrophy
- Enlarged calves because of fat infiltration into the muscle
- Posture changes
- Lordosis with abdominal protrusion
- Scapular "winging" or flaring when raising arms
- Contractures
- Tachypnea and shortness of breath

LANDOUZY-DEJERINE
- Pendulous lower lip
- Possible disappearance of nasolabial fold
- Diffuse facial flattening leading to a masklike expression
- Inability to suckle (infants)
- Scapulae with a winglike appearance; inability to raise arms above head

ERB'S
- Muscle weakness and wasting
- Winging of the scapulae
- Lordosis with abdominal protrusion
- Waddling gait
- Poor balance
- Inability to raise arms

Test results

LABORATORY
- Urine creatinine, serum creatine kinase, lactate dehydrogenase, alanine aminotransferase, and aspartate aminotransferase levels are elevated.

DIAGNOSTIC PROCEDURES
- Muscle biopsy result confirms the diagnosis.
- Immunologic and biological results facilitate prenatal and postnatal diagnosis.
- Electromyography shows abnormal muscle movements.
- Amniocentesis detects sex of fetus for high-risk family.
- Genetic testing may be used to detect the gene defect that leads to muscular dystrophy in some families.

◆ TREATMENT

General
- No known treatment to stop progression
- Orthopedic appliances

Diet
- Low-calorie, high-protein, high-fiber

Activity
- Exercise, as tolerated
- Physical therapy

Medication
- Stool softeners
- Possible steroids

Surgery
- Surgery to correct contractures

Nursing diagnoses

- Activity intolerance
- Bathing or hygiene self-care deficit
- Disabled family coping
- Disturbed body image
- Impaired physical mobility
- Ineffective breathing pattern
- Ineffective coping
- Risk for disuse syndrome
- Risk for injury

Key outcomes

The patient will:

- perform activities of daily living without muscle fatigue or intolerance
- participate in self-care activities to the fullest extent possible
- demonstrate adaptive coping behaviors
- express positive feelings about body image
- achieve the highest degree of mobility possible within the confines of the disease
- maintain respiratory rate within 5 breaths of baseline
- use support measures and exhibit adaptive coping behaviors
- maintain muscle strength, joint mobility, and range of motion
- remain free from injury.

Nursing interventions

- Encourage coughing and deep-breathing exercises.
- Take steps to prevent muscle atrophy.
- Promote use of splints, braces, grab bars, and overhead slings.
- Provide a footboard or high-topped shoes and a foot cradle.
- Provide a low-calorie, high-protein, high-fiber diet.

Monitoring

- Intake and output
- Respiratory status
- Joint mobility
- Muscle weakness
- Complications

Be sure to cover:

- disorder, diagnostic tests, and treatment
- maintenance of peer relationships
- how to maintain mobility and independence
- possible complications and prevention
- signs and symptoms of respiratory tract infections
- need for a low-calorie, high-protein, high-fiber diet
- need to avoid long periods of bed rest and inactivity.

Discharge planning

Refer the patient to:

- sexual counseling, if indicated
- physical therapy, vocational rehabilitation, social services, and financial assistance
- the Muscular Dystrophy Association
- genetic counseling.

Organizations

American Academy of Pediatrics: *www.aap.org*
Muscular Dystrophy Association: *www.mda.org*
National Institutes of Health: *www.nih.gov*

Selected references

Bostrom K., and Ahistrom, G. "Quality of Life in Patients with Muscular Dystrophy and Their Next of Kin," *Internal Journal of Rehabilitation Research* 28(2):103-109, June 2005.

Hoogerwaard, F.M., et al. "Dystrophin Analysis in Carriers of Duchenne and Becker Muscular Dystrophy Population," *Neurology* 65(12):1984-986, December 2005.

Parker, A.E., et al. "Analysis of an Adult Duchenne Musular Dystrophy Population," *QJM* 98(10):729-36, October 2005.

Myasthenia gravis

● OVERVIEW

Description
- Abnormal fatigability of striated (skeletal) muscles
- Sporadic but progressive muscle weakness, which is exacerbated by exercise and repetitive movement
- Initial symptoms related to cranial nerves
- With respiratory system involvement, may be life-threatening
- Spontaneous remissions in about 25% of patients

Pathophysiology
- Blood cells and thymus gland produce antibodies that block, destroy, or weaken neuroreceptors (which transmit nerve impulses).
- The result is failure in transmission of nerve impulses at the neuromuscular junction.

Causes
- Autoimmune disorder associated with the thymus gland
- Other immune and thyroid disorders
- Rheumatoid arthritis
- Systemic lupus erythematosus
- Thyrotoxicosis

Incidence
- Occurs at any age
- Three times more common in women than men
- Highest in women ages 18 to 25
- Highest in men ages 50 to 60
- Transient myasthenia in about 20% of infants born to myasthenic mothers

Common characteristics
- Weak eye closure; ptosis
- Diplopia
- Skeletal muscle weakness; paralysis

Complications
- Respiratory distress
- Pneumonia
- Aspiration

✳ ASSESSMENT

History
- Variable assessment findings
- Extreme muscle weakness and fatigue (cardinal symptoms)
- Ptosis and diplopia (most common sign)
- Difficulty chewing and swallowing
- Jaw hanging open (especially when tired)
- Head bobbing
- Symptoms milder on awakening; worsen as the day progresses
- Short rest periods that temporarily restore muscle function
- Symptoms that become more intense during menses, after emotional stress, after prolonged exposure to sunlight or cold, and with infections

Physical findings
- Sleepy, masklike expression
- Drooping jaw
- Ptosis
- Decreased breath sounds
- Decreased tidal volume
- Respiratory distress and myasthenic crisis
- Limb weakness

Test results
IMAGING
- Chest X-rays or computed tomography scan shows thymoma.

DIAGNOSTIC PROCEDURES
- Positive Tensilon test shows temporary improved muscle function and confirms the diagnosis.
- Electrodiagnostic testing shows a rapid reduction of more than 10% in the amplitude of evoked responses.

◆ TREATMENT

General
- Plasmapheresis
- Emergency airway and ventilation management

Diet
- As tolerated

Activity
- As tolerated

Medication
- Anticholinesterase drugs
- Corticosteroids
- I.V. immune globulin

Surgery
- Thymectomy

❖ NURSING CONSIDERATIONS

Nursing diagnoses
- Activity intolerance
- Anxiety
- Bathing or hygiene self-care deficit
- Chronic low self-esteem
- Disturbed body image
- Dressing or grooming self-care deficit
- Fatigue
- Feeding self-care deficit
- Impaired gas exchange
- Impaired physical mobility
- Ineffective airway clearance

Key outcomes
The patient will:
- peform activities of daily living within the confines of the disease process
- identify strategies to reduce anxiety
- perform bathing and hygiene activities to the fullest extent possible
- voice feelings related to increased self-esteem
- express positive feelings about body image
- perform dressing and grooming activities to the fullest extent possible
- verbalize the importance of balancing activity with adequate rest periods
- perform self-care needs related to feeding to the fullest extent possible
- maintain adequate ventilation and oxygenation
- maintain range of motion and joint mobility
- maintain a patent airway.

Nursing interventions
- Provide psychological support.
- Provide frequent rest periods.
- Maintain nutritional management program.
- Administer medications, as ordered.

Monitoring
- Neurologic and respiratory function
- Response to medications

NURSING ALERT Monitor for signs of impending myasthenic crisis including increased muscle weakness, respiratory distress, and difficulty talking or chewing.

▶ PATIENT TEACHING

Be sure to cover:
- disorder, diagnostic tests, and treatment
- surgery (preoperative and postoperative teaching)
- energy conservation techniques
- medication administration, dosage, and possible adverse effects
- avoidance of strenuous exercise, stress, infection, needless exposure to the sun or cold weather
- nutritional management program
- swallowing therapy program.

Discharge planning
- Refer the patient to the Myasthenia Gravis Foundation.

✳ RESOURCES

Organizations
Myasthenia Gravis Foundation of America: *www.myasthenia.org*
National Institutes of Health: *www.nih.gov*

Selected references
Burch, J., et al. "Myasthenia Gravis—A Rare Presentation with Tongue Atrophy and Fasciulation," *Age and Aging* 35(1):87-88, January 2006.

Diseases, 4th ed. Philadelphia: Lippincott Williams & Wilkins, 2005.

Handbook of Pathophysiology, 2nd ed. Lippincott Williams & Wilkins, 2005.

Hughes, T. "The Early History of Myasthenia Gravis," *Neuromuscular Disorders* 15(12):878-86, December 2005.

Wagner, A.J., et al. "Long-Term Follow-Up after Thymectomy for Myasthenia Gravis: Thoracoscopic vs. Open," *Journal of Pediatric Surgery* 41(1):50-54, January 2006.

Myocardial infarction

● OVERVIEW

Description
- Myocardial ischemia and necrosis caused by reduced blood flow through one or more coronary arteries
- Infarction site dependent on the vessels involved
- Also called *MI* and *heart attack*; may be classified as an acute coronary syndrome

Pathophysiology
- One or more coronary arteries becomes occluded.
- If coronary occlusion causes prolonged ischemia lasting longer than 30 to 45 minutes, irreversible myocardial cell damage and muscle death occur.
- Every MI has a central area of necrosis surrounded by an area of hypoxic injury. This injured tissue is potentially viable and may be salvaged if circulation is restored, or it may progress to necrosis.

Causes
- Atherosclerosis
- Thrombosis
- Platelet aggregation
- Coronary artery stenosis or spasm

Risk factors
- Increased age (40 to 70)
- Diabetes mellitus
- Elevated serum triglyceride, low-density lipoprotein, and cholesterol levels, and decreased serum high-density lipoprotein levels
- Excessive intake of saturated fats, carbohydrates, or salt
- Hypertension
- Obesity
- Positive family history of coronary artery disease (CAD)
- Sedentary lifestyle
- Smoking
- Stress or a type A personality
- Use of drugs, such as amphetamines or cocaine

Incidence
- Men more susceptible than premenopausal women
- Increasing among women who smoke and take oral contraceptives
- In postmenopausal women, similar to incidence in men

Common characteristics
- Substernal chest pain with radiation in men
- Atypical symptoms such as fatigue and nausea in women

Complications
- Arrhythmias
- Cardiogenic shock
- Heart failure causing pulmonary edema
- Pericarditis
- Rupture of the atrial or ventricular septum or ventricular wall
- Ventricular aneurysm
- Cerebral or pulmonary emboli
- Extensions of the original infarction
- Mitral insufficiency

✳ ASSESSMENT

History
- Possible CAD with increasing anginal frequency, severity, or duration
- Cardinal symptom of MI: persistent, crushing substernal pain possibly radiating to the left arm, jaw, neck, and shoulder blades, and possibly persisting for 12 or more hours
- In elderly patient or one with diabetes, pain possibly absent; in others, pain possibly mild and confused with indigestion
- A feeling of impending doom, fatigue, nausea, vomiting, and shortness of breath
- Sudden death (may be the first and only indication of MI)

Physical findings
- Extreme anxiety and restlessness
- Dyspnea
- Diaphoresis
- Tachycardia
- Hypertension
- Bradycardia and hypotension, in inferior MI
- An S_4, an S_3, and paradoxical splitting of S_2 with ventricular dysfunction
- Systolic murmur of mitral insufficiency
- Pericardial friction rub with transmural MI or pericarditis
- Low-grade fever possibly developing during the next few days

Test results
LABORATORY
- Serum creatine kinase (CK) levels are elevated, especially the CK-MB isoenzyme, the cardiac muscle fraction of CK.
- Serum lactate dehydrogenase (LD) levels are elevated; higher LD_1 isoenzyme (found in cardiac tissue) than LD_2 (in serum).
- White blood cell count is elevated, usually appearing on the second day and lasting 1 week.
- Myoglobin (the hemoprotein found in cardiac and skeletal muscle) is detected and is released with muscle damage as soon as 2 hours after MI.
- Troponin I a structural protein found in cardiac muscle, is elevated, only in cardiac muscle damage; it's more specific than the CK-MB level. (Troponin levels increase within 4 to 6 hours of myocardial injury and may remain elevated for 5 to 11 days.)

IMAGING
- Nuclear medicine scans, using I.V. technetium 99m pertechnetate, can identify acutely damaged muscle by picking up accumulations of radioactive nucleotide, which appears as a "hot spot" on the film. Myocardial perfusion imaging with thallium 201 reveals a "cold spot" in most patients during the first few hours after a transmural MI.
- Echocardiography shows ventricular wall dyskinesia with a transmural MI and helps to evaluate the ejection fraction.

DIAGNOSTIC PROCEDURES
- Serial 12-lead electrocardiography (ECG) readings may be normal or inconclusive during the first few hours after an MI. Characteristic abnormalities include serial ST-segment depression in subendocardial MI and ST-segment elevation and Q waves, representing scarring and necrosis, in transmural MI.
- Pulmonary artery catheterization may be performed to detect left- or right-sided heart failure and to monitor response to treatment.

TREATMENT

General
- Pacemaker, or electrical cardioversion for arrhythmias
- Intra-aortic balloon pump for cardiogenic shock

Diet
- Low-fat, low-cholesterol
- Calorie restriction, if indicated

Activity
- Bed rest with bedside commode
- Gradual increase in activity, as tolerated

Medication
- I.V. thrombolytic therapy started within 3 hours of the onset of symptoms
- Aspirin
- Antiarrhythmics
- Antianginals
- Calcium-channel blockers
- Heparin I.V.
- Morphine I.V.
- Inotropic drugs
- Beta-adrenergic blockers
- Angiotensin-converting inhibitors
- Stool softeners
- Oxygen

Surgery
- Surgical revascularization
- Percutaneous revascularization

NURSING CONSIDERATIONS

Nursing diagnoses
- Activity intolerance
- Acute pain
- Anxiety
- Decreased cardiac output
- Excess fluid volume
- Fatigue
- Ineffective coping
- Ineffective denial
- Ineffective sexuality patterns
- Ineffective tissue perfusion: Cardiopulmonary

Key outcomes
The patient will:
- perform activities of daily living without excessive fatigue or exhaustion
- express feelings of increased comfort and decreased pain and anxiety
- maintain adequate cardiac output
- remain free of complications of fluid volume excess
- demonstrate a balance of rest and activity
- exhibit adequate coping skills
- recognize the acuity of the illness and accept lifestyle changes that need to be made
- verbalize feelings about changes in sexual patterns
- maintain hemodynamic stability without arrhythmias.

Nursing interventions
- Assess pain and give analgesics as ordered. Record the severity, location, type, and duration of pain. Avoid I.M. injections.
- Check the patient's blood pressure before and after giving nitroglycerin.
- Obtain ECG during episodes of chest pain.
- Organize patient care and activities to provide periods of uninterrupted rest.
- Provide a low-cholesterol, low-sodium diet without caffeine-containing beverages.
- Allow the patient to use a bedside commode.
- Assist with range-of-motion exercises.
- Provide emotional support, and help to reduce stress and anxiety.
- If the patient has undergone percutaneous transluminal coronary angioplasty, sheath care is necessary. Watch for bleeding. Keep the leg with the sheath insertion site immobile. Maintain strict bed rest. Check peripheral pulses in the affected leg frequently.

Monitoring
- Serial ECGs
- Vital signs and heart and breath sounds
- **NURSING ALERT** Watch for crackles, cough, tachypnea, and edema, which may indicate impending left-sided heart failure.
- Daily weight; intake and output
- Cardiac enzyme levels; coagulation studies
- Cardiac rhythm for reperfusion arrhythmias (treat according to facility protocol)

PATIENT TEACHING

Be sure to cover:
- disorder, diagnostic tests, and treatment
- procedures (answering questions for the patient and family members)
- medication administration, dosage, possible adverse effects and signs of toxicity to watch for and report
- dietary restrictions
- progressive resumption of sexual activity
- appropriate responses to new or recurrent symptoms
- types of chest pain to report.

Discharge planning
Refer the patient to a:
- cardiac rehabilitation program
- smoking-cessation program, if needed
- weight-loss program, if needed.

RESOURCES

Organizations
American Heart Association: *www.americanheart.org*

Selected references
DeVon, H.A., and Ryan, C.J. "Chest Pain and Associated Symptoms of Acute Coronary Syndrome," *Journal of Cardiovascular Nursing* 20 (4):232-38, July-August 2005.

Gershlick, A.H., et al. "Rescue Angioplasty after Failed Thrombolytic Therapy for Acute Myocardial Infarction," *New England Journal of Medicine* 353(26):2758-768, December 2005.

Quinn, T. "The Role of Nurses in Improving Emergency Cardiac Care," *Nursing Standard* 19(48):41-48, August 2005.

Vorchheimer, D.A., and Becker, R. "Platelets in Atherothrombosis," *Mayo Clinic Proceedings* 81(1):59-68, January 2006.

Myocarditis

● OVERVIEW

Description
- Focal or diffuse inflammation of the myocardium that's typically uncomplicated and self-limiting
- Recovery usually spontaneous and without residual defects
- May be acute or chronic

Pathophysiology
- An infectious organism triggers an autoimmune, cellular, and humoral reaction.
- Inflammation may lead to hypertrophy, fibrosis, and inflammatory changes of the myocardium and conduction system.
- Heart muscle weakens and contractility is reduced.

Causes
- Viruses
- Bacteria
- Hypersensitive immune reactions such as acute rheumatic fever
- Radiation therapy
- Chronic alcoholism
- Parasitic infections
- Helminthic infections such as trichinosis

Incidence
- Can occur at any age

Common characteristics
- Mild, continuous chest soreness or pressure

Complications
- Left-sided heart failure
- Cardiomyopathy
- Chronic valvulitis (when it results from rheumatic fever)
- Arrhythmias
- Thromboembolism

✱ ASSESSMENT

History
- Possible recent upper respiratory tract infection with fever, viral pharyngitis, or tonsillitis
- Nonspecific symptoms, such as fatigue, dyspnea, palpitations, persistent tachycardia, and persistent fever
- Mild, continuous pressure or soreness in the chest

Physical findings
- S_3 and S_4 gallops, muffled S_1
- Pericardial friction rub

Test results
LABORATORY
- Cardiac enzyme levels, including creatine kinase (CK), CK-MB, aspartate aminotransferase, and lactate dehydrogenase, are elevated.
- White blood cell count and erythrocyte sedimentation rate are elevated.
- Antibody titers, such as antistreptolysin-O titer in rheumatic fever, are elevated.
- Cultures of stool, throat, pharyngeal washings, or other body fluids show the causative bacteria or virus.

DIAGNOSTIC PROCEDURES
- Endomyocardial biopsy can be used to confirm diagnosis.
- Electrocardiography typically shows diffuse ST-segment and T-wave abnormalities as in pericarditis, conduction defects (prolonged PR interval), and other ventricular and supraventricular ectopic arrhythmias.

◆ TREATMENT

General
- Hospitalization until stabilized, for patient with signs and symptoms of heart failure
- Oxygen therapy, if indicated

Diet
- Avoidance of alcohol
- Low sodium

Activity
- Modified bed rest
- Activity, as tolerated

Medication
- Anti-infectives
- Antiarrhythmics
- Anticoagulants
- Anti-inflammatory agents
- Angiotensin-converting enzyme inhibitors
- Diuretics
- Inotropic agents

Surgery
- Pacemaker implantation
- Ventricular assist device implantation
- Heart transplantation

❖ NURSING CONSIDERATIONS

Nursing diagnoses
- Activity intolerance
- Anxiety
- Decreased cardiac output
- Deficient diversional activity
- Impaired gas exchange
- Ineffective role performance

Key outcomes
The patient will:
- carry out activities of daily living with little or no weakness or fatigue
- cope with condition without demonstrating severe signs of anxiety
- maintain hemodynamic stability and adequate cardiac output without arrhythmia
- express interest in using leisure time meaningfully
- maintain adequate ventilation and oxygenation
- express feelings about diminished capacity to perform usual roles

Nursing interventions
- Stress the importance of bed rest. Provide a bedside commode.
- Allow the patient to express his concerns about the effects of activity restrictions on his responsibilities and routines.
- Administer oxygen, as needed.
- Administer parenteral anti-infectives and other medications, as ordered.

Monitoring
- Vital signs
- Cardiovascular status
- Intake and output
- Signs and symptoms of heart failure
- Signs and symptoms of digoxin toxicity
- Cardiac rhythm
- Arterial blood gas levels
- Daily weight
- Response to treatment

▶ PATIENT TEACHING

Be sure to cover:
- disorder, diagnostic tests, and treatment
- medication administration, dosage, and possible adverse effects
- prevention of myocarditis
- signs and symptoms of heart failure
- (for a patient taking cardiac glycosides at home) how to check the pulse for 1 full minute before taking the dose, and the need to withhold the dose and notify the physician if the heart rate falls below the predetermined rate (usually 60 beats/minute)
- when to notify the physician.

✱ RESOURCES

Organizations
American Heart Association
  www.americanherat.org
Mayo Health Clinic: *www.mayohealth.org*
National Heart, Lung, and Blood Institute: *www.nhlbi.hih.gov/*

Selected references
Kasper, D.L., et al., eds. *Harrison's Principles of Internal Medicine*, 16th ed. New York: McGraw-Hill Book Co., 2005.

The Merck Manual of Diagnosis & Therapy, 18th ed, Whitehouse Station, N.J.: Merck & Co., Inc., 2006.

Pulerwitz, T.C., et al. "Mortality in Primary and Secondary Myocarditis," *American Heart Journal* 147(4):746-50, April 2005.

Takkenberg, J., et al. "Eosinophilic Myocarditis in Patients Awaiting Heart Transplantation," *Critical Care Medicine* 32(3):714-21, March 2004.

Williams, P., and Lainchbury, J. "Enteritis-associated Myocarditis," *Heart, Lung & Circulation* 13(1):106-109, March 2004.

Near drowning

Description
- Victim surviving physiologic effects of submersion
- Hypoxemia and acidosis primary problems
- "Dry" near drowning: fluid not aspirated; respiratory obstruction or asphyxia
- "Wet" near drowning: fluid aspirated; asphyxia or secondary changes from fluid aspiration
- "Secondary" near drowning: recurrence of respiratory distress

Pathophysiology
- Immersion stimulates hyperventilation.
- Voluntary apnea occurs.
- Laryngospasm develops.
- Hypoxemia can lead to brain damage and cardiac arrest.

Causes
- Inability to swim
- Panic
- Boating accident
- Sudden acute illness
- Blow to the head while in the water
- Venomous stings from aquatic animals
- Excessive alcohol consumption before swimming
- Decompression sickness from deep-water diving
- Dangerous water conditions
- Suicide attempt

Incidence
- Most common cause of injury and death in children ages 1 month to 14 years
- Incidence greater in males

Common characteristics
- Altered vital signs
- Dyspnea
- Hypoxia
- Altered level of consciousness
- Cardiopulmonary arrest

Complications
- Neurologic impairment
- Seizure disorder
- Pulmonary edema
- Renal damage
- Bacterial aspiration
- Pulmonary complications
- Cardiac complications

ASSESSMENT

History
- Victim found in water

Physical findings
- Fever or hypothermia
- Rapid, slow, or absent pulse
- Shallow, gasping, or absent respirations
- Confusion
- Seizures
- Apprehension
- Irritability
- Restlessness
- Lethargy
- Cyanosis or pink, frothy sputum or both
- Abdominal distention
- Crackles, rhonchi, wheezing, or apnea
- Tachycardia
- Irregular heartbeat

Test results
LABORATORY
- Arterial blood gas (ABG) level shows degree of hypoxia, intrapulmonary shunt, and acid-base balance.
- Electrolyte levels are imbalanced.
- Complete blood count shows hemolysis.
- Blood urea nitrogen and creatinine levels reveal impaired renal function.
- Urinalysis showing signs of impaired renal function.

IMAGING
- Cervical spine X-ray may show evidence of fracture.
- Serial chest X-rays may show pulmonary edema.

DIAGNOSTIC PROCEDURES
- Electrocardiogram (ECG) may show myocardial ischemia or infarct or cardiac arrhythmias.

TREATMENT

General
- Neck stabilization
- Endotracheal intubation and mechanical ventilation if necessary
- Warming measures if hypothermic
- Fluid replacement
- Dialysis (with renal failure)

Diet
- Nothing by mouth until swallowing ability has returned

Activity
- Based on extent of injury and success of resuscitation

Medication
- Bronchodilators
- Cardiac drug therapy, if appropriate
- Prophylactic antibiotics

Nursing diagnoses
- Anxiety
- Compromised family coping
- Decreased cardiac output
- Hypothermia
- Impaired gas exchange
- Ineffective airway clearance
- Ineffective breathing pattern
- Risk for aspiration
- Risk for infection

Key outcomes
The patient (and family) will:
- report decreased anxiety
- develop effective individual and family coping mechanisms
- maintain cardiac output
- achieve a normal body temperature
- maintain adequate ventilation and oxygenation
- have a patent airway at all times
- maintain an effective breathing pattern
- remain free from signs or symptoms of aspiration
- remain free from signs and symptoms of infection.

Nursing interventions
- Perform cardiopulmonary rescusitation, as indicated.
- Perform active external rewarming and passive rewarming measures for mild hypothermia (93.2° to 96.8° F [34° C to 36° C]); active external rewarming of truncal areas only and passive rewarming measures for moderate hypothermia (86° F [30° C] to 93.2° F); and active internal rewarming measures for severe hypothermia (less than 86° F).
- Protect the cervical spine.
- Provide fluid resuscitation.
- Administer medications, as ordered.

Monitoring
- Electrolyte and ABG measurement results
- Cardiac rhythm
- Vital signs
- Neurologic status
- Respiratory status
- Core body temperature
- Psychological state

Be sure to cover:
- injury, diagnostic tests, and treatment
- need to avoid using alcohol or drugs before swimming
- water safety measures (such as the "buddy system").

Discharge planning
- Recommend a water safety course given by the Red Cross, YMCA, or YWCA.
- Refer the patient for psychological counseling.
- Refer the patient to resource and support services.

Organizations
American Academy of Neurology: *www.aan.com*
Brain Injury Association: *www.biausa.org*
Harborview Injury Prevention and Research Center: *www.depts.washington.edu/hiprc/*
National Center for Injury Prevention and Control: *www.cdc.gov/ncipc/*

Selected references
Buford, A.E., et al. "Drowning and Near-drowning in Children and Adolescents: A Succint Review for Emergency Physicians and Nurses," *Pediatric Emergency Care* 21(9):610-16, September, 2005.

Pierro, M.M., et al. "Anoxic Brain Injury Following Near-Drowning in Children. Rehabilitation Outcome: Three Case Reports," *Brain Injury* 19(13):1147-155, December 2005.

Robles, L.A., and Curiel, A. "Posttraumatic Cervical Disc Herniation: An Unusual Cause of Near Drowning," *American Journal of Emergency Medicine* 23(7):905-907, November 2005.

Ross, J.L. "Summer Injuries: Near Drowning," *RN* 68(7):36-38, July 2005.

Necrotizing fasciitis

● OVERVIEW

Description
- Progressive, rapidly spreading inflammatory infection of the deep fascia
- High mortality (70% to 80%)
- Most commonly called *"flesh-eating bacteria"*
- Also called *hemolytic streptococcal gangrene, acute dermal gangrene, suppurative fasciitis,* and *synergistic necrotizing cellulitis*

Pathophysiology
- Infecting bacteria enter the host through a local tissue injury or a breach in a mucous membrane barrier.
- Organisms proliferate in an environment of tissue hypoxia caused by trauma, recent surgery, or a medical condition that compromises the patient.
- Necrosis of the surrounding tissue results, which accelerates the disease process by creating a favorable environment for organisms.
- The fascia and fat tissues are destroyed, with secondary necrosis of subcutaneous tissue.

Causes
- Group A beta-hemolytic *Streptococcus* (GAS) and *Staphylococcus aureus,* alone or together, most common primary infecting bacteria (more than 80 types of the causative bacteria, *Streptococcus pyogenes,* makes epidemiology of GAS infections complex)

Risk factors
- Elderly
- Immunocompromised state
- Chronic illness
- Steroid use

Incidence
- Three times more likely in men than women
- Rarely occurs in children except in countries with poor hygiene practices
- Mean age is 38 to 44

Common characteristics
- Pain out of proportion to the size of the wound or injury
- Rapid deterioration in overall clinical status

Complications
- Renal failure
- Septic shock
- Scarring with cosmetic deformities
- Myositis
- Myonecrosis
- Amputation

✻ ASSESSMENT

History
- Associated risk factors
- Pain

Physical findings
- Rapidly progressing erythema at the site of insult
- Fluid-filled blisters and bullae (indicate rapid progression of the necrotizing process)
- By days 4 and 5, large areas of gangrenous skin
- By days 7 to 10, extensive necrosis of the subcutaneous tissue
- Fever, sepsis
- Hypovolemia, hypotension
- Respiratory insufficiency
- Deterioration in level of consciousness

Test results
LABORATORY
- Cultures of microorganisms from the periphery of the spreading infection or from deeper tissues during surgical debridement identify the causative organism.
- Gram stain and culture of biopsied tissue identify the causative organism.
IMAGING
- Radiographic studies can pinpoint the presence of subcutaneous gases.
- Computed tomography scans can show the anatomic site of involvement by locating necrosis.
- Magnetic resonance imaging shows areas of necrosis and areas that require surgical debridement.

DIAGNOSTIC PROCEDURES
- Tissue biopsy shows infiltration of the deep dermis, fascia, and muscular planes with bacteria and polymorphonuclear cells, and necrosis of fatty and muscular tissue.

◆ TREATMENT

General
- Hyperbaric oxygen therapy
- Wound care

Diet
- High-protein, high-calorie
- Increased fluid intake

Activity
- Bed rest until treatment effective

Medication
- Antimicrobials
- Analgesics

Surgery
- Immediate surgical debridement, fasciectomy, or amputation

❖ NURSING CONSIDERATIONS

Nursing diagnoses
- Acute pain
- Decreased cardiac output
- Deficient fluid volume
- Hyperthermia
- Impaired tissue integrity
- Ineffective tissue perfusion: Cardiopulmonary, peripheral

Key outcomes
The patient will:
- express feelings of increased comfort and decreased pain
- maintain adequate cardiac output
- maintain adequate fluid volume
- remain afebrile
- achieve adequate healing of wounds
- maintain collateral circulation and attain hemodynamic stability.

Nursing interventions
- Administer medications, as ordered.
- Provide supportive care and supplemental oxygen, as appropriate.
- Provide emotional support.
- Provide wound care

Monitoring
- Signs and symptoms of complications
- Vital signs
- Mental status
- Wound status
- Pain level

▶ PATIENT TEACHING

Be sure to cover:
- disorder, diagnostic tests, and treatment
- importance of good hand washing
- medication administration, dosage, and possible adverse effects
- importance of recognizing and reporting signs and symptoms of complications.
- wound care

Discharge planning
- Refer the patient for follow up with an infectious disease specialist and surgeon, as indicated.
- Refer the patient to physical rehabilitation, if indicated.
- For education and support, refer the patient to organizations such as the National Necrotizing Fasciitis Foundation.

✷ RESOURCES

Organizations
Centers for Disease Control and Prevention: *www.cdc.gov*
Harvard University Consumer Health Information: *www.intelihealth.com*
National Health Information Center: *www.health.gov/nhic/*
National Institute of Allergy and Infectious Diseases: *www.niaid.nih.gov*
National Library of Medicine: *www.nlm.nih.gov*

Selected references
Kasper, D.L., et al., eds. *Harrison's Principles of Internal Medicine*, 16th ed. New York: McGraw-Hill Book Co., 2005.

McGee, E.J. "Necrotizing Fasciitis Review of Pathophysiology, Diagnosis and Treatment," *Critical Care Nursing Quarterly* 28(1):80-84, January-March 2005.

Rodreguez, R.M., et al. "A Pilot Study of Cytokine Levels and White Blood Cell Counts in the Diagnosis of Necrotizing Fasciitis," *American Journal of Emergency Medicine* 24(1):58-61, January 2006.

Young, M.H., et al. "Therapies for Necrotising Fasciitis," *Expert Opinion on Biological Therapy* 6(2):155-65, February 2006.

Nephrotic syndrome

Description
- Characterized by marked proteinuria, hypoalbuminemia, hyperlipidemia, increased coagulation, and edema
- Results from a glomerular defect that affects permeability, indicating renal damage
- Prognosis highly variable, depending on underlying cause
- Some forms possibly progressing to end-stage renal failure
- Classified as primary or secondary

Pathophysiology
- Glomerular protein permeability increases.
- Urinary excretion of protein, especially albumin, increases.
- Hypoalbuminemia develops and causes decreased colloidal oncotic pressure.
- Leakage of fluid into interstitial spaces leads to acute, generalized edema.
- Vascular volume loss leads to increased blood viscosity and coagulation disorders.
- The renin-angiotensin system is triggered, causing tubular reabsorption of sodium and water and contributing to edema.

Causes
- Primary (idiopathic) glomerulonephritis (about 75% of cases)
- Lipid nephrosis (nil lesions) (main cause in children under age 8)
- Membranous glomerulonephritis (most common lesion in adult idiopathic nephrotic syndrome)
- Focal glomerulosclerosis (can develop spontaneously at any age, occur after kidney transplantation, or result from heroin injection; develops in about 10% of childhood cases and up to 20% of adult cases)
- Membranoproliferative glomerulonephritis (may follow infection, particularly streptococcal infection; occurs primarily in children and young adults)
- Metabolic diseases
- Collagen-vascular disorders
- Circulatory diseases
- Certain neoplastic diseases such as multiple myeloma

Risk factors
- Nephrotoxins
- Infection
- Allergic reactions
- Pregnancy
- Hereditary nephritis
- Chronic analgesic abuse

Incidence
- In children, 1 in 50,000 new cases per year
- In adults, 1 or 2 in 50,000 new cases per year
- In children, peak incidence between ages 2 and 3
- Slightly more common in males than in females
- Incidence higher in Native American, Hispanic, and Black populations

Common characteristics
- Fluid retention
- Anorexia
- Hypertension
- Decreased urine output

Complications
- Malnutrition
- Infection
- Coagulation disorders
- Thromboembolic vascular occlusion
- Accelerated atherosclerosis
- Acute renal failure

History
- Evidence of risk factors
- Lethargy
- Depression
- Anorexia

Physical findings
- Periorbital edema
- Mild to severe dependent edema
- Orthostatic hypotension
- Ascites
- Swollen external genitalia
- Signs of pleural effusion
- Pallor
- Decreased urination
- Frothy urine

Test results
LABORATORY
- Urinalysis reveals an increased number of hyaline, granular, waxy, fatty casts and oval fat bodies; consistent, heavy proteinuria (levels over 3.5 mg/dl for 24 hours) strongly suggests nephrotic syndrome.
- Serum cholesterol, serum phospholipid, and serum triglyceride levels are increased; and serum albumin levels are decreased.

DIAGNOSTIC PROCEDURES
- Renal biopsy allows histologic identification of the lesion.

General
- Correction of the underlying cause, if possible

Diet
- 0.6 g of protein per kilogram of body weight
- Restricted sodium intake

Activity
- Frequent rest periods, as needed

Medication
- Diuretics
- Antibiotics for infection
- Glucocorticoids
- Possible alkylating agents
- Possible cytotoxic agents
- I.V. albumin
- Angiotensin-converting enzyme inhibitors (cornerstone of treatment in adults)

Nursing diagnoses
- Activity intolerance
- Disturbed body image
- Excess fluid volume
- Imbalanced nutrition: Less than body requirements
- Ineffective tissue perfusion: Renal
- Risk for infection
- Risk for injury

Key outcomes
The patient will:
- verbalize measures to balance activity and pain
- express positive feelings about self
- maintain fluid balance
- demonstrate adequate nutritional intake
- exhibit urine output within acceptable range
- remain free from infection, injury, and complications.

Nursing interventions
- Offer the patient reassurance and support, especially during the acute phase, when severe edema changes body image.
- Provide information about dietary and fluid restrictions.

Monitoring
- Urine for protein
- Intake and output
- Daily weight
- Plasma albumin and transferrin levels
- Edema

Be sure to cover:
- disorder, diagnostic tests, and treatment
- signs of infection to report
- adherence to diet
- medication administration, dosage, and possible adverse effects.

Discharge planning
- Refer the patient to resource and support services.

Organizations
American Association of Kidney Patients:
www.aakp.org
National Institute of Diabetes and Digestive and Kidney Diseases:
www.niddk.nih.gov

Selected references
Broom, L.F. "Treating Pediatric Nephrotic Syndrome: A Clinical Challenge," *Nephrology Nursing Journal* 30(6):662-63, 667, December 2003.
Diseases, 4th ed. Philadelphia: Lippincott Williams & Wilkins, 2006.
Papez, K.E., and Smoyer, W.E. "Recent Advances in Congenital Nephrotic Syndrome," *Current Opinions in Pediatrics* 16(2):165-70, April 2004.
Yakupoglu, U., et al. "Post-Transplant Nephrotic Syndrome: A Comprehensive Clinicopathologic Study," *Kidney International* 65(6):2360-370, June 2004.

Neural tube defects

OVERVIEW

Description
- Birth defects that involve the spine or skull
- Result from neural tube's failure to close about 28 days after conception
- Different forms: spina bifida occulta (50% of cases), anencephaly (40%), and encephalocele (10%)

Pathophysiology
- Spina bifida occulta, the least severe and most common neural tube defect (NTD), is characterized by incomplete closure of one or more vertebrae without protrusion of the spinal cord or meninges. When defects of neural tube closure occur, such as meningocele and myelomeningocele, an accompanying vertebral defect allows the protrusion of the neural tube contents. (See *Types of spinal cord defects.*)
- In encephalocele, a saclike portion of the meninges and brain protrudes through a defective opening in the skull. Usually, it occurs in the occipital area, but it may also occur in the parietal, nasopharyngeal, or frontal area.
- In anencephaly, the closure defect occurs at the cranial end of the neuraxis and, as a result, part or the entire top of the skull is missing, severely damaging the brain. Portions of the brain stem and spinal cord may also be missing. This condition is fatal.

Causes
- A combination of genetic and environmental factors (possibly a lack of folic acid in the mother's diet)
- Exposure to a teratogen
- Trisomy 18 or trisomy 13 syndrome, or another multiple malformation syndrome

Incidence
- Incidence in North Carolina and South Carolina at least twice that than in the rest of the United States
- More common in Whites than in Blacks

Common characteristics
- Saclike protrusion or dimpling
- Paralysis

Complications
- Paralysis below the level of the defect
- Infection such as meningitis
- Hydrocephalus
- Death

ASSESSMENT

History
- Maternal history revealing factors that cause defect

Physical findings
SPINA BIFIDA OCCULTA
- Possibly a depression or dimple, tuft of hair, soft fatty deposit, port wine nevi, or a combination of these abnormalities on the skin over the spinal area
- Saclike protrusion over the spinal cord
- Flaccid or spastic paralysis
ENCEPHALOCELE
- Saclike protrusion through a defective opening in the skull
- Paralysis
ANENCEPHALY
- Part or entire top of skull missing

Test results
LABORATORY
- Levels of maternal alpha-fetoprotein (AFP), amniotic fluid AFP, and amniotic fluid acetylcholinesterase are elevated, indicating the need for further testing.
- Results of fetal karyotype analysis detect chromosomal abnormalities (present in 5% to 7% of NTDs).
- Results of maternal serum AFP screening, combined with screening for other serum markers, such as human chorionic gonadotropin (hCG), free beta-hCG, and unconjugated estriol (for patients with a lower risk of NTDs and those who will be younger than age 34 at the time of delivery), estimate the risk of fetal NTD and possible perinatal complications (premature rupture of the membranes, abruptio placentae, and fetal death).
IMAGING
- Ultrasonography (used when family history or abnormal serum screening results indicate an increased risk of open NTD) isn't conclusive for open NTDs or ventral wall defects.
- Spinal X-rays reveal spina bifida occulta.
- Myelography results differentiate spina bifida occulta from other spinal abnormalities, especially spinal cord tumors.

TYPES OF SPINAL CORD DEFECTS

There are three major types of spinal cord defects. *Spina bifida occulta* is characterized by a depression or raised area and a tuft of hair over the defect. In *myelomeningocele*, an external sac contains meninges, cerebrospinal fluid, and a portion of the spinal cord or nerve roots. *Meningocele* is characterized by an external sac containing only meninges and cerebrospinal fluid.

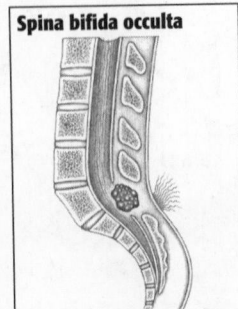
Spina bifida occulta

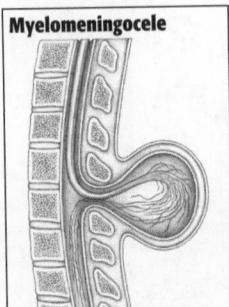
Myelomeningocele

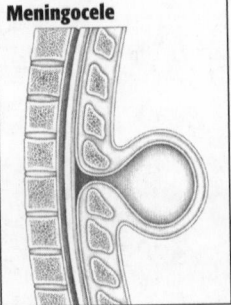
Meningocele

- Skull X-rays, cephalic measurements, and computed tomography (CT) scan demonstrate associated hydrocephalus.
- X-rays show a basilar, bony skull defect (CT scan and ultrasonography results further define the defect [for encephalocele]).

DIAGNOSTIC PROCEDURES
- Transillumination of the protruding sac distinguishes between myelomeningocele (typically doesn't transilluminate) and meningocele (typically transilluminates).

◆ TREATMENT

General
- Symptomatic based on neurologic effects of defect
- Assessment of growth and development throughout lifetime

Diet
- As tolerated

Activity
- Physical therapy

Medications
- Antibiotics, as indicated

Surgery
- Surgical closure of the protruding sac
- Shunt placement to relieve associated hydrocephalus
- Surgery during infancy to place protruding tissues back in the skull, excise the sac, and correct associated craniofacial abnormalities (for encephalocele)

❖ NURSING CONSIDERATIONS

Nursing diagnoses
- Decreased intracranial adaptive capacity
- Delayed growth and development
- Impaired physical mobility
- Impaired skin integrity
- Impaired urinary elimination
- Ineffective tissue perfusion: Peripheral
- Risk for impaired parenting
- Risk for impaired parent/infant/child attachment
- Risk for infection
- Risk for injury

Key outcomes
The patient (or family) will:
- maintain a stable head circumference and soft, flat fontanels
- achieve age-appropriate growth, skills, and behaviors to the fullest extent possible and identify realistic goals for their child
- maintain joint mobility and range of motion
- maintain adequate skin integrity
- maintain balance in intake and output
- exhibit signs of adequate peripheral perfusion
- show signs of bonding with their infant and participate in his care
- remain free from signs and symptoms of infection and injury.

Nursing interventions
- Provide psychological support.

BEFORE SURGERY
- Clean the defect gently with sterile saline solution or other solutions as ordered.
- Handle the infant carefully, and do not allow any pressure on the defect.
- Provide adequate time for parent-child bonding, if possible.

AFTER SURGERY
- Change the dressing regularly, as ordered, and check and report any signs of drainage, wound rupture, and infection.
- Place the infant prone to protect and assess the site.
- If leg casts have been applied, watch for signs that the child is outgrowing the cast. Regularly check distal pulses to ensure adequate circulation.

Monitoring
BEFORE SURGERY
- Neurologic status
- Feeding ability
- Nutritional status

AFTER SURGERY
- Signs of infection
- Signs of increased intracranial pressure
- Intake and output
- Vital signs

▶ PATIENT TEACHING

Be sure to cover:
- disorder, diagnostic tests, and treatment
- how to prevent contractures, pressure ulcers, and urinary tract infections.

Discharge planning
- Refer the prospective parents to a genetic counselor when a NTD has been diagnosed prenatally.
- Refer the family for psychological and support services.

✷ RESOURCES

Organizations
American Academy of Neurology: *www.aan.com*
Centers for Disease Control and Prevention: *www.cdc.gov*
The Merck Manual of Medical Information - Second Home Edition, Online Version: *www.merck.comlmmhe*

Selected references
Mowatt, D.J., et al. "Tissue Expansion for the Delayed Closure of Large Myelomeningoceles," *Journal of Neurosurgery* 103(6 Suppl):544-48, December 2005.
Neville-Jan, A. "The Problem with Prevention: The Case of Spina Bifida," *American Journal of Occupational Therapy* 59(5):527-39, September-October 2005.
Ryan, M. "Folic Acid to Prevent Neural Tube Defects: A Potential Pharmacy Initiative with Public Health Implications," *Hospital Pharmacy* 39(10):962-69, October 2004.

Obesity

● OVERVIEW

Description
- Excess of body fat, generally 20% above ideal body weight
- Body mass index (BMI) of 30 or greater (see *BMI measurements*)
- Second-leading cause of preventable deaths

Pathophysiology
- Fat cells increase in size in response to dietary intake.
- When the cells can no longer expand, they increase in number.
- With weight loss, the size of the fat cells decreases, but the number of cells doesn't.

Causes
- Excessive caloric intake combined with inadequate energy expenditure
- Theories that may explain obesity include:
  - hypothalamic dysfunction of hunger and satiety centers
  - genetic predisposition
  - abnormal absorption of nutrients
  - impaired action of GI and growth hormones and of hormonal regulators, such as insulin
  - socioeconomic status
  - environmental factors
  - psychological factors

Incidence
- Affects more than 50% of U.S. residents
- Affects one in five children.

Common characteristics
- Increased weight
- Increased BMI

Complications
- Respiratory difficulties
- Hypertension
- Cardiovascular disease
- Diabetes mellitus
- Renal disease
- Gallbladder disease
- Psychosocial difficulties
- Premature death

✳ ASSESSMENT

History
- Increasing weight
- Complications of obesity

Physical findings
- BMI of 30 or greater

Test results
DIAGNOSTIC PROCEDURES
- Height is compared to weight using a standard table.
- Measurement of the thickness of subcutaneous fat folds are measured with calipers to approximate total body fat. (See *Taking anthropometric arm measurements*.)
- BMI is calculated.

◆ TREATMENT

General
- Hypnosis and behavior modification techniques
- Psychological counseling

Diet
- Reduction in daily caloric intake

Activity
- Increase in daily activity level

Surgery
- Vertical banded gastroplasty
- Gastric bypass

✛ NURSING CONSIDERATIONS

Nursing diagnoses
- Chronic low self-esteem
- Disturbed body image
- Imbalanced nutrition: More than body requirements
- Ineffective coping
- Sedentary lifestyle

Key outcomes
The patient will:
- voice feelings related to self-esteem
- express positive feelings about self
- safely reduce weight and reduce BMI to a normal level
- demonstrate effective coping mechanisms to deal with long-term compliance
- state the need to increase activity level.

BMI MEASUREMENTS

Use these steps to calculate body mass index (BMI):
- Multiply weight in pounds by 705.
- Divide this number by height in inches.
- Then divide this by height in inches again.
- Compare results to these standards:
  - 18.5 to 24.9: normal
  - 25 to 29.9: overweight
  - 30 to 39.9: obese
  - 40 or greater: morbidly obese.

Nursing interventions

- Obtain an accurate diet history to identify the patient's eating patterns and the importance of food to his lifestyle.
- Promote increased physical activity, as appropriate.

Monitoring

- Diet
- Intake and output
- Vital signs
- Weight and BMI

▶ **PATIENT TEACHING**

Be sure to cover:
- need for long-term maintenance after desired weight is achieved
- dietary guidelines
- safe weight loss practices.

Discharge planning

- Refer the patient to a weight-reduction program.

✳ **RESOURCES**

Organizations

American Obesity Association: *www.obesity.org*
Obesity Help, Inc.: *www.obesityhelp.com*
The Obesity Society: *www.naaso.org*

Selected references

Brown, I. "Nurses' Attitudes Towards Adult Patients Who are Obese: Literature Review," *Journal of Advanced Nursing* 53(2):221-32, January 2006.

Dietz, W.H., and Robinson, T.N. "Clinical Practice. Overweight Children and Adolescents," *New England Journal of Medicine* 352(20):2100-2109, May 2005.

Lapane, K.L., and Resnik, L. "Obesity in Nursing Homes: An Escalating Problem," *Journal of the American Geriatrics Society* 53(8):1386-391, August 2005.

Yensel, C.S., et al. "Childhood Obesity and Insulin-resistant Syndrome," *Journal of Pediatric Nursing* 19(4):238-46, August 2004.

TAKING ANTHROPOMETRIC ARM MEASUREMENTS

Follow these steps to determine triceps skin-fold thickness, midarm circumference, and midarm muscle circumference.

Triceps skin-fold thickness

- Find the midpoint circumference of the arm by placing the tape measure halfway between the axilla and the elbow. Grasp the patient's skin with your thumb and forefinger, aboout ⅜" (1 cm) above the midpoint, as shown below left.
- Place calipers at the midpoint, and squeeze for 3 seconds.
- Record the measurement to the nearest millimeter.
- Take two more readings, and use the average.

Midarm circumference and midarm muscle circumference

- At the midpoint, measure the midarm circumference, as shown below right. Record the measurement in centimeters.

- Calculate the midarm muscle circumference by multiplying the triceps skin-fold thickness—measured in millimeters—by 3.14.
- Subtract this number from the midarm circumference.

Recording the measurements

Record all three measurements as a percentage of the standard measurements (see table below), using this formula:

$$\frac{\text{Actual measurement}}{\text{Standard measurement}} \times 100\%$$

Remember, a measurement less than 90% of the standard indicates caloric deprivation. A measurement over 90% indicates adequate or more-than-adequate energy reserves.

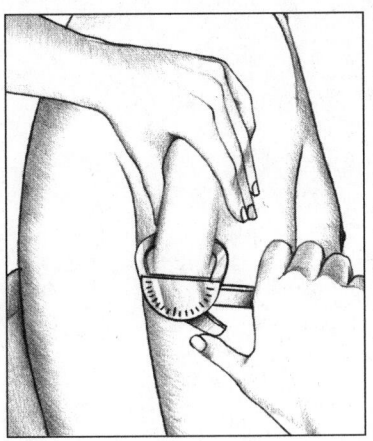
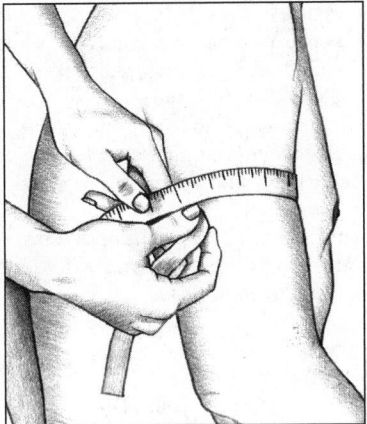

Measurement	Standard	90%
Triceps skin-fold thickness	Men: 12.5 mm Women: 16.5 mm	Men: 11.3 mm Women: 14.9 mm
Midarm circumference	Men: 29.3 cm Women: 28.5 cm	Men: 26.4 cm Women: 25.7 cm
Midarm muscle circumference	Men: 25.3 cm Women: 23.3 cm	Men: 22.8 cm Women: 20.9 cm

Obsessive-compulsive disorder

● OVERVIEW

Description
- Obsessive thoughts and compulsive behaviors that impair everyday functioning
- May be simple or complex and ritualized
- Also known as *OCD*

Pathophysiology
- This anatomic-physiologic disturbance is thought to involve an alteration in the frontal-subcortical neural circuitry of the brain.

Causes
- Decrease in caudate nucleus volume

Risk factors
- Coexisting mental disorder
- Tic disorders

Incidence
- Affects 1 in 50 Americans
- Can occur at any age
- More common in males and first-born children

Common characteristics
- Repetitive behaviors and activities that comprise more than 1 hour per day
- Activities that alleviate anxiety triggered by a core fear

Complications
- Impairment of occupational and social functioning
- Endangerment of health and safety

✳ ASSESSMENT

History
- Presence of obsessive thoughts, words, or mental images that persistently and involuntarily invade the consciousness
- Moderate to severe impairment of social and occupational functioning
- Patient usually rigid and conscientious, with great aspirations
- Patient taking responsibility seriously and finding decision making difficult
- Patient lacking creativity and the ability to find alternate solutions to problems

Physical findings
- Formal, reserved manner
- Patient accurate and complete, carefully qualifying statements and anticipating every move and gesture of person to whom he speaks
- Flat and unemotional affect, except for controlled anxiety
- Self-awareness that's intellectual, without accompanying emotion or feeling

DSM-IV-TR criteria
Diagnosis is confirmed when the patient meets these criteria:

OBSESSIONS
- Patient experiences recurrent and persistent ideas, thoughts, impulses, or images as intrusive and senseless.
- Patient attempts to ignore or suppress such thoughts or impulses or to neutralize them with some other thought or action.
- Patient recognizes that the obsessions are products of his mind, not externally imposed.
- Patient's obsession is unrelated to another Axis I disorder.

COMPULSIONS
- Patient performs repetitive, purposeful, and intentional behaviors in response to an obsession or according to certain rules or in a stereotypical manner.
- Behavior is intended to neutralize or prevent discomfort or some dreaded event or situation, but the behavior isn't connected in a realistic way with intended outcome, or is clearly excessive.
- Patient recognizes that the behavior is excessive or unreasonable.

Test results
- No specific test exists for diagnosis
- Diagnosis is confirmed by *DSM-IV-TR* criteria.

◆ TREATMENT

General
- Behavioral therapy
- Increasing exposure to stressful situations and learning to manage response in appropriate manner
- Keeping a diary of daily stressors
- Substituting new activities for compulsive behavior

Diet
- No restrictions

Activity
- No restrictions

Medication
- Selective serotonin-reuptake inhibitors

♣ NURSING CONSIDERATIONS

Nursing diagnoses
- Anxiety
- Chronic low self-esteem
- Fear
- Impaired social interaction
- Ineffective coping
- Ineffective role performance
- Risk for injury
- Social isolation

Key outcomes
The patient will:
- express feelings of anxiety as they occur
- express positive feelings about self
- express fears and concerns
- maintain family and peer relationships
- cope with stress without excessive obsessive-compulsive behavior
- reduce the amount of time spent each day on obsessing and ritualizing
- produce no harmful effects from ritualistic behavior
- demonstrate effective social interaction skills.

Nursing interventions
- Provide an accepting, patient atmosphere.
- Allow time for ritualistic behavior (unless it's dangerous) until distraction occurs.
- Provide for basic needs.
- Make reasonable demands and set reasonable limits; make the patient's purpose clear.
- Explore patterns leading to the behavior or recurring problems.
- Encourage active diversional resources.
- Assist with individualized problem solving.
- Identify insight and improved behavior.

Monitoring
- Behavioral changes
- Disturbing topics of conversation
- Effective interventions
- Effects of pharmacologic therapy

▶ PATIENT TEACHING

Be sure to cover:
- disorder, diagnostic tests, and treatment
- how to identify progress
- importance of realistic expectations of self and others
- stress relief by channeling emotional energy
- relaxation and breathing techniques.

Discharge planning
Refer the patient to:
- social services
- support services.

✴ RESOURCES

Organizations
American Psychiatric Association:
www.psych.org
American Psychological Association:
www.helping.apa.org
Anxiety Disorders Association of America:
www.adaa.org
Obsessive Compulsive Foundation:
www.ocfoundation.org

Selected references
Diagnostic and Statistical Manual of Mental Disorders, Fourth Edition, Text Revision. Washington, D.C.: American Psychiatric Association, 2000.

Grover, S., and Gupta, N. "Shared Obsessive-Compulsive Disorder," *Psychopathology* 39(2):99-101, January, 2006.

Hohenhaus, S.M. "Caring for OCD Patients in the Emergency Department," *Journal of Emergency Nursing* 30(3):249, June 2004.

Mancebo, M.C., et al. "Obsessive-Complsive Personality Disorder and Obsessive-Compulsive Disorder: Clinical Characteristics, Diagnostic Difficulties, and Treatment," *Annals of Clinical Psychiatry* 18(4):197-204, October-December 2005.

Moritz, S., et al. "Quality of Life in Obessive-Compulsive Disorder Before and After Treatment," *Comprehensive Psychiatry* 46(6):453-59, November-December 2005.

Shoval, G., et al. "Clinical Characterstics of Inpatient Adolescents with Severe Obsessive-Compulsive Disorder," *Depression and Anxiety* 23(2):62-70, 2006.

Osgood-Schlatter disease

● OVERVIEW

Description
- Partial separation of the epiphysis of the tibial tubercle from the tibial shaft, leading to tendinitis
- Affects one or both knees
- Also known as *osteochondrosis*

Pathophysiology
- Bone growth is faster than soft-tissue growth.
- Muscle tendon tighteness occurs across the joint.
- Flexibility is decreased.
- Mechanical inefficiency of the extensor mechanism follows incomplete separation of the epiphysis from the shaft.
- Tendinitis of the knee results.

Causes
- Traumatic avulsion of the proximal tibial tuberosity at the patellar tendon insertion
- Locally deficient blood supply
- Genetic factors
- Exercise

Incidence
- Most common in active adolescent boys

Common characteristics
- Frequent fractures
- Pain at inferior aspect of patella

Complications
- Irregular growth of the proximal tibial epiphysis
- Partial avascular necrosis of the proximal tibial epiphysis
- Chronic pain
- Patellar tendon avulsion

✳ ASSESSMENT

History
- Constant aching, pain, swelling, and tenderness below the kneecap
- Pain that worsens during activity
- Symptoms that are relieved with rest
- Precipitating trauma

Physical findings
- Soft-tissue swelling
- Localized heat and tenderness
- Decreased flexibility and restriction in the hamstrings, triceps surae, and quadriceps muscle
- Pain at 30-degree flexion with tibia starting at 90 degrees in internal rotation
- Palpabale firm mass

Test results
IMAGING
- X-rays show epiphyseal closings, soft tissue swelling, and bone fragments.
- Bone scan may reveal increased uptake in the area of the tibial tuberosity.

◆ TREATMENT

General
- Ice application for 20 minutes every 2 to 4 hours
- Reinforced elastic knee support, plaster cast, or splint

Diet
- No restrictions

Activity
- Reduction of sports activities or exercise
- Avoidance of exercises that demand quadriceps contraction
- In severe cases, immobilization for 6 to 8 weeks
- Rehabilitation exercises

Medication
- Nonsteroidal anti-inflammatory drugs
- Analgesics

Surgery
- Removal or fixation of the epiphysis

❖ NURSING CONSIDERATIONS

Nursing diagnoses
- Acute pain
- Delayed growth and development
- Disturbed body image
- Dressing or grooming self-care deficit
- Fear
- Impaired physical mobility

Key outcomes
The patient will:
- express feelings of increased comfort and decreased pain
- exhibit developmental milestones within the confines of the disease process.
- express positive feelings about self
- perform activities of daily living within the confines of the disease
- discuss fears and concerns
- maintain joint mobility and range of motion.

Nursing interventions
- Administer analgesics and assess response.
- Ensure proper application of knee support or splint.
- Provide the patient with crutches if needed.
- Promote and allow adequate time for self-care.
- Encourage verbalization and provide support.

Monitoring
- Limitation of movement
- Muscle atrophy
- After surgery: circulation, sensation, and pain
- Excessive bleeding

▶ PATIENT TEACHING

Be sure to cover:
- disorder, diagnostic tests, and treatment
- prescribed exercise program
- use of crutches, if needed
- protection of the injured knee
- avoidance of activities that require deep knee bending for 2 to 4 months.

Discharge planning
- Refer the patient for occupational and physical therapy, as appropriate.

✳ RESOURCES

Organizations
American Orthopaedic Association: *www.aoassn.org*
National Institutes of Health: *www.nih.gov*
WebMD: *www.webmd.com*

Selected references
Diseases, 4th ed. Philadelphia: Lippincott Williams & Wilkins, 2006.
Handbook of Pathophysiology, 2nd ed. Philadelphia: Lippincott Williams & Wilkins, 2005.
Ishida, K., et al. "Infrapatellar Bursal Osteochondromatosis Associated with Unresolved Osgood-Schlatter Disease. A Case Report," *Journal of Bone and Joint Surgery* 87(12):2780-783, December 2005.

Osteoarthritis

● OVERVIEW

Description
- Chronic degeneration of joint cartilage
- Most common form of arthritis
- Disability from minor limitation to near immobility
- Variable progression rates

Pathophysiology
- Deterioration of the joint cartilage occurs.
- Reactive new bone forms at the margins and subchondral areas.
- Breakdown of chondrocytes occurs in the hips and knees.
- Cartilage flakes irritate synovial lining.
- The cartilage lining becomes fibrotic.
- Joint movement is limited.
- Synovial fluid leaks into bone defects, causing cysts.

Causes
- Advancing age
- Hereditary, possibly
- Secondary osteoarthritis
- Traumatic injury
- Congenital abnormality
- Endocrine disorders such as diabetes mellitus
- Metabolic disorders such as chondrocalcinosis

Incidence
- Occurs equally in both sexes
- Occurs after age 40

Common characteristics
- Deep, aching joint pain
- Stiffness, especially in morning and after exercise
- Crepitus of the joint during motion
- Heberden's nodes (bony enlargements of distal interphalangeal joints)
- Altered gait
- Decreased range of motion (ROM)
- Localized headaches

Complications
- Flexion contractures
- Subluxation
- Deformity
- Ankylosis
- Bony cysts
- Gross bony overgrowth
- Central cord syndrome
- Nerve root compression
- Cauda equina syndrome

✳ ASSESSMENT

History
- Predisposing traumatic injury
- Deep, aching joint pain
- Pain after exercise or weight bearing
- Pain possibly relieved by rest
- Stiffness in morning and after exercise
- Aching during changes in weather
- "Grating" feeling when the joint moves
- Limited movement

Physical findings
- Contractures
- Joint swelling
- Muscle atrophy
- Deformity of the involved areas
- Gait abnormalities
- Hard nodes that may be red, swollen, and tender on the distal and proximal interphalangeal joints (see *Signs of osteoarthritis*)
- Loss of finger dexterity
- Muscle spasms, limited movement, and joint instability

Test results
LABORATORY
- Synovial fluid analysis rules out inflammatory arthritis.
IMAGING
- X-rays of the affected joint may show a narrowing of the joint space or margin, cystlike bony deposits in the joint space and margins, sclerosis of the subchondral space, joint deformity or articular damage, bony growths at weight-bearing areas, and possible joint fusion.
- Radionuclide bone scan may be used to rule out inflammatory arthritis by showing normal uptake of the radionuclide.
- Magnetic resonance imaging shows affected joint, adjacent bones, and disease progression.
DIAGNOSTIC PROCEDURES
- Neuromuscular tests may show reduced muscle strength.
- Arthroscopy shows internal joint structures and identifies soft-tissue swelling.

◆ TREATMENT

General
- Relieving pain
- Improving mobility
- Minimizing disability

Diet
- No restrictions

Activity
- As tolerated
- Physical therapy
- Assistive mobility devices

Medication
- Analgesics

Surgery
- Arthroplasty (partial or total)
- Arthrodesis
- Osteoplasty
- Osteotomy

Nursing diagnoses

- Acute pain
- Anxiety
- Disturbed body image
- Disturbed sleep pattern
- Dressing or grooming self-care deficit
- Impaired physical mobility
- Ineffective coping
- Risk for injury

Key outcomes

The patient will:

- express feelings of increased comfort and decreased pain
- identify strategies to reduce anxiety
- express positive feelings about self
- report feeling well-rested
- perform activities of daily living within confines of the disease
- maintain joint mobility and ROM
- exhibit positive coping behaviors
- remain free from injury.

Nursing interventions

- Allow adequate time for self-care.
- Adjust pain medications to allow maximum rest.
- Identify techniques that promote rest and relaxation.
- Administer anti-inflammatory medication.
- For affected hand joints, use hot soaks and paraffin dips.
- For affected lumbosacral spinal joints, provide a firm mattress.
- For affected cervical spinal joints, apply a cervical collar.
- For an affected hip, apply moist heat pads and administer antispasmodic drugs.
- For an affected knee, help with ROM exercises.
- Apply elastic supports or braces.
- Check crutches, cane, braces, or walker for proper fit.

Monitoring

- Pain pattern
- Response to analgesics
- ROM

Be sure to cover:

- disorder, diagnostic tests, and treatment
- need for adequate rest during the day, after exertion, and at night
- energy conservation methods
- need to take medications exactly as prescribed
- adverse reactions to medication
- wearing support shoes that fit well and repairing worn heels
- installation of safety devices at home
- ROM exercises, performing them as gently as possible
- need to maintain proper body weight
- use of crutches or other orthopedic devices.

Discharge planning

- Refer the patient to occupational or physical therapist, as indicated.

Organizations

Arthrtiis Foundation: *www. arthritis.org*
National Institutes of Health: *www.nih.gov*
WebMD: *www.webmd.com*

Selected references

Cuddy, M.I. "Geriatric Pharmacology: Osteoarthritis," *Journal of Practical Nursing* 55(1):6-15, Spring 2005.

Diseases, 4th ed. Philadelphia: Lippincott Williams & Wilkins, 2006.

Handbook of Pathophysiology, 2nd ed. Philadelphia: Lippincott Williams & Wilkins, 2005.

Sharma, L., et al. "Epidemiology of Osteoarthritis: An Update," *Current Opinion in Rheumatology* 18(2):147-56, March 2006.

Wang, T.J. "A Theoretical Model for Preventing Osteoarthritis-related Disability," *Rehabilitation Nursing* 30(2):63-67, March-April 2005.

SIGNS OF OSTEOARTHRITIS

Heberden's nodes appear on the dorsolateral aspect of the distal interphalangeal joints. These bony and cartilaginous enlargements are usually hard and painless. They typically occur in middle-aged and elderly patients with osteoarthritis. Bouchard's nodes are similar to Heberden's nodes but are less common and appear on the proximal interphalangeal joints.

Heberden's nodes

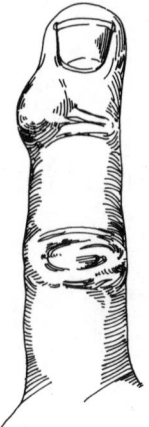

Bouchard's nodes

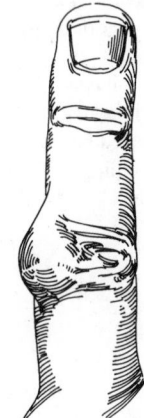

Osteomyelitis

● OVERVIEW

Description
- Pyogenic bone infection
- May be acute or chronic
- For acute form, good prognosis with prompt treatment
- For chronic form, poor prognosis

Pathophysiology
- Organisms settle in a hematoma or weakened area and spread directly to bone.
- Pus is produced and pressure builds within the rigid medullary cavity.
- Pus is forced through the haversian canals.
- Subperiosteal abscess forms.
- Bone is deprived of its blood supply.
- Necrosis results and new bone formation is stimulated.
- Dead bone detaches and exits through an abscess or the sinuses.
- Osteomyelitis becomes chronic.

Causes
- Minor traumatic injury
- Acute infection originating elsewhere in the body
- *Staphylococcus aureus*
- *Streptococcus pyogenes*
- *Pseudomonas aeruginosa*
- *Escherichia coli*
- *Proteus vulgaris*
- Fungi or viruses

Incidence
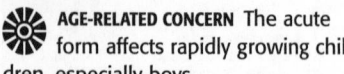 **AGE-RELATED CONCERN** The acute form affects rapidly growing children, especially boys.
- Incidence of both types declining, except in drug abusers

Common characteristics
- Sudden pain in affected bone
- Tenderness, heat, swelling
- Restricted movement
- Chronic infection

Complications
- Chronic infection
- Skeletal deformities
- Joint deformities
- Disturbed bone growth in children
- Differing leg lengths
- Impaired mobility

✳ ASSESSMENT

History
- Previous injury, surgery, or primary infection
- Sudden, severe pain in the affected bone
- Pain unrelieved by rest and worse with motion
- Related chills, nausea, and malaise
- Refusal to use the affected area

Physical findings
- Tachycardia and fever
- Swelling and restricted movement over the infection site
- Tenderness and warmth over the infection site
- Persistent pus drainage from an old pocket in a sinus tract

Test results
LABORATORY
- White blood cell (WBC) count shows leukocytosis.
- Erythrocyte sedimentation rate is increased.
- Blood culture identifies pathogen.
IMAGING
- X-rays may show bone involvement.
- Bone scans may detect early infection.
- Computed tomography scan and magnetic resonance imaging can show extent of infection.

◆ TREATMENT

General
- Decreasing internal bone pressure
- Preventing bone necrosis
- Hyperbaric oxygen therapy
- Free tissue transfers
- I.V. fluids, as needed

Diet
- High-protein, rich in vitamin C

Activity
- Bed rest
- Immobilization of involved bone and joint with a cast or traction

Medication
- I.V. antibiotics
- Analgesics
- Intracavitary instillation of antibiotics for open wounds

Surgery
- Surgical drainage
- Local muscle flaps
- Sequestrectomy
- Amputation for chronic and unrelieved symptoms

❖ NURSING CONSIDERATIONS

Nursing diagnoses
- Activity intolerance
- Acute and chronic pain
- Anxiety
- Deficient knowledge (osteomyelitis)
- Excess fluid volume
- Fear
- Impaired physical mobility
- Impaired tissue integrity
- Powerlessness

Key outcomes
The patient will:
- perform activities of daily living without excessive pain or fatigue
- express feelings of increased comfort and decreased pain
- demonstrate a decrease in anxiety
- exhibit adequate fluid volume
- express fears and concerns
- maintain joint mobility and range of motion as much as possible
- exhibit adequate tissue perfusion and pulses distally
- express feelings of control over situation.

Nursing interventions
- Control infection.
- Protect the bone from injury.
- Provide support.
- Promote and allow adequate time for self-care.
- Promote activities that promote rest and relaxation.
- Use strict sterile technique.
- With skeletal traction, cover the pin insertion points with small, dry dressings.
- Provide firm pillows.
- Provide thorough skin care.
- Provide complete cast care.
- Give analgesics, as ordered.

Monitoring
- Vital signs
- Wound appearance
- Pain control
- Drainage and suctioning equipment
- Sudden malpositioning of the limb

▶ PATIENT TEACHING

Be sure to cover:
- disorder, diagnostic tests, and treatment
- medication administration, dosage, and, possible adverse effects
- techniques for promoting rest and relaxation
- wound site care
- signs of recurring infection
- importance of follow-up examinations.

Discharge planning
- Refer the patient for occupational therapy, as appropriate.

✴ RESOURCES

Organizations
American Orthopaedic Association: *www.aoassn.org*
Cleveland Clinic Health Information Center: *www.clevelandclinic.org/health*
The Merck Manuals Online Medical Library: *www.merck.com/mmhe*

Selected references
Diseases, 4th ed. Philadelphia: Lippincott Williams & Wilkins, 2006.
Embli, J.M., and Trepman, E. "Microbiological Evaluation of Diabetic Foot Osteomyelitis," *Clinical Infectious Diseases* 42(1):63-65, January 2006.
Gamble, K., et al. "Osteomyelitis of the Pubic Symphysis in Pregnancy," *Obstetrics and Gynecology* 107(2):477-81, February 2006.
Handbook of Pathophysiology, 2nd ed. Philadelphia: Lippincott Williams & Wilkins, 2005.
Singh, G., et al. "Cervical Osteomyelitis Associated with Intravenous Drug Use," *Emergency Medicine Journal* 23(2):e16, February 2006.

Osteoporosis

OVERVIEW

Description
- Loss of calcium and phosphate from bones, leaving bone abnormally vulnerable to fractures
- Primary or secondary to underlying disease
- Types of primary osteoporosis: postmenopausal osteoporosis (Type I) and age-associated osteoporosis (Type II)
- Secondary osteoporosis: caused by an identifiable agent or disease

Pathophysiology
- The rate of bone resorption accelerates as the rate of bone formation decelerates.
- Decreased bone mass results and bones become porous and brittle.

Causes
- Exact cause unknown
- Prolonged therapy with steroids or heparin
- Bone immobilization
- Alcoholism
- Malnutrition
- Rheumatoid arthritis
- Liver disease
- Malabsorption
- Scurvy
- Lactose intolerance
- Hyperthyroidism
- Osteogenesis imperfecta
- Sudeck's atrophy (localized in hands and feet, with recurring attacks)

Risk factors
- Mild, prolonged negative calcium balance
- Declining gonadal adrenal function
- Faulty protein metabolism (caused by estrogen deficiency)
- Sedentary lifestyle

Incidence
- Idiopathic form affecting children and adults
- Type I affecting women ages 51 to 75
- Type II most common between ages 70 and 85

Common characteristics
- Sudden pain associated with bending or lifting
- Back pain (if vertebral collapse occurs)
- Increasing deformity
- Kyphosis
- Loss of height
- Decreased exercise tolerance
- Spontaneous wedge fractures

Complications
- Bone fractures (vertebrae, femoral neck, and distal radius)

ASSESSMENT

History
- Postmenopausal patient
- Condition known to cause secondary osteoporosis
- Snapping sound or sudden pain in lower back when bending down to lift something
- Possible slow development of pain (over several years)
- With vertebral collapse, backache and pain radiating around the trunk
- Pain aggravated by movement or jarring

Physical findings
- Humped back
- Markedly aged appearance
- Loss of height
- Muscle spasm
- Decreased spinal movement with flexion more limited than extension

Test results
LABORATORY
- Serum calcium, phosphorus, and alkaline levels are normal.
- Parathyroid hormone level is elevated.
IMAGING
- X-ray studies show characteristic degeneration in the lower thoracolumbar vertebrae.
- Computed tomography scan accurately assesses spinal bone loss.
- Bone scans show injured or diseased areas.
- Dual or single photon absorptiometry (measurement of bone mass) shows loss of bone mass.
DIAGNOSTIC PROCEDURES
- Bone biopsy shows thin, porous, but otherwise normal bone.

◆ TREATMENT

General
- Controling bone loss
- Preventing additional fractures
- Controlling pain
- Reduction and immobilization of fractures

Diet
- Rich in vitamin D, calcium, and protein

Activity
- Physical therapy program of gentle exercise and activity
- Supportive devices

Medication
- Estrogen
- Sodium fluoride
- Calcium and vitamin D supplements
- Calcitonin

Surgery
- Open reduction and internal fixation for femur fractures

❖ NURSING CONSIDERATIONS

Nursing diagnoses
- Acute pain and chronic pain
- Disturbed body image
- Dressing or grooming self-care deficit
- Imbalanced nutrition: Less than body requirements
- Impaired physical mobility
- Risk for impaired skin integrity
- Risk for injury

Key outcomes
The patient will:
- express feelings of increased comfort and decreased pain
- report a decrease in episodes of chronic pain
- express positive feelings about self
- perform activities of daily living within the limits of the disease
- maintain adequate dietary intake
- maintain joint mobility and range of motion (ROM)
- maintain skin integrity
- demonstrate measures to prevent injury.

Nursing interventions
- Encourage careful positioning, ambulation, and prescribed exercises.
- Promote self-care while allowing adequate time.
- Encourage mild exercise.
- Assist with walking.
- Perform passive ROM exercises.
- Promote physical therapy sessions.
- Use safety precautions.
- Administer analgesia, as ordered.
- Apply heat.

Monitoring
- Skin for redness, warmth, and new pain sites
- Response to analgesia
- Nutritional status
- Height
- Exercise tolerance
- Joint mobility

▶ PATIENT TEACHING

Be sure to cover:
- disorder, diagnostic tests, and treatment
- medication administration, dosage, and possible adverse effects
- performing monthly breast self-examination while on estrogen therapy
- need to report vaginal bleeding promptly
- need to report new pain sites immediately
- sleeping on a firm mattress
- avoiding excessive bed rest
- use of back brace, if appropriate
- proper body mechanics
- home safety devices
- diet rich in calcium.

Discharge planning
- Refer the patient for physical and occupational therapy as appropriate.

✹ RESOURCES

Organizations
National Institutes of Health—Osteoporosis and Related Bone Diseases National Resource Center: *www.osteo.org*
National Osteoporosis Foundation: *www.nof.org*

Selected references
Chang, S. "A Cross-sectional Survey of Calcium Intake in Relation to Knowledge of Osteoporosis and Beliefs in Young Adult Women," *International Journal of Nursing Practice* 12(1):21-27, February 2006.

Diseases, 4th ed. Philadelphia: Lippincott Williams & Wilkins, 2006.

Handbook of Pathophysiology, 2nd ed. Philadelphia: Lippincott Williams & Wilkins, 2005.

Kessenich, C.R. "Osteoporosis: New Options for Pain Relief," *Nurse Practitioner* 31(2):44-47, February 2006.

Reginster, J., and Sarlet, N. "The Treatment of Severe Postmenopausal Osteoporosis: A Review of Current and Emerging Therapeutic Options," *Treatments in Endocrinology* 5(1):15-23, 2006.

Otitis media

OVERVIEW

Description
- Inflammation of the middle ear associated with fluid accumulation
- May be acute, chronic, suppurative, or secretory

Pathophysiology
- Differs with otitis media type.

SUPPURATIVE FORM
- Nasopharyngeal flora reflux through the eustachian tube and colonize the middle ear.
- Respiratory tract infections, allergic reactions, and position changes allow reflux of nasopharyngeal flora through the eustachian tube and colonization in the middle ear.

SECRETORY FORM
- Obstruction of the eustachian tube promotes transudation of sterile serous fluid from blood vessels in the middle ear membrane.

Causes
- Acute otitis media: disruption of eustachian tube patency
- Suppurative otitis media: bacterial infection with pneumococci, group A beta-hemolytic streptococci, staphylococci, and gram-negative bacteria
- Chronic suppurative otitis media: inadequate treatment of acute otitis episodes or infection by resistant strains of bacteria
- Secretory otitis media: viral infection, allergy, or barotrauma
- Chronic secretory otitis media: adenoidal tissue overgrowth, edema, chronic sinus infection, or inadequate treatment of acute suppurative otitis media

Incidence
- Most common in infants and children
- Peaks between ages 6 and 24 months
- Subsides after age 3 years
- Most common during winter months

AGE-RELATED CONCERN Acute otitis media is an emergency in an immunocompromised child.

Common characteristics
- Severe, deep, throbbing ear pain
- Mild to high fever

Complications
- Spontaneous rupture of the tympanic membrane
- Persistent perforation
- Chronic otitis media
- Mastoiditis
- Meningitis
- Cholesteatomas
- Abscesses, septicemia
- Lymphadenopathy, leukocytosis
- Permanent hearing loss and tympanosclerosis
- Vertigo

ASSESSMENT

History
- Upper respiratory tract infection
- Allergies
- Severe, deep, throbbing ear pain
- Dizziness
- Nausea, vomiting

ACUTE SECRETORY OTITIS MEDIA
- Sensation of fullness in the ear
- Popping, crackling, or clicking sounds on swallowing or moving the jaw
- Describes hearing an echo when speaking

TYMPANIC MEMBRANE RUPTURE
- Pain that suddenly stops
- Recent air travel or scuba diving

Physical findings
- Sneezing and coughing with upper respiratory tract infection
- Mild to high fever
- Painless, purulent discharge in chronic suppurative otitis media
- Obscured or distorted bony landmarks of the tympanic membrane in acute suppurative otitis media
- Tympanic membrane retraction in acute secretory otitis media
- Clear or amber fluid behind the tympanic membrane
- Blue-black tympanic membrane with hemorrhage into the middle ear
- Pulsating discharge with tympanic perforation
- Conductive hearing loss (varies with the size and type of tympanic membrane perforation and ossicular destruction)

CHRONIC OTITIS MEDIA
- Thickening and scarring of tympanic membrane
- Decreased or absent tympanic membrane mobility
- Cholesteatoma

Test results

LABORATORY
- Culture and sensitivity tests of exudate show the causative organism.
- Complete blood count shows leukocytosis.

IMAGING
- Radiographic studies demonstrate mastoid involvement.

DIAGNOSTIC PROCEDURES
- Pneumatoscopy shows decreased tympanic membrane mobility.
- Tympanometry detects hearing loss and evaluates the condition of the middle ear.
- Audiometry shows degree of hearing loss.
- Pneumatic otoscopy may show decreased tympanic membrane mobility.

NURSING ALERT In adults, unilateral serous otitis media should always be evaluated for a nasopharyngeal-obstructing lesion such as carcinoma.

TREATMENT

General
- In acute secretory otitis media, Valsalva's maneuver several times per day (may be the only treatment required)
- Concomitant treatment of the underlying cause
- Elimination of eustachian tube obstruction

Diet
- No restrictions

Activity
- No restrictions

Medication
- Antibiotics
- Aspirin or acetaminophen
- Analgesics
- Sedatives (small children)
- Nasopharyngeal decongestant therapy

Surgery

- Myringotomy and aspiration of middle ear fluid, followed by insertion of a polyethylene tube into the tympanic membrane
- Myringoplasty
- Tympanoplasty
- Mastoidectomy
- Cholesteatoma excision
- Stapedectomy for otosclerosis

❖ NURSING CONSIDERATIONS

Nursing diagnoses

- Acute pain
- Disturbed sensory perception: Auditory
- Disturbed sleep pattern
- Impaired verbal communication
- Risk for infection
- Risk for injury

Key outcomes

The patient will:

- express feelings of increased comfort and decreased pain
- regain hearing or develop compensatory mechanisms
- resume normal sleep patterns
- communicate feelings and needs
- remain free from signs and symptoms of infection and injury.

Nursing interventions

- Answer all questions.
- Encourage discussion of concerns about hearing loss.

WITH HEARING LOSS

- Offer reassurance, when appropriate, that hearing loss caused by serious otitis media is temporary.
- Provide clear, concise explanations.
- Face the patient when speaking and enunciate clearly and slowly.
- Allow time for the patient to grasp what was said.
- Provide a pencil and paper.
- Alert the staff to the patient's communication problem.

AFTER MYRINGOTOMY

- Wash hands before and after ear care.
- Maintain drainage flow.
- Place sterile cotton loosely in the external ear to absorb drainage and prevent infection. Change the cotton when damp. Avoid placing cotton or plugs deep in ear canal.
- Administer analgesics, as ordered.
- Administer antiemetics after tympanoplasty and reinforce dressings.

Monitoring

- Pain level
- Excessive bleeding or discharge
- Auditory acuity
- Response to treatment
- Complications

◉ **NURSING ALERT** Watch for and immediately report pain and fever due to acute secretory otitis media.

▶ PATIENT TEACHING

Be sure to cover:

- proper instillation of ointment, drops, and ear wash, as ordered
- medication administration, dosage, and possible adverse effects
- importance of taking antibiotics
- adequate fluid intake
- correct instillation of nasopharyngeal decongestants
- use of fitted earplugs for swimming after myringotomy and tympanostomy tube insertion
- notification of the physician if tube falls out and for ear pain, fever, or pus-filled discharge
- preventing recurrence. (See *Preventing otitis media.*)

☀ RESOURCES

Organizations

American Academy of Allergy, Asthma and Immunology: *www.aaaai.org*
American Academy of Audiology: *www.audiology.org*

Selected references

Carlson, L., and Scudder, L. "Controversies in the Management of Pediatric Otitis Media. Are More Definitive Answers On the Horizon?" *Advance for Nurse Practitioners* 12(2):73-77, February 2004.

Friedman, N.R., et al. "Development of a Practical Tool for Assessing the Severity of Acute Otitis Media," *Pediatric Infectious Disease Journal* 25(2):101-107, February 2006.

Leskinen, K., and Jero, J. "Acute Complications of Otitis Media in Adults," *Clinical Otolaryngology* 30(6):511-16, December 2005.

Montgomery, D. "A New Approach to Treating Acute Otitis Media," *Journal of Pediatric Health Care* 19(1):505-502, January-February 2005.

PREVENTING OTITIS MEDIA

For a patient recovering from otitis media at home, follow these guidelines to help prevent a recurrence:

- Teach the patient how to recognize upper respiratory tract infections, and encourage early treatment of them.
- Instruct parents not to feed an infant in a supine position and not to put him to bed with a bottle. Explain that doing so could cause reflux of nasopharyngeal flora.
- Teach the patient to promote eustachian tube patency by performing Valsalva's maneuver several times per day, especially during airplane travel.
- After tympanoplasty, advise the patient not to blow his nose or get his ear wet when bathing.
- Explain adverse reactions to the prescribed medication, emphasizing those that require immediate medical attention.

Otosclerosis

Description
- Bone disease that occurs only in the middle ear and results in an overgrowth of abnormal bone, usually involving the stapes bone
- Most common cause of conductive hearing loss
- With surgery, good prognosis
- Also known as *hardening of the ear* and *otospongiosis*

Pathophysiology
- Normal bone of otic capsule is gradually replaced with highly vascular spongy bone.
- Spongy bone immobilizes the footplate of the normally mobile stapes.
- Conduction of vibrations from the tympanic membrane to the cochlea is disrupted and conductive hearing loss results.
- If the inner ear is involved, sensorineural hearing loss may develop.

Causes
- Genetic factor transmitted as an autosomal dominant trait
- Pregnancy (may trigger the onset)

Risk factors
- Pregnancy
- Family history

Incidence
- Occurs in at least 10% of whites
- Twice as common in women as in men
- Usually occurs between ages 15 and 50

Common characteristics
- Slow, progressive hearing loss in one ear, with progression to both ears, without middle ear infection
- Tinnitus

Complications
- Bilateral conductive hearing loss
- Taste disturbance

ASSESSMENT

History
- Family history of hearing loss (excluding presbycusis)
- Tinnitus
- Ability to hear a conversation better in a noisy environment than in a quiet one (paracusis of Willis)
- Vertigo, especially after bending over

Physical findings
- Tympanic membrane that appears normal
- Schwartze's sign (faint pink blush throughout the tympanic membrane from vascularity of active otosclerotic bone)

Test results
DIAGNOSTIC PROCEDURES
- Rinne test results show bone-conducted tone that's heard longer than air-conducted tone.
- Weber's test results show that sound lateralizes to more damaged ear.
- Audiometric testing reveals hearing loss.

TREATMENT

General
- Hearing aids

Diet
- No restrictions

Activity
- Avoidance of activities that provoke dizziness

Medication
- Antibiotics
- Sodium fluoride (may prevent further worsening of hearing)

Surgery
- Stapedectomy
- Prosthesis insertion to restore partial or total hearing
- Fenestration
- Stapes mobilization

✤ NURSING CONSIDERATIONS

Nursing diagnoses
- Anxiety
- Deficient knowledge (otosclerosis)
- Disturbed sensory perception: Auditory
- Fear
- Impaired verbal communication
- Ineffective coping
- Risk for infection
- Risk for injury

Key outcomes
The patient will:
- identify measures to reduce anxiety.
- express understanding of illness and treatment
- regain hearing or develop alternative ways of communicating
- verbalize fears and concerns
- communicate needs and feelings
- demonstrate effective coping strategies
- remain free from signs and symptoms of infection
- remain free from injury.

Nursing interventions
- Encourage discussion of concerns about hearing loss.
- Offer reassurance with hearing loss, when appropriate.
- Give clear, concise explanations.
- Face the patient when speaking.
- Enunciate clearly and slowly, in a normal tone.
- Allow adequate time to grasp what was said.
- Provide a pencil and paper to aid communication.
- Alert the staff to communication problem.

AFTER SURGERY
- Position, as ordered.
- Assist with ambulation, when indicated.
- Administer prescribed pain medication.
- Reassure the patient that taste disturbance is common and usually subsides in a few weeks.

Monitoring
- For vertigo
- Response to medication
- Hearing loss

◈ **NURSING ALERT** Watch for and report postoperative facial drooping, which may indicate swelling of or around the facial nerve.

▶ PATIENT TEACHING

Be sure to cover:
- disorder, diagnostic tests, and treatment
- preoperative and postoperative teaching, if indicated
- slow movement to prevent vertigo
- medication administration, dosage, and possible adverse effects
- importance of protecting ears against cold
- need to avoid activities that provoke dizziness
- avoidance of anyone with upper respiratory tract infection
- changing external ear dressing and incision care
- completion of prescribed antibiotic regimen
- need for follow-up care
- how hearing may be masked by packing, dressing, and postoperative edema
- why hearing may not be noticeably improved for 1 to 4 weeks after surgery
- avoidance of loud noises and sudden pressure changes until healing is complete
- avoidance of blowing nose for at least 1 week to prevent contaminated air and bacteria from entering the eustachian tube
- avoidance of sudden movements
- avoidance of wetting head in shower or swimming for about 6 weeks
- avoidance of getting water in the ear for an additional 4 weeks
- prevention of constipation and avoidance of straining while defecating.

✱ RESOURCES

Organizations
Alexander Graham Bell Association for the Deaf and Hard of Hearing: *www.agbell.org/index.html*
Hearing Loss Association of America: *www.shhh.org*

Selected references
Karosi, T., et al. "Two Subgroups of Stapes Fixation: Otosclerosis and Pseudo-Otosclerosis," *Laryngoscope* 115(11):1968-973, November 2005.

Knox, G.W., and Reitan, H. "Shape-memory Stapes Prosthesis for Otosclerosis Surgery," *Laryngoscope* 115(8):1340-346, August 2005.

Menger, D.J., et al. "The Genetics of Otosclerosis," *Clinical Otolaryngology & Allied Sciences* 29(4):435, August 2004.

Rama-Lopez, J., et al. "Cochlear Implantation of Patients with Far-Advanced Otosclerosis," *Otology & Neurology* 27(2):153-58, February 2006.

Ovarian cancer

● OVERVIEW

Description
- Malignancy arising from the ovary; a rapidly progressing cancer that's difficult to diagnose
- Prognosis varying with histologic type and stage
- 90% primary epithelial tumors
- Other tumor types: stromal and germ cell tumors

Pathophysiology
- Ovarian cancer spreads rapidly intraperitoneally by local extension or surface seeding and, occasionally, through the lymphatics and the bloodstream.
- Metastasis to the ovary can occur from breast, colon, gastric, and pancreatic cancers.

Causes
- Exact cause unknown

Risk factors
- Infertility problems or nulliparity
- Celibacy
- Exposure to asbestos and talc
- History of breast or uterine cancer
- Family history of ovarian cancer
- Diets high in saturated fat

Incidence
- After lung, breast, and colon cancer, primary ovarian cancer most common cause of cancer death among American women (about 40% surviving for 5 years)
- More common after age 50
- Women in industrialized nations at greater risk
- Metastatic ovarian cancer more common than cancer at any other site in women with previously treated breast cancer

Common characteristics
- Initially no signs
- Weight loss
- Abdominal pain

Complications
- Fluid and electrolyte imbalance
- Leg edema
- Ascites
- Intestinal obstruction
- Profound cachexia
- Recurrent malignant effusions

✳ ASSESSMENT

History
- Lack of obvious signs, or signs and symptoms that vary with tumor size and extent of metastasis (disease usually metastasized before diagnosis is made)
- In later stages: urinary frequency, constipation, pelvic discomfort, distention, weight loss, and pain

Physical findings
- Gaunt appearance
- Grossly distended abdomen accompanied by ascites
- Palpable abdominal mass with rocky hardness or rubbery or cystlike quality

Test results
LABORATORY
- Laboratory tumor marker studies (such as ovarian carcinoma antigen, carcinoembryonic antigen, and human chorionic gonadotropin) show abnormalities that may indicate complications.

IMAGING
- Abdominal ultrasonography, computed tomography scan, or X-rays delineate tumor size.

DIAGNOSTIC PROCEDURES
- Aspiration of ascitic fluid can reveal atypical cells.
- Exploratory laparotomy, including lymph node evaluation and tumor resection is required for accurate diagnosis and staging.

◆ TREATMENT

General
- Radiation therapy (not commonly used because it causes myelosuppression, which limits effectiveness of chemotherapy)
- Radioisotopes as adjuvant therapy

Diet
- High-protein
- Small, frequent meals

Activity
- No restrictions

Medication
- Chemotherapy after surgery
- Immunotherapy (under investigation)
- Hormone replacement therapy in prepubertal girl who had bilateral salpingo-oophorectomy

Surgery
- Total abdominal hysterectomy and bilateral salpingo-oophorectomy with tumor resection
- Omentectomy, appendectomy, lymph node palpation with probable lymphadenectomy, tissue biopsies, and peritoneal washings
- Resection of involved ovary
- Biopsies of omentum and uninvolved ovary
- Peritoneal washings for cytologic examination of pelvic fluid

❖ NURSING CONSIDERATIONS

Nursing diagnoses
- Acute pain
- Anticipatory grieving
- Anxiety
- Excess fluid volume
- Fear
- Hopelessness
- Imbalanced nutrition: Less than body requirements
- Impaired skin integrity
- Ineffective coping
- Risk for infection
- Sexual dysfunction

Key outcomes
The patient will:
- express feelings of increased comfort and decreased pain
- express feelings about the potential loss
- express feelings of decreased anxiety
- maintain appropriate fluid balance
- verbalize fears and concerns related to the diagnosis and treatment
- begin to make decisions on own behalf
- maintain weight within an acceptable range
- maintain skin integrity
- demonstrate positive coping behaviors
- remain free from signs of infection
- verbalize concerns about actual or potential impairment in sexual function.

Nursing interventions
- Encourage verbalization and provide support.
- Administer medications, as ordered.
- Provide abdominal support and be alert for abdominal distention.
- Encourage coughing and deep breathing.

Monitoring
- Vital signs
- Intake and output
- Wound site
- Pain control
- Effects of medication
- Hydration and nutrition status

▶ PATIENT TEACHING

Be sure to cover:
- disorder, diagnostic tests, and treatment
- dietary needs
- relaxation techniques
- importance of preventing infection, emphasizing good hand-washing technique
- medication administration, dosage, and possible adverse effects.

Discharge planning
- Refer the patient to resource and support services.

✷ RESOURCES

Organizations
American Cancer Society: *www.cancer.org*
Guide to Internet Resources for Cancer: *www.cancerindex.org*
National Cancer Institute: *www.nci.nih.gov*

Selected references
Atlas of Pathophysiology, 2nd ed. Philadelphia: Lippincott Williams & Wilkins, 2005.

Brooks, S.E., et al. "Ovarian Cancer: A Clinician's Perspective," *Pathology Case Reviews* 11(1):3-8, January-February 2006.

Ferrell, B., et al. "Perspectives on the Impact of Ovarian Cancer: Women's Views of Quality of Life," *Oncology Nursing Forum* 32(6):1143-149, November 2005.

Lecuru, F., et al. "Impact of Initial Surgical Access on Staging and Survival of Patients with Stage I Ovarian Cancer," *International Journal of Gynecological Cancer* 16(1):87-94, January-February 2006.

Schildkraut, J.M., et al, "Analgesic Drug Use and Risk of Ovarian Cancer," *Epidemiology* 18(1):104-107, January 2006.

Paget's disease

Description
- Bone disorder that causes an irregular bone formation
- Affects one or several skeletal areas (spine, pelvis, femur, and skull)
- Slow and progressive
- Causes malignant bone changes in about 5% of patients
- Can be fatal, particularly when associated with heart failure, bone sarcoma, or giant cell tumors
- Also known as *osteitis deformans*

Pathophysiology
- In the initial phase (osteoclastic phase) excessive bone resorption occurs.
- The second phase (osteoblastic phase) involves excessive abnormal bone formation.
- The affected bones enlarge and soften.
- New bone structure is chaotic, fragile, and weak.

Causes
- Exact cause unknown
- Theory: slow or dormant viral infection (possibly mumps)

Incidence
- More common after age 40
- More common in men

Common characteristics
- Severe, persistent pain that worsens with weight-bearing activities
- Cranial enlargement
- Barrel-shaped chest
- Kyphosis
- Asymmetric bowing of the tibia and femur
- Pathologic fractures
- Muscle weakness

Complications
- Fractures
- Paraplegia
- Blindness and hearing loss with tinnitus and vertigo
- Osteoarthritis
- Sarcoma
- Hypertension
- Renal calculi
- Hypercalcemia
- Gout
- Heart failure

History
- Severe, persistent pain
- Impaired mobility
- Pain that worsens with weight bearing
- Increased hat size
- Headaches

Physical findings
- Cranial enlargement over frontal and occipital areas
- Kyphosis
- Barrel-shaped chest
- Asymmetrical bowing of the tibia and femur
- Warmth and tenderness over affected sites

Test results
LABORATORY
- Red blood cell count shows anemia.
- Serum alkaline phosphatase levels are elevated.
- 24-hour urine hydroxyproline levels are elevated.
IMAGING
- X-ray studies show bone expansion and increased bone density.
- Bone scans clearly show early pagetic lesions.
DIAGNOSTIC PROCEDURES
- Bone biopsy shows a characteristic mosaic pattern of bone tissue.

General
- Heat therapy
- Massage
- Weight management

Diet
- Adequate intake of calcium and vitamin D

Activity
- As tolerated
- Pacing of activities
- Use of assistive devices
- Regular exercise

Medication
- Calcitonin
- Nonsteroidal anti-inflammatory drugs
- Biphosphonates
- Calcium supplements
- Vitamin D

Surgery
- Reduction of pathologic fractures
- Correction of secondary deformities
- Relief of neurologic impairment

✥ NURSING CONSIDERATIONS

Nursing diagnoses
- Chronic pain
- Deficient knowledge (Paget's disease)
- Dressing or grooming self-care deficit
- Impaired physical mobility
- Risk for impaired skin integrity
- Risk for injury

Key outcomes
The patient will:
- express feelings of increased comfort and decreased pain
- verbalize understanding of condition and treatment
- perform activities of daily living to the extent possible
- maintain joint mobility and range of motion
- maintain adequate skin integrity
- remain free from injury.

Nursing interventions
- Take measures to prevent pressure ulcers.
- Instruct the patient with footdrop to wear high-topped sneakers or use a footboard.

Monitoring
- Pain level, response to analgesic therapy
- New areas of pain
- New movement restrictions
- Sensory and motor disturbances
- Serum calcium and alkaline phosphatase levels
- Intake and output

▶ PATIENT TEACHING

Be sure to cover:
- disorder, diagnostic tests, and treatment
- pacing of activities
- use of assistive devices
- exercise program
- use of a firm mattress or a bed board
- home safety measures
- medication administration, dosage, and possible adverse effects.

Discharge planning
- Refer the patient to community resource and support sources, as appropriate.

✹ RESOURCES

Organizations
Arthritis Foundation: *www.arthritis.org*
National Institutes of Health: *www.nih.gov*
Paget Foundation for Paget's Disease of Bone and Related Disorders: *www.paget.org*

Selected references
Handbook of Pathophysiology, 2nd ed. Philadelphia: Lippincott Williams & Wilkins, 2005.
Hosking, D. "Pharmacological Therapy of Paget's and Other Metabolic Bone Disease," *Bone* 38(2 Suppl 2):3-7, February 2006.
Lee, G.C., et al. "Total Knee Arthroplasty in Patients with Paget's Disease of Bone at the Knee," *Journal of Arthroplasty* 20(6):689-93, September 2005.
Professional Guide to Diseases, 8th ed. Philadelphia: Lippincott Williams & Wilkins, 2005.
Rendina, D., et al, "Paget's Disease and Bisphosphonates," *New England Journal of Medicine* 353(24):2616-618, December 2005.

Pancreatic cancer

● OVERVIEW

Description
- Proliferation of cancer cells in the pancreas
- Fifth most lethal type of carcinoma
- Poor prognosis (most patients dying within 1 year of diagnosis)

Pathophysiology
- Pancreatic cancer is almost always adenocarcinoma.
- Nearly two-thirds of tumors appear in the head of the pancreas; islet cell tumors are rare.
- Two main tissue types form fibrotic nodes. Cylinder cells arise in ducts and degenerate into cysts; large, fatty, granular cells arise in parenchyma.
- A high-fat or excessive protein diet induces chronic hyperplasia of the pancreas, with increased cell turnover.

Causes
- Possible link to inhalation or absorption of carcinogens, which the pancreas then excretes (such as cigarette smoke, excessive fat and protein, food additives, and industrial chemicals)

Risk factors
- Chronic pancreatitis
- Diabetes
- Chronic alcohol abuse
- Smoking
- Occupational exposure to chemicals
- High-fat diet

Incidence
- Three to four times more common in smokers than nonsmokers
- Highest in black men between ages 35 and 70
- Highest in Israel, United States, Sweden, and Canada; lowest in Switzerland, Belgium, and Italy

Common characteristics
- Intermittent epigastric pain
- Weight loss
- Anorexia, nausea, and vomiting

Complications
- Nutrient malabsorption
- Type 1 diabetes
- Liver and GI problems
- Mental status changes
- Depression
- Hemorrhage
- Pulmonary congestion

✳ ASSESSMENT

History
- Colicky, dull, or vague intermittent epigastric pain, which may radiate to the right upper quadrant or dorsolumbar area; unrelated to posture or activity and aggravated by meals
- Anorexia, nausea, and vomiting
- Rapid, profound weight loss

Physical findings
- Jaundice
- Large, palpable, well-defined mass in the subumbilical or left hypochondrial region
- Abdominal bruit or pulsation

Test results
LABORATORY
- Pancreatic enzymes are absent.
- Serum bilirubin levels are elevated.
- Serum lipase and amylase levels may be increased.
- Thrombin time is prolonged.
- Aspartate aminotransferase and alanine aminotransferase levels are elevated (if liver cell necrosis present).
- Alkaline phosphatase levels are markedly elevated (in biliary obstruction).
- Serum insulin is measurable (if islet cell tumor present).
- Hypoglycemia or hyperglycemia is present.
- Specific tumor markers for pancreatic cancer are elevated, including carcinoembryonic antigen, pancreatic oncofetal antigen, alpha-fetoprotein, and serum immunoreactive elastase.

IMAGING
- Barium swallow, retroperitoneal insufflation, cholangiography, and scintigraphy can locate the neoplasm and detect changes in the duodenum or stomach.
- Ultrasonography and computed tomography scans can identify a mass.
- Magnetic resonance imaging scan discloses tumor location and size.
- Angiography reveals tumor vascularity.
- Endoscopic retrograde cholangiopancreatography allows tumor visualization and specimen biopsy.

DIAGNOSTIC PROCEDURES
- Percutaneous fine-needle aspiration biopsy may detect tumor cells.
- Laparotomy with biopsy allows definitive diagnosis.

◆ TREATMENT

General
- Palliative
- Radiation therapy as adjunct to fluorouracil chemotherapy

Diet
- Well-balanced; as tolerated
- Small, frequent meals

Activity
- Postoperative avoidance of lifting and contact sports
- After recovery, no restriction

Medication
- Chemotherapy
- Antibiotics
- Anticholinergics
- Antacids
- Diuretics
- Insulin
- Analgesics
- Pancreatic enzymes

Surgery
- Total pancreatectomy
- Cholecystojejunostomy, choledochoduodenostomy, and choledochojejunostomy
- Gastrojejunostomy
- Whipple's operation or radical pancreatoduodenectomy

Nursing diagnoses
- Acute pain
- Anxiety
- Constipation
- Deficient fluid volume
- Imbalanced nutrition: Less than body requirements
- Impaired skin integrity
- Ineffective coping
- Risk for injury

Key outcomes
The patient will:
- express increased comfort and decreased pain
- express feelings of reduced anxiety
- regain normal bowel movements
- maintain normal fluid volume status
- maintain an adequate weight
- maintain skin integrity
- demonstrate positive coping behaviors
- remain free from injury.

Nursing interventions
- Administer medications and blood transfusions, as ordered.
- Provide small, frequent meals.
- Ensure adequate rest and sleep.
- Assist with range-of-motion and isometric exercises, as appropriate.
- Perform scrupulous skin care.
- Apply antiembolism stockings.
- Encourage verbalization and provide emotional support.

Monitoring
- Fluid balance and nutrition
- Abdominal girth, metabolic state, and daily weight
- Blood glucose levels
- Complete blood count
- Pain control
- Signs and symptoms of hemorrhage

Be sure to cover:
- disorder, diagnostic tests, and treatment
- end-of-life issues
- medication administration, dosage, and possible adverse effects
- expected postoperative care
- information about diabetes, including signs and symptoms of hypoglycemia and hyperglycemia
- adverse effects of radiation therapy and chemotherapy.

Discharge planning
Refer the patient to:
- community resource and support services
- hospice care, if indicated
- the American Cancer Society.

Organizations
American Cancer Society: *www.cancer.org*
American Diabetes Association: *www.diabetes.org*
Guide to Internet Resources for Cancer: *www.cancerindex.org*
National Cancer Institute: *www.nci.org*
National Institute of Diabetes & Digestive & Kidney Diseases: *www.niddk.nih.gov*

Selected references
Handbook of Pathophysiology, 2nd ed. Philadelphia: Lippincott Williams & Wilkins, 2005.
Leonard, G.D., et al. "Metastases to the Breast from Primary Pancreatic Cancer," *Breast Journal* 11(6):503, November-December 2005.
Lerch, M.M. "Anticipating Disaster: The Genetics of Familial Pancreatic Cancer," *Gut* 55(2):150-51, February 2006.
Wasan, S.M., and Ross, W.A. "Use of Expandable Metallic Biliary Stents in Resectable Pancreatic Cancer," *Journal of Vascular & Interventional Radiology* 17(1):192, January 2006.

Pancreatitis

OVERVIEW

Description
- Inflammation of the pancreas
- Occurs in acute and chronic forms
- With acute form, 10% mortality
- With chronic form, irreversible tissue damage, which tends to progress to significant pancreatic function loss
- May be idiopathic but sometimes associated with biliary tract disease, alcoholism, trauma, and certain drugs

Pathophysiology
- Enzymes normally excreted into the duodenum by the pancreas are activated in the pancreas or its ducts and start to autodigest pancreatic tissue.
- Consequent inflammation causes intense pain, third spacing of large fluid volumes, pancreatic fat necrosis with consumption of serum calcium and, occasionally, hemorrhage.

Causes
- Biliary tract disease
- Alcoholism
- Abnormal organ structure
- Metabolic or endocrine disorders
- Pancreatic cysts or tumors
- Penetrating peptic ulcers
- Penetrating trauma
- Viral or bacterial infection

Risk factors
- Use of glucocorticoids, sulfonamides, thiazides, and oral contraceptives
- Renal failure and kidney transplantation
- Endoscopic retrograde cholangiopancreatography (ERCP)
- Heredity
- Emotional or neurogenic factors

Incidence
- Acute form: 2 of every 10,000 people
- Chronic form: 2 of every 25,000 people
- Affects more men than women
- Four times more common in Blacks than in Whites.

Common characteristics
- Intense epigastric pain
- History of predisposing factors

Complications
- Diabetes mellitus
- Massive hemorrhage
- Diabetic acidosis
- Shock and coma
- Acute respiratory distress syndrome
- Atelectasis and pleural effusion
- Pneumonia
- Paralytic ileus
- GI bleeding
- Pancreatic abscess and cancer
- Pseudocysts

ASSESSMENT

History
- Intense epigastric pain centered close to the umbilicus and radiating to the back, between the tenth thoracic and sixth lumbar vertebrae
- Pain aggravated by fatty foods, alcohol consumption, or recumbent position
- Weight loss with nausea and vomiting
- Predisposing factor

Physical findings
- Hypotension
- Tachycardia
- Fever
- Dyspnea, orthopnea
- Generalized jaundice
- Cullen's sign (bluish periumbilical discoloration)
- Turner's sign (bluish flank discoloration)
- Steatorrhea (with chronic pancreatitis)
- Abdominal tenderness, rigidity, and guarding

Test results
LABORATORY
PANCREATITIS
- Serum amylase and lipase levels are elevated.
- White blood cell count is elevated.
- Serum bilirubin levels are elevated.
- Hyperglycemia and glycosuria are transient.
CHRONIC PANCREATITIS
- Serum alkaline phosphatase, amylase, and bilirubin levels are elevated.
- Serum glucose levels are transiently elevated.
- Lipid and trypsin levels are elevated (in stool).

IMAGING
- Abdominal and chest X-rays differentiate pancreatitis from other diseases that cause similar symptoms; they also detect pleural effusions.
- Computed tomography scans and ultrasonography show increased pancreatic diameter, pancreatic cysts, and pseudocysts.
DIAGNOSTIC PROCEDURES
- ERCP shows pancreatic anatomy, identifies ductal system abnormalities, and differentiates pancreatitis from other disorders.

TREATMENT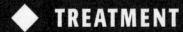

General
- Emergency treatment of shock, as needed; vigorous I.V. replacement of fluid, electrolytes, and proteins
- Blood transfusions (for hemorrhage)
- Nasogastric suctioning

Diet
- Nothing by mouth
- Once crisis starts to resolve, oral low-fat, low-protein feedings implemented gradually
- Alcohol and caffeine abstention

Activity
- As tolerated

Medication
- Analgesics
- Antacids
- Histamine antagonists
- Antibiotics
- Anticholinergics
- Total parenteral nutrition
- Pancreatic enzymes
- Insulin
- Albumin

Surgery
- Not indicated in acute pancreatitis unless complications occur
- Sphincterotomy, for chronic pancreatitis
- Pancreaticojejunostomy

❖ NURSING CONSIDERATIONS

Nursing diagnoses
- Acute pain
- Deficient fluid volume
- Disturbed body image
- Hopelessness
- Imbalanced nutrition: Less than body requirements
- Ineffective breathing pattern
- Risk for impaired skin integrity
- Risk for injury

Key outcomes
The patient will:
- verbalize feelings of increased comfort and decreased pain
- maintain normal fluid volume
- express positive feelings about self
- participate in decisions about care
- achieve adequate caloric and nutritional intake
- maintain an effective breathing pattern
- maintain skin integrity
- remain free from injury.

Nursing interventions
- Administer medications and I.V. therapy, as ordered.
- Encourage the patient to express feelings.
- Provide emotional support.

Monitoring
- Vital signs
- Nasogastric tube function and drainage
- Respiratory status
- Acid-base balance
- Serum glucose level
- Fluid and electrolyte balance
- Daily weight
- Pain level
- Nutritional status and metabolic requirements

▶ PATIENT TEACHING

Be sure to cover:
- disorder, diagnostic tests, and treatment
- identification and avoidance of acute pancreatitis triggers
- dietary needs
- medication administration, dosage, and possible adverse effects.

Discharge planning
- Refer the patient to community resource and support services, as needed.

✷ RESOURCES

Organizations
Alcoholics Anonymous: *www.aa.org*
Digestive Disease National Coalition: *www.ddnc.org*
National Digestive Diseases Information Clearinghouse: *www.niddk.nih.gov/health/digest/nddic.htm*

Selected references
Handbook of Diseases, 3rd ed. Philadelphia: Lippincott Williams & Wilkins, 2004.

Hughes, E. "Understanding the Care of Patients with Acute Pancreatitis," *Nursing Standard* 18(18):45-52, January 2004.

Shrikhande, S.V., et al. "Management of Pain in Small Duct Chronic Pancreatitis," *Journal of Gastrointestinal Surgery* 10(2):227-33, February 2006.

Swaroop, V.S., et al. "Severe Acute Pancreatitis," *JAMA* 291(23):2865-868, June 2004.

Tierney, I., et al. *Current Medical Diagnosis & Treatment 2006.* New York: McGraw-Hill Book Co., 2006.

Parkinson's disease

● OVERVIEW

Description
- Brain disorder that causes progressive deterioration, with muscle rigidity, akinesia, and involuntary tremors
- Aspiration pneumonia usual cause of death
- One of the most common crippling diseases in the United States

Pathophysiology
- Dopaminergic neurons degenerate, causing loss of available dopamine.
- Dopamine deficiency prevents affected brain cells from performing their normal inhibitory function.
- Excess excitatory acetylcholine occurs at synapses.
- Nondopaminergic receptors are also involved.
- Motor neurons are depressed. (See *Understanding Parkinson's disease.*)

Causes
- Exact cause unknown
- Exposure to such toxins as manganese dust and carbon monoxide

Incidence
- Affects more men than women
- Occurs in middle age or later

Common characteristics
- Muscle rigidity
- Tremor
- Resistance to passive muscle stretching
- Akinesia
- High-pitched, monotonous voice
- Drooling
- Loss of posture control
- Dysarthria
- Excessive sweating
- Decreased GI motility
- Orthostatic hypotension
- Oily skin
- Eyes fixed upward

Complications
- Injury from falls
- Food aspiration
- Urinary tract infections
- Skin breakdown
- Pneumonia
- Depression
- Sexual dysfunction
- Sleep problems

✳ ASSESSMENT

History
- Muscle rigidity
- Akinesia
- Dysphagia
- Fatigue with activities of daily living (ADLs)
- Muscle cramps of legs, neck, and trunk
- Oily skin
- Increased perspiration
- Insomnia
- Mood changes
- Dysarthria

Physical findings
- Insidious (unilateral pill-roll) tremor, which increases during stress or anxiety and decreases with purposeful movement and sleep
- High-pitched, monotonous voice
- Drooling
- Masklike facial expression
- Difficulty walking
- Lack of parallel motion in gait
- Loss of posture control with walking
- Oculogyric crises (eyes fixed upward, with involuntary tonic movements)
- Muscle rigidity causing resistance to passive muscle stretching
- Difficulty pivoting
- Loss of balance

Test results
IMAGING
- Computed tomography scan or magnetic resonance imaging can rule out other disorders such as intracranial tumors.

◆ TREATMENT

General
- Environmental safety measures
- Assistance with ADLs

Diet
- Small, frequent meals
- High-bulk foods

Activity
- Physical therapy
- Assistive devices to aid ambulation
- Occupational therapy

Medication
- Dopamine replacement drugs
- Anticholinergics
- Antihistamines
- Antiviral agents
- Enzyme-inhibiting agents
- Tricyclic antidepressants
- Dopamine agonists

Surgery
- Used when drug therapy fails
- Stereotaxic neurosurgery
- Destruction of ventrolateral nucleus of thalamus
- Deep brain stimulation

UNDERSTANDING PARKINSON'S DISEASE

New research on the pathogenesis of Parkinson's disease focuses on damage to the substantia nigra from oxidative stress. Oxidative stress is believed to:
- alter the brain's iron content
- impair mitochondrial function
- alter antioxidant and protective systems
- reduce glutathione
- damage lipids, proteins, and deoxyribonucleic acid.

❖ NURSING CONSIDERATIONS

Nursing diagnoses
- Bathing or hygiene self-care deficit
- Chronic low self-esteem
- Constipation
- Disturbed body image
- Dressing or grooming self-care deficit
- Feeding self-care deficit
- Imbalanced nutrition: Less than body requirements
- Impaired physical mobility
- Impaired social interaction
- Impaired verbal communication
- Ineffective coping
- Interrupted family processes
- Risk for injury

Key outcomes
The patient (or family) will:
- perform bathing and hygiene activities to the fullest extent possible
- verbalize feelings regarding self-esteem
- resume a normal bowel elimination pattern
- express positive feelings about self
- perform dressing and grooming activities to the fullest extent possible
- perform self-care needs related to feeding to the fullest extent possible
- consume adequate daily calories, as requierd
- maintain maximal mobility within the confines of the disorder
- maintain family and peer relationships
- develop alternative means of communication
- demonstrate effective coping skills
- discuss the impact of the patient's condition on the family unit
- remain free from injury.

Nursing interventions
- Take measures to prevent aspiration.
- Protect the patient from injury.
- Stress the importance of rest periods between activities.
- Ensure adequate nutrition.
- Provide frequent warm baths and massage.
- Encourage the patient to enroll in a physical therapy program.
- Provide emotional and psychological support.
- Encourage the patient to be independent.

Monitoring
- Vital signs
- Intake and output
- Drug therapy
- Adverse reactions to medications
- Postoperatively: signs of hemorrhage and increased intracranial pressure
- Swallowing
- Self-care abilities

▶ PATIENT TEACHING

Be sure to cover:
- disorder, diagnostic tests, and treatment
- medication administration, dosage, and possible adverse effects
- measures to prevent pressure ulcers and contractures
- household safety measures
- importance of daily bathing
- methods to improve communication
- swallowing therapy regimen (aspiration precautions).

Discharge planning
- Refer the patient for occupational and physical rehabilitation, as indicated.

✸ RESOURCES

Organizations
American Parkinson Disease Association: *www.apdaparkinson.com*
National Institutes of Health: *www.nih.gov*
National Parkinson Foundation: *www.parkinson.org*
Parkinson Disease Foundation: *www.pdf.com*

Selected references
Aarsland, D., et al. "Neuroleptic Sensitvity in Parkinson's Disease and Parkinsonian Dementias," *Journal of Clinical Psychiatry* 66(5):633-37, May 2005.

Diseases, 4th ed. Philadelphia: Lippincott Williams & Wilkins, 2006.

Eriksen, J.L., et al. "Molecular Pathogenesis of Parkinson Disease," *Archives of Neurology* 62(3):353-57, March 2005.

Grosser, K.A., et al. "Measuring Therapy Adherence in Parkinson's Disease: A Comparison of Methods," *Journal of Neurology, Neurosurgery & Psychiatry* 77(2):249-51, February 2006.

Habermann, B., and Davis, I. "Caring for Family with Alzheimer's Disease and Parkinson's Disease: Needs, Challenges, and Satisfaction," *Journal of Gerontological Nursing* 31(6):49-54, June 2005.

Handbook of Pathophysiology, 2nd ed. Philadelphia: Lippincott Williams & Wilkins, 2005.

Pelvic inflammatory disease

● OVERVIEW

Description
- Umbrella term that refers to any acute, subacute, recurrent, or chronic infection of the oviducts and ovaries, with adjacent tissue involvement
- Includes inflammation of the cervix (cervicitis), uterus (endometritis), fallopian tubes (salpingitis), and ovaries (oophoritis)
- Possible extension of the inflammation to connective tissue lying between the broad ligaments (parametritis)
- Commonly called *PID*

Pathophysiology
- Various conditions, procedures, or instrumentation can alter or destroy the cervical mucus, which normally serves as a protective barrier.
- As a result, bacteria enter the uterine cavity, causing inflammation of various structures.

Causes
- Aerobic or anaerobic organisms (commonly, overgrowth of one or more of the bacterial species found in the cervical mucus)
- Sexually transmitted infections (*Neisseria gonorrhea* and *Chlamydia trachomatis*)
- Septicemia
- Infected drainage from a chronically infected fallopian tube
- Ruptured appendix
- Diverticulitis of the sigmoid colon
- Pelvic abscess
- Use of intrauterine device

Risk factors
- Multiple sex partners
- Conditions or procedures that alter or destroy cervical mucus
- Sexual intercourse at an early age
- Procedures that risk transfer of contaminated cervical mucus into the endometrial cavity by an instrument
- Infection during or after pregnancy
- Cigarette smoking
- Multiparity
- Douching
- Intercourse during menses
- Therapeutic abortion

Incidence
- Primarily affects women ages 16 to 40
- **AGE-RELATED CONCERN** Adolescents are at high risk for sexually transmitted diseases, including PID.

Common characteristics
- Profuse, purulent vaginal discharge
- Lower abdominal pain
- Vaginal bleeding

Complications
- Septicemia (potentially fatal)
- Pulmonary embolism
- Infertility
- Peritonitis
- Shock
- Death
- Ectopic pregnancy

✳ ASSESSMENT

History
- Profuse, purulent vaginal discharge
- Low-grade fever
- Malaise
- Lower abdominal pain
- Vaginal bleeding

Physical findings
- Pain with cervical movement or adnexal palpation
- Vaginal discharge
- Unilaterally or bilaterally tender adnexal mass

Test results
LABORATORY
- Culture and sensitivity and Gram stain of endocervix or cul-de-sac secretions shows the causative agent.
- Urethral and rectal secretions show the causative agent.
- C-reactive protein levels are elevated.
IMAGING
- Transvaginal ultrasonography may show the presence of thickened, fluid-filled fallopian tubes.
- Computed tomography scan may show complex tubo-ovarian abscesses and is useful in diagnosing PID.
- Magnetic resonance imaging provides images of soft tissue; useful not only for establishing the diagnosis of PID, but also for detecting other processes responsible for symptoms.

DIAGNOSTIC PROCEDURES
- Culdocentesis obtains peritoneal fluid or pus for culture and sensitivity testing.
- Diagnostic laparoscopy identifies cul-de-sac fluid, tubal distention, and masses in pelvic abscess.

◆ TREATMENT

General
- Frequent perineal care if vaginal discharge occurs

Diet
- No restrictions

Activity
- Bed rest

Medication
- Antibiotics
- Analgesics
- I.V. fluids, as needed

Surgery
- Drainage of pelvic abscess

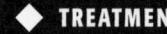 **NURSING ALERT** A ruptured pelvic abscess is a life-threatening condition. The patient may need a total abdominal hysterectomy with bilateral salpingo-oophorectomy.

Nursing diagnoses
- Acute pain
- Anxiety
- Deficient fluid volume
- Deficient knowledge (PID)
- Ineffective coping
- Ineffective sexuality patterns
- Risk for infection

Key outcomes
The patient will:
- express feelings of increased comfort and decreased pain
- identify strategies to reduce anxiety
- maintain fluid balance
- demonstrate understanding of condition and treatment
- demonstrate positive coping strategies
- express feelings about potential or actual changes in sexual activity
- remain free from signs or symptoms of infection.

Nursing interventions
- Administer antibiotics and analgesics as ordered.
- Provide frequent perineal care.
- Use meticulous hand-washing technique.
- Encourage the patient to discuss her feelings, and offer emotional support.
- Help the patient develop effective coping strategies.
- Inspect vaginal discharge.

Monitoring
- Vital signs
- Fluid intake and output
- Signs and symptoms of dehydration

◈ **NURSING ALERT** Watch for and report abdominal rigidity and distention. These signs may indicate developing peritonitis.

Be sure to cover:
- disorder, diagnostic tests, and treatment
- ways to prevent a recurrence
- importance of avoiding multiple sexual partners
- need for the patient's sexual partner to be examined and, if necessary, treated for infection
- condom use
- causes of PID, such as dyspareunia and sexual activity
- signs and symptoms of infection after a minor gynecologic procedure

◈ **NURSING ALERT** Tell the patient to immediately report fever, increased vaginal discharge, or pain—especially after a minor gynecologic procedure.
- avoidance of douching or intercourse for at least 7 days after a minor gynecologic procedure.

Discharge planning
Refer the patient to:
- infertility counseling, if indicated.
- a smoking-cessation program, if indicated.

Organizations
American College of Obstetricians and Gynecologists: *www.acog.org*
American Society for Reproductive Medicine: *www.asrm.org*
American Fertility Association: *www.theafa.org*

Selected references
Banikarim, C., and Chacko, M.R. "Pelvic Inflammatory Disease in Adolescents," *Seminars in Pediatric Infectious Diseases* 16(3):175-80, July 2005.
Dahlberg, D.L., et al. "Differential Diagnosis of Abdominal Pain in Women of Childbearing Age. Appendicitis or Pelvic Inflammatory Disease?" *Advance for Nurse Practitioners* 12(1):40-45, January 2004.
Mahoon, B.E., et al. "Pelvic Inflammatory Disease During the Post-partum Year," *Infectious Diseases in Obstetrics and Gynecology* 13(4):191-96, December 2005.
Ness, R.B., et al. "Effectiveness of Treatment Strategies of Some Women with Pelvic Inflammatory Disease: A Randomized Trial," *Obstetrics and Gynecology* 106(3):573-80, September 2005.

Peptic ulcer disease

● OVERVIEW

Description
- Development of circumscribed lesions in the mucosal membrane of the lower esophagus, stomach, duodenum, or jejunum
- Occurs in two major forms: gastric ulcer and duodenal ulcer (both forms are chronic)
- Duodenal ulcers representing about 80% of peptic ulcers; affect the proximal part of the small intestine and follow a chronic course characterized by remissions and exacerbations (about 5% to 10% of patients with duodenal ulcers developing complications that necessitate surgery)

Pathophysiology
- *Helicobacter pylori* releases a toxin that promotes mucosal inflammation and ulceration.
- In a peptic ulcer resulting from *H. pylori*, acid isn't the dominant cause of bacterial infection but contributes to the consequences.
- Ulceration stems from inhibition of prostaglandin synthesis, increased gastric acid and pepsin secretion, reduced gastric mucosal blood flow, or decreased cytoprotective mucus production.

Causes
- *H. pylori*
- Use of nonsteroidal anti-inflammatory drugs (NSAIDs) or glucocorticoids
- Pathologic hypersecretory states

Risk factors
- Type A blood (for gastric ulcer)
- Type O blood (for duodenal ulcer)
- Other genetic factors
- Exposure to irritants
- Cigarette smoking
- Trauma
- Psychogenic factors
- Normal aging

Incidence
- Gastric ulcers: most common in middle-aged and elderly men, especially those who are poor and undernourished; prevalence higher in chronic users of aspirin or alcohol
- Duodenal ulcers: most common in men ages 20 to 50

Common characteristics
- Left epigastric or abdominal pain, with exacerbations and remissions
- History of predisposing factor

Complications
- GI hemorrhage
- Abdominal or intestinal infarction
- Ulcer penetration into attached structures

✱ ASSESSMENT

History
- Periods of symptom exacerbation and remission, with remissions lasting longer than exacerbations
- History of predisposing factor
- Left epigastric pain described as heartburn or indigestion, accompanied by feeling of fullness or distention

GASTRIC ULCER
- Recent weight or appetite loss
- Nausea
- Pain triggered or worsened by eating

DUODENAL ULCER
- Pain relieved by eating; may occur 1½ to 3 hours after food intake
- Pain that awakens the patient from sleep
- Weight gain

Physical findings
- Pallor
- Epigastric tenderness
- Hyperactive bowel sounds
- Vomiting

Test results
LABORATORY
- Complete blood count shows anemia.
- Occult blood is present in stools.
- Venous blood sample shows *H. pylori* antibodies.
- White blood cell count is elevated.
- In urea breath test, exhaled carbon 13 (^{13}C) levels are low.
- Serum gastrin level is fasting (rules out Zollinger-Ellison syndrome).

IMAGING
- Barium swallow or upper GI and small-bowel series may reveal the ulcer.
- Upper GI tract X-rays reveal mucosal abnormalities.

DIAGNOSTIC PROCEDURES
- Upper GI endoscopy or esophagogastroduodenoscopy confirm the ulcer and permit cytologic studies and biopsy to rule out *H. pylori* or cancer.
- Gastric secretory studies show hyperchlorhydria.

◆ TREATMENT

General
- Symptomatic
- Iced saline lavage, possibly containing norepinephrine
- Laser or cautery during endoscopy
- Stress reduction
- Smoking cessation

Diet
- Avoidance of dietary irritants
- Nothing by mouth (NPO) if GI bleeding evident

Activity
- No restrictions

Medication
FOR *H. PYLORI*
- Amoxicillin, clarithromycin, and omeprazole

GASTRIC OR DUODENAL ULCER
- Proton pump inhibitors
- Antacids
- Histamine-receptor antagonists or gastric acid pump inhibitor
- Coating agents (for duodenal ulcer)
- Antisecretory agents, if ulcer resulted from NSAID use; NSAIDs must be continued
- Sedatives and tranquilizers (for gastric ulcer)
- Anticholinergics (for duodenal ulcers; usually contraindicated in gastric ulcers)
- Prostaglandin analogs

Surgery
- Indicated for perforation, lack of response to conservative treatment, suspected cancer, or other complications

- Type of surgery dependent on ulcer location and extent; major operations: bilateral vagotomy, pyloroplasty, and gastrectomy

❖ NURSING CONSIDERATIONS

Nursing diagnoses
- Acute or chronic pain
- Anxiety
- Deficient fluid volume
- Deficient knowledge (peptic ulcer)
- Disturbed sleep pattern
- Imbalanced nutrition: Less than body requirements
- Risk for injury

Key outcomes
The patient will:
- express feelings of increased comfort and decreased pain
- identify strategies to reduce anxiety
- maintain adequate fluid volume
- verbalize an understanding of the illness and treatment regimen
- regain regular sleep patterns
- achieve adequate nutritional intake
- remain free of injury.

Nursing interventions
- Administer medications, as ordered.
- Provide six small meals or small hourly meals as ordered.
- Offer emotional support.

Monitoring
- Medication effects
- Vital signs
- Signs and symptoms of bleeding
- Pain control

IF PATIENT HAD SURGERY
- Nasogastric tube function and drainage
- Bowel function
- Fluid and nutritional status
- Wound site
- Signs and symptoms of metabolic alkalosis or perforation

▶ PATIENT TEACHING

Be sure to cover:
- disorder, diagnostic tests, and treatment
- medication administration, dosage, and possible adverse effects
- warnings against avoid over-the-counter medications, especially aspirin, aspirin-containing products, and NSAIDs, unless the doctor approves
- warnings against caffeine and alcohol intake during exacerbations
- appropriate lifestyle changes
- smoking-cessation program, if indicated.

Discharge planning
- Refer the patient to a smoking-cessation program, if indicated.

✴ RESOURCES

Organizations
Digestive Disease National Coalition: *www.ddnc.org*
National Digestive Diseases Information Clearinghouse: *www.niddk.nih.gov/health/digest/nddic.htm*

Selected references
Gisbert, J.P., et al. "Risk Assessment and Outpatient Management in Bleeding Peptic Ulcer," *Journal of Clinical Gastroenterology* 40(2):129-34, February 2006.

Goldstein, J.L., et al. "Healing of Gastric Ulcers with Esomeprazole versus Ranitidine in Patients who Continued to Receive NSAID Therapy: A Randomized Trial," *American Journal of Gastroenterology* 100(12):2650-657, December 2005.

Handbook of Diseases, 3rd ed. Philadelphia: Lippincott Williams & Wilkins, 2004.

Krumberger, J.M. "How to Manage an Acute Upper GI Bleed," *RN* 68(3):34-39, March 2005.

Tierney, L., et al. *Current Medical Diagnosis & Treatment 2006.* New York: McGraw-Hill Book Co., 2006.

Yuan, Y., et al. "Peptic Ulcer Disease Today," *Nature Clinical Practice—Gastroenterology & Hepatology* 3(2):80-89, February 2006.

Pericarditis

● OVERVIEW

Description
- Inflammation of the pericardium— the fibroserous sac that envelops, supports, and protects the heart
- Occurs in acute and chronic forms
- Acute form: can be fibrinous or effusive; characterized by serous, purulent, or hemorrhagic exudate
- Chronic form (called *constrictive pericarditis*): characterized by dense fibrous pericardial thickening

Pathophysiology
- Pericardial tissue is damaged by bacteria or another substance that releases chemical mediators of inflammation into surrounding tissue.
- Friction occurs as the inflamed layers rub against each other.
- Chemical mediators dilate blood vessels and increase vessel permeability.
- Vessel walls leak fluids and proteins, causing extracellular edema.

Causes
- Bacterial, fungal, or viral infection (in infectious pericarditis)
- Neoplasms (primary or metastatic)
- High-dose chest radiation
- Uremia
- Hypersensitivity or autoimmune disease
- Drugs, such as hydralazine or procainamide
- Idiopathic factors
- Myocardial infarction (MI)
- Chest trauma
- Aortic aneurysm with pericardial leakage
- Myxedema with cholesterol deposits in pericardium
- Radiation
- Rheumatic conditions
- Tuberculosis

Incidence
- Most common in men ages 20 to 50

Common characteristics
- Pericardial friction rub
- Chest pain

Complications
- Pericardial effusion
- Cardiac tamponade

✳ ASSESSMENT

History
- Predisposing factor
- Sharp, sudden pain, usually starting over the sternum and radiating to the neck, shoulders, back, and arms
- Pleuritic pain, increasing with deep inspiration and decreasing when the patient sits up and leans forward
- Dyspnea
- Chest pain (may mimic MI pain)

Physical findings
- Pericardial friction rub
- Diminished apical impulse
- Fluid retention, ascites, hepatomegaly (resembling those of chronic right-sided heart failure)
- With pericardial effusion: tachycardia
- With cardiac tamponade: pallor, clammy skin, hypotension, pulsus paradoxus, neck vein distention, and dyspnea

Test results
LABORATORY
- White blood cell count is elevated (especially in infectious pericarditis).
- Erythrocyte sedimentation rate is elevated.
- Serum creatine kinase-MB levels are slightly elevated (with associated myocarditis).
- Pericardial fluid culture may identify a causative organism in bacterial or fungal pericarditis.
- Blood urea nitrogen is elevated in uremia.
- Elevated antistreptolysin-O titers may indicate rheumatic fever.
- Positive reaction in purified protein derivative skin test indicates tuberculosis.

IMAGING
- Echocardiography showing an echo-free space between the ventricular wall and the pericardium indicates pericardial effusion.
- High-resolution computed tomography and magnetic resonance imaging reveal pericardial thickness.

DIAGNOSTIC PROCEDURES
- Electrocardiography shows initial ST-segment elevation across the precordium.

◆ TREATMENT

General
- Management of rheumatic fever, uremia, tuberculosis, or other underlying disorder

Diet
- Restrictions, based on underlying disorder

Activity
- Bed rest as long as fever and pain persist

Medication
- Nonsteroidal anti-inflammatory drugs
- Corticosteroids
- Antibiotics, antifungals, or antiviral therapy

Surgery
- Surgical drainage
- Pericardiocentesis
- Partial pericardectomy (for recurrent pericarditis)
- Total pericardectomy (for constrictive pericarditis)

♣ NURSING CONSIDERATIONS

Nursing diagnoses
- Acute pain
- Anxiety
- Decreased cardiac output
- Deficient diversional activity
- Impaired gas exchange
- Ineffective breathing pattern
- Ineffective role performance

Key outcomes
The patient will:
- express feelings of increased comfort and decreased pain
- cope with the medical condition without demonstrating serious signs of anxiety
- maintain hemodynamic stability and adequate cardiac output
- avoid arrhythmias
- express an interest in using leisure time meaningfully
- maintain adequate ventilation and oxygenation
- maintain adequate breathing pattern
- express feelings about diminished capacity to perform usual roles.

Nursing interventions
- Administer analgesics and oxygen, as ordered.
- Give prescribed antibiotics on time.
- Stress the importance of bed rest. Provide a bedside commode.
- Place the patient upright to relieve dyspnea and chest pain.

  ◆ **NURSING ALERT** Keep a pericardiocentesis set readily available whenever you suspect pericardial effusion.

- Encourage the patient to express concerns about the effects of activity restrictions on responsibilities and routines.
- Review the patient's allergy history.
- Provide appropriate postoperative care.

Monitoring
- Vital signs
- Heart rhythm
- Heart sounds
- Hemodynamic values

▶ PATIENT TEACHING

Be sure to cover:
- disorder, diagnostic tests, and treatment
- how to perform deep-breathing and coughing exercises
- need to resume daily activities slowly and to schedule rest periods into daily routine, as instructed by the physician.

Discharge planning
- Refer patient to community resources, as indicated.

✳ RESOURCES

Organizations
Mayo Clinic: *www.mayohealth.org*
National Heart, Lung and Blood Institute: *www.nhlbi.hih.gov/nhlbi/cardio*

Selected references
Demmler, G.J. "Infectious Pericarditis in Children," *Pediatric Infectious Disease Journal* 25(2):165-66, February 2006.

Imazio, M., et al. "Management, Risk Factors, and Outcomes in Recurrent Pericarditis," *American Journal of Cardiology* 96(5):763-69, September 2005.

Kasper, D. L., et al., eds. *Harrison's Principles of Internal Medicine,* 16th ed. New York: McGraw-Hill Book Co., 2005.

Mayosi, B.M., et al. "Tuberculosis Pericarditis," *Circulation* 112(23):3608-616, December 2005.

The Merck Manual of Diagnosis & Therapy, 18th ed., Whitehouse Station, N.J.: Merck and Co., Inc., 2006.

Rheuban, K.S. "Pericarditis," *Current Treatment Options in Cardiovascular Medicine* 7(5):419-27, October 2005.

Peritonitis

Description

- Inflammation of the peritoneum; may extend throughout the peritoneum or localize as an abscess
- Commonly decreases intestinal motility and causes intestinal distention with gas
- Lethal in 10% of cases, with bowel obstruction the usual cause of death
- Can be acute or chronic

Pathophysiology

- Bacteria invade the peritoneum after inflammation and perforation of the GI tract.
- Fluid containing protein and electrolytes accumulates in the peritoneal cavity; normally transparent, the peritoneum becomes opaque, red, inflamed, and edematous.
- Infection may localize as an abscess rather than disseminate as a generalized infection.

Causes

- GI tract perforation (from appendicitis, diverticulitis, peptic ulcer, or ulcerative colitis)
- Bacterial or chemical inflammation
- Ruptured ectopic pregnancy
- Peritoneal dialsysis
- Ascites

Incidence

- Affects more men than women

Common characteristics

- Abdominal pain
- Fever

Complications

- Abscess
- Septicemia
- Respiratory compromise
- Bowel obstruction
- Shock

History

EARLY PHASE

- Vague, generalized abdominal pain
- If localized: pain over a specific area (usually the inflammation site)
- If generalized: diffuse pain over the abdomen

WITH PROGRESSION

- Increasingly severe and constant abdominal pain that increases with movement and respirations
- Possible referral of pain to shoulder or thoracic area
- Anorexia, nausea, and vomiting
- Inability to pass stools and flatus
- Hiccups

Physical findings

- Fever
- Tachycardia
- Hypotension
- Shallow breathing
- Signs of dehydration
- Positive bowel sounds (early); absent bowel sounds (later)
- Abdominal rigidity
- General abdominal tenderness
- Rebound tenderness
- Typical patient positioning: lying very still with knees flexed

Test results

LABORATORY

- Complete blood count shows leukocytosis.

IMAGING

- Abdominal X-rays show edematous and gaseous distention of the small and large bowel. With perforation of a visceral organ, X-rays show air in the abdominal cavity.
- Chest X-rays may reveal elevation of the diaphragm.
- Computed tomography reveals fluid and inflammation.

DIAGNOSTIC PROCEDURES

- Paracentesis shows the nature of the exudate and permits bacterial culture testing.

General

- I.V. fluids
- Nasogastric (NG) intubation

Diet

- Nothing by mouth until bowel function returns
- Gradual increase in diet
- Parenteral nutrition, if necessary

Activity

- Bed rest until condition improves
- Semi-Fowler's position
- Avoidance of lifting for at least 6 weeks postoperatively

Medication

- Antibiotics, based on infecting organism
- Electrolyte replacement
- Analgesics

Surgery

- Procedure dependent on the cause of peritonitis

✤ NURSING CONSIDERATIONS

Nursing diagnoses
- Acute pain
- Anxiety
- Deficient fluid volume
- Fear
- Imbalanced nutrition: Less than body requirements
- Ineffective tissue perfusion: GI

Key outcomes
The patient will:
- express feelings of increased comfort and decreased pain
- identify measures to reduce anxiety
- maintain normal fluid volume
- verbalize fears and concerns
- achieve adequate caloric intake
- exhibit signs of adequate GI perfusion and regain normal bowel function.

Nursing interventions
- Administer medications as ordered.
- Encourage early postoperative ambulation.
- Encourage the patient to express feelings.
- Provide emotional support.

Monitoring
- Fluid and nutritional status
- Pain control
- Vital signs
- NG tube function and drainage
- Bowel function
- Wound site
- Signs and symptoms of dehiscence

◈ **NURSING ALERT** Watch for signs and symptoms of abscess formation, including persistent abdominal tenderness and fever.

▶ PATIENT TEACHING

Be sure to cover:
- disorder, diagnostic tests, and treatment
- preoperatively, coughing and deep-breathing techniques
- postoperative care procedures
- signs and symptoms of infection
- proper wound care
- medication administration, dosage, and possible adverse effects
- dietary and activity limitations (depending on type of surgery).

Discharge planning
- Refer the patient for appropriate community resources for follow up.

✳ RESOURCES

Organizations
National Digestive Diseases Information Clearinghouse: *www.niddk.nih.gov/health/digest/nddic.htm*
Digestive Disease National Coalition: *www.ddnc.org*

Selected references
Akman, S., et al. "Value of the Urine Strip Test in the Early Diagnosis of Bacterial Peritonitis," *Pediatrics International* 47(5):523-27, October 2005.

Courtney, A.E., and Doherty, C.C. "Fulminant Sclerosing Peritonitis Immediately Following Acute Bacterial Peritonitis," *Nephrology Dialysis Transplantation* 21(2):532-34, February 2006.

Handbook of Diseases, 3rd ed. Philadelphia: Lippincott Williams & Wilkins, 2004.

McNally, P. *GI/Liver Secrets,* 3rd ed. Philadelphia: Hanely & Belfus, Inc., 2006.

Yamamoto, N., et al. "Gastrointestinal Sclerosing Encapsulating Peritonitis," *Journal of Gastroenterology & Hepatology* 20(6):952, June 2005.

Pertussis

● OVERVIEW

Description
- Highly contagious respiratory infection
- Typically causes an irritating cough that becomes paroxysmal and ends in a high-pitched, inspiratory whoop
- Follows a 6- to 8-week course that includes three 2-week stages with varying symptoms
- Also called *whooping cough*

Pathophysiology
- The infecting organism adheres to ciliated epithelial cells and multiplies.
- The resulting local mucosal damage induces paroxysmal coughing, which enhances disease transmission.
- Various toxins produced during the infection impair local defenses, cause local tissue damage, and may cause direct central nervous system injury.

Causes
- Nonmotile, gram-negative coccobacillus *Bordetella pertussis;* occasionally, *B. parapertussis* or *B. bronchiseptica* (see Bordetella pertussis)
- Typically transmitted by direct inhalation of contaminated droplets from someone in the acute disease stage
- Spreads indirectly through soiled linen and other articles contaminated by respiratory secretions

Incidence
- 50% of cases seen in underimmunized children younger than age 1
- Commonly occurs in schools, nursing homes, and residential facilities
- Epidemics occurring every 3 to 5 years without seasonal variation

Common characteristics
CATARRHAL (INITIAL) STAGE
- Hacking nocturnal cough
- Anorexia
- Sneezing, lacrimation, and rhinorrhea
PAROXYSMAL (SECOND) STAGE
- Spasmodic, recurrent cough with tenacious mucus that typically ends in a loud, crowing, inspiratory whoop
- Vomiting if the patient chokes on mucus

CONVALESCENT (THIRD) STAGE
- Gradual subsidence of paroxysmal coughing and vomiting

Complications
- Increased venous pressure
- Anterior eye chamber hemorrhage
- Detached retina and blindness
- Rectal prolapse
- Inguinal or umbilical hernia
- Encephalopathy, seizures
- Atelectasis, pneumonitis, or pneumonia
- Apnea, anoxia (in infants)
- Otitis media
- Cerebral hemorrhage

✱ ASSESSMENT

History
- Possible lack of immunization coupled with exposure to pertussis during previous 3 weeks

Physical findings
- Low or normal body temperature
- Mild conjunctivitis
- Listlessness
- Engorged neck veins
- Epistaxis during paroxysmal coughing
- Exhaustion and cyanosis after coughing spell
- Diminished breath sounds, upper airway wheezing
- Cough producing high-pitched "whooping" sound
- Vomiting from repeated coughing
- Choking spells (in infants)

Test results
LABORATORY
- White blood cell count and differential show lymphocytosis.
- *B. pertussis* is found in nasopharyngeal swabs and sputum culture in early disease stages.
- Direct immunofluorescence shows antigen.

◆ TREATMENT

General
- For infants and elderly patients: hospitalization with vigorous supportive therapy and fluid and electrolyte replacement

Diet
- Adequate nutrition with small, frequent meals
- Increased fluid intake

Activity
- Rest periods when fatigued

Medication
- Antibiotics
- Oxygen

BORDETELLA PERTUSSIS

This microscopic enlargement shows *Bordetella pertussis,* the nonmotile, gram-negative coccobacillus that commonly causes whooping cough. After entering the tracheobronchial tree, pertussis causes mucus to become increasingly tenacious. The classic 6-week course of whooping cough follows.

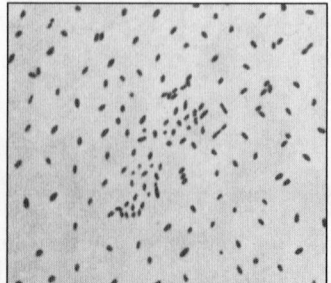

❖ NURSING CONSIDERATIONS

Nursing diagnoses
- Activity intolerance
- Acute pain
- Anxiety
- Deficient fluid volume
- Impaired gas exchange
- Ineffective airway clearance
- Ineffective breathing pattern
- Risk for infection
- Risk for injury

Key outcomes
The patient will:
- return to a normal activity level as patient recovers
- report increased comfort and decreased pain
- identify strategies to reduce anxiety
- attain and maintain normal fluid and electrolyte balance
- maintain adequate ventilation and oxygenation
- maintain a patent airway
- remain free from adventitious breath sounds
- remain free from signs and symptoms of infection
- remain free from injury.

Nursing interventions
- Maintain respiratory isolation (mask only) for 5 to 7 days after antibiotic therapy begins.
- Provide oxygen and moist air as ordered; if needed, assist respiration.
- Suction secretions as necessary. Elevate the head of the bed to ease breathing.
- Create a quiet environment to decrease coughing stimulation.
- Assess for complications caused by excessive coughing.
- Provide emotional support to the patient and parents as appropriate.
- Report pertussis cases to local public health authorities.

Monitoring
- Respiratory status
- Acid-base balance
- Fluid and electrolyte balance

▶ PATIENT TEACHING

Be sure to cover (with the patient or parents as appropriate):
- disorder, diagnostic tests, and treatment
- need for the patient's close contacts to get medical care
- when to notify the physician
- importance of immunization and vaccinations and the need to notify the physician of adverse reactions to the vaccine.

Discharge planning
- Refer the patient to a pulmonologist for follow-up care, as indicated.

✷ RESOURCES

Organizations
American Lung Association: *www.lungusa.org*
Centers for Disease Control and Prevention: *www.cdc.gov*
Harvard Medical School's Consumer Health Information: *www.intelihealth.com*
National Health Information Center: *www.health.gov/nhic/*
National Institute of Allergy and Infectious Diseases: *www.niaid.nih.gov*
National Library of Medicine: *www.nlm.nih.gov*

Selected references
Casey, J.R., and Pichichero, M.E. "Acellular Pertussis Vaccine Safety and Efficacy in Children, Adolescents and Adults," *Drugs* 65(10):1367-389, 2005.

Edwards, K., and Freeman, D.M. "Adolescent and Adult Pertussis: Disease Burden and Prevention," *Current Opinion in Pediatrics* 18(1):77-80, February 2006.

Hu, J.J., et al. "Survey of Pertussis in Patients with Prolonged Cough," *Journal of Microbiology, Immunology, and Infection* 39(1):54-58, February 2006.

Kasper, D.L., et al., eds. *Harrison's Principles of Internal Medicine,* 16th ed. New York: McGraw-Hill Book Co., 2005.

Pharyngitis

● OVERVIEW

Description
- Acute or chronic inflammation of the pharynx
- Most common throat disorder
- Usually subsides in 3 to 10 days, unless complications occur

Pathophysiology
- Cellular damage caused by a virus or bacteria causes an inflammatory response, resulting in hyperemia and fluid exudation.

Causes
- Viral or bacterial infection
- Beta-hemolytic streptococci (15% to 20% of acute pharyngitis cases)
- Mononucleosis
- Streptococcal bacteria infections (in children)

GONOCOCCAL PHARYNGITIS
- Release of a toxin produced by *Corynebacterium diphtheria*

FUNGAL PHARYNGITIS
- Prolonged antibiotic use (in immunosuppressed patients)

Incidence
Widespread among adults who:
- live or work in dusty or dry environments
- use their voices excessively
- use tobacco or alcohol habitually
- suffer from chronic sinusitis, persistent coughs, or allergies

Common characteristics
- Sore throat
- Pharyngeal edema

Complications
- Otitis media
- Sinusitis
- Mastoiditis
- Rheumatic fever
- Nephritis

✳ ASSESSMENT

History
- Sore throat
- Slight difficulty swallowing (swallowing saliva more painful than swallowing food)
- Sensation of a lump in the throat
- Constant, aggravating urge to swallow
- Headache
- Muscle and joint pain

Physical findings
- Mild fever
- Fiery red appearance of the posterior pharyngeal wall
- Swollen, exudate-flecked tonsils
- Lymphoid follicles

BACTERIAL PHARYNGITIS
- Acutely inflamed throat, with patches of white and yellow follicles
- Strawberry red tongue
- Enlarged, tender cervical lymph nodes

Test results

LABORATORY
- Throat culture identifies the causative organism.
- Rapid strep test shows group A beta-hemolytic streptococcal infection.
- White blood cell count and differential show atypical lymphocytes.

IMAGING
- Computed tomography scans locate abscesses.

◆ TREATMENT

General
- Warm saline gargles
- Hospitalization for dehydration
- Elimination of the underlying cause
- Adequate humidification

Diet
- Adequate fluids
- Avoidance of citrus juices
- Easy to swallow foods

Activity
- Bed rest while febrile

Medication
- Anesthetic throat lozenges
- Analgesics, as needed
- Antibiotics
- Antifungal agents (for fungal pharyngitis)
- Antipyretics
- Equine antitoxins (for diphtherial pharyngitis)

Surgery
- Abscess drainage

NURSING CONSIDERATIONS

Nursing diagnoses
- Acute pain
- Fatigue
- Imbalanced nutrition: Less than body requirements
- Impaired oral mucous membrane
- Risk for deficient fluid volume

Key outcomes
The patient will:
- express feelings of increased comfort decreased pain
- verbalize importance of adequate rest periods
- achieve adequate daily calorie intake
- maintain intact mucous membranes
- maintain normal fluid volume.

Nursing interventions
- Administer medications, as ordered.
- Obtain throat cultures, as ordered.
- Instruct the patient to use warm saline gargles.
- Encourage adequate oral fluid intake.
- Perform meticulous mouth care.
- Maintain a restful environment.

Monitoring
- Intake and output
- Signs and symptoms of dehydration

NURSING ALERT Examine the patient's skin twice per day for rashes caused by drug sensitivity or rashes that could indicate a communicable disease.

PATIENT TEACHING

Be sure to cover:
- disorder, diagnostic tests, and treatment
- importance of completing prescribed antibiotic therapy
- adverse reactions to medications
- preventive measures
- avoidance of excessive exposure to air conditioning
- smoking cessation
- ways to minimize environmental sources of throat irritation
- importance of throat cultures for all family members if the patient has a streptococcal infection.

Discharge planning
- Refer the patient to a smoking cessation program, if indicated.

RESOURCES

Organizations
American Academy of Allergy, Asthma and Immunology: *www.aaaai.org*
National Institute of Allergy and Infectious Disease: *www.niad.nih.gov*

Selected references
Linder, J.A., et al. "Antibiotic Treatment of Children with Sore Throat," *JAMA* 294(18)2315-322, November 2005.

Moukarel, R.V., et al. "Acute Pharyngitis: An Unusual Presentation of Acute Enemic Typhus," *Otolaryngology-Head and Neck Surgery* 133(4):645, October 2005.

Summers, A. "Sore Throats," *Accident and Emergency Nursing* 13(1):15-17, January 2005.

Woolley, S.L., et al. "Sore Throat in Adults—Does the Introduction of a Clinical Scoring System Improve the Management of these Patients in a Secondary Care Setting?" *Journal of Laryngology and Otology* 119(7):550-55, July 2005.

Pheochromocytoma

OVERVIEW

Description
- Catecholamine-producing tumor that's typically benign; usually derived from adrenal medullary cells
- Most common cause of adrenal medullary hypersecretion
- Usually produces norepinephrine, with large tumors secreting both epinephrine and norepinephrine
- Potentially fatal, but with treatment carries a good prognosis
- Also known as *chromaffin tumor*

Pathophysiology
- Pheochromocytoma causes excessive catecholamine production from autonomous tumor functioning.
- The tumor stems from a chromaffin cell tumor of the adrenal medulla or sympathetic ganglia (more commonly in the right adrenal gland than in the left).
- Extra-adrenal pheochromocytomas may occur in the abdomen, thorax, urinary bladder, and neck and in association with the ninth and tenth cranial nerves.

Causes
- May be inherited as an autosomal dominant trait

Incidence
- Rare; seen in about 0.5% of newly diagnosed hypertensive patients
- Seen in all races
- Affects both sexes equally
- Typically familial
- Most common in patients ages 30 to 50

Common characteristics
- Paroxysmal or sustained hypertension
- Hypertensive crises triggered by conditions that displace the abdominal contents or by use of opiates, histamine, glucagon, or corticotropin
- Headache
- Flushing
- Diaphoresis
- Tachycardia

Complications
- Stroke
- Retinopathy
- Irreversible kidney damage
- Acute pulmonary edema
- Cholelithiasis
- Cardiac arrhythmias
- Heart failure

> **NURSING ALERT** Pheochromocytoma may occur during pregnancy when uterine pressure on the tumor causes more frequent hypertensive crises. These crises carry a high risk for spontaneous abortion and can be fatal for both the mother and fetus.

ASSESSMENT

History
- Unpredictable episodes of hypertensive crisis
- Paroxysmal symptoms suggesting a seizure disorder or anxiety attack
- Hypertension that responds poorly to conventional treatment
- Hypotension or shock after surgery or diagnostic procedures

DURING PAROXYSMS OR CRISES
- Throbbing headache
- Palpitations
- Visual blurring
- Nausea and vomiting
- Severe diaphoresis
- Feelings of impending doom
- Precordial or abdominal pain
- Moderate weight loss
- Dizziness or light-headedness when moving to an upright position

Physical findings
DURING PAROXYSMS OR CRISES
- Hypertension
- Tachypnea
- Pallor or flushing
- Profuse sweating
- Tremor
- Seizures
- Tachycardia

Test results
LABORATORY
- In 24-hour urine specimen, vanillylmandelic acid and metanephrine levels are increased.
- Total plasma catecholamine levels are 10 to 50 times higher than normal on direct assay.

IMAGING
- Computed tomography (CT) scan or magnetic resonance imaging of adrenal glands may show intra-adrenal lesions.
- CT scan, chest X-ray, or abdominal aortography may reveal extra-adrenal pheochromocytoma.
- Iodine-131-meta-iodobenzyl-guanindine scan locates or confirms disease.

TREATMENT

General
- Blood pressure control

Diet
- High-protein, with adequate calories

Activity
- Rest during acute attacks

Medication
- Alpha-adrenergic blockers
- Catecholamine-synthesis antagonists
- Beta-adrenergic blockers
- Calcium-channel blockers
- I.V. phentolamine or nitroprusside during paroxysms or crises

> **NURSING ALERT** Because severe and occasionally fatal paroxysms have been induced by opioids, histamine, and other drugs, all medications should be considered carefully and administered cautiously in patients with known or suspected pheochromocytoma.

Surgery
- Removal of pheochromocytoma

✦ NURSING CONSIDERATIONS

Nursing diagnoses
- Acute pain
- Anxiety
- Fear
- Imbalanced nutrition: Less than body requirements
- Ineffective coping
- Ineffective tissue perfusion: Cardiopulmonary, renal
- Risk for infection

Key outcomes
The patient will:
- express feelings of increased comfort and decreased pain
- identify strategies to reduce anxiety
- discuss fears and concerns
- identify appropriate food choices according to a prescribed diet
- demonstrate adaptive coping behaviors
- exhibit signs of adequate cardiopulmonary and renal perfusion
- remain free from signs and symptoms of infection.

Nursing interventions
- Administer medications, as ordered.
- Ensure the reliability of urine catecholamine measurements.
- Provide comfort measures.
- Consult a dietitian, as needed.
- Tell the patient to report symptoms of an acute attack.
- Encourage the patient to express feelings.
- Help the patient develop effective coping strategies.

AFTER ADRENALECTOMY

⬥ **NURSING ALERT** Be aware that postoperative hypertension is common because the stress of surgery and adrenal gland manipulation stimulate catecholamine secretion.

Monitoring
- Vital signs, especially blood pressure
- Serum glucose level
- Daily weight
- Neurologic status
- Renal function
- Cardiovascular status
- Adverse reactions to medications

AFTER ADRENALECTOMY
- Vital signs

- Bowel sounds
- Dressings
- Incision
- Signs and symptoms of hemorrhage
- Pain

▶ PATIENT TEACHING

Be sure to cover:
- disorder, diagnostic tests, and treatment
- medication administration, dosage, and possible adverse effects
- when to notify the physician
- way to prevent paroxysmal attacks
- signs and symptoms of adrenal insufficiency
- importance of wearing medical identification.

Discharge planning
- Refer family members for genetic counseling if autosomal dominant transmission of pheochromocytoma is suspected.

✱ RESOURCES

Organizations
American Association of Clinical Endocrinologist: *www.aace.com*
American Society of Human Genetics: *www.faseb.org/genetics*
Endocrine Society: *www.endo-society.org.*
Pheochromocytoma Support and Awareness Group: *www.ndrf.org/pheochro.htm*

Selected references
Dahia, P.L. "Evolving Concepts in Pheochromocytoma and Paraganglioma," *Current Opinion in Oncology* 18(1):1-8, January 2006.

Guller, U., et al. "Detecting Pheochromocytoma: Defining the Most Sensitive test," *Annals of Surgery* 243(1):102-107, January 2006.

Ilias, I., and Pacak, K. "Diagnosis and Management of Tumors of the Adrenal Medulla," *Hormone and Metabolic Research* 37(12):717-21, December 2005.

Nettina, S.M. *Lippincott Manual of Nursing Practice*, 8th ed. Philadelphia: Lippincott Williams & Wilkins, 2006.

Sullivan, J., et al. "Presenting Signs and Symptoms of Pheochromocytoma in Pediatric-aged Patients," *Clinical Pediatrics* 44(8):715-19, October 2005.

Pituitary tumor

● OVERVIEW

Description
- Nonmalignant intracranial tumor; accounts for 10% of all intracranial neoplasms
- Most common tumor tissue types: chromophobe adenoma (90%), basophil adenoma, and eosinophil adenoma
- Most common site: anterior pituitary (adenohypophysis)
- Considered a neoplastic condition because of the tumor's invasive growth
- Carries a fair to good prognosis, depending on how far the tumor spreads beyond the sella turcica

Pathophysiology
- As a pituitary adenoma grows, it replaces normal glandular tissue and enlarges the sella turcica (which houses it).
- Chromophobe adenoma may be associated with production of corticotropin, melanocyte-stimulating hormone, growth hormone, and prolactin.
- Basophil adenoma may be associated with excess corticotropin production and, consequently, Cushing's syndrome.
- Eosinophil adenoma may be associated with excessive growth hormone.

Causes
- Exact cause unknown

Risk factors
- Autosomal dominant trait

Incidence
- Affects adults of both sexes between ages 30 and 40
- Twice as common in females as in males

Common characteristics
- Headache, visual changes, double vision, and drooping eyelids
- Nipple discharge
- Gynecomastia
- Menses cessation
- Decreased libido, male impotence
- Cold intolerance
- Nausea, vomiting, and constipation
- Personality changes
- Skin changes
- Hair loss
- Seizures
- Hypotension

Complications
- Endocrine abnormalities throughout the body, unless lost hormones are replaced
- Diabetes insipidus from tumor compression of the hypothalamus

✳ ASSESSMENT

History
- Neurologic and endocrine abnormalities
- Personality changes or dementia
- Amenorrhea
- Decreased libido
- Impotence
- Lethargy, weakness, increased fatigability
- Sensitivity to cold
- Constipation
- Seizures
- With cranial nerve involvement: diplopia and dizziness

Physical findings
- Rhinorrhea
- Head tilting during physical exam
- Skin changes
- Strabismus

Test results
LABORATORY
- Protein levels are increased in cerebrospinal fluid (CSF).
IMAGING
- Skull X-rays with tomography may show an enlarged sella turcica or erosion of its floor; if growth hormone secretion predominates, X-rays show enlargement of the paranasal sinuses and mandible, thickened cranial bones, and separated teeth.
- Carotid angiography may identify displacement of the anterior cerebral and internal carotid arteries from tumor enlargement and may rule out intracerebral aneurysm.
- Computed tomography scan may confirm an adenoma and accurately depict its size.
- Magnetic resonance imaging scan differentiates healthy, benign, and malignant tissues and blood vessels.

◆ TREATMENT

General
- Radiation therapy used for small, nonsecretory tumors confined to the sella turcica or for patients considered poor surgical risks

Diet
- Individualized according to tumor manifestations; possible sodium or caloric restriction

Activity
INITIAL POSTOPERATIVE PERIOD
- Avoidance of coughing, sneezing, bending, and other movements that may increase intracranial pressure (ICP) or cause CSF leakage
AFTER RECOVERY
- No restrictions

Medication
- Corticosteroids or thyroid or sex hormones
- Electrolyte replacement
- Insulin
- Bromocriptine (dopamine agent)

Surgery
- Transfrontal removal of a large tumor impinging on the optic apparatus
- Transsphenoidal resection for a smaller tumor confined to the pituitary fossa
- Cryohypophysectomy

❖ NURSING CONSIDERATIONS

Nursing diagnoses
- Acute pain
- Constipation
- Disturbed sensory perception: Visual
- Fatigue
- Ineffective coping
- Risk for injury
- Sexual dysfunction

Key outcomes
The patient will:
- express feelings of increased comfort and decreased pain
- report a normal elimination pattern
- maintain optimal functioning within the limits of the visual impairment
- exhibit increased energy
- demonstrate adaptive coping behaviors
- remain free from injury
- maintain a positive attitude toward his sexuality and sexual performance.

Nursing interventions
- Administer medications, as ordered.
- Maintain patient safety.
- Provide rest periods to avoid fatigue.
- Establish a supportive, trusting relationship with the patient.

Monitoring
AFTER SUPRATENTORIAL OR TRANSSPHENOIDAL HYPOPHYSECTOMY
- Proper positioning (head of the bed elevated 30 degrees)
- Intake and output
- Signs and symptoms of infection
- Blood glucose level

AFTER CRANIOTOMY
- Vital signs
- Neurologic status
- Signs and symptoms of increased ICP

▶ PATIENT TEACHING

Be sure to cover:
- disorder, diagnostic tests, and treatment
- preoperative instructions on surgery, treatments, and postoperative course
- avoidance of coughing, sneezing, and bending
- importance of immediately reporting persistent postnasal drip or constant swallowing.

Discharge planning
- Encourage the patient to wear medical identification that indicates his medical condition and its proper treatment.

✳ RESOURCES

Organizations
American Brain Tumor Association: *www.abta.org*
American Cancer Society: *www.cancer.org*
Guide to Internet Resources for Cancer: *www.cancerindex.org*
National Cancer Institute: *www.nci.org*
Pituitary Network Association: *www.pituitary.org*

Selected references
Akabane, A., et al. "Gamma Knife Radiosurgery for Pituitary Adenomas," *Endocrine* 28(1):87-92, October 2005.

Atlas of Pathophysiology, 2nd ed. Philadelphia: Lippincott Williams & Wilkins, 2005.

Barahona, M.J., et al. "Determinants of Neurosurgical Outcome in Pituitary Tumors," *Journal of Endocrinological Investigation* 28(9)787-94, October 2005.

Kontogeorgos, G. "Classification and Pathology of Pituitary Tumors," *Endocrine* 28(1):27-35, October 2005.

Seilicovich, A., et al. "Gene Therapy for Pituitary Tumors," *Current Gene Therapy* 5(6):539-72, December 2005.

Placenta previa

Description
- Placental implantation in the lower uterine segment, encroaching on the internal cervical os
- Common cause of bleeding during the second half of pregnancy; among patients who develop placenta previa during the second trimester, less than 15% have persistent previa at term
- Carries good maternal prognosis if hemorrhage can be controlled
- Usually necessitates pregnancy termination if bleeding is heavy
- Fetal prognosis dependent on gestational age and amount of blood lost; frequent monitoring and prompt management greatly reducing risk for death

Pathophysiology
- The placenta covers all or part of the internal cervical os. (See *Three types of placenta previa.*)

Causes
- Exact cause unknown

Risk factors
- Defective vascularization of the decidua
- Multiple pregnancy
- Previous uterine surgery
- Multiparity
- Advanced maternal age
- Endometriosis
- Smoking

Incidence
- About 1 in every 200 pregnancies
- More common in multigravidas than primigravidas

Common characteristics
- Painless, bright red, vaginal bleeding
- Vaginal bleeding after 20th week of pregnancy

Complications
- Anemia
- Hemorrhage
- Disseminated intravascular coagulation
- Shock
- Renal damage
- Cerebral ischemia
- Maternal or fetal death

ASSESSMENT

History
- Onset of painless, bright red, vaginal bleeding after 20th week of pregnancy
- Vaginal bleeding before labor onset, typically episodic and stopping spontaneously
- May be asymptomatic

Physical findings
- Soft, nontender uterus
- Fetal malpresentation
- Minimal descent of fetal presenting part
- Good fetal heart tones

Test results
LABORATORY
- Maternal hemoglobin levels are decreased.
IMAGING
- Transvaginal ultrasound scanning determines placental position.
DIAGNOSTIC PROCEDURES
- Pelvic examination confirms diagnosis.

NURSING ALERT Pelvic examination isn't commonly performed because it increases maternal bleeding and can dislodge more of the placenta.

TREATMENT

General
- Control of blood loss, blood replacement
- Delivery of viable neonate
- Prevention of coagulation disorders
- With premature fetus, careful observation to give fetus more time to mature
- With complete placenta previa, hospitalization
- Possible vaginal delivery if bleeding is minimal and placenta previa is marginal, or when labor is rapid

NURSING ALERT Because of possible fetal blood loss through the placenta, a pediatric team should be on hand during delivery to immediately assess and treat neonatal shock, blood loss, and hypoxia.

Diet
- Nothing by mouth initially, then as guided by clinical status

Activity
- Bed rest

Medication
- I.V. fluids, using large-bore catheter

Surgery
- Immediate cesarean delivery in case of severe hemorrhage or as soon as fetus is sufficiently mature

NURSING CONSIDERATIONS

Nursing diagnoses
- Acute pain
- Anxiety
- Deficient fluid volume
- Dysfunctional grieving
- Fear
- Ineffective coping
- Risk for injury

Key outcomes
The patient will:
- express feelings of increased comfort and decreased pain
- express feelings of decreased anxiety
- maintain normal fluid volume
- express feelings about the current condition
- discuss fears and concerns
- use available support systems, such as family and friends, to aid coping
- remain free from injury.

Nursing interventions
- Obtain blood specimens for complete blood count and blood type and cross match.
- Initiate external electronic fetal monitoring.
- Administer I.V. fluids and blood products, as ordered.
- If the patient is Rh-negative, give $Rh_O(D)$ immune globulin (RhoGAM) after every bleeding episode, as ordered.
- Offer emotional support during labor.
- Provide information about labor progress and the condition of the fetus.
- Encourage the patient to express her feelings.
- Help the patient develop effective coping strategies.

Monitoring
- Vital signs
- Vaginal bleeding
- Central venous pressure
- Intake and output
- Fetal heart tones
- Signs and symptoms of hemorrhage and shock

PATIENT TEACHING

Be sure to cover:
- disorder, diagnostic tests, and treatment
- signs and symptoms of placenta previa
- possibility of emergency cesarean delivery
- possibility of the birth of a premature neonate
- possibility of neonatal death
- postpartum physical and emotional changes to expect.

Discharge planning
- Refer the patient for professional counseling, if necessary.

RESOURCES

Organizations
American College of Obstetricians and Gynecologists: *www.acog.org*
American Society for Reproductive Medicine: *www.asrm.org*

Selected references
Luo, G., et al. "Failure of Conservative Management of Placenta Previa-Percreta," *Journal of Perinatal Medicine* 33(6):564-68, 2005.

MacMullen, N.J., et al. "Red Alert: Perinatal Hemorrhage," *American Journal of Maternal Child Nursing* 30(1):46-51, January-February 2005.

Wu, S., et al. "Abnormal Placentation: Twenty-Year Analysis," *American Journal of Obstetrics & Gynecology* 192(5):1458-461, May 2005.

Zlatnik, M., et al. "Placenta Previa & the Attributable Risk of Preterm Delivery," *American Journal of Obstetrics & Gynecology* 193(Suppl 6):S122, February 2006.

THREE TYPES OF PLACENTA PREVIA

The degree of placenta previa depends largely on the extent of cervical dilation at the time of examination because the dilating cervix gradually uncovers the placenta, as shown below.

Marginal placenta previa
If the placenta covers just a fraction of the internal cervical os, the patient has marginal, or low-lying, placenta previa.

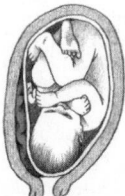

Partial placenta previa
The patient has the partial, or incomplete, form of the disorder if the placenta caps a larger part of the internal os.

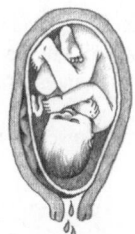

Total placenta previa
If the placenta covers all of the internal os, the patient has total, complete, or central placenta previa.

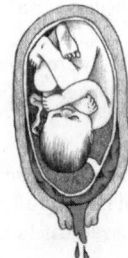

Plague

● OVERVIEW

Description
- Acute, febrile, zoonotic infection caused by the gram-negative, non-sporulating bacillus *Yersinia pestis*
- Usually transmitted to humans through the bite of a flea from an infected rodent host, such as a rat or squirrel; occasional transmission from handling infected animals or their tissues (see *Bubonic plague carrier*)
- Potential bioterrorism and biological warfare agent

FORMS OF PLAGUE
- *Bubonic:* most common form; causes swollen and sometimes suppurating, lymph glands (buboes)
- *Septicemic:* rapid, severe systemic form
- *Pneumonic:* can be primary or secondary to the other two forms; highly contagious, with secondary spread a serious concern
  - primary pneumonic plague: an acutely fulminant form causing acute prostration, respiratory distress, and death, possibly within 2 to 3 days after onset
  - secondary pneumonic plague: transmitted by contaminated respiratory droplets
- Without treatment, 60% mortality in bubonic plague and nearly 100% in septicemic and pneumonic plague; with treatment, 18% mortality

Pathophysiology
- *Y. pestis* is one of the most invasive bacterium known; mechanisms by which it causes disease aren't fully understood.
- Once inoculated through the skin or mucous membranes, *Y. pestis* usually invades cutaneous lymphatic vessels and regional lymph nodes; direct bloodstream inoculation may also occur.
- Organisms probably are phagocytized by mononuclear phagocytes without being destroyed and are then disseminated to distant sites in the body.
- Plague can involve almost any organ, and usually results in massive and widespread tissue destruction, especially if left untreated.

Causes
- *Yersinia pestis*

Incidence
- Becoming more prevalent in the United States
- Most common between May and September; in hunters who skin wild animals, between October and February
- Affects males and females equally

Common characteristics
- Fever
- Chills
- Weakness
- Headache

BUBONIC PLAGUE
- Characteristic buboes
- History of exposure to rodents

Complications
- Peritoneal or pleural effusions
- Septicemia
- Fulminant pneumonia
- Pericarditis
- Seizures
- Diffuse interstitial myocarditis
- Multifocal hepatic necrosis
- Diffuse hemorrhagic splenic necrosis
- Respiratory failure
- Cardiovascular collapse
- Disseminated intravascular coagulation
- Meningitis
- Death

✳ ASSESSMENT

History
MILDER FORM OF BUBONIC PLAGUE
- History of exposure to rodents
- Malaise
- Excruciatingly painful bubo

SEVERE FORM OF BUBONIC PLAGUE
- Sudden high fever of 103° to 106° F (39.4° to 41.1° C)
- Chills, myalgia, and headache
- Restlessness, disorientation
- Abdominal pain, nausea, and vomiting
- Constipation followed by bloody diarrhea

Physical findings
MILDER FORM OF BUBONIC PLAGUE
- Fever
- Pain or tenderness in regional lymph nodes
- Painful, inflamed, and possibly suppurative buboes (usually in the axillary or inguinal areas)
- Necrotization of hemorrhagic areas
- Moribund state within hours after onset

SEVERE FORM OF BUBONIC PLAGUE
- Fever
- Prostration
- Restlessness, disorientation, delirium
- Toxemia
- Staggering gait
- Skin mottling, petechiae
- Circulatory collapse

Test results
LABORATORY
- *Y. pestis* found in capsular antigen testing, Wayson stain, or fluorescent antibody stain
- White blood cell count above 20,000/µl, with increased polymorphonuclear leukocytes and hemoagglutination reaction
- *Y. pestis* present in culture and Gram stain of skin-lesion needle aspirate or lymph node aspirate

IMAGING
- Chest X-ray shows fulminating pneumonia in pneumonic plague.

◆ TREATMENT

General
- Supportive management to control fever, shock, and seizures and maintain fluid balance
- Warm, moist compresses on buboes

Diet
- As tolerated
- Tube feedings or total parenteral nutrition if required
- Supplemental I.V. fluids

Activity
- Bed rest during the acute phase

Medication

- Antibiotics
- Oxygen
- Corticosteroids
- Benzodiazepines
- Anticonvulsants
- Antipyretics

Surgery

- Incision and drainage of necrotic buboes

✤ NURSING CONSIDERATIONS

Nursing diagnoses

- Acute pain
- Anxiety
- Decreased cardiac output
- Fatigue
- Fear
- Hyperthermia
- Imbalanced nutrition: Less than body requirements
- Impaired gas exchange
- Impaired skin integrity
- Ineffective coping
- Ineffective tissue perfusion: Cerebral, cardiopulmonary, peripheral
- Risk for imbalanced fluid volum
- Risk for infection
- Risk for injury

Key outcomes

The patient will:

- express feelings of comfort and decreased pain
- use support systems to assist with anxiety and fear
- maintain adequate cardiac output and hemodynamic stability
- verbalize the importance of balancing activity, as tolerated, with rest
- verbalize feelings of fear and anxiety
- achieve adequate nutritional intake
- maintain adequate ventilation and oxygenation
- maintain skin integrity
- demonstrate effective coping mechanisms
- maintain acceptable tisse perfusion and cellular oxygenation
- maintain fluid balance
- experience no further signs or symptoms of infection
- avoid complications

Nursing interventions

- Administer medications, I.V. fluids, and oxygen as ordered and needed.
- Use standard precautions.
- Provide adequate nutrition.
- Maintain a patent airway and adequate oxygenation.
- Apply warm, moist compresses to buboes.
- Provide meticulous skin care.
- Prevent further injury to necrotic tissue areas.
- Institute seizure precautions.
- Report suspected plague cases to local public health department.

Monitoring

- Vital signs
- Intake and output
- Skin integrity
- Pulmonary status
- Cardiovascular status
- Nutritional status
- Seizures
- Complications
- Abnormal bleeding
- Mentation

▶ PATIENT TEACHING

Be sure to cover:

- disorder, diagnostic tests, and treatment
- medications and possible adverse reactions
- isolation procedures
- personal protective measures
- avoidance of contact with sick or dead wild animals and wearing gloves when handling animal carcasses
- importance of insect and rodent population control
- use of repellents, insecticides, and protective clothing when at risk for exposure to rodents' fleas
- elimination of rodent food and habitats
- insecticide control of fleas.

Discharge planning

- Refer the patient for appropriate community support services as indicated.

✳ RESOURCES

Organizations

Centers for Disease Control and Prevention (CDC), National Center for Infectious Diseases: www.cdc.gov

National Centers for Infectious Diseases: www.cdc.gov/ncidod

Selected references

Dennis, D.T. and Chow, C.C. "Plague," Pediatric Infectious Disease Journal 23(1):69-71, January 2004.

Drumm, C., et al. "Plague Comes to New York: Visitors from New Mexico Test a Big-City Hospital's Emergency Preparedness," AJN 104(8):61-64, Augsut 2004.

Khasnis, A.A., and Nettleman, M.D. "Global Warning and Infectious Disease," Archives of Medical Research 36(6):689-96, November-December 2005.

Mwengee, W., et al. "Treatment of Plaque with Gentamicin or Doxycycline in a Randomized Clinical Trial in Tanzania," Clinical Infectious Diseases 42(5):614-21, March 2006.

Snow, M. "Preparing for a Plaque Outbreak," Nursing 35(12):14, December 2005.

BUBONIC PLAGUE CARRIER

Bubonic plague is usually transmitted to humans through the bite of an infected flea (*Xenopsylla cheopis*), shown here.

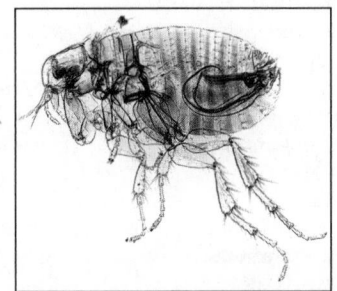

Pleural effusion

● OVERVIEW

Description
- Fluid accumulation in the pleural space, which may be extracellular, pus (empyema), blood (hemothorax), chyle (chylothorax), or bilious
- Classified as transudative or exudative

Pathophysiology
- Typically, fluid and other blood components migrate through the walls of intact capillaries bordering the pleura.
- In *transudative* effusion, fluid is watery and diffuses out of the capillaries if hydrostatic pressure increases or capillary oncotic pressure decreases.
- In *exudative* effusion, inflammatory processes increase capillary permeability. Exudative effusion is less watery and contains high concentrations of white blood cells and plasma proteins.
- *Empyema* occurs when pulmonary lymphatics become blocked, leading to outpouring of contaminated lymphatic fluid into the pleural space.

Causes
TRANSUDATIVE PLEURAL EFFUSION
- Cardiovascular disease
- Hepatic disease
- Renal disease
- Hypoproteinemia
EXUDATIVE PLEURAL EFFUSION
- Pleural infection
- Pleural inflammation
- Pleural malignancy
EMPYEMA
- Pulmonary infection
- Lung abscess
- Infected wound
- Intra-abdominal infection
- Thoracic surgery

Incidence
- Can occur at any age
- Affects males and females equally

Common characteristics
- Shortness of breath
- Chest pain
- Malaise

Complications
- Atelectasis
- Infection
- Hypoxemia
- Pneumothorax

✳ ASSESSMENT

History
- Underlying pulmonary disease
- Shortness of breath
- Chest pain
- Malaise

Physical findings
- Fever
- Trachea deviated away from the affected side
- Dullness and decreased tactile fremitus over the effusion
- Diminished or absent breath sounds
- Pleural friction rub
- Bronchial breath sounds

Test results
LABORATORY
PLEURAL FLUID ANALYSIS FINDINGS
- In transudative effusion, specific gravity is below 1.015; less than 3 g/dl of protein.
- In exudative effusion, there's a 0.5 or higher ratio of protein in pleural fluid to protein in serum; there's a lactate dehydrogenase (LDH) level of 200 IU or higher; and there's a 0.6 or higher ratio of LDH in pleural fluid to LDH in serum.
- In empyema, microorganisms are present, white blood cell count is increased, glucose levels are decreased.
- In esophageal rupture or pancreatitis, pleural fluid amylase levels exceed serum amylase levels
IMAGING
- Chest X-ray may show pleural effusions; lateral decubitus films may show loculated pleural effusions or small pleural effusions not visible on standard chest X-rays.
- Computed tomography scan of the thorax shows small pleural effusions.
DIAGNOSTIC PROCEDURES
- Thoracentesis obtains pleural fluid specimens for analysis.
- Tuberculin skin test may be positive for tuberculosis.
- Pleural biopsy may be positive for carcinoma.

◆ TREATMENT

General
- Thoracentesis, to remove fluid
- Possible chest tube insertion
- Possible chemical pleurodesis

Diet
- High-calorie

Activity
- As tolerated

Medication
- Antibiotics
- Oxygen

Surgery
- Removal of thick coating over lung (decortication)

Nursing diagnoses

- Acute pain
- Anxiety
- Fatigue
- Impaired gas exchange
- Ineffective airway clearance
- Ineffective breathing pattern
- Ineffective coping
- Risk for infection

Key outcomes

The patient will:

- report feelings of increased comfort and decreased pain
- report reduced levels of anxiety
- verbalize the importance of balancing activity with adequate rest periods
- maintain adequate ventilation and oxygenation
- maintain a patent airway
- maintain an effective breathing pattern
- use support systems and develop adequate coping mechanisms
- remain free from signs and symptoms of infection.

Nursing interventions

- Administer medications and oxygen, as ordered.
- Assist during thoracentesis.
- Encourage the patient to use incentive spirometry.
- Encourage deep-breathing exercises.
- Provide meticulous chest tube care.
- Use sterile technique.
- Ensure chest tube patency.
- Keep petroleum gauze at the bedside.

Monitoring

- Vital signs
- Intake and output
- Respiratory status
- Pulse oximetry
- Signs and symptoms of pneumothorax
- Chest tube drainage

Be sure to cover:

- disorder, diagnostic tests, and treatment
- medication administration, dosage, and possible adverse effects
- how thoracentesis is performed
- chest tube insertion and drainage
- signs and symptoms of infection
- signs and symptoms of pleural fluid reaccumulation
- when to notify the physician.

Discharge planning

- Provide a home health referral for follow-up care.
- Refer the patient to a smoking-cessation program, if indicated.

Organizations

American Association for Respiratory Care: www.aarc.org
American Thoracic Society: www.thoracic.org

Selected references

Guyton, A.C., and Hall, J.E. *Textbook of Medical Physiology,* 11th ed. Philadelphia: W.B. Saunders Co., 2006.

Kunyuski, V., et al. "Complicated Pneumonias with Empyema and/or Pneumatocele in Children," *Pediatric Surgery International* 22(2):186-90, February 2006.

Ruiz, E., et al. "Angiogenic Factors and Pleural Effusions," *Lung* 183(3):185-95, May-June 2005.

Schiza, S.F., et al. "Pharmacotherapy in Complicated Parapneumonic Pleural Effusions and Thoracic Empyema," *Pulmonary Pharmacology & Therapeutics* 18(6):381-89, 2005.

Soriano, T., et al. "Factors Influencing Length of Hospital Stay in Patients with Bacterial Pleural Effusion," *Respiration* 72(6):587-93, November-December 2005.

Pleurisy

Description
- Inflammation of the visceral and parietal pleurae that line the inside of the thoracic cage and envelop the lungs
- Also called *pleuritis*

Pathophysiology
- The pleurae become swollen and congested.
- As a result, pleural fluid transport is hampered and friction between the pleural surfaces increases.

Causes
- Pneumonia
- Tuberculosis
- Viruses
- Systemic lupus erythematosus
- Rheumatoid arthritis
- Uremia
- Dressler's syndrome
- Cancer
- Pulmonary embolism
- Chest trauma
- Pathologic rib fractures
- Pneumothorax
- Certain drugs, such as methotrexate or penicillin
- Heart failure
- Human immunodeficiency virus
- Kidney disease
- Radiation therapy
- Sickle cell disease

Incidence
- Affects males and females equally

Common characteristics
- Sudden dull, aching, burning, or sharp pain that worsens on inspiration
- Limited movement on the affected side during breathing
- Shortness of breath

Complications
- Adhesions
- Pleural effusion
- Chronic pain

History
- Sudden dull, aching, burning, or sharp pain that worsens on inspiration
- Predisposing factor
- Cough
- Shortness of breath

Physical findings
- Fever
- Characteristic late-inspiration and early-expiration pleural friction rub
- Coarse vibration on palpation of the affected area

Test results
IMAGING
- Chest X-ray shows absence of pneumonia.
DIAGNOSTIC PROCEDURES
- Electrocardiography shows absence of ischemic heart disease.

General
- Possible intercostal nerve block
- Symptomatic

Diet
- As tolerated

Activity
- Bed rest

Medication
- Anti-inflammatory agents
- Analgesics
- Antibiotics, if cause is infection

Surgery
- Thoracentesis

Nursing diagnoses
- Activity intolerance
- Acute pain
- Anxiety
- Impaired gas exchange
- Ineffective airway clearance
- Ineffective breathing pattern
- Ineffective coping

Key outcomes
The patient will:
- demonstrate energy conservation techniques
- express feelings of increased comfort and decreased pain
- report reduced anxiety
- maintain adequate ventilation and oxygenation
- maintain a patent airway
- maintain respiratory rate within 5 breaths of baseline
- use support systems to assist with coping.

Nursing interventions
- Administer medications, as ordered.
- Encourage deep breathing and coughing.
- Encourage the patient to use incentive spirometry.
- Assist the patient in splinting the affected side.
- Position the patient in high Fowler's position.
- Plan care to allow frequent rest periods.
- Assist with passive range-of-motion (ROM) exercises.
- Encourage active ROM exercises.
- Provide comfort measures.

Monitoring
- Vital signs
- Intake and output
- Response to treatment
- Pain level
- Complications
- Breath sounds
- Respiratory status

Be sure to cover:
- disorder, diagnostic tests, and treatment
- medication administration, dosage, and possible adverse effects
- how to perform splinting and deep-breathing exercises
- importance of regular rest periods
- when to notify the physician.

Discharge planning
- Refer patient to appropriate community resources, as necessary.

Organizations
American Association for Respiratory Care: *www.aarc.org*
National Heart, Lung and Blood Institute: *www.nhlbi.gov*

Selected references
Diseases, 4th ed. Philadelphia: Lippincott Williams & Wilkins, 2006.
Gorg, C., et al. "Contrast-enhanced Sonography for Differential Diagnosis of Pleurisy and Focal Pleural Lesions of Unknown Cause," *Chest* 128(6):3894-899, December 2005.
Guyton, A.C., and Hall, J.E. *Textbook of Medical Physiology,* 11th ed. Philadelphia: W.B. Saunders Co., 2006.
Yoshida, H., et al. "Imidapril-induced Eosinophilic Pleurisy Case Report and Review of the Literature," *Respiration* 72(4):423-26, July-August 2005.

Pneumocystis jiroveci (carinii) pneumonia

● OVERVIEW

Description
- Communicable, opportunistic infection frequently associated with human immunodeficiency virus (HIV)
- Leading cause of opportunistic infection and death among patients with acquired immunodeficiency syndrome (AIDS) in industrialized countries

Pathophysiology
- The infecting organism invades the lungs bilaterally, multiplies extracellularly, and fills alveoli with organisms and exudate.
- As a result, gas exchange is impaired.
- Alveoli hypertrophy and thicken, eventually leading to extensive consolidation.

Causes
- *P. jiroveci* that spreads mainly through the air (although part of the normal flora in most healthy people, organism becoming an aggressive pathogen in immunocompromised patients)
- Possible role of B-cell function defects

Incidence
- Most common in premature or malnourished infants, children with primary immunodeficiency disease, patients receiving immunosuppressive therapy, and those with AIDS

Common characteristics   .
- Insidious onset, with increasing shortness of breath and nonproductive cough
- Hypoxemia and hypercapnia (may not cause significant clinical symptoms)

Complications
- Disseminated infection
- Hypoxemia
- Respiratory failure
- Pneumothorax
- Death

✳ ASSESSMENT

History
- Immunodepression, as from HIV infection, leukemia, lymphoma, or organ transplantation

Physical findings
- Low-grade, intermittent fever
- Tachypnea, dyspnea, and accessory muscle use
- Cyanosis (with acute illness)
- Dullness on percussion (with consolidation)
- Crackles, decreased breath sounds

Test results
LABORATORY
- *P. jiroveci* is found on histologic sputum specimen studies
- Arterial blood gas (ABG) values reveal hypoxia and increased A-a gradient.
IMAGING
- Chest X-ray may show slowly progressing, fluffy infiltrates, occasional nodular lesions, or spontaneous pneumothorax.
- Gallium scan may show increased uptake over the lungs.
DIAGNOSTIC PROCEDURES
- Fiber-optic bronchoscopy helps confirm diagnosis (most common).
- Transbronchial biopsy helps confirm diagnosis (less common).
- Open lung biopsy may be done in rare cases to confirm diagnosis.

◆ TREATMENT

General
- Supportive care
- Mechanical ventilation

Diet
- High-calorie, high-protein
- Nutritional supplements, as needed
- Small, frequent meals
- Increased fluid intake

Activity
- Rest periods when fatigued

Medication
- Oxygen
- Co-trimoxazole (may be given prophylactically or to AIDS patients and other high-risk patients)
- Immunosuppressants
- Antibiotics

❖ NURSING CONSIDERATIONS

Nursing diagnoses
- Activity intolerance
- Deficient fluid volume
- Fear
- Hyperthermia
- Imbalanced nutrition: Less than body requirements
- Impaired gas exchange
- Impaired social interaction
- Ineffective breathing pattern
- Powerlessness

Key outcomes
The patient will:
- perform activities of daily living to the fullest extent possible
- maintain adequate fluid volume
- verbalize fears, feelings, and concerns
- remain afebrile
- experience no further weight loss
- regain normal ABG values and maintain adequate ventilation and oxygenation
- demonstrate effective social interaction skills
- maintain an effective breathing pattern
- participate in self-care and make decisions about care.

Nursing interventions
- Implement standard precautions.
- Administer medications and oxygen, as ordered.
- Encourage ambulation, deep-breathing exercises, and use of incentive spirometry.
- Provide adequate rest periods.
- Encourage the patient to express fears, feelings, and concerns.
- Provide emotional support.

Monitoring
- Respiratory status
- ABG values
- Fluid and electrolyte status

▶ PATIENT TEACHING

Be sure to cover:
- disorder, diagnostic tests, and treatment
- medication administration, dosage, and possible adverse effects
- energy conservation techniques
- prevention (for HIV-infected patients and other immunocompromised individuals)
- home oxygen therapy, if indicated.

Discharge planning
- Refer the patient to a pulmonologist or an infectious diseases specialist for follow-up care as needed.
- If the patient has AIDS or HIV, provide information about resources and support organizations.

✹ RESOURCES

Organizations
Centers for Disease Control and Prevention: *www.cdc.gov*
Harvard Medical School's Consumer Health Information: *www.intelihealth.com*
National Health Information Center: *www.health.gov/nhic/*
National Institute of Allergy and Infectious Diseases: *www.niaid.nih.gov*
National Library of Medicine: *www.nlm.nih.gov*

Selected references
Ioannidis, J., and Wilkinson, D. "HIV: Prevention of Opportunistic Infections," *Clinical Evidence* (13):834-53, June 2005.
Kasper, D.L., et al., eds. *Harrison's Principles of Internal Medicine,* 16th ed. New York: McGraw-Hill Book Co., 2005.
Pop, S.M., et al. "Pneumocystis: Immune Recognition and Evasion," *International Journal of Biochemistry & Cell Biology* 38(1):17-22, January 2006.
Wells, J., et al. "Complement and Fc Function Are Required for Optimal Antibody Prophlyaxis against *Pneumocytis carinii* Pneumonia," *Infection and Immunity* 74(1):390-93, January 2006.

Pneumonia

● OVERVIEW

Description
- Acute infection of the lung parenchyma that impairs gas exchange
- May be classified by etiology, location, or type

Pathophysiology
- A gel-like substance forms as microorganisms and phagocytic cells break down.
- This substance consolidates within the lower airway structure.
- Inflammation involves the alveoli, alveolar ducts, and interstitial spaces surrounding the alveolar walls.
- In lobar pneumonia, inflammation starts in one area and may extend to the entire lobe. In bronchopneumonia, it starts simultaneously in several areas, producing patchy, diffuse consolidation. In atypical pneumonia, inflammation is confined to the alveolar ducts and interstitial spaces.

Causes
ASPIRATION PNEUMONIA
- Casutic substance entering airway
BACTERIAL AND VIRAL PNEUMONIA
- Chronic illness and debilitation
- Cancer
- Abdominal and thoracic surgery
- Atelectasis
- Bacterial or viral respiratory infections
- Chronic respiratory disease
- Influenza
- Endotracheal intubation or mechanical ventilation
- Malnutrition
- Alcoholism
- Sickle cell disease
- Tracheostomy
- Exposure to noxious gases
- Aspiration
- Immunosuppressive therapy

Risk factors
- Advanced age
- Debilitation
- Nasogastric (NG) tube feedings
- Impaired gag reflex
- Poor oral hygiene
- Decreased level of consciousness
- Immobility
- History of smoking

AGE-RELATED CONCERN Incidence and mortality are highest in elderly patients.

Incidence
- Affects both sexes and all ages
- More than 3 million cases annually in the United States

Common characteristics
- Pleuritic chest pain
- Cough
- Excessive sputum production
- Chills

Complications
- Septic shock
- Hypoxemia
- Respiratory failure
- Empyema
- Bacteremia
- Endocarditis
- Pericarditis
- Meningitis
- Lung abscess (see *Lung abscess*)
- Pleural effusion

✳ ASSESSMENT

History
ASPIRATION PNEUMONIA
- Fever
- Weight loss
- Malaise
BACTERIAL PNEUMONIA
- Sudden onset of pleuritic chest pain, cough, purulent sputum production, and chills
VIRAL PNEUMONIA
- Nonproductive cough
- Constitutional symptoms

Physical findings
- Fever
- Sputum production
- Dullness over the affected area
- Crackles, wheezing, or rhonchi
- Decreased breath sounds
- Decreased fremitus
- Tachypnea
- Accessory muscle use

Test results
LABORATORY
- Complete blood count shows leukocytosis.
- Blood cultures are positive for causative organism.
- Arterial blood gas (ABG) values show hypoxemia.
- Fungal or acid-fast bacilli cultures identify the etiologic agent.
- Assay for legionella soluble antigen in urine detects presence of antigen.
- Sputum culture, Gram stain, and smear reveal the infecting organism.

LUNG ABSCESS

Lung abscess is a localized bacterial infection that causes purulence and tissue destruction. Bacteria may spread and cause multiple abscesses throughout the lungs.

Lung abscess may occur secondary to localized pneumonia or necrosis from a neoplasm that can't drain. Other causes include necrotizing infections or cysts, cavitary infarctions or cancers, and necrotic lesions from pneumoconiosis.

History findings
The patient's history typically reveals coughing (sometimes with bloody or purulent sputum), pleuritic chest pain, and dyspnea. Headache, anorexia, malaise, diaphoresis, chills, fever, and finger clubbing may occur. You may detect dullness over the affected lung, crackles, and decreased breath sounds.

Diagnostic findings
Blood and sputum cultures and Gram staining identify the causative organism. White blood cell count is elevated.

Chest X-rays show a solid mass or localized infiltrate with clear spaces that contain air and fluid. Computed tomography scan helps determine the lesion type. Bronchoscopy may be done later to collect specimens and identify obstruction.

Treatment
Treatment involves extensive antibiotic therapy and, possibly, postural drainage and oxygen therapy. Massive hemoptysis, cancer, or bronchiectasis may necessitate lesion or lobe resection. All patients require rigorous follow-up and serial chest X-rays.

IMAGING
- Chest X-rays generally show patchy or lobar infiltrates.

DIAGNOSTIC PROCEDURES
- Bronchoscopy or transtracheal aspiration specimens identify the etiologic agent.
- Pulse oximetry may reveal decreased oxygen saturation.

TREATMENT

General
- Mechanical ventilation (positive end-expiratory pressure) for respiratory failure

Diet
- High-calorie
- Adequate fluids

Activity
- Bed rest

Medication
- Antibiotics
- Humidified oxygen
- Antitussives
- Analgesics
- Bronchodilators

Surgery
- Drainage of parapneumonic pleural effusion or lung abscess

❖ NURSING CONSIDERATIONS

Nursing diagnoses
- Acute pain
- Anxiety
- Hyperthermia
- Imbalanced nutrition: Less than body requirements
- Impaired gas exchange
- Ineffective airway clearance
- Ineffective coping
- Risk for deficient fluid volume
- Risk for infection

Key outcomes
The patient will:
- express feelings of increased comfort and decreased pain
- identify measures to reduce anxiety

- maintain a normal body temperature
- maintain adequate calorie intake
- maintain adequate ventilation and oxygenation
- maintain a patent airway
- demonstrate effective coping strategies
- maintain fluid balance
- remain free from signs and symptoms of infection.

Nursing interventions
- Administer medications, as ordered.
- Administer I.V. fluids and electrolyte replacement, as ordered.
- Maintain a patent airway and adequate oxygenation.
- Administer supplemental oxygen as ordered. Give oxygen cautiously if the patient has chronic lung disease.
- Suction the patient, as needed.
- Obtain sputum specimens, as needed.
- Provide a high-calorie, high-protein diet of soft foods.
- Administer supplemental oral feedings, NG tube feedings or parenteral nutrition, if needed.
- Take steps to prevent aspiration during NG feedings.
- Dispose of secretions properly.
- Provide a quiet, calm environment with frequent rest periods.
- Include the patient in care decisions whenever possible.

Monitoring
- Vital signs
- Intake and output
- Daily weight
- Sputum production
- Respiratory status
- Breath sounds
- Pulse oximetry
- ABG values

▶ PATIENT TEACHING

Be sure to cover:
- disorder, diagnostic tests, and treatment
- medication administration, dosage, and possible adverse effects
- need for adequate fluid intake
- importance of adequate rest
- deep-breathing and coughing exercises
- adequate fluid intake
- chest physiotherapy
- avoidance of irritants
- when to notify the physician
- home oxygen therapy, if required
- ways to prevent pneumonia. (See *Preventing pneumonia*.)

Discharge planning
- Refer the patient to a smoking-cessation program, if indicated.

✳ RESOURCES

Organizations
American Lung Association: *www.lungusa.org*
Centers for Disease Control and Prevention: *www.cdc.gov*

Selected references
Andriesse, G.I., and Verhoef, J. "Nosocomial Pneumonia: Rationalizing the Approach to Empircal Therapy," *Treatments in Respiratory Medicine* 5(1):11-30, 2006.
Micek, S.T., et al. "Optimizing Antibiotic Treatment for Ventilator-associated Pneumonia," *Pharmacotherapy* 26(2):204-13, February 2006.

PREVENTING PNEUMONIA

To help prevent pneumonia, teach the patient these measures:
- Urge bedridden and postoperative patients to perform deep-breathing and coughing exercises frequently. Position these patients properly to promote full aeration and secretion drainage.
- Advise the patient to avoid using antibiotics indiscriminately for minor infections. Doing so could produce upper airway colonization with antibiotic-resistant bacteria. If pneumonia develops, the causative organisms may require treatment with more toxic antibiotics.
- Encourage the high-risk patient to ask the doctor about an annual influenza vaccination and pneumococcal pneumonia vaccination. A single dose of pneumococcal vaccine is recommended for most patients age 54 or older; certain patients may need one booster dose after 5 years.
- Discuss ways to avoid spreading the infection to others. Remind the patient to sneeze and cough into tissues and to dispose of tissues in a waxed or plastic bag. Advise the patient to wash his hands thoroughly after handling contaminated tissues.

Pneumothorax

● OVERVIEW

Description
- Accumulation of air or gas between the parietal and visceral pleurae, leading to lung collapse
- Amount of trapped air or gas determines degree of lung collapse
- Most common pneumothorax types: open, closed, and tension

Pathophysiology
- Air accumulates and separates the visceral and parietal pleurae.
- Negative pressure is eliminated, affecting elastic recoil forces.
- The lung recoils and collapses toward the hilus.
- In open pneumothorax, atmospheric air flows directly into the pleural cavity, collapsing the lung on the affected side.
- In closed pneumothorax, air enters the pleural space from within the lung, increasing pleural pressure and preventing lung expansion.
- In tension pneumothorax, air in the pleural space is under higher pressure than air in the adjacent lung. Air enters the pleural space from a pleural rupture only on inspiration. This air pressure exceeds barometric pressure, causing compression atelectasis. Increased pressure may displace the heart and great vessels and cause mediastinal shift.

Causes
OPEN PNEUMOTHORAX
- Penetrating chest injury
- Central venous catheter insertion
- Chest surgery
- Transbronchial biopsy
- Thoracentesis
- Percutaneous lung biopsy

CLOSED PNEUMOTHORAX
- Blunt chest trauma
- Rib fracture
- Clavicle fracture
- Congenital bleb rupture
- Emphysematous bullae rupture
- Barotrauma
- Erosive tubercular or cancerous lesions
- Interstitial lung disease

TENSION PNEUMOTHORAX
- Penetrating chest wound
- Lung or airway puncture from positive-pressure ventilation
- Mechanical ventilation after chest injury
- High positive end-expiratory pressures, causing rupture of alveolar blebs
- Chest tube occlusion or malfunction

Incidence
- Occurs in 9,000 Americans annually

Common characteristics
- Sudden, sharp, pleuritic pain
- Pain exacerbated by chest movement
- Shortness of breath

Complications
- Pulmonary and circulatory impairment
- Death

✱ ASSESSMENT

History
- Possibly asymptomatic (with small pneumothorax)
- Sudden, sharp, pleuritic pain
- Pain that worsens with chest movement, breathing, and coughing
- Shortness of breath

Physical findings
- Asymmetrical chest wall movement
- Overexpansion and rigidity on the affected side
- Possible cyanosis
- Subcutaneous emphysema
- Hyperresonance on the affected side
- Decreased or absent breath sounds on the affected side
- Decreased tactile fremitus over the affected side

TENSION PNEUMOTHORAX
- Distended neck veins
- Pallor
- Anxiety
- Tracheal deviation away from the affected side
- Weak, rapid pulse
- Hypotension
- Tachypnea
- Cyanosis

Test results
LABORATORY
- Arterial blood gas analysis may show hypoxemia.

IMAGING
- Chest X-rays may show air in the pleural space and, possibly, a mediastinal shift.

DIAGNOSTIC PROCEDURES
- Pulse oximetry may show decreased oxygen saturation.

◆ TREATMENT

General
- Conservative treatment of spontaneous pneumothorax with no signs of increased pleural pressure, less than 30% lung collapse, and no obvious physiologic compromise
- Chest tube insertion
- Needle thoracotomy

Diet
- As tolerated

Activity
- Bed rest

Medication
- Oxygen
- Analgesics
- Doxycycline or talc instillation into pleural space

Surgery
- Thoracotomy, pleurectomy for recurring spontaneous pneumothorax
- Repair of traumatic pneumothorax

❖ NURSING CONSIDERATIONS

Nursing diagnoses
- Acute pain
- Anxiety
- Deficient knowledge (pneumothorax)
- Fear
- Impaired gas exchange
- Ineffective breathing pattern
- Ineffective coping
- Ineffective tissue perfusion: Cardio-pulmonary
- Risk for infection

Key outcomes
The patient will:
- express feelings of increased comfort and decreased pain
- identify measures to reduce anxiety
- verbalize an understanding of the disorder
- discuss fears and concerns
- maintain adequate ventilation and oxygenation
- maintain a respiratory rate within five breaths of baseline
- use support systems to assist with coping
- maintain adequate cardiopulmonary perfusion
- remain free from signs and symptoms of infection.

Nursing interventions
- Administer medications, as ordered.
- Assist with chest tube insertion.

◆ **NURSING ALERT** If the chest tube dislodges, immediately place a petroleum gauze dressing over the opening.
- Provide comfort measures.
- Encourage deep-breathing and coughing exercises.
- Offer reassurance as appropriate.
- Include the patient and family members in care decisions whenever possible.

Monitoring
- Vital signs
- Intake and output
- Respiratory status
- Breath sounds
- Chest tube system
- Complications
- Pneumothorax recurrence

◆ **NURSING ALERT** Watch for signs and symptoms of tension pneumothorax, which can be fatal. These include anxiety, hypotension, tachycardia, tachypnea, and cyanosis.

▶ PATIENT TEACHING

Be sure to cover:
- disorder, diagnostic tests, and treatment
- medication administration, dosage, and possible adverse effects
- chest tube insertion
- deep-breathing exercises
- signs and symptoms of recurrent spontaneous pneumothorax and when to notify the physician.

Discharge planning
- Refere the patient to a smoking cessation prgoram, if appropriate.
- Refer the patient to community support services, as indicated.

✴ RESOURCES

Organizations
American Lung Association: *www.lungusa.org*
National Heart, Lung and Blood Institute: *www.nhlbi.nih.gov*

Selected references
Jenner, R., and Sen, A. "Chest Drains in Traumatic Occult Pneumothorax," *Emergency Medicine Journal* 23(2):138-39, February 2006.

Ong, Y.E., et al. "Radiotherapy: A Novel Treatment for Pneumothorax," *European Respiratory Journal* 27(2):427-29, February 2006.

Trevisanuto, D., et al. "Neonatal Pneumothorax: Comparison Between Neonatal Transfers and Inborn Infants," *Journal of Perinatal Medicine* 33(5):449-54, October 2005.

Yamamoto, L., et al. "Thoracic Trauma: The Deadly Dozen," *Critical Care Nursing Quarterly* 28(1):22-40, January-March 2005.

Zhan, C., et al. "Accidental Iatrogenic Pneumothorax in Hospitalized Patients," *Medical Care* 44(2):182-86, February 2006.

Poisoning

● OVERVIEW

Description
- Contact with a harmful substance by inhalation, ingestion, injection, or skin contact
- Prognosis dependent on the amount of poison absorbed, its toxicity, and the time lapse between poisoning and treatment

Pathophysiology
- The course of the disorder varies with the type of poison.

Causes
- Accidental poisoning or overdose
- Improper cooking, canning, or storage of food
- Suicide attempt
- Homicide attempt

Risk factors
- Employment in chemical plant

Incidence
- Affects 1 million people annually; fatal in about 800 cases
- Fourth most common cause of death in children

Common characteristics
- Hypotension
- Altered neurologic status
- Changes in skin temperature and color
- Cardiopulmonary arrest

Complications
- Cardiac arrhythmias
- Seizures
- Coma and death

✳ ASSESSMENT

History
- Poison exposure
- Drug overdose

Physical findings
- Vary with type of poison; may include:
  - central nervous system depression or excitability
  - respiratory depression
  - cardiovascular depression
  - cardiovascular excitation
  - cardiac arrhythmias
  - acute renal failure
  - liver failure

Test results
LABORATORY
- Lactate levels may be increased or decreased.
- Serum calcium levels are increased.
- Serum magnesium levels are increased.
- Toxicology studies show poison levels in the patient's mouth, vomitus, urine, feces, or blood or on the patient's hands or clothing.
- Arterial blood gas values identify hypoxemia or metabolic derangements.
- Serum electrolyte levels are imbalanced, possibly revealing hypokalemia; may show anion-gap metabolic acidosis.

IMAGING
- Chest X-rays may show pulmonary infiltrates or edema in inhalation poisoning; may show aspiration pneumonia in petroleum distillate inhalation.
- Abdominal X-rays may show the presence of iron pills or other radiopaque substances.

DIAGNOSTIC PROCEDURES
- Electrocardiogram may show arrhythmias or QRS- and QT-interval prolongation.

◆ TREATMENT

General
- Emergency resuscitation as needed
- Recommendations of local poison control center
- Symptomatic care
- Airway and ventilation maintenance

Diet
- Nothing by mouth until the episode resolves

Activity
- No restrictions
- Safety measures

Medication
- Specific antidote, if available
- Activated charcoal, if appropriate
- Oxygen

NURSING CONSIDERATIONS

Nursing diagnoses
- Acute pain
- Deficient fluid volume
- Deficient knowledge (poisoning)
- Disturbed thought processes
- Impaired gas exchange
- Ineffective breathing pattern
- Risk for aspiration
- Risk for injury

Key outcomes
The patient will:
- express feelings increased comfort and decreased pain
- maintain an adequate fluid volume
- verbalize an understanding of condition and treatment
- maintain orientation to time, place, and person
- maintain adequate ventilation and oxygenation
- maintain an effective respiratory rate within acceptable parameters
- remain free of signs and symptoms of aspiration
- remain free from injury

Nursing interventions
- Perform cardiopulmonary resuscitation if needed.
- Induce emesis (unless a corrosive acid is involved).
- Perform gastric lavage and administer a cathartic as ordered.
- Provide supplemental oxygen as ordered and needed.
- Send vomitus and aspirate for analysis.
- In severe poisoning, provide peritoneal dialysis or hemodialysis.

Monitoring
- Vital signs
- Level of consciousness
- Respiratory status
- Suicidal ideations (if indicated)

PATIENT TEACHING

Be sure to cover:
- importance of reading all labels before taking medication
- proper medication and chemical storage
- dangers of taking medications prescribed for someone else
- dangers of transferring medications or chemicals from their original container
- dangers of telling children that medication is "candy"
- importance of keeping ipecac syrup available at home
- use of childproof caps on medication containers.

Discharge teaching
- Refer the patient for psychological counseling in case of suicide attempt.
- Refer the patient to the proper authorities in case of deliberate poisoning.

RESOURCES

Organizations
National Center for Injury Prevention and Control: *www.cdc.ncipc*
National Institutes of Health: *www.nih.gov*
Poison Control: *www.poisoncontrol.org*

Selected references
Balch, C. "Critical Care-Carbon Monoxide Poisoning: Too Easily Overlooked," *Nursing* 34(5):32cc10-32cc12, May 2004.

Centers for Disease Control and Prevention (CDC). "Toxicology Testing and Results for Suicide Victims—13 States, 2004," *Morbidity, Mortality Weekly Report* 55(46):1245-248, November 2006.

"Important Information You Need to Know," *Home Healthcare Nurse* 22(8):518-19, August 2004.

Kress, T., and Krueger, D. "Eye on Diagnostics: Identifying Carbon Monoxide Poisoning," *Nursing* 34(11):68-69, November 2004.

Risser, N., and Murphy, M. "Literature Review: Syrup of Ipecac Use," *The Nurse Practitioner: The American Journal of Primary Health Care* 29(3):48, March 2004.

Smith, D. "Action Stat: Methylene Chloride Inhalation," *Nursing* 36(6):90, June 2006.

White, M.L., and Liebelt, E.L. "Update on Antidotes for Pediatric Poisoning," *Pediatric Emergency Care* 22(11):747-49, November 2006.

Poliomyelitis

Description
- Acute communicable disease caused by the polio virus
- Ranges in severity from inapparent infection to fatal paralytic illness (mortality 5% to 10%)
- Excellent prognosis if central nervous system (CNS) is spared
- Also called *polio* or *infantile paralysis*

Pathophysiology
- The poliovirus has three antigenically distinct serotypes (types I, II, and III) that cause poliomyelitis.
- The incubation period ranges from 5 to 35 days (7 to 14 days on average).
- The virus usually enters the body through the alimentary tract, multiplies in the oropharynx and lower intestinal tract, and then spreads to regional lymph nodes and the blood.
- Factors that increase the risk of paralysis include pregnancy; old age; localized trauma, such as a recent tonsillectomy, tooth extraction, or inoculation; and unusual physical exertion at or just before the clinical onset of poliomyelitis.

Causes
- Contraction of the virus from direct contact with infected oropharyngeal secretions or feces

Incidence
- Minor polio outbreaks, usually among nonimmunized groups
- Onset during the summer and fall
- Mostly occurs in people over age 15
- Adults and girls at greater risk for infection; boys, for paralysis

Common characteristics
- Fever
- Muscle weakness
- Tripod positioning when sitting

Complications
- Hypertension
- Urinary tract infection
- Urolithiasis
- Atelectasis
- Pneumonia
- Myocarditis
- Cor pulmonale
- Skeletal and soft-tissue deformities
- Paralytic ileus

✳ ASSESSMENT

History
- Exposure to polio virus
- Fever

Physical findings
- Muscle weakness
- Resistance to neck flexion (nonparalytic and paralytic poliomyelitis)
- Patient "tripods" (extends his arms behind him for support) when sitting up
- Head falls back when supine and shoulders are elevated (Hoyne's sign)
- Unable to raise legs 90 degrees when in a supine position
- Kernig's and Brudzinski's signs (paralytic poliomyelitis)

Test results
LABORATORY
- Polio virus is isolated from throat washings early in the disease, from stools throughout the disease, and from cerebrospinal fluid cultures in CNS infection.
- Convalescent serum antibody titers are four times greater than acute titers.
- Tests to rule out coxsackievirus and echovirus infections must be performed.

◆ TREATMENT

General
- Supportive
- Moist heat applications

Diet
- Well-balanced diet

Activity
- As tolerated
- Physical therapy
- Assistive devices

Medication
- Analgesics
- Antipyretics

✿ NURSING CONSIDERATIONS

Nursing diagnoses
- Activity intolerance
- Delayed growth and development
- Fatigue
- Impaired gas exchange
- Impaired physical mobility
- Impaired skin integrity
- Impaired urinary elimination
- Ineffective airway clearance
- Ineffective breathing pattern
- Ineffective coping
- Interrupted family processes
- Risk for aspiration
- Risk for infection

Key outcomes
The patient (or family) will:
- demonstrate skill in conserving energy while carrying out daily activities to his tolerance level
- demonstrate age-appropriate skills and behaviors to the extent possible
- report increased energy levels
- maintain adequate ventilation and oxygenation
- retain physical mobility to the highest level possible
- maintain skin integrity
- exhibit adequate urine output by voiding spontaneously or with catheterization
- cough and expectorate mucous effectively
- maintain respiratory rate within five breaths of baseline
- demonstrate effective coping mechanisms
- agree to seek help from peer support groups or professional counselors to increase adaptive and coping behaviors
- remain free from aspiration
- remain free from further signs or symptoms of infection.

Nursing interventions
- Provide emotional support.
- Provide good skin care, reposition the patient often, and keep the bed dry.
- Maintain contact isolation.

Monitoring
- Signs of paralysis
- Respiratory status
- Vital signs
- Nutritional status

▶ PATIENT TEACHING

Be sure to cover:
- disorder, diagnostic tests, and treatment
- physical therapy
- avoiding complications of limited mobility
- proper hand-washing and contact isolation techniques.

Discharge planning
- Refer the patient to support services, as appropriate.

✹ RESOURCES

Organizations
Global Polio Eradication Initiative: *www.polioeradication.org*
National Institutes of Health: *www.nih.gov*
World Health Organization: *www.who.int*

Selected references
Huycke, L. "Postpolio Syndrome – Care in the Workplace," *AAOHN Journal* 53(11): 472-76, November 2005.

Kramasz, V.C. "Polio Patients take a Second Hit," *RN* 68(11):33-37, November 2005.

Laassri, M., et al. "Effect of Different Vaccination Schedules on Excretion of Oral Poliovirus Vaccine Strains," *Journal of Infectious Diseases* 192(12):2092-2098, December 2005.

Racaniello, V.R. "One Hundred Years of Poliovirus Pathogenesis," *Virology* 344(1):9-16, January 2006.

Polycystic kidney disease

⬤ OVERVIEW

Description
- Growth of multiple, bilateral, grape-like clusters of fluid-filled cysts in the kidneys
- May progress slowly even after renal insufficiency symptoms appear
- Has two distinct forms: *infantile* form, which causes stillbirth or early neonatal death; and *adult* form, which has insidious onset but usually becomes obvious between ages 30 and 50
- Usually fatal within 4 years of uremic symptom onset, unless dialysis begins
- Carries a widely varying prognosis in adults
- Also known as *PKD*

Pathophysiology
- Cysts enlarge the kidneys, compressing and eventually replacing functioning renal tissue.
- Renal deterioration results; deterioration is more gradual in adults than in infants.
- The condition progresses relentlessly to fatal uremia.

Causes
- Familial
- Infantile form inherited as an autosomal recessive trait
- Adult form inherited as an autosomal dominant trait

Risk factors
- 50% chance of acquiring disease with autosomal dominant PKD
- If one parent has autosomal dominant PKD, 50% chance that the disease will pass to a child
- In autosomal recessive PKD, nonaffected parents may have child with the disease if both parents carry the abnormal gene and both pass the gene to their child — one in four chance

Incidence
- Affects males and females equally
- Infantile form: 1 in 6,000 to 40,000 infants
- Adult form: 1 in 50 to 1,000 adults

Common characteristics
- Enlarged kidneys
- Signs and symptoms of renal failure

Complications
- Hepatic failure
- Renal failure
- Respiratory failure
- Heart failure
- Recurrent hematuria
- Life-threatening retroperitoneal bleeding
- Proteinuria

✱ ASSESSMENT

History
ADULT POLYCYSTIC DISEASE
- Family history
- Polyuria
- Urinary tract infections
- Headaches
- Pain in back or flank area
- Gross hematuria
- Abdominal pain, usually worsened on exertion and eased by lying down

Physical findings
INFANTILE FORM
- Pronounced epicanthal folds
- Pointed nose
- Small chin
- Floppy, low-set ears (Potter facies)
- Huge, bilateral, symmetrical flank masses that are tense and can't be transilluminated
- Signs of respiratory distress, heart failure and, eventually, uremia and renal failure
- Signs of portal hypertension (bleeding varices)

ADULT FORM
- Hypertension
- Signs of an enlarging kidney mass
- Grossly enlarged kidneys (in advanced stages)

Test results
LABORATORY
- Urinalysis may show hematuria or bacteria or protein.
- Creatinine clearance test results may show renal insufficiency or failure.
- Blood or urine tests may show sodium loss or retention.

IMAGING
- Excretory or retrograde urography reveals enlarged kidneys, with pelvic elongation, flattening of the calyces, and indentations caused by cysts. In a neonate, excretory urography shows poor excretion of contrast medium.
- Ultrasonography, tomography, and radioisotopic scans show kidney enlargement and cysts.
- Tomography, computed tomography scan, and magnetic resonance imaging show multiple areas of cystic damage.

◆ TREATMENT

General
- Monitoring of renal function
- Dialysis

Diet
- Low-protein
- Fluid restriction (in renal failure)

Activity
- Avoidance of contact sports

Medication
- Analgesics
- Antibiotics for urinary tract infection
- Antihypertensives for hypertension

Surgery
- Kidney transplantation
- Surgical drainage for cystic abscess or retroperitoneal bleeding

Nursing diagnoses

- Acute pain
- Deficient fluid volume
- Fatigue
- Impaired urinary elimination
- Ineffective coping
- Ineffective tissue perfusion: Renal
- Interrupted family processes
- Risk for infection
- Risk for injury

Key outcomes

The patient will:

- report feelings of increased comfort and decreased pain
- maintain fluid balance
- verbalize the importance of balancing activity with adequate rest periods
- demonstrate skill in managing the urinary elimination problem
- demonstrate adaptive coping behaviors
- modify lifestyle to minimize risk of decreased tissue perfusion
- discuss the impact of the patient's condition on the family unit
- remain free from signs and symptoms of infection
- remain free from injury.

Nursing interventions

- Administer medications, as ordered.
- Provide supportive care to minimize symptoms.
- Individualize patient care accordingly.

Monitoring

- Urine (for blood, cloudiness, calculi, and granules)
- Intake and output
- Electrolytes
- Vital signs
- Access site for dialysis

Be sure to cover:

- disorder, diagnostic tests, and treatment
- medication administration, dosage, and possible adverse effects
- follow-up with the physician for severe or recurring headaches
- signs and symptoms of urinary tract infection and prompt notification of the physician
- importance of blood pressure control
- possible need for dialysis or transplantation.

Discharge planning

- Refer a young adult patient or the parents of an infant with polycystic kidney disease for genetic counseling.

Organizations

American Association of Kidney Patients: *www.aakp.org*
National Institute of Diabetes & Digestive & Kidney Diseases: *www.niddk.nih.gov*
Polycystic Kidney Research Foundation: *www.pkdcure.org*

Selected references

Bisceglia, M., et al. "Renal Cystic Diseases: A Review," 13(1):26-56, January 2006.

Diseases, 4th ed. Philadelphia: Lippincott Williams & Wilkins, 2006.

Fuller, T.F., et al. "End Stage Polycystic Kidney Disease: Indications and Timing of Native Nephrectomy Relative to Kidney Transplantation," *Journal of Urology* 174(6):2284-288, December 2005.

Thiveirge, C., et al. "Overexpression of PKD1 Causes Polycystic Kidney Disease," *Molecular and Cellular Biology* 26(4);1538-548, February 2006.

Torres, V.E. "Vasopressin Antagonists in Polycystic Kidney Disease," *Kidney International* 68(5):2405-418, November 2005.

Polycystic ovarian syndrome

● OVERVIEW

Description
- Metabolic disorder characterized by multiple ovarian cysts
- Good prognosis for ovulation and fertility with appropriate treatment

Pathophysiology
- A general feature of all anovulation syndromes is a lack of pulsatile release of gonadotropin-releasing hormone.
- Initial ovarian follicle development is normal.
- Many small follicles begin to accumulate because there's no selection of a dominant follicle.
- These follicles may respond abnormally to the hormonal stimulation, causing an abnormal pattern of estrogen secretion during the menstrual cycle.
- Endocrine abnormalities may be the cause of polycystic ovarian syndrome or cystic abnormalities; muscle and adipose tissue are resistant to the effects of insulin, and lipid metabolism is abnormal.

Causes
- Exact cause unknown, but theories include:
  - abnormal enzyme activity that triggers excess androgen secretion
  - endocrine abnormalities

Incidence
- Occurs in 6% to 10% of women in the United States; 50% to 80%, of which, are obese
- Among women who seek treatment for infertility, more than 75% having some degree of polycystic ovarian syndrome, usually manifested by anovulation alone
- Affects women of reproductive age

Common characteristics
- Pelvic discomfort
- Dyspareunia

Complications
- Malignancy
- Increased risk for cardiovascular disease and type 2 diabetes mellitus
- Secondary amenorrhea
- Oligomenorrhea
- Infertility
- Addison's disease
- Ovarian atrophy

✳ ASSESSMENT

History
- Diabetes
- Mild pelvic discomfort
- Lower back pain
- Dyspareunia
- Abnormal uterine bleeding secondary to disturbed ovulatory pattern

Physical findings
- Obesity
- Hirsutism
- Acne
- Male-pattern hair loss
- Hyperpigmentation of the skin

Test results
LABORATORY
- Urinary 17-ketosteroid levels are slightly elevated.
- Anovulation
- Estrogen action is unopposed during menstrual cycle (due to anovulation).
- Ratio of luteinizing hormone to follicle-stimulating hormone is elevated (usually 3:1 or greater).
- Testosterone and androstenedione levels are elevated.

IMAGING
- Ultrasound (abdominal or transvaginal) permits visualization of the ovary, which may reveal multiple ovarian cysts.

DIAGNOSTIC PROCEDURES
- Laparoscopy provides direct visualization of cysts.

◆ TREATMENT

General
- Lifestyle modifications
- Hair removal

Diet
- Low-calorie

Activity
- Daily exercise program

Medication
- Clomiphene
- Medroxyprogesterone
- Low-dose hormonal contraceptives
- Metformin
- Antiandrogens (for hirsutism)

Surgery
- Ovarian wedge resection
- Laparoscopic surgery to create focal areas of damage in the ovarian cortex and stroma

❖ NURSING CONSIDERATIONS

Nursing diagnoses
- Acute pain
- Anxiety
- Deficient fluid volume
- Ineffective coping
- Ineffective sexuality pattern
- Risk for infection

Key outcomes
The patient will:
- report feelings of increased comfort and decreased pain
- identify strategies to reduce anxiety
- maintain a normal fluid volume
- demonstrate effective coping mechanisms
- express feelings with partner about the condition and its effect on their sexual relationship
- remain free from signs and symptoms of infection.

Nursing interventions
- Postoperatively, encourage frequent movement in bed and early ambulation.
- Provide emotional support.
- Encourage weight reduction, if appropriate.
- Provide guidelines for exercise program.

Monitoring
PREOPERATIVELY
- Signs of cyst rupture

POSTOPERATIVELY
- Vital signs
- Signs of infection

▶ PATIENT TEACHING

Be sure to cover:
- disorder, diagnostic tests, and treatment
- diabetic diet, if appropriate
- low-calorie diet
- importance of regular follow-up care.

Discharge planning
- Refer the patient to a reproductive endocrinologist.
- Refer the patient to supportive services, as appropriate.

✱ RESOURCES

Organizations
The Hormone Foundation: *www.hormone.org/learn/pcos.html*
Mayo Health Clinic: *www.mayohealth.org*
The Polycystic Ovarian Syndrome Association: *www.pcosupport.org*

Selected references
Allemand, M.C., et al. "Diagnosis of Polycystic Ovaries by Three-Dimensional Transvaginal Ultrasound," *Fertility and Sterility* 85(1):214-19, January 2006.
Franks, S., et al. "Development of Polycystic Ovary Syndrome: Involvement of Genetic and Environmental Factors," *International Journal of Andrology* 29(1):278-85, February 2006.
Lane, D.E. "Polycystic Ovary Syndrome and its Differential Diagnosis," *Obstetrical & Gynecological Survey* 61(2):125-35, February 2006.
Mohlig, M., et al. "Predictors Of Abnormal Glucose Metabolism In Women With Polycystic Ovary Syndrome," *European Journal of Endocrinology* 154(2):295-301, February 2006.
Snyder, B.S. "Polycystic Ovary Syndrome (PCOS) in the Adolescent Patient: Recommendations for Practice," *Pediatric Nursing* 31(5):416-21, September-October 2005.

Polycythemia vera

Description
- Chronic, myeloproliferative disorder of increased red blood cell (RBC) mass, leukocytosis, thrombocytosis, and increased hemoglobin concentration
- Also called *primary polycythemia, erythema, polycythemia rubra vera, splenomegalic polycythemia,* and *Vasquez-Osler disease*

Pathophysiology
- Uncontrolled and rapid cellular reproduction and maturation cause proliferation or hyperplasia of all bone marrow cells.
- Increased RBC mass makes the blood abnormally viscous and inhibits blood flow to the microcirculation.
- Diminished blood flow and thrombocytosis set the stage for intravascular thrombosis.

Causes
- Exact cause unknown

Incidence
- Onset usually between ages 50 and 70
- Most common among Jewish men, but affects all ethnic groups
- Rare in children and blacks

Common characteristics
- Joint pain
- Hypertension

Complications
- Hemorrhage
- Vascular thromboses
- Uric acid calculi
- Myelofibrosis
- Acute leukemia

History
- Vague feeling of fullness in the head or rushing in the ears
- Tinnitus
- Headache
- Dizziness, vertigo
- Epistaxis
- Night sweats
- Epigastric and joint pain
- Vision alterations, such as scotomas, double vision, and blurred vision
- Pruritus
- Abdominal fullness

Physical findings
- Congestion of the conjunctiva, retina, and retinal veins
- Oral mucous membrane congestion
- Hypertension
- Ruddy cyanosis
- Ecchymosis
- Hepatosplenomegaly

Test results
LABORATORY
- Increased uric acid level
- Increased RBC mass and normal arterial oxygen saturation confirm the diagnosis, in association with splenomegaly or two of the following:
  - platelet count above 400,000/mm³ (thrombocytopenia)
  - white blood cell count above 12,000/mm³ in adults
  - elevated leukocyte alkaline phosphatase level
  - elevated serum vitamin B_{12} levels or unbound B_{12}-binding capacity.
IMAGING
- Computed tomography of abdomen shows enlarged spleen.
DIAGNOSTIC PROCEDURES
- Bone marrow biopsy shows panmyelosis.

General
- Phlebotomy
- Pheresis
- Sequential compression stockings (if no deep vein thrombosis)

Diet
- No restrictions

Activity
- No restrictions

Medication
- Myelosuppressive agents
- Radioactive phosphorus
- Chemotherapy

Surgery
- Splenectomy, as necessary

Nursing diagnoses
- Activity intolerance
- Acute pain
- Anxiety
- Fatigue
- Imbalanced nutrition: Less than body requirements
- Ineffective tissue perfusion: Peripheral
- Risk for impaired skin integrity
- Risk for infection
- Risk for injury

Key outcomes
The patient will:
- verbalize the importance of balancing activity, as tolerated, with rest
- express feelings of increased comfort and decreased pain
- verablize measures to reduce anxiety level
- express feelings of increased energy
- maintain daily calorie requirements
- maintain strong peripheral pulses
- maintain skin integrity
- remain free from signs and symptoms of infection
- remain free from injury.

Nursing interventions
- Keep the patient active and ambulatory.

- If bed rest is necessary, implement a daily program of active and passive range-of-motion exercises.
- Encourage additional fluid intake.
- If the patient has symptomatic splenomegaly, suggest or provide small, frequent meals followed by a rest period.
- If the patient has pruritus, give medications as ordered.
- Encourage the patient to express concerns about the disease and its treatment.

◆ **NURSING ALERT** Report acute abdominal pain immediately. It may signal splenic infarction, renal calculus formation, or abdominal organ thrombosis.

DURING AND AFTER PHLEBOTOMY
- Make sure the patient is lying down comfortably. Stay alert for tachycardia, clamminess, and complaints of vertigo. If these effects occur, the procedure should be stopped.
- Immediately after phlebotomy, have the patient sit up for about 5 minutes before allowing ambulation. Administer 24 oz (710 ml) of juice or water.

DURING MYELOSUPPRESSIVE CHEMOTHERAPY
- If nausea and vomiting occur, begin antiemetic therapy and adjust the patient's diet.
- For treatment with radioactive phosphorus, obtain a blood sample for complete blood cell (CBC) count and platelet count before starting treatment. (Personnel who administer radioactive phosphorous should take radiation precautions to prevent contamination.)
- Have the patient lie down during I.V. administration and for 15 to 20 minutes afterward.

Monitoring
- Vital signs
- Adverse reactions to medications
- CBC and platelet count before and during therapy
- Complications
- Signs and symptoms of impending stroke
- Hypertension
- Signs and symptoms of heart failure
- Signs and symptoms of bleeding

▶ **PATIENT TEACHING**

Be sure to cover:
- disorder, diagnostic tests, and treatment
- importance of staying as active as possible
- use of an electric razor to prevent accidental cuts
- ways to minimize falls and contusions at home
- avoidance of high altitudes
- common bleeding sites, if the patient has thrombocytopenia
- importance of reporting abnormal bleeding promptly
- phlebotomy procedure (if scheduled) and its effects
- symptoms of iron deficiency to report
- possible adverse reactions to myelosuppressive therapy
- instructions on infection prevention for an outpatient who develops leukopenia (including avoiding crowds and watching for infection symptoms)
- radioactive phosphorus administration procedure (if scheduled) and the possible need for repeated phlebotomies
- dental care
- use of gloves (when outdoors) if the temperature is below 50° F (10° C).

Discharge planning
- Refer the patient to appropriate community support services as necessary.

✷ **RESOURCES**

Organizations
The Leukemia and Lymphoma Society: *www.leukemia. org*
Mayo Clinic: *www.mayoclinic.org*
The Merck Manuals Online Medical Library: *www.merck.com/mmhe*
National Heart, Lung and Blood Institute: *www.nhlbi.nih.gov*

Selected references
Kasper, D.L., et al., eds. *Harrison's Principles of Internal Medicine,* 16th ed. New York: McGraw-Hill Book Co., 2005.
Munson, B.I. "Myths & Facts...About Polycythemia Vera," *Nursing* 35(5):28, May 2005.
Silver, R.T. "Treatment of Polycythemia Vera with Recombinant Interferon Alpha (rIFNalpha) or Imatinib Mesylate," *Current Hematology Reports* 4(3):235-37, May 2005.
Tierney, L., et al. *Current Medical Diagnosis and Treatment 2006.* New York: McGraw-Hill Book Co., 2006.
Wu, C.F., et al. "Polycythemia Vera Presenting as ST-Elevation Myocardial Infarction," *Heart, Lung & Circulation* 14(1):51-53, March 2005.

Porphyrias

● OVERVIEW

Description
- Umbrella term for a group of metabolic disorders that affect the biosynthesis of heme (a hemoglobin component), resulting in excessive porphyrin production
- Classified by the site of excessive porphyrin production as erythropoietic, hepatic, or erythrohepatic porphyria

Pathophysiology
- Various metabolic disorders affect heme biosynthesis, leading to excessive production and excretion of porphyrins or their precursors.

Causes
- Inherited as an autosomal dominant trait, except Günther's disease (inherited as an autosomal recessive trait)
- Lead ingestion or exposure (toxic-acquired porphyria)

Risk factors
- Certain medications
- Hormonal changes
- Infection
- Malnutrition

Incidence
- More common in Whites than Blacks or Asians

Common characteristics
- Neuropsychiatric, dermatologic, and abdominal symptoms

Complications
- With erythropoietic porphyria: hemolytic anemia
- With hepatic porphyria: neurologic and hepatic dysfunction
- With acute intermittent porphyria: flaccid paralysis, respiratory paralysis, and death

✳ ASSESSMENT

History
- Mild or severe abdominal pain
- Photosensitivity
- Paresthesia, hypothesia
- Neuritic pain

Physical findings
- Wide variation, depending on the type of porphyria
- Psychosis
- Seizures
- Skin lesions
- Darkening of urine left in the light or air
- Neurologic signs of wristdrop or footdrop
- Muscle weakness
- Fever (with an acute attack)
- Splenomegaly (if hemolytic anemia is present)
- Wheezing and dyspnea (with acute intermittent porphyria)

Test results
LABORATORY
- The ion-exchange chromotography test reveals urine aminolevulinic acid.
- In acute intermittent porphyria, the Watson-Schwartz test reveals urine porphobilinogen, leukocytosis, elevated bilirubin and alkaline phosphatase levels, and hyponatremia.
- In variegate porphyria, protoporphyrin and coproporphyrin are present in stools.
- In hereditary coproporphyria, there's abundant coproporphyrin in stools and, to a lesser extent, in urine.
- In porphyria cutanea tarda, uroporphyrin excretion is increased, with varying amounts of fecal porphyrins.
- In Günther's disease, urine porphyrins are present.
- In erythropoietic protoporphyria, protoporphyrin is present in red blood cells.
- In toxic acquired porphyria, urine lead level is 0.2 mg/L or higher.
- In porphyria cutanea tarda, serum iron levels are increased.

◆ TREATMENT

General
- Avoidance of sun-exposure

Diet
- High-carbohydrate
- Fluid restriction

Activity
- As tolerated

Medication
- Betacarotene supplements
- Chlorpromazine I.V.
- Analgesics
- Hematin
- Sunscreen preparations

Surgery
- Splenectomy (in hemolytic anemia)

✤ NURSING CONSIDERATIONS

Nursing diagnoses
- Acute pain
- Constipation
- Impaired gas exchange
- Impaired skin integrity
- Risk for injury

Key outcomes
The patient will:
- express feelings of increased comfort and decreased pain
- regain normal bowel movements
- maintain adequate ventilation and oxygenation
- maintain skin integrity
- remain free from injury.

Nursing interventions:
- Check the patient's history for use of medications that can trigger an acute attack. (See *Drugs that aggravate porphyria.*)
- Administer hemin and analgesics, as ordered.
- Perform passive and active range-of-motion exercises.
- Encourage the patient to express feelings and concerns about the disease.
- Provide emotional support.

Monitoring
- Respiratory status
- GI motility
- Vital signs
- Response to treatment

▶ PATIENT TEACHING

Be sure to cover:
- disorder, diagnostic tests, and treatment
- avoidance of excessive sun exposure
- importance of wearing medical identification
- lead sources (if the patient has toxic-acquired porphyria)
- precipitating factors, including crash diets, fasting, and use of alcohol, estrogens, and barbiturates
- stress-management techniques
- ways to prevent infection
- value of a high-carbohydrate diet.

Discharge planning
- For toxic-acquired porphyria, refer the patient and family to resources that can help identify lead sources in the home.

✶ RESOURCES

Organizations
American Porphyria Foundation: *www.porphyria foundation.com*
National Organization for Rare Disorders: *www.rarediseases.org*

Selected references

Chen, H.W., et al. "Effects of Diabetes on the ED Presentation of Acute Intermittent Porphyria," *American Journal of Emergency Medicine* 23(4):571-72, July 2005.

Dombeck, T.A., and Satonik, R.C. "The Porphyrias," *Emergency Medicine Clinics of North America* 23(3):885-99, August 2005.

Herrick, A.L., and McColl, K.F. "Acute Intermittent Porphyria," *Best Practice & Research–Clinical Gastroenterology* 19(2):235-49, April 2005.

Milward, I.M., et al. "Anxiety and Depression in the Acute Porphyrias," *Journal of Inherited Metabolic Disease* 28(6):1099-1107, 2005.

DRUGS THAT AGGRAVATE PORPHYRIA

Make sure the patient with porphyria doesn't receive any of the following drugs, which are known to trigger signs and symptoms of porphyria:
- barbiturates
- carbamazepine
- carisoprodol
- chloramphenicol
- chlordiazepoxide
- danazol
- diazepam
- ergot alkaloids
- estrogens
- glutethimide
- griseofulvin
- imipramine
- meprobamate
- methsuximide
- methyldopa
- pentazocine
- phenytoin
- progesterones
- sulfonamides
- tolbutamide.

Posttraumatic stress disorder

● OVERVIEW

Description
- Development of psychological symptoms, such as intense fear and feelings of hopelessness and loss of control, after exposure to extreme trauma
- Can be acute, chronic, or delayed
- Also known as *PTSD*

Pathophysiology
- The alpha$_2$-adrenergic receptor response that inhibits stress-induced release of norepinephrine is impaired.
- Progressive behavioral sensitization results, with generalization to stimulus cues from the original trauma.
- Consequently, responses of increased sympathetic activity occur.

Causes
- An event that the patient views as traumatic (typically an event outside the range of usual human experience)

Risk factors
- History of psychopathology
- Neurotic and extroverted characteristics
- History of child abuse or neglect

Incidence
- Affects 30% of trauma victims
- Occurs in up to 15% of Americans at some time in their lives
- More common in women than men
- Occurs at any age

Common characteristics
- Detachment and loss of emotional response
- Feelings of depersonalization
- Inability to recall specific aspects of the traumatic event
- Flashbacks within dreams or thoughts when cues to the event occur
- Nightmares of the traumatic event

Complications
- Increased risk for other anxiety, mood, and substance-related disorders
- Substance abuse
- Feelings of detachment or estrangement, which may damage interpersonal relationships
- Suicide

✳ ASSESSMENT

History
- Difficulty falling or staying asleep
- Aggressive outbursts on awakening
- Panic attacks
- Phobic avoidance of situations that arouse memories of the traumatic event
- Early life experiences, interpersonal factors, military experiences, or other incidents that suggest the traumatic event
- Symptoms that began immediately or soon after the trauma (although in some cases, symptoms don't develop until months or years later)
- Pangs of painful emotions and unwelcome thoughts
- Traumatic reexperiencing of the traumatic event
- Chronic anxiety
- Rage and survivor guilt
- Use of violence to solve problems
- Depression and suicidal thoughts
- Fantasies of retaliation

Physical findings
- Emotional numbing (diminished or constricted response)
- Memory impairment
- Difficulty concentrating
- Substance abuse
- Physiologic reactivity on exposure to internal or external cues that symbolize or resemble an aspect of the traumatic event

DSM-IV-TR criteria
Diagnosis is confirmed when the patient meets the following criteria:
- Exposure to a traumatic event that included both of the following:
  - actual or threatened death or serious injury or threat to the physical integrity of self or others
  - a response of intense fear, helplessness, or horror.
- Persistent reexperiencing of this traumatic event in at least one of these criteria:
  - recurrent and intrusive distressing recollections of the event
  - recurrent distressing dreams of the event
  - flashbacks of the event

- intense psychological distress at exposure to events
- physiologic reactivity on exposure to events.
- Persistent avoidance of stimuli associated with the trauma, or numbing of general responsiveness not present before the trauma, as indicated by at least three of these criteria:
  - efforts to avoid thoughts or feelings associated with the traumatic event
  - efforts to avoid activities or situations that arouse recollections of the traumatic event
  - inability to recall an important aspect of the event
  - sharply decreased interest in significant activities
  - feeling of detachment or estrangement from others
  - restricted range of affect
  - sense of a foreshortened future.
- Persistent symptoms of increased arousal (not previously present) as indicated by two or more of these criteria:
  - difficulty falling or staying asleep
  - irritability or outbursts of anger
  - difficulty concentrating
  - hypervigilance
  - exaggerated startle response.

The disturbance must have lasted at least 1 month and must cause significant distress or impairment of social, occupational, or other important areas of functioning.

◆ TREATMENT

General
- Supportive or expressive psychotherapy
- Behavior therapies
- Support groups
- Rehabilitation programs in physical, social, and occupational areas
- Treatment of alcohol or drug abuse, as needed
- Active avoidance of stimuli that trigger memories of the traumatic event

Diet
- No restrictions

Activity
- No restrictions

Medication

- Benzodiazepines (short-term use)
- Tricyclic antidepressants
- Monoamine oxidase inhibitors
- Selective serotonin-reuptake inhibitors
- Sedating antidepressants
- Anticonvulsants

❖ NURSING CONSIDERATIONS

Nursing diagnoses

- Anxiety
- Chronic low self-esteem
- Disturbed personal identity
- Disturbed sleep pattern
- Fear
- Impaired social interaction
- Ineffective coping
- Ineffective role performance
- Powerlessness
- Risk for posttrauma syndrome

Key outcomes

The patient will:

- verbalize strategies to reduce anxiety
- use available support systems
- express feelings related to personal identity
- report feeling well-rested
- use effective coping mechanisms to reduce fear
- maintain or reestablish adaptive social interactions with family members
- use effective coping mechanisms
- resume usual roles and responsibilities
- participate in self-care and the decision-making process
- express feelings and fears related to the traumatic event.

Nursing interventions

- Encourage the patient to express feelings of grief, mourning, and anger.
- Practice crisis intervention techniques, as needed.
- Assume a positive, consistent, honest, and nonjudgmental attitude.
- Help the patient evaluate behavior.

Monitoring

- Response to drug therapy
- Suicidal tendencies or thoughts

▶ PATIENT TEACHING

Be sure to cover:

- disorder, diagnostic tests, and treatment
- healing process
- importance of identifying and avoiding cues that worsen symptoms
- problem-solving skills
- relaxation and breathing techniques
- medication administration, dosage, and possible adverse effects.

Discharge planning

Refer the patient to:

- support services
- psychotherapy
- physical, social, and occupational rehabilitation programs, as indicated
- drug treatment programs, as appropriate.

✱ RESOURCES

Organizations

American Psychiatric Association: *www.helping.apa.org*
American Psychological association: *www.psych.org*
National Center for Posttraumatic Stress Disorder: *www.ncptsd.org*

Selected references

Diagnostic and Statistical Manual of Mental Disorders, Fourth Edition, Text Revision. Washington, D.C.: American Psychiatric Association, 2000.

Gross, R., and Neria, Y. "Posttraumatic Stress among Survivors of Bioterrorism," *JAMA* 292(5):566, August 2004.

Kashdan, T.B., et al. "Anhedonia and Emotional Numbing in Combat Veterans with PTSD," *Behaviour Research and Therapy* 44(3):457-56, March 2006.

Kasper, D.L,. et al., eds. *Harrison's Principles of Internal Medicine,* 16th ed. New York: McGraw-Hill Book Co., 2005.

Olszewski, T.M., and Varrasse, J.F. "The Neurology of PTSD: Implications for Nurses," *Journal of Psychosocial Nursing and Mental Health Services* 43(6):40-47, June 2005.

Premenstrual syndrome

● OVERVIEW

Description
- Group of somatic, behavioral, cognitive, and mood-related symptoms occurring 1 to 14 days before menses and usually subsiding with menses onset
- Causes effects that range from minimal discomfort to severe, disruptive symptoms
- Also known as *PMS*
- Severe form known as *premenstrual dysphoric disorder (PMDD)* (see *Premenstrual dysphoric disorder*)

Pathophysiology
- PMS may result from a progesterone deficiency during the luteal phase of the ovarian cycle.
- Hormone levels and patterns in women with PMS don't differ significantly from women who don't experience PMS.

Causes
- Physiologic, psychological, and sociocultural factors
- Possible progesterone deficiency in the luteal phase
- Possible serotonin or norepinephrine deficiency

Incidence
- Affects 30% of women in the United States
- Moderate to severe symptoms that occur in 14% to 88% of adolescent girls
- Usually occurs between ages 25 and 45
- Affects women in their 40s most severely
- Resolves completely at menopause

Common characteristics
- Anxiety
- Irritability
- Depression
- Multiple somatic complaints

Complications
- Psychosocial problems
- Reduced self-esteem
- Depression
- Inability to function (in PMDD)

✳ ASSESSMENT

History
- Behavioral changes
- Breast tenderness or swelling
- Abdominal tenderness or bloating
- Joint pain
- Headache
- Edema
- Diarrhea or constipation
- Exacerbations of skin, respiratory, or neurologic problems
- Lower back pain

Physical findings
- Possible edema

Test results
LABORATORY
- Blood studies rule out anemia, thyroid disease, or other hormonal imbalances.
DIAGNOSTIC PROCEDURES
- A daily symptom calendar aids diagnosis of PMS.
- Psychological evaluation may be used to rule out or detect an underlying psychiatric disorder.

◆ TREATMENT

General
- Symptom relief
- Stress reduction
- Relaxation techniques

Diet
- Low in simple sugars
- Low in caffeine intake
- Low-sodium
- Low-fat
- Increased calcium and complex carbohydrate intake

Activity
- Aerobic exercise

Medication
- Antidepressants
- Vitamins (such as B complex)
- Progestins
- Prostaglandin inhibitors
- Monophasic birth control pills
- Nonsteroidal anti-inflammatory drugs
- Pituitary-ovarian axis supplements
- Gonadotropin-releasing hormone agonists

PREMENSTRUAL DYSPHORIC DISORDER

Premenstrual dysphoric disorder (PMDD) is a severe form of premenstrual syndrome (PMS) that has a cyclical occurrence of psychiatric symptoms that starts after ovulation (usually the week before the onset of menstruation) and ends within the first day or two of menses. Its underlying cause and pathophysiology remain unclear. However, researchers theorize that normal cyclic changes in the body cause abnormal responses to neurotransmitters, such as serotonin, resulting in physical and behavioral signs and symptoms.

PMDD affects as many as 1 in 20 American women who have regular menstrual periods. It's unclear why some women are affected whereas others aren't.

How PMDD and PMS differ
PMDD is characterized by severe monthly mood swings and physical signs and symptoms that interfere with everyday life. Compared with PMS, its signs and symptoms are abnormal and unmanageable. Although depression, anxiety, and sadness are common with PMS, in patients with PMDD, these symptoms are extreme. Some women may feel the urge to hurt or kill themselves or others.

The *DSM-IV-TR* sets these criteria for diagnosing PMDD:
- functional impairment
- predominant mood symptoms, with one being affective
- symptoms beginning 1 week before the onset of menstruation
- symptoms that don't result from any underlying primary mood disorder.

In addition, at least five of the following symptoms must be present:
- appetite changes
- decreased interests
- difficulty concentrating
- fatigue
- feelings of being overwhelmed
- insomnia or hypersomnia
- irritability
- "low mood"
- mood swings
- physical symptoms
- tension.

Nursing diagnoses
- Acute pain
- Anxiety
- Disturbed body image
- Excess fluid volume
- Hopelessness
- Impaired social interaction
- Ineffective coping
- Ineffective role performance
- Inefective sexuality patterns
- Interrupted family processes
- Situational low self-esteem

Key outcomes
The patient will:
- express feelings of increased comfort and decreased pain
- identify strategies to reduce anxiety
- express positive feelings about self
- maintain a normal fluid balance
- become actively involved in planning own care
- use available support systems, such as family, friends, and groups, to develop and maintain effective coping skills
- identify effective and ineffective coping skills
- resume usual roles and responsibilities
- express the effects of the condition on sexuality patterns
- express the effects of the condition on the family unit
- express feelings about self-esteem.

Nursing interventions
- Encourage adequate fluid intake.
- Provide comfort measures.
- Offer emotional support and reassurance.
- Encourage the patient to express feelings.
- Help the patient develop effective coping strategies.
- Urge the patient to chart symptoms daily for two cycles.

Monitoring
- Response to treatment
- Coping skills

Be sure to cover:
- disorder, diagnostic tests, and treatment
- physiologic basis of PMS
- beneficial lifestyle changes
- relaxation and stress-reduction techniques
- dietary management.

Discharge planning
- Refer the patient to a self-help group for women with PMS.
- Refer the patient for psychological counseling, as indicated.
- Refer the patient to a dietitian, as needed.

Organizations
American College of Obstetricians and Gynecologists: *www.acog.org*
National Association for Premenstrual Syndrome: *www.pms.org.uk*
Women's Health America: *www.womenshealth.com*

Selected references
Chou, P.B., and Morse, C.A. "Understanding Premenstrual Syndrome from a Chinese Medicine perspective," *Journal of Alternative and Complementary Medicine* 11(92)355-61, April 2005.

Dowd, S.M. "Premenstrual Dysphoric Disorder. A Clinical Trial Approach to Assessment," *Advance for Nurse Practitioners* 13(2):57-59, February 2005.

Martin, V.T., et al. "Symptoms of Premenstrual Syndrome and Their Association with Migraine Headache," *Headache* 46(1):125-37, January 2006.

Steiner, M., et al. "Expert Guidelines for the Treatment of Severe PMS, PMDD, and Comorbidities: The Role of SSRIs," *Journal of Women's Health* 15(1):57-69, January-February 2006.

Pressure ulcers

Description
- Localized areas of ischemic tissue caused by pressure, shearing, or friction
- Most common over bony prominences, especially the sacrum, ischial tuberosities, greater trochanter, heels, malleoli, and elbows
- May be superficial, caused by localized skin irritation (with subsequent surface maceration), or deep, arising in underlying tissue (may go undetected until they penetrate the skin)
- Also called *decubitus ulcers, pressure sores,* or *bedsores*

Pathophysiology
- Impaired skin capillary pressure results in local tissue anoxia.
- Anoxia leads to edema and multiple capillary thromboses.
- An inflammatory reaction results in ulceration and necrosis of ischemic cells.

Causes
- Local tissue compression
- Shearing force
- Friction

Risk factors
- Poor nutrition
- Diabetes mellitus
- Immobility or paralysis
- Cardiovascular disorders
- Advanced age
- Incontinence
- Obesity
- Edema
- Anemia
- Poor hygiene
- Exposure to chemicals
- Steroids

Incidence
- Affect roughly 10% of hospitalized patients and 20% to 40% of patients in long-term care facilities

Common characteristics
- Vary with the ulcer stage (see *Stages of pressure ulcers*)

Complications
- Secondary bacterial infection
- Septicemia
- Gangrene

History
- One or more risk factors

Physical findings
- Shiny, erythematous superficial lesion (early)
- Small blisters or erosions with progression of superficial erythema
- Possible necrosis and ulceration with deeper erosions and ulcerations
- Malodorous, purulent discharge (suggesting secondary bacterial infection)

STAGES OF PRESSURE ULCERS

The National Pressure Ulcer Advisory Panel has updated the staging of pressure ulcers to include the original four stages but also has added two other stages.

Suspected deep tissue injury
Suspected deep tissue injury involves maroon or purple intact skin or a blood-filled blister due to damage from shearing or pressure on the underlying soft tissue. Before the discoloration occurs, the area may be painful, mushy or firm or boggy, warmer or cooler as compared to other tissue.

Stage I
A stage I pressure ulcer is an area of intact skin that does not blanch and is usually over a bony prominence. Skin that is darkly pigmented may not show blanching but its color may differ from surrounding area. The area may be painful, firm or soft, or warmer or cooler when compared to the surrounding tissue.

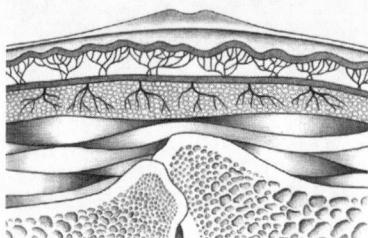

Stage II
A stage II pressure ulcer is a superficial partial-thickness wound that presents clinically a shallow and open ulcer without slough and with a red and pink wound bed. This term should not be used to describe perineal dermatitis, maceration, tape burns, skin tears or excoriation. n abrasion, a blister, or a shallow crater involving the epidermis and dermis.

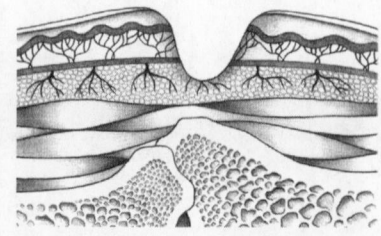

Stage III
A stage III pressure ulcer is a full-thickness wound with tissue loss. The subcutaneous tissue may be visible but muscle, tendon or bone is not exposed. Slough may be present but it does not hide the depth of the tissue loss. Undermining and tunneling may be present.

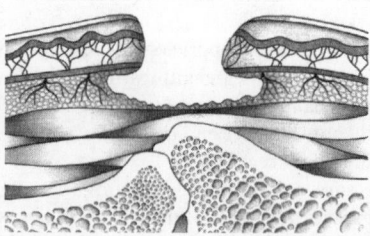

Stage IV
A stage IV pressure ulcer involves full-thickness skin loss with exposed muscle, bone, and tendon. Eschar and sloughing may be present as well as undermining and tunneling.

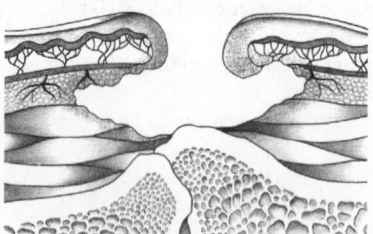

Unstageable
An unstageable pressure ulcer involves full thickness tissue loss. The base of the ulcer is covered by yellow, tan, gray, green, or brown slough or tan, brown or black eschar. Some may have both slough and eschar. The pressure cannot be staged until enough eschar or slough is removed to expose the base of the wound.

- Black eschar around and over the lesion

Test results
- Diagnosis is typically based on physical inspection.

LABORATORY
- Infecting organism is identified by wound culture and sensitivity testing of exudate.
- Total serum protein is decreased.

◆ TREATMENT

General
- Measures to prevent pressure ulcers
- Relief of pressure on the affected area
- Meticulous skin care
- Devices such as pads, mattresses, and special beds
- Moist wound therapy dressings
- Gelatin-type wafers
- Whirlpool baths
- Granular and absorbent dressings

Diet
- High in protein, iron, and vitamin C (unless contraindicated)

Activity
- As tolerated
- Active and passive range-of-motion (ROM) exercises
- Frequent turning and repositioning

Medication
- Enzymatic ointments
- Healing ointments
- Antibiotics, if indicated

Surgery
- Debridement of necrotic tissue
- Skin grafting (in severe cases)

❖ NURSING CONSIDERATIONS

Nursing diagnoses
- Imbalanced nutrition: Less than body requirements
- Impaired physical mobility
- Impaired skin integrity
- Impaired tissue integrity
- Risk for infection

Key outcomes
The patient will:
- maintain adequate daily calorie intake
- maintain joint mobility and ROM
- exhibit signs indicating improved or healed lesions or wounds
- demonstrate reduced redness, swelling, and pain at impaired tissue site
- remain free from infection.

Nursing interventions
- Administer medications, as ordered.
- Apply dressings appropriate for the ulcer stage.
- Encourage adequate food and fluid intake.
- Reposition the bedridden patient at least every 2 hours.
- Elevate the head of the bed 30 degrees or less.
- Perform passive ROM exercises.
- Encourage active ROM exercises if possible.
- Use pressure-relief aids on the bed.
- Provide meticulous skin care.

Monitoring
- Changes in skin color, turgor, temperature, and sensation
- Change in the ulcer stage
- Laboratory results
- Complications
- Response to treatment
- Intake and output

▶ PATIENT TEACHING

Be sure to cover:
- disorder, diagnostic tests, and treatment
- techniques for changing positions
- active and passive ROM exercises
- proper hygiene
- avoidance of skin-damaging agents
- debridement procedures
- skin graft surgery, if required
- signs and stages of healing
- importance of a well-balanced diet and adequate fluid intake
- medication administration, dosage, and possible adverse effects
- importance of notifying the physician immediately of signs and symptoms of infection.

Discharge planning
- Refer the patient to a wound care specialist if indicated.

✴ RESOURCES

Organizations
American Academy of Dermatology: *www.aad.org*
Dermatology Foundation: *www.dermfnd.org*
National Decubitus Foundation: *www.decubitus.org*
U.S. Agency for Healthcare Research and Quality (Clinical Practice Guidelines): *www.ahcpr.gov/clinic/cpgonline.htm*

Selected references
Domini, L.M., et al. "Nutritional Status and Evolution of Pressure Sores in Geriatric Patients," *Journal of Nutrition, Health & Aging* 9(6):446-54, November-December 2005.

Jones, J. "Evaluation of Pressure Ulcer Prevention Devices: A Critical Review of the Literature," *Journal of Wound Care* 14(9):422-25, October 2005.

Lepisto, M., et al. "Developing a Pressure Ulcer Risk Assessment Scale for Patients in Long-Term Care," *Ostomy/Wound Management* 52(2):34-46, February 2006.

Moore, Z. "Pressure Ulcer Grading," *Nursing Standard* 19(52):56-64, September 2005.

Thomas, D.R. "Prevention and Treatment of Pressure Ulcers," *Journal of the American Medical Directors Association* 7(1):46-59, January-February 2006.

Prostatic cancer

● OVERVIEW

Description
- Usually takes the form of adenocarcinoma, and typically originates in the posterior prostate gland
- May progress to widespread bone metastases and death
- Leading cause of cancer deaths in men

Pathophysiology
- Slow-growing prostatic cancer seldom causes signs and symptoms until it's well advanced.
- Typically, when a primary prostatic lesion spreads beyond the prostate gland, it invades the prostatic capsule and spreads along ejaculatory ducts in the space between the seminal vesicles or perivesicular fascia.
- Endocrine factors may play a role, leading researchers to suspect that androgens speed tumor growth.
- Malignant prostatic tumors seldom result from the benign hyperplastic enlargement that commonly develops around the prostatic urethra in older men.

Causes
- Exact cause unknown

Risk factors
- Over age 40
- Infection
- Vasectomy
- Family history
- Heavy metal exposure

Common characteristics
- Urinary problems

Incidence
- Most common among Blacks; least common among Asians
- Incidence not affected by socioeconomic status or fertility
- Most common neoplasm in men over age 50

Complications
- Spinal cord compression
- Deep vein thrombosis
- Pulmonary emboli
- Myelophthisis
- Death

✳ ASSESSMENT

History
- Symptoms rare in early stages
- Later, urinary problems, such as difficulty initiating a urinary stream, dribbling, and urine retention

Physical findings
- In early stages: nonraised, firm, nodular mass with a sharp edge
- In advanced disease: edema of the scrotum or leg; a hard lump in the prostate region

Test results
LABORATORY
- Serum prostate-specific antigen (PSA) level is elevated (may indicate cancer with or without metastases).

IMAGING
- Transrectal prostatic ultrasonography shows prostate size and presence of abnormal growths.
- Bone scan and excretory urography can determine the extent of disease.
- Magnetic resonance imaging and computed tomography scan can define the extent of the tumor.

DIAGNOSTIC PROCEDURES
- Standard screening testis the digital rectal examination (recommended yearly by the American Cancer Society for men over age 40).

◆ TREATMENT

General
- Varies with cancer stage
- Radiation therapy or internal beam radiation

Diet
- Well-balanced; no restrictions

Activity
- As tolerated

Medication
- Hormonal therapy
- Chemotherapy

Surgery
- Prostatectomy
- Orchiectomy
- Radical prostatectomy
- Transurethral resection of prostate
- Crysosurgical ablation

❖ NURSING CONSIDERATIONS

Nursing diagnoses
- Acute pain
- Antcipatory grieving
- Anxiety
- Fear
- Impaired urinary elimination
- Ineffective coping
- Risk for infection
- Sexual dysfunction

Key outcomes
The patient will:
- express felings of increased comfort and decreased pain
- verbalize feelings related to diagnosis and potential loss
- use support systems to assist with anxiety and fear
- verbalize fears and concerns
- maintain an adequate urine output
- demonstrate effective coping mechanisms
- remain free from signs and symptoms of infection
- express feelings about potential or actual changes in sexual activity.

Nursing interventions
- Administer medications, as ordered.
- Encourage the patient to express his feelings.
- Provide emotional support.

Monitoring
- Pain level
- Wound site
- Postoperative complications
- Medication effects

▶ PATIENT TEACHING

Be sure to cover:
- disorder, diagnostic tests, and treatment
- perineal exercises that decrease incontinence
- follow-up care
- medication administration, dosage, and possible adverse effects.

Discharge planning
- Refer the patient to appropriate resources and support services.

✴ RESOURCES

Organizations
American Cancer Society: *www.cancer.org*
Guide to Internet Resources for Cancer: *www.cancerindex.org*
National Cancer Institute: *www.nci.org*

Selected references
Atlas of Pathophysiology, 2nd ed. Philadelphia: Lippincott Williams & Wilkins, 2005.

Baillargeon, J., and Rose, D.P. "Obesity, Adipokines, and Prostate Cancer (Review)," *International Journal of Oncology,* 28(3):737-45, March 2006.

Mitchell, R.E., et al. "Does Year of Radical Prostatectomy Independently Predict Outcomes in Prostate Cancer?" *Urology* 67(2):368-72, February 2006.

Nishiyama, T., et al. "Stepping Stone to the Further Advancement of Androgen-Deprivation Therapy for Prostate Cancer," *Expert Review of Anticancer Therapy* 6(2):259-68, February 2006.

Yu, G., et al. "CSRI Suppresses Tumor Growth and Metastasis of Prostate Cancer," *American Journal of Pathology* 168(2):597-607, February 2006.

Prostatitis

● OVERVIEW

Description
- Inflammation of the prostate gland
- Occurs in acute, chronic, and several other forms

ACUTE PROSTATITIS
- Easily recognized and treated

CHRONIC PROSTATITIS
- Most common cause of recurrent urinary tract infection in men
- More difficult to recognize than acute prostatitis

OTHER PROSTATITIS FORMS
- Granulomatous prostatitis (also called *tuberculous prostatitis)*
- Nonbacterial prostatitis
- Prostatodynia (painful prostate)

Pathophysiology
- Infectious organism spreads to the prostate gland by the hematogenous route, an ascending urethral infection, invasion of rectal bacteria via lymphatic vessels, or reflux of infected bladder urine into prostate ducts.
- Inflammation results.

Causes
- Bacterial prostatitis: *Escherichia coli* (80% of cases); *Klebsiella, Enterobacter, Proteus, Pseudomonas, Serratia, Streptococcus, Staphylococcus,* and diphtheroids (20% of cases)
- Chronic prostatitis: bacterial invasion from urethra
- Granulomatous prostatitis: miliary spread of *Mycobacterium tuberculosis*
- Nonbacterial prostatitis: *Mycoplasma, Ureaplasma, Chlamydia,* or *Trichomonas vaginalis* or a virus
- Prostatodynia: exact cause unknown

Risk factors
- Invasive urethral procedures
- Infrequent or excessive sexual intercourse

Incidence
CHRONIC PROSTATITIS
- Affects up to 35% of men over age 50
- Seen in 5 of every 1,000 outpatient visits

BACTERIAL PROSTATITIS
- Seen in 2 of every 10,000 outpatient visits

NONBACTERIAL PROSTATITIS
- Seen in 5 of every 10,000 outpatient visits

Common characteristics
- Urinary frequency and urgency
- Fever

Complications
- Urinary tract infection
- Prostatic abscess
- Acute urinary retention
- Pyelonephritis
- Epididymitis

✳ ASSESSMENT

History
- Sudden fever, chills
- Lower back pain
- Perineal fullness
- Arthralgia, myalgia
- Urinary urgency and frequency
- Dysuria, nocturia
- Transient erectile dysfunction

CHRONIC PROSTATITIS
- May be asymptomatic
- Usually causes same urinary symptoms as the acute form, but to a lesser degree
- Hemospermia
- Persistent urethral discharge
- Painful ejaculation

NONBACTERIAL PROSTATITIS
- Dysuria
- Mild perineal or lower back pain
- Frequent nocturia

PROSTATODYNIA
- Perineal, lower back, or pelvic pain

Physical findings
- Cloudy urine
- Distended bladder
- Prostatic tenderness, induration, swelling, firmness, and warmth
- Crepitation (if prostatic calculi are present)

CHRONIC PROSTATITIS
- Stony, hard induration of the prostate

Test results
LABORATORY
- Infectious organism is identified by urine culture.
- In nonbacterial prostatitis, inflammatory cells are found in smears of prostatic secretion.
- In prostatodynia, urine cultures are negative and absence of inflammatory cells are found in smears of prostatic secretions.

DIAGNOSTIC PROCEDURES
- In granulomatous prostatitis, prostate tissue biopsy shows *M. tuberculosis.*
- Urodynamic evaluation reveals detrusor hyperreflexia and pelvic floor myalgia (from chronic spasms).
- Rectal examination findings may suggest prostatitis.

◆ TREATMENT

General
- Sitz baths
- Prostatic massage

Diet
- Increased oral fluids

Activity
- Best until the condition improves
- Regular, protected sexual intercourse

AFTER SURGERY
- Avoidance of lifting, strenuous exercise, and long automobile rides
- Avoidance of sexual activity for several weeks after discharge

Medication
- Analgesics
- Antipyretics

ACUTE PROSTATITIS
- Systemic antibiotics

CHRONIC PROSTATITIS
- Oral antibiotics

GRANULOMATOUS PROSTATITIS
- Antitubercular drug combinations

NONBACTERIAL PROSTATITIS
- Oral antibiotics
- Anticholinergics

PROSTATODYNIA
- Muscle relaxants
- Alpha-adrenergic blocking agents

Surgery
- Transurethral resection of the prostate or total prostatectomy, if drug therapy unsuccessful

❖ NURSING CONSIDERATIONS

Nursing diagnoses
- Acute pain
- Impaired urinary elimination
- Ineffective coping
- Ineffective sexuality patterns
- Risk for infection
- Sexual dysfunction
- Situational low self-esteem

Key outcomes
The patient will:
- express feelings of increased comfort and decreased pain
- demonstrate skill in managing urinary elimination problems
- use available counseling, referrals, or support groups for coping
- resume sexual activity to the fullest extent possiblet
- remain free from signs and symptoms of infection
- express feelings about potential or actual changes in sexual activity
- express feelings related to self-esteem.

Nursing interventions
- Administer medications, as ordered.
- Ensure bed rest and adequate hydration.
- Administer sitz baths, as ordered.
- Avoid rectal examinations.

Monitoring
AFTER SURGERY
- Intake and output
- Catheter function and drainage
- Signs of infection
- Pain control

▶ PATIENT TEACHING

Be sure to cover:
- disorder, diagnostic tests, and treatment
- medication administration, dosage, and possible adverse effects
- importance of increased fluid intake
- benefits of regular sexual activity (with chronic prostatitis)
- prescribed activity limits
- importance of getting immediate medical attention for fever, inability to void, or bloody urine.

Discharge planning
- Refer the patient to appropriate community support services, as indicated.

✳ RESOURCES

Organizations
American Association of Kidney Patients: *www.aakp.org*
National Institute of Diabetes & Digestive & Kidney Diseases: *www.niddk.nih.gov*

Selected references
Chen, W.M., et al. "Combination Regimen in the Treatment of Chronic Prostatitis," *Archives of Andrology* 52(2):117-21, March-April 2006.
Diseases, 4th ed. Philadelphia: Lippincott Williams & Wilkins, 2006.
Habermacher, G.M., et al. "Prostatitis/Chronic Pelvic Pain Syndrome," *Annual Review of Medicine* 57:195-206, 2006.
Propert, K.J., et al. "A Prospective Study of Symptoms and Quality of Life in Men with Chronic Prostatitis/Chronic Pelvic Pain Syndrome: The National Institutes of Health Chronic Prostatitis Cohort Study," *Journal of Urology* 175(2):619-23, February 2006.

Psoriasis

● OVERVIEW

Description
- Hereditary chronic skin disease marked by epidermal proliferation
- Causes lesions of erythematous papules and plaques covered with silvery scales; lesions varying widely in severity and distribution
- Involves recurring remissions and exacerbations
- Exacerbations unpredictable, but usually can be controlled with therapy

Pathophysiology
- Psoriatic skin cells have a shortened maturation time as they migrate from the basal membrane to the surface or stratum corneum.
- As a result, the stratum corneum develops thick, scaly plaques (the cardinal manifestation of psoriasis).

Causes
- Genetic predisposition
- Possible autoimmune process
- Physical trauma
- Beta-hemolytic streptococci infection

Risk factors
- Pregnancy
- Endocrine changes
- Cold weather
- Emotional stress

Incidence
- Affects about 2% of the U.S. population
- Affects males and females equally
- Can occur at any age
- More frequent among whites
- Two periods of onset: early (young adulthood) and late (middle adulthood)

Common characteristics
- Silvery scales on red plaques
- Pruritus
- Knee-elbow-scalp distribution

Complications
- Infection
- Altered self-image
- Social isolation
- Depression

✳ ASSESSMENT

History
- Family history of psoriasis
- Risk factors
- Pruritus and burning
- Arthritic symptoms such as morning joint stiffness
- Remissions and exacerbations

Physical findings
- Erythematous, well-demarcated papules and plaques covered with silver scales, typically appearing on the scalp, chest, elbows, knees, back, and buttocks
- In mild psoriasis: plaques scattered over a small skin area
- In moderate psoriasis: plaques more numerous and larger (up to several centimeters in diameter)
- In severe psoriasis: plaques covering at least half the body
- Friable or adherent scales
- Fine bleeding points or Auspitz sign after attempts to remove scales
- Thin, erythematous guttate lesions, alone or with plaques, and with few scales (see *Identifying types of psoriasis*)
- Small indentations or pits, and yellow or brown discoloration of fingernails or toenails
- In severe cases, separation of nail from nail bed

Test results
LABORATORY
- Serum uric acid level is elevated.
- In early-onset familial psoriasis, human leukocyte antigens Cw6, B13, and Bw-57 are preset.
DIAGNOSTIC PROCEDURES
- Skin biopsy helps rule out other diseases.

◆ TREATMENT

General
- Dependent on the psoriasis type, extent, and effect on the patient's quality of life
- Lesion management
- Lukewarm baths
- Ultraviolet B light or natural sunlight
- Smoking cessation
- Avoidance of aggravating medications

Diet
- No alcohol

Activity
- No restrictions

Medication
- Topical corticosteroid creams and ointments
- Antihistamines
- Analgesics
- Nonsteroidal anti-inflammatory agents
- Occlusive ointment bases
- Urea or salicylic acid preparations
- Coal tar preparations
- Vitamin D analogs
- Emollients
- Kerolytic agents
- Methotrexate for severe, unresponsive psoriasis
- Potent retinoic acid derivative for resistant psoriasis
- Cyclosporine for severe, widespread psoriasis

Surgery
- Surgical nail removal to treat severely disfigured or damaged nails caused by psoriasis

Nursing diagnoses
- Acute pain
- Disturbed body image
- Impaired skin integrity
- Ineffective therapeutic regimen management
- Powerlessness
- Social isolation

Key outcomes
The patient will:
- report feelings of increased comfort and decreased pain
- verbalize feelings about changed body image
- exhibit improved or healed lesions
- demonstrate understanding of proper skin care
- express feelings of control over his condition and well-being
- maintain family and peer relationships.

Nursing interventions
- Administer medications, as ordered.
- Apply topical medications using a downward motion.
- Encourage the patient to verbalize his feelings.
- Provide emotional support.
- Involve family members in the treatment regimen.

Monitoring
- Response to treatment
- Lipid profile results
- Liver function tests
- Renal function
- Blood pressure
- Signs and symptoms of hepatic or bone marrow toxicity

Be sure to cover:
- disorder, diagnostic tests, and treatment
- risk factors
- incommunicability of psoriasis
- likelihood of exacerbations and remissions
- medication administration, dosage, and possible adverse effects
- how to apply prescribed ointments, creams, and lotions
- importance of avoiding scratching plaques
- measures to relieve pruritus
- importance of avoiding sun exposure
- stress-reduction techniques
- safety precautions
- relationship between psoriasis and arthritis
- when to notify the physician.

Discharge planning
- Refer the patient to the National Psoriasis Foundation.

Organizations
National Psoriasis Foundation:
  www.psoriasis.org
The Psoriasis Association:
  www.psoriasis-association.org.uk
Psoriasis Support:
  www.psoriassupport.com

Selected references
Cooper, M. "Diseases of the Epidermis: Psoriasis," *Dermatology Nursing* 17(5):381, October 2005.

Melton, L.P. "Psoriasis in the War Zone," *AJN* 105(3):52-56, March 2005.

Nemeth, M., et al. "Psoriatic Arthritis: A Holistic Approach to Management," *Advance for Nurse Practitioners* 13(11):29-34, November 2005.

Van de Kerkhof, P.C. "Perceptions on the Treatment of Psoriasis," *Journal of Dermatological Treatment* 16(5-6):255-56, 2005.

IDENTIFYING TYPES OF PSORIASIS

Psoriasis occurs in various forms, ranging from one or two localized plaques that seldom require long-term medical attention to widespread lesions and crippling arthritis.

Erythrodermic psoriasis
This type is marked by extensive flushing all over the body, which may result in scaling. The rash may develop rapidly, signaling new psoriasis or gradually in chronic psoriasis. Sometimes the rash occurs as an adverse drug reaction.

Guttate psoriasis
This type typically affects children and young adults. Erupting in drop-sized plaques over the trunk, arms, legs and, sometimes, the scalp, this rash generalizes in several days. It's commonly associated with upper respiratory streptococcal infections.

Inverse psoriasis
Smooth, dry, bright red plaques characterize inverse psoriasis. Located in skin folds (armpits and groin, for example), the plaques fissure easily.

Psoriasis vulgaris
This psoriasis type is the most common. It begins with red, dotlike lesions that gradually enlarge and produce dry, silvery scales. The plaques usually appear symmetrically on the knees, elbows, extremities, genitalia, scalp, and nails.

Pustular psoriasis
This type features an eruption of local or extensive small, raised, pus-filled plaques. Possible triggers include emotional stress, sweating, infections, and adverse drug reactions.

Pulmonary edema

● OVERVIEW

Description
- Accumulation of fluid in the extravascular spaces of the lung
- Common complication of cardiovascular disorders
- May be chronic or acute
- Can become fatal rapidly

Pathophysiology
- Pulmonary edema results from either increased pulmonary capillary hydrostatic pressure or decreased colloid osmotic pressure. Normally, the two pressures are in balance.
- If pulmonary capillary hydrostatic pressure increases, the compromised left ventricle needs higher filling pressures to maintain adequate output; these pressures are transmitted to the left atrium, pulmonary veins, and pulmonary capillary bed. Fluids and solutes are then forced from the intravascular compartment into the lung interstitium. With fluid overloading the interstitium, some fluid floods peripheral alveoli and impairs gas exchange.
- If colloid osmotic pressure decreases, the pulling force that contains intravascular fluids is lost, and nothing opposes the hydrostatic force. Fluid flows freely into the interstitium and alveoli, causing pulmonary edema.

Causes
- Cardiac disease or injury
- Pulmonary disease or injury

Risk factors
- Left-sided heart failure
- Diastolic dysfunction
- Valvular heart disease
- Arrhythmias
- Fluid overload
- Acute myocardial ischemia and infarction
- Barbiturate or opiate poisoning
- Impaired pulmonary lymphatic drainage
- Inhalation of irritating gases
- Left atrial myxoma
- Pneumonia
- Pulmonary veno-occlusive disease

Incidence
- More common in middle-aged and elderly people
- Affects male and females equally

Common characteristics
- Persistent cough
- Dyspnea on exertion
- Orthopnea
- Paroxysmal nocturnal dyspnea

Complications
- Respiratory and metabolic acidosis
- Cardiac or respiratory arrest
- Death

✳ ASSESSMENT

History
- Predisposing factor
- Persistent cough
- Dyspnea on exertion
- Paroxysmal nocturnal dyspnea
- Orthopnea

Physical findings
- Restlessness and anxiety
- Rapid, labored breathing
- Intense, productive cough
- Frothy, bloody sputum
- Mental status changes
- Neck vein distention
- Sweaty, cold, clammy skin
- Wheezing
- Crackles
- S_3 gallop
- Tachycardia
- Hypotension
- Thready pulse
- Peripheral edema
- Hepatomegaly

Test results
LABORATORY
- Arterial blood gas (ABG) analysis shows hypoxemia, hypercapnia, or acidosis.
IMAGING
- Chest X-rays show diffuse haziness of the lung fields, cardiomegaly, and pleural effusion.
DIAGNOSTIC PROCEDURES
- Pulse oximetry may show decreased oxygen saturation.
- Pulmonary artery catheterization may reveal increased pulmonary artery wedge pressures.
- Electrocardiography may show valvular disease and left ventricular hypokinesis or akinesis.

◆ TREATMENT

General
- Fluid overload reduction
- Improved gas exchange and myocardial function
- Correction of underlying condition
- Mechanical ventilation

Diet
- Sodium restriction
- Fluid restriction

Activity
- As tolerated

Medication
- Supplemental oxygen
- Diuretics
- Antiarrhythmics
- Morphine sulfate
- Preload-reducing agents
- Afterload-reducing agents
- Bronchodilators
- Positive inotropic agents
- Vasopressors

◈ **NURSING ALERT** Be aware that morphine sulfate can further compromise respirations in a patient with respiratory distress. Keep resuscitation equipment at hand in case the patient stops breathing.

Surgery
- Valve repair or replacement or myocardial revascularization, if appropriate, to correct the underlying cause

Nursing diagnoses
- Anxiety
- Excess fluid volume
- Fear
- Impaired gas exchange
- Ineffective coping
- Ineffective tissue perfusion: Cardiopulmonary

Key outcomes
The patient will:
- verbalize decreased anxiety
- maintain adequate fluid balance
- discuss fears and concerns
- maintain adequate ventilation and oxygenation
- demonstrate adequate coping mechanisms
- maintain adequate cardiac output and circulation.

Nursing interventions
- Administer medications and oxygen, as ordered.
- Place the patient in high Fowler's position.
- Restrict fluids and sodium intake.
- Promote rest and relaxation.
- Provide emotional support.

Monitoring
- Vital signs
- Intake and output
- Daily weight
- Respiratory status
- Response to treatment
- Complications
- Heart rhythm
- ABG values
- Pulse oximetry values
- Hemodynamic values

Be sure to cover:
- disorder, diagnostic tests, and treatment
- medication administration, dosage, and possible adverse effects
- fluid and sodium restrictions
- daily weight
- signs and symptoms of fluid overload
- energy conversation strategies
- avoidance of alcohol
- when to notify the physician.

Discharge planning
Refer the patient to a:
- cardiac rehabilitation program, if indicated
- smoking-cessation program, if indicated.

Organizations
American Thoracic Society:
www.thoracic.org
National Heart, Lung and Blood Institute:
www.nhlbi.nih.gov

Selected references
Patroniti, N., et al. "Measurement of Pulmonary Edema in Patients with Acute Respiratory Distress Syndrome," *Critical Care Medicine* 33(11):2547-554, November 2005.

Poole,. J.H., and Spreen, D.T. "Acute Pulmonary Edema in Pregnancy," *Journal of Perinatnal & Neonatal Nursing* 19(4):316-31, October-December 2005.

Remo, E.F. "Heart Failure Management. Prevention of Pulmonary Edema is Essential," *Advance for Nurse Practitioners* 13(12):27-28, 30, 62, December 2005.

Ware, L.B., and Mattay, M.A. "Clinical Practice. Acute Pulmonary Edema," *New England Journal of Medicine* 353(26):2788-796, December 2005.

Pulmonary embolism

● **OVERVIEW**

Description
- Obstruction of the pulmonary arterial bed occurring when a mass (such as a dislodged thrombus) lodges in the main pulmonary artery or branch, partially or completely obstructing it
- Most thrombi originating in deep veins of the leg
- Can be asymptomatic, but sometimes causes rapid death from pulmonary infarction

Pathophysiology
- Thrombus formation results from vascular wall damage, venous stasis, or blood hypercoagulability.
- Trauma, clot dissolution, sudden muscle spasm, intravascular pressure changes, or peripheral blood flow changes can cause the thrombus to loosen or fragmentize.
- The thrombus (now an embolus) floats to the heart's right side and enters the lung through the pulmonary artery. There, the embolus may dissolve, continue to fragment, or grow.
- By occluding the pulmonary artery, the embolus prevents alveoli from producing enough surfactant to maintain alveolar integrity. Alveoli collapse and atelectasis develops.
- If the embolus enlarges, it may occlude most or all of the pulmonary vessels and cause death.

Causes
- Deep vein thrombosis
- Pelvic, renal, and hepatic vein thrombosis
- Right heart thrombus
- Upper extremity thrombosis
- Valvular heart disease
- Rarely, other types of emboli, such as bone, air, fat, amniotic fluid, tumor cells, or a foreign body

Risk factors
- Various disorders and treatments (See *Who's at risk for pulmonary embolism?*)

Incidence
- 600,000 to 700,000 cases annually
- Affects males and females equally
- More common with advancing age

Common characteristics
- Shortness of breath for no apparent reason
- Tachycardia
- Anxiety
- Pleuritic or anginal pain

Complications
- Respiratory failure
- Pulmonary infarction
- Pulmonary hypertension
- Embolic extension
- Hepatic congestion and necrosis
- Pulmonary abscess
- Shock
- Acute respiratory distress syndrome
- Massive atelectasis
- Right-sided heart failure
- Ventilation-perfusion mismatch
- Death

✳ **ASSESSMENT**

History
- Predisposing factor
- Shortness of breath for no apparent reason
- Pleuritic pain or angina

Physical findings
- Tachycardia
- Low-grade fever
- Weak, rapid pulse
- Hypotension
- Productive cough, possibly with blood-tinged sputum
- Warmth, tenderness, and edema of the lower leg
- Restlessness
- Transient pleural friction rub
- Crackles
- S_3 and S_4 gallop with increased intensity of the pulmonic component of S_2
- With a large embolus: cyanosis, syncope, distended neck veins

Test results
LABORATORY
- Arterial blood gas (ABG) values show hypoxemia.
- D-dimer level is elevated.
IMAGING
- Lung ventilation perfusion scan shows a ventilation-perfusion mismatch.
- Pulmonary angiography shows a pulmonary vessel filling defect or an abrupt vessel ending and reveals the location and extent of pulmonary embolism.
- Chest X-rays may show a small infiltrate or effusion.
- Spiral chest computed tomography scan may show central pulmonary emboli.
DIAGNOSTIC PROCEDURES
- Electrocardiography may reveal right axis deviation and right bundle-branch block; it also may show atrial fibrillation.

◆ **TREATMENT**

General
- Maintenance of adequate cardiovascular and pulmonary function
- Mechanical ventilation

Diet
- Possible fluid restriction

Activity
- Bed rest during the acute phase

Medication
- Oxygen therapy
- Thrombolytics
- Anticoagulants
- Corticosteroids (controversial)
- Diuretics
- Antiarrhythmics
- Vasopressors (for hypotension)
- Antibiotics (for septic embolus)

Surgery
- Vena caval interruption
- Vena caval filter placement
- Pulmonary embolectomy

NURSING CONSIDERATIONS

Nursing diagnoses

- Acute pain
- Anxiety
- Decreased cardiac output
- Fear
- Imbalanced nutrition: Less than body requirements
- Impaired gas exchange
- Ineffective airway clearance
- Ineffective coping
- Ineffective tissue perfusion: Cardiopulmonary
- Risk for injury

Key outcomes

The patient will:

- express feelings of increased comfort and decreased pain
- identify strategies to reduce anxiety
- discuss fears and concerns
- consume required daily caloric intake
- maintain adequate ventilation and oxygenation
- maintain a patent airway
- use support systems to assist with coping
- maintain adequate cardiopulmonary perfusion
- remain free from injury.

Nursing interventions

- Administer medications, as ordered.
- Avoid I.M. injections.
- Encourage active and passive range-of-motion exercises, unless contraindicated.
- Avoid massage of the lower legs.
- Apply antiembolism stockings.
- Provide adequate nutrition.
- Assist with ambulation as soon as the patient is stable.
- Encourage use of incentive spirometry.

Monitoring

- Vital signs
- Intake and output
- Respiratory status
- Pulse oximetry
- ABG values
- Signs of deep vein thrombosis
- Complications
- Coagulation study results
- Abnormal bleeding
- Stools for occult blood

PATIENT TEACHING

Be sure to cover:

- disorder, diagnostic tests, and treatment
- medication administration, dosage, and possible adverse effectss
- ways to prevent deep vein thrombosis and pulmonary embolism
- signs and symptoms of abnormal bleeding
- prevention of abnormal bleeding
- how to monitor anticoagulant effects
- dietary sources of vitamin K
- when to notify the physician.

Discharge planning

- Refer the patient to a weight management program, if indicated.

RESOURCES

Organizations

American Lung Association: *www.lungusa.org*
National Heart, Lung and Blood Institute: *www.nhlbi.nih.gov*

Selected references

Bonde, P., and Graham, A. "Surgical Management of Pulmonary Embolism," *Journal of Thoracic and Cardiovascular Surgery* 131(2):503-504, February 2006.

Kucher, N., et al. "Massive Pulmonary Embolism," *Circulation* 113(4):577-82, January 2006.

Roy, P.M., et al. "Appropriateness of Diagnostic Management and Outcomes of Suspected Pulmonary Embolism" *Annals of Internal Medicine* 144(3):157-64, February 2006.

Yang, J.C. "Prevention and Treatment of Deep Vein Thrombosis and Pulmonary Embolism in Critically Ill Patients," *Critical Care Nursing Quarterly* 28(1):72-79, January-March 2005.

WHO'S AT RISK FOR PULMONARY EMBOLISM?

Many disorders and treatments heighten the risk for pulmonary embolism. At particular risk are surgical patients. The anesthetic used during surgery can injure lung vessels, and surgery or prolonged bed rest can promote venous stasis, which compounds the risk.

Predisposing disorders

- Lung disorders, especially chronic types
- Cardiac disorders
- Infection
- Diabetes mellitus
- History of thromboembolism, thrombophlebitis, or vascular insufficiency
- Sickle cell disease
- Autoimmune hemolytic anemia
- Polycythemia
- Osteomyelitis
- Long-bone fracture
- Manipulation or disconnection of central lines

Venous stasis

- Prolonged bed rest or immobilization
- Obesity
- Over age 40
- Burns
- Recent childbirth
- Orthopedic casts

Venous injury

- Surgery, particularly of the legs, pelvis, abdomen, or thorax
- Leg or pelvic fractures or injuries
- I.V. drug abuse
- I.V. therapy

Increased blood coagulability

- Cancer
- Use of high-estrogen oral contraceptives

Pulmonary hypertension

● OVERVIEW

Description
- Occurs in a primary form (rare) and a secondary form
- In both forms, resting systolic pulmonary artery pressure (PAP) above 30 mm Hg and mean PAP above 18 mm Hg
- In primary or idiopathic form, increased PAP and pulmonary vascular resistance for no obvious cause
- Primary form also known as *PPH*

Pathophysiology
- In primary pulmonary hypertension, the intimal lining of the pulmonary arteries thickens for no apparent reason. This narrows the artery and impairs distensibility, increasing vascular resistance.
- Secondary pulmonary hypertension occurs from hypoxemia caused by conditions involving alveolar hypoventilation, vascular obstruction, or left-to-right shunting.

Causes
PRIMARY PULMONARY HYPERTENSION
- Exact cause unknown
- Possible hereditary factors
- Possible altered autoimmune mechanisms
- Associated with portal hypertension

SECONDARY PULMONARY HYPERTENSION
- Lung disease

Risk factors
SECONDARY PULMONARY HYPERTENSION
- Chronic obstructive pulmonary disease
- Sarcoidosis
- Diffuse interstitial pneumonia
- Malignant metastases
- Scleroderma
- Use of some diet drugs
- Obesity
- Sleep apnea
- Hypoventilation syndromes
- Kyphoscoliosis
- Pulmonary embolism
- Vasculitis
- Left atrial myxoma
- Congenital cardiac defects
- Mitral stenosis

Incidence
PRIMARY PULMONARY HYPERTENSION
- Most common in women ages 20 to 40
- More prevalent in people with collagen disease

Common characteristics
- Dyspnea on exertion
- Weakness, fatigue
- Syncope

Complications
- Cor pulmonale
- Heart failure
- Cardiac arrest
- Death

✳ ASSESSMENT

History
- Shortness of breath with exertion
- Weakness, fatigue
- Pain during breathing
- Near-syncope

Physical findings
- Ascites
- Neck vein distention
- Peripheral edema
- Restlessness and agitation
- Mental status changes
- Decreased diaphragmatic excursion
- Apical impulse displaced beyond midclavicular line
- Right ventricular lift
- Reduced carotid pulse
- Hepatomegaly
- Tachycardia
- Systolic ejection murmur
- Widely split S_2
- S_3 and S_4
- Hypotension
- Decreased breath sounds
- Tubular breath sounds

Test results
LABORATORY
- Arterial blood gas (ABG) values show hypoxemia.

IMAGING
- Ventilation-perfusion lung scan may show a ventilation-perfusion mismatch.
- Pulmonary angiography may reveal filling defects in the pulmonary vasculature.

DIAGNOSTIC PROCEDURES
- Electrocardiography may reveal right axis deviation.
- Pulmonary artery catheterization shows increased PAP, with systolic pressure above 30 mm Hg; increased pulmonary artery wedge pressure; decreased cardiac output; and decreased cardiac index.
- Pulmonary function tests may show decreased flow rates and increased residual volume or reduced total lung capacity.
- Echocardiography may show valvular heart disease or atrial myxoma.
- Lung biopsy may show tumor cells.

◆ TREATMENT

General
- Based on underlying disease
- Symptom relief
- Smoking cessation

Diet
- Low-sodium
- Fluid restriction (in right-sided heart failure)

Activity
- Bed rest during acute phase

Medication
- Oxygen therapy
- Cardiac glycosides
- Diuretics
- Vasodilators
- Calcium-channel blockers
- Bronchodilators
- Beta-adrenergic blockers
- Epoprostenol

Surgery
- Heart-lung transplantation, if indicated

♣ NURSING CONSIDERATIONS

Nursing diagnoses
- Activity intolerance
- Anxiety
- Decreased cardiac output
- Fatigue
- Fear
- Impaired gas exchange
- Ineffective coping

Key outcomes
The patient will:
- demonstrate skill in conserving energy while carrying out daily activities to tolerance level
- verbalize strategies to reduce anxiety
- maintain adequate cardiac output
- express feelings of energy and decreased fatigue
- discuss fears and concerns
- maintain adequate ventilation and oxygenation
- use support systems to assist with coping.

Nursing interventions
- Administer medications and oxygen, as ordered.
- Implement comfort measures.
- Provide adequate rest periods.
- Offer emotional support.

Monitoring
- Vital signs
- Intake and output
- Daily weight
- Respiratory status
- Signs and symptoms of right-sided heart failure
- Heart rhythm
- ABG values
- Hemodynamic values

▶ PATIENT TEACHING

Be sure to cover:
- disorder, diagnostic tests, and treatment
- medication administration, dosage, and possible adverse effects
- dietary restrictions
- frequent rest periods
- signs and symptoms of right-sided heart failure
- when to notify the physician.

Discharge planning
- Refer the patient to a smoking-cessation program, if indicated.

✳ RESOURCES

Organizations
American Lung Association:
www.lungusa.org
American Thoracic Society:
www.thoracic.org
National Heart, Lung and Blood Institute:
www.nhlbi.nih.gov

Selected references
Holcomb, S.S. "Understanding Pulmonary Arterial Hypertension," *Nursing* 34(9):50-54, September 2004.
Steinbis, S."What You Should Know about Pulmonary Hypertension," *Nurse Practitioner* 29(4):8, April 2004.
Thistlethwaite, P.A., et al. "Outcomes of Pulmonary Endarterectomy for Treatment of Extreme Thromboembolic Pulmonary Hypertension," *Journal of Thoracic and Cardiovascular Surgery* 131(2):307-13, February 2006.

Radiation exposure

● OVERVIEW

Description
- Exposure to excessive radiation
- Causes tissue damage that varies with the amount of body area exposed, length of exposure, dosage absorbed, distance from the source, and presence of protective shielding
- Can result from cancer radiotherapy, working in a radiation facility, or other exposure to radioactive materials
- Can be acute or chronic

Pathophysiology
- Ionization occurs in the molecules of living cells.
- Electrons are removed from atoms, resulting in charged atoms or ions that form and react with other atoms to cause cell damage.
- Rapidly dividing cells are the most susceptible to radiation damage, whereas highly differentiated cells are more resistant to radiation.

Causes
- Exposure to radiation through inhalation, ingestion, or direct contact

Risk factors
- Cancer
- Employment in a radiation facility

Incidence
- Unknown

Common characteristics
- Nausea
- Diarrhea
- General weakness
- Immunosuppression
- Infections

Complications
- Leukemia
- Thyroid cancer
- Fetal growth retardation or genetic defects in offspring (from exposure during childbearing years)
- Decreased fertility
- Shortened life span
- Anemia
- Malignant neoplasms
- Bone necrosis and fractures

✳ ASSESSMENT

History
ACUTE HEMATOPOIETIC RADIATION TOXICITY
- Bleeding from the skin, genitourinary tract, and GI tract
- Nosebleeds
- Hemorrhage
- Increased susceptibility to infection

GI RADIATION TOXICITY
- Intractable nausea, vomiting, and diarrhea

CEREBRAL RADIATION TOXICITY
- Nausea, vomiting, and diarrhea
- Lethargy

CARDIOVASCULAR RADIATION TOXICITY
- Hypotension, shock, and cardiac arrhythmias

Physical findings
ACUTE HEMATOPOIETIC RADIATION TOXICITY
- Petechiae
- Pallor
- Weakness
- Oropharyngeal abscesses

GI RADIATION TOXICITY
- Mouth and throat ulcers and infection
- Circulatory collapse and death

CEREBRAL RADIATION TOXICITY
- Tremors
- Seizures
- Confusion
- Coma and death

GENERALIZED RADIATION EXPOSURE
- Signs of hypothyroidism
- Cataracts
- Skin dryness, erythema, atrophy, and malignant lesions
- Alopecia
- Brittle nails

CARDIOVASCULAR RADIATION TOXICITY
- Irregular pulse rate and rhythm
- Pallor
- Hypotension

Test results
LABORATORY
- White blood cell, platelet, and lymphocyte counts are decreased.
- Serum potassium and chloride levels are decreased.

IMAGING
- X-rays may reveal bone necrosis.

DIAGNOSTIC PROCEDURES
- Bone marrow studies may show blood dyscrasias.
- Geiger counter helps determine if radioactive material was ingested or inhaled and evaluates the amount of radiation in open wounds.

◆ TREATMENT

General
- Management of life-threatening injuries
- Symptomatic and supportive treatment
- Based on the type and extent of radiation injury

Diet
- High-protein, high-calorie

Activity
- As tolerated by clinical status

Medication
- Chelating agents
- Potassium iodide
- Aluminum phosphate gel
- Barium sulfate

❖ NURSING CONSIDERATIONS

Nursing diagnoses
- Anxiety
- Decreased intracranial adaptive capacity
- Deficient fluid volume
- Imbalanced nutrition: Less than body requirements
- Impaired oral mucous membrane
- Impaired skin integrity
- Risk for infection

Key outcomes
The patient will:
- verbalize feelings of anxiety and fear
- remain oriented to person, place, and time
- maintain normal fluid volume; output should equal intake
- maintain an acceptable weight
- remain free from complications related to trauma to oral mucous membranes
- experience skin healing without complications
- remain free from signs and symptoms of infection.

Nursing interventions
- Implement appropriate respiratory and cardiac support measures.
- Administer I.V. fluids and electrolytes, as ordered.
- For skin contamination, wash the patient's body thoroughly with mild soap and water.
- Debride and irrigate open wounds, as ordered.
- For ingested radioactive material, perform gastric lavage and whole-bowel irrigation, and administer activated charcoal, as ordered.
- Dispose of contaminated clothing properly.
- Dispose of contaminated excrement and body fluids according to facility policy.
- Use strict sterile technique.

Monitoring
- Intake and output
- Fluid and electrolyte balance
- Vital signs
- Signs and symptoms of hemorrhage
- Fluid and nutritional status

▶ PATIENT TEACHING

Be sure to cover:
- disorder, diagnostic tests, and treatment
- effects of radiation exposure
- how to prevent a recurrence
- skin care
- wound care
- need for follow-up care.

Discharge planning
- Refer the patient to resource and support services.
- If the patient was exposed to significant amounts of radiation, provide a referral to genetic counseling resources.

✳ RESOURCES

Organizations
Environmental Protection Agency: *www.epa.gov/radiation*
National Center for Injury Prevention and Control: *www.cdc.gov/ncipc*
National Institutes of Health: *www.nih.gov*
United States Nuclear Regulatory Commission—Radiation Exposure Information and Reporting System (REIRS) for Radiation Workers: *www.reirs.com*

Selected references
Hendrix, C. "Radiation Guidelines for Radioimmunotherapy with Yttrium 90 Ibritumomab Tiuxetan," *Clinical Journal of Oncology Nursing* 8(1):31-34, February 2004.

Thieden, E. , et al. "Ultraviolet Radiation Exposure Pattern in Winter Compared with Summer Based on Time-Stamped Personal Dosimeter Readings," *British Journal of Dermatology* 154(1):133-38, January 2006.

Valentin, J. International Commission on Radiological Protection. "Protecting People Against Radiation Exposure in the Event of a Radiological Attack. A Report of The International Commission on Radiological Protection," *Annals of the ICRP* 35(1):1-110, iii-iv, 2005.

Wolfson, A.B., et al. *Harwood-Nuss' Clinical Practice of Emergency Medicine,* 4th ed. Philadelphia: Lippincott Williams & Wilkins, 2005.

Rape-trauma syndrome

● OVERVIEW

Description
- Occurs during the period after rape (illicit sexual intercourse without consent) or attempted rape, which causes varying degrees of physical and psychological trauma
- Refers to the victim's short- and long-term reactions and the methods used to cope with trauma
- Good prognosis if the victim receives physical and emotional support and counseling to help deal with feelings

Pathophysiology
- Rape causes psychological and physiologic reactions, resulting in early-stage (short-term) and later-stage (long-term) reactions.

Causes
- Rape or attempted rape

Incidence
- Known victims of rape ranging in age from 2 months to 97 years
- Rape most common in women ages 16 to 19 (roughly 8% of American women victims of rape or attempted rape)
- In children, rapist usually a family member

Common characteristics
- Signs of physical trauma, depending on length of the attack and whether additional physical violence occurred
- Tearfulness, crying
- Withdrawal
- Anxiousness

Complications
- Lasting psychiatric problems, such as depression, guilt, anxiety, and suicidal ideation
- Sexually transmitted disease (STD)
- Unwanted pregnancy

✳ ASSESSMENT

History
- Rape or attempted rape
- Early stage of rape-trauma syndrome:
  - Disbelief
  - Panic
  - Severe anxiety
  - Anger
  - Self-blame
  - Humiliation
  - Depression
- Late stage of rape-trauma syndrome:
  - Anxiety
  - Nightmares
  - Flashbacks
  - Depression
  - Anger
  - Disinterest in sex
  - Anorgasmia
  - Suicidal ideation
- History that includes:
  - Whether she was pregnant at the time of the attack
  - Date of her last menstrual period
  - Details of her obstetric and gynecologic history
  - The victim's statements (recorded in the first person, using quotation marks)
  - Objective information provided by others
- Assessment notes that include:
  - Time the victim arrived at the facility
  - Date and time of the alleged rape
  - Time the victim was examined

> 🔲 **NURSING ALERT** Be aware that your assessment notes may be used as evidence if the rapist goes to a trial.

Physical findings
- Sore throat
- Difficulty swallowing
- Vaginal pain
- Rectal pain
- Pain from other injuries incurred during the assault
- Early stage of rape-trauma syndrome:
  - Reddened (sore) throat
  - Mouth irritation
  - Ecchymoses
  - Rectal pain and bleeding
  - Lacerations, contusions, and abrasions to the vulva, cervix, and vaginal walls (in female victims)
  - Lacerations, contusions (in male victims)
  - Outward calm
  - Compliance
  - Glibness
  - Talkativeness

Test results
LABORATORY
- STD screening test results are positive.
- Syphilis on rapid plasma reagin card test results are positive.
- Urine pregnancy test 0 to 3 weeks after missed period is positive.
- Serum human chorionic gonadotropin 24 to 48 hours after implantation is positive.
- Drug screens are positive (if symptoms warrant).
- Serum ethanol level is elevated (if symptoms warrant).

> 🔲 **NURSING ALERT** If the rape occurred in the past 7 days, the following specimens may be obtained for legal purposes: blood samples; evidence for deoxyribonucleic acid testing (should be collected within 48 hours); hair samples that are of a different color from the victim's or that are obviously out of place; fiber samples; soiled or torn material; body fluids, such as blood or semen that don't belong to the victim; and specimens from the cervical canal, throat, or rectum.

◆ TREATMENT

General
- Treatment of physical injuries
- Crisis intervention and counseling
- Follow-up gynecologic examination after 7 to 14 days; for male patient, follow-up urologic examination
- Emergency contraception such as the Copper-T intrauterine device

Diet
- No restrictions

Activity
- Based on injuries

Medication
- Tetanus prophylaxis
- STD prophylaxis
- Emergency contraceptive pills

NURSING CONSIDERATIONS

Nursing diagnoses
- Acute pain
- Anxiety
- Disturbed body image
- Disturbed sleep pattern
- Impaired oral mucous membrane
- Ineffective coping
- Powerlessness
- Rape-trauma syndrome
- Risk for infection
- Situational low self-esteem

Key outcomes
The patient will:
- express feelings of increased comfort and decreased pain
- report absence of or reduction in anxiety
- express positive feelings about self
- appear well rested and verbalize feeling as such
- not exhibit complications related to trauma to oral mucous membranes
- use support systems and exhibit adequate coping behaviors
- identify methods to achieve control over personal situation
- recognize signs and symptoms of rape-trauma syndrome and demonstrate healthy coping behaviors
- remain free from signs and symptoms of infection
- discuss feelings related to the rape and its effect on self-esteem.

Nursing interventions
- Don't leave the patient alone unless requested.
- Place the patient's clothing in paper, *not plastic,* bags. Label each bag and its contents.
- Collect and label fingernail scrapings and foreign material obtained by combing the patient's pubic hair.
- Label all specimens with the patient's name, physician's name, and site from which the specimen was obtained.
- Note the name of the person to whom specimens were given.
- Report the rape if required by state law.
- Encourage the patient to express feelings.
- Provide emotional support.

Monitoring
- Mental status
- Vital signs
- Signs and symptoms of shock

PATIENT TEACHING

Be sure to cover:
- disorder, diagnostic tests, and treatment
- verbal and written instructions regarding treatment
- medication administration, dosage, and possible adverse effects.

Discharge planning
- Encourage the patient to get follow-up care.
- Refer the patient to resource and support services.

RESOURCES

Organizations
Arming Women Against Rape and Endangerment: *www.aware.org*
National Institutes of Health: *www.nih.gov*
Women Organized Against Rape: *www.woar.org*

Selected references
Burgess, A.W., et al. "Forensic Markers in Elder Female Sexual Abuse Cases," *Clinics in Geriatric Medicine* 21(2):399-412, May 2005.
Lessing, J.E. "Primary Care Provider Interventions for the Delayed Disclosure of Adolescent Sexual Assault," *Journal of Pediatric Health Care* 19(1):17-24, January-February 2005.
Mancino, P., et. al. "Introducing Colposcopy and Vulvovaginoscopy as Routine Examinations for Victims of Sexual Assault," *Clinical and Experimental Obstetrics & Gynecology* 30(1):40-42, 2003.
Wolfson, A.B., et al. *Harwood-Nuss' Clinical Practice of Emergency Medicine,* 4th ed. Philadelphia: Lippincott Williams & Wilkins, 2005.

Raynaud's phenomenon

Description
- Primary arteriospastic disorder
- Causes episodic vasospasms in the small peripheral arteries and arterioles in response to cold exposure or stress
- Typically occurs in three phases
- Also called *vasospastic arterial disease*

Pathophysiology
- Blood flow to digits decreases in response to stress or cold.
- Proposed explanations for decreased digital blood flow include an antigen-antibody immune response (most probable theory); intrinsic vascular wall hyperactivity to cold; ineffective basal heat production; and increased vasomotor tone from sympathetic stimulation or stress.

Causes
SECONDARY CAUSES
- Collagen vascular disease
- Arterial occlusive disease
- Neurologic disorders
- Blood dyscrasias
- Trauma
- Drugs
- Pulmonary hypertension

(see *Causes of Raynaud's phenomenon*)

Incidence
- More common in females, particularly between late adolescence and age 40

Common characteristics
- Occurs bilaterally
- Usually affects the hands or, less often, the feet; rarely, the earlobes and tip of nose

Complications
- Ischemia
- Gangrene
- Amputation

History
- Skin color changes, numbness and tingling (during second stage), or throbbing, burning painful sensation (during third stage) in response to cold or stress

Physical findings
- First phase: marked pallor of affected skin areas
- Second phase: cyanosis of affected skin areas
- Third phase: red, warm skin
- Between attacks, normal appearance of affected areas (occasionally, coolness and excessive perspiration of these areas)
- In long-standing disease, trophic changes, such as sclerodactylia and ulcerations

Test results
DIAGNOSTIC PROCEDURES
- Arteriography and digital photo-plethysmography may aid diagnosis.

General
- Smoking cessation
- Biofeedback therapy

Diet
- No restrictions

Activity
- Avoidance of activities involving exposure to cold and mechanical or chemical injury

Medication
- Calcium-channel blockers
- Alpha blockers
- Vasodilators

Surgery
- Sympathectomy, if conservative treatment fails to prevent ischemic ulcers
- Amputation of fingers or toes if gangrene develops (rare)

Nursing diagnoses

- Acute pain
- Impaired skin integrity
- Impaired tissue integrity
- Ineffective coping
- Ineffective role performance
- Ineffective thermoregulation
- Ineffective tissue perfusion: Peripheral

Key outcomes

The patient will:

- express feelings of increased comfort and decreased pain
- maintain skin integrity
- experience reduced tissue redness, swelling, and pain
- demonstrate effective coping skills
- perform normal activities and function in usual roles to the extent possible
- maintain adequate skin temperature in affected areas
- maintain adequate collateral circulation, tissue perfusion, and oxygenation.

Nursing interventions

- Evaluate the patient's occupation and its effect on symptom occurrence.
- Help the patient identify stress triggers and use effective coping strategies.
- Provide psychological support and reassurance

Monitoring

- Response to treatment
- Signs and symptoms of skin breakdown
- Signs and symptoms of infection

Be sure to cover:

- avoidance of exposure to cold
- importance of wearing mittens or gloves in cold weather and when handling cold items or defrosting the freezer
- avoidance of stress and cigarette smoking
- how to inspect the skin frequently and to seek immediate care for signs of skin breakdown or infection
- medication administration, dosage, and possible adverse effects, including which ones to report to the physician
- importance of follow-up care.

Discharge planning

Refer the patient to a:

- smoking-cessation program, if indicated
- support group, as needed.

Organizations

Mayo Clinic: *www.mayoclinic.com*
National Institute of Arthritis, Musculoskeletal and Skin Diseases: *www.nih.gov/niams/healthinfo*

Selected references

Cooke, J.P., and Marshall, J.M. "Mechanisms of Raynaud's Disease," *Vascular Medicine* 10(4):293-307, November 2005.

Fries, R., et al. "Sildenafil in the Treatment of Raynaud's Phenomenon Resistant to Vasodilatory Therapy," *Circulation* 112(19):2980-985, November 2005.

Kasper, D.L., et al., eds. *Harrison's Principles of Internal Medicine*, 16th ed. New York: McGraw-Hill Book Co., 2005.

The Merck Manual of Diagnosis & Therapy, 18th ed. Whitehouse Station, N.J.: Merck & Co., Inc. 2006.

Summers, A. "From White to Blue to Red: Raynaud's Phenomenon," *Emergency Nurse* 13(7):18-20, November 2005.

CAUSES OF RAYNAUD'S PHENOMENON

In primary or idiopathic Raynaud's phenomenon, more than 50% of patients have Raynaud's disease. Raynaud's phenomenon may also occur secondary to the following diseases and conditions as well as with the use of certain drugs.

Collagen vascular disease

- Dermatomyositis
- Polymyositis
- Rheumatoid arthritis
- Scleroderma
- Systemic lupus erythematosus

Arterial occlusive disease

- Acute arterial occlusion
- Atherosclerosis of the extremities
- Thoracic outlet syndrome
- Thromboangiitis obliterans

Neurologic disorders

- Carpal tunnel syndrome
- Stroke
- Invertebral disk disease
- Poliomyelitis
- Spinal cord tumors
- Syringomyelia

Blood dyscrasias

- Cold agglutinins
- Cryofibrinogenemia
- Myeloproliferative disorders
- Waldenström's disease

Trauma

- Cold injury
- Electric shock
- Hammering
- Keyboarding
- Piano playing
- Vibration injury

Drugs

- Beta-adrenergic blockers
- Bleomycin
- Cisplatin
- Ergot derivatives such as ergotamine
- Methysergide
- Vinblastine

Other

- Pulmonary hypertension

Reiter's syndrome

● OVERVIEW

Description
- Self-limiting syndrome associated with polyarthritis, urethritis, mucocutaneous lesions, and conjunctivitis (or, less commonly, uveitis)

Pathophysiology
- Infection is thought to trigger an aberrant and hyperactive immune response that causes inflammation in involved target organs.

Causes
- Exact cause unknown

Risk factors
- Typically follows venereal or enteric infection, especially with *Mycoplasma*, *Shigella*, *Campylobacter*, *Salmonella*, *Yersinia*, and *Chlamydia* organisms
- May involve genetic susceptibility

Incidence
- Most common in men ages 20 to 40, especially those who are human immunodeficiency virus–positive
- Rare in women and children

Common characteristics
- Polyarthritis (dominant feature)

Complications
- Ankylosing spondylitis
- Persistent joint pain and swelling
- Anterior uveitis, glaucoma, blindness
- Prostatitis and hemorrhagic cystitis
- Cardiomyopathy, pericarditis
- Pulmonary edema
- Vertebral inflammation
- Foot deformity and chronic heel pain

✳ ASSESSMENT

History
- Initially: dysuria, hematuria, urinary urgency and frequency, and mucopurulent penile discharge with swelling and reddening of the urethral meatus
- Possible suprapubic pain, fever, and anorexia with weight loss

Physical findings
- Small, painless ulcers on glans penis
- Asymmetrical and extremely variable polyarticular arthritis, usually in weight-bearing joints of the legs and sometimes in the lower back or sacroiliac joints
- Warm, erythematous, painful joints
- Muscle wasting near affected joints
- Swollen, sausagelike appearance of fingers and toes
- Skin lesions (keratoderma blennorrhagicum)
- Thick, opaque, brittle nails with keratic debris accumulation under nails
- Painless, transient ulcerations on the buccal mucosa, palate, and tongue
- Patches of scaly skin on the palms, soles, scalp, or trunk
- Ophthalmalogic signs, such as photophobia, eye pain, excessive tearing, erythema, and burning

Test results
LABORATORY
- Human leukocyte antigen (HLA) is positive for HLA B27.
- White blood cell (WBC) count and erythrocyte sedimentation rate are elevated.
- Complete blood count and anemia panel show mild anemia.
- Many WBCs (mostly polymorphonuclear leukocytes) are found in urethral discharge and synovial fluid.
- Synovial fluid is grossly purulent with high complement and protein levels.
- Cultures of urethral discharge and synovial fluid rule out other possible causes of symptoms.

IMAGING
- During the first few weeks of the syndrome, X-rays are normal. Later, they may show osteoporosis in inflamed areas. If inflammation persists, X-rays may show small joint erosion, periosteal proliferation (new bone formation) of involved joints, and calcaneal spurs.

◆ TREATMENT

General
- Physical therapy
- Padded or supportive shoes

Diet
- No restrictions
- High-calorie, high-protein

Activity
- During acute stages, weight-bearing restrictions or complete bed rest

Medication
- Nonsteroidal anti-inflammatory drugs (NSAIDs)
- Cytotoxic agents
- Analgesics
- Corticosteroids
- Antibiotics (for underlying infection)

Surgery
- In patients where medical management doesn't prevent severe joint damage, surgical reconstruction of the joints

NURSING CONSIDERATIONS

Nursing diagnoses
- Acute pain
- Disturbed sensory perception: Visual
- Fatigue
- Imbalanced nutrition: Less than body requirements
- Impaired oral mucous membrane
- Impaired physical mobility
- Impaired skin integrity
- Impaired tissue integrity
- Impaired urinary elimination
- Ineffective role performance
- Ineffective sexuality patterns
- Risk for infection

Key outcomes
The patient will:
- express feelings of increased comfort and decreased pain
- maintain optimal functioning within the confines of the vision impairment
- express feelings of increased energy
- maintain weight or achieve ideal weight
- maintain adequate oral mucous membranes
- attain the highest degree of mobility possible within confines of the disease
- experience healing of wounds and lesions without complications
- experience reduced tissue pain, redness, and swelling
- maintain adequate urine output
- recognize limitations imposed by the illness and express feelings about these limitations
- verbalize feelings about altered sexuality patterns
- remain free from signs or symptoms of infection.

Nursing interventions
- Follow standard precautions.
- Administer analgesics, as ordered and needed.
- Provide a high-calorie, high-protein diet.
- Provide frequent rest periods.
- Develop an exercise regimen with the physical therapist.
- Maintain a nonjudgmental attitude.

Monitoring
- Response to medications
- Complications
- Pain control
- Joint mobility

PATIENT TEACHING

Be sure to cover:
- disorder, diagnostic tests, and treatment
- importance of using condoms and avoiding multiple sex partners
- how to avoid exposure to enteric pathogens (such as via anal intercourse)
- medication administration, dosage, and possible adverse effects
- importance of taking NSAIDs with meals or milk
- maintaining normal daily activities and moderate exercise
- good posture and body mechanics
- use of a firm mattress.

Discharge planning
- If the patient has severe or chronic joint impairment, arrange for occupational counseling.

RESOURCES

Organizations
Arthritis Foundation: *www.arthritis.org*
National Institute of Arthritis, Musculoskeletal and Skin Disorders: *www.nih.gov/niams*
Reiter's Information and Support Group: *www.risg.org*

Selected references
Kohnke, S.J. "Reactive Arthritis: A Clinical Approach," *Orthopaedic Nursing* 23(4):274-80, July-August 2004.
Liao, C.H., et al. "Juvenile Reiter's Syndrome: A Case Report," *Journal of Microbiology, Immunology and Infection* 37(6):379-81, December 2004.
The Merck Manual of Diagnosis & Therapy, 18th ed. Whitehouse Station, N.J.: Merck & Co., Inc. 2006.

Renal calculi

● OVERVIEW

Description
- Formation of calculi ("stones") any-where in the urinary tract
- Most common in the renal pelvis or calyces
- Vary in size; may be solitary or multi-ple (see *Variations in renal calculi*)
- Require hospitalization in roughly 1 of every 1,000 Americans

Pathophysiology
- Calculi form when substances nor-mally dissolved in the urine, such as calcium oxalate and calcium phos-phate, precipitate.
- Large, rough calculi may occlude the opening to the ureteropelvic junction.
- The frequency and force of peristaltic contractions increase, causing pain.

Causes
- Exact cause unknown

Risk factors
- Dehydration
- Infection
- Urine pH changes
- Urinary tract obstruction
- Immobilization
- Metabolic factors
- Family history of renal calculi

Incidence
- Affect more men than women
- Rare in blacks and children
- Can occur at any age, but most com-mon between ages 35 and 45

Common characteristics
- Flank pain
- Nausea, vomiting

Complications
- Renal parenchymal damage
- Renal cell necrosis
- Hydronephrosis
- Complete ureteral obstruction

✳ ASSESSMENT

History
- Classic renal colic pain: severe pain that travels from the costovertebral angle to the flank and then to the suprapubic region and external geni-talia
- Calculi in the renal pelvis and calcyes: relatively constant, dull pain
- Pain of fluctuating intensity; may be excruciating at its peak
- Nausea, vomiting
- Fever, chills
- Anuria (rare)

Physical findings
- Hematuria
- Abdominal distention
- Costovertebral tenderness on palpa-tion
- Tachycardia
- Elevated blood pressure

Test results
LABORATORY
- 24-hour urine collection shows cal-cium oxalate, phosphorus, and uric acid excretion levels.
- Urinalysis shows increased urine spe-cific gravity, hematuria, crystals, casts, and pyuria.
IMAGING
- Kidney-ureter-bladder (KUB) radiog-raphy reveals most renal calculi.
- Excretory urography helps confirm the diagnosis and determines calculi size and location.
- Kidney ultrasonography can detect obstructive changes and radiolucent calculi not seen on KUB.

◆ TREATMENT

General
- Percutaneous ultrasonic lithotripsy
- Extracorporeal shock wave lithotripsy

Diet
- Vigorous hydration (more than 3 qt [3 L]/day)
- Adequate calcium intake

Activity
- No restriction

Medication
- Antibiotics
- Analgesics
- Diuretics
- Methenamine mandelate
- Allopurinol (for uric acid calculi)
- Ascorbic acid
- Ketorolac (Toradol)
- Desmopressin (DDAVP)

Surgery
- Cystoscopy
- Ureteral stent
- Percutaneous nephrostomy

Nursing diagnoses

- Acute pain
- Impaired urinary elimination
- Ineffective tissue perfusion: Renal
- Risk for imbalanced fluid volume
- Risk for infection
- Risk for injury

Key outcomes

The patient will:

- express feelings of increased comfort and decreased pain
- demonstrate the ability to manage urinary elimination problems
- maintain adequate urine output
- maintain fluid balance
- remain free from signs and symptoms of infection and injury.

Nursing interventions

- Provide I.V. fluids, as ordered; force fluids, as needed.
- Strain all urine and save solid material for analysis.
- Encourage ambulation to aid spontaneous calculus passage.

Monitoring

- Intake and output
- Daily weight
- Pain control
- Catheter function and drainage
- Signs and symptoms of infection

Be sure to cover:

- disorder, diagnostic tests, and treatment
- prescribed diet and importance of compliance
- drug therapy
- ways to prevent recurrences
- how to strain urine for stones
- immediate return visit to hospital for fever, uncontrolled pain, or vomiting.

Discharge planning

- Refer patients who don't meet admission critieria for follow-up with a urologist.

Organizations

American Association of Kidney Patients: *www.aakp.org*
National Institute of Diabetes & Digestive & Kidney Diseases: *www.niddk.nih.gov*
National Kidney Foundation: *www.kidney.org*

Selected references

Colella, J., et al. "Urolithiasis/Nephrolithiasis: What's It All About?" *Urologic Nursing* 25(6):427-48, 449, 475, December 2005.

Diseases, 4th ed. Philadelphia: Lippincott Williams & Wilkins, 2006.

Moe, O.W. "Kidney Stones: Pathophysiology and Medical Management," *Lancet* 367(9507):333-44, January 2006.

Thomas, J.C., et al. "Pediatric Ureteroscopic Stone Management," *Journal of Urology* 174(3):1072-1074, September 2005.

VARIATIONS IN RENAL CALCULI

Renal calculi vary in size and type. Small calculi may remain in the renal pelvis or pass down the ureter. A staghorn calculus (a cast of the calyceal and pelvic collecting system) may develop from a calculus that stays in the kidney.

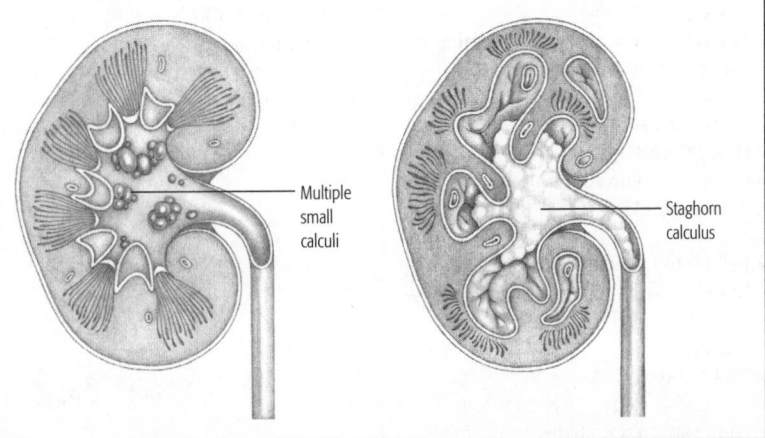

Multiple small calculi

Staghorn calculus

Renal failure, acute

● OVERVIEW

Description
- Sudden interruption of renal function resulting from obstruction, reduced circulation, or renal parenchymal disease
- Classified as prerenal failure, intrarenal failure (also called *intrinsic* or *parenchymal failure*), or postrenal failure
- Usually reversible with medical treatment
- If not treated, may progress to end-stage renal disease, uremia, and death
- Normally occurs in three distinct phases: oliguric, diuretic, and recovery

OLIGURIC PHASE
- May last a few days or several weeks
- Urine output dropping below 400 ml/day
- Evidence of fluid volume excess, azotemia, and electrolyte imbalance
- Release of local mediators, causing intrarenal vasoconstriction
- Medullary hypoxia causing cellular swelling and adherence of neutrophils to capillaries and venules
- Hypoperfusion, cellular injury, and necrosis occurring
- Reperfusion causing reactive oxygen species to form, leading to further cellular injury

DIURETIC PHASE
- Renal function recovered
- Urine output gradually increasing
- Glomerular filtration rate improving, although tubular transport systems remain abnormal

RECOVERY PHASE
- May last 3 to 12 months, or even longer
- Renal function gradually returning to normal or near normal function

Pathophysiology
PRERENAL FAILURE
- Glomerular filtration rate declines because of the decrease in filtration pressure.
- Failure to restore blood volume or blood pressure may cause acute tubular necrosis (ATN) or acute cortical necrosis.

INTRARENAL FAILURE
- A severe episode of hypotension, commonly associated with hypovol-emia, is a significant contributing event.
- Ischemia generates toxic oxygen–free radicals and anti-inflammatory mediators that cause cell swelling, injury, and necrosis— a form of reperfusion injury that may also be caused by nephrotoxins.

POSTRENAL FAILURE
- Postrenal failure usually occurs with urinary tract obstruction that affects the kidneys bilaterally, such as with prostatic hyperplasia.

Causes
PRERENAL FAILURE
- Hypovolemia
- Impaired blood flow
- Hemorrhagic blood loss
- Loss of plasma volume
- Water and electrolyte losses
- Hypotension or hypoperfusion

INTRARENAL FAILURE
- ATN
- Glomerulopathies
- Malignant hypertension
- Coagulation defects

POSTRENAL FAILURE
- Obstructive uropathies, usually bilateral
- Ureteral destruction
- Bladder neck obstruction

Incidence
- Seen in 5% of hospitalized patients

Common characteristics
- Vary with renal failure phase

Complications
- Renal shutdown
- Electrolyte imbalance
- Metabolic acidosis
- Acute pulmonary edema
- Hypertensive crisis
- Infection
- Death

✳ ASSESSMENT

History
- Predisposing disorder
- Recent fever, chills, or central nervous system problem
- Recent GI problem

Physical findings
- Oliguria or anuria, depending on renal failure phase
- Tachycardia
- Bibasilar crackles
- Irritability, drowsiness, or confusion
- Altered level of consciousness
- Bleeding abnormalities
- Dry, pruritic skin
- Dry mucous membranes
- Uremic breath odor

Test results
LABORATORY
- Blood urea nitrogen, serum creatinine, and potassium levels are elevated.
- Blood pH, bicarbonate, hematocrit, and hemoglobin levels are decreased.
- Urine casts, cellular debris, and specific gravity are decreased.
- In glomerular disease, proteinuria and urine osmolality are close to serum osmolality level.
- Urine sodium level is below 20 mEq/L, in oliguria caused by decreased perfusion.
- Urine sodium level is above 40 mEq/L, in oliguria from an intrarenal problem.
- Urine creatinine clearance measures glomerular filtration rate and estimates number of remaining functioning nephrons.

IMAGING
The following imaging tests may show the cause of renal failure:
- kidney ultrasonography
- kidney-ureter-bladder radiography
- excretory urography renal scan
- retrograde pyelography
- computed tomography scan
- nephrotomography

DIAGNOSTIC PROCEDURES
- Electrocardiography shows tall, peaked T waves; a widening QRS complex; and disappearing P waves, if hyperkalemia is present.

◆ TREATMENT

General
- Hemodialysis or peritoneal dialysis, as appropriate

Diet
- High-calorie
- Low in protein, sodium, and potassium
- Fluid restriction

Activity
- Rest periods, as appropriate

Medication
- Diuretics
- Hypertonic glucose-and-insulin infusions, sodium bicarbonate, and sodium polystyrene sulfonate, in hyperkalemia

Surgery
- Creation of vascular access for hemodialysis

❖ NURSING CONSIDERATIONS

Nursing diagnoses
- Activity intolerance
- Decreased cardiac output
- Fatigue
- Fear
- Imbalanced nutrition: Less than body requirements
- Impaired urinary elimination
- Ineffective tissue perfusion: Renal
- Interrupted family processes
- Risk for imbalanced fluid volume
- Risk for infection
- Risk for injury

Key outcomes
The patient (or family) will:
- perform activities of daily living without excessive fatigue or exhaustion
- maintain hemodynamic stability
- express the importance of balancing activities with adequate rest periods
- discuss fears or concerns
- verbalize appropriate food choices
- demonstrate the ability to manage urinary elimination problems
- maintain adequate urine output

- verbalize the effect the patient's condition has on the family unit
- maintain fluid balance; output should equal intake
- remain free from signs and symptoms of infection
- remain free from injury.

Nursing interventions
- Administer medications, as ordered.
- Encourage the patient to express feelings.
- Provide emotional support.
- Identify patients at risk for and take steps to prevent ATN. (See *Preventing acute tubular necrosis.*)

Monitoring
- Intake and output
- Daily weight
- Renal function studies
- Vital signs
- Effects of excess fluid volume
- Dialysis access site

▶ PATIENT TEACHING

Be sure to cover:
- disorder, diagnostic tests, and treatment
- medication administration, dosage, and possible adverse effects
- recommended fluid allowance
- compliance with diet and medication regimen
- daily weight and importance of immediately reporting changes of 3 lb or more
- signs and symptoms of edema and importance of reporting them to the physician.

✳ RESOURCES

Organizations
American Association of Kidney Patients: *www.aakp.org*
National Institute of Diabetes & Digestive & Kidney Diseases: *www.niddk.nih.gov*
National Kidney Foundation: *www.kidney.org*

Selected references
Chan, V,. et al. "Valve Replacement Surgery Complicated by Acute Renal Failure—Predictors of Early Mortality," *Journal of Cardiac Surgery* 21(2):139-43, March-April 2006.
Diseases, 4th ed. Philadelphia: Lippincott Williams & Wilkins, 2006.
Francisco., A.L., and Pinera, C. "Challenges and Future of Renal Replacement Therapy," *Hemodialysis International* 10(Suppl 1):519-23, January 2006.
Perkins, C., and Kisel, M. "Utilizing Physiological Knowledge to Care for Acute Renal Failure," *British Journal of Nursing* 14(14):768-73, July-August 2005.
Uchino, S. , et al. "Acute Renal Failure in Critically Ill Patients: A Multinational Multicenter Study," *JAMA* 294(7):813-18, August 2005.

PREVENTING ACUTE TUBULAR NECROSIS

Patients at risk for acute tubular necrosis need to be identified. Because it occurs predominantly in elderly hospitalized patients, be aware of contributing causes. These include aminoglycoside therapy and exposure to industrial chemicals, heavy metals, and contrast media. Patients who have been exposed must receive adequate hydration; monitor their urinary output closely.

To prevent acute tubular necrosis, make sure every patient is well hydrated before surgery or after X-rays that use a contrast medium. Administer mannitol, as ordered, to the high-risk patient before and during these procedures. Carefully monitor a patient receiving a blood transfusion, and discontinue the transfusion immediately if early signs of transfusion reaction (fever, rash, and chills) occur.

Renal failure, chronic

● OVERVIEW

Description
- Usually the end result of gradually progressive loss of renal function
- Symptoms sparse until more than 75% of glomerular filtration lost; symptoms worsening as renal function declines
- Fatal unless treated; sustaining life possibly requiring maintenance dialysis or kidney transplantation

Pathophysiology
- Nephron destruction eventually causes irreversible renal damage.
- Disease course may progress through the following stages: reduced renal reserve, renal insufficiency, renal failure, and end-stage renal disease.

Causes
- Chronic glomerular disease
- Chronic infections such as chronic pyelonephritis
- Congenital anomalies such as polycystic kidney disease
- Vascular diseases
- Obstructive processes such as calculi
- Collagen diseases such as systemic lupus erythematosus
- Nephrotoxic agents
- Endocrine disease

Incidence
- Affects about 2 of every 100,000 people
- Can occur at all ages but more common in adults
- Affects more men than women
- Affects more Blacks than Whites

Common characteristics
- Fatigue
- Decreasing urine output
- Increasing edema
- Electrolyte imbalance
- Fluid overload

Complications
- Anemia
- Peripheral neuropathy
- Lipid disorders
- Platelet dysfunction
- Pulmonary edema
- Electrolyte imbalances
- Sexual dysfunction

✳ ASSESSMENT

History
- Predisposing factor
- Dry mouth
- Fatigue
- Nausea
- Hiccups
- Muscle cramps
- Fasciculations, twitching
- Infertility, decreased libido
- Amenorrhea
- Impotence
- Pathologic fractures

Physical findings
- Decreased urine output
- Hypotension or hypertension
- Altered level of consciousness
- Peripheral edema
- Cardiac arrhythmias
- Bibasilar crackles
- Pleural friction rub
- Gum ulceration and bleeding
- Uremic fetor
- Abdominal pain on palpation
- Poor skin turgor
- Pale, yellowish bronze skin color
- Thin, brittle fingernails and dry, brittle hair
- Growth retardation (in children)

Test results
LABORATORY
- Blood urea nitrogen, serum creatinine, sodium, and potassium levels are elevated.
- Arterial blood gas (ABG) values show decreased arterial pH and bicarbonate levels.
- Hematocrit and hemoglobin level are low; red blood cell (RBC) survival time is decreased.
- Thrombocytopenia is mild, with evidence of platelet defects.
- Aldosterone secretion is increased.
- Hyperglycemia and hypertriglyceridemia are present.
- High-density lipoprotein levels are decreased.
- ABG values show metabolic acidosis.
- Urine specific gravity is fixed at 1.010.
- Proteinuria, glycosuria; and urinary RBCs, leukocytes, casts, and crystals are present.

IMAGING
- Kidney-ureter-bladder radiography, excretory urography, nephrotomography, renal scan, and renal arteriography show reduced kidney size.

DIAGNOSTIC PROCEDURES
- Renal biopsy allows histologic identification of the underlying pathology.
- Electroencephalography shows changes suggesting metabolic encephalopathy.

◆ TREATMENT

General
- Hemodialysis or peritoneal dialysis

Diet
- Low-protein (with peritoneal dialysis, high-protein)
- High-calorie
- Low in sodium, phosphorus, and potassium
- Fluid restriction

Activity
- Rest periods, as appropriate

Medication
- Loop diuretics
- Cardiac glycosides
- Antihypertensives
- Antiemetics
- Iron and folate supplements
- Erythropoietin
- Antipruritics
- Supplementary vitamins and essential amino acids

Surgery
- Creation of vascular access for dialysis
- Possible kidney transplant

NURSING CONSIDERATIONS

Nursing diagnoses
- Acute pain
- Decreased cardiac output
- Disabled family coping
- Excess fluid volume
- Imbalanced nutrition: Less than body requirements
- Impaired gas exchange
- Impaired oral mucous membrane
- Impaired urinary elimination
- Ineffective coping
- Ineffective sexuality patterns
- Ineffective tissue perfusion: Renal
- Interrupted family processes
- Powerlessness
- Risk for infection
- Risk for injury

Key outcomes
The patient will:
- express feelings of increased comfort and decreased pain
- maintain hemodynamic stability
- demonstrate adaptive coping behaviors
- maintain fluid balance
- verbalize appropriate food choices according to the prescribed diet
- maintain adequate ventilation and oxygenation
- maintain intact oral mucous membranes
- demonstrate the ability to manage the urinary elimination problems
- use support resources and exhibit adaptive coping beahviors
- resume sexual activity to the fullest extent possible
- maintain adequate urine output
- verbalize the effect the patient's condition has on the family unit
- verbalize feelings of control over condition and own well-being
- remain free from signs or symptoms of infection
- remain free from injury.

Nursing interventions
- Administer medications, as ordered.
- Perform meticulous skin care.
- Encourage the patient to express feelings.
- Provide emotional support.

Monitoring
- Renal function studies
- Laboratory results
- Vital signs
- Intake and output
- Daily weight
- Signs and symptoms of fluid overload
- Signs and symptoms of bleeding

PATIENT TEACHING

Be sure to cover:
- disorder, diagnostic tests, and treatment
- dietary changes
- fluid restrictions
- dialysis site care as appropriate
- importance of wearing medical identification.

Discharge planning
- Refer the patient to resource and support services.

RESOURCES

Organizations
American Association of Kidney Patients: *www.aakp.org*
National Institute of Diabetes & Digestive & Kidney Diseases: *www.niddk.nih.gov*
National Kidney Foundation: *www.kidney.org*

Selected references
Campoy, S., and Elwell, R. "Pharmacology and CKD: How Chronic Kidney Disease and Its Complications Alter Drug Response," *AJN* 105(9):60-71, September 2005.
Castner, D., and Douglas, C. "Now on Stage: Chronic Kidney Disease," *Nursing* 35(12):58-63, December 2005.
Diseases, 4th ed. Philadelphia: Lippincott Williams & Wilkins, 2006.
Harwood, L., et al. "Preparing for Hemodialysis: Patient Stressors and Responses," *Nephrology Nursing Journal* 32(3):295-302, May-June 2005.
Lim, W.H., et al. "Renal Transplantation Reverses Functional Deficiencies in Circulating Dendritic Cell Subsets in Chronic Renal Failure Patients," *Transplantation* 81(2):160-68, January 2006.

Respiratory distress syndrome

● OVERVIEW

Description
- Involves widespread alveolar collapse
- Most common cause of neonatal death
- If mild, subsides slowly after about 3 days
- Also called *RDS* or *hyaline membrane disease*

Pathophysiology
- In neonates born before the 27th week of gestation, immaturity of alveoli and capillary blood supply lead to alveolar collapse from lack of surfactant (a lipoprotein normally present in alveoli and respiratory bronchioles).
- Surfactant deficiency causes widespread atelectasis, resulting in inadequate alveolar ventilation and shunting of blood through collapsed lung areas.
- Hypoxia and acidosis result.
- Compensatory grunting occurs, producing positive end-expiratory pressure (PEEP) that helps prevent further alveolar collapse.

Causes
- Surfactant deficiency stemming from preterm birth

Risk factors
- Diabetes in mother during pregnancy
- Stress during preterm labor

Incidence
- Almost exclusively affects neonates born before the 37th gestational week; occurs in about 60% of those born before the 28th week
- Most common in neonates of mothers with diabetes, neonates delivered by cesarean delivery, and neonates delivered suddenly after antepartum hemorrhage

Common characteristics
- Labored breathing within minutes to hours after birth

Complications
- Respiratory insufficiency
- Shock
- Bronchopulmonary dysplasia
- Death

✳ ASSESSMENT

History
- Preterm birth
- Cesarean delivery
- Maternal history of diabetes or antepartum hemorrhage

Physical findings
- Rapid, shallow respirations
- Intercostal, subcostal, or sternal retractions
- Nasal flaring
- Audible expiratory grunting
- Pallor
- Frothy sputum
- Low body temperature
- Diminished air entry and crackles
- Possible hypotension, peripheral edema, and oliguria
- Possible apnea, bradycardia, and cyanosis

Test results
LABORATORY
- Partial pressure of arterial oxygen (PaO_2) is decreased; partial pressure of arterial carbon dioxide is normal, decreased, or increased; and arterial pH is reduced.
- Lecithin-sphingomyelin ratio shows prenatal lung development and RDS risk.
IMAGING
- Chest X-rays may show a fine reticulonodular pattern and dark streaks, indicating air-filled, dilated bronchioles.

◆ TREATMENT

General
- Aggressive management, assisted by mechanical ventilation with PEEP or continuous positive airway pressure (CPAP) administered by a tight-fitting face mask or, when necessary, an endotracheal tube
- For a neonate who can't maintain adequate gas exchange, high-frequency oscillation ventilation
- Radiant warmer or Isolette

Diet
- Tube feedings or total parenteral nutrition

Activity
- Bed rest

Medication
- I.V. fluids and sodium bicarbonate
- Pancuronium bromide
- Prophylactic antibiotics
- Diuretics
- Surfactant replacement therapy
- Vitamin E
- Antenatal corticosteroids
- Oxygen therapy

Surgery
- Possible tracheostomy

❖ NURSING CONSIDERATIONS

Nursing diagnoses
- Compromised family coping
- Impaired gas exchange
- Impaired skin integrity
- Ineffective airway clearance
- Risk for infection
- Risk for injury

Key outcomes
The patient (or family) will:
- communicate feelings about neonate's decision
- maintain adequate ventilation and oxygenation
- maintain skin integrity
- maintain a patent airway
- remain free from signs and symptoms of infection
- remain free from injury.

Nursing interventions
- Administer medications, as ordered.
- Check the umbilical catheter for arterial or venous hypotension, as appropriate.
- Suction, as necessary.
- Change the transcutaneous PaO_2 monitor lead placement site every 2 to 4 hours.
- Adjust PEEP or CPAP settings as indicated by arterial blood gas (ABG) values.
- Implement measures to prevent infection.
- Provide mouth care every 2 hours.
- Encourage the parents to participate in the infant's care.
- Encourage the parents to ask questions and to express their fears and concerns.
- Advise parents that full recovery may take up to 12 months.
- Offer emotional support.

◆ **NURSING ALERT** In a neonate on a mechanical ventilator, watch carefully for signs of barotrauma and accidental disconnection from the ventilator. Check ventilator settings frequently. Stay alert for signs of complications of PEEP or CPAP therapy, such as decreased cardiac output, pneumothorax, and pneumomediastinum.

Monitoring
- Vital signs
- ABG values
- Intake and output
- Central venous pressure
- Signs and symptoms of infection
- Thrombosis
- Decreased peripheral circulation
- Pulse oximetry
- Daily weight
- Skin color
- Respiratory status
- Skin integrity

◆ **NURSING ALERT** Watch for indications of oxygen therapy complications: lung capillary damage, decreased mucus flow, impaired ciliary functioning, and widespread atelectasis. Also stay alert for signs of patent ductus arteriosus, heart failure, retinopathy, pulmonary hypertension, necrotizing enterocolitis, and neurologic abnormalities.

▶ PATIENT TEACHING

Be sure to cover (with the parents):
- disorder, diagnosis, and treatment
- medication administration, dosage, and possible adverse effects
- explanations of respiratory equipment, alarm sounds, and mechanical noise
- potential complications
- when to notify the physician.

Discharge planning
- Refer the parents to pastoral counselors and social workers, as indicated.
- Refer the patient for follow-up care with a neonatal ophthalmologist, as indicated.

✴ RESOURCES

Organizations
American Academy of Pediatrics: *www.aap.org*
American Association for Respiratory Care: *www.aarc.org*
American Lung Association: *www.lungusa.org*
National Heart, Lung and Blood Institute: *www.nhlbi.nih.gov*

Selected references
Boyd, S. "Causes and Treatment of Neonatal Respiratory Distress Syndrome," *Nursing Times* 100(30):40-44, July-August 2004.

Burnes, S.M. "Mechanical Ventilation of Patients with Acute Respiratory Distress Syndrome and Patients Requiring Weaning: The Evidence Guiding Practice," *Critical Care Nurse* 25(4):14-23, August 2005.

Fan, E., et al. "Ventilatory Management of Acute Lung Injury and Acute Respiratory Distress Syndrome," *JAMA* 294(22):2889-896, December 2005.

Rebmann, Y. "Severe Acute Respiratory Distress Syndrome: Implications for Perinatal and Neonatal Nurses," *Journal of Perinatal & Neonatal Nursing* 19(4):332-45, October-December 2005.

Respiratory syncytial virus infection

● OVERVIEW

Description
- Leading cause of lower respiratory tract infection in infants and young children
- Suspected cause of fatal respiratory diseases in infants
- Can cause serious illness in immuno-compromised adults, institutionalized elderly people, and patients with underlying cardiopulmonary disease

Pathophysiology
- Virus attaches to cells, eventually resulting in necrosis of the bronchiolar epithelium; in severe infection, peribronchiolar infiltrate of lymphocytes and mononuclear cells occurs.
- Intra-alveolar thickening and filling of the alveolar spaces with fluid results.

Causes
- Respiratory syncytial virus, a subgroup of myxoviruses resembling paramyxovirus
- Transmitted from person to person by respiratory secretions

Risk factors
- Day care attendance
- Contact with school-age children
- Low birth weight
- Crowded living conditions
- Environmental air pollutants

Incidence
- Almost exclusively affects infants and young children, especially those in day-care settings
- Highest among infants ages 1 to 6 months; peaking incidence between ages 2 and 3 months
- Annual epidemics during winter and spring

Common characteristics
- Rhinorrhea, low-grade fever, and mild systemic symptoms accompanied by cough and wheezing
- Reinfection common; produces milder symptoms than primary infection

Complications
- Pneumonia and progressive pneumonia
- Bronchiolitis
- Croup
- Otitis media
- Respiratory failure
- Sudden infant death syndrome
- Residual lung damage

✳ ASSESSMENT

History
- Nasal congestion
- Coughing
- Wheezing
- Malaise
- Sore throat
- Earache
- Dyspnea
- Fever

Physical findings
- Nasal and pharyngeal inflammation
- Otitis media
- Severe respiratory distress (nasal flaring, retraction, cyanosis, and tachypnea)
- Wheezes, rhonchi, and crackles

Test results
LABORATORY
- Cultures of nasal and pharyngeal secretions show respiratory syncytial virus.
- Serum respiratory syncytial virus antibody titers are elevated.
- Arterial blood gas values show hypoxemia.
- Blood urea nitrogen is elevated in dehydration.

◆ TREATMENT

General
- Respiratory support
- Symptomatic treatment

Diet
- Adequate nutrition
- Avoidance of overhydration

Activity
- Rest periods, as appropriate

Medication
- Ribavirin
- Oxygen (for severe infection)
- I.V. fluids (for severe infection)

Surgery
- Possible tracheostomy

♣ NURSING CONSIDERATIONS

Nursing diagnoses
- Activity intolerance
- Compromised family coping
- Imbalanced nutrition: Less than body requirements
- Impaired gas exchange
- Impaired social interaction
- Ineffective airway clearance
- Risk for aspiration
- Risk for deficient fluid volume
- Risk for infection

Key outcomes
The patient (or parents) will:
- return to previous activity level
- demonstrate effective coping strategies for handling their child's illness
- maintain adequate nutritional intake
- express or indicate feelings of comfort while maintaining adequate air exchange
- demonstrate effective social interactions in both one-on-one and group settings
- maintain a patent airway, cough effectively, and expectorate mucus
- maintain effective breathing pattern and a respiratory rate within 5 breaths/minute of baseline
- not develop aspiration pneumonia
- maintain adequate fluid volume
- remain free from further signs or symptoms of infection.

Nursing interventions
- Institute contact isolation.
- Perform percussion, drainage, and suction, when necessary.
- Administer oxygen, as ordered.
- Use a croup tent, as needed.
- Place the patient in semi-Fowler's position.
- Observe for signs and symptoms of dehydration, and administer I.V. fluids accordingly.
- Promote bed rest.
- Offer diversional activities tailored to the patient's condition and age.

Monitoring
- Respiratory status
- Fluid and electrolyte status

▶ PATIENT TEACHING

Be sure to cover with the parents:
- disorder, diagnostic tests, and treatment
- how the infection spreads
- avoidance of taking infants into crowds
- medication administration, dosage, and possible adverse effects
- importance of a nonsmoking environment in the home
- when to notify the physician
- follow-up care.

✴ RESOURCES

Organizations
American Lung Association: *www.lungusa.org*
Mayo Clinic: *www.mayoclinic.com*
National Center for Infectious Diseases: *www.cdc.gov/ncidod*
National Institute of Allergy and Infectious Diseases: *www.niaid.nih.gov*
The RSV Info Center: *www.rsvinfo.com*

Selected references
Blanco, J.C., et al. "Prospects of Antiviral and Anti-Inflammatory Therapy for Respiratory Syncytial Virus Infection," *Expert Review of Anti-Infective Therapy* 3(6):945-55, December 2005.

Kasper, D. L., et. al., eds. *Harrison's Principles of Inernal Medicine,* 16th ed. New York: McGraw-Hill Book Co., 2005.

Lauts, N.M. "RSV: Protecting the Littlest Patients," *RN* 68(12):46-51, December 2005.

Mejias, A., et al. "Respiratory Syncytial Virus Infections: Old Challenges and New Opportunities," *Pediatric Infectious Disease Journal* 24(11 Suppl) S189-96, November 2005.

Nagayama, Y., et al. "Gender Analysis in Acute Bronchiolitis Due to Respiratory Syncytial Virus," *Pediatric Allergy and Immunology* 17(1):29-36, February 2006.

Pruitt, B. "Keeping Respiratory Syncytial Virus at Bay," *Nursing* 35(11):62-64, November 2005.

Retinal detachment

● OVERVIEW

Description
- Separation of the sensory retina from the underlying pigment epithelium
- May be primary or secondary
- Usually involves only one eye; may occur in the contralateral eye later
- Rarely heals spontaneously; usually can be reattached successfully with surgery
- Prognosis dependent on the retinal area affected

Pathophysiology
- A hole or tear in the retina allows the liquid vitreous to seep between the retinal layers.
- Liquid separates the sensory retinal layer from its choroidal blood supply. (See *Understanding retinal detachment*.)

Causes
- Intraocular inflammation
- Trauma
- Age-related degenerative changes
- Tumors
- Systemic disease
- Traction placed on the retina by vitreous bands or membranes
- Hereditary factors, usually in association with myopia

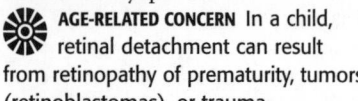 **AGE-RELATED CONCERN** In a child, retinal detachment can result from retinopathy of prematurity, tumors (retinoblastomas), or trauma.

Risk factors
- Myopia
- Cataract surgery
- Trauma
- History of uncontrolled diabetes

Incidence
- Affects twice as many men as women
- More common with increased age

Common characteristics
- Painless vision loss
- Sensation of floaters or of looking through a veil, curtain, or cobweb

Complications
- Severe vision impairment
- Blindness

✳ ASSESSMENT

History
- Sensation of seeing floaters and flashes
- Painless vision loss, described as sensation of looking through a veil, curtain, or cobweb (which may obscure objects in a particular visual field)

Physical findings
- Visual field loss

Test results
IMAGING
- Ocular ultrasonography may be used to examine the retina if the lens is opaque and shows intraocular and intraorbital pathology. It also commonly detects retinal detachments, characteristically producing a dense, sheetlike echo or a B-mode scan.

DIAGNOSTIC PROCEDURES
- Direct ophthalmoscopy shows folds or discoloration in the usually transparent retina.
- Indirect ophthalmoscopy shows retinal tears.

◆ TREATMENT

General
- Dependent on location and severity of detachment

Diet
- Nothing by mouth before surgery

Activity
- Bed rest before surgery
- Restriction of eye movements before surgery
- Positioning of the patient's head to allow gravity to pull the detached retina closer to the choroid

Medication
- Antiemetics
- Analgesics
- Mydriatics
- Cycloplegics
- Steroidal eyedrops
- Antibiotic eyedrops

Surgery
- Cryothermy
- Laser therapy
- Scleral buckling (may be followed by vitreous replacement with silicone, oil, air, or gas)
- Diathermy

UNDERSTANDING RETINAL DETACHMENT

Traumatic injury or degenerative changes cause retinal detachment by allowing the retina's sensory tissue layers to separate from the retinal pigment epithelium. This permits fluid—from the vitreous, for example—to seep into the space between the retinal pigment epithelium and the rods and cones of the tissue layers.

The pressure, which results from the fluid entering the space, balloons the retina into the vitreous cavity away from choroidal circulation. Separated from its blood supply, the retina can't function. Without prompt repair, the detached retina can cause permanent vision loss.

Nursing diagnoses

- Anxiety
- Disturbed sensory perception: Visual
- Impaired tissue integrity
- Ineffective health maintenance
- Risk for infection

Key outcomes

The patient will:

- verbalize strategies to reduce anxiety
- regain the previous level of visual functioning
- regain adequate perfusion to the retina
- maintain current health status
- remain free from signs or symptoms of infection
- remain free from injury.

Nursing interventions

- Prepare the patient for surgery.
- Administer antibiotics and cycloplegic or mydriatic eyedrops, as ordered.
- In macular involvement, maintain bed rest to prevent further retinal detachment.
- Postoperatively, position the patient, as directed.
- Administer antiemetics, as indicated and ordered.
- Administer analgesics, as ordered.
- Discourage activities that increase intraocular pressure.
- With retrobulbar injection, apply a protective eye patch.
- Apply cold compresses.
- Avoid putting pressure on the eye.
- Provide encouragement and emotional support.

Monitoring

- Localized corneal edema and perilimbal congestion after laser therapy
- Persistent pain
- Vital signs
- Visual acuity
- Response to treatment

Be sure to cover:

- disorder, diagnostic tests, and treatment
- leg and deep-breathing exercises
- possible persistence of blurred vision for several days after laser therapy
- importance of avoiding driving, bending, heavy lifting, and other activities that affect intraocular pressure for several days after surgery
- avoidance of activities that could cause eye trauma
- how to instill eyedrops
- importance of wearing sunglasses
- applying cold compresses
- medication administration, dosage, and possible adverse effects
- signs and symptoms of increasing ocular pressure and infection
- early symptoms of retinal detachment.

Organizations

American Academy of Ophthalmology: *www.aao.org*
National Eye Institute: *www.nei.nih.gov*

Selected references

Boyd-Monk, H. "Bringing Common Eye Emergencies into Focus," *Nursing* 35(12):46-51, December 2005.

Church, J.R., and Winder, S.M., "Surgical Repair of a Retinal Detachment in a Patient with Osteogenesis Imperfecta," *Retina* 26(2):242-43, February 2006.

Sonoda, Y., et al. "Endoscopy-Guided Subretinal Fluid Drainage in Vitrectomy for Retinal Detachment," *Ophthalmologica* 220(2):83-86, 2006.

Yuen, K.S., et al. "Bilateral Exudative: Retinal Detachments as the Presenting Feature of Idiopathic Orbital Inflammation," *Clinical & Experimental Ophthalmology* 33(6):671-74, December 2005.

Rhabdomyolysis

OVERVIEW

Description
- Breakdown of muscle tissue, causing myoglobinuria
- Usually follows major muscle trauma, especially a muscle crush injury
- Good prognosis if contributing causes are stopped or disease is checked before damage becomes irreversible

Pathophysiology
- Muscle trauma that compresses tissue causes ischemia and necrosis.
- The ensuing local edema further increases compartment pressure and tamponade; pressure from severe swelling causes blood vessels to collapse, leading to tissue hypoxia, muscle infarction, neural damage in the area of the fracture, and release of myoglobin from the necrotic muscle fibers into the circulation.

Causes
- Traumatic injury
- Prescription and nonprescription drugs (see *Drugs that may cause rhabdomyolysis*)
- Familial tendency
- Strenuous exertion, such as long-distance running
- Infection, especially severe infection
- Anesthetics that cause intraoperative rigidity
- Heat stroke
- Electrolyte disturbances
- Cardiac arrhythmias
- Excessive muscular activity associated with status epilepticus, electroconvulsive therapy, or high-voltage electrical shock

Risk factors
- Alcohol use
- Recent soft tissue compression
- Seizure activity

Incidence
- More common in males than females
- May occur at any age

Common characteristics
- Muscle pain
- Reddish-brown urine

Complications
- Renal failure
- Amputation

ASSESSMENT

History
- Muscle trauma or breakdown
- Muscle pain
- Presence of any risk factors

Physical findings
- Dark, reddish-brown urine
- Tense, tender muscle compartment (compartment syndrome)

Test results
LABORATORY
- Urine myoglobin level exceeds 0.5 mg/dl (evident with only 200 g of muscle damage).
- Creatinine kinase level is elevated (0.5 to 0.95 mg/dl) from muscle damage.
- Serum potassium, phosphate, creatinine, and creatine levels are elevated.
- Hypocalcemia occurs in early stages, hypercalcemia in later stages.
- Intracompartmental venous pressure measurements (using a wick catheter, needle, or slit catheter inserted into the muscle) are elevated.

IMAGING
- Computed tomography, magnetic resonance imaging, and bone scintigraphy are used to detect muscle necrosis.

TREATMENT

General
- For underlying disorder
- Prevention of renal failure

Diet
- As tolerated

Activity
- Bed rest

Medication
- Anti-inflammatory agents
- Corticosteroids (in extreme cases)
- Analgesics

Surgery
- Immediate fasciotomy and debridement if compartment venous pressure exceeds 25 mm Hg

DRUGS THAT MAY CAUSE RHABDOMYOLYSIS

The use of these drugs may cause rhabdomyolysis:
- amphetamines
- antilipemics
- antipsychotics
- anesthetic and paralytic agents
- antihistamines
- cocaine
- corticosteroids
- cyclic antidepressants
- emetics
- fibric acid derivatives
- laxatives
- neuroleptics
- salicylates
- sedative-hypnotics
- selective serotonin reuptake inhibitors

Nursing diagnoses
- Acute pain
- Excess fluid volume
- Hyperthermia
- Impaired urinary elimination

Key outcomes
The patient will:
- express feelings of increased comfort and decreased pain
- exhibit signs of normal fluid balance
- maintain a normal body temperature
- maintain normal renal function and urine output.

Nursing interventions
- Give prescribed I.V. fluids and diuretics.
- Measure intake and output accurately.
- Promote comfort measures.

Monitoring
- Intake and output
- Urine myoglobins
- Renal studies
- Pain control

Be sure to cover:
- disorder, diagnostic tests, and treatment
- need for prolonged, low-intensity exercise as opposed to short bursts of intense activity.

Organizations
American Association of Kidney Patients: *www.aakp.org*
National Institute of Diabetes & Digestive & Kidney Diseases: *www.niddk.nih.gov*
Rhabdomyolysis Kidney Failure and Damage: *www.rhabdomyolysis.org*

Selected references
Betten, D.P., et al. "Massive Honey Bee Invenomation-Induced Rhabdomyolysis in an Adolescent," *Pediatrics* 117(1):231-35, January 2006.
Hansen, K.E., et al. "Outcomes of 45 Patients with Statin-Associated Myopathy," *Archives of Internal Medicine* 165(22):2671-676, December 2005.
Kring, D. "Outmuscling Rhabdomyolysis," *Nursing Management* Suppl:24, 26, 29, 2005.
Ocana, J., et al. "Rhabdomyolysis," *American Journal of Kidney Diseases* 47(1):A32, e1-2, January 2006.
Vasudevan, A.R., et al. "Safety of Statins: Effects on Muscle and the Liver," *Cleveland Clinic Journal of Medicine* 72(11):990-93, 996-1001, November 2005.

Rheumatic fever and rheumatic heart disease

● OVERVIEW

Description
- Systemic inflammatory disease of childhood that follows upper respiratory tract infection with group A beta-hemolytic streptococci and commonly recurs
- Principally involves the heart, joints, central nervous system, skin, and subcutaneous tissues
- Rheumatic heart disease (cardiac manifestations of rheumatic fever): may affect the endocardium, myocardium, or pericardium during the early acute phase; later, may affect the heart valves, causing chronic valvular disease

Pathophysiology
- Rheumatic fever appears to be a hypersensitivity reaction in which antibodies produced to combat streptococci react and produce lesions at specific tissue sites.
- Antigens of group A streptococci bind to receptors in the heart, muscle, brain, and synovial joints, causing an autoimmune response.
- Because the antigens are similar to the body's own cells, antibodies may attack healthy body cells by mistake.

Causes
- Group A beta-hemolytic streptococcal pharyngitis

Incidence
- In the United States, most common in northern states
- Worldwide, 15 to 20 million new cases annually

Common characteristics
- Tends to be familial
- Most common during cool, damp weather in winter and early spring

Complications
- Destruction of mitral and aortic valves
- Severe pancarditis
- Pericardial effusion
- Heart failure
- Systemic emboli

✴ **AGE-RELATED CONCERN** In children, mitral insufficiency is the major consequence of rheumatic heart disease.

✳ ASSESSMENT

History
- Recent streptococcal infection
- Recent history of low-grade fever spiking to at least 100.4° F (38° C) in late afternoon, along with unexplained epistaxis and abdominal pain
- Migratory joint pain (polyarthritis)

Physical findings
- Swelling, redness, and signs of effusion, most commonly in the knees, ankles, elbows, and hips
- With pericarditis: sharp, sudden pain that usually starts over the sternum and radiates to the neck, shoulders, back, and arms; increases with deep inspiration and decreases when the patient sits up and leans forward
- With heart failure caused by severe rheumatic carditis: dyspnea; right upper quadrant pain; and a hacking, nonproductive cough
- With left-sided heart failure: edema and tachypnea, bibasilar crackles, and ventricular or atrial gallop
- Skin lesions, such as erythema marginatum, typically appearing on the trunk and extremities
- Subcutaneous nodules, 3 mm to 2 cm in diameter, that are firm, movable, and nontender occurring near tendons or bony prominences of joints, persisting for several days to weeks
- Transient Huntington's disease up to 6 months after original streptococcal infection
- Pericardial friction rub
- Heart murmurs and gallops

Test results
LABORATORY
- White blood cell count and erythrocyte sedimentation rate are elevated (during acute phase).
- Complete blood count shows slight anemia (during inflammation).
- C-reactive protein is positive (especially during acute phase).

- Cardiac enzyme levels are increased (in severe carditis).
- Antistreptolysin-O titer is elevated (seen in 95% of patients within 2 months of onset).
- Throat cultures show group A beta-hemolytic streptococci.

IMAGING
- Chest X-rays show normal heart size (except with myocarditis, heart failure, and pericardial effusion).
- Echocardiography helps evaluate valvular damage, chamber size, and ventricular function and detects pericardial effusion.

DIAGNOSTIC PROCEDURES
- Electrocardiography reveals no diagnostic changes, but 20% of patients show a prolonged PR interval.
- Cardiac catheterization evaluates valvular damage and left ventricular function in severe cardiac dysfunction.

◆ TREATMENT

General
- Symptomatic treatment

Diet
- Sodium restriction, if indicated

Activity
- Bed rest during acute phase
- Gradual activity increase, as tolerated

Medication
- Antibiotics
- Anti-inflammatories

Surgery
- Commissurotomy, valvuloplasty, or heart valve replacement

NURSING CONSIDERATIONS

Nursing diagnoses
- Activity intolerance
- Acute pain
- Anxiety
- Decreased cardiac output
- Deficient diversional activity
- Fatigue
- Impaired gas exchange
- Ineffective role performance
- Risk for infection

Key outcomes
The patient will:
- carry out activities of daily living without weakness or fatigue
- express feelings of increased comfort and decreased pain
- cope with medical condition without demonstrating severe signs of anxiety
- maintain hemodynamic stability, have no arrhythmias, and maintain adequate cardiac output
- identify appropriate diversionary activities to partake in while on bed rest
- verbalize the importance of balancing activity with adequate rest periods
- maintain adequate ventilation and oxygenation
- express feelings about diminished capacity to perform usual roles
- remain free from signs and symptoms of infection.

Nursing interventions
- Find out if the patient has ever had a hypersensitivity reaction to penicillin. Warn the parents (if appropriate) that such a reaction is possible.
- Administer antibiotics on time, as ordered.
- Stress the importance of bed rest. Provide a bedside commode.
- Position the patient upright.
- Provide analgesics and oxygen, as needed.
- Allow the patient to express feelings and concerns.
- Help the parents overcome any feelings of guilt that they may harbor about their child's illness.
- Encourage the parents and child to vent their frustrations during the long recovery. If the child has severe carditis, help them prepare for permanent changes in the child's lifestyle.

Monitoring
- Vital signs
- Heart rhythm
- Heart and breath sounds

PATIENT TEACHING

Be sure to cover:
- disorder, diagnostic tests, and treatment
- importance of slowly resuming activities of daily living and scheduling frequent rest periods, as instructed by the physician
- what to do if signs of an allergic reaction to penicillin occur
- importance of reporting early signs and symptoms of left-sided heart failure, such as dyspnea and a hacking, nonproductive cough, and immediately reporting signs of recurrent streptococcal infection
- keeping the child away from people with respiratory tract infections.
- transient nature of Huntington's disease
- compliance with prolonged antibiotic therapy and follow-up care
- need for prophylactic antibiotics before any dental work or invasive procedures.

Discharge planning
- Refer patient and family to appropriate support services, as indicated.

RESOURCES

Organizations
American Heart Association:
www.americanheart.org
National Heart, Lung and Blood Institute:
www.nhlbi.nih.gov/nhlbi/cardio

Selected references
Carapetis, J.R., et al. "Acute Rheumatic Fever," *Lancet* 366(9480):155-68, July 2005.

Kasper, D.L., et al., eds. *Harrison's Principles of Internal Medicine*, 16th ed. New York: McGraw-Hill Book Co., 2005.

Lee, G.M., and Wessels, M.R. "Changing Epidemiology of Acute Rheumatic Fever in the United States," *Clinical Infectious Diseases* 42(4):448-50, February 2005.

The Merck Manual of Diagnosis & Therapy, 18th ed. Whitehouse Station, N.J.: Merck & Co., Inc. 2006.

Mota, C. "Limitations and Perspectives with the Approach to Rheumatic Fever and Rheumatic Heart Disease," *Cardiology in the Young* 15(6):580-82, December 2005.

Rheumatoid arthritis

● OVERVIEW

Description
- Chronic, systemic, symmetrical inflammatory disease
- Primarily attacks peripheral joints and surrounding muscles, tendons, ligaments, and blood vessels
- Marked by spontaneous remissions and unpredictable exacerbations
- Potentially crippling

Pathophysiology
- Cartilage damage resulting from inflammation triggers further immune responses, including complement activation.
- Complement, in turn, attracts polymorphonuclear leukocytes and stimulates release of inflammatory mediators, which exacerbates joint destruction.

Causes
- Exact cause unknown
- Possible influence of infection (viral or bacterial), hormonal factors, and lifestyle

Incidence
- Strikes three times as many women as men
- Can occur at any age; peak onset between ages 35 and 50

Common characteristics
- Stiff, swollen joints

Complications
- Fibrous or bony ankylosis
- Soft-tissue contractures
- Joint deformities
- Sjögren's syndrome
- Spinal cord compression
- Carpal tunnel syndrome
- Osteoporosis
- Recurrent infections
- Hip joint necrosis

✳ ASSESSMENT

History
- Insidious onset of nonspecific symptoms, including fatigue, malaise, anorexia, persistent low-grade fever, weight loss, and vague articular symptoms
- Later, more specific localized articular symptoms, commonly in the fingers
- Bilateral and symmetrical symptoms, which may extend to the wrists, elbows, knees, and ankles
- Painful, red, swollen arms
- Stiff joints
- Stiff, weak, or painful muscles
- Numbness or tingling in the feet or weakness or loss of sensation in the fingers
- Pain on inspiration
- Shortness of breath

Physical findings
- Joint deformities and contractures
- Foreshortened hands
- Boggy wrists
- Rheumatoid nodules
- Leg ulcers
- Eye redness
- Joints that are warm to the touch
- Pericardial friction rub
- Positive Babinski's sign

Test results
LABORATORY
- Rheumatoid factor test is positive (in 75% to 80% of patients), as indicated by titer of 1:160 or higher.
- Synovial fluid analysis shows increased volume and turbidity but decreased viscosity and complement (C3 and C4) levels, with white blood cell count possibly exceeding 10,000/mm³.
- Serum globulin levels are elevated.
- Erythrocyte sedimentation rate is elevated.
- Complete blood count shows moderate anemia and slight leukocytosis.

IMAGING
- In early stages, X-rays show bone demineralization and soft-tissue swelling. Later, they help determine the extent of cartilage and bone destruction, erosion, subluxations, and deformities and show the characteristic pattern of these abnormalities.
- Magnetic resonance imaging and computed tomography scan may provide information about the extent of damage

◆ TREATMENT

General
- Adequate sleep
- Splinting
- Moist heat application

Diet
- No restrictions

Activity
- Frequent rest periods between activities
- Range-of-motion (ROM) exercises and carefully individualized therapeutic exercises

Medication
- Salicylates
- Nonsteroidal anti-inflammatory drugs
- Antimalarials (hydroxychloroquine)
- Gold salts
- Penicillamine
- Corticosteroids
- Antineoplastics
- Monoclonal antibody therapy, such as infliximab (Remicacle)

Surgery
- Metatarsal head and distal ulnar resectional arthroplasty and insertion of silastic prosthesis between the metacarpophalangeal and proximal interphalangeal joints
- Arthrodesis (joint fusion)
- Synovectomy
- Osteotomy
- Repair of ruptured tendon
- Joint reconstruction or total joint arthroplasty (in advanced disease)

❖ NURSING CONSIDERATIONS

Nursing diagnoses
- Activity intolerance
- Bathing or hygiene deficit
- Chronic pain
- Energy field disturbance
- Fatigue
- Hopelessness
- Impaired physical mobility
- Ineffective health maintenance
- Ineffective role performance
- Ineffective tissue perfusion: Peripheral
- Powerlessness
- Risk for impaired skin integrity
- Risk for infection

Key outcomes
The patient will:
- verbalize the importance of balancing activity, as tolerated, with rest.
- participate in activities of daily living, to the fullest extent possible
- express feelings of increased comfort and decreased pain
- express an increased sense of well-being with less fatigue
- express feelings of increased energy
- make decisions on own behalf
- attain the highest degree of mobility possible within the confines of the disease
- continue to receive treatments that promote relaxation and inner well-being
- recognize limitations imposed by the illness and express feelings about these limitations
- maintain adequate peripheral perfusion, as evidenced by palpable pulses and warm extremities
- express feelings of control over condition
- maintain skin integrity
- remain free from signs or symptoms of infection.

Nursing interventions
- Administer analgesics as ordered, and watch for adverse reactions.
- Perform meticulous skin care.
- Supply adaptive devices, such as a zipper-pull, easy-to-open beverage cartons, lightweight cups, and unpackaged silverware.

AFTER TOTAL KNEE OR HIP ARTHROPLASTY
- Administer blood replacement products, antibiotics, and pain medication, as ordered.
- Have the patient perform active dorsiflexion; immediately report inability to do so.
- Supervise isometric exercises every 2 hours.
- After total hip arthroplasty, check traction for pressure areas and keep the head of the bed raised 30 to 45 degrees.
- Change or reinforce dressings, as needed, using sterile technique.
- Have the patient turn, cough, and breathe deeply every 2 hours.
- After total knee arthroplasty, keep the leg extended and slightly elevated.
- After total hip arthroplasty, keep the hip in abduction. Watch for and immediately report inability to rotate the hip or bear weight on it, increased pain, or a leg that appears shorter.
- Help the patient with activities, keeping the weight on the unaffected side.

Monitoring
- Joint stiffness
- Skin integrity
- Vital signs
- Daily weight
- Sensory disturbances
- Pain level
- Serum electrolyte, hemoglobin, and hematocrit levels
- Complications of corticosteroid therapy

▶ PATIENT TEACHING

Be sure to cover:
- chronic nature of rheumatoid arthritis and possible need for major lifestyle changes
- diagnostic tests and treatment
- importance of a balanced diet and weight control
- sexual concerns.
  If the patient requires total knee or hip arthroplasty, be sure to cover:
- preoperative and surgical procedures
- postoperative exercises, with supervision of the patient's practice

- deep-breathing and coughing exercises to perform after surgery
- performing frequent ROM leg exercises after surgery
- use of a constant-passive-motion device after total knee arthroplasty, or placement of an abduction pillow between the legs after total hip arthroplasty
- how to use a trapeze to move about in bed
- medication administration, dosage, and possible adverse effects.

Discharge planning
- Refer the patient for physical and occupational therapy.
- Refer the patient to the Arthritis Foundation.

✷ RESOURCES

Organizations
Arthritis Foundation: *www.arthritis.org*
The Arthritis Society: *www.arthritis.ca*
John Hopkins Arthritis Center: *www.hopkins-arthritis.som.jhmi.edu*
National Institute of Arthritis and Musculoskeletal and Skin Diseases: *www.nih.gov/niams/healthinfo*

Selected references
Bathon, J.M., et. al. "Safety and Efficacy of Etanercept Treatment in Elderly Subjects with Rheumatoid Arthritis," *Journal of Rheumatology* 33(2);234-43, February 2006.

Firestein, G.S. "Inhibiting Inflammation in Rheumatoid Arthritis," *New England Journal of Medicine* 354(1):80-82, January 2006.

Kasper, D.L., et al., eds. *Harrison's Principles of Internal Medicine*, 16th ed. New York: McGraw-Hill Book Co., 2005.

Mitka, M. "Early Rheumatoid Arthritis Treatments Weighed," *JAMA* 294(24):3073-3074, December 2005.

Rocky Mountain spotted fever

● OVERVIEW

Description
- Acute infectious, febrile, rash-producing illness associated with outdoor activities
- Fatal in about 5% of patients

Pathophysiology
- Infecting organism multiplies within endothelial cells and spreads via the bloodstream.
- Focal areas of infiltration lead to thrombosis and leakage of red blood cells into surrounding tissue.

Causes
- *Rickettsia rickettsii*, transmitted by the wood tick *(Dermacentor andersoni)* in the western United States and by the dog tick *(D. variabilis)* in the eastern United States (*R. rickettsii* entering humans or small animals with the prolonged bite [4 to 6 hours] of an adult tick)
- Occasionally acquired through inhalation or contact of abraded skin with tick excreta or tissue juices

Risk factors
- Recent hiking

Incidence
- Endemic throughout continental United States, but most common in southeastern and south-central regions
- Particularly prevalent in children ages 5 to 9 years
- Increased occurrence in spring and summer

Common characteristics
- Usual incubation period of 7 days
- Fever, headache, mental confusion, and myalgia
- Macular papular rash on palms and soles (in about 90% of patients)
- Rash evident in about 15% of patients on day 1 and in nearly half of patient by day 3; rash starts at the wrists, ankles, or forehead and spreads to remainder of extremities and trunk
- Within 2 days, rash seen over the entire body (including scalp, palms, and soles)

Complications
- Lobar pneumonia
- Disseminated intravascular coagulation
- Renal failure
- Meningoencephalitis
- Hepatic injury
- Death
- Cardiac or respiratory failure

✳ ASSESSMENT

History
- Recent exposure to ticks or tick-infested areas, or a known tick bite
- Abrupt symptom onset, including persistent fever (temperature of 102° to 104° F [38.9° to 40° C]); generalized, excruciating headache; and aching in bones, muscles, joints, and back

Physical findings
- Erythematous macules, 1 to 5 mm in diameter, becoming maculopapules that blanch on pressure
- Frank hemorrhage at the center of maculopapules, creating petechia that does not blanch on pressure
- Bronchial cough
- Tachypnea
- Altered level of consciousness
- Decreased urine output; dark urine
- Tachycardia
- Hypotension
- Hepatomegaly; splenomegaly
- Generalized pitting edema
- Abdominal tenderness

Test results
LABORATORY
- Serologic test results may be negative in initial stages.
- Indirect immunofluorescence assay diagnostic titer of 64 or greater is detectable between days 7 and 14 of the illness.
- Latex agglutination diagnostic titer of 128 or greater is detectable 1 week after onset.
- Platelet count, white blood cell count, and fibrinogen levels are decreased.
- Prothrombin time and partial thromboplastin time are prolonged.
- Serum protein levels are decreased (especially albumin).
- Hyponatremia and hypochloremia are associated with increased aldosterone excretion.
- Hepatic function is abnormal.
- Cerebrospinal fluid analysis shows mild mononuclear pleocytosis with slightly elevated protein content.
- Immunohistologic examination of cutaneous biopsy of a rash lesion shows *R. rickettsii*.

◆ TREATMENT

General
- Careful tick removal
- Intubation and mechanical ventilation, if needed
- Hemodialysis, if needed
- Treatment of hemorrhage and thrombocytopenia, if needed

Diet
- Careful fluid administration
- Small, frequent meals
- Parenteral nutrition if the patient can't receive oral intake

Activity
- Bed rest until condition improves

Medication
- Doxycycline (drug of choice)
- Anticonvulsants
- Oxygen therapy

✤ NURSING CONSIDERATIONS

Nursing diagnoses
- Activity intolerance
- Acute pain
- Decreased cardiac output
- Deficient fluid volume
- Hyperthermia
- Imbalanced nutrition: Less than body requirements
- Impaired skin integrity
- Ineffective tissue perfusion: Peripheral
- Risk for infection

Key outcomes
The patient will:
- resume normal activity level during recovery
- express feelings of increased comfort and decreased pain
- maintain adequate cardiac output
- maintain adequate fluid volume
- remain afebrile
- maintain adequate nutritional intake
- exhibit improved or healed lesions or wounds
- maintain hemodynamic stability
- remain free from signs and symptoms of infection.

Nursing interventions
- Administer medication, as ordered.
- Provide oxygen therapy and assisted ventilation for pulmonary complications, as ordered.
- Offer mentholated lotions if the rash itches.
- Turn the patient frequently.
- Encourage incentive spirometry and deep breathing.
- Plan care to promote adequate rest periods.

Monitoring
- Vital signs
- Fluid and electrolyte status
- Respiratory status
- Neurologic status
- Skin integrity

▶ PATIENT TEACHING

Be sure to cover:
- disorder, diagnostic tests, and treatment
- importance of reporting recurrent symptoms immediately
- preventive strategies, including avoiding tick-infested areas, whole-body inspection (including scalp) every 3 to 4 hours for attached ticks, protective clothing, and insect repellent
- correct tick removal technique using tweezers or forceps and steady traction.

Discharge planning
- Refer the patient to an infectious disease specialist, if needed.

✴ RESOURCES

Organizations
Centers for Disease Control and Prevention: www.cdc.gov
Harvard University Consumer Health Information: www.intelihealth.com
Mayo Clinic: www.mayoclinic.com
The Merck Manuals Online Medical Library: www.merck.com/mmhe
National Center for Infectious Diseases: www.cdc.gov/ncidod
National Health Information Center: www.health.gov/nhic

Selected references
Gunther, G., and Haglund, M. "Tick-bourne Encephalopathies: Epidemiology, Diagnosis, Treatment and Prevention," *CNS Drugs* 19(12):1009-1032, 2005.

Kasper, D. L., et al., eds. *Harrison's Principles of Internal Medicine,* 16th ed. New York: McGraw-Hill Book Co., 2005.

Paddock, C.D., et al. "*Rickettsia Parkeri:* A Newly Recognized Cause of Spotted Fever Rickettsiosis in the United States," *Clinical Infectious Diseases* 38(6):805-11, March 2004.

Raoult, D., and Paddock, C.D. "*Rickettsia Parkeri* Infection and Other Spotted Fevers in the United States," *New England Journal of Medicine* 353(6):626-27, August 2005.

Razzaq, S., and Schutze, G.E. "Rocky Mountain Spotted Fever: A Physician's Challenge," *Pediatrics in Review/American Academy of Pediatrics* 26(4):125-30, April 2005.

Rosacea

● OVERVIEW

Description
- Chronic adult skin disorder that affects the skin and eyes
- Produces flushing and dilation of small blood vessels in the face, especially the nose and cheeks
- May cause papules and pustules, but without the characteristic comedones of acne vulgaris
- Usually spreads slowly; rarely subsides spontaneously
- Usually associated with rhinophyma (dilated follicles and thickened, bulbous skin on the nose)

Pathophysiology
- Vascular reactivity leads to varying degrees of papules, pustules, and hyperplasia of the sebaceous glands.

Causes
- Exact cause unknown

Risk factors
- Drinking hot beverages
- Tobacco or alcohol use
- Spicy food intake
- Exposure to extreme heat or cold or to sunlight
- Stress

Incidence
- Most common in white women ages 30 to 50; however, commonly more severe in men

Common characteristics
- Flushed areas on cheeks, nose, forehead, and chin
- Ocular involvement (50% of cases)

Complications
- Decreased self-esteem
- Rosacea fulminans

WITH OCULAR INVOLVEMENT
- Blepharitis
- Conjunctivitis
- Uveitis
- Keratitis
- Recurrent chalazion

✳ ASSESSMENT

History
- Facial flushing
- Gritty feeling in eyes
- Facial edema
- Predisposing or aggravating factors
- Complaints of burning or stinging of face

Physical findings
- Flushed areas on the cheeks, nose, forehead, and chin; flushing usually starting across the central oval of the face (see *Lupoid or granolomatous rosacea*)
- Telangiectasia with pustules and papules
- Rhinophyma (in severe rosacea)
- Facial edema
- Ocular roscacea
  - Conjunctival infection
  - Chalazion
  - Episcleritis

Test results
- Diagnosis is usually confirmed by observation of typical vascular and acneiform lesions without comedones.

DIAGNOSTIC PROCEDURES
- Skin biopsy may rule out other diseases such as lupus erythematosus.

◆ TREATMENT

General
- Identification and avoidance of aggravating factors

Diet
- Avoidance of hot beverages, alcohol, and spicy foods

Activity
- Avoidance of physical activities involving sunlight or exposure to extreme heat or cold

Medication
- Topical azelaic acid
- Topical sodium sulfacetamide
- Topical metronidazole
- Oral doxycycline (for ocular involvement)
- Topical corticosteroids

Surgery
- Electrosurgery
- Laser therapy

LUPOID OR GRANULOMATOUS ROSACEA

Firm yellow, brownish, or reddish cutaneous papules or nodules characterize the variant form called lupoid or granulomatous rosacea. The lesions are less inflammatory than those of rosacea. Often the surrounding skin is relatively normal looking, but sometimes it's red and thickened diffusely. Usually, the lesions are monomorphic in each patient, affecting the cheeks and periorificial areas. Other signs or symptoms of rosacea aren't needed to make the diagnosis of this form of rosacea. Diascopy with a glass spatula reveals the lupoid character of the infiltrations. Lupoid or granulomatous rosacea may scar the skin.

✦ NURSING CONSIDERATIONS

Nursing diagnoses
- Disturbed body image
- Impaired skin integrity
- Risk for infection
- Situational low self-esteem

Key outcomes
The patient will:
- verbalize feelings about change in body image
- exhibit improved or healed wounds or lesions
- remain free from signs and symptoms of secondary infection
- report feelings of improved self-image.

Nursing interventions
- Administer medications, as ordered.
- Encourage the patient to express feelings.
- Offer emotional support and reassurance.
- Assist with trigger identification.

Monitoring
- Adverse reactions to medications
- Complications
- Response to treatment

▶ PATIENT TEACHING

Be sure to cover:
- disorder, diagnostic tests, and treatment
- medication administration, dosage, and possible adverse effects
- aggravating factors
- stress reduction techniques
- meticulous hand washing and personal hygiene
- ways to prevent infection
- signs and symptoms of infection
- when to notify the physician
- use of non-comedogenic, high-actor sunscreen when exposed to sunlight and wind.

✺ RESOURCES

Organizations
American Academy of Dermatology: *www.aad.org*
Dermatology Foundation: *www.dermfnd.org*
International Rosacea Foundation: *www.internationalrosaceafoundation.org*
National Rosacea Society: *www.rosacea.org*

Selected references
Butterwick, K.J., et al. "Laser and Light Therapies for Acne Rosacea," *Journal of Drugs in Dermatology* 5(1):35-39, January 2006.

Katz, B., and Patel, V. "Photodynamic Therapy for the Treatment of Erythema, Papules, Pustules, and Severe Flushing Consistent with Rosacea," *Journal of Drugs in Dermatology* 5(2 Suppl):6-8, February 2006.

Lindow, K.B. "Rosacea. An Overview of Diagnosis and Management," *Advance for Nurse Practitioners* 12(12):27-32, December 2004.

Lindow, K.B., et al. "Perception of Self in Persons with Rosacea," *Dermatology Nursing* 17(4):249-54, 314, August 2005.

Roebuck, H.L. "Face Up to Rosacea," *Nurse Practitioner* 30(9):24-30, 35, September 2005.

Roseola infantum

Description
- Common acute, benign, presumably viral illness characterized by fever with subsequent rash
- Also known as *exanthema subitum*

Pathophysiology
- Human herpesvirus (HHV) type 6B, which causes the disorder, is similar to cytomegalovirus.
- HHV-6B shows persistent and intermittent or chronic shedding in the normal population, resulting in the unusually early infection of children.
- HHV-6B is thought to be latent in salivary glands and blood.

Causes
- HHV-6B
- May be transmitted by saliva and, possibly, by genital secretions

Incidence
- Affects infants and young children, typically from age 6 months to 3 years
- Affects both sexes equally
- Occurs year-round, but most common in spring and fall

Common characteristics
- Incubation period of 10 to 15 days
- High fever, with rash appearing after the fever breaks

Complications
- Encephalopathy
- Thrombocytopenic purpura
- Febrile seizures
- Meningitis
- Hepatitis

History
- Abruptly increasing, unexplainable fever that peaks between 103° and 105° F (39.4° and 40.5° C) for 3 to 5 days and then drops suddenly
- Anorexia, irritability, and listlessness
- Cough

Physical findings
- When temperature drops abruptly, maculopapular, nonpruritic rash that blanches with pressure
- Profuse rash on the trunk, arms, and neck; mild rash on the face and legs; rash fading within 24 hours
- Nagayama spots (red papules on soft palate and uvula)
- Periorbital edema

Test results
- Diagnosis is usually confirmed from clinical observation.

LABORATORY
- Causative organism is present in saliva.
- HHV-6B is isolated in peripheral blood.
- Complete blood count shows leukopenia and relative lymphocytosis as temperature increases.
- Immunofluorescence or enzyme immunoassays may show seroconversion during the convalescent phase.

General
- Supportive and symptomatic

Diet
- Increased fluid intake

Activity
- Rest until fever subsides

Medication
- Antipyretics
- Anticonvulsants

✿ NURSING CONSIDERATIONS

Nursing diagnoses
- Deficient fluid volume
- Hyperthermia
- Imbalanced nutrition: Less than body requirements
- Impaired skin integrity

Key outcomes
The patient will:
- maintain adequate fluid volume
- regain a normal body temperature
- maintain adequate nutritional intake
- exhibit improved or healed lesions or wounds.

Nursing interventions
- Give tepid sponge baths and administer antipyretics, as ordered.
- Replace fluids and electrolytes, as needed.
- Institute seizure precautions.
- Provide emotional support to parents.

Monitoring
- Neurologic status
- Fluid and electrolyte status
- Vital signs, especially temperature

▶ PATIENT TEACHING

Be sure to cover:
- disorder, diagnostic tests, and treatment
- methods to reduce fever (tepid sponge baths, dressing the child in lightweight clothing, keeping a comfortable room temperature, and use of antipyretics)
- importance of adequate fluid intake
- how isolation isn't necessary
- reassurance that brief febrile seizures won't cause brain damage and will stop as the fever subsides.

✱ RESOURCES

Organizations
American Academy of Dermatology: *www.aad.org*
American Academy of Neurology *www.aan.org*
American Academy of Pediatrics: *www.aap.org*
Dermatology Foundation: *www.dermfnd.org*
National Health Information Center: *www.health.gov/nhic*
National Institute of Allergy and Infectious Diseases: *www.niaid.nih.gov*

Selected references
Kasper, D. L., et al., eds. *Harrison's Principles of Internal Medicine,* 16th ed. New York: McGraw-Hill Book Co., 2005.

Ohsaka, M., et al. "Acute Necrotizing Encephalopathy Associated with Human Herpesvirus-6 Infection," *Pediatric Neurology* 34(2):160-63, February 2006.

Tamiya, H., et al. "Generalized Eruptive Histiocytoma with Rapid Progression and Resolution Following Exanthema Subitum," *Clinical and Experimental Dermatology* 30(3):300-301, May 2005.

Zerr, D.M., et al. "A Population-Based Study of Primary Human Herpesvirus 6 Infection," *New England Journal of Medicine* 352(8):768-76, February 2005.

Rotavirus

● OVERVIEW

Description
- Self-limiting illness that causes mild to severe diarrhea in children
- Requires hospitalization for approximately 55,000 children each year in the United States and causes death of more than 600,000 children worldwide

Pathophysiology
- Rotavirus invades the cells of the intestinal mucosa, which damages these cells.
- Damage decreases viable absorptive surface, causing an imbalance of secretion and absorption that results in diarrhea.

Causes
- Infection with rotavirus, a member of the *Reoviridae* family
- Transmitted primarily by the fecal-oral route through ingestion of contaminated water or food or through contact with contaminated surfaces (see *Spreading rotavirus infection*)

Incidence
- Highest among infants and young children; affects most children in the United States by age 2
- Winter seasonal pattern seen in the United States and other temperate climate countries, with annual epidemics from November to April

Common characteristics
- Vomiting and watery diarrhea for 3 to 8 days
- Fever
- Abdominal pain

Complications
- Severe dehydration and shock
- Skin breakdown
- Worsening of other conditions such as cystic fibrosis

✳ ASSESSMENT

History
- Fever, nausea, and vomiting followed by diarrhea

Physical findings
- Diarrhea
- Signs of dehydration, such as tachycardia, hypotension, dry mucous membranes, concentrated urine, poor tear production, poor skin turgor, oliguria, sunken eyeballs, and sunken anterior fontanel
- Rectal excoriation

Test results
LABORATORY
- Rapid antigen test detects rotavirus in stool.

◆ TREATMENT

General
- Skin care
- Symptomatic treatment

Diet
- Small, frequent meals
- Increased fluid intake

Activity
- Rest periods, as appropriate

Medication
- None (antibiotics and antimotility drugs contraindicated)

SPREADING ROTAVIRUS INFECTION

Rotavirus infection is contagious. Rotavirus particles pass in the stool of infected persons before and after they have symptoms of the illness. A child can catch a rotavirus infection if he puts his fingers in his mouth after touching something that has been contaminated by the stool of an infected person. Usually this happens when the child forgets to wash his hands often enough, especially before eating and after using the toilet. Because of the widespread nature of rotavirus and the fact that almost 100% of children get rotavirus illness, total prevention of the spread of rotavirus is nearly impossible.

✦ NURSING CONSIDERATIONS

Nursing diagnoses
- Activity intolerance
- Acute pain
- Fatigue
- Hyperthermia
- Imbalanced nutrition: Less than body requirements
- Impaired skin integrity
- Risk for deficient fluid volume

Key outcomes
The patient will:
- return to previous activity level
- express feelings of increased comfort and decreased pain
- verbalize or demonstrate increased energy
- remain afebrile
- maintain adequate nutritional status
- exhibit improved or healed lesions or wounds
- maintain normal fluid volume and electrolyte balance.

Nursing interventions
- Institute contact precautions if patient is incontinent or using diapers.
- Enforce strict hand washing and careful cleaning of all equipment, including toys.
- Implement measures to ensure adequate hydration.
- Clean the patient's perineum thoroughly to prevent skin breakdown.
- Be aware that breast-fed infants can continue to breast-feed without restrictions. Bottle-fed infants can use lactose-free soybean formulas.

Monitoring
- Intake and output (including stools)
- Skin integrity

▶ PATIENT TEACHING

Be sure to cover (with the parents):
- disorder, diagnostic testing, and treatment
- proper hand-washing technique
- instructions on diaper changing and thorough cleaning of the perineum and all affected surfaces
- importance of notifying the physician of increased diarrhea or signs of dehydration.

✱ RESOURCES

Organizations
National Center for Infectious Diseases: *www.cdc.gov/ncidod*
National Institute of Allergy and Infectious Diseases: *www.niaid.nih.gov*
Rotavirus Vaccine Program: *www.rotavirusvaccine.org*
World Health Organization: *www.who.int*

Selected references
Haupt, R.M., et al. "Physician's Knowledge and Attitudes about Rotavirus Gastroenteritis and Rotavirus Vaccine," *Pediatric Annals* 35(1):54-61, January 2006.

Kasper, D. L., et al., eds. *Harrison's Principles of Internal Medicine,* 16th ed. New York: McGraw-Hill Book Co., 2005.

Lowenthal, A., et al. "Secondary Bacteremia after Rotavirus Gastroenteritis in Infancy," *Pediatrics* 117(1):224-26, January 2006.

Parashar, U.D. "Rotavirus and Severe Childhood Diarrhea," *Emerging Infectious Diseases* 12(2):304-306, February 2006.

Ruiz-Palacios, G.M., et al. "Safety and Efficacy of an Attenuated Vaccine Against Severe Rotavirus Gastroenteritis," *New England Journal of Medicine* 354(1):11-22, January 2006.

Rubella

Description

- Acute, mildly contagious viral disease that causes a distinctive maculopapular rash (resembling measles or scarlet fever) and lymphadenopathy
- Self-limiting with an excellent prognosis, except for congenital rubella, which can have disastrous consequences
- Transmitted through contact with blood, urine, stools, or nasopharyngeal secretions of an infected person; can also be transmitted transplacentally
- Communicable from about 10 days before until 5 days after rash appears
- Also called *German measles*

Pathophysiology

- A ribonucleic acid virus enters the bloodstream, usually through the respiratory route.
- The rash is thought to be a result of virus dissemination to the skin.

Causes

- Rubella virus (a togavirus)

Risk factors

- Exposure to active case without immunization

Incidence

- Occurs worldwide
- Most common among children ages 5 to 9, adolescents, and young adults
- Epidemics seen in institutions, colleges, and military populations
- Flourishes during spring, with limited outbreaks in schools and workplaces

Common characteristics

- Incubation period of 18 days, with duration of 12 to 23 days
- Rash covering the trunk and body; by the end of day 2, rash beginning to fade in the opposite order in which it appeared
- Rash subsiding on the face by end of day 2
- Rash disappearing by day 3

Complications

- Arthritis
- Postinfectious encephalitis
- Thrombocytopenic purpura
- Congenital rubella

IN FETAL INFECTION (RARE AFTER 20TH WEEK OF GESTATION)

- Intrauterine death
- Spontaneous abortion
- Congenital malformations of major organ systems

✳ ASSESSMENT

History

- Inadequate immunization, exposure to a person with rubella infection within the previous 2 to 3 weeks, or recent travel to an endemic area without reimmunization
- Absence of prodromal symptoms in a child
- Headache, malaise, anorexia, coryza, sore throat, and cough preceding rash onset (in adolescent or adult)
- Polyarthralgias and polyarthritis (in some adults)

Physical findings

- Rash accompanied by low-grade fever (99° to 101° F [37.2° to 38.3° C); fever may reach 104° F (40° C)
- Exanthematous, maculopapular, mildly pruritic rash; typically begins on the face and spreads rapidly, covering the trunk and extremities within hours
- Small, red, petechial macules on the soft palate (Forschheimer spots) preceding or accompanying the rash
- Coryza
- Conjunctivitis
- Suboccipital, postauricular, and postcervical lymph node enlargement

Test results

- Diagnosis is usually made from clinical observation.

LABORATORY

- Cultures of throat, blood, urine, and cerebrospinal fluid, show isolation of rubella virus; convalescent serum shows a fourfold increase in antibody titers.
- ELISA for immunoglobulin (Ig) M antibodies reveals rubella-specific IgM antibody.
- In congenital rubella, the rubella-specific IgM antibody is present in umbilical cord blood.

◆ TREATMENT

General

- Skin care
- Infection control precautions

Diet

- Small, frequent meals
- Increased fluid intake

Activity

- Rest until fever subsides

Medication

- Antipyretics
- Analgesics

Nursing diagnoses
- Activity intolerance
- Acute pain
- Compromised family coping
- Hyperthermia
- Impaired skin integrity
- Risk for infection

Key outcomes
The patient will:
- perform self-care activities to tolerance level
- express feelings of increased comfort and decreased pain
- demonstrate adaptive coping behaviors
- remain afebrile
- exhibit improvement or healing of lesions or wounds
- remain free from further signs or symptoms of infection

Nursing interventions
- Administer medications, as ordered.
- Institute infection control precautions until 5 days after the rash disappears. Keep an infant with congenital rubella in isolation for 3 months, until three throat cultures are negative.
- Keep the patient's skin clean and dry.
- Ensure that the patient receives care only from nonpregnant hospital workers who are not at risk for rubella. As ordered, administer immune globulin to nonimmunized people who visit the patient. (See *Preventing rubella.*)
- Report confirmed rubella cases to local public health officials.

Monitoring
- Vital signs
- Skin for signs of exanthem
- If congenital rubella, auditory impairment

Be sure to cover (with the parents):
- disorder, diagnostic tests, and treatment
- ways to reduce fever
- devastating effects of rubella on an unborn neonate
- importance of people with rubella avoiding pregnant women
- avoidance of aspirin in a child receiving rubella vaccine.

Discharge planning
- Refer the patient to an infectious disease specialist, if congenital rubella is confirmed.
- Provide parents of an infant with congenital rubella with support, counseling, and referrals, as needed.

Organizations
Centers for Disease Control and Prevention: *www.cdc.gov*
Mayo Clinic: *www.mayoclinic.com*
National Institute of Allergy and Infectious Diseases: *www.niaid.nih.gov*
World Health Organization: *www.who.int*

Selected references
Bedford, H., and Tookey, P. "Rubella and the MMR Vaccine," *Nursing Times* 102(5):55-57, January-February 2006.
Corcoran, C., and Hardie, D.R., "Serologic Diagnosis of Congenital Rubella: A Cautionary Tale," *Pediatric Infectious Disease Journal* 24(3):286-87, March 2005.
Kasper, D. L., et al., eds. *Harrison's Principles of Internal Medicine,* 16th ed. New York: McGraw-Hill Book Co., 2005.
Singh, R., et al. "Measles, Mumps and Rubella—The Urologist's Perspective," *International Journal of Clinical Practice* 60(3):335-339, March 2006.

PREVENTING RUBELLA

Know how to manage rubella immunization before giving the vaccine. First, ask about allergies, especially to neomycin. If the patient has this allergy or if he has had a reaction to any immunization in the past, check with the physician before giving the vaccine.

If the patient is a woman of childbearing age, ask her if she's pregnant. If she is or thinks she may be, don't give the vaccine.

Give the vaccine at least 3 months after any administration of immune globulin or blood. These substances may have antibodies that could neutralize the vaccine.

Don't vaccinate an immunocompromised patient, a patient with immunodeficiency diseases, or a patient receiving immunosuppressant, radiation, or corticosteroid therapy. Instead, administer immune serum globulin, as ordered, to prevent or reduce infection.

Rubeola

● OVERVIEW

Description
- Acute, highly contagious infection causing a characteristic rash
- One of the most common and most serious communicable childhood diseases
- In the United States, usually carries an excellent prognosis
- Can be severe or fatal in patients with impaired cell-mediated immunity
- Mortality highest in children under age 2 and in adults
- Also called *measles* or *morbilli*

Pathophysiology
- Virus invades the respiratory epithelium and spreads via the blood stream to the reticuloendothelial system, infecting all types of white blood cells.
- Viremia and viruria develop, leading to infection of the entire respiratory tract, which spreads to the integumentary system.
- In measles encephalitis, focal hemorrhage, congestion, and perivascular demyelination occur.

Causes
- Rubeola virus
- Spread by direct contact or by contaminated airborne respiratory droplets, with portal of entry in the upper respiratory tract

Risk factors
- Lack of immunization

Incidence
- Affects mostly preschool children
- In temperate zones, most commonly seen in late winter and early spring

Common characteristics
- Fever, Koplik's spots, and characteristic red, blotchy, rash that begins on the face and becomes generalized
- Peak communicability 1 to 2 days before symptom onset until 4 days after the rash appears

Complications
- Secondary bacterial infection
- Autoimmune reaction
- Bronchitis
- Otitis media
- Pneumonia
- Encephalitis

✳ ASSESSMENT

History
- Inadequate immunization and exposure to someone with measles within the past 10 to 14 days
- Photophobia
- Malaise
- Anorexia
- Coryza
- Hoarseness
- Hacking cough

Physical symptoms
- Temperature peaking at 103° to 105° F (39.4° C to 40.5° C)
- Periorbital edema, conjunctivitis
- Koplik's spots (tiny, bluish-gray specks, surrounded by red halo) on oral mucosa opposite the molars, which may bleed
- Pruritic rash that starts as faint macules behind the ears and on the neck and cheeks, becoming papular and erythematous, and rapidly spreading over the face, neck, eyelids, arms, chest, back, abdomen, and thighs
- Rash usually fading once it reaches the feet 2 to 3 days later; occurs in the same sequence the rash appeared, leaving brown discoloration that disappears in 7 to 10 days
- Severe cough
- Rhinorrhea
- Lymphadenopathy

Test results
LABORATORY
- Measles virus is isolated from blood, nasopharyngeal secretions, and urine during the febrile period.
- Serum antibodies appear within 3 days after rash onset and reach peak titers 2 to 4 weeks later.

◆ TREATMENT

General
- Infection control precautions
- Use of vaporizer
- Warm environment
- Skin care

Diet
- Small, frequent meals
- Increased fluid intake

Activity
- Rest until symptoms improve

Medication
- Antipyretics

❖ NURSING CONSIDERATIONS

Nursing diagnoses
- Activity intolerance
- Disturbed sensory perception: Visual
- Hyperthermia
- Imbalanced nutrition: Less than body requirements
- Impaired oral mucous membrane
- Impaired skin integrity
- Risk for infection

Key outcomes
The patient will:
- perform self-care activities to tolerance level
- maintain level of visual acuity
- remain afebrile
- communicate an understanding of the patient's special dietary needs
- remain free from complications related to trauma to oral mucous membranes
- exhibit improved or healed lesions or wounds
- remain free from further signs or symptoms of infection.

Nursing interventions
- Institute respiratory infection control measures for 4 days after rash onset.
- Follow standard precautions.
- Administer medications, as ordered.
- Encourage bed rest during the acute period.
- If photophobia occurs, darken the room or provide sunglasses.
- To prevent the disease from spreading, administer measles vaccine, as ordered and needed.
- Report measles cases to local health authorities.

Monitoring
- Vital signs
- Skin for signs of exanthem
- Eyes for conjunctivitis
- Ears for otitis media
- Mental status
- Signs and symptoms of pneumonia

▶ PATIENT TEACHING

Be sure to cover (with the parents):
- disorder, diagnostic tests, and treatment
- supportive measures, isolation, bed rest, and increased fluids
- instructions on cleaning a vaporizer (if used) and the importance of changing the water every 8 hours
- early signs and symptoms of complications that should be reported.

✱ RESOURCES

Organizations
Centers for Disease Control and Prevention: *www.cdc.gov*
Mayo Clinic: *www.mayoclinic.com*
National Center for Infectious Diseases: *www.cdc.gov/ncidod*
National Institute of Allergy and Infectious Diseases: *www.niaid.nih.gov*
World Health Organization: *www.who.int*

Selected references
Bedford, H. "Measles and the Importance of Maintaining Vaccination Levels," *Nursing Times* 100(26):53-55, June-July 2004.

Kasper, D. L., et al., eds. *Harrison's Principles of Internal Medicine,* 16th ed. New York: McGraw-Hill Book Co., 2005.

Ovsyannikova, I.G., et al. "Human Leukocyte Antigen Haplotypes in the Genetic Control of Immune Response to Measles-Mumps-Rubella Vaccine," *Journal of Infectious Diseases* 193(5): 655-63, March 2006.

Yoshida, M., et al. "Development of Follicular Rash in Measles," *British Journal of Dermatology* 153(6):1226-228, December 2005.

Salmonella infection

Description
- One of the most common infections in the United States
- Occurs as enterocolitis, bacteremia, localized infection, typhoid fever, or paratyphoid fever
- Nontyphoid forms: usually produce mild to moderate illness with low mortality
- Typhoid fever: most severe form of salmonella infection; usually lasts from 1 to 4 weeks; attack confers life-long immunity, although the patient may become a carrier

Pathophysiology
- Invasion occurs across the small intestinal mucosa, altering the plasma membrane and entering the lamina propria.
- The invasion activates cell-signaling pathways, which alter electrolyte transport and may cause diarrhea.
- Some salmonella produce a molecule that increases electrolyte and fluid secretion.

Causes
- Gram-negative bacilli of the genus *Salmonella* (member of the Enterobacteriaceae family)
  - Enterocolitis: *S. enteritidis*
  - Bacteremia: *S. choleresis*
  - Typhoid fever: *S. typhi*

Risk factors
- Nontyphoid forms: usually, ingestion of contaminated water or food or inadequately processed food, especially eggs, chicken, turkey, and duck
- Typhoid fever: usually, drinking water contaminated by excretions of a carrier
- Contact with infected person or animal
- Ingestion of contaminated dry milk, chocolate bars, or pharmaceuticals of animal origin

✲ AGE-RELATED CONCERN Salmonella infection may occur in children under age 5 from fecal-oral spread.

Incidence
- Increasing incidence in the United States due to travel to endemic areas, especially the borders of Mexico
- Paratyphoid fever rare in the United States

Common characteristics
- Enterocolitis and bacteremia: especially common (and more virulent) among infants, elderly people, and those already weakened by other infections, especially human immunodeficiency virus infection
- Nontyphoid forms: usually, mild to moderate illness, with low mortality

Complications
- Dehydration
- Hypovolemic shock
- Abscess formation
- Sepsis
- Toxic megacolon

History
- With enterocolitis, possible report of contaminated food eaten 6 to 48 hours before onset of symptoms
- With bacteremia, the patient usually revealing immunocompromised condition, especially acquired immunodeficiency syndrome
- With typhoid fever, possible ingestion of contaminated food or water, typically 1 to 2 weeks before symptoms develop

Physical findings
- Fever
- Abdominal pain
- With enterocolitis, severe diarrhea
- With typhoid fever, headache, increasing fever, and constipation

Test results
LABORATORY
- Blood culture in typhoid or paratyphoid fever and bacteremia shows causative organism in most cases.
- Stool culture in typhoid or paratyphoid fever and enterocolitis shows causative organism.
- Other culture specimens (urine, bone marrow, pus, and vomitus) show causative organism.
- Presence of *S. typhi* in stools 1 or more years after treatment indicates that the patient is a carrier (about 3% of patients).
- Widal's test, an agglutination reaction against somatic and flagellar antigens, suggests typhoid fever with a fourfold increase in titer.
- Complete blood count (CBC) shows transient leukocytosis during the first week of typhoidal salmonella infection.
- CBC shows leukopenia during the third week of typhoidal salmonella infection.

General
- Usually no treatment
- Possible hospitalization for severe diarrhea

Diet
- Fluid and electrolyte replacement
- High-calorie fluids

Activity
- Bed rest

Medication
- Antimicrobials

⬥ NURSING ALERT Avoid giving antidiarrheals. Their use may prolong the infectious process.

Surgery
- Surgical drainage of localized abscesses

✣ NURSING CONSIDERATIONS

Nursing diagnoses
- Activity intolerance
- Acute pain
- Deficient fluid volume
- Diarrhea
- Hyperthermia
- Imbalanced nutrition: Less than body requirements
- Risk for infection

Key outcomes
The patient will:
- demonstrate measures to conserve energy while carrying out daily activities to tolerance level
- express feelings of increased comfort and decreased pain
- regain and maintain fluid and electrolyte balance
- return to a normal elimination pattern
- remain afebrile
- experience no further weight loss
- remain free from further signs and symptoms of infection.

Nursing interventions
- Follow contact precautions.
- Continue enteric precautions until three consecutive stool cultures are negative—the first one 48 hours after antibiotic treatment ends, followed by two more at 24-hour intervals.
- Observe closely for signs of bowel perforation.
- Maintain adequate I.V. fluid and electrolyte therapy, as ordered.
- Provide good skin and mouth care.
- Apply mild heat to relieve abdominal cramps.

  ◆ **NURSING ALERT** Don't administer antipyretics. They may mask fever and lead to hypothermia. Instead, promote heat loss by applying tepid, wet towels to the patient's groin and axillae.
- Report salmonella cases to public health officials.

Monitoring
- Fluid and electrolyte status
- Vital signs
- Daily weight

▶ PATIENT TEACHING

Be sure to cover:
- disorder, diagnostic tests, and treatment
- need for close contacts to obtain a medical examination and treatment if cultures are positive
- how to prevent salmonella infections
- need to be vaccinated (for those at high risk for contracting typhoid fever, such as laboratory workers and travelers)
- importance of proper hand washing
- need to avoid preparing food or pouring water for others until salmonella infection is eliminated.

Discharge planning
- Arrange for follow-up with an infectious disease specialist or a gastroenterologist, as needed. (See *Preventing recurrence of salmonella infection.*)

✳ RESOURCES

Organizations
Centers for Disease Control and Prevention: *www.cdc.gov*
The Merck Manuals Online Medical Library: *www.merck.com/mmhe*
National Center for Infectious Diseases: *www.cdc.gov/ncidod*
World Health Organization: *www.who.int*

Selected references
Feder, H.M., and Zempsky, W. "Neonatal Salmonella Orchitis," *Infectious Diseases in Clinical Practice* 13(6):313-14, November 2005.

Hosoglu, S., et al. "Risk Factors for Enteric Perforation in Patients with Typhoid Fever," *American Journal of Epidemiology* 160(1):46-50, July 2004.

Kilby, J.M. "Salmonella Infections in the Setting of AIDS: A Serpentine Course," *Southern Medical Journal* 98(11):1066-67, November 2005.

Kasper, D. L., et al., eds. *Harrison's Principles of Internal Medicine,* 16th ed. New York: McGraw-Hill Book Co., 2005.

PREVENTING RECURRENCE OF SALMONELLA INFECTION
To prevent salmonella infection from recurring, follow these teaching guidelines:
- Explain the causes of salmonella infection.
- Show the patient how to wash his hands by wetting them under running water, lathering with soap and scrubbing, rinsing under running water with his fingers pointing down, and drying with a clean towel or paper towel.
- Tell the patient to wash his hands after using the bathroom and before eating.
- Tell him to cook foods thoroughly — especially eggs and chicken — and to refrigerate them at once.
- Teach him how to avoid cross-contaminating foods by cleaning preparation surfaces with hot, soapy water and drying them thoroughly after use; cleaning surfaces between foods when preparing more than one food; and washing his hands before and after handling each food.
- Tell the patient with a positive stool culture to avoid handling food and to use a separate bathroom or clean the bathroom after each use.
- Tell the patient to report dehydration, bleeding, or recurrence of signs of salmonella infection.

Sarcoidosis

● OVERVIEW

Description
- Multisystemic, granulomatous disorder
- Characteristically produces lymphadenopathy, pulmonary infiltration, and skeletal, liver, eye, or skin lesions
- May be acute (usually resolves within 2 years) or chronic
- Chronic, progressive sarcoidosis (uncommon) associated with pulmonary fibrosis and progressive pulmonary disability

Pathophysiology
- An excessive inflammatory process is initiated in the alveoli, bronchioles, and blood vessels of the lungs.
- Monocyte-macrophages accumulate in the target tissue where they induce the inflammatory process.
- $CD4^+$ T lymphocytes and sensitized immune cells form a ring around the inflamed area.
- Fibroblasts, mast cells, collagen fibers, and proteoglycans encase the inflammatory and immune cells, causing granuloma formation.

Causes
- Exact cause unknown
- Possible causes:
  - Hypersensitivity response to atypical mycobacteria, fungi, and pine pollen
  - Chemicals
  - T-cell abnormalities
  - Lymphokine production abnormalities

Incidence
- Most common in young adults ages 20 to 40
- In the United States, occurs predominantly among blacks
- Affects twice as many women as men
- Incidence slightly higher in families, suggesting genetic predisposition

Common characteristics
- Pain in the wrists, ankles, and elbows
- Malaise
- Unexplained weight loss
- Shortness of breath on exertion
- Substernal pain

Complications
- Pulmonary fibrosis
- Pulmonary hypertension
- Cor pulmonale

✳ ASSESSMENT

History
- Pain in the wrists, ankles, and elbows
- General fatigue and malaise
- Unexplained weight loss
- Breathlessness and dyspnea
- Nonproductive cough
- Substernal pain

Physical findings
- Erythema nodosum
- Punched out lesions on the fingers and toes
- Cranial or peripheral nerve palsies
- Extensive nasal mucosal lesions
- Anterior uveitis
- Glaucoma and blindness occasionally in advanced disease
- Bilateral hilar and paratracheal lymphadenopathy
- Splenomegaly
- Arrhythmias

Test results
LABORATORY
- Arterial blood gas (ABG) analysis shows a decreased partial pressure of arterial oxygen.

IMAGING
- Chest X-rays show bilateral hilar and right paratracheal adenopathy, with or without diffuse interstitial infiltrates.

DIAGNOSTIC PROCEDURES
- Kveim-Siltzbach skin test shows granuloma development at the injection site in 2 to 4 weeks when positive.
- Lymph node, skin, or lung biopsy shows noncaseating granulomas with negative cultures for mycobacteria and fungi.
- Pulmonary function tests show decreased total lung capacity and compliance and reduced diffusing capacity.

◆ TREATMENT

General
- No treatment required, if asymptomatic
- Protection from sunlight

Diet
- Low-calcium, for hypercalcemia
- Reduced-sodium
- High-calorie
- Adequate fluids

Activity
- As tolerated

Medication
- Corticosteroids

✤ NURSING CONSIDERATIONS

Nursing diagnoses
- Activity intolerance
- Anxiety
- Dysfunctional grieving
- Fear
- Imbalanced nutrition: Less than body requirements
- Impaired gas exchange
- Risk for infection

Key outcomes
The patient will:
- perform activities of daily living within confines of the illness
- identify strategies to reduce anxiety
- use support systems to assist with coping
- discuss fears and concerns
- maintain adequate nutrition and hydration
- maintain adequate ventilation and oxygenation
- remain free from signs and symptoms of infection.

Nursing interventions
- Administer medications, as ordered.
- Administer supplemental oxygen.
- Provide a nutritious, high-calorie diet.
- Encourage oral fluid intake.
- Provide a low-calcium diet for hypercalcemia.
- Provide emotional support.
- Provide comfort measures.
- Include the patient in care decisions whenever possible.

Monitoring
- Vital signs
- Intake and output
- Daily weight
- Respiratory status
- Chest X-ray results
- Sputum production
- ABG results
- Cardiac rhythm

◈ **NURSING ALERT** Because corticosteroids may induce or worsen diabetes mellitus, test the patient's blood by fingersticks for glucose and acetone at least every 12 hours at the beginning of corticosteroid therapy. Also, watch for other adverse effects, such as fluid retention, electrolyte imbalance (especially hypokalemia) moon face, hypertension, and personality changes.

▶ PATIENT TEACHING

Be sure to cover:
- disorder, diagnostic tests, and treatment
- medication administration, dosage, and possible adverse effects
- when to notify the physician
- steroid therapy
- need for regular follow-up examinations
- importance of wearing a medical identification bracelet
- infection prevention.

Discharge planning
- Refer the patient with failing vision to community support and resource groups such as the American Foundation for the Blind, if necessary.

✺ RESOURCES

Organizations
American Lung Association:
  www.lungusa.org
American Thoracic Society:
  www.thoracic.org
National Sarcoidosis Resource Center:
  www.nsrc-global.net
Sarcoidosis Center: *www.sarcoidcenter.com*

Selected references
Alazemi, S., and Campos, M.A. "Interferon-induced Sarcoidosis," *International Journal of Clinical Practice* 60(2):201-11, February 2006.

Caca, L., et al. "Conjunctival Deposits as the First Sign of Systemic Sarcoidosis in a Pediatric Patient," *European Journal of Ophthalmology* 45(2):169-70, January-February 2006.

Choi, H.J., et al. "Papular Sarcoidosis Limited to the Knees: A Clue for Systemic Sarcoidosis," *International Journal of Dermatology* 45(2):169-70, February 2006.

Doughan, A.R., and Williams, B.R., "Cardiac Sarcoidosis," *Heart* 92(2):282-88, February 2006.

Gurrieri, C., et al. "Cytokines, Chemokines, and Other Biomolecular Markers in Sarcoidosis," *Sarcoidosis, Vasculitis, and Diffuse Lung Diseases* 22(Suppl 1):S9-14, December 2005.

Scabies

Description
- Transmissible skin infestation with *Sarcoptes scabiei* var. *hominis* (itch mite)

Pathophysiology
- Mites burrow into the skin on contact, progressing 2 to 3 mm per day.
- Females live about 4 to 6 weeks and lay about 40 to 50 eggs, which hatch in 3 to 4 days.
- Pruritus occurs only after sensitization to the mite develops. With initial infestation, sensitization requires several weeks. With reinfestation, sensitization develops within 24 hours.
- Dead mites, eggs, larvae, and their excrement trigger an inflammatory eruption of the skin in infested areas.

Causes
- Transmissible by direct (skin to skin) contact or contact with contaminated articles for up to 48 hours (see *Scabies: Cause and effect*)

Risk factors
- Overcrowding
- Poor hygiene
- Sexual promiscuity
- Day care or institutional settings

Incidence
- Common in children and young adults
- Common in elderly and debilitated patients
- Occurs worldwide
- Can be endemic

Common characteristics
- Burrows
- Severe pruritus
- Excoriations

Complications
- Secondary bacterial infection
- Abscess formation
- Septicemia

History
- Predisposing factor
- May be asymptomatic initially
- Intense pruritus that's more severe at night

Physical findings
- Characteristic gray-brown threadlike burrows (0.5 to 1 cm long) with tiny papule or vesicle at one end
- Common sites including flexor surfaces of wrists, elbows, axillary folds, waistline, nipples in females, and genitalia

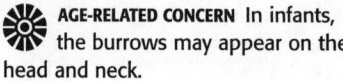 **AGE-RELATED CONCERN** In infants, the burrows may appear on the head and neck.

- Papules, vesicle, crusting, abscess formation, and cellulites with secondary infection

Test results
LABORATORY
- Wound culture demonstrates secondary bacterial infection.

DIAGNOSTIC PROCEDURES
- Mineral oil burrow-scraping reveals mites, nits, or eggs, and feces or scybala.
- Punch biopsy may help to confirm the diagnosis.
- Resolution of infestation with therapeutic trial of a pediculicide confirms the diagnosis.

General
- Bathing with soap and water
- Skin care
- Environmental and clothing decontamination

Diet
- No restrictions

Activity
- No restrictions

Medication
- Scabicides
- 6% to 10% sulfur solution
- Systemic antibiotics
- Antipruritics

⬙ **NURSING ALERT** Avoid the use of topical steroids, which may potentiate the infection.

✳ **AGE-RELATED CONCERN** When treating infants, include the head in treatment.

SCABIES: CAUSE AND EFFECT

Infestation with *Sarcoptes scabiei* – the itch mite – causes scabies. This mite (shown enlarged below) has a hard shell and measures a microscopic 0.1 mm.

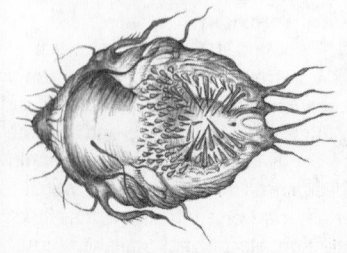

❖ NURSING CONSIDERATIONS

Nursing diagnoses
- Acute pain
- Disturbed body image
- Impaired skin integrity
- Ineffective therapeutic regimen management
- Risk for infection

Key outcomes
The patient will:
- express feelings of increased comfort and decreased pain
- voice feelings about change in body image
- exhibit improved or healed wounds or lesions and resolution of the infestation
- demonstrate understanding of proper skin care regimen
- remain free from secondary infection.

Nursing interventions
- Trim fingernails short.
- Administer medications, as ordered.
- Isolate the patient until treatment is completed.
- Use meticulous hand washing.
- Sterilize blood pressure cuffs in a gas autoclave before using on other patients.
- Decontaminate linens, towels, clothing, and personal articles.
- Disinfect the patient's room after discharge.
- Notify a child's school of infestation.
- Encourage verbalization of feelings.
- Observe contact precautions for 24 hours after treatment with a scabicide.

Monitoring
- Response to treatment
- Complications
- Neurologic status

⬥ **NURSING ALERT** Prolonged use of scabicides may lead to excessive central nervous system stimulation and seizures.

▶ PATIENT TEACHING

Be sure to cover:
- disorder, diagnostic tests, and treatment
- identification of characteristic lesions
- modes of transmission
- mite resistance to scabicides
- assessment of close personal contacts for infestation
- successful treatment for infestation with good hygiene and scabicides
- prevention of transmission and recurrence
- proper application of the prescribed scabicide.

✱ RESOURCES

Organizations
American Academy of Dermatology: *www.aad.org*
Dermatology Foundation: *www.dermfnd.org*
National Center for Infectious Diseases: *www.cdc.gov/ncidod*

Selected references

Almeida, H.I., Jr. "Treatment of Steroid-Resistant Nodular Scabies with Topical Primecrolimus," *Journal of the American Academy of Dermatology* 53(2):357-58, August 2005.

Cestari, T.F., and Martignago, B.F. "Scabies, Pediculosis, Bedbugs, and Stinkbugs: Uncommon Presentations," *Clinical Dermatology* 23(6):545-54, November-December 2005.

Krohn, B. "Scabies in Long-Term Care Settings: Expedient Diagnosis and Treatment Are Essential," *Advance for Nurse Practitioners* 12(12):35-36, December 2004.

Pannell, R.S., et al. "The Incidence of Molluscum Contagiosum, Scabies, and Lichen Planus," *Epidemiology and Infection* 133(6):985-91, December 2005.

Siderits, R., et al. "Preparation and Use of a Scabies Skin Scraping Kit," *Advances in Skin & Wound Care* 19(1):22-25, January-February 2006.

Scarlet fever

Description

- A hypersensitivity reaction that usually follows streptococcal pharyngitis
- May follow other streptococcal infections, such as wound infections, urosepsis, and puerperal sepsis
- Also known as *scarlatina*

Pathophysiology

- After infection, an erythrogenic toxin is produced, resulting in a hypersensitivity reaction.
- Replication sites include the tonsils and pharynx.
- Inflammatory reaction occurs.

Causes

- Group A beta-hemolytic streptococci transmitted by direct contact with infected person or droplet spread; indirectly by contact with contaminated articles or ingestion of contaminated food

Incidence

- Most common in children ages 3 to 15, peaking in those ages 4 to 8
- Increased infection rate in overcrowded situations
- Affects males and females equally

Common characteristics

- Incubation period commonly lasting 2 to 4 days, but may last 1 to 7 days
- High fever, pharyngitis, and rash

Complications

- Severe disseminated toxic illness
- Septicemia
- Rheumatic heart disease
- Liver damage
- Otitis media
- Peritonsillar and retropharyngeal abscess
- Sinusitis
- Glomerulonephritis
- Meningitis
- Brain abscess

ASSESSMENT

History

- Possible sore throat, headache, chills, anorexia, abdominal pain, and malaise
- Likely high temperature (100° to 103° F [37.8° to 39.4° C])
- Onset of rash 12 to 48 hours after fever

Physical findings

- Inflamed and heavily coated tongue, progressing to strawberry-like tongue
- Tongue that peels and becomes beefy red, returning to normal by the end of the second week
- Red and edematous uvula, tonsils, and posterior oropharynx, with mucopurulent exudate
- Fine, erythematous rash that appears first on the upper chest and back, spreading to the neck, abdomen, legs, and arms
- Rash that resembles sunburn with goose bumps; blanches with pressure
- Flushed face; circumoral pallor
- Tachycardia

Test results
LABORATORY

- Pharyngeal culture is positive for group A beta-hemolytic streptococci.
- Complete blood count reveals granulocytosis and reduced red blood cell count.

TREATMENT

General

- Infection control precautions
- Skin care

Diet

- No restrictions

Activity

- Rest periods, as appropriate

Medication

- Antibiotics
- Antipyretics

❖ NURSING CONSIDERATIONS

Nursing diagnoses
- Acute pain
- Hyperthermia
- Impaired oral mucous membrane
- Impaired skin integrity
- Impaired swallowing
- Risk for infection

Key outcomes
The patient will:
- express feelings of increased comfort and decreased pain
- achieve a normal temperature
- have moist and pink mucous membranes without lesions
- maintain skin integrity
- chew and swallow without discomfort
- remain free from further signs or symptoms of infection.

Nursing interventions
- Implement droplet precautions for 24 hours after starting antibiotic therapy.
- Offer frequent oral fluids and oral hygiene.
- Administer medication, as ordered.
- Provide skin care to relieve discomfort from the rash.
- Provide warm liquids or cold foods to ease sore throat pain.
- Use a cool mist humidifier to keep the air moist and prevent the throat from getting too dry and more sore.

Monitoring
- Adverse drug reactions
- Response to treatment
- Complications
- Body temperature
- Rash
- Nutritional status
- Signs and symptoms of dehydration

▶ PATIENT TEACHING

Be sure to cover:
- disorder, diagnostic tests, and treatment
- need to take oral antibiotics for the prescribed length of time to prevent serious complications
- proper disposal of purulent discharge
- follow-up care
- when to notify the physician
- medication administration, dosage, and possible adverse effects
- prevention of scarlet fever and strep throat.

✱ RESOURCES

Organizations
American Academy of Dermatology: *www.aad.org*
American Academy of Pediatrics: *www.aap.org*
Harvard University Consumer Health Information: *www.intelihealth.com*
National Center for Infectious Diseases *www.cdc.gov/ncidod*

Selected references
Diseases, 4th ed. Philadelphia: Lippincott Williams & Wilkins, 2006.

Kasper, D. L., et al., eds. *Harrison's Principles of Internal Medicine,* 16th ed. New York: McGraw-Hill Book Co., 2005.

Vargas, M.H. "Ecological Association Between Scarlet Fever and Asthma," *Respiratory Medicine* 100(2):363-66, February 2006.

Schizophrenia

● OVERVIEW

Description
- Disturbances occurring for at least 6 months in thought content and form, perception, affect, language, social activity, sense of self, volition, interpersonal relationships, and psychomotor behavior
- Five types recognized by *DSM-IV-TR:* catatonic, paranoid, disorganized, residual, and undifferentiated
- Insidious onset with poor outcome
- Can progress to social withdrawal, perceptual distortions, chronic delusions, and hallucinations
- Up to one-third of patients having only one psychotic episode
- Some patients having no disability between periods of exacerbation; others needing continuous institutional care
- Worsening prognosis with each acute episode

Pathophysiology
- A biochemical hypothesis holds that schizophrenia results from excessive activity at dopaminergic synapses.
- Other neurotransmitter alterations may also contribute to schizophrenic symptoms.
- Structural abnormalities of the intraventricular system, temporal lobe abnormalities, decreased volume of the amygdala and hippocampus of the limbic system, structural changes in prefrontal white matter, and increased volume of the basal ganglia have been found.

Causes
- Exact cause unknown
- May result from a combination of genetic, biological, cultural, and psychological factors

Risk factors
- Family history
- Gestational and birth complications
- Prenatal nutritional deficiencies

Incidence
- Affects approximately 0.85% of individuals worldwide, with a lifetime prevalence of 1% to 1.5%
- Close relatives of patients up to 50 times more likely to develop schizophrenia; the closer the degree of biological relatedness, the higher the risk
- Higher incidence among lower socioeconomic groups

🌀 AGE-RELATED CONCERN The onset of schizophrenia usually occurs during late adolescence.

Common characteristics
- Change in emotional expression
- Inappropriate behavior
- Inaccurate interpretation of events
- Ineffective communication

Complications
- Suicide
- Impairment of health
- Impairment of social functioning

✳ ASSESSMENT

History
- Possible long-standing psychiatric illness with repeated episodes
- Decreased social functioning

Physical findings
- Decreased emotional expression
- Impaired concentration

DSM-IV-TR criteria
Diagnosis depends on identifying two or more of the following signs and symptoms for a significant portion of time during a 1-month period (or only one symptom if delusions are bizarre, hallucinations consist of a voice issuing a running commentary, or hallucinations consist of two or more voices conversing with each other):
- delusions
- prominent hallucinations
- disorganized speech
- grossly disorganized or catatonic behavior
- negative symptoms (flat affect or inability to make decisions or speak).

In addition, one or more major areas of functioning (work, relationships, and self-care) are markedly below previous level, and the disturbance isn't due to a substance, medical condition, or schizoaffective or mood disorder.

Test results
- Diagnosis is based on *DSM-IV-TR* criteria.

◆ TREATMENT

General
- Psychotherapy
- Psycho-education
- Social skills training
- Family therapy
- Vocational counseling

Diet
- No restrictions

Activity
- Monitored for safety

Medication
- Antipsychotics (neuroleptic drugs)
- Antidepressants
- Anxiolytics

❖ NURSING CONSIDERATIONS

Nursing diagnoses

- Anxiety
- Bathing or hygiene self-care deficit
- Disabled family coping
- Disturbed personal identity
- Disturbed sensory perception: Auditory, kinesthetic, visual
- Disturbed sleep pattern
- Dressing or grooming self-care deficit
- Fear
- Hopelessness
- Imbalanced nutrition: Less than body requirements
- Impaired home maintenance
- Impaired verbal communication
- Ineffective coping
- Ineffective role performance
- Powerlessnses
- Risk for injury
- Risk for other-directed violence
- Risk for self-directed violence
- Social isolation

Key outcomes

The patient will:

- consider an alternative interpretation of a situation without becoming unduly hostile or anxious
- perform bathing and hygiene activities to the fullest extent possible
- demonstrate adaptive coping behavior
- verbalize positive feelings about self
- identify internal and external feelings that trigger delusional episodes
- maintain maximal functioning within the limits of his auditory, kinesthetic, or visual impairment
- resume appropriate rest and activity patterns
- perform dressing and grooming activities to the fullest extent possible
- express fears and concerns
- participate in care and prescribed therapies
- remain free from signs of malnutrition
- maintain usual roles and responsibilities to the fullest extent possible
- express needs
- develop effective social interaction skills in both one-on-one and group settings
- demonstrate effective coping behaviors

- recognize limitations imposed by the illness and express feelings about these limitations
- gradually join in self-care and the decision-making process
- remain free from injury
- not harm others
- not harm self
- maintain family and peer relationships.

Nursing interventions

- Evaluate the patient's ability to carry out activities of daily living.
- Maintain a safe environment, minimizing stimuli.
- Administer prescribed medications to decrease symptoms and anxiety.
- Adopt an accepting and consistent approach.
- Avoid promoting dependence.
- Reward positive behavior.
- Provide reality-based explanations for distorted body images or hypochondriacal complaints.
- Set limits on inappropriate behavior.
- Offer simple and matter-of-fact explanations about environmental safeguards, medications, and policies.
- Build trust; be honest and dependable. Don't threaten, and don't promise what you can't fulfill.

Monitoring

- Suicidal ideation
- Homicidal ideation
- Effect of medication regimen
- Weight

▶ PATIENT TEACHING

Be sure to cover:

- disorder, diagnostic tests, and treatment
- medication administration, dosage, and possible adverse effects
- how family members can recognize an impending relapse, and ways to manage symptoms.

Discharge planning

- Refer the patient to appropriate community resources and support services.

✴ RESOURCES

Organizations

American Psychiatric Association:
www.helping.apa.org
American Psychological Association:
www.psych.org
National Alliance for the Mentally Ill:
www.nami.org
National Alliance for Research on Schizophrenia and Depression:
www.narsad.org

Selected references

Bilder, R.M., et al. "Cognitive Development in Schizophrenia: Follow-Back from the First Episode," *Journal of Clinical and Experimental Neuropsychology* 28(2):270-82, February 2006.

Chur-Hansen, A., et al. "Mental Health Nurses' and Psychiatrists' Views on the Prognosis of Schizophrenia and Depression: An Exploratory Qualitative Investigation," *Journal of Psychiatric and Mental Health Nursing* 12(5):607-13, October 2005.

Diagnostic and Statistical Manual of Mental Disorders, 4th ed, Text Revision, Washington, D.C.: American Psychiatric Association, 2000.

Honer, W.G., et al. "Clozapine Alone Versus Clozapine and Risperidone with Refractory Schizophrenia," *New England Journal of Medicine* 354(5):472-82, February 2006.

Moser, D.J., et al. "Informed Consent in Medication-Free Schizophrenia Research," *American Journal of Psychiatry* 162(2):1209-11, June 2005.

Scleroderma

● OVERVIEW

Description

- Connective tissue disease characterized by inflammatory, degenerative, and fibrotic changes in skin, blood vessels, synovial membranes, skeletal muscles, and internal organs; thickening of tissues
- May affect the visceral organs or remain localized to the skin when the connective tissues of many organs, including the kidney, GI tract, and lungs, are involved
- Cutaneous lesions usually appearing on the face, hands, neck, and upper chest
- Also known as *systemic sclerosis*

Pathophysiology

- The skin atrophies, and infiltrates containing CD4+ T cells surround the blood vessels; inflamed collagen fibers become edematous, losing strength and elasticity.
- The dermis becomes tightly bound to the underlying structures, resulting in atrophy of the affected dermal appendages and destruction of the distal phalanges by osteoporosis.
- As the disease progresses, atrophy can affect other areas.

Causes

- Exact cause unknown
- Possible causes:
  - Systemic exposure to silica dust or polyvinyl chloride
  - Anticancer agents such as bleomycin (Blenoxane) or nonopioid analgesics such as pentazocine (Talwin)
  - Fibrosis due to an abnormal immune system response
  - Underlying vascular cause with tissue changes initiated by a persistent perfusion

Incidence

- Affects women three to four times more often than men, especially between ages 30 and 50
- Peak incidence between ages 50 to 60
- Rare in children and men younger than age 35

Common characteristics

- Skin thickening in face and fingers

Complications

- Related to thickening of tissues:
  - Slowly healing ulcerations on fingertips or toes leading to gangrene
  - Decreased food intake and weight loss due to GI symptoms
  - Arrhythmias and dyspnea
  - Malignant hypertension
  - Respiratory failure
  - Renal failure
  - Esophageal or intestinal obstruction or perforation
- Raynaud's phenomenon
- Pulmonary fibrosis

✳ ASSESSMENT

History

- Pain, stiffness, and swelling of fingers and joints (later symptoms)
- Frequent reflux, heartburn, dysphagia, and bloating after meals due to GI dysfunction
- Diarrhea, constipation, and malodorous floating stool

Physical findings

- Skin thickening, commonly limited to the distal extremities and face, but possibly involving internal organs
- CREST syndrome (a benign subtype of limited systemic sclerosis): calcinosis, Raynaud's phenomenon, esophageal dysfunction, sclerodactyly, and telangiectasia
- Patchy skin changes with a teardrop-like appearance known as morphea (localized scleroderma)
- Band of thickened skin on the face or extremities that severely damages underlying tissues, causing atrophy and deformity (linear scleroderma)
- Raynaud's phenomenon (blanching, cyanosis, and erythema of the fingers and toes); progressive phalangeal resorption that may shorten the fingers (early symptoms)
- Taut, shiny skin over the entire hand and forearm due to skin thickening
- Tight and inelastic facial skin, causing a masklike appearance and "pinching" of the mouth
- Thickened skin over proximal limbs and trunk (diffuse systemic sclerosis)
- Abdominal distention

Test results

LABORATORY

- Erythrocyte sedimentation rate is slightly elevated, rheumatoid factor is positive in 25% to 35% of patients, and antinuclear antibody is positive.
- Urinalysis shows proteinuria, microscopic hematuria, and casts.

IMAGING

- Hand X-rays show terminal phalangeal tuft resorption, subcutaneous calcification, and joint space narrowing and erosion.
- Chest X-rays show bilateral basilar pulmonary fibrosis.
- GI X-rays show distal esophageal hypomotility and stricture, duodenal loop dilation, small-bowel malabsorption pattern, and large diverticula.

DIAGNOSTIC PROCEDURES

- Pulmonary function studies show decreased diffusion and vital capacity.
- Electrocardiogram shows nonspecific abnormalities related to myocardial fibrosis and possible arrhythmias.
- Skin biopsy shows changes consistent with disease progression, such as marked thickening of the dermis and occlusive vessel changes.

◆ TREATMENT

General

- Physical therapy
- Heat therapy
- Hemodialysis
- Skin care with lanolin emollients

Diet

- Soft, bland foods
- Possible enteral feedings

Activity

- Regular exercise, as tolerated
- Frequent rest periods

Medication

- Immunosuppressants
- Vasodilators
- Antihypertensives
- Antacids
- Histamine-2 receptor antagonist or proton pump inhibitor
- Broad-spectrum antibiotics
- Vasodilators

- Angiotensin-converting enzyme inhibitor
- Oxygen therapy

Surgery
- Digital sympathectomy or, rarely, cervical sympathetic blockade
- Digital plaster cast
- Possible surgical debridement
- Renal transplant

❖ NURSING CONSIDERATIONS

Nursing diagnoses
- Activity intolerance
- Acute pain
- Decreased cardiac output
- Diarrhea
- Disabled family coping
- Disturbed body image
- Fatigue
- Fear
- Imbalanced nutrition: Less than body requirements
- Impaired gas exchange
- Impaired physical mobility
- Impaired skin integrity
- Ineffective coping
- Ineffective tissue perfusion: Peripheral
- Risk for infection

Key outcomes
The patient (or family) will:
- verbalize the importance of balancing activity, as tolerated, with rest
- express feelings of increased comfort and decreased pain
- maintain adequate cardiac output
- regain normal bowel function
- demonstrate effective coping behaviors
- express positive feelings about self
- express feelings of increased energy
- discuss fears and concerns
- achieve adequate nutritional intake
- maintain adequate ventilation and oxygenation
- attain the highest degree of mobility possible within the confines of disability
- exhibit improved or healed wounds or lesions
- use support systems to help cope with the disease

- maintain adequate peripheral perfusion, as evidenced by palpable pulses and warm extremities
- remain free from signs or symptoms of infection.

Nursing interventions
- Avoid using fingersticks for blood tests.
- Provide heat therapy to relieve joint stiffness.
- Elevate the head of the bed to help relieve GI symptoms.
- Provide meticulous skin care.
- Encourage oral fluid intake.
- Provide a soft, bland diet with frequent small meals.
- Administer oxygen, as ordered, for pulmonary complications.

Monitoring
- Intake and output
- Adverse reactions to medications
- Daily weight
- End organ damage such as renal failure
- Skin integrity
- Nutritional status
- Vital signs, especially blood pressure
- Renal function
- Electrocardiograms
- Pulmonary function
- Abdominal distention

▶ PATIENT TEACHING

Be sure to cover:
- disorder, diagnostic tests, and treatment
- avoiding cold weather and cigarette smoking
- reporting abnormal bleeding or bruising and any nonhealing abrasions
- importance of staying as active as possible, balanced with frequent rest periods
- follow-up care.

Discharge planning
Refer the patient to:
- physical therapy and occupational therapy, as needed
- smoking-cessation programs, as indicated
- the Scleroderma Foundation.

✱ RESOURCES

Organizations
American Academy of Dermatology: *www.aad.org*
Arthritis Foundation: *www.arthritis.org*
National Institute of Allergy and Infectious Diseases: *www.niaid.nih.gov/publications*
Raynaud's & Scleroderma Association: *www.raynauds.org.uk*
The Scleroderma Foundation: *www.scleroderma.org*
Scleroderma Research Foundation: *www.srfcure.org*

Selected references
Chang, B., et al. "Natural History of Mild-Moderate Pulmonary Hypertension and the Risk Factors for Severe Pulmonary Hypertension in Scleroderma," *Journal of Rheumatology* 33(2)269-74, February 2006.
Joslin, N. "Early Identification Key to Scleroderma Treatment," *Nurse Practitioner* 29(7):24-39, July 2004.
Kasper, D. L., et al., eds. *Harrison's Principles of Internal Medicine,* 16th ed. New York: McGraw-Hill Book Co., 2005.
Melani, L., et al. "A Case of Nodular Scleroderma," *Journal of Dermatology* 32(12):1028-31, December 2005.
The Merck Manual of Diagnosis & Therapy, 18th ed. Whitehouse Station, N.J.: Merck and Co., Inc., 2006.
Pope, J.E., et al. "Scleroderma Treatment Differs Between Experts and General Rheumatologists," *Arthritis and Rheumatism* 55(1):138-45, February 2006.

Scoliosis

● OVERVIEW

Description
- Lateral curvature of the spine
- Right thoracic curve most common
- Classified as nonstructural (flexible spinal curve, with temporary straightening when patient leans sideways) or structural (fixed deformity)

Pathophysiology
- The vertebrae rotate, forming the convex part of the curve.
- The rotation causes rib prominence along the thoracic spine and waistline asymmetry in the lumbar spine.
- Severity of the deformity dictates physiological impairment

Causes
- Nonstructural scoliosis:
  - Leg-length discrepancies
  - Poor posture
  - Paraspinal inflammation
  - Acute disk disease
- Structural scoliosis: no known cause
- Neuromuscular scoliosis: may be caused by muscular dystrophy, polio, cerebral palsy, or spinal muscular atrophy
- Neurofibromatosis (Recklinghausen's disease)
- Traumatic scoliosis: may result from vertebral fractures or disk disease

  ✵ AGE-RELATED CONCERN Degenerative scoliosis may develop in older patients with osteoporosis and degenerative joint disease of the spine.

Risk factors
- Congenital or neuromuscular problem
- Aging process

Incidence
- Affects less than 1% of school-age children
- Seen at growth spurts between ages 10 and 13
- Affects boys and girls equally
- Infantile scoliosis: most common in boys ages 1 to 3
- Juvenile scoliosis: affects boys and girls ages 3 to 10 equally
- Adolescent scoliosis: occurs after age 10 and during adolescence

Common characteristics
- Fatigue
- Backache
- Dyspnea
- Change in appearance
- Kyphosis

Complications
- Debilitating back pain
- Severe deformity
- With thoracic curve exceeding 60 degrees, possible reduced pulmonary function
- With thoracic curve exceeding 80 degrees, increased risk of cor pulmonale in middle age

✲ ASSESSMENT

History
- Family history of scoliosis
- Detected during community or school scoliosis screening
- Pant legs that appear unequal in length
- One hip that rises higher than the other
- Backache, fatigue, and dyspnea

Physical findings
- Signs of scoliosis (see *Testing for scoliosis*)

Test results
IMAGING
- Spinal X-rays confirm scoliosis and determine the degree of curvature and flexibility of the spine; they also determine skeletal maturity, predict remaining bone growth, and differentiate nonstructural from structural scoliosis.

DIAGNOSTIC PROCEDURES
- Bone growth studies may help determine skeletal maturity.

◆ TREATMENT

General
- Close observation
- Brace
- Spinal orthoses
- Functional strengthening program

Diet
- No restrictions

Activity
- Prescribed exercise regimen, characterized by a gradual increase
- Swimming, but no diving
- No vigorous sports

TESTING FOR SCOLIOSIS

When assessing the patient for an abnormal spinal curve, use this screening test for scoliosis. Have the patient remove her shirt and stand as straight as she can with her back to you. Instruct her to distribute her weight evenly on each foot. While the patient does this, observe both sides of her back from neck to buttocks. Look for these signs:
- uneven shoulder height and shoulder blade prominence
- unequal distance between the arms and the body
- asymmetrical waistline
- uneven hip height
- a sideways lean.

  With the patient's back still facing you, ask the patient to do the "forward-bend" test. In this test, the patient places her palms together and slowly bends forward, remembering to keep her head down. As she complies, check for these signs:
- asymmetrical thoracic spine or prominent rib cage (rib hump) on either side
- asymmetrical waistline.

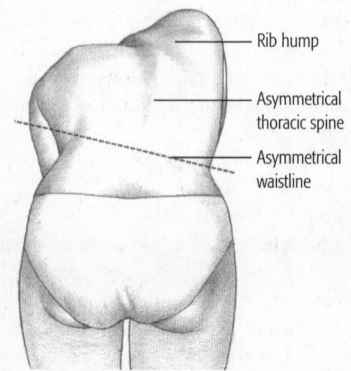

- Rib hump
- Asymmetrical thoracic spine
- Asymmetrical waistline

Surgery

- Posterior spinal fusion and internal stabilization (rods and spinal hardware)

NURSING CONSIDERATIONS

Nursing diagnoses

- Anxiety
- Chronic pain
- Disturbed body image
- Fear
- Impaired physical mobility
- Risk for injury

Key outcomes

The patient will:

- identify strategies to reduce anxiety
- express feelings of increased comfort and decreased pain
- express positive feelings about self
- discuss fears and concerns
- maintain joint mobility and range of motion (ROM)
- achieve the highest level of mobility possible
- remain free from injury.

Nursing interventions

- Promote self-care while allowing adequate time.
- Administer pain medications, as ordered.
- Encourage deep-breathing exercises.
- Promote active ROM arm exercises.

Monitoring

- Sensation, movement, color, and pulses
- Intake and output
- Activity level
- Pain management

▶ PATIENT TEACHING

Be sure to cover:

- disorder, diagnostic tests, and treatment
- brace care
- prevention of skin breakdown
- safe body mechanics
- cast care, if needed
- signs of cast syndrome
- medication administration, dosage, and possible adverse effects
- relaxation techniques.

✳ RESOURCES

Organizations

American Academy of Orthopaedic Surgeons: *www.aaos.org*
American College of Obstetricians and Gynecologists: *www.acog.org*
National Scoliosis Foundation: *www.scoliosis.org*
Scoliosis Association, Inc.: *www.scoliosisassoc.org*
Scoliosis Research Society: *www.srs.org*

Selected references

Diseases, 4th ed. Philadelphia: Lippincott Williams & Wilkins, 2006.
Gillingham, B.I., et al. "Early Onset Idiopathic Scoliosis," *Journal of the American Academy of Orthopaedic Surgeons* 14(2):101-12, February 2006.
Handbook of Pathophysiology, 2nd ed. Philadelphia: Lippincott Williams & Wilkins, 2005.
Larsson, E.L., et al. "Long-Term Follow-Up of Functioning after Spinal Surgery in Patients with Neuromuscular Scoliosis," *Spine* 30(19):2145-152, October 2005.
Lonstein, J.E. "Scoliosis: Surgical Versus Nonsurgical Treatment," *Clinical Orthopaedics and Related Research* 443:248-59, February 2006.

Septic arthritis

● OVERVIEW

Description
- Inflammation of synovial membrane
- Usually affects a single joint
- Possible sudden onset
- Also known as *infectious arthritis*

Pathophysiology
- Bacteria invade a joint, and inflammation of the synovial lining results.
- Organisms invade the joint cavity, and effusion and pyogenesis follow.
- Eventual bone and cartilage destruction result.

Causes
- Bacteria spread from a primary site of infection
- *Staphylococcus aureus*
- *Streptococcus pyogenes*
- *Streptococcus pneumoniae*
- *Streptococcus viridans*
- Gram-positive or -negative cocci
- *Neisseria gonorrhoeae*
- *Haemophilus influenzae*
- Gram-negative bacilli
- *Escherichia coli*
- Salmonella
- Pseudomonas
- Fungi or mycobacteria (rare cause)

Risk factors
- Concurrent bacterial infection
- Serious chronic illness
- Alcoholism
- Advanced age
- Immune system depression
- History of immunosuppressive therapy
- I.V. drug abuse
- Recent articular trauma
- Joint surgery
- Intra-articular injections
- Local joint abnormalities

Incidence
- Gram-positive cocci more common in children older than age 2 and adults
- *H. influenzae* most common in children younger than age 2

Common characteristics
- Joint inflammation
- Severe pain
- Pseudoparalysis of affected area
- Warmth and erythema of affected area

Complications
- Osteomyelitis
- Loss of joint cartilage
- Ankylosis
- Fatal septicemia

✳ ASSESSMENT

History
- Abrupt onset of intense pain in the affected joint
- Fever and chills

Physical findings
- Affected joint kept in a flexed position
- Redness and edema over the affected joint
- Severely reduced range of motion
- Warmth and extreme tenderness over the involved joint

Test results
LABORATORY
- Synovial fluid analysis shows pus or watery, cloudy fluid of decreased viscosity, typically with 50,000 µl or more of white blood cells (WBCs) containing primarily neutrophils; glucose level is also low.
- Gram stain or culture of the fluid identifies causative organism.
- Countercurrent immunoelectrophoresis measures bacterial antigens in body fluids and guides treatment.
- Positive blood cultures confirm the diagnosis even with negative synovial culture.
- WBC count is elevated with many polymorphonuclear cells.
- Erythrocyte sedimentation rate is increased.
- C-reactive protein is elevated.
- Lactic assay distinguishes septic from nonseptic arthritis.
IMAGING
- X-rays may show distention of the joint capsule, narrowing of the joint space, and erosion of bone.
- Radioisotope joint scan may show infection or inflammation, especially in less accessible joints.

DIAGNOSTIC PROCEDURES
- Arthrocentesis allows collection of a synovial fluid specimen for analysis.
- Biopsy of the synovial membrane confirms the diagnosis and identifies the causative organism.

◆ TREATMENT

General
- Based on antimicrobial susceptibilities and the patient's age
- Drainage by repeated closed-needle aspiration, arthroscopy, or arthrotomy

Diet
- No restrictions

Activity
- Exercise
- Joint immobilization

Medication
- Analgesics
- Parenteral antibiotic

Surgery
- Reconstructive surgery for severe joint damage
- Possible open surgical drainage

Nursing diagnoses

- Acute pain
- Anxiety
- Dressing or grooming self-care deficit
- Fear
- Impaired physical mobility
- Risk for infection

Key outcomes

The patient will:

- express feelings of increased comfort and decreased pain
- identify measures to reduce anxiety
- perform activities of daily living within confines of the disorder
- discuss concerns and fears related to the diagnosis
- maintain joint mobility and range of motion (ROM)
- remain free from signs and symptoms of infection.

Nursing interventions

- Use strict sterile technique.
- Check splints or traction regularly.
- Maintain proper alignment.
- Assist with ROM exercises.
- Provide pain medication.
- Allow adequate time for and promote self-care.

Monitoring

- Signs and symptoms of joint inflammation
- Vital signs and fever pattern
- Pain levels
- Response to pain medications
- Condition after joint aspiration

Be sure to cover:

- disorder, diagnostic tests, and treatment
- role of I.V. drug use
- prevention of recurrence
- medication administration, dosage, and possible adverse effects
- exercise regimen
- rest periods
- home I.V. therapy, if required.

Discharge planning

- Refer the patient to drug counseling or Alcoholics Anonymous, if appropriate.

Organizations

Arthritis Foundation: *www.arthritis.org*
National Institute of Arthritis and Musculoskeletal and Skin Diseases: *www.nih.gov/niams/healthinfo*

Selected references

Butbul-Aviel, Y., et al. "Procalcitonin as a Diagnostic Aid in Osteomyelitis and Septic Arthritis," *Pediatric Emergency Care* 21(12):828-32, December, 2005.

Diseases, 4th ed. Philadelphia: Lippincott Williams & Wilkins, 2006.

Handbook of Pathophysiology, 2nd ed. Philadelphia: Lippincott Williams & Wilkins, 2005.

Lu, J.J., et al. "Septic Arthritis Caused by Vancomycin-Intermediate *Staphylococcus Aureus,*" *Journal of Clinical Microbiology* 43(8):4156-158, August 2005.

Ross, J.J. "Septic Arthritis," *Infectious Disease Clinics of North America* 19(4):799-817, December 2005.

Zicat, B., et al. "Septic Arthritis of the Acromioclavicular Joint: Tc-99m Leukocyte Imaging," *Clinical Nuclear Medicine* 31(3):145-46, March 2006.

Severe acute respiratory syndrome

● OVERVIEW

Description
- Severe viral infection that may progress to pneumonia
- Believed to be less infectious than influenza
- Incubation period ranging from 2 to 7 days (average, 3 to 5 days)
- Not highly contagious when protective measures are used
- Also known as *SARS*

Pathophysiology
- Coronaviruses cause the disease in pigs, birds, and other animals.
- One theory suggests that a coronavirus may have mutated, allowing transmission to and infection of humans.

Causes
- A new type of coronavirus known as SARS-associated coronavirus (SARS-CoV)

Risk factors
- Close contact with an infected person
- Contact with aerosolized (exhaled) droplets and bodily secretions from an infected person
- Travel to endemic areas

Incidence
- More common in adults than children
- Outbreaks in China, Hong Kong, Toronto, Singapore, Taiwan, and Vietnam, with many other countries reporting smaller numbers of cases
- Affects all races and both sexes equally

Common characteristics
- Flulike symptoms
- Cough
- Fever
- Progressive respiratory distress

Complications
- Respiratory difficulties
- Severe thrombocytopenia (low platelet count)
- Death

✳ ASSESSMENT

History
- Contact with a person known to have SARS
- Travel to an endemic area
- Flu-like symptoms
- Headache

Physical findings
- Non-productive cough
- Rash
- High fever
- Diarrhea
- Respiratory distress (in later stages)

Test results
LABORATORY
- Antibodies to coronavirus are detected.
- Sputum Gram's stain and culture isolates coronavirus.
- Platelet count may be low.

IMAGING
- Changes in chest X-rays indicate pneumonia (infiltrates).

DIAGNOSTIC PROCEDURES
- SARS-specific polymerase chain reaction test detects SARS-CoV RNA.

◆ TREATMENT

General
- Symptomatic treatment
- Isolation for hospitalized patients
- Strict respiratory and mucosal barrier precautions
- Quarantine of exposed people to prevent spread
- Global surveillance and reporting of suspected cases to national health authorities

Diet
- As tolerated

Activity
- As tolerated

Medication
- Antivirals
- Combination of steroids and antimicrobials

❖ NURSING CONSIDERATIONS

Nursing diagnoses
- Activity intolerance
- Anxiety
- Dysfunctional grieving
- Fear
- Imbalanced nutrition: Less than body requirements
- Impaired gas exchange
- Risk for infection

Key outcomes
The patient will:
- perform activities of daily living, as tolerated
- identify strategies to reduce anxiety
- use support systems to assist with coping
- discuss fears and concerns
- maintain adequate nutrition and hydration
- maintain adequate ventilation and oxygenation
- remain free from signs and symptoms of infection.

Nursing interventions
- Give prescribed drugs.
- Encourage adequate nutritional intake.
- Observe, record, and report nature of rash.
- Maintain proper isolation technique.
- Collect laboratory specimens, as needed.

Monitoring
- Vital signs
- Nutritional status
- Respiratory status
- Complications

▶ PATIENT TEACHING

Be sure to cover:
- importance of frequent hand-washing
- covering mouth and nose when coughing or sneezing
- avoiding close personal contact with friends and family
- importance of not going to work, school, or other public places until 10 days after fever and respiratory symptoms resolve
- wearing a surgical mask when around other people or, if the patient can't wear one, having those in close contact with patient wear masks
- not sharing silverware, towels, or bedding until they have been washed in soap and hot water
- using disposable gloves and household disinfectant to clean any surface that might have been exposed to the patient's bodily fluids.

Discharge planning
- Refer the patient for follow-up, as needed.

✳ RESOURCES

Organizations
Centers for Disease Control and Prevention: *www.cdc.gov*
Occupational Safety & Health Administration: *www.osha.gov/dep/sars/*
World Health Organization: *www.who.int*

Selected references
Chan, P.K., et al. "SARS: Clinical Presentation, Transmission, Pathogenesis, and Treatment Options," *Clinical Science* 110(2):193-204, February 2006.

Chu, C.M., et al. "Viral Load Distribution in SARS Outbreak," *Emerging Infectious Diseases* 11(12):1882-886, December 2005.

Rebmann, T. "Severe Acute Respiratory Syndrome: Implications for Perinatal and Neonatal Nurses," *Journal of Perinatal & Neonatal Nursing* 19(4):332-45, October-December 2005.

Tseng, H.C., et al. "SARS: Key Factors in Crisis Management," *Journal of Nursing Research* 13(1):58-65, March 2005.

Severe combined immunodeficiency disease

● OVERVIEW

Description
- Deficient or absent cell-mediated (T-cell) and humoral (B-cell) immunity
- Predisposes patient to infection from all classes of microorganisms during infancy
- Also known as *SCID* and *bubble-boy disease*

Pathophysiology
- Three types of SCID have been identified:
  - reticular dysgenesis, the most severe type, in which the hematopoietic stem cell fails to differentiate into lymphocytes and granulocytes
  - Swiss-type agammaglobulinemia, in which the hematopoietic stem cell fails to differentiate into lymphocytes alone
  - enzyme deficiency, such as adenosine deaminase deficiency, in which the buildup of toxic products in the lymphoid tissue causes damage and subsequent dysfunction.

Causes
- Transmitted as autosomal recessive trait but may be X-linked
- Possibly, enzyme deficiency
- Thymus or bursa equivalent may fail to develop normally or possible defect in thymus and bone marrow (responsible for T- and B-cell development)

Risk factors
- Family history of SCID

Incidence
- Affects more males than females
- Occurs in 1 in every 100,000 to 500,000 births
- Usual onset at about age 2 months

Common characteristics
- Frequent infections in the first few months of life

Complications
- Without treatment, death due to infection within 1 year of birth
- Pneumonia
- Oral ulcers
- Failure to thrive
- Dermatitis

✳ ASSESSMENT

History
- Extreme susceptibility to infection within the first few months of life but probably no signs of any gram-negative infections until about age 6 months because of protection by maternal immunoglobulin G

Physical findings
- Emaciated appearance and failure to thrive
- Assessment findings dependent on the type and site of infection
- Signs of chronic otitis media and sepsis
- Signs of the usual childhood diseases such as chickenpox

Test results
- Defective humoral immunity is difficult to detect before an infant reaches age 5 months.

LABORATORY
- Tests show a severely diminished or absent T-cell number and function.

IMAGING
- Chest X-ray shows characteristic bilateral pulmonary infiltrates.

DIAGNOSTIC PROCEDURES
- Lymph node biopsy that shows an absence of lymphocytes can be used to confirm a diagnosis of SCID.

◆ TREATMENT

General
- Strict protective isolation (germ-free environment)
- Gene therapy (experimental)

Diet
- No restrictions

Activity
- No restrictions

Medication
- Immunoglobulin
- Antibiotics

Surgery
- Histocompatible bone marrow transplantation
- Fetal thymus and liver transplantation
- Stem cell transplant

❖ NURSING CONSIDERATIONS

Nursing diagnoses
- Acute pain
- Anxiety
- Delayed growth and development
- Diarrhea
- Disabled family coping
- Impaired gas exchange
- Impaired oral mucous membrane
- Impaired skin integrity
- Ineffective protection
- Risk for impaired parent/infant/child attachment
- Risk for infection

Key outcomes
The patient (or parents) will:
- express feelings of increased comfort and decreased pain
- verbalize strategies to reduce anxiety.
- demonstrate age-appropriate skills and behaviors
- regain normal bowel function
- develop adequate coping mechanisms and support systems
- maintain adequate ventilation and oxygenation
- maintain intact oral mucous membranes
- maintain skin integrity
- demonstrate protective measures, including conserving energy, maintaining a balanced diet, and getting plenty of rest
- establish eye, physical, and verbal contact with the infant or child
- remain free from signs or symptoms of infection.

Nursing interventions
- If infection develops, provide prompt and aggressive drug therapy and supportive care, as ordered.
- Watch for adverse effects of any medications given.
- Avoid vaccinations, and give only irradiated blood products, if a transfusion is ordered.
- ✹ **AGE-RELATED CONCERN** Although SCID infants must remain in strict protective isolation, try to provide a stimulating atmosphere to promote growth and development.
- Encourage parents to visit their child often, to hold him, and to bring him toys that can be easily sterilized.

- Maintain a normal day and night routine, and talk to the child as much as possible. If parents can't visit, call them often to report on the infant's condition.
- Provide emotional support for the family.

Monitoring
- Signs and symptoms of infection
- Growth and development
- Skin integrity
- Respiratory status
- Response to treatment
- Complications
- Signs and symptoms of transplant rejection
- Social interaction

▶ PATIENT TEACHING

Be sure to cover:
- disorder, diagnostic tests, and treatment
- proper technique for strict protective isolation
- signs and symptoms of infection and importance of notifying the physician promptly
- medication administration, dosage, and possible adverse effects.

Discharge planning
- Encourage the parents to seek genetic counseling.

✷ RESOURCES

Organizations
The Merck Manuals Online Medical Library: *www.merck.com/mmhe*
National Center for Biotechnology Information: *www.ncbi.nlm.nih.gov/diseases*

Selected references
Grunebaum, E., et al. "Bone Marrow Transplantation for Severe Combined Immune Deficiency," *JAMA* 295(5):508-18, February 2006.

Kasper, D. L., et al., eds. *Harrison's Principles of Internal Medicine,* 16th ed. New York: McGraw-Hill Book Co., 2005.

McGhee, S.A., et al. "Potential Costs and Benefits of Newborn Screening for Severe Combined Immunodeficiency," *Journal of Pediatrics* 147(5):603-608, November 2005.

The Merck Manual of Diagnosis & Therapy, 18th ed. Whitehouse Station, N.J.: Merck and Co., Inc., 2006.

Pesu, M., et al. "Jak3, Severe Combined Immunodeficiency and a New Class of Immunosuppressive Drugs," *Immunological Review* 203:127-42, February 2005.

Shock, cardiogenic

Description
- Condition of diminished cardiac output that severely impairs tissue perfusion
- Most lethal form of shock
- Sometimes called *pump failure*

Pathophysiology
- Left ventricular dysfunction initiates a series of compensatory mechanisms that attempt to increase cardiac output.
- As cardiac output decreases, aortic and carotid baroreceptors activate sympathetic nervous responses.
- Responses increase heart rate, left ventricular filling pressure, and peripheral resistance to flow to enhance venous return to the heart.
- This action initially stabilizes the patient but later causes deterioration with increasing oxygen demands on the already compromised myocardium.
- These events consist of a cycle of low cardiac output, sympathetic compensation, myocardial ischemia, and even lower cardiac output.

Causes
- Myocardial infarction (MI): most common
- Myocardial ischemia
- Papillary muscle dysfunction
- End-stage cardiomyopathy
- Myocarditis
- Acute mitral or aortic insufficiency
- Ventricular septal defect
- Ventricular aneurysm

Incidence
- Typically affects patients with area of infarction involving 40% or more of left ventricular muscle mass (in such patients, mortality may exceed 85%)

Common characteristics
- Previous disorder that decreases left ventricular function

Complications
- Multisystem organ failure
- Death

History
- Disorder, such as MI or cardiomyopathy, that severely decreases left ventricular function
- Anginal pain

Physical findings
- Urine output less than 20 ml/hour
- Pale, cold, and clammy skin
- Decreased sensorium
- Rapid, shallow respirations
- Rapid, thready pulse
- Mean arterial pressure of less than 60 mm Hg in adults
- Gallop rhythm, faint heart sounds and, possibly, a holosystolic murmur
- Jugular vein distention
- Pulmonary crackles

Test results
LABORATORY
- Serum enzyme measurements show elevated levels of creatine kinase, lactate dehydrogenase, aspartate aminotransferase, and alanine aminotransferase, pointing to MI or ischemia and suggesting heart failure or shock; CK-MB isoenzyme and tropinin levels may confirm acute MI.

IMAGING
- Cardiac catheterization and echocardiography reveal other conditions that can lead to pump dysfunction and failure, such as cardiac tamponade, papillary muscle infarct or rupture, ventricular septal rupture, pulmonary emboli, venous pooling (associated with venodilators and continuous intermittent positive-pressure breathing), and hypovolemia.

DIAGNOSTIC PROCEDURES
- Pulmonary artery pressure monitoring reveals increased pulmonary artery pressure and pulmonary artery wedge pressure, reflecting an increase in left ventricular end-diastolic pressure (preload) and heightened resistance to left ventricular emptying (afterload) caused by ineffective pumping and increased peripheral vascular resistance.
- Invasive arterial pressure monitoring shows systolic arterial pressure less than 80 mm Hg caused by impaired ventricular ejection.

- Arterial blood gas (ABG) analysis may show metabolic and respiratory acidosis and hypoxia.
- Electrocardiography demonstrates possible evidence of acute MI, ischemia, or ventricular aneurysm.

General
- Intra-aortic balloon pump (IABP)
- Symptomatic treatment
- Intubation and mechanical ventilation, if necessary

Diet
- Possible parenteral nutrition or tube feedings

Activity
- Bed rest

Medication
- Vasopressors
- Inotropics
- Vasoconstrictors
- Analgesics; sedatives
- Antiarrhythmics
- Diuretics
- Vasodilators
- Oxygen

Surgery
- Possible ventricular assist device
- Possible heart transplant

NURSING CONSIDERATIONS

Nursing diagnoses
- Anxiety
- Decreased cardiac output
- Excess fluid volume
- Fear
- Hopelessness
- Impaired gas exchange
- Impaired physical mobility
- Ineffective coping
- Ineffective tissue perfusion: Cardio-pulmonary

Key outcomes
The patient will:
- verbalize strategies to reduce anxiety
- maintain adequate cardiac output and hemodynamic stability
- develop no complications of fluid volume excess
- discuss fears and concerns
- make decisions on own behalf
- maintain adequate ventilation and oxygenation
- maintain joint mobility and muscle strength
- express feelings and develop adequate coping mechanisms
- maintain adequate cardiopulmonary perfusion.

Nursing interventions
- Institute IABP according to protocol and policies.
- Administer oxygen, adjusting the flow rate to a higher or lower level, guided by ABG measurements.
- **NURSING ALERT** When a patient is on the IABP, move him as little as possible. Never place the patient in a sitting position higher than 45 degrees (including for chest X-rays) because the balloon may tear through the aorta and cause immediate death. Assess pedal pulses and skin temperature and color. Check the dressing on the insertion site frequently for bleeding, and change it according to facility protocol. Also check the site for hematoma or signs of infection, and culture any drainage.
- If the patient becomes hemodynamically stable, gradually reduce the frequency of balloon inflation to wean him from the IABP. During weaning, carefully watch for monitor changes, chest pain, and other signs of recurring cardiac ischemia and shock.
- Monitor for arrhythmias, such as atrial fibrillation, which further decrease cardiac output. Electrical cardioversion or antiarrhythmics may be necessary.
- Plan your care to allow frequent rest periods, and provide for as much privacy as possible. Allow family members to visit and comfort the patient as much as possible.
- Allow the family to express their anger, anxiety, and fear.
- Provide explanations and reassurance for patient and family members, as appropriate.
- Prepare the patient and family members for a probable fatal outcome and help them find effective coping strategies.

Monitoring
- ABG levels (acid-base balance)
- Complete blood count and electrolyte levels
- Vital signs and peripheral pulses
- Cardiac rate and rhythm continuously
- Hemodynamics
- Hourly urine output with an indwelling urinary catheter
- Heart sounds and breath sounds
- Level of consciousness

PATIENT TEACHING

Be sure to cover:
- disorder, diagnostic tests, and treatment options
- explanations and reassurance for patient and family members
- probability of fatal outcome.

Discharge planning
- Assist with referrals for community support services.

RESOURCES

Organizations
American Heart Association: *www.americanheart.org*
National Heart, Lung and Blood Institute: *www.nhlbi.nih.gov/nhlbi/cardio*

Selected references
Ellis, T.C., et al. "Therapeutic Strategies for Cardiogenic Shock, 2006," *Current Treatment Options in Cardiovascular Medicine* 8(1):79-94, February 2006.

Jolly, S., et al. "Effects of Vasopressin in Hemodynamics in Patients with Refractory Cardiogenic Shock Complicating Acute Myocardial Infarction," *American Journal of Cardiology* 96(12):1617-20, December 2005.

Nanda, U., et al. "Modified Release Verapamil Induced Cardiogenic Shock," *Emergency Medicine Journal* 22(11):832-33, November 2005.

Nettina, S.M. *Lippincott Manual of Nursing Practice*, 8th ed. Philadelphia: Lippincott Williams & Wilkins, 2006.

Revelly, J.P., et al. "Lactate and Glucose Metabolism in Severe Sepsis and Cardiogenic Shock," *Critical Care Medicine* 33(10):2235-240, October 2005.

Shock, hypovolemic

● OVERVIEW

Description
- Reduced intravascular blood volume that causes circulatory dysfunction and inadequate tissue perfusion
- Potentially life-threatening

Pathophysiology
- When fluid is lost from the intravascular space, venous return to the heart is reduced.
- This decreases ventricular filling, which leads to a drop in stroke volume.
- Cardiac output falls, causing reduced perfusion to tissues and organs.
- Tissue anoxia prompts a shift in cellular metabolism from aerobic to anaerobic pathways.
- This produces an accumulation of lactic acid, resulting in metabolic acidosis.

Causes
- Acute blood loss (about one-fifth of total volume)
- Intestinal obstruction
- Burns
- Peritonitis
- Acute pancreatitis
- Ascites
- Dehydration from excessive perspiration, severe diarrhea or protracted vomiting, diabetes insipidus, diuresis, and inadequate fluid intake
- Diuretic abuse

Incidence
- Depends on cause
- Affects all ages
- More frequent and less well-tolerated in elderly patients
- Affects males and females equally

Common characteristics
- Pallor, tachycardia
- Decreased urine output

Complications
- Acute respiratory distress syndrome
- Acute tubular necrosis and renal failure
- Disseminated intravascular coagulation (DIC)
- Multisystem organ dysfunction

✳ ASSESSMENT

History
- Disorders or conditions that reduce blood volume, such as GI hemorrhage, trauma, and severe diarrhea and vomiting
- With existing cardiac disease, possible anginal pain because of decreased myocardial perfusion and oxygenation

Physical findings
- Pale, cool, and clammy skin; mottling as shock progresses
- Decreased sensorium
- Rapid, shallow respirations
- Urine output usually less than 20 ml/ hour
- Rapid, thready pulse
- Mean arterial pressure normal to less than 60 mm Hg narrowing pulse pressure
- Blood pressure possibly normal initially; hypotension, as shock progresses
- Orthostatic vital signs and tilt test results consistent with hypovolemic shock (see *Checking for early hypovolemic shock*)

Test results
LABORATORY
- Hematocrit is low and decreased hemoglobin levels and red blood cell and platelet counts are decreased.
- Serum potassium, sodium, lactate dehydrogenase, creatinine, and blood urea nitrogen levels are elevated.
- Urine specific gravity (greater than 1.020) and urine osmolality are increased.
- pH and partial pressure arterial oxygen are decreased; partial pressure of arterial carbon dioxide is increased.
- Aspiration of gastric contents through a nasogastric tube identifies internal bleeding.
- Occult blood tests are positive.
- Coagulation studies show coagulopathy from DIC.

IMAGING
- X-rays (chest or abdominal) help to identify internal bleeding sites.

DIAGNOSTIC PROCEDURES
- Gastroscopy helps to identify internal bleeding sites.

- Invasive hemodynamic monitoring shows reduced central venous pressure, right atrial pressure, pulmonary artery pressure, pulmonary artery wedge pressure (PAWP), and cardiac output.

◆ TREATMENT

General
- In severe cases, an intra-aortic balloon pump, ventricular assist device, or pneumatic antishock garment
- Mechanical ventilation, if necessary
- Control of bleeding by direct application of pressure and related measures

Diet
- Possible parenteral nutrition or tube feedings

Activity
- Bed rest

Medication
- Prompt and vigorous blood and fluid replacement
- Positive inotropes
- Oxygen therapy

Surgery
- Possibly, to correct underlying problem

NURSING CONSIDERATIONS

Nursing diagnoses
- Anxiety
- Decreased cardiac output
- Deficient fluid volume
- Disabled family coping
- Impaired gas exchange
- Ineffective tissue perfusion: Cardiopulmonary, cerebral, renal
- Risk for infection
- Risk for injury

Key outcomes
The patient (or family) will:
- verbalize strategies to reduce anxiety
- maintain adequate cardiac output and hemodynamic stability
- maintain adequate fluid volume
- express feelings and develop adequate coping mechanisms
- maintain adequate ventilation and oxygenation
- maintain adequate cardiopulmonary, cerebral, and renal perfusion as evidenced by palpable pulses, no signs of respiratory distress, normal urine output, and normal mentation
- remain free from signs and symptoms of infection
- remain free from injury.

Nursing interventions
- Check for a patent airway and adequate circulation. If blood pressure and heart rate are absent, start cardiopulmonary resuscitation.
- Obtain type and crossmatch, as ordered.

NURSING ALERT When there isn't time for cross-matching, give type O-negative blood, which can be given to anyone.

- Start an I.V. infusion with normal saline solution or lactated Ringer's solution, using a large-bore (14G to 18G) catheter, which allows easier administration of later blood transfusions.
- Notify the physician and increase the infusion rate if the patient has a progressive drop in blood pressure accompanied by a thready pulse.
- Insert an indwelling urinary catheter, if necessary, to measure hourly urine output. If output is less than 30 ml/hour in adults, increase the fluid infu-

sion rate, but watch for signs of fluid overload. Notify the physician if urine output doesn't improve.
- Determine fluid replacement goal by monitoring urine output and hemodynamics or PAWP.
- Administer oxygen by face mask or endotracheal tube to ensure adequate tissue oxygenation.
- Provide emotional support to the patient and family members.

Monitoring
- Vital signs and peripheral pulses
- Cardiac rhythm continuously
- Coagulation studies for signs of impending coagulopathy
- Complete blood count and electrolyte measurements
- Arterial blood gas levels
- Intake and output
- Hemodynamics

▶ PATIENT TEACHING

Be sure to cover:
- disorder, diagnostic tests, and treatment
- procedures and their purpose
- risks associated with blood transfusions
- purpose of all equipment such as mechanical ventilation
- dietary restrictions
- medication administration, dosage, and possible adverse effects.

✷ RESOURCES

Organizations
American Heart Association:
www.americanheart.org
National Heart, Lung and Blood Institute:
www.nhlbi.nih.gov/nhlbi/cardio

Selected references
Kelley, D.M. "Hypovolemic Shock: An Overview," *Critical Care Nursing Quarterly* 28(1):2-19, January-March 2005.
Muhlberg, A.H., and Ruth-Sahd, L. "Holistic Care: Treatment and Interventions for Hypovolemic Shock Secondary to Hemorrhage," *Dimensions of Critical Care Nursing* 23(2):55-59, March-April 2004.
Nettina, S.M. *Lippincott Manual of Nursing Practice,* 8th ed. Philadelphia: Lippincott Williams & Wilkins, 2006.
Yanagawa, Y., et al. "Early Diagnosis of Hypovolemic Shock by Sonographic Measurement of Inferior Vena Cava in Trauma Patients," *Journal of Trauma Injury Infection & Critical Care* 58(4):825-29, April 2005.

CHECKING FOR EARLY HYPOVOLEMIC SHOCK

Orthostatic vital signs and tilt test results can help in assessing for the possibility of impending hypovolemic shock.

Orthostatic vital signs
Measure the patient's blood pressure and pulse rate while he's lying in a supine position, sitting, and standing. Wait at least 1 minute between each position change. A systolic blood pressure decrease of 10 mm Hg or more between positions or a pulse rate increase of 10 beats/minute or more is a sign of volume depletion and impending hypovolemic shock.

Tilt test
With the patient lying in a supine position, raise his legs above heart level. If his blood pressure increases significantly, the test is positive, indicating volume depletion and impending hypovolemic shock.

Shock, septic

OVERVIEW

Description
- Low systemic vascular resistance and an elevated cardiac output
- Likely response to infections that release microbes or an immune mediator

Pathophysiology
- Initially, the body's defenses activate chemical mediators in response to the invading organisms.
- The release of these mediators results in low systemic vascular resistance and increased cardiac output.
- Blood flow is unevenly distributed in the microcirculation, and plasma leaking from capillaries causes functional hypovolemia.
- Diffuse increase in capillary permeability occurs.
- Eventually, cardiac output decreases, and poor tissue perfusion and hypotension cause multisystem dysfunction syndrome and death.

Causes
- Any pathogenic organism
- Gram-negative bacteria, such as *Escherichia coli, Klebsiella pneumoniae, Serratia, Enterobacter,* and *Pseudomonas* (most common causes; up to 70% of cases)

Risk factors
- Any person with impaired immunity

  ✸ **AGE-RELATED CONCERN** Neonates and elderly people are at greatest risk for septic shock.

Incidence
- About two-thirds of cases in hospitalized patients (most have underlying diseases)

Common characteristics
- Hyperdynamic (or warm) phase
- Hypodynamic (or cold) phase

Complications
- Disseminated intravascular coagulation
- Renal failure
- Heart failure
- GI ulcers
- Abnormal liver function
- Death

ASSESSMENT

History
- Possible disorder or treatment that can cause immunosuppression
- Possibly, previous invasive tests or treatments, surgery, or trauma
- Possible fever and chills (although 20% of patients possibly hypothermic)

Physical findings
HYPERDYNAMIC (OR WARM) PHASE
- Peripheral vasodilation
- Skin possibly pink and flushed or warm and dry
- Altered level of consciousness (LOC) reflected by agitation, anxiety, irritability, and shortened attention span
- Rapid and shallow respirations
- Urine output below normal
- Rapid, full, bounding pulse
- Normal or slightly elevated blood pressure

HYPODYNAMIC (OR COLD) PHASE
- Peripheral vasoconstriction and inadequate tissue perfusion
- Pale skin and possible cyanosis
- Decreased LOC; possible obtundation and coma
- Possible rapid and shallow respirations
- Urine output possibly less than 25 ml/hour or absent
- Rapid pulse that's weak and thready
- Irregular pulse if arrhythmias are present
- Cold and clammy skin
- Hypotension
- Crackles or rhonchi, if pulmonary congestion present

Test results
LABORATORY
- Blood cultures are positive for the causative organism.
- Complete blood count shows the presence or absence of anemia and leukopenia, severe or absent neutropenia, and usually the presence of thrombocytopenia.
- Blood urea nitrogen and creatinine levels are increased, and creatinine clearance is decreased.
- Prothrombin time and partial thromboplastin time are abnormal.
- Serum lactate dehydrogenase levels are elevated with metabolic acidosis.
- Urine studies show increased specific gravity (more than 1.020) and osmolality and decreased sodium.
- Arterial blood gas (ABG) analysis demonstrates elevated blood pH and partial pressure of arterial oxygen and decreased partial pressure of arterial carbon dioxide with respiratory alkalosis in early stages.

DIAGNOSTIC PROCEDURES
- Invasive hemodynamic monitoring shows:
  - increased cardiac output and decreased systemic vascular resistance in warm phase
  - decreased cardiac output and increased systemic vascular resistance in cold phase.

TREATMENT

General
- Removal of I.V., intra-arterial, or urinary drainage catheters whenever possible
- In patients who are immunosuppressed because of drug therapy, drugs discontinued or reduced if possible
- Mechanical ventilation, if respiratory failure occurs
- Fluid volume replacement

Diet
- Possible parenteral nutrition or tube feedings

Activity
- Bed rest

Medication
- Antimicrobials
- Granulocyte transfusions
- Colloid or crystalloid infusions
- Oxygen
- Diuretics
- Vasopressors
- Antipyretics
- Drotrecogin alpha (Xigris)

Nursing diagnoses

- Anxiety
- Decreased cardiac output
- Deficient fluid volume
- Disabled family coping
- Impaired gas exchange
- Ineffective tissue perfusion: Cardiopulmonary, renal
- Risk for imbalanced body temperature
- Risk for infection
- Risk for injury

Key outcomes

The patient (or family) will:

- verbalize strategies to reduce anxiety
- maintain adequate cardiac output and hemodynamic stability
- maintain adequate fluid volume
- express feelings and develop adequate coping mechanisms
- maintain adequate ventilation and oxygenation
- maintain adequate cardiopulmonary and renal perfusion
- maintain a normal body temperature
- remain free from signs and symptoms of infection
- remain free from injury.

Nursing interventions

- Remove any I.V., intra-arterial, or urinary drainage catheters, and send them to the laboratory to culture for the presence of the causative organism. New catheters can be inserted in the intensive care unit.
- Give I.V. fluids and blood products, as ordered.

NURSING ALERT A progressive drop in blood pressure accompanied by a thready pulse generally signals inadequate cardiac output from reduced intravascular volume. Notify the physician immediately and increase the infusion rate.

- Administer appropriate antimicrobials I.V.
- If urine output is less than 30 ml/hour in adults, increase the fluid infusion rate, but watch for signs of fluid overload. Notify the physician if urine output doesn't improve.
- Administer oxygen and adjust the oxygen flow rate, as blood gas measurements indicate.
- Provide emotional support to the patient and family members.
- Document the occurrence of a nosocomial infection, and report it to the infection-control practitioner.

Monitoring

- ABG levels
- Hourly intake and urine output
- Vital signs and peripheral pulses
- Hemodynamics
- Cardiac rhythm continuously
- Heart and breath sounds

Be sure to cover:

- disorder, diagnostic tests, and treatment
- all procedures and their purpose (to ease the patient's anxiety)
- risks associated with blood transfusions
- all equipment and its purpose
- medication administration, dosage, and possible adverse effects
- possible complications.

Organizations

American Heart Association:
www.americanheart.org
National Heart, Lung and Blood Institute:
www.nhlbi.nih.gov/nhlbi/cardio

Selected references

Hernandez, G., et al. "Implementation of a Norepinephrine-Based Protocol for Management of Septic Shock: A Pilot Feasibility Study," *Journal of Trauma* 60(1):77-81, January 2006.

Nettina, S.M. *Lippincott Manual of Nursing Practice,* 8th ed. Philadelphia: Lippincott Williams & Wilkins, 2006.

Rivers, E.P. "Early Goal-Directed Therapy in Severe Sepsis and Septic Shock: Converting Science to Reality," *Chest* 129(2):217-18, February 2006.

Sutherland, A.M., et al. "Are Vasopressin Levels Increased or Decreased in Septic Shock?" *Critical Care Medicine* 34(2):542-43, February 2006.

Silicosis

● OVERVIEW

Description
- Most common form of pneumonoconiosis
- Progressive disease characterized by nodular lesions, commonly leading to fibrosis
- Classified according to severity of pulmonary disease and rapidity of its onset and progression
- Usually a simple, asymptomatic illness
- Good prognosis unless complications occur

Pathophysiology
- Small particles of mineral dust are inhaled and deposited in the respiratory bronchioles, alveolar ducts, and alveoli.
- The surface of these particles generates silicon-based radicals that lead to the production of hydroxy, hydrogen peroxide, and other oxygen radicals that damage cell membranes and inactivate essential cell proteins.
- Alveolar macrophages ingest the particles, become activated, and release cytokines, such as tumor necrosis factor and others, that attract other inflammatory cells.
- Inflammation damages resident cells and the extracellular matrix.
- Fibroblasts are stimulated to produce collagen, resulting in fibrosis.

Causes
- Silica dust due to:
  - manufacture of ceramics (flint) and building materials (sandstone)
  - mixed form in construction materials (cement)
  - powder form (silica flour), in paints, porcelain, scouring soaps, and wood fillers
  - mining of gold, lead, zinc, and iron

Risk factors
- Occupational exposure to silica dust

Incidence
- Highest incidence in those who work around silica dust, such as foundry workers, boiler scalers, and stone cutters
- Acute silicosis possible after 1 to 3 years in sand blasters, tunnel workers, and others exposed to high concentrations of respirable silica
- Accelerated silicosis possible in those exposed to lower concentrations of free silica, usually after about 10 years of exposure
- Most common in those ages 40 to 75
- More common in males than females

Common characteristics
- Long-term history of exposure to silica dust
- Dyspnea on exertion
- Dry cough, especially in the morning

Complications
- Lung infection
- Pneumothorax
- Pulmonary fibrosis
- Cor pulmonale
- Cardiac or respiratory failure
- Pulmonary tuberculosis

✳ ASSESSMENT

History
- Long-term exposure to silica dust
- Dyspnea on exertion
- Dry cough, especially in the morning

Physical findings
- Decreased chest expansion
- Tachypnea
- Lethargy
- Decreased mentation
- Areas of increased and decreased resonance
- Medium crackles
- Diminished breath sounds

◈ **NURSING ALERT** Assess for the presence of an intensified ventricular gallop on inspiration, which is a hallmark of cor pulmonale.

Test results
LABORATORY
- Arterial blood gas analysis shows:
  - normal partial pressure of arterial oxygen in simple silicosis; may be significantly decreased in late stages or complicated disease
  - normal partial pressure of arterial carbon dioxide in the early stages of the disease; hyperventilation may cause it to decrease; restrictive lung disease may cause it to increase.

IMAGING
- Chest X-rays in simple silicosis show small, discrete, nodular lesions distributed throughout both lung fields, although they typically concentrate in the upper lung.
- Lung nodes may appear enlarged and show eggshell calcification.
- Chest X-rays in complicated silicosis show one or more conglomerate masses of dense tissue.

DIAGNOSTIC PROCEDURES
- Pulmonary function tests show:
  - reduced forced vital capacity (FVC) in complicated silicosis
  - reduced forced expiratory volume in 1 second (FEV_1) with obstructive disease
  - reduced FEV_1 with a normal or high ratio of FEV_1 to FVC in complicated silicosis
  - reduced diffusing capacity for carbon monoxide when fibrosis destroys alveolar walls and obliterates pulmonary capillaries or when it thickens the alveocapillary membrane.

◆ TREATMENT

General
- Symptomatic relief
- Management of hypoxia and cor pulmonale
- Prevention of respiratory tract infections
- Steam inhalation and chest physiotherapy

Diet
- Increased fluid intake
- High-calorie, high-protein

Activity
- Regular exercise program, as tolerated

Medication
- Bronchodilators
- Oxygen
- Antibiotics
- Anti-inflammatories

Surgery
- Possible tracheostomy
- Possible lung transplantation
- Whole lung lavage

✤ NURSING CONSIDERATIONS

Nursing diagnoses
- Fatigue
- Imbalanced nutrition: Less than body requirements
- Impaired gas exchange
- Ineffective breathing pattern
- Interrupted family processes
- Risk for infection

Key outcomes
The patient will:
- use energy conservation techniques
- maintain adequate caloric intake
- maintain adequate ventilation and oxygenation
- maintain a respiratory rate within acceptable parameters
- identify appropriate resources for support
- remain free from signs and symptoms of infection.

Nursing interventions
- Administer medications, as ordered.
- Perform chest physiotherapy.
- Provide a high-calorie, high-protein diet.
- Provide small, frequent meals.
- Provide frequent mouth care.
- Ensure adequate hydration.
- Encourage daily exercise, as tolerated.
- Provide diversional activities, as appropriate.
- Provide frequent rest periods.
- Help with adjustment to the lifestyle changes associated with a chronic illness.
- Include the patient and family members in care decisions whenever possible.

Monitoring
- Vital signs
- Intake and output
- Daily weight
- Respiratory status
- Activity tolerance
- Complications
- Changes in mentation
- Sputum production
- Breath sounds

▶ PATIENT TEACHING

Be sure to cover:
- disorder, diagnostic tests, and treatment
- medication administration, dosage, and possible adverse effects
- when to notify the physician
- need to avoid crowds and people with known infections
- home oxygen therapy, if needed
- transtracheal catheter care, if needed
- postural drainage and chest percussion
- coughing and deep-breathing exercises
- need to consume a high-calorie, high-protein diet
- adequate hydration
- risk of tuberculosis
- energy conservation techniques.

Discharge planning
Refer the patient:
- for influenza and pneumococcus immunizations, as needed
- to a smoking-cessation program, if indicated
- for tuberculosis testing, if indicated.

✳ RESOURCES

Organizations
Mine Safety and Health Administration: *www.msha.gov*
National Institute for Occupational Safety and Health: *www.cdc.gov/maso/nioshfs.htm*
World Health Organization: *www.who.int*

Selected references

Collins, J.F., et al. "Development of a Chronic Inhalation Reference Level for Respirable Crystalline Silica," *Regulatory Toxicology and Pharmacology* 43(3)292-300, December 2005.

Lahiri, S., et al. "The Cost Effectivenesss of Occupational Health Interventions: Prevention of Silicosis," *American Journal of Industrial Medicine* 48(6):503-14, December 2005.

McDonald, J.C., et al. "Mortality from Lung and Kidney Disease in a Cohort of North American Industrial Sand Workers: An Update," A*nnals of Occupational Hygiene* 49(5):367-73, July 2005.

Rosenberg, B., et al. "Change in the World of Occupational Health: Silica Control, Then and Now," *Journal of Public Health Policy* 26(2):192-202, July 2005.

Sjögren's syndrome

● OVERVIEW

Description
- Most common autoimmune disorder after rheumatoid arthritis
- May be primary disorder or associated with inflammatory connective tissue disorders

Pathophysiology
- Lymphocytic infiltration of exocrine glands causes tissue damage that results in xerostomia and dry eyes.
- Immunologic system is activated.

Causes
- Exact cause unknown
- Possible genetic and environmental factors

Incidence
- Affects more women (about 90%) than men
- Typically strikes around age 50

Common characteristics
- Dry eyes and mouth

Complications
- Corneal ulceration or perforation
- Epistaxis
- Deafness
- Otitis media
- Splenomegaly
- Renal tubular necrosis

✳ ASSESSMENT

History
- Xerophthalmia or xerostomia
- Complaints of gritty, sandy eye along with redness, burning, photosensitivity, eye fatigue, itching, and mucoid discharge
- Difficulty swallowing and talking; an abnormal taste or smell sensation (or both); thirst; ulcers of the tongue, mouth, and lips (especially at the corners of the mouth); and severe dental caries
- Possible epistaxis, hoarseness, chronic nonproductive cough, recurrent otitis media, and frequent respiratory tract infections
- Possible dyspareunia
- Generalized itching, fatigue, recurrent low-grade fever, and arthralgia or myalgia

Physical findings
- Mouth ulcers, dental caries and, possibly, enlarged salivary glands
- Palpable purpura
- Palpable lymph node enlargement
- Dry, crusty erythematous oral mucosa

Test results
LABORATORY
- Elevated erythrocyte sedimentation rate occurs in more than 90% of patients.
- Complete blood count shows mild anemia and leukopenia in about 30% of patients.
- Serum protein electrophoresis shows hypergammaglobulinemia in about 50% of patients.
- Typically, 75% to 90% of patients test positive for rheumatoid factor, and between 50% and 80% of patients test positive for antinuclear antibodies.

DIAGNOSTIC PROCEDURES
- For a diagnosis of Sjögren's syndrome, symptoms must meet specific criteria. (See *Diagnosing Sjögren's syndrome.*)
- Tests supporting the diagnosis include measuring eye involvement with the Schirmer's test and a slit-lamp examination with rose bengal dye.
- Labial biopsy (to detect lymphoid foci), a simple procedure with minimal risk is the only specific diagnostic technique.
- Salivary gland involvement may be evaluated by measuring the volume of parotid saliva, by secretory sialography, and by salivary scintigraphy.
- Salivary gland biopsy results typically show lymphocytic infiltration; lower lip biopsy findings show salivary gland infiltration by lymphocytes.

◆ TREATMENT

General
- Meticulous oral hygiene
- Humidifier
- Unscented skin lotions
- Frequent dental care

Diet
- Avoidance of sugar, tobacco, alcohol, and spicy, salty, or highly acidic foods
- Increased oral fluid intake for mouth dryness

Activity
- No restrictions

Medication
- Pilocarpine and cevimeline
- Preservative-free artificial tears and sustained-release cellulose capsules
- Artificial salivas
- Glucocorticoids or other immunosuppressive agents for extraglandular manifestations such as systemic vasculitis
- Saline nasal sprays
- Vaginal lubricants
- Nonsteroidal anti-inflammatory drugs
- Antifungals
- Ophthalmic lubricants
- Cyclosporin eye drops (Restasis)
- Antimalarials such as hydroxychloroquine (Plaquenil)

DIAGNOSING SJÖGREN'S SYNDROME

For a diagnosis of Sjögren's syndrome, the patient must have the following:
- keratoconjunctivitis sicca
- diminished salivary gland flow
- positive salivary gland biopsy, showing mononuclear cell infiltration
- presence of autoantibodies in a serum sample, indicating a systemic autoimmune process.

✿ NURSING CONSIDERATIONS

Nursing diagnoses
- Acute pain
- Disturbed body image
- Disturbed sensory perception: Visual
- Fatigue
- Impaired oral mucous membrane
- Impaired skin integrity
- Impaired swallowing
- Impaired tissue integrity
- Ineffective sexuality patterns
- Risk for deficient fluid volume
- Risk for infection
- Risk for injury
- Sexual dysfunction

Key outcomes
The patient will:
- express feelings of increased comfort and decreased pain
- verbalize feelings regarding a change in body image
- maintain optimal functioning within the limits of the vision impairment
- express feelings of increased energy
- have pink and moist oral mucosa
- exhibit improved or healed wounds or lesions
- exhibit no signs of aspiration
- experience reduced redness, swelling, and pain at the site of impaired tissue
- express feelings related to altered sexuality patterns
- maintain adequate fluid balance
- remain free from signs and symptoms of infection
- remain free from injury
- acknowledge problems in sexual function.

Nursing interventions
- Instill artificial tears as often as every 30 minutes to prevent eye damage, and instill an eye ointment at bedtime.
- Provide plenty of fluids—especially water—for the patient to drink, and sugarless chewing gum or candy.

Monitoring
- Response to treatment
- Extraglandular manifestations
- Complications

▶ PATIENT TEACHING

Be sure to cover:
- disorder, diagnostic tests, and treatment
- instillation of eye drops and ointments
- need for sunglasses to protect the eyes
- need to keep the face clean and to avoid rubbing the eyes
- avoidance of saliva-decreasing drugs, such as atropine derivatives, antihistamines, anticholinergics, and antidepressants
- meticulous oral hygiene
- high-calorie, protein-rich liquid supplements to prevent malnutrition if mouth lesions make eating painful
- need to consume a nutritious diet
- avoidance of sugar, tobacco, alcohol, and spicy, salty, or highly acidic foods
- need to humidify the home and work environments (suggest use of normal saline solution [in drop or spray form] to relieve nasal dryness).
- avoidance of prolonged hot showers and baths and the use of moisturizing lotions on dry skin (suggest use of a water-soluble gel as a vaginal lubricant).

✳ RESOURCES

Organizations
American College of Rheumatology: *www.rheumatology.org*
Arthritis Foundation: *www.arthritis.org*
National Institute of Neurological Disorders and Stroke: *www.ninds.nih.gov*
Sjögren's Syndrome Foundation: *www.sjogrens.org*

Selected references
Hansen, A. , et al. "Immunopathologies of Primary Sjögren's Syndrome: Implications for Disease Management and Therapy," *Current Opinion in Rheumatology* 17(5):558-65, September 2005.
Larche, M.J. "A Short Review of the Pathogenesis of Sjögren's Syndrome," *Autoimmunity Reviews* 5(2):132-35, February 2006.
Ohlsson, V., et al. "Renal Tubular Necrosis, Arthritis, and Autoantibodies: Primary Sjögren's Syndrome in Childhood," *Rheumatology* 45(2):238-40, February 2006.

Smallpox

● OVERVIEW

Description
- Acute, highly contagious infectious disease caused by *Poxvirus variola*
- Two related viruses:
  – *Variola major* (classic smallpox), with a mortality rate of 20% to 50%
  – *Variola minor* (alastrim), a clinically milder form with a mortality rate less than 1%
- Eliminated worldwide in 1980 (World Health Organization declaration) due to global vaccination and eradication program
- Potential for use in bioterrorism and biological warfare; classified as category-A biological disease; transmits human to human with no known treatment
- Also known as *variola*

Pathophysiology
- Poxviruses are characterized by a large double-stranded deoxyribonucleic acid (DNA) genome and a brick-shaped morphology.
- Poxviruses are the only DNA viruses that replicate in cytoplasm.
- The virus is spread through direct contact or inhalation of respiratory droplets.
- The incubation period is 7 to 19 days. Illness onset is in 10 to 14 days, with onset of the characteristic rash in 2 to 4 days. Fever and macular rash appear after an average incubation period of 12 days, with a progression to typical vesicular and pustular lesions over 1 or 2 weeks.
- It's most contagious before the eruptive period and from the time between lesion development and scab disappearance.

Causes
- *P. variola*

Risk factors
- Lack of immunization with exposure to active virus

Incidence
- Last known case in United States reported in 1949
- Last case of endemic smallpox reported in Africa in 1977
- Affected people of all ages
- In temperate zones, incidence was highest during winter
- In tropics, incidence was highest during hot, dry months

Common characteristics
- Fever
- Maculopapular rash

Complications
- Secondary bacterial infections
- Encephalitis
- Bleeding abnormalities
- Blindness
- Death (rare)

✳ ASSESSMENT

History
- Influenza-type symptoms
- High fever, chills
- Rash
- Malaise
- Headache, backache
- Abdominal pain
- Nausea, vomiting

Physical findings
- After average incubation period of 12 days:
  – Fever
  – Macular rash
  – Progression to typical vesicular and pustular lesions, and then crusted scabs
  – Centrifugal distribution to rash; starts on the face and extremities, eventually spreading to the trunk

Test results
LABORATORY
- Culture of aspirate from vesicles and pustules shows presence of variola.
- Electron microscopy of vesicular scrapings shows presence of variola.

◆ TREATMENT

General
- Home treatment, if possible, to reduce spread
- No current treatment other than supportive
- Strict isolation

Diet
- As tolerated

Activity
- As tolerated

Medication
- Antibiotics
- Antipruritics
- Antihistamines
- Analgesics
- I.V. fluids

✤ NURSING CONSIDERATIONS

Nursing diagnoses
- Acute pain
- Anxiety
- Disturbed body image
- Imbalanced nutrition: Less than body requirements
- Impaired skin integrity
- Ineffective coping

Key outcomes
The patient will:
- express feelings of increased comfort and decreased pain
- verbalize feelings of fear and anxiety
- verbalize positive feelings regarding self and body image
- remain afebrile
- maintain adequate nutrition and hydration
- exhibit healed or improved lesions or wounds
- demonstrate effective coping mechanisms.

Nursing interventions
- Administer medications, as ordered.
- Report any case of smallpox to the appropriate public health office.
- Institute strict exposure precautions, including isolation and airborne, contact, and standard precautions.
- Autoclave all laundry and hospital waste before laundering or incinerating.
- Provide meticulous skin care.
- Encourage verbalization of fears and concerns.
- Provide adequate hydration.
- Provide a well-balanced diet.
- Assist in the development of effective coping mechanisms.
- Provide adequate rest periods.

Monitoring
- Vital signs
- Intake and output
- Complications
- Fluid and electrolyte status
- Signs and symptoms of secondary bacterial infection

▶ PATIENT TEACHING

Be sure to cover:
- disorder, diagnostic tests, and treatment
- medication administration, dosage, and possible adverse effects
- when to notify the physician
- isolation
- hydration
- skin lesion care.

Discharge planning
- Refer those in direct contact with infected individual for preexposure and postexposure vaccination if more than 3 years since last vaccine.

✴ RESOURCES

Organizations
National Center for Infectious Diseases: *www.cdc.gov/ncidod*
United States Department of Health & Human Services: *www.hhs.gov*
World Health Organization: *www.who.int*

Selected references
Beasley, A., et al. "Treating Patients with Smallpox in the Operating Room," *AORN Journal* 80(4):681-85, 688-89, October 2004.

Jahrling, P.B., et al. "Countermeasures to the Bioterrorist Threat of Smallpox," *Current Molecular Medicine* 5(8):817-26, December 2005.

Mack, K. "Oncology Nursing Implications Related to Smallpox Bioterrorism Preparations," *Clinical Journal of Oncology Nursing* 8(1):51-55, February 2004.

Milgrom, H., et al. "Smallpox Vaccination: A Conundrum of Risks and Outcomes," *Current Opinion in Allergy & Clinical Immunology* 5(3):207-209, June 2005.

Moore, Z.S., et al. "Smallpox," *Lancet* 367(9508):425-35, February 2006.

Murphy, F.A., and Osburn, B.J. "Adventitious Agents and Smallpox Vaccine in Strategic National Stockpile," *Emerging Infectious Diseases* 11(7):1086-1089, July 2005.

Seguin, D., and Stoner, H.J. "Triage of a Febrile Patient with a Rash: A Comparison of Chickenpox, Monkeypox, and Smallpox," *Disaster Management & Response* 2(3):81-86, July-September 2004.

Spinal injury

Description
- Fractures, contusions, and compressions of the spine
- Most common sites: C5, C6, C7, T12, and L1 vertebrae

Pathophysiology
- Injury causes microscopic hemorrhages.
- All of the gray matter is filled with blood, resulting in necrosis.
- Edema causes spinal cord compression, further decreasing blood supply.
- Long-term scarring and meningeal thickening occur.
- Nerves are blocked or tangled.
- Sensory and motor deficits occur.

Causes
- Trauma to spine

Risk factors
- Motor vehicle crash
- Fall
- Diving into shallow water
- Gunshot and related wound
- Improper lifting of heavy object
- Minor fall
- Neoplastic lesion
- Osteoporosis

Incidence
- Most common between ages 15 and 35

Common characteristics
- Based on severity and location of injury:
  - Muscle spasm or back pain (worsens with movement)
  - Mild paresthesia to quadriplegia
  - Shock
  - Loss of motor function, muscle flaccidity
  - Bladder and bowel atony
  - Loss of perspiration below the level of the injury
  - Respiratory impairment

Complications
- Paralysis
- Death
- Autonomic dysreflexia
- Spinal shock
- Neurogenic shock

History
- Muscle spasm
- Back or neck pain
- Point tenderness (in cervical fractures)
- Back or neck pain
- Risk factors

Physical findings
- Level of injury and any spinal cord damage located by neurologic assessment
- Limited movement and activities that cause pain
- Surface wounds
- Pain location
- Loss of sensation below the level of injury
- Deformity

Test results
IMAGING
- Spinal X-rays, myelography, computed tomography, and magnetic resonance imaging scans can indicate the location of the fracture and the site of the compression.

General
- Stabilization of spine and prevention of cord damage
- Hemodynamic support
- Application of a hard cervical collar
- Wound care, if appropriate
- Chemotherapy and radiation for neoplastic lesion
- Aspiration precautions
- Intubation and mechanical ventilation, if necessary

Diet
- Nothing by mouth; or, as tolerated, based on clinical status

Activity
- Skeletal traction with skull tongs
- Bed rest on a firm surface
- Rotation bed with cervical traction, if appropriate

Medication
- Corticosteroids
- Analgesics
- Muscle relaxants
- Chemotherapy for neoplastic lesion

Surgery
- Decompression of spinal cord
- Stabilization of spinal column

Nursing diagnoses

- Acute pain
- Anxiety
- Autonomc dysreflexia
- Deficient diversional activity
- Deficient fluid volume
- Disturbed body image
- Dressing or grooming self-care deficit
- Hopelessness
- Impaired physical mobility
- Ineffective airway clearance
- Ineffective breathing pattern
- Ineffective coping
- Risk for aspiration
- Risk for disuse syndrome
- Risk for impaired skin integrity
- Risk for infection
- Risk for posttrauma syndrome

Key outcomes

The patient will:

- express a feelings of increased comfort and decreased pain
- express feelings of decreased anxiety
- show no signs or symptoms of autonomic dysreflexia
- participate in interests and activities unrelated to the illness or confinement
- maintain adequate fluid volume
- express positive feelings about self
- participate in self-care activities at the highest level possible within the confines of the injury
- recognize choices and alternatives and make decisions on own behalf
- attain the highest degree of mobility possible within the confines of the injury
- maintain a patent airway
- maintain adequate ventilation and oxygenation
- develop effective coping mechanisms
- show no signs of aspiration
- maintain muscle strength and joint range of motion to the highest degree possible within the confines of the injury
- maintain skin integrity with no signs or symptoms of breakdown
- remain free from signs and symptoms of infection
- express fears and feelings about the traumtic event.

Nursing interventions

- Apply a hard cervical collar.
- Immobilize the patient.
- Offer the patient comfort and reassurance.
- Administer medications, as ordered.
- Provide wound care, if appropriate.
- Provide diversionary activities.
- Provide proper skin care.

Monitoring

- Neurologic changes
- Respiratory status
- Changes in skin sensation and loss of muscle strength
- Skin integrity
- Hydration and nutritional status
- Pain control

▶ PATIENT TEACHING

Be sure to cover:

- disorder, diagnostic tests, and treatment
- traction methods used
- exercises to maintain physical mobility
- medication administration, dosage, and possible adverse effects
- prescribed home care regimen
- importance of follow-up examinations.

Discharge planning

- Refer the patient to an appropriate rehabilitation center and resource and support services.

Organizations

American Academy of Neurology:
www.aan.com
American Spinal Injury Association:
www.asia-spinalinjury.org
Christopher Reeve Foundation:
www.apacure.com
National Spinal Cord Injury Association:
www.spinalcord.org

Selected references

Atlas of Pathophysiology, 2nd ed. Philadelphia: Lippincott Williams & Wilkins, 2005.
Cotton, B.A., et al. "Respiratory Complications and Mortality Risk Associated with Thoracic Spine Injury," *Journal of Trauma* 59(6):1400-407, December 2005.
Hayes, J.S., and Arriola, T. "Pediatric Spinal Injuries," *Pediatric Nursing* 31(6):464-67, November-December 2005.
Lemke, D.M. "Vertebroplasty and Kyphoplasty for Treatment of Painful Osteoporotic Compression Fractures," *Journal of the American Academy of Nurse Practitioners* 17(7):268-76, July 2005.
Wilson, J.B., et al. "Spinal Injuries in Contact Sports," *Current Sports Medicine Reports* 5(1):50-55, February 2006.

Sprains and strains

● OVERVIEW

Description
- Sprain: complete or incomplete tear in supporting ligaments surrounding a joint
- Strain: acute or chronic injury to a muscle or tendinous attachment
- Both classified as mild, moderate, or severe (see *Classifying sprains and strains*)

Pathophysiology
SPRAIN
- A ligament tear causes bleeding, resulting in a hematoma, followed by formation of inflammatory exudates.
- Granulation tissue develops, and collagen forms.
- Swelling or stretching of nerves or vessels occurs.
- Persistent laxity and chronic joint instability result.

STRAIN
- Strains result from the same process as sprains.
- New tendon or muscle eventually becomes strong enough to withstand normal muscle strain.

Causes
- Fall
- Motor vehicle accident
- Trauma
- Excessive exercise

Common characteristics
SPRAIN
- Localized pain
- Swelling and warmth
- Progressive loss of motion
- Ecchymosis

STRAIN
- Pain
- Inflammation
- Erythema
- Ecchymosis
- Elevated skin temperature

Risk factors
- Participation in sports
- Strenuous exercise

Incidence
- More common in athletes (occurs in 80% of athletes)
- More common in men than in women

Complications
SPRAIN
- Avulsion fracture

STRAIN
- Complete rupture of muscle tendon unit
- Deep vein thrombosis

✳ ASSESSMENT

History
- Physical activity
- Similar injury in past
- Systemic disease with high risk factors
- Local pain that worsens during joint movement
- Loss of mobility
- Sharp, transient pain and rapid swelling
- Stiffness, soreness, and generalized tenderness

Physical findings
- Ecchymosis
- Swelling
- Point tenderness

Test results
IMAGING
- X-rays rule out fractures and confirm damage to ligaments.

◆ TREATMENT

General
- "RICE" (rest, ice, compression [wrapping in an elastic bandage], and elevation) to affected area

Diet
- Nothing by mouth if surgery scheduled
- No restrictions

Activity
- Limited activity and weight bearing to injured area, based on extent of injury
- Elevation of affected joint above the level of the heart for 48 to 72 hours
- Rehabilitation or exercise program
- Range-of-motion (ROM) exercises

Medication
- Vitamin C supplements
- Nonsteroidal anti-inflammatory drugs
- Analgesics
- COX-2 inhibitors

Surgery
- Based on extent of injury

CLASSIFYING SPRAINS AND STRAINS

The guide below will help you classify the severity of sprains and strains.

Sprains
- Grade 1 (mild): minor or partial ligament tear with normal joint stability and function
- Grade 2 (moderate): partial tear with mild joint laxity and some function loss
- Grade 3 (severe): complete tear or incomplete separation of ligament from bone, causing total joint laxity and function loss

Strains
- Grade I (mild): microscopic muscle or tendon tear (or both) with no loss of strength
- Grade 2 (moderate): incomplete tear with bleeding into muscle tissue and some loss of strength
- Grade 3 (severe): complete rupture, usually resulting from separation of muscle from muscle, muscle from tendon, or tendon from bone (This type of strain usually stems from sudden, violent movement or direct injury.)

NURSING CONSIDERATIONS

Nursing diagnoses
- Acute pain
- Impaired physical mobility
- Risk for injury

Key outcomes
The patient will:
- express feelings of increased comfort and decreased pain
- attain the highest possible level of mobility
- remain free from injury.

Nursing interventions
- Apply ice intermittently.
- Apply an elastic bandage or air cast.
- Administer medications, as ordered.
- Elevate the extremity.

Monitoring
- Circulation and sensation
- Edema
- Response to treatment
- Pain level
- Complications
- Adverse effects of medications
- ROM

PATIENT TEACHING

Be sure to cover:
- disorder, diagnostic tests, and treatment
- how to apply ice intermittently for the first 12 to 48 hours
- how to reapply elastic bandage
- crutch-gait training
- avoidance of further injury to the joint
- medication administration, dosage, and possible adverse effects
- resources.

RESOURCES

Organizations
American Academy of Orthopaedic Surgeons: *www.aaos.org*
American Orthopaedic Society for Sports Medicine: *www.sportsmed. org*
National Institute of Arthritis and Musculoskeletal and Skin Diseases: *www.niams.nih.gov*

Selected references
Atlas of Pathophysiology, 2nd ed. Philadelphia: Lippincott Williams & Wilkins, 2005.
Crites, B.M. "Ankle Sprains," *Current Opinion in Orthopedics* 16(2):117-19, April 2005.
Paget, S.A., et al. *Hospital for Special Surgery Manual of Rheumatology and Outpatient Orthopedic Disorders,* 5th ed. Philadelphia: Lippincott Williams & Wilkins, 2006.
Willems, T.M., et al. "Intrinsic Risk Factors for Inversion Ankle Sprains in Females—A Prospective Study," *Scandinavian Journal of Medicine & Science in Sports* 15(5):336-45, October 2005.

Squamous cell carcinoma

● OVERVIEW

Description
- Invasive tumor that arises from keratinizing epidermal cells

Pathophysiology
- Transformation from a premalignant lesion to squamous cell carcinoma may begin with induration and inflammation of the preexisting lesion.
- When squamous cell carcinoma arises from normal skin, the nodule grows slowly on a firm, indurated base. If untreated, this nodule eventually ulcerates and invades underlying tissues. (See *Squamous cell carcinoma nodule.*)

Causes
- Exact cause unknown
- Actinic damage from solar ultraviolet (UV) radiation
- Burns, scars
- Chemical carcinogens
- Ionizing radiation
- Ulcerations

Risk factors
- Overexposure to the sun's UV rays
- Radiation therapy
- Ingestion of herbicides containing arsenic
- Chronic skin irritation and inflammation
- Exposure to local carcinogens (such as tar and oil)
- Hereditary diseases (such as xeroderma pigmentosum and albinism)
- Presence of premalignant lesions (such as actinic keratosis or Bowen's disease)
- Rarely, develops on site of smallpox vaccination, psoriasis, or chronic discoid hippus erythematosus

Common characteristics
- Chronic skin ulceration

Incidence
- Most common in fair-skinned white men over age 60
- Risk greatly increased by outdoor employment and residence in sunny, warm climate

Complications
- Lymph node involvement
- Visceral metastasis

✳ ASSESSMENT

History
- Areas of chronic ulceration, especially on sun-damaged skin
- Pain, malaise, anorexia, fatigue, and weakness

Physical findings
- Lesions on the face, ears, or dorsa of the hands and forearms, and on other sun-damaged skin areas (lesions possibly scaly and keratotic with raised, irregular borders; in late disease, lesions growing outward or are exophytic and friable and tending toward chronic crusting)

Test results
DIAGNOSTIC PROCEDURES
- Excisional biopsy allows a definitive diagnosis.

◆ TREATMENT

General
- Treatment determined by size, shape, location, and invasiveness of tumor and condition of underlying tissue
- Radiation therapy for older or debilitated patients

Diet
- High-protein, high-calorie

Activity
- No restrictions

Medication
- Chemotherapy
- Topical corticosteroids
- Analgesics

Surgery
- Wide surgical excision, curettage, and electrodesiccation
- Cryosurgery

SQUAMOUS CELL CARCINOMA NODULE

An ulcerated nodule with an indurated base and a raised, irregular border is a typical lesion in squamous cell carcinoma.

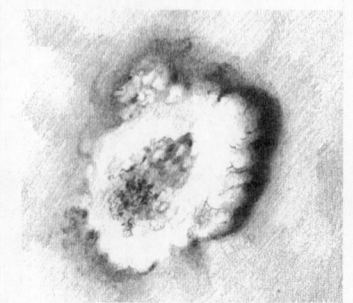

Nursing diagnoses

- Acute pain
- Anxiety
- Disturbed body image
- Fatigue
- Fear
- Imbalanced nutrition: Less than body requirements
- Impaired skin integrity
- Ineffective coping

Key outcomes

The patient will:

- express feelings of increased comfort and decreased pain
- use support systems to assist with anxiety and fear
- express positive feelings about self
- experience feelings of increased energy
- express concerns and fears related to the diagnosis and condition
- maintain adequate nutrition and hydration
- exhibit improved or healed lesions or wounds
- demonstrate positive coping behaviors.

Nursing interventions

- Encourage verbalization and provide support.
- Provide appropriate wound care.
- Provide periods of rest between procedures if the patient fatigues easily.
- Provide small, frequent meals of a high-protein, high-calorie diet.

Monitoring

- Wound site
- Adverse effects of radiation therapy, such as nausea, vomiting, hair loss, malaise, and diarrhea
- Pain control

Be sure to cover:

- disorder, diagnostic tests, and treatment
- medications administration, dosage, and possible adverse effects
- information about skin examination
- importance of follow-up skin surveillance
- avoidance of excessive sun exposure to prevent recurrence and need to use strong sunscreen.

Discharge planning

- Refer the patient to resource and support services.

Organizations

American Academy of Dermatology: *www.aad.org*
American Cancer Society: *www.cancer.org*
Guide to Internet Resources for Cancer: *www.cancerindex.org*
National Cancer Institute: *www.cancer.gov*

Selected references

Atlas of Pathophysiology, 2nd ed. Philadelphia: Lippincott Williams & Wilkins, 2005.

Casciato, D.A. *Manual of Clinical Oncology,* 5th ed. Philadelphia: Lippincott Williams & Wilkins, 2004.

Kanitakis, J., et al. "Squamous Cell Carcinoma of the Skin Complicating Lupus Vulgaris," *Journal of the European Academy of Dermatology & Venereology* 20(1):114-16, January 2006.

Kurt, M., et al. "Malignant Fibrous Histiocytoma, Malignant Melanoma, and Squamous Cell Carcinoma Arising from Different Areas in an Adult," *Southern Medical Journal* 98(12):1228-229, December 2005.

Lim, Y.C., et al. "Level IIb Lymph Node Metastasis in Laryngeal Squamous Cell Carcinoma," *Laryngoscope* 116(2):268-72, February 2006.

Stomatitis

● OVERVIEW

Description
- Common infection occurring alone or as part of systemic disease
- Inflammation of oral mucosa; may extend to the buccal mucosa, lips, and palate
- Two main types: acute herpetic stomatitis and aphthous stomatitis
- Usually heals spontaneously, without scarring, in 10 to 14 days

Pathophysiology
- An inflammatory reaction occurs that may cause loss of the oral epithelium as a protective barrier.

Causes
ACUTE HERPETIC STOMATITIS
- Herpes simplex virus
APHTHOUS STOMATITIS
- Exact cause unknown (autoimmune and psychosomatic causes under investigation)

Risk factors
- Smoking
- Poor oral hygiene
- Stress
- Poor nutrition
- Chemotherapy
- Immunosuppression

Incidence
ACUTE HERPETIC STOMATITIS
- Common in children between ages 1 and 3
APHTHOUS STOMATITIS
- Common in young girls and female adolescents

Common characteristics
- Painful gums
- Ulcers on gum papillae

Complications
- Dysphagia
- Sepsis (in immunocompromised patient)
- Ocular or central nervous system involvement (acute herpetic stomatitis)

✳ ASSESSMENT

History
- Burning mouth pain
- Malaise
- Lethargy
- Anorexia
- Irritability
- Fever
- Extreme tenderness of the oral mucosa

Physical findings
ACUTE HERPETIC STOMATITIS
- Bleeding and swollen gums
- Papulovesicular ulcers in the mouth and throat
- Submaxillary lymphadenitis
APHTHOUS STOMATITIS
- Slight swelling of the mucous membrane
- Single or multiple shallow ulcers with whitish centers and red borders, about 2 to 5 mm diameter (see *Looking at aphthous stomatitis*)

Test results
LABORATORY
- Smear of ulcer exudate identifies the causative organism in Vincent's angina (painful pseudomembranous ulceration of gums, oral mucous membranes, pharynx, and tonsils).
- Viral cultures performed on fluid and herpetic vesicles in acute herpetic stomatitis identify the virus.

◆ TREATMENT

General
- Symptomatic relief
- Nonantiseptic warm-water mouth rinses
- Smoking cessation
- Ice
- Soft-bristled toothbrush

Diet
- Soft, pureed, or liquid diet
- Avoidance of salty, spicy foods

Activity
- As tolerated

Medication
- I.V. fluids (severe cases)
ACUTE HERPETIC STOMATITIS
- Topical anesthetic solutions
- Topical corticosteroids
- Acyclovir
APHTHOUS STOMATITIS
- Topical anesthetic coating agent

LOOKING AT APHTHOUS STOMATITIS

In aphthous stomatitis, numerous small, round vesicles appear. They soon break and leave shallow ulcers with red areolae.

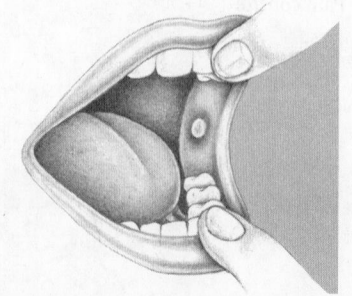

✣ NURSING CONSIDERATIONS

Nursing diagnoses
- Acute pain
- Imbalanced nutrition: Less than body requirements
- Impaired oral mucous membrane
- Ineffective health maintenance
- Risk for infection

Key outcomes
The patient will:
- express feelings of increased comfort and decreased pain
- maintain adequate nutritional intake
- show improvement or complete healing of lesions or wounds
- describe routine oral care
- demonstrate good oral hygiene practices
- remain free from further signs and symptoms of infection.

Nursing interventions
- Advise using a sponge instead of a toothbrush to clean the teeth.
- Suggest rinsing with hydrogen peroxide or normal saline mouthwash.
- Administer prescribed analgesics.
- Develop a meal plan based on soft, liquid, or pureed foods.
- Offer iced drinks.

Monitoring
- Lesion state
- Response to treatment
- Complications

▶ PATIENT TEACHING

Be sure to cover:
- infection and expected course
- importance of good oral hygiene
- proper application of topical medications
- recommended dietary changes
- medication administration, dosage, and possible adverse effects
- (with aphthous stomatitis) need to avoid such precipitating factors as stress and fatigue.

Discharge planning
- Refer the patient to a smoking-cessation program, if appropriate.

✳ RESOURCES

Organizations
National Digestive Diseases Information Clearinghouse (NDDIC): *www.niddk. nih.gov/health/digest/nddic.htm*
National Institute of Diabetes & Digestive & Kidney Diseases: *www.niddk.nih.gov*

Selected references
Albanidou-Farmaki, E., et al. "Outcomes Following Treatment for *Helicobacter Pylori* in Patients with Recurrent Aphthous Stomatitis," *Oral Diseases* 11(1):22-26, January 2005.

Handbook of Diseases, 3rd ed. Philadelphia: Lippincott Williams & Wilkins, 2004.

Jurge, S., et al. "Number VI Recurrent Aphthous Stomatitis," *Oral Diseases* 12(1):1-21, January 2006.

Shulman, J.D., et al. "Risk Factors Associated With Denture Stomatits in the United States," *Journal of Oral Pathology & Medicine* 34(6):340-46, July 2005.

Stroke

● OVERVIEW

Description

- Third most common cause of death in the United States
- Affects 500,000 persons each year and half result in death
- Most common cause of neurologic disability
- About 50% of stroke survivors permanently disabled
- Recurrences possible within weeks, months, or years
- Also known as *cerebrovascular accident* or *brain attack*

Pathophysiology

- The oxygen supply to the brain is interrupted or diminished due to sudden impairment of cerebral circulation in blood vessels to the brain.
- In thrombotic or embolic stroke, neurons die from lack of oxygen.
- In hemorrhagic stroke, impaired cerebral perfusion causes infarction.

Causes
CEREBRAL THROMBOSIS
- Most common cause of stroke
- Obstruction of a blood vessel in the extracerebral vessels
- Site possibly intracerebral
CEREBRAL EMBOLISM
- Second most common cause of stroke
- Cardiac arrhythmias
- Endocarditis
- History of rheumatic heart disease
- Open heart surgery
- Posttraumatic valvular disease
CEREBRAL HEMORRHAGE
- Third most common cause of stroke
- Arteriovenous malformation
- Cerberal aneurysms
- Chronic hypertension

Risk factors

- Uncontrolled hypertension
- History of transient ischemic attack
- Heart disease
- Obesity
- Alcohol
- High red blood cell count
- Arrhythmias
- Diabetes mellitus
- Gout
- High serum triglyceride levels
- Use of oral contraceptives in conjunction with smoking and hypertension
- Smoking
- Family history of stroke

Incidence

- Mostly affects older adults but can strike at any age
- More common in men than women
- Affects Blacks and Hispanics more commonly than other groups

Common characteristics

- Unilateral limb weakness
- Speech difficulties
- Numbness on one side
- Vision disturbances
- Ataxia, gait disturbance
- Altered level of consciousness (LOC)

Complications

- Malnutrition
- Infections
- Sensory impairment
- Altered LOC
- Aspiration
- Contractures
- Skin breakdown
- Deep vein thrombosis
- Pulmonary emboli
- Depression

✳ ASSESSMENT

History

- Varying clinical features, depending on:
  - Artery affected
  - Severity of damage
  - Extent of collateral circulation
- One or more risk factors present
- Sudden hemiparesis or hemiplegia
- Gradual onset of dizziness, mental disturbances, or seizures
- Loss of consciousness or sudden aphasia

Physical findings

- With stroke in left hemisphere, signs and symptoms seen on right side
- With stroke in right hemisphere, signs and symptoms seen on left side
- With stroke that causes cranial nerve damage, signs and symptoms seen on same side
- Unconsciousness or changes in LOC
- With conscious patient, anxiety along with communication and mobility difficulties
- Urinary incontinence
- Loss of voluntary muscle control
- Hemiparesis or hemiplegia
- Decreased deep tendon reflexes
- Hemianopia on the affected side
- With left-sided hemiplegia, problems with visuospatial relations
- Sensory losses

Test results
LABORATORY
- Laboratory tests (including anticardiolipin antibodies, antiphospholipid, factor V [Leiden] mutation, antithrombin III, protein S and C) may show increased thrombotic risk.
IMAGING
- Magnetic resonance imaging and magnetic resonance angiography evaluates the lesion's location and size.
- Cerebral angiography details the disruption of cerebral circulation and is the test of choice for examining the entire cerebral blood flow.
- Computed tomography scan is used to detect structural abnormalities.
- Positron emission tomography provides data on cerebral metabolism and on cerebral blood flow changes.
DIAGNOSTIC PROCEDURES
- Transcranial Doppler studies are used to evaluate the velocity of blood flow.
- Carotid Doppler is used to measure flow through the carotid arteries.
- Two-dimensional echocardiogram is used to evaluate the heart.
- Cerebral blood flow studies are used to measure blood flow to the brain.
- EEG shows reduced electrical activity in an area of cortical infarction.

◆ TREATMENT

General

- Careful blood pressure management
- Varies, depending on cause and clinical manifestations

Diet

- Pureed dysphagia diet or tube feedings if indicated
- Thickened liquids, as indicated

Activity
- Physical, speech, and occupational therapy
- Care measures to help the patient adapt to specific deficits

Medication
- Tissue plasminogen activator (emergency care within 3 hours of onset of the symptoms)
- Anticonvulsants
- Stool softeners
- Anticoagulants
- Analgesics
- Antidepressants
- Antiplatelets
- Lipid-lowering agents
- Antihypertensives

Surgery
- Craniotomy
- Endarterectomy
- Extracranial-intracranial bypass
- Ventricular shunts

❖ NURSING CONSIDERATIONS

Nursing diagnoses
- Anxiety
- Bathing, toileting, or hygiene self-care deficit
- Disturbed sensory perception: Tactile
- Dressing or grooming self-care deficit
- Impaired gas exchange
- Impaired physical mobility
- Impaired verbal communication
- Ineffective airway clearance
- Ineffective coping
- Ineffective tissue perfusion: Cerebral
- Powerlessness
- Risk for aspiration
- Risk for disuse syndrome
- Risk for impaired skin integrity
- Risk for infection
- Risk for injury
- Situational low self-esteem

Key outcomes
The patient (or family) will:
- identify strategies to reduce anxiety
- perform bathing, toileting, and hygiene activities to the fullest extent possible
- report signs and symptoms of impaired sensation

- perform dressing and grooming activities to the fullest extent possible
- maintain adequate ventilation and oxygenation
- achieve maximum mobility possible
- effectively communicate needs verbally or through an alternate means of communication
- maintain a patent airway
- develop adequate coping mechanisms
- exhibit signs of adequate cerebral perfusion
- express feelings of control over health and well-being
- remain free from signs of aspiration
- maintain intact skin
- remain free from infection and injury
- verbalize feelings about self-esteem

Nursing interventions
- Maintain a patent airway and oxygenation.
- Offer urinal or bedpan every 2 hours.
- Insert an indwelling urinary catheter, if necessary.
- Ensure adequate nutrition.
- Provide careful eye and mouth care.
- Follow the physical therapy program, and assist the patient with exercise.
- Establish and maintain communication with the patient.
- Provide psychological support.
- Set realistic short-term goals.
- Protect the patient from injury.
- Provide careful positioning to prevent aspiration and contractures.
- Take steps to prevent complications.
- Administer medications, as ordered.

Monitoring
- Continuous neurologic assessment
- Continuous respiratory support
- Continuous monitoring of vital signs
- Continuous monitoring of GI problems
- Fluid, electrolyte, and nutritional intake
- Development of deep vein thrombosis and pulmonary embolus
- Response to medication

▶ PATIENT TEACHING

Be sure to cover:
- disorder, diagnostic tests, and treatment
- occupational and speech therapy programs
- dietary regimen
- medication administration, dosage, and possible adverse effects
- stroke prevention measures.

Discharge planning
Refer the patient to:
- home care services
- outpatient services and speech and occupational rehabilitation programs, as indicated.

✳ RESOURCES

Organizations
American Academy of Neurology: *www.aan.com*
American Heart Association: *www.americanheart.org*
American Neurological Association: *www.aneuroa.org*
American Stroke Association: *www.stroke-association.org*
National Aphasia Association: *www.aphasia.org*
National Institutes of Health: *www.nih.gov*
National Stroke Association: *www.stroke.org*

Selected references
Bakas, T., et al. "Outcomes Among Family Caregivers of Aphasic versus Nonaphasic Stroke Survivors," *Rehabilitation Nursing* 31(1):33-42, January-February 2006.

Kasper, D. L., et al., eds. *Harrison's Principles of Internal Medicine,* 16th ed. New York: McGraw-Hill Book Co., 2005.

Koenig, M.A., et al. "Safety of Induced Hypertension Therapy in Patients with Acute Ischemic Stroke, " *Neurocritical Care* 4(1):3-7, 2006.

Subarachnoid hemorrhage

OVERVIEW

Description
- Rupture of a cerebral or intracranial aneurysm
- Causes death in about one-half of cases
- Also called *SAH*

Pathophysiology
- Rupture of the arterial wall allows blood to spill into brain tissue, leading to increased intracranial pressure (ICP) and pressure exerted on surrounding structures including cranial nerves.
- Increased ICP leads to disruption in respiratory control centers.
- Dilation of third ventricle exerts mechanical pressure on hypothalamus, causing progressive loss of nerve tissue, ultimately leading to hypothalamic dysfunction.
- Hypothalamic dysfunction leads to impaired synthesis and transport or release of antidiuretic hormone (ADH).
- ADH can't respond to changes in plasma osmolality, and the kidneys' inability to reabsorb water leads to excretion of large amounts of dilute urine.

Causes
- Spontaneous rupture
- Overstretching of aneurysm
- Trauma

Incidence
- Can occur at any age or in either sex
- SAH due to cerebral aneurysm development slightly higher in women than men
- Effects of hemorrhage (if untreated) proving fatal in 40% of cases; recurrent hemorrhage causing death in an additional 20% of cases
- Blacks at higher risk than Whites

Common characteristics
- Neurologic changes
- Sudden severe headache

Complications
- Diabetes insipidus
- Respiratory failure
- Vasospasm

ASSESSMENT

- Severity of symptoms dependent on the site and amount of bleeding (see *Classification for subarachnoid hemorrhage*)

History
- Known history of cerebral or intracranial aneurysm
- Headache; sudden and severe with rupture
- Intermittent nausea

Physical findings
- Projectile vomiting
- Altered level of consciousness
- Nuchal rigidity
- Hemiparesis
- Hemisensory defects
- Dilated pupils

Test results
IMAGING
- Cerebral angiography reveals altered cerebral blood flow, vessel lumen dilation, and differences in arterial filling.
- Computed tomography scan identifies evidence of aneurysm and possible hemorrhage.
- Magnetic resonance imaging may help to locate the site of bleeding.
- Positron-emission tomography shows chemical activity of the brain and extent of tissue damage.

DIAGNOSTIC PROCEDURES
- Lumbar puncture (LP) and cerebrospinal fluid (CSF) analysis reveal blood in the CSF; elevated CSF pressure, protein, and white blood cell count; and decreased glucose level.

NURSING ALERT Because LP increases the risk for herniation and rebleeding in patients with SAH and increased ICP, the procedure is performed only if the results of the CT scan are inconclusive.

TREATMENT

General
- Emergency management of airway, breathing, and circulation
- Supportive treatment
- Electrothrombosis, if surgical repair is contraindicated

Diet
- Avoidance of stimulants such as coffee
- Nothing by mouth before surgery

Activity
- Bed rest in a quiet darkened room

Medication
- Oxygen therapy
- Analgesics
- Antihypertensives
- Vasoconstrictors
- Sedatives
- Anticonvulsants

Surgery
- Clipping, ligation, or wrapping of aneurysm
- Interventional radiology with endovascular balloon therapy

CLASSIFICATION FOR SUBARACHNOID HEMORRHAGE

The classification below identifies five grades that characterize an SAH from a ruptured cerebral aneurysm:
- *Grade I (minimal bleeding)* – The patient is alert and oriented without symptoms.
- *Grade II (mild bleeding)* – The patient is alert and oriented, with a mild to severe headache and nuchal rigidity.
- *Grade III (moderate bleeding)* – The patient is lethargic and confused or drowsy, with nuchal rigidity and, possibly, a mild focal deficit such as hemiparesis.
- *Grade IV (severe bleeding)* – The patient is stuporous, with nuchal rigidity and, possibly, moderate to severe focal deficits, hemiparesis, early decerebrate rigidity, and vegetative disturbances.
- *Grade V: (moribund; often fatal)* – If the rupture is nonfatal, the patient is in a deep coma, with such severe neurological deficits as decerebrate rigidity and moribund appearance.

❖ NURSING CONSIDERATIONS

Nursing diagnoses
- Acute pain
- Anxiety
- Decreased intracranial adaptive capacity
- Impaired gas exchange
- Ineffective breathing pattern
- Ineffective tissue perfusion: Cerebral
- Risk for imbalanced fluid volume
- Risk for injury

Key outcomes
The patient will:
- express feelings of increased comfort and decreased pain
- identify strategies to reduce anxiety
- exhibit a level of consciousness within acceptable parameters
- maintain adequate ventilation and oxygenation
- exhibit a respiratory rate and pattern within acceptable parameters
- demonstrate signs of adequate cerebral perfusion
- maintain adequate fluid balance
- remain free from signs and symptoms of injury.

Nursing interventions
- Maintain a patent airway.
- Institute bedrest in a quiet, darkened room with head of bed flat or raised slightly, but less than 30 degrees.
- Give prescribed drugs.
- Prepare patient for surgical repair, as indicated.
- Administer oxygen therapy, as ordered.
- Institute aneurysm precautions.
- Provide frequent turning and skin care measures.
- Provide postoperative care, as indicated.

Monitoring
- Airway
- Level of consciousness and neurologic status
- Vital signs
- Intake and output
- Signs and symptoms of rebleeding
- Signs and symptoms of increased intracranial pressure
- Skin integrity

© PATIENT TEACHING

Be sure to cover:
- disorder, diagnostic tests, and treatment
- medication administration, dosage, possible adverse effects
- activity limitations, if indicated
- signs and symptoms to report to the physician
- signs and symptoms of rebleeding.

Discharge planning
- Refer the patient to home care services or rehabilitation services, as necessary.

✴ RESOURCES

Organizations
American Academy of Neurology: *www.aan.com*
American Neurological Association: *www.aneuroa.org*
National Institute of Neurological Disorders and Stroke: *www.ninds.nih.gov*

Selected references
Dooling, E., and Winkelman, C. "Hyponatremia in the Patient with Subarachnoid Hemorrhage," *Journal of Neuroscience Nursing* 36(3):130-35, 2004.

Kazzi, A.A., and Zebian, R. "Subarachnoid Hemorrhage," Updated October 2006. Available at: *http://www.emedicine.com/EMERG/topic559.htm.* Accessed 12/20/06.

Nettina, S.M. *Lippincott's Manual of Nursing Practice,* 8th ed. Philadelphia: Lippincott Williams & Wilkins, 2005.

Walling, A.D. "Management of Unruptured Intracranial Aneurysms – Tips," *American Family Physician* 69(4):939, February, 2004.

Zhang, J.H. "Introduction: Experimental Therapies for Cerebral Vascular Diseases," *Neurological Research* 27(3):227-28, April 2005.

Substance abuse and dependence

● OVERVIEW

Description
- Use of a legal or an illegal drug that causes physical, mental, emotional, or social harm, such as opioids, stimulants, depressants, anxiolytics, and hallucinogens
- Number one health problem in the United States

Pathophysiology
- Tolerance develops when a drug is administered chronically (such as an opioid for a cancer patient), with cross-tolerance developing.
- Withdrawal occurs with abrupt discontinuation or administration of an antagonist due to rebound noradrenergic activity in the central nervous system (CNS).

Causes
- Combination of low self-esteem, peer pressure, inadequate coping skills, and curiosity
- May follow the use of drugs to relieve physical pain

Risk factors
- Male gender
- History of depression
- History of other substance abuse disorders
- Family history
- Peer pressure
- Low socioeconomic status

Incidence
- Can occur at any age
- Experimentation common beginning in adolescence and preadolescence
- Affects more than 18 million Americans who use alcohol and 5 million who use illicit drugs (fewer than one-quarter get treatment)

Common characteristics
- Nutritional deficiency
- Mood swings, anxiety, impaired memory, sleep disturbances, flashbacks, slurred speech, depression, and thought disorders
- Physical signs of substance abuse (based on substance)
- Withdrawal signs when substance not used

Complications
- Cardiac and respiratory arrest
- Intracranial hemorrhage
- Acquired immunodeficiency syndrome
- Subacute bacterial endocarditis
- Hepatitis
- Cirrhosis
- Vasculitis
- Septicemia
- Thrombophlebitis
- Pulmonary emboli
- Gangrene
- Malnutrition and GI disturbances
- Respiratory infections
- Musculoskeletal dysfunction
- Trauma
- Depression and increased risk of suicide
- Psychosis
- Toxic or allergic reactions
- Impaired social and occupational functioning

✳ ASSESSMENT

History
- Abdominal pain, nausea, or vomiting
- Painful injury or chronic illness
- Feigned illnesses
- Overdose
- High tolerance to potentially addictive drugs
- Amenorrhea
- Suggestive behavior patterns or the presence of known risk factors
- Mood swings, anxiety, impaired memory, sleep disturbances, flashbacks, slurred speech, depression, and thought disorders

Physical signs
- Lacrimation of eyes (with opiate withdrawal)
- Nystagmus (with central nervous system depressants and phencyclidine intoxication)
- Drooping eyelids (with opiate or CNS depressant use)
- Constricted pupils (with opiate use or withdrawal)
- Dilated pupils (with hallucinogens or amphetamines)
- Rhinorrhea (with opiate withdrawal or cocaine abuse)
- Inflammation, atrophy, or perforation of the nasal mucosa (with drug sniffing)
- Sweating (with opiates or CNS stimulants or drug withdrawal)
- Sensation of bugs crawling on the skin (with alcohol withdrawal)
- Excoriated skin
- Needle marks or tracks
- Cellulitis or abscesses
- Thrombophlebitis
- Fascial infection
- Bilateral crackles and rhonchi (with smoking and inhaling drugs or by opioid overdose)
- Cardiopulmonary signs of overdose (respiratory depression and hypotension)
- Acute-onset hypertension
- Cardiac arrhythmias
- Hemorrhoids
- Tremors, hyperreflexia, hyporeflexia, and seizures
- Uncooperative, disruptive, or violent behavior

DSM-IV-TR criteria
- Diagnosis is confirmed with at least three of the the following criteria (some symptoms must have persisted for at least 1 month or have occurred repeatedly over a longer time):
  - substance often taken in larger amounts or for a longer time than the patient intended
  - persistent desire or one or more unsuccessful efforts to cut down or control substance use
  - excessive time devoted to activities necessary to obtain the substance
  - frequent intoxication or withdrawal symptoms when expected to fulfill major obligations at work, school, or home or when substance use is physically hazardous
  - impaired social, occupational, or recreational activities
  - continued substance use despite the recognition of a persistent or recurrent social, psychological, or physical problem that's caused or exacerbated by the use of the substance
  - marked tolerance
  - characteristic withdrawal symptoms
  - substance often taken to relieve or avoid withdrawal symptoms

Test results

LABORATORY

- Serum or urine drug screen indicate the substance.
- Serum protein electrophoresis shows elevated serum globulin levels.
- Serum glucose shows hypoglycemia.
- Complete blood count (CBC) shows leukocytosis.
- Liver function abnormalities are present.
- CBC shows elevated mean corpuscular hemoglobin levels.
- Uric acid levels are elevated.
- Blood urea nitrogen levels are reduced.

◆ TREATMENT

General

- Symptomatic treatment based on the drug ingested
- Fluid replacement therapy
- Symptomatic treatment for complications
- Gastric lavage, induced emesis, activated charcoal, forced diuresis and, possibly, hemoperfusion or hemodialysis
- Detoxification (inpatient or outpatient)
- Psychotherapy
- Exercise
- Relaxation techniques
- Rehabilitation

Diet

- Well-balanced

Activity

- Monitored for safety

Medication

- Detoxification with the same drug or a pharmacologically similar drug
- Sedatives
- Anticholinergics
- Antidiarrheals
- Antianxiety drugs
- Anticonvulsants
- Nutritional and vitamin supplements

❖ NURSING CONSIDERATIONS

Nursing diagnoses

- Anxiety
- Compromised family coping
- Dysfunctional family processes: Alcoholism
- Hopelessness
- Imbalanced nutrition: Less than body requirements
- Impaired social interaction
- Ineffective coping
- Ineffective role performance
- Powerlessness
- Risk for deficient fluid volume
- Risk for injury
- Risk for other-directed violence
- Situational low self-esteem

Key outcomes

The patient will:

- verbalize strategies to reduce anxiety
- develop adequate coping mechanisms and support systems
- acknowledge that he has a problem and needs treatment
- consume regular, nutritious meals
- engage in social interactions with others and identify coping strategies
- acknowledge the effects of his condition on his usual roles and responsibilities
- gradually join in self-care and the decision-making process
- maintain an adequate fluid balance
- remain free from injury
- not harm others
- express his feelings related to self-esteem.

Nursing interventions

- Maintain a quiet, safe environment.
- Institute seizure precautions.
- Set limits for dealing with demanding, manipulative behavior.

Monitoring

- Vital signs
- Suicidal ideation
- Visitors
- Signs of complications
- Nutrition
- Effects of pharmacologic therapy

▶ PATIENT TEACHING

Be sure to cover:

- disorder, diagnostic tests, and treatment
- detoxification and rehabilitation, as appropriate
- measures for preventing human immunodeficiency virus infection and hepatitis
- measures for safer sex and birth control.

Discharge planning

- Recommend participation in a drug-oriented self-help group.
- Refer the patient to support services.

✳ RESOURCES

Organizations

Alcoholics Anonymous: *www.alcoholics-anonymous.org*
Nar-Anon: *www.naranon.com*
Narcotics Anonymous: *www.na.org*
National Council on Alcoholism and Drug Abuse: *www.ncadd.org*

Selected references

Collins, E.D., et al. "Anesthesia-Assisted vs. Buprenorphine- or Clonidine-Assisted Heroin Detoxification and Naltrexone Induction: A Randomized Trial," *JAMA* 294(8)903-13, August 2005.

Diagnostic and Statistical Manual of Mental Disorders, 4th edition, Text Revision. Washington, D.C.: American Pyschiatric Association, 2000.

Fazel, S., et al. "Substance Abuse and Dependence in Prisoners: A Systematic Review," *Addiction* 10(2):181-91, February 2006.

Letizia M., and Reinbolz, M. "Identifying and Managing Acute Alcohol Withdrawal in the Elderly," *Geriatric Nursing* 26(3):176-83, May-June 2005.

McClelland, G.T. "The Effects and Management of Crack Cocaine Dependency," *Nursing Times* 101(29):26-27, July 2005.

Sudden infant death syndrome

Description

- Leading cause of death among apparently healthy infants ages 1 month to 1 year
- Also known as *SIDS* and *crib death*

Pathophysiology

HYPOTHESES

- The infant may have damage to the respiratory control center in the brain from chronic hypoxemia.
- The infant may have periods of sleep apnea and eventually die during one of these episodes.
- The infant may not respond to increasing carbon dioxide levels. During an episode of apnea, carbon dioxide levels increase, but the child isn't stimulated to breathe. As apnea continues, high levels of carbon dioxide further suppress the ventilatory effort until the infant stops breathing.

Causes

- Possibly viral
- Hypoxia theory
- Apnea theory
- Possible *Clostridium botulinum* toxin
- Possibly associated with diphtheria, tetanus, and pertussis vaccines

Incidence

- Significant decline in number of SIDS deaths since mid-1990s; however, approximately 2,295 fatalities under age 1 year in 2004
- Male to female ratio of 60% of 40%
- Greatest number occurring between ages 2 and 4 months; most by end of 6 months
- Rare during first month of life
- Increased incidence in non–breast-fed infants
- Occurs most often in fall and winter
- Slightly higher incidence in:
  - preterm neonates
  - Inuit neonates
  - disadvantaged black neonates
  - neonates of mothers under age 20
  - neonates of multiple births

Common characteristics

- Respiratory tract infections
- Apnea

Complications

- Death (always)

History

- Occasionally, respiratory tract infection
- Possible abnormal hepatic or pancreatic function
- Previous near-miss respiratory event in 60% of cases
- With infant wedged in a crib corner or with blankets wrapped around head, suffocation ruled out by autopsy as the cause of death
- With frothy, blood-tinged sputum found around infant's mouth or on crib sheets revealing a patent airway, aspiration of vomitus ruled out by autopsy as cause of death
- No crying and signs of disturbed sleep by infant

PHYSICAL FINDINGS

- Postmortem examination may show:
  - changes indicating chronic hypoxia, hypoxemia, and large airway obstruction
  - bruising; possible fractured ribs
  - blood in the infant's mouth, nose, or ears
  - mottled complexion; extremely cyanotic lips and fingertips
  - pooled blood in legs and feet
  - diaper possibly wet and full of stool

Test results

DIAGNOSTIC PROCEDURES

- Autopsy may show:
  - small or normal adrenal glands
  - enlarged thymus
  - petechiae over the visceral surfaces of the pleura, within the thymus, and in the epicardium
  - well-preserved lymphoid structures
  - signs of chronic hypoxemia
  - increased pulmonary artery smooth muscle
  - edematous, congestive, and fully expanded lungs
  - liquid blood in the heart
  - stomach curd inside the trachea.

General

- Emotional support for the family
- Prevention for any surviving infant found apneic and any sibling with apnea; assessment with home apnea monitor until the at-risk infant passes age of vulnerability

Nursing diagnoses

- Dysfunctional grieving
- Fear
- Hopelessness
- Interrupted family processes
- Risk for sudden infant death syndrome
- Spiritual distress

Key outcomes

The family will:

- seek appropriate persons for assistance
- use available support systems to assist in coping
- identify feelings of hopelessness regarding the current situation
- share feelings about the event as a family
- verbalize measures to prevent SIDS
- use effective coping strategies to ease spiritual discomfort.

Nursing interventions

- Ensure that both parents are present when the child's death is confirmed.
- Stay calm and allow the parents to express their feelings.
- Reassure the parents that they aren't to blame.
- Allow the parents to see the infant in a private room and to express their grief. Stay in the room with them, if appropriate.
- Offer to call clergy, friends, or relatives.
- Return the infant's belongings to the parents.
- Ensure that the parents receive the autopsy report promptly.

Monitoring

- Parents' reactions and coping mechanisms

Be sure to cover:

- need for an autopsy to confirm the diagnosis
- basic facts about SIDS
- information to help parents cope with pregnancy and the first year of a new infant's life if they decide to have another child.

Discharge planning

- Refer the parents and family to community and health care facility support services.
- Refer the parents to a local SIDS parents' group.
- Advise the parents to contact the SIDS hot line (1-800-221-SIDS).
- Refer the parents to cardiopulmonary resuscitation classes, if appropriate.
- Refer the family to a home health nurse for continued support, if indicated.

Organizations

American Academy of Pediatrics: *www.aap.org*
Association of Sudden Infant Death Syndrome and Infant Mortality Programs: *www.asip1.org*
National Institute of Child Health and Human Development: *www.nichd.nih.gov*
SIDS Alliance: *www.sidsalliance.org*

Selected references

Heinig, M.J., and Banuelos, J. "American Academy of Pediatrics Task Force on Sudden Infant Death Syndrome (SIDS) Statement on SIDS Reduction: Friend or Foe of Breastfeeding?" *Journal of Human Lactation* 22(1):7-10, November 2005.

Maindonald, F., "Helping Parents Reduce the Risk of SIDS," *Nursing* 35(7):50-52, July 2005.

Makielski, J.C. "SIDS: Genetic and Environmental Influences May Cause Arrhythmia in This Silent Killer," *Journal of Clinical Investigation* 116(2):297-99, February 2006.

Menihan, C.A., et al. "Fetal Heart Rate Patterns and Sudden Infant Death Syndrome," *Journal of Obstetrics, Gynecologic, and Neonatal Nursing* 35(1):116-22, January-February 2006.

Thompson, D.G. "Safe Sleep Practices for Hospitalized Infants," *Pediatric Nursing* 31(5):400-403, 409, September-October 2005.

Syndrome of inappropriate antidiuretic hormone secretion

● OVERVIEW

Description
- Disease of the posterior pituitary
- Marked by excessive release of antidiuretic hormone (ADH) (vasopressin)
- Prognosis dependent on underlying disorder and response to treatment
- Also known as *SIADH*

Pathophysiology
- Excessive ADH secretion occurs in the absence of normal physiologic stimuli for its release.
- Excessive water reabsorption from the distal convoluted tubule and collecting ducts results in hyponatremia and normal to slightly increased extracellular fluid volume. (See *Understanding SIADH.*)

Causes
- Oat cell carcinoma of the lung
- Neoplastic diseases
- Central nervous system disorders
- Pulmonary disorders
- Drugs
- Miscellaneous conditions, such as myxedema and psychosis

Incidence
- Common complication of surgery or critical illness
- Common cause of hospital-acquired hyponatremia

Common characteristics
- Increased water retention
- Fluid and electrolyte imbalance
- Hyponatremia

Complications
- Water intoxication
- Cerebral edema
- Severe hyponatremia
- Heart failure
- Seizures
- Coma
- Death

✱ ASSESSMENT

History
- Possible clue to the cause
- Cerebrovascular disease
- Cancer
- Pulmonary disease
- Recent head injury
- Anorexia, nausea, vomiting
- Weight gain
- Lethargy, headaches, emotional and behavioral changes

Physical findings
- Tachycardia associated with increased fluid volume
- Disorientation
- Seizures and coma
- Sluggish deep tendon reflexes
- Muscle weakness

Test results
LABORATORY
- Serum osmolality levels less than 280 mOsm/kg of water confirm SIADH.
- Serum sodium levels less than 123 mEq/L confirm SIADH.
- Urine sodium levels more than 20 mEq/L (without diuretics) support the diagnosis.
- Renal function tests are normal.

◆ TREATMENT

General
- Based primarily on symptoms
- Correction of the underlying cause

Diet
- Restricted water intake (500 to 1,000 ml/day)

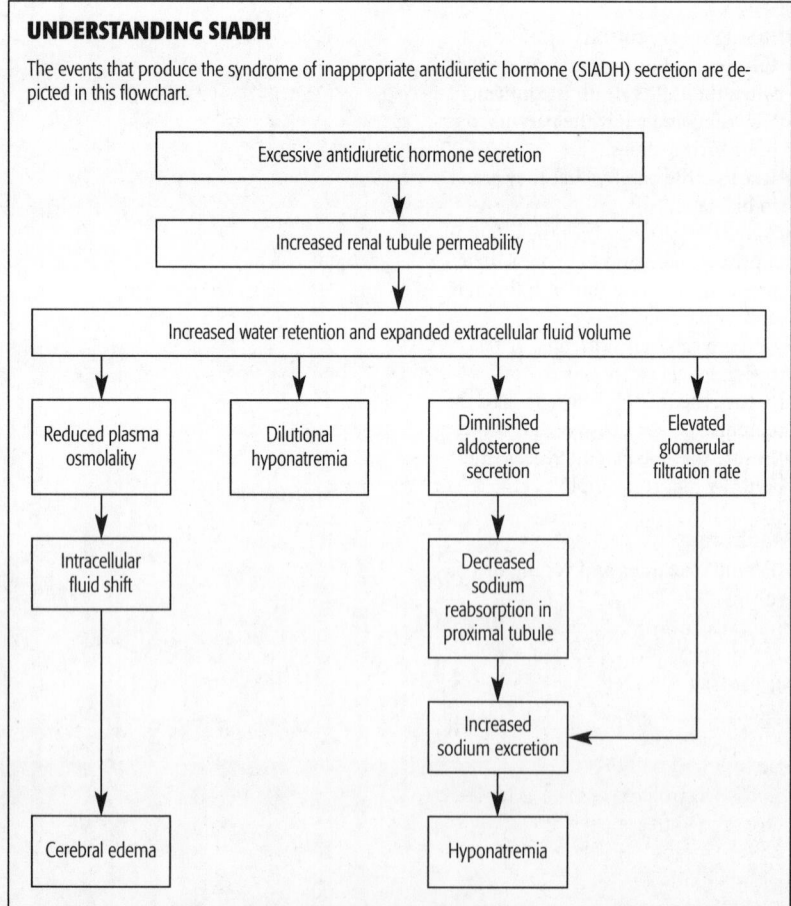

UNDERSTANDING SIADH

The events that produce the syndrome of inappropriate antidiuretic hormone (SIADH) secretion are depicted in this flowchart.

- High-salt, high-protein diet or urea supplements to enhance water excretion

Activity
- As tolerated

Medication
- Demeclocycline or lithium for chronic treatment
- Loop diuretics, if fluid overload, history of heart failure, or resistance to treatment
- 3% sodium chloride solution, if serum sodium less than 120 or if the patient is seizing

Surgery
- To treat underlying cause such as cancer

❖ NURSING CONSIDERATIONS

Nursing diagnoses
- Anxiety
- Fear
- Excess fluid volume
- Risk for injury

Key outcomes
The patient will:
- identify strategies to reduce anxiety
- discuss fears and concerns
- maintain adequate fluid balance
- remain free from injury.

Nursing interventions
- Restrict fluids.
- Provide comfort measures for thirst.
- Reduce unnecessary environmental stimuli.
- Orient the patient, as needed.
- Provide a safe environment.
- Institute seizure precaution, as needed.
- Administer medications, as ordered.

Monitoring
- Intake and output
- Vital signs
- Daily weight
- Serum electrolytes, especially sodium
- Response to treatment
- Breath sounds
- Heart sounds
- Neurologic checks

- Changes in level of consciousness

NURSING ALERT Watch closely for signs and symptoms of heart failure, which may occur because of fluid overload.

▶ PATIENT TEACHING

Be sure to cover:
- disorder, diagnostic tests, and treatment
- fluid restriction
- methods to decrease discomfort from thirst
- medication administration, dosage, and possible adverse effects
- self-monitoring techniques for fluid retention such as daily weight
- signs and symptoms that require immediate medical intervention.

✱ RESOURCES

Organizations
American Cancer Society: *www.cancer.org*
Endocrine and Metabolic Diseases Information Service: *www.endocrine.niddk.nih.gov*
Endocrine Society: *www.edo-society.org*

Selected references
Diseases, 4th ed. Philadelphia: Lippincott Williams & Wilkins, 2006.
Feidman, B.J., et al. "Nephrogenic Syndrome of Inappropriate Antidiuresis," *New England Journal of Medicine* 352(18):1884-890, May 2005.
Huang, E.A., et al. "Oral Urea for the Treatment of Chronic Syndrome of Inappropriate Antidiuresis in Children," *Journal of Pediatrics* 148(1):128-31, January 2006.
Nakazato, Y., et al. "Unpleasant Sweet Taste: A Symptom of SIADH Caused by Lung Cancer," *Journal of Neurology, Neurosurgery & Psychiatry* 77(3):405-406, March 2006.
Nettina, S.M. *Lippincott Manual of Nursing Practice,* 8th ed. Philadelphia: Lippincott Williams & Wilkins, 2006.

Syntax

Syphilis

OVERVIEW

Description
- Chronic, infectious, sexually transmitted disease
- Untreated, progresses in four stages: primary, secondary, latent, and late (formerly called tertiary)

Pathophysiology
- The infecting organism penetrates intact mucous membranes or abrasions in the skin, entering lymphatics and blood.
- Systemic infection and systemic foci precede primary lesion development at the site of inoculation.
- Organ involvement occurs from dissemination.

Causes
- Spirochete, *Treponema pallidum*
- Transmission primarily through sexual contact during the primary, secondary, and early latent stages of infection
- Prenatal transmission possible
- Transmission by way of fresh blood transfusion (rare)

Incidence
- In the United States, incidence highest in urban populations, especially between ages 15 and 39, drug users, and those infected with human immunodeficiency virus (HIV)
- About 34,000 cases, in primary and secondary stages, reported in the United States annually

Common characteristics
- Appearance of chancre or lesions
- History of unprotected sex

Complications
- Cardiovascular disease
- Irreversible neurologic disease
- Irreversible organ damage
- Membranous glomerulonephritis
- Death
- With fetal infection:
  - Spontaneous abortion
  - Stillbirth
  - Low birth weight
  - Deafness

ASSESSMENT

History
- Unprotected sexual contact with an infected person or with multiple or anonymous sexual partners

Physical findings
PRIMARY SYPHILIS
- One or more chancres (small, fluid-filled lesions) on the genitalia; others on the anus, fingers, lips, tongue, nipples, tonsils, or eyelids
- In female patient, possible chancres on cervix or vaginal wall
- Unilateral or bilateral adenopathy

SECONDARY SYPHILIS
- Headache, malaise
- Nausea, vomiting
- Anorexia, weight loss
- Sore throat, slight fever
- Symmetrical mucocutaneous lesions
- Rash possibly macular, papular, pustular, or nodular
- Lesions uniform, well defined, and generalized
- Macules typically erupting between rolls of fat on the trunk and proximally on the arms, palms, soles, face, and scalp
- In warm, moist body areas, lesions enlarged and eroding, producing highly contagious, pink or grayish-white lesions (condylomata lata)
- Alopecia
- Brittle and pitted nails
- Generalized lymphadenopathy

LATENT SYPHILIS
- Physical signs and symptoms absent except for possible recurrence of mucocutaneous lesions that resemble those of secondary syphilis

LATE SYPHILIS
- Findings dependent on the involved organ
- With three subtypes (neurosyphilis, late benign, and cardiovascular):
  - Neurosyphilis affecting meningovascular tissues: headache, vertigo, insomnia, hemiplegia, seizures, and psychological difficulties; if parenchymal tissue affected: paresis, alteration in intellect, paranoia, illusions, and hallucinations; in addition, Argyll Robertson pupil (a small, irregular pupil that's nonreactive to light but accommodates for vision),

ataxia, slurred speech, trophic joint changes, positive Romberg's sign, and a facial tremor
  - Late benign: gummas (lesions that develop between 1 and 10 years after infection and may be a chronic, superficial nodule or a deep, granulomatous lesion that's solitary, asymmetrical, painless, indurated, and large or small), visible on the skin and mucocutaneous tissues and commonly affect bones and can develop in any organ
  - Cardiovascular: decreased cardiac output that may cause decreased urine output and decreased sensorium related to hypoxia and pulmonary congestion

Test results
LABORATORY
- Dark-field microscopy identifies *T. pallidum* from lesion exudate and provides an immediate syphilis diagnosis. (See *Identifying syphilis by dark-field microscopy.*)
- Non-treponemal serologic tests, which include the Venereal Disease Research Laboratory (VDRL) slide test, the rapid plasma reagin (RPR) test, and the automated reagin test, detect nonspecific antibodies.
- Treponemal serologic studies, which include the fluorescent treponemal antibody absorption test, the *T. pallidum* hemagglutination assay, and the microhemagglutination assay, detect the specific antitreponemal antibody and confirm positive screening results.
- Cerebrospinal fluid examination identifies neurosyphilis when the total protein level is above 40 mg/dl, the VDRL slide test is reactive, and the white blood cell count exceeds five mononuclear cells/mm^3.

◆ TREATMENT

General
- Immediate examination of all sexual contacts
- Avoidance of pregnancy until a good response to therapy is demonstrated
- Hospitalization for symptomatic late syphilis

Diet
- No restrictions

Activity
- No sexual activity until cured

Medication
- Antibiotics (Penicillin)

♣ NURSING CONSIDERATIONS

Nursing diagnoses
- Acute pain
- Disturbed body image
- Impaired physical mobility
- Impaired skin integrity
- Ineffective sexuality patterns
- Risk for infection
- Risk for injury
- Sexual dysfunction

Key outcomes
The patient will:
- express feelings of increased comfort and decreased pain
- express concern about self-concept, esteem, and body image
- maintain joint mobility and muscle strength
- exhibit improved or healed lesions or wounds
- voice feelings about potential or actual changes in sexual activity
- remain free from further signs or symptoms of infection
- remain free from injury
- verbalize methods to protect against future STD infection.

Nursing interventions
- Follow standard precautions.
- Administer medications, as ordered.
- Promote rest and adequate nutrition.

- In secondary syphilis, keep lesions clean and dry; dispose of contaminated materials properly.
- Report all syphilis cases to the appropriate health authorities.

Monitoring
- Neurologic status
- Cardiovascular status
- Complications
- Response to treatment
- Compliance with treatment

▶ PATIENT TEACHING

Be sure to cover:
- disorder, diagnostic tests, and treatment
- importance of completing the prescribed course of therapy even after symptoms subside
- importance of informing, testing, and treating of sexual partners
- need to refrain from sexual activity until treatment is completed and follow-up VDRL/RPR test results are normal
- information for patient and sexual partners about HIV infection
- risks to the fetus if the patient is contemplating pregnancy.

Discharge planning
- As needed, obtain a physical or occupational therapy consultation.
- Refer the patient for contact tracing.
- Refer the patient to a specialist, if congenital syphilis is suspected.
- Consult a social worker to determine home care needs.

✳ RESOURCES

Organizations
Centers for Disease Control and Prevention: www.cdc.gov
Harvard University Consumer Health Information: www.intelihealth.com
Mayo Clinic: www.mayoclinic.com
National Health Information Center: www.health.gov/nhic

Selected references
Ferguson, L.A., and Varnado, J.W. "Syphilis: An Old Enemy Still Lurks," *Journal of the American Academy of Nurse Practitioners* 18(2):49-55, Febraury 2006.

Ghanem, K.G., et al. "Doxycycline Compared with Benzathine Penicillin for the Treatment of Early Syphilis," *Clinical Infectious Diseases* 42(6):e45-49, March 2006.

Heymann, W.R. "The History of Syphilis," *Journal of the American Academy of Dermatology* 54(2):322-23, February 2006.

Hyman, E.L. "Syphilis," *Pediatrics in Review* 27(1):37-39, January 2006.

Kasper, D. L., et al., eds. *Harrison's Principles of Internal Medicine,* 16th ed. New York: McGraw-Hill Book Co., 2005.

Taylor, M.L., et al. "Prostate Cancer and Sexually Transmitted Diseases: A Meta-Analysis," *Family Medicine* 37(7):506-12, July-August 2005.

IDENTIFYING SYPHILIS BY DARK-FIELD MICROSCOPY

The presence of spiral-shaped bacteria (*Treponema pallidum*) on dark-field examination confirms the diagnosis of syphilis.

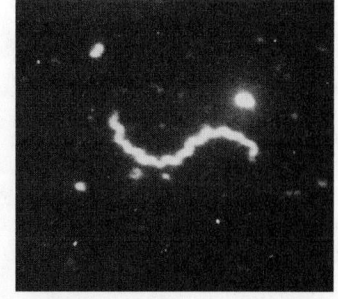

Systemic inflammatory response syndrome

● OVERVIEW

Description
- Characterized by excessive production of inflammatory mediators
- Known as sepsis, when caused by an infection
- Also known as *SIRS*

Pathophysiology
- The body receives an insult from a chemical, traumatic, or infectious stimulus.
- Cytokine is produced to promote an inflammatory response, which is then released into the circulation.
- Growth factor is stimulated along with recruitment of macrophages and platelets.
- Without homeostasis, cytokine release leads to the activation of numerous humoral responses and activation of the reticuloendothelial system.
- Circulatory integrity is lost leading to end organ dysfunction.

Causes
- Ischemia
- Inflammation
- Trauma
- Infection
- Combination of causes

Risk factors
- Severe illness or presence of comorbid conditions
- Age extremes
- Immunodeficiency

Incidence
- Highly variable
- Affects men and women equally

Common characteristics
- Fever
- Tachycardia
- Tachypnea

Complications
- Acute respiratory distress syndrome
- Renal failure
- Respiratory failure
- Mulitple organ dysfunction syndrome
- Disseminated intravascular coagulation (DIC)

✳ ASSESSMENT

History
- Presence of risk factor
- Pain

Physical findings
Two or more of the following:
- Temperature greater than 38° C or less than 36° C
- Heart rate greater than 90 beats/minute
- Respiratory rate greater than 24 breaths/minute
- $PaCO_2$ level less than 32 mm Hg

Test results
LABORATORY
- White blood cell count is greater than 12,000/uL or less than 4000/uL or greater than 10% bands.
- Complete blood count may show thrombocytopenia.
- Coagulation studies may reveal prolonged thrombin time, decreased fibrinogen, and possible D-dimer suggesting DIC.
- Blood cultures may identify infectious organism.

◆ TREATMENT

General
- Treatment of underlying cause
- Supportive therapy

Diet
- As tolerated
- Enteral feedings (possibly)

Activity
- Bed rest with activity as tolerated based on condition

Medication
- Oxygen therapy
- Antibiotics (if infectious cause)
- I.V. fluids
- Vasopressors
- Insulin (if hyperglycemic)

Surgery
- Incision and drainage of abscess or infectious cause

❖ NURSING CONSIDERATIONS

Nursing diagnoses
- Anxiety
- Activity intolerance
- Impaired gas exchange
- Ineffective tissue perfusion: Cardiopulmonary, renal
- Risk for imbalanced body temperature
- Risk for imbalanced fluid volume
- Risk for infection
- Risk for injury

Key outcomes
The patient will:
- verbalize strategies to reduce anxiety
- demonstrate measures to conserve energy while carrying out daily activities
- maintain adequate ventilation and oxygenation
- demonstrate adequate tissue perfusion
- achieve a body temperature within acceptable parameters
- maintain adequate fluid balance
- remain free from signs and symptoms of infection
- remain free from injury and complications

Nursing interventions
- Admininster medications, as ordered.
- Provide supplemental oxygen.
- Give tepid sponge baths and antipyretics for fever.
- Notify physician of vital signs outside accepted parameters.
- Provide wound care, as indicated, after drainage of infectious source.
- Provide emotional support to patient and family.

Monitoring
- Vital signs
- ABG and pulse oximetry
- Fluid status, intake and output
- Laboratory tests, including cultures
- Cardiac and respiratory status
- Signs and symptoms of infection

▶ PATIENT TEACHING

Be sure to cover:
- disorder, diagnostic tests, and treatment
- medication administration, dosage, and possible adverse effects
- wound care, if indicated
- possible complications.

Discharge planning
- Refer the patient for follow up with community support services, as necessary.

✹ RESOURCES

Organizations
National Center for Infectious Diseases: *www.cdc.gov/ncidod*
National Heart, Lung, and Blood Institute: *www.nhlbi.nih.gov*

Selected references
Burdette, S.D., et al. "Systemic Inflammatory Response Syndrome," Updated October 2006. Available at: *http://www.emedicine.com/med/topic2227.htm.* Accessed 12/21/06.

Hoover, L., et al. "Systemic Inflammatory Response Syndrome and Nosocomial Infection in Trauma," *Journal of Trauma* 61(2): 310-16, 2006.

Kasper, D.L., et al., eds. *Harrison's Manual of Medicine,* 16th ed. New York: McGraw-Hill Book Co., 2005.

Kliger, E., et al. "Stress Doses of Hydrocortisone Reduce Severe Systemic Inflammatory Response Syndrome and Improve Early Outcome in a Risk Group of Patients after Cardiac Surgery," *Critical Care Medicine* 31(4):1068-1073, 2003.

Nettina, S.M. *Lippincott Manual of Nursing Practice,* 8th ed. Philadelphia: Lippincott Williams & Wilkins, 2006.

Systemic lupus erythematosus

● OVERVIEW

Description
- Chronic inflammatory autoimmune disorder that affects connective tissues
- Two forms: discoid lupus erythematosus, which affects the skin only; and systemic lupus erythematosus (SLE)

Pathophysiology
- The body produces antibodies, such as antinuclear antibodies (ANAs), against its own cells such as red blood cells (RBCs), neutrophils, platelets, lymphocytes, and almost any organ or tissue in the body.
- The formed antigen-antibody complexes suppress the body's normal immunity and damage tissues.

Causes
- Exact cause unknown

Risk factors
- Stress
- Streptococcal or viral infections
- Exposure to sunlight or ultraviolet light
- Injury
- Surgery
- Exhaustion
- Emotional upsets
- Immunization
- Pregnancy
- Abnormal estrogen metabolism

Incidence
- Affects women eight times more often than men (15 times more often during childbearing years)
- Occurs worldwide; most prevalent among Asians and Blacks

Common characteristics
- Recurrent seasonal remissions and exacerbations, especially during spring and summer

Complications
- Pleurisy
- Pleural effusions
- Pericarditis, myocarditis, endocarditis
- Coronary atherosclerosis
- Renal failure
- Seizures and mental dysfunction

✳ ASSESSMENT

History
- Onset acute or insidious; no characteristic clinical pattern
- Possible fever, anorexia, weight loss, malaise, fatigue, abdominal pain, nausea, vomiting, rash, and polyarthralgia
- Possible drug history with one of 25 drugs that can cause SLE-like reaction
- Irregular menstruation or amenorrhea, particularly during flare-ups
- Chest pain and dyspnea
- Emotional instability, psychosis, organic brain syndrome, headaches, irritability, and depression
- Oliguria, urinary frequency, dysuria, and bladder spasms

Physical findings
- Joint involvement that resembles rheumatoid arthritis
- Raynaud's phenomenon
- Skin eruptions provoked or aggravated by sunlight or ultraviolet light
- Tachycardia, central cyanosis, and hypotension
- Altered level of consciousness, weakness of the extremities, and speech disturbances
- Skin lesions
- Butterfly rash over nose and cheeks
- Patchy alopecia (common)
- Vasculitis
- Lymph node enlargement
- Pericardial friction rub

Test results
LABORATORY
- Complete blood count with differential shows anemia and a reduced white blood cell (WBC) count; decreased platelet count; elevated erythrocyte sedimentation rate; and serum electrophoresis showing hypergammaglobulinemia.
- ANA, anti-DNA, and lupus erythematosus cell test findings are positive in most patients with active SLE but only slightly useful in diagnosing the disease (the ANA test is sensitive but not specific for SLE).
- Urine studies show RBCs, WBCs, urine casts and sediment, and significant protein loss (more than 3.5 g in 24 hours).
- Blood studies demonstrate decreased serum complement (C3 and C4) levels, indicating active disease (leukopenia, mild thrombocytopenia, and anemia also are seen during active disease).
- C-reactive protein is increased during flare-ups.
- Rheumatoid factor is positive in 30% to 40% of patients.

IMAGING
- Chest X-rays may disclose pleurisy or lupus pneumonitis.

DIAGNOSTIC PROCEDURES
- Central nervous system (CNS) involvement may account for abnormal EEG results in about 70% of patients. However, brain and magnetic resonance imaging scans may be normal in patients with SLE despite CNS disease. (See *Diagnostic signs of SLE.*)
- Electrocardiography may show a conduction defect with cardiac involvement or pericarditis.
- Renal biopsy shows progression of SLE and the extent of renal involvement.
- Skin biopsy shows immunoglobulin and complement deposition in the dermal-epidermal junction.

◆ TREATMENT

General
- Use of sunscreen with sun protection factor of at least 15

Diet
- No restrictions unless renal failure

Activity
- Regular exercise program

Medication
- Nonsteroidal anti-inflammatory drugs
- Fluorinated steroids
- Antimalarials
- Corticosteroids (including topical)
- Cytotoxic drugs
- Antihypertensives

Surgery
- Possible joint replacement

❖ NURSING CONSIDERATIONS

Nursing diagnoses
- Acute pain
- Constipation
- Decreased cardiac output
- Diarrhea
- Disturbed body image
- Fatigue
- Imbalanced nutrition: Less than body requirements
- Impaired oral mucous membrane
- Impaired physical mobility
- Impaired tisue and skin integrity
- Impaired urinary elimination
- Ineffective breathing pattern
- Risk for infection
- Risk for peripheral neurovascular dysfunction

Key outcomes
The patient will:
- express feelings of increased comfort and decreased pain
- pass soft, regular stools without straining
- maintain adequate cardiac output
- resume a normal bowel elimnation pattern
- verbalize feelings about a changed body image
- express feelings of increased energy
- maintain daily calorie requirements
- maintain intact oral mucous membranes
- maintain joint mobility and range of motion (ROM)
- maintain skin integrity
- have reduced pain, redness, and swelling of the site of impaired tissue
- maintain fluid balance: intake will equal output
- maintain a respiratory rate within 5 breaths/minute of baseline
- remain free from signs and symptoms of infection
- report alterations in sensation or pain in the extremities.

Nursing interventions
- Provide a balanced diet, with bland, cool foods if the patient has a sore mouth.
- Provide a normal saline mouth rinse after meals to help heal oral lesions.
- Apply heat packs to relieve joint pain and stiffness.
- Encourage regular exercise to maintain full ROM.
- Institute seizure precautions if you suspect CNS involvement.
- Warm and protect the patient's hands and feet if she has Raynaud's phenomenon.
- Support the patient's self-image.

Monitoring
- Signs and symptoms of organ involvement
- Urine, stools, and GI secretions for blood
- Scalp for hair loss and skin and mucous membranes for petechiae, bleeding, ulceration, pallor, and bruising
- Response to treatment
- Complications
- Nutritional status
- Joint mobility
- Seizure activity

▶ PATIENT TEACHING

Be sure to cover:
- disorder, diagnostic tests, and treatment
- ROM exercises and body alignment and postural techniques
- ways to avoid infection (avoiding crowds and people with infections)
- need to notify the physician if fever, cough, or rash occurs or if chest, abdominal, muscle, or joint pain worsens
- importance of balanced diet and restrictions of medications
- medication administration, dosage, and possible adverse effects
- importance of good skin care
- benefits of exercise, such as aerobics, swimming, walking, bicycling, and ROM exercises
- importance of keeping regular follow-up appointments and contacting the physician if flare-ups occur
- need to wear protective clothing and use a sunscreen
- how to perform mouth care.

Discharge planning
- Arrange for a physical therapy and occupational therapy consultation if musculoskeletal involvement compromises mobility.
- Refer to a rheumatology specialist if the patient becomes pregnant.

✺ RESOURCES

Organizations
Arthritis Foundation: *www.arthritis.org*
Lupus Foundation of America: *www.lupus.org*

Selected references
Burt, R.K., et al. "Nonmyeloablative Hematopoietic Stem Cell Transplantation for Systemic Lupus Erythematosus," *JAMA* 295(5):527-35, February 2006.

Kasper, D. L., et al., eds. *Harrison's Principles of Internal Medicine,* 16th ed. New York: McGraw-Hill Book Co., 2005.

Kyttaris, V.C., et al. "Gene Therapy in Systemic Lupus Erythematosus," *Current Gene Therapy* 5(6):677-84, December 2005.

The Merck Manual of Diagnosis & Therapy, 18th ed. Whitehouse Station, N.J.: Merck and Co., Inc., 2006.

Petri, M. "Systemic Lupus Erythematosus: 2006 Update," *Journal of Clinical Rheumatology* 12(1):37-40, February 2006.

DIAGNOSTIC SIGNS OF SLE

Diagnosing systemic lupus erythematosus (SLE) isn't easy because the disease so often mimics other disorders. Signs may be vague and vary from patient to patient. The American College of Rheumatology has devised the following criteria for identifying SLE (usually four or more of the following signs must appear at some time in the disease course):
- discoid rash
- facial erythema (butterfly rash)
- hematologic abnormality (hemolytic anemia, leukopenia, lymphopenia, or thrombocytopenia)
- immune dysfunction (identified by positive lupus erythematosus cell, anti-DNA, or anti-Sm tests; or false-positive test results for syphilis for more than 6 months)
- neurologic disorder
- nonerosive arthritis
- oral ulcers
- photosensitivity
- positive antinuclear antibody test results
- renal disorder
- serositis

Tay-Sachs disease

● OVERVIEW

Description
- Most common lipid storage disease
- Results from a congenital enzyme deficiency
- Leads to progressive mental and motor deterioration
- Always fatal, usually before age 5
- No known cure

Pathophysiology
- In this autosomal recessive disorder, the enzyme hexosaminidase A is absent or deficient.
- Without hexosaminidase A, lipid pigments accumulate and progressively destroy and demyelinate central nervous system cells.
- The juvenile form generally appears between ages 2 and 5 as a progressive deterioration of psychomotor skills and gait.

Causes
- Autosomal recessive disorder

Incidence
- Affects fewer than 100 infants born yearly in the United States
- About 100 times more common (about 1 in 3,600 live births) in those with Ashkenazic Jewish ancestry than in the general population
- About 1 in 30 Ashkenazi Jews, French Canadians, and American Cajuns heterozygous carriers of gene for this disorder

Common characteristics
- Progressive mental and motor deterioration

Complications
- Recurrent bronchopneumonia
- Dementia
- Blindness
- Seizures
- Paralysis
- Death

✳ ASSESSMENT

History
- Family history of Tay-Sachs disease
- Normal appearance at birth (but with possible exaggerated Moro's reflex)
- Onset of clinical signs and symptoms between ages 5 and 6 months
- Progressive deterioration
- Psychomotor retardation
- Blindness
- Dementia

Physical findings
- In 3- to 6-month-old infant:
  - Apathetic appearance
  - Displays augmented response to loud sounds
  - Progressive weakness of the neck, trunk, arm, and leg muscles that prevents child from sitting up or lifting head
  - Difficulty turning over
  - Can't grasp objects
  - Progressive vision loss
- By 18 months:
  - Possible seizures
  - Generalized paralysis
  - Spasticity
  - Blindness
  - May hold eyes wide open and roll eyeballs
  - Pupils always dilated
  - Decerebrate rigidity
  - Complete vegetative state follows
  - Head circumference possibly showing enlargement
  - Pupils nonreactive to light
  - Ophthalmoscopic examination possibly showing optic nerve atrophy and a distinctive cherry-red spot on the retina
- In a child who survives bouts of recurrent bronchopneumonia, possible ataxia and progressive motor retardation between ages 2 and 8

Test results
LABORATORY
- Serum analysis shows deficient hexosaminidase A.
- Amniocentesis or chorionic villus sampling allows prenatal diagnosis of hexosaminidase A deficiency.

◆ TREATMENT

General
- Supportive care
- Suctioning
- Postural drainage to remove secretions
- Meticulous skin care
- Long-term care in special facility

Diet
- Tube feedings with nutritional supplements

Activity
- As tolerated
- Active and passive range-of-motion exercises

Medication
- Mild laxatives
- Anticonvulsants

Nursing diagnoses
- Anticipatory grieving
- Deficient knowledge (Tay-Sachs disease)
- Disabled family coping
- Impaired physical mobility
- Ineffective airway clearance
- Risk for impaired skin integrity
- Risk for injury

Key outcomes
The patient (or family) will:
- express feelings of guilt and loss
- express understanding of the disease process and treatment regimen
- seek outside sources to assist with coping and adjustment to the patient's situation
- maintain muscle strength and joint mobility
- maintain a patent airway
- maintain skin integrity
- remain free from injury.

Nursing interventions
- Help family members deal with progressive illness and death.
- Stress the importance of amniocentesis in future pregnancies.
- Prevent skin breakdown.
- Provide adequate nutrition.
- Maintain a patent airway.
- Implement seizure precautions.
- Administer medications, as ordered.

Monitoring
- Vital signs
- Intake and output
- Respiratory status
- Nutritional status
- Neurologic status
- Response to treatment

Be sure to cover:
- disorder, diagnostic tests, and treatment
- suctioning
- postural drainage
- tube feedings
- skin care.

Discharge planning
- Refer the parents for genetic counseling.
- Refer the parents to the National Tay-Sachs and Allied Diseases Association.
- Refer the parents for psychological counseling, if indicated.
- Refer the siblings for screening to determine whether they're carriers.
- If the siblings are adult carriers, refer them for genetic counseling; stress that the disease isn't transmitted to offspring unless both parents are carriers.

Organizations
National Institute of Neurological Disorders and Stroke: *www.ninds.nih.gov*
National Organization for Rare Disorders: *www.rarediseases.org*
National Tay-Sachs and Allied Diseases Association: *www.ntsad.org*

Selected references
Bembi, B., et al. "Substrate Reduction Therapy in the Infantile Form of Tay-Sachs Disease," *Neurology* 66(2):278-80 January 2006.

Gason, A.A., et al. "Tay Sachs Disease Carrier Screening in Schools: Educational Alternatives and Cheekbrush Sampling," *Genetics in Medicine* 7(9):626-32, November-December 2005.

Leib, J.R., et al. "Carrier Screening Panels for Ashkenazi Jews: Is More Better?" *Genetics in Medicine* 7(3):185-90, March 2005.

Neudorfer, O., et al. "Late-Onset Tay Sachs Disease: Phenotype Characterization and Genotypic Correlations in 21 Affected Patients," *Genetics in Medicine* 7(2):119-23, February 2005.

Rucker, J.C., et al. "Neuro-ophthalmology of Late-Onset Tay-Sachs Disease (LOTS)," *Neurology* 63(10):1918-926, November 2004.

Tendinitis and bursitis

● OVERVIEW

Description

TENDINITIS
- Inflammation affecting the tendons and tendon-muscle attachments
- Most common sites:
  - Shoulder rotator cuff
  - Hip
  - Achilles tendon
  - Hamstring
  - Elbow

BURSITIS
- Painful inflammation of one or more bursae
- Most common sites:
  - Subdeltoid
  - Subacromial
  - Olecranon
  - Trochanteric
  - Calcaneal
  - Prepatellar
- May be septic, calcific, acute, or chronic

Pathophysiology

TENDINITIS
- Inflammation causes localized pain around the affected area.
- Joint movement is restricted.
- Swelling results from fluid accumulation.
- Calcium deposits form in and around the tendon.
- Further swelling and immobility result.

BURSITIS
- Bursae sacs hold lubricating synovial fluid.
- Inflammation of the sac causes gradual pain and limits joint motion.

Causes

TENDINITIS
- Trauma (such as a strain during sports activity)
- Musculoskeletal disorders (rheumatic diseases and congenital defects)
- Postural malalignment
- Abnormal body development
- Hypermobility in calcific tendonitis

BURSITIS
- Recurring trauma from an inflammatory joint disease
- Common stressors:
  - Repetitive kneeling

- Jogging in worn-out shoes on hard asphalt surfaces
- Prolonged sitting with crossed legs on hard surfaces
- Septic bursitis: wound infection or from bacterial invasion (see *Anatomy of tendons and bursae*)

Incidence
- More common in elderly people
- Common in those who perform activities that overstress a tendon or repeatedly stress a joint

Common characteristics
- Localized pain
- Interrupted sleep
- Limited movement
- Crepitus over involved area
- Swelling over involved area

Complications
- Scar tissue with subsequent disability

✳ ASSESSMENT

History

TENDINITIS
- Traumatic injury or strain associated with athletic activity
- Concurrent musculoskeletal disorder
- Palpable tenderness over the affected site
- Referred tenderness in the related segment
- Shoulder:
  - Localized pain that's most severe at night and usually interferes with sleep
  - Heat that aggravates shoulder pain
- Elbow: pain when grasping objects or twisting the elbow
- Hamstring: pain in the posterolateral aspect of the knee
- Foot: pain over the Achilles tendon and on dorsiflexion

BURSITIS
- Unusual strain or injury 2 to 3 days before pain began
- Pain that develops suddenly or gradually
- Pain that may limit movement
- Work or leisure activity that may involve repetitive action

Physical findings

TENDINITIS
- Shoulder: restricted shoulder movement (especially abduction)
- Elbow: tenderness over the lateral epicondyle
- Hamstring: palpable tenderness when knee flexed at a 90-degree angle
- Foot: crepitus when patient moves his foot

BURSITIS
- Tenderness over the site
- Swelling with severe bursitis

Test results

LABORATORY
- Various serum and urine test results rule out other disorders.

IMAGING
- X-rays in tendinitis may show bony fragments, osteophyte sclerosis, or calcium deposits.
- X-rays in calcific bursitis may show calcium deposits in the joint.
- Arthrography is usually normal in tendinitis with only minor irregularities on the tendon under the surface.

DIAGNOSTIC PROCEDURES
- Arthrocentesis may identify causative microorganisms and other causes of inflammation.

◆ TREATMENT

General
- Cold, heat, or ultrasound applications

Diet
- No restrictions

Activity
- Resting the joint
- Range-of-motion (ROM) exercises, as tolerated

Medication
- Nonsteroidal anti-inflammatory drugs (NSAIDs)
- Local anesthetics
- Corticosteroids
- Oral anti-inflammatory agents
- Short-term analgesics

❖ NURSING CONSIDERATIONS

Nursing diagnoses
- Acute and chronic pain
- Anxiety
- Impaired physical mobility
- Bathing or hygiene or dressing or grooming self-care deficit

Key outcomes
The patient will:
- express feelings of increased comfort and decreased pain
- develop adequate coping mechanisms and exhibit a decrease in anxiety
- maintain joint mobility and ROM
- perform activities of daily living.

Nursing interventions
- Promote self-care while allowing adequate time.
- Administer medications, as ordered.
- Apply cold or heat therapies, as ordered.
- Encourage use of active ROM exercises.

Monitoring
- Severity and pattern of pain
- Response to treatment
- ROM

▶ PATIENT TEACHING

Be sure to cover:
- disorder, diagnostic tests, and treatment
- minimization of GI distress from NSAID use
- medication administration, dosage, and possible adverse effects
- activities that promote rest and relaxation
- strengthening exercises
- the prescribed exercise regimen
- sports equipment, cushioned shoes, and playing surfaces
- cold packs
- proper body mechanics.

Discharge planning
- Refer the patient to a weight management program, as appropriate.

✹ RESOURCES

Organizations
American College of Rheumatology: www.rheumatology. org

American Orthopaedic Association: www.aoassn.org

Arthritis Foundation: www.arthritis.org

Selected references

Chen, M.J., et al. "Ultrasound-guided Shoulder Injections in the Treatment of Subcaromial Bursitis," *American Journal of Physical Medicine & Rehabilitation* 85(1):31-35, January 2005.

Diseases, 2nd ed. Philadelphia: Lippincott Williams & Wilkins, 2006.

Handbook of Pathophysiology, 2nd ed. Philadelphia: Lippincott Williams & Wilkins, 2005.

Llinas, L., et al. "Osteomyelitis Resulting from Chronic Filamentous Fungus Olecranon Bursitis," *Journal of Clinical Rheumatology* 11(5):280-82, October 2005.

Meislin, R.J., et al. "Persistent Shoulder Pain: Epidemiology, Pathophysiology, and Diagnosis," *American Journal of Orthopedics* 34(12 Suppl):5-9, December 2005.

Small, L.N., and Ross, J.J. "Suppurative Tenosynovitis and Septic Bursitis," *Infectious Disease Clinics of North America* 19(4):991-1005, xi, December 2005.

ANATOMY OF TENDONS AND BURSAE

Tendons, like stiff rubber bands, hold the muscles in place and enable them to move the bones. Bursae are located at friction points around joints and between tendons, cartilage, or bone. Bursae keep these body parts lubricated so they move freely.

Shoulder joint

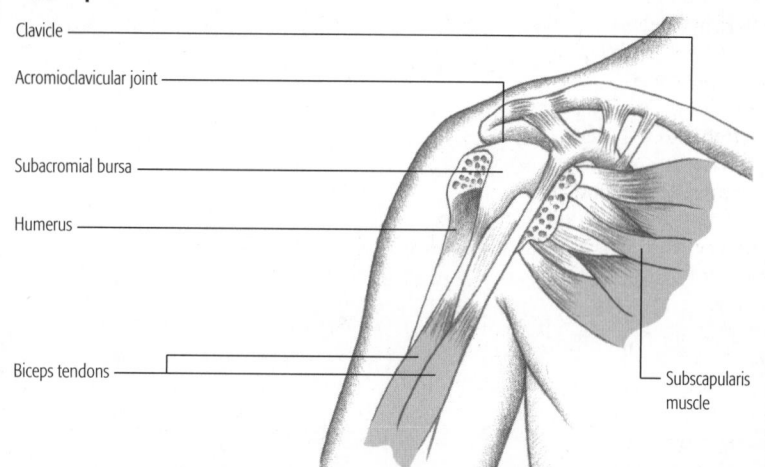

Clavicle

Acromioclavicular joint

Subacromial bursa

Humerus

Biceps tendons

Subscapularis muscle

Testicular cancer

Description
- Proliferation of cancer cells in the testicles
- Most originate from germinal cells and about 40% become seminomas
- Prognosis dependent on cancer cell type and stage (with treatment, a more than 5-year survival rate)

Pathophysiology
- Testicular cancer spreads through the lymphatic system to the iliac, para-aortic, and mediastinal nodes.
- Metastases affect the lungs, liver, viscera, and bone.

Causes
- Exact cause unknown

Risk factors
- Cryptorchidism (see *Cryptorchidism and testicular cancer*)
- Mumps orchitis
- Inguinal hernia in childhood
- Maternal use of diethylstilbestrol (DES) or other estrogen-progestin combinations during pregnancy

Common characteristics
- Fullness in testes
- Lump in testes

Incidence
- Most common in men ages 20 to 40
- Rare in nonwhite men
- Accounts for less than 1% of all male cancer deaths
- Rare in children

Complications
- Back or abdominal pain from retroperitoneal adenopathy
- Metastasis
- Ureteral obstruction

History
- Previous injuries to the scrotum
- Viral infection (such as mumps)
- Use of DES or other estrogen-progestin drugs by the patient's mother during pregnancy
- Feeling of heaviness or a dragging sensation in the scrotum
- Swollen testes or a painless lump
- Weight loss (late sign)
- Fatigue and weakness (late sign)

Physical findings
- Enlarged testes
- Gynecomastia
- Lethargic, thin, and pallid appearance (later stages)
- Palpable firm, smooth testicular mass
- Enlarged lymph nodes in surrounding areas

Test results
LABORATORY
- Elevated human chorionic gonadotropin (HCG) and alpha-fetoprotein (AFP) levels suggest testicular cancer and can differentiate a seminoma from a nonseminoma.
- Elevated HCG and AFP levels indicate a nonseminoma.
- Elevated HCG but normal AFP levels indicate a seminoma.
DIAGNOSTIC PROCEDURES
- Biopsy can confirm the diagnosis and stage the disease.

General
- Varies with tumor cell type and stage
- Radiation therapy
- Autologous bone marrow transplantation for patients nonresponsive to standard therapy

Diet
- Well-balanced; no restrictions

Activity
- No restrictions

Medication
- Chemotherapy
- Hormonal therapy

Surgery
- Orchiectomy and retroperitoneal node dissection

CRYPTORCHIDISM AND TESTICULAR CANCER

In men with cryptorchidism (the failure of a testicle to descend into the scrotum), testicular tumors are about 50 times more common than in men with normal anatomic structure. A simple surgical procedure, called orchiopexy, can bring the testicle to its normal position in the scrotum and reduce the testicular cancer risk. Nevertheless, testicular tumors occur more commonly in a surgically descended testicle than in a naturally descended one.

What happens in orchiopexy
In orchiopexy, the surgeon incises the groin area and separates the testicle and its blood supply from surrounding abdominal structures. Then, he creates a "tunnel" into the scrotum to accommodate the descent of the testicle.

Reducing the risk further
After orchiopexy, urge the patient to examine himself monthly to detect a tumor at its earliest stage.

❖ NURSING CONSIDERATIONS

Nursing diagnoses

- Acute pain
- Anxiety
- Disturbed body image
- Fear
- Impaired oral mucous membrane
- Ineffective coping
- Ineffective role performance
- Risk for infection
- Sexual dysfunction

Key outcomes

The patient will:

- express feelings of increased comfort and decreased pain
- express feelings of decreased anxiety
- express positive feelings about himself
- express concerns and fears related to his diagnosis and condition
- maintain intact oral mucous membranes
- demonstrate positive coping mechanisms
- continue to function in usual roles to the greatest degree possible
- remain free from signs and symptoms of infection
- express feelings and perceptions about change in sexual performance.

Nursing interventions

- Encourage verbalization and provide support.
- Administer medications, as ordered.
- Apply an ice pack to the scrotum.

Monitoring

- Wound site
- Vital signs
- Hydration and nutritional status
- Pain control
- Effects of medication
- Postoperative complications

▶ PATIENT TEACHING

Be sure to cover:

- disorder, diagnostic tests, and treatments
- reassurance that sterility and impotence usually don't follow unilateral orchiectomy
- (as suitable), sperm-banking procedures before the patient begins treatment, especially if infertility and impotence may result from surgery
- testicular self-examination.

Discharge planning

- Refer the patient to resource and support services.

✷ RESOURCES

Organizations

American Cancer Society: *www.cancer.org*
Guide to Internet Resources for Cancer: *www.cancerindex.org*
National Cancer Institute: *www.nci.org*
Testicular Cancer Information & Support: *www.tc-cancer.com*
The Testicular Cancer Resource Center: *www.tcrc.acor.org/*

Selected references

Atlas of Pathophysiology, 2nd ed. Philadelphia: Lippincott Williams & Wilkins, 2005.
Gleason, A.M. "Racial Disparities in Testicular Cancer: Impact on Health Promotion," *Journal of Transcultural Nursing* 17(1):58-64, January 2006.
Kleier, J.A. "Nurse Practitioners' Behavior Regarding Teaching Testicular Self-examination," *Journal of the American Academy of Nurse Practitioners* 16(5):206-208, 210, 212 passim, May 2004.
Richie, J.P. "Fertility Gonadal and Sexual Function in Survivors of Testicular Cancer," *Journal of Urology* 175(3 pt 1):961-62, March 2006.
Stevenson, T.D., and McNeill, J.A. "Surgical Management of Testicular Cancer," *Clinical Journal of Oncology Nursing* 8(4):355-60, August 2004.
van den Belt-Dusebout, A.W., et al. "Long-term Risk of Cardiovascular Disease in 5-year Survivors of Testicular Cancer," *Journal of Clinical Oncology* 24(3):467-75, January 2006.

Tetanus

● OVERVIEW

Description
- Acute exotoxin-mediated infection
- Usually systemic, but possibly localized
- Up to 60% fatal in unimmunized patients
- Also known as *lockjaw*

Pathophysiology
- After the organism enters the body, local infection and tissue necrosis result.
- Toxins enter the bloodstream and lymphatics, eventually spreading to central nervous system tissue.
- The incubation period is 3 to 21 days.

Causes
- Anaerobic, spore-forming, gram-positive bacillus *Clostridium tetani*
- Transmission through puncture wounds, burns, or minor wounds contaminated by soil, dust, or animal excreta containing *C. tetani*

Incidence
- Occurs worldwide, but more prevalent in agricultural regions and developing countries that lack mass immunization programs
- One of the most common causes of neonatal deaths in developing countries
- In the United States, approximately 110 cases each year, all in patients who aren't immunized or whose immunization has expired
- About 75% of cases occurring between April and September

Common characteristics
- Usually, a normal body temperature or a slight fever in the early stages; fever possibly rising as disease progresses
- Despite pronounced neuromuscular symptoms, assessment showing normal cerebral and sensory function

Complications
- Pneumonia
- Airway obstruction
- Respiratory arrest
- Heart failure
- Fractures
- Cardiac arrhythmias
- Rhabdomyolysis
- Death

✳ ASSESSMENT

History
- Possible inadequate immunization, and recent skin wound or burn
- Possible pain or paresthesia at the site of injury
- Possible early complaints of difficulty chewing or swallowing food

Physical findings
- Spasm and increased muscle tone near the wound (local infection)
- Irregular heartbeat, and tachycardia
- Marked muscle hypertonicity
- Hyperactive deep tendon reflexes
- Profuse sweating, low-grade fever
- Painful, involuntary muscle contractions
- Rigid neck and facial muscles, resulting in lockjaw (trismus) and a grotesque, grinning expression (risus sardonicus)
- Rigid somatic muscles, causing arched-back rigidity (opisthotonos)
- Intermittent tonic seizures

Test results
LABORATORY
- Blood cultures and tetanus antibody tests are negative.
- Wound culture is positive in one-third of patients.

DIAGNOSTIC PROCEDURES
- Lumbar puncture (spinal tap) may show elevated cerebrospinal fluid pressure.

◆ TREATMENT

General
- Airway maintenance

Diet
- Enteral or parenteral feeding

Activity
- Bed rest until recovery

Medication
- Tetanus immune globulin
- Tetanus antitoxin
- Tetanus toxoid immunization
- Muscle relaxants
- Neuromuscular blockers
- Antibiotics

❖ NURSING CONSIDERATIONS

Nursing diagnoses
- Acute pain
- Imbalanced nutrition: Less than body requirements
- Impaired physical mobility
- Ineffective airway clearance
- Ineffective breathing pattern
- Ineffective tissue perfusion: Cerebral, peripheral
- Risk for deficient fluid volume
- Risk for injury

Key outcomes
The patient will:
- express feelings of increased comfort and decreased pain
- maintain adequate nutrition and hydration
- resume normal physical mobility during therapy
- maintain a patent airway
- maintain adequate ventilation and oxygenation
- maintain tissue perfusion and cellular oxygenation
- maintain adequate fluid balance
- remain free from injury during severe spasming or seizure activity.

Nursing interventions
- Debride and clean the injury site.
- Check the immunization history.
- Maintain an adequate airway and ventilation.
- Keep emergency airway equipment on standby.
- Administer I.V. therapy, as prescribed.
- Minimize stimulation.
- Perform range-of-motion exercises.

Monitoring
- Response to treatment
- Fluid and electrolyte status
- Respiratory status
- Cardiovascular status
- Injury site
- Complications
- Deep tendon reflexes
- Muscle tone

▶ PATIENT TEACHING

Be sure to cover:
- disorder, diagnostic tests, and treatment
- importance of maintaining active immunization with a booster dose of tetanus toxoid every 10 years
- need to receive tetanus prophylaxis in case of a skin injury or burn
- need to avoid minimal external stimulation (evokes muscle spasms) and to keep the room dark and quiet
- potential outcomes.

✷ RESOURCES

Organizations
Centers for Disease Control and Prevention: *www.cdc.gov*
Harvard University Consumer Health Information: *www.intelihealth.com*
National Health Information Center: *www.health.gov/nhic*
National Library of Medicine: *www.nlm.nih.gov*
U.S. Food and Drug Administration: *www.fda.gov*

Selected references
Burton, T., and Crane, S. "Unnecessary Tetanus Boosters in the ED," *Emergency Medicine Journal* 22(8):609-10, August 2005.

Gonzalez-Forero, D., et al. "Transynaptic Effects of Tetanus Neurotoxin in the Oculomotor System," *Brain* 128(9):2175-188, September 2005.

Hoel, T., et al. "Combined Diphtheria-Tetanus-Pertussis Vaccine for Tetanus-Prone Wound Management in Adults," *European Journal of Emergency Medicine* 13(2):67-71, April 2006.

Kasper, D.I., et al., eds. *Harrison's Principles of Internal Medicine*, 16th ed. New York: McGraw-Hill Book Co., 2005.

Rhee, P., et al. "Tetanus and Trauma: A Review and Recommendations," *Journal of Trauma-Injury Infection & Critical Care* 58(5):1082-1088, May 2005.

Sheffield, J.S., and Ramin, S.M. "Tetanus in Pregnancy," *American Journal of Perinatology* 21(4):173-82, May 2004.

Thalassemia

● OVERVIEW

Description
- Group of genetic disorders
- Characterized by defective synthesis in one or more of the polypeptide chains necessary for hemoglobin production
- Most commonly occurs as a result of reduced or absent production of alpha or beta chains
- Affects hemoglobin production and impairs red blood cell (RBC) synthesis

Pathophysiology
ALPHA-THALASSEMIA
- Four forms exist:
  - alpha trait (the carrier trait): a single alpha-chain-forming gene is defective
  - alpha-thalassemia minor: two genes are defective
  - hemoglobin H disease: three genes are defective
  - alpha-thalassemia major: all four alpha-chain-forming genes are defective; death is inevitable because alpha chains are absent and oxygen can't be released to the tissues.

BETA-THALASSEMIA
- The fundamental defect is the uncoupling of alpha- and beta-chain synthesis.
- Beta-chain production is depressed— moderately in beta-thalassemia minor and severely in beta-thalassemia major (also called *Cooley's anemia*).
- Depression of beta-chain synthesis results in erythrocytes with reduced hemoglobin and accumulations of free-alpha chains.
- The free-alpha chains are unstable and easily precipitate in the cell; most erythroblasts that contain precipitates are destroyed by mononuclear phagocytes in the marrow, resulting in ineffective erythropoiesis and anemia.
- Some precipitate-carrying cells mature and enter the bloodstream but are destroyed prematurely in the spleen, resulting in mild hemolytic anemia.

Causes
- Inherited autosomal recessive disorder

Incidence
- Second most common cause of microcytic anemia
- Alpha-thalassemia more common in Blacks and Asians
- Beta-thalassemia more common in Mediterranean populations

Common characteristics
- Anemia

Complications
- Iron overload from RBC transfusions
- Pathologic fractures
- Cardiac arrhythmias
- Liver failure
- Heart failure
- Death

✳ ASSESSMENT

History
- Severity of anemia and symptoms ranging from mild to severe, including:
  - fatigue
  - shortness of breath
  - headache
  - angina

Physical findings
- Pallor or bronze appearance
- Dyspnea on exertion
- Splenomegaly
- Hepatomegaly
- Tachycardia
- Systolic murmur (in moderate or severe anemia)

Test results
LABORATORY
- Complete blood count shows decreased hemoglobin, hematocrit, and mean corpuscular volum.
- Serum iron is normal or increased.
- Serum ferritin is normal or increased.
- Total iron-binding capacity is normal.
- Reticulocyte count is normal or inceased.
- Hemoglobin electrophoresis shows decreased alpha- or beta-hemoglobulin chains.

IMAGING
- In thalassemia major, X-rays of the skull and long bones show thinning and widening of the marrow space because of overactive bone marrow. Long bones may show areas of osteoporosis. The phalanges may also be deformed (rectangular or biconvex). The bones of the skull and vertebrae may appear granular. (See *Skull changes in thalassemia major.*)

◆ TREATMENT

General
- No treatment for mild or moderate forms
- Iron supplements contraindicated in all forms

Diet
- Avoidance of iron-rich foods

Activity
- Avoidance of strenuous activities

Medication
- Transfusions of packed RBCs
- Desferal (chelation therapy)

Surgery
- Splenectomy
- Bone marrow transplantation

SKULL CHANGES IN THALASSEMIA MAJOR

This illustration of an X-ray shows a characteristic skull abnormality in thalassemia major: diploetic fibers extending from internal lamina and resembling hair standing on end.

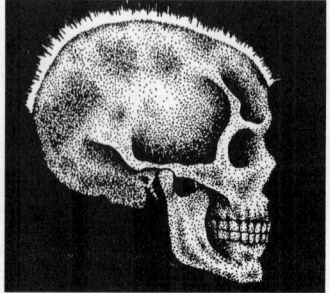

Nursing diagnoses

- Activity intolerance
- Delayed growth and development
- Disturbed body image
- Ineffective tissue perfusion: Cardiopulmonary
- Interrupted family processes
- Risk for infection

Key outcomes

The patient (or family) will:

- verbalize the importance of balancing activity, as tolerated, with frequent rest periods
- demonstrate age-appropriate skills and behaviors to the extent possible
- express positive feelings about himself
- maintain hemodynamic stability and develop no arrhythmias
- discuss how the patient's condition has affected the family's daily life
- remain free from signs and symptoms of infection.

Nursing interventions

- Administer blood transfusions, as ordered; observe for adverse reactions.
- Provide an adequate diet and encourage oral fluid intake.
- Provide emotional support to help the patient and family cope with the chronic nature of the illness and the need for lifelong transfusions.

Monitoring

- Transfusion reaction
- Signs and symptoms of iron overload
- Complications
- Cardiac arrhythmias
- Anemia symptom severity
- Response to treatment

Be sure to cover:

- disorder, diagnostic tests, and treatment
- importance of good nutrition
- signs and symptoms of iron overload
- follow-up care
- (with the parents of a young patient) various options for healthy physical and creative outlets. Such a child must avoid strenuous athletic activity. Reassure the parents that the child may be allowed to participate in less stressful activities.

Discharge planning

- Refer the patient to a hematologist and for genetic counseling, as appropriate.

Organizations

Cooleys Anemia Foundation:
www.cooleysanemia.org
Iron Disorders Institute:
www.irondisorders.org
National Heart, Lung and Blood Institute
www.nhlbi.nih.gov
Thalassaemia International Federation:
www.thalssaemia.org.cy

Selected references

Aessopos, A., et al. "Cardiac Status in Well-Treated Patients with Thalassemia Major," *European Journal of Haematology* 73(5):359-66, November 2004.

Aydinok, Y., et. al. "Psychosocial Implications of Thalassemia Major," *Pediatrics International* 47(1):84-89, February 2005.

Chui, D.J., et al. "Screening and Counseling for Thalassemia," *Blood* 107(4):1735-737, February 2005.

Kasper, D.L., et al., eds. *Harrison's Principles of Internal Medicine*, 16th ed. New York: McGraw-Hill Book Co., 2005.

Tierney, L., et al. *Current Medical Diagnosis & Treatment 2006.* New York: McGraw-Hill Book Co., 2006.

Thrombocytopenia

● OVERVIEW

Description
- Most common cause of hemorrhagic disorders
- Characterized by a deficient number of circulating platelets

Pathophysiology
- Lack of platelets can cause inadequate hemostasis.
- Four mechanisms are responsible: decreased platelet production, decreased platelet survival, pooling of blood in the spleen, and intravascular dilation of circulating platelets.
- Megakaryocytes are giant cells in bone marrow that produce the marrow. Platelet production decreases when the number of megakaryocytes is reduced or when platelet production becomes dysfunctional.

Causes
- May be congenital or acquired
- Decreased or defective platelet production in the bone marrow
- Increased platelet destruction outside the marrow caused by an underlying disorder (such as cirrhosis of the liver, disseminated intravascular coagulation, and severe infection)
- Sequestration (hypersplenism, hypothermia) or platelet loss
- Transient occurrence after a viral infection (such as Epstein-Barr) or infectious mononucleosis

Incidence
- Acquired form more common

Common characteristics
- Sudden onset of petechiae or ecchymoses on skin
- Bleeding into any mucous membrane

Complications
- In severe thrombocytopenia, hemorrhage or death

✱ ASSESSMENT

History
- Sudden onset of petechiae and ecchymoses or bleeding into mucous membranes (GI, urinary, vaginal, or respiratory)
- Malaise, fatigue, and general weakness (with or without accompanying blood loss)
- In acquired thrombocytopenia, possible use of one or several offending drugs
- Menorrhagia

Physical findings
- Petechiae and ecchymoses, along with slow, continuous bleeding from any injuries or wounds
- In adults, blood-filled bullae in the mouth

Test results
LABORATORY
- Platelet count is decreased (in adults, less than 100,000/mm³).
- Bleeding time is prolonged.
- Prothrombin and partial thromboplastin times are normal.

DIAGNOSTIC PROCEDURES
- In severe thrombocytopenia, a bone marrow study shows the number, size, and cytoplasmic maturity of the megakaryocytes (bone marrow cells that release mature platelets); may show ineffective platelet production as the cause of thrombocytopenia and be used to rule out a malignant disease process.

◆ TREATMENT

General
- Removal of the offending agents in drug-induced thrombocytopenia

Diet
- Well-balanced

Activity
- Rest periods between activities
- During active bleeding, strict bed rest

Medication
- Platelet transfusions
- Corticosteroids
- Immune globulin

Surgery
- Splenectomy

Nursing diagnoses

- Activity intolerance
- Anxiety
- Disturbed body image
- Fatigue
- Impaired skin integrity
- Ineffective coping
- Ineffective protection
- Risk for infection
- Risk for injury

Key outcomes

The patient will:

- verbalize the importance of balancing activity, as tolerated, with rest
- state measures to reduce levels of anxiety
- express positive feelings about self
- express feelings of increased energy
- exhibit improved or healed wounds or lesions
- demonstrate effective coping skills
- demonstrate use of protective measures, including conserving energy, maintaining a balanced diet, and getting adequate rest
- remain free from signs and symptoms of infection and avoid injury.

Nursing interventions

- Provide emotional support as necessary. Encourage the patient to discuss his concerns about his condition.
- Provide rest periods between activities if the patient tires easily.
- Provide a stool softener, if necessary.
- Protect all areas of ecchymosis and petechiae from further injury.
- Take precautions against bleeding; protect the patient from trauma.
- Avoid invasive procedures, such as venipuncture and urinary catheterization, if possible. When venipuncture is unavoidable, exert pressure on the puncture site for at least 20 minutes or until the bleeding stops.
- During active bleeding, maintain strict bed rest; keep the head of the bed elevated.
- When administering platelet concentrate, remember that platelets are extremely fragile; infuse them quickly using the administration set recommended by the blood bank.

- During platelet transfusion, monitor for a febrile reaction. Such reactions are common, and a fever will destroy the blood products.
- If the patient has a history of minor reactions, consider administration of acetaminophen and diphenhydramine before the transfusion.
- About 1 or 2 hours after administering platelet concentrate, monitor the patient's platelet count to assess his response to the infusion.

Monitoring

- Daily platelet count
- Bleeding
- Ecchymoses and petechiae
- Occult blood in stool, urine, and emesis
- During corticosteroid therapy, fluid and electrolyte balance and signs and symptoms of infection, pathologic fractures, and mood changes

▶ PATIENT TEACHING

Be sure to cover:

- disorder and its cause, if known, and, if appropriate, reassurance that thrombocytopenia commonly resolves spontaneously
- how to recognize and report signs of intracranial bleeding and other signs of bleeding
- avoidance of straining with stools and coughing (both can lead to increased intracranial pressure)
- function of platelets and warning that the lower the platelet count falls, the more cautious the patient must be in activities
- (in severe thrombocytopenia) an understanding that even minor bumps or scrapes may result in bleeding
- how to control local bleeding
- (if thrombocytopenia is drug induced) importance of avoiding the offending drug
- (if the patient must receive long-term steroid therapy) need to watch for and report cushingoid symptoms and to discontinue corticosteroids gradually
- avoidance of taking aspirin in any form as well as other drugs that impair coagulation

- how to recognize aspirin compounds and nonsteroidal anti-inflammatory drugs listed on labels of over-the-counter remedies
- (if the patient experiences frequent nosebleeds) recommendations for using a humidifier at night
- how to monitor the condition by examining the skin for ecchymoses and petechiae
- how to test stools for occult blood
- importance of wearing a medical identification bracelet.

☀ RESOURCES

Organizations

Harvard University Consumer Health Information: *www.intelihealth.com*
Mayo Clinic: *www.mayohealth.org*
The Merck Manuals Online Medical Library: *www.merck.com/mmhe*
National Heart, Lung and Blood Institute: *www.nhlbi.nih.gov*

Selected references

Begelman, S.M., et al. "Heparin-induced Thrombocytopenia from Venous Thromboembolism Treatment," *Journal of Internal Medicine* 258(6):563-72, December 2005.

Francis, J.L., and Drexler, A.J. "Striking Back at Heparin-induced Thrombocytopenia," *Nursing* 35(9):48-51, September 2005.

Gyamfi, C., and Eddleman, K.A. "Alloimmune Thrombocytopenia," *Clinical Obstetrics & Gynecology* 48(4):897-909, December 2005.

Kasper, D.L., et al., eds. *Harrison's Principles of Internal Medicine*, 16th ed. New York: McGraw-Hill Book Co., 2005.

Tierney, L., et al. *Current Medical Diagnosis and Treatment 2006.* New York: McGraw-Hill Book Co., 2005.

Thrombophlebitis

Description

- Acute condition characterized by inflammation and thrombus formation, which may lead to vessel occlusion or embolization
- May occur in deep or superficial veins (see *Major venous pathways of the leg*)
- Typically occurs at the valve cusps because venous stasis encourages accumulation and adherence of platelet and fibrin

Pathophysiology

- Alteration in epithelial lining causes platelet aggregation and fibrin entrapment of red blood cells, white blood cells, and additional platelets.
- The thrombus initiates a chemical inflammatory process in the vessel epithelium that leads to fibrosis.

Causes

- May be idiopathic
- Prolonged bed rest
- Trauma
- Surgery
- Pregnancy and childbirth
- Oral contraceptives such as estrogens
- Neoplasms
- Fracture of the spine, pelvis, femur, or tibia
- Venous stasis
- Venulitis

Incidence

- Increasing with the use of subclavian vein catheters
- Risk for developing deep vein thrombophlebitis dramatically increased after age 40

Common characteristics

- Tenderness, erythema, and warmth over affected area

Complications

- Pulmonary embolism
- Chronic venous insufficiency

History

- Asymptomatic in up to 50% of patients with deep vein thrombophlebitis
- Possible tenderness, aching, or severe pain in the affected leg or arm; fever, chills, and malaise

Physical findings

- Redness, swelling, and tenderness of the affected leg or arm
- Possible positive Homans' sign
- Positive cuff sign
- Possible warm feeling in affected leg or arm
- Lymphadenitis in case of extensive vein involvement

Test results
DIAGNOSTIC PROCEDURES

- Doppler ultrasonography shows reduced blood flow to a specific area and any obstruction to venous flow, particularly in iliofemoral deep vein thrombophlebitis.
- Plethysmography shows decreased circulation distal to the affected area and is more sensitive than ultrasonography in detecting deep vein thrombophlebitis.
- Phlebography also shows filling defects and diverted blood flow.

General

- Application of warm, moist compresses to the affected area
- Antiembolism stockings, pneumatic compression devices

Diet

- No restrictions

Activity

- Bed rest, with elevation of the affected extremity

Medication

- Anticoagulants
- Thrombolytics
- Analgesics

Surgery

- Simple ligation to vein plication, or clipping
- Embolectomy
- Caval interruption with transvenous placement of a vena cava filter

---

MAJOR VENOUS PATHWAYS OF THE LEG

Thrombophlebitis can occur in any leg vein. It most commonly occurs at valve sites.

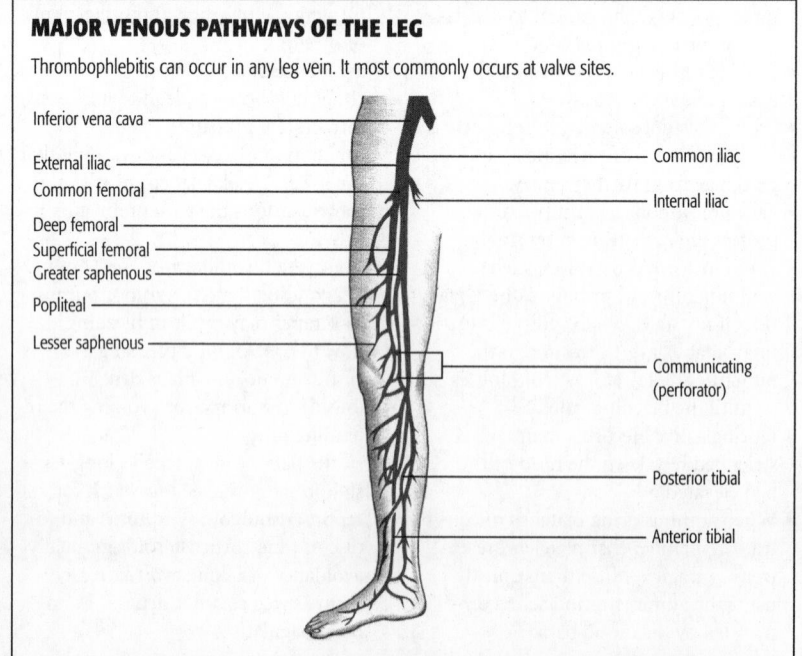

Inferior vena cava — External iliac — Common femoral — Deep femoral — Superficial femoral — Greater saphenous — Popliteal — Lesser saphenous — Common iliac — Internal iliac — Communicating (perforator) — Posterior tibial — Anterior tibial

NURSING CONSIDERATIONS

Nursing diagnoses
- Activity intolerance
- Acute pain
- Impaired skin integrity
- Ineffective tissue perfusion: Cardiopulmonary, peripheral
- Risk for infection
- Risk for injury

Key outcomes
The patient will:
- reduce metabolic demands
- express feelings of increased comfort and decreased pain
- exhibit skin color and temperature within acceptable limits
- maintain collateral circulation
- maintain tissue perfusion and cellular oxygenation
- remain free from signs or symptoms of infection
- remain free from injury.

Nursing interventions
- Enforce bed rest as ordered and elevate the patient's affected arm or leg, but avoid compressing the popliteal space of the leg.
- Apply warm compresses or a covered aquathermia pad.
- Give analgesics as ordered.
- Mark, measure, and record the circumference of the affected arm or leg daily, and compare this measurement with that of the other arm or leg.
- Administer anticoagulation as ordered.
- To prevent thrombophlebitis in high-risk patients, perform range-of-motion exercises while the patient is on bed rest, use pneumatic compression devices during lengthy surgical or diagnostic procedures, apply antiembolism stockings postoperatively, and encourage early ambulation.

Monitoring
- Signs and symptoms of bleeding
- Vital signs
- Partial thromboplastin time for patient on heparin therapy
- Prothrombin time for patient on warfarin
- Signs and symptoms of heparin-induced thrombocytopenia
- Signs and symptoms of pulmonary embolism
- Response to treatment

PATIENT TEACHING

Be sure to cover:
- disorder, diagnostic tests, and treatment
- importance of follow-up blood studies to monitor anticoagulant therapy
- how to give injections (if the patient is being discharged on subcutaneous anticoagulation therapy)
- need to avoid prolonged sitting or standing to help prevent a recurrence
- proper application and use of antiembolism stockings
- importance of adequate hydration
- proper use of an electric razor and avoidance of medications that contain aspirin (to prevent bleeding).

RESOURCES

Organizations
Harvard University Consumer Health Information: *www.intelihealth.com*
Mayo Clinic: *www.mayohealth.org*
The Merck Manuals Online Medical Library: *www.merck.com/mmhe*
National Heart, Lung and Blood Institute: *www.nhlbi.hih.gov/nhlbi/cardio*

Selected references
Chirinos, J.A., et al. "Septic Thrombophlebitis: Diagnosis and Management," *American Journal of Cardiovascular Drugs* 6(1):9-14, 2006.

Comp, P.C. "Should Coagulation Tests be Used to Determine which Oral Contraceptive Users Have an Increased Risk of Thrombophlebitis," *Contraception* 73(1):4-5, January 2006.

Craig, A. "Pain, Inflammation, and a Nodule after I.V. Medication," *Advance for Nurse Practitioners* 13(7):21-22, July 2005.

Decousus, H., and Leizorowicz, A. "Superficial Thrombophlebitis of the Legs: Still a Lot to Learn," *Journal of Thrombosis and Haemostasis* 3(6):1149-151, June 2005.

Kasper, D.L., et al., eds. *Harrison's Principles of Internal Medicine*, 16th ed. New York: McGraw-Hill Book Co., 2005.

The Merck Manual of Diagnosis & Therapy, 18th ed. Whitehouse Station, N.J.: Merck and Co., Inc., 2006.

Thyroid cancer

● OVERVIEW

Description
- Most common endocrine malignancy
- Papillary carcinomas: 50% of all cases
- Medullary cancer: may be associated with pheochromocytoma; curable when detected before it causes symptoms

Pathophysiology
- Papillary cancer is usually multifocal and bilateral. It metastasizes slowly into regional nodes of the neck, mediastinum, lungs, and other distant organs.
  - It's the least virulent form of thyroid cancer.
- Follicular cancer is less common but is more likely to recur and metastasize to the regional lymph nodes and spread through blood vessels into the bones, liver, and lungs.
- Medullary (solid) carcinoma originates in the parafollicular cells derived from the last branchial pouch and contains amyloid and calcium deposits.
  - It can produce calcitonin, histaminase, corticotropin (producing Cushing's syndrome), and prostaglandins (producing diarrhea).
  - Untreated medullary cancer grows rapidly, frequently metastasizing to bones, liver, and kidneys.
- Anaplastic carcinoma (giant and spindly cell cancer) resists radiation and is almost never curable by resection.
  - This cancer metastasizes rapidly, causing death by invading the trachea and compressing adjacent structures.

Causes
- Previous exposure to radiation treatment in the neck area
- Prolonged secretion of thyroid-stimulating hormone (radiation or heredity)

Risk factors
- Familial predisposition (possibly inherited as an autosomal dominant trait)
- Chronic goiter

Incidence
- 1 to 3 per 100,000 cases in men
- 2 to 4 per 100,000 cases in women
- Nearly twice the number of cases in Iceland and Hawaii compared with Canada and the United States
- Particularly common among Chinese males and Filipino females
- Rare in children

Common characteristics
- Painless, hard nodule in an enlarged thyroid gland
- Palpable lymph nodes with an enlarged thyroid
- Hoarseness
- Dysphagia

Complications
- Dysphagia
- Stridor
- Hormone alterations
- Distant metastasis

✳ ASSESSMENT

History
- Sensitivity to cold and mental apathy (hypothyroidism)
- Sensitivity to heat, restlessness, and overactivity (hyperthyroidism)
- Diarrhea
- Dysphagia
- Anorexia
- Irritability
- Ear pain

Physical findings
- Hard, painless nodule in an enlarged thyroid gland or palpable lymph nodes with thyroid enlargement
- Hoarseness and vocal stridor
- Disfiguring thyroid mass
- Bruits

Test results
LABORATORY
- Calcitonin assay identifies silent medullary carcinoma; calcitonin level is measured during a resting state and during a calcium infusion (15 mg/kg over a 4-hour period) and shows an elevated fasting calcitonin level and an abnormal response to calcium stimulation—a high release of calcitonin from the node in comparison with the rest of the gland—indicating medullary cancer.

IMAGING
- Thyroid scan differentiates functional nodes, which are rarely malignant, from hypofunctional nodes, which are commonly malignant.
- Ultrasonography shows changes in the size of thyroid nodules after thyroxine suppression therapy and is used to guide fine-needle aspiration and to detect recurrent disease.
- Magnetic resonance imaging and computed tomography scans provide a basis for treatment planning because they establish the extent of the disease within the thyroid and in surrounding structures.

DIAGNOSTIC PROCEDURES
- Fine-needle aspiration biopsy differentiates benign from malignant thyroid nodules.
- Histologic analysis stages the disease and thereby guides treatment plans.

◆ TREATMENT

General
- Radioisotope (^{131}I) therapy with external radiation (sometimes postoperatively in lieu of radical neck excision) or alone (for metastasis)

Diet
- Soft diet with small frequent meals if dysphagia occurs

Activity
- No limitations

Medication
- Suppressive thyroid hormone therapy
- Chemotherapy

Surgery
- Total or subtotal thyroidectomy with modified node dissection (bilateral or homolateral) on the side of the primary cancer (for papillary or follicular cancer)
- Total thyroidectomy and radical neck excision (for medullary or anaplastic cancer)

❖ NURSING CONSIDERATIONS

Nursing diagnoses
- Acute pain
- Anxiety
- Diarrhea
- Disturbed body image
- Imbalanced nutrition: Less than body requirements
- Impaired gas exchange
- Impaired skin integrity
- Impaired swallowing
- Impaired verbal communication
- Ineffective airway clearance
- Risk for aspiration

Key outcomes
The patient will:
- express feelings of increased comfort and decreased pain
- express feelings of decreased anxiety
- resume a normal elimination pattern
- express positive feelings about self
- maintain current weight without further loss
- maintain adequate ventilation and oxygenation
- maintain skin integrity
- maintain the ability to swallow
- express feeelings and needs without frustration
- maintain a patent airway
- not aspirate.

Nursing interventions
- Encourage verbalization and provide support.

BEFORE SURGERY
- Prepare the patient for scheduled surgery.
- Establish a way to communicate postoperatively.

AFTER SURGERY
- Keep the patient in semi-Fowler's position, with adequate neck support.
- Keep a tracheotomy set and oxygen equipment handy for use if respiratory obstruction occurs.

Monitoring
- Vital signs
- Wound site
- Pain control
- Serum calcium levels (if the parathyroid glands were removed)
- Postoperative complications
- Hydration and nutritional status

▶ PATIENT TEACHING

Be sure to cover:
- disorder, diagnostic tests, and treatment
- (before surgery) the operation and postoperative procedures and positioning
- home care
- medication administration, dosage, and possible adverse effects.

Discharge planning
- Refer the patient to resource and support services.

✳ RESOURCES

Organizations
American Cancer Society: *www.cancer.org*
Guide to Internet Resources for Cancer: *www.cancerindex.org*
National Cancer Institute: *www.nci.org*

Selected references
Atlas of Pathophysiology, 2nd ed. Philadelphia: Lippincott Williams & Wilkins, 2005.

Clark, J.R., et al. "Variables Predicting Distant Metastases in Thyroid Cancer," *Laryngoscope* 115(4):661-67, April 2005.

Hameed, R., and Zacharin, M.R. "Changing Face of Paediatric and Adolescent Thyroid Cancer," *Journal of Paediatrics & Child Health* 41(11):572-74, November 2005.

Kumar, V., et al. "Anaplastic Thyroid Cancer and Hyperthyroidism," *Endocrine Pathology* 16(3):245-50, Fall 2005.

Pacilio, M., et al. "Management of [131]I Therapy for Thyroid Cancer: Cumulative Dose from In-Patients, Discharge Planning and Personnel Requirements," *Nuclear Medicine Communications* 26(7):623-31, July 2005.

Patel, K.N., and Shaha, A.R. "Locally Advanced Thyroid Cancer," *Current Opinion in Otolaryngology & Head & Neck Surgery* 13(2):112-16, April 2005.

Thyroiditis

● OVERVIEW

Description
- Several disorders that involve inflammation of the thyroid gland
- Autoimmune thyroiditis or Hashimoto's thyroiditis: most common chronic inflammatory disease of the thyroid gland
- Postpartum thyroiditis: form of autoimmune thyroiditis that occurs within 1 year of delivery
- Subacute thyroiditis: transient inflammation of the thyroid gland that's probably viral in origin
- Riedel's thyroiditis: rare condition with unknown etiology that may be a variant of Hashimoto's thyroiditis
- Supportive thyroiditis: uncommon bacterial or fungal infection of the thyroid that's potentially very serious
- Silent thyroiditis: transient hyperthyroid condition that's characterized by a small painless goiter and may be autoimmune in origin

Pathophysiology
- The inflammatory process has varying effects on thyroid hormone levels (may be low, normal, or high). There may also be thyroid tissue infiltration by lymphocytes and leukocytes.
- Hashimoto's thyroiditis may result from lymphocytic infiltration of the thyroid gland and formation of antibodies to thyroid antigens in the blood.
- Riedel's thyroiditis causes intense fibrosis of the thyroid and surrounding structures.

Causes
- Mumps
- Influenza, coxsackievirus, or adenovirus infections
- Tuberculosis
- Syphilis
- Actinomycosis
- Bacterial infection
- Sarcoidosis and amyloidosis

Incidence
- More common in women than men
- Autoimmune thyroiditis or Hashimoto's thyroiditis occurring most often in middle-aged women; most common cause of sporadic goiter in children

Common characteristics
- Signs and symptoms of hyperthyroidism or hypothyroidism

Complications
- Dependent on type of inflammation:
  - Non-Hodgkin's lymphoma of the thyroid gland
  - Permanent hypothyroid or hyperthyroid condition
  - Abscess formation and rupture
  - Tracheal or esophageal compression, necrosis, and hemorrhage

✳ ASSESSMENT

History
- Recent viral or bacterial infection
- Disorder, such as systemic lupus erythematosus, rheumatoid arthritis, pernicious anemia, or Graves' disease
- Gradual onset of hypothyroid-like symptoms
- Occasionally, symptoms of hyperthyroidism
- Local pain or pain referred to the lower jaw, ear, or occiput
- Dysphagia
- Dyspnea
- Asthenia; malaise

Physical findings
- Enlargement of the thyroid gland (goiter)
- Reddened skin over the thyroid gland
- Indurated neck tissues
- Small, firm, and finely nodular thyroid gland with a characteristic band-like depression circling the gland
- Small lymph node found in the midline above the isthmus
- Swelling and warmth of the overlying skin
- Woody, hard enlargement that feels "anchored" to surrounding structures
- Stridor

Test results
LABORATORY
- Serum thyroglobulin levels and microsomal antibodies are increased in autoimmune processes.

HASHIMOTO'S THYROIDITIS
- Thyroid-stimulating hormone (TSH) levels are increased.

- Triiodothyronine and thyroxine levels are normal or decreased.
- Antimicrosomal and antithyroglobulin antibodies are increased.

SUBACUTE THYROIDITIS
- Thyroid hormone levels may be elevated, suppressed, or normal depending on the phase of the disorder.
- Protein-bound iodine levels are elevated.
- TSH levels are decreased in the thyrotoxic phase, failing to respond to thyrotropin-releasing hormone; TSH levels are increased in the hypothyroid phase.
- Radioactive iodine (^{131}I) uptake is increased.
- Erythrocyte sedimentation rate, white blood cell count, and hepatic enzyme levels are increased.
- Thyroid antibodies are transiently low.
- Thyroglobin levels are elevated.

RIEDEL'S THYROIDITIS
- ^{131}I uptake is normal or decreased.
- Antimicrosomal antibodies are increased.

IMAGING
- Thyroid scan may show isolated areas of function or total failure to visualize the gland.

DIAGNOSTIC PROCEDURES
- Fine-needle thyroid gland biopsy shows histologic confirmation.

◆ TREATMENT

General
- Varies with the type of thyroiditis

Diet
- No restrictions

Activity
- As tolerated

Medication
- Thyroid hormone
- Analgesics
- Anti-inflammatory drugs
- Beta-adrenergic antagonists
- Steroids
- Antibiotics

Surgery
- Partial thyroidectomy

✤ NURSING CONSIDERATIONS

Nursing diagnoses
- Acute pain
- Disturbed body image
- Imbalanced nutrition: Less than body requirements
- Impaired swallowing
- Ineffective airway clearance
- Ineffective coping

Key outcomes
The patient will:
- express feelings of increased comfort and decreased pain
- express positive feelings about self
- consume adequate daily calorie requirements
- swallow without coughing or choking
- maintain a patent airway
- demonstrate adaptive coping behaviors.

Nursing interventions
- Administer medications as ordered.
- Elevate the head of the bed 90 degrees during mealtimes and for 30 minutes afterward.
- Keep suction equipment readily available.
- Consult the dietitian.
- Provide frequent mouth care.
- Provide meticulous skin care.
- Provide comfort measures.
- Encourage oral fluid intake.
- Encourage verbalization of feelings.
- Offer emotional support.
- Help the patient develop effecting coping strategies.

◆ **NURSING ALERT** After thyroidectomy, watch for signs of tetany secondary to accidental parathyroid injury during surgery. Keep 10% calcium gluconate available for I.V. use, if needed. Check dressings frequently for excessive bleeding. Watch for signs of airway obstruction, such as difficulty talking or increased swallowing, and keep tracheotomy equipment handy.

Monitoring
- Vital signs
- Intake and output
- Daily weight
- Respiratory status
- Signs and symptoms of hyperthyroidism or hypothyroidism
- Neck circumference

▶ PATIENT TEACHING

Be sure to cover:
- disorder, diagnostic tests, and treatment
- medication administration, dosage, and possible adverse effects
- when to notify the physician
- signs and symptoms of respiratory distress
- signs and symptoms of hyperthyroidism and hypothyroidism
- long-term hormone replacement therapy after thyroidectomy
- importance of wearing a medical identification bracelet.

Discharge planning
- Refer the patient to a mental health professional for additional counseling, if indicated.

✱ RESOURCES

Organizations
American Foundation of Thyroid Patients: *www.thyroidfoundation.org*
American Thyroid Association: *www.thyroid.org*
Endocrine and Metabolic Diseases Information Service: *www.endocrine.niddk.nih.gov*
Endocrine Society: *www.endo-society.org*
Thyroid Foundation of America, Inc.: *www.clark.net/puB/tfa*

Selected references

Cipolla, C., et al. "Hashimoto Thyroiditis Coexistent with Papillary Thyroid Carcinoma," *The American Surgeon* 71(10):874-78, October 2005.

Erdem, F., et al. "Autoimmune Thyroiditis during Thalidomide Treatment," *American Journal of Hematology* 81(2):152, February 2006.

Goldani, I.Z., et al. "Fungal Thyroiditis: An Overview," *Mycopathologia* 161(3):129-39, March 2006.

Lucas, A., et al. "Postpartum Thyroiditis: Long-term Follow-up," *Thyroid* 15(10):1177-181, October 2005.

Stagi, S., et al. "Thyroid Function, Autoimmune Thyroiditis and Coeliac Disease in Juvenile Idiopathic Arthritis," *Rheumatology* 44(4):517-20, April 2005.

Thyrotoxicosis

● OVERVIEW

Description
- Alteration in thyroid function in which thyroid hormones (TH) exert greater than normal responses
- Management determined by cause
- Graves' disease (also known as *toxic diffuse goiter*); autoimmune disease; most common form of thyrotoxicosis
- Hyperthyroidism: form of thyrotoxicosis in which excess thyroid hormones are secreted by the thyroid gland
- Thyrotoxicoses not associated with hyperthyroidism: subacute thyroiditis, ectopic thyroid tissue, and ingestion of excessive TH
- Also known as *hyperthyroidism*

Pathophysiology
- In Graves' disease, thyroid-stimulating antibodies bind to and stimulate the thyroid-stimulating hormone (TSH) receptors of the thyroid gland.
- The trigger for Graves' disease is unclear.
- It's associated with the production of autoantibodies possibly caused by a defect in suppressor T-lymphocyte function that allows the formation of these autoantibodies.

Causes
- Diseases that can cause hyperthyroidism:
  - Graves' disease
  - Toxic multinodular goiter
  - Thyroid cancer
  - Increased TSH secretion
  - Genetic and immunologic factors

Risk factors
- Excessive intake of iodine
- Stress
- Surgery
- Infection
- Toxemia of pregnancy
- Diabetic ketoacidosis

Incidence
- Graves' disease: most common between ages 30 and 60; more common in women
- Increased among monozygotic twins
- More common with family history of thyroid abnormalities
- Only 5% of hyperthyroid patients younger than age 15

Common characteristics
- Increased metabolic rate
- Heat intolerance
- Increased tissue sensitivity to sympathetic nervous system stimulation
- Goiter (almost always present)
- Exophthalmos

Complications
- Arrhythmias
- Left ventricular hypertrophy
- Heart failure
- Muscle weakness and atrophy
- Paralysis
- Osteoporosis
- Vitiligo
- Skin hyperpigmentation
- Corneal ulcers
- Myasthenia gravis
- Impaired fertility
- Decreased libido
- Gynecomastia
- Thyrotoxic crisis or thyroid storm
- Hepatic or renal failure

✱ ASSESSMENT

History
GRAVES' DISEASE
- Nervousness, tremor
- Heat intolerance
- Weight loss despite increased appetite
- Sweating
- Frequent bowel movements
- Palpitations
- Poor concentration
- Shaky handwriting
- Clumsiness
- Emotional instability and mood swings
- Thin, brittle nails
- Hair loss
- Nausea and vomiting
- Weakness and fatigue
- Oligomenorrhea or amenorrhea
- Fertility problems
- Diminished libido
- Diplopia

Physical findings
GRAVES' DISEASE
- Enlarged thyroid (goiter)
- Exophthalmos
- Tremor
- Smooth, warm, flushed skin
- Fine, soft hair
- Premature graying and increased hair loss
- Friable nails and onycholysis
- Pretibial myxedema
- Thickened skin
- Accentuated hair follicles
- Tachycardia at rest
- Full, bounding pulses
- Arrhythmias, especially atrial fibrillation
- Wide pulse pressure
- Possible systolic murmur
- Dyspnea
- Hepatomegaly
- Hyperactive bowel sounds
- Weakness, especially in proximal muscles, and atrophy
- Possible generalized or localized paralysis
- Gynecomastia in males
- Increased tearing

◆ **NURSING ALERT** When thyrotoxicosis escalates to thyroid storm, these signs and symptoms can be accompanied by extreme irritability, hypertension, vomiting, temperature up to 106° F (41.1° C), delirium, and coma.

Test results
LABORATORY
- Radioimmunoassay shows increased serum triiodothyronine and thyroxine concentrations.
- Serum protein-bound iodine is increased.
- Serum cholesterol and total lipid levels are decreased.
- TSH levels are decreased.

IMAGING
- Thyroid scan shows increased uptake of radioactive iodine (^{131}I).
- Ultrasonography shows subclinical ophthalmopathy.

◆ TREATMENT

General
- Symptom relief

Diet
- Adequate caloric intake

Activity
- As tolerated

Medication
- Treatment with ^{131}I: a single oral dose; treatment of choice for post-menopausal women or men and women not planning to have children
- Thyroid hormone antagonists
- Beta-adrenergics
- Corticosteroids
- Sedatives

✳ AGE-RELATED CONCERN During pregnancy, antithyroid medication should be kept at the minimum dosage required to maintain normal maternal thyroid function and to minimize the risk for fetal hypothyroidism.

Surgery
- Subtotal (partial) thyroidectomy
- Surgical decompression

✣ NURSING CONSIDERATIONS

Nursing diagnoses
- Decreased cardiac output
- Diarrhea
- Disturbed body image
- Imbalanced nutrition: Less than body requirements
- Ineffective coping
- Risk for deficient fluid volume
- Risk for imbalanced body temperature

Key outcomes
The patient will:
- maintain normal cardiac output
- have normal bowel movements
- express positive feelings about body
- maintain adequate nutrition and hydration with no further weight loss
- demonstrate adaptive coping behaviors
- maintain an adequate fluid balance
- remain normothermic.

Nursing interventions
- Minimize physical and emotional stress.
- Balance rest and activity periods.
- Keep the patient's room cool and quiet and the lights dim.
- Encourage the patient to dress in loose-fitting, cotton clothing.
- Consult a dietitian to ensure a nutritious diet with adequate calories and fluids.
- Offer frequent, small meals.
- Provide meticulous skin care.
- Reassure the patient and family members that mood swings and nervousness usually subside with treatment.
- Encourage verbalization of feelings.
- Help the patient identify and develop coping strategies.
- Offer emotional support.
- Administer medications as ordered.
- Avoid excessive palpation of the thyroid.

AFTER THYROIDECTOMY
- Change dressings and perform wound care as ordered.
- Keep the patient in semi-Fowler's position.
- Support his head and neck with sandbags.

◈ NURSING ALERT After thyroidectomy, assess for respiratory distress and keep a tracheotomy tray at the bedside.

Monitoring
- Vital signs
- Daily weight
- Intake and output
- Daily neck circumference
- Serum electrolyte results
- Hyperglycemia and glycosuria
- Electrocardiogram for arrhythmias and ST-segment changes
- Complete blood count results
- Signs and symptoms of heart failure
- Frequency and characteristics of stools

AFTER THYROIDECTOMY
- Dressings
- Signs and symptoms of hemorrhage into the neck
- Surgical incision
- Dysphagia or hoarseness
- Signs and symptoms of hypocalcemia

▶ PATIENT TEACHING

Be sure to cover:
- disorder, diagnostic tests, and treatment
- medication administration, dosage, and possible adverse effects
- when to notify the physician
- need for regular medical follow-up visits
- need for lifelong thyroid hormone replacement
- importance of wearing a medical identification bracelet
- precautions with ^{131}I therapy
- signs and symptoms of hypothyroidism and hyperthyroidism
- eye care for ophthalmopathy.

Discharge planning
- Refer the patient and family members to a mental health counselor, if necessary.

✶ RESOURCES

Organizations
American Association of Clinical Endocrinologists: www.aace.com
Endocrine and Metabolic Diseases Information Service: www.endocrine.niddk.nih.gov
Endocrine Society: www.endo-society.org

Selected references
Amer, K.S. "Advances in Assessment, Diagnosis, and Treatment of Hyperthyroidism in Children," *Journal of Pediatric Nursing* 20(2):119-25, April 2005.
Franklyn, J.A., et al. "Thyroid Function and Mortality in Patients Treated for Hyperthyroidism," *JAMA* 294(1):71-80, July 2005.
Holcomb, S.S. "Detecting Thyroid Disease," *Nursing* 35(10 Suppl):4-8, October 2005.
Strategies for Managing Multisystem Disorders, Philadelphia: Lippincott Williams & Wilkins, 2006.
Waltman, P.A., et al. "Thyroid Storm During Pregnancy: A Medical Emergency," *Critical Care Nurse* 24(2):74-79, April 2004.

Tonsillitis

Description
- Acute or chronic inflammation of the tonsils
- Common viral infection that's mild and of limited duration

Pathophysiology
- The inflammatory response to cell damage by viruses or bacteria results in hyperemia and fluid exudation.

Causes
- Bacterial infection (group A beta-hemolytic streptococci) or viral infection

Incidence
- Commonly affects children between ages 5 and 10
- Tonsils tend to hypertrophy during childhood and atrophy after puberty

Common characteristics
- Sore throat
- Enlarged tonsils

Complications
- Chronic upper airway obstruction
- Sleep disturbance, sleep apnea
- Cor pulmonale
- Failure to thrive
- Eating or swallowing disorders
- Speech abnormalities
- Febrile seizures
- Otitis media
- Cardiac valvular disease
- Peritonsillar abscesses
- Glomerulonephritis
- Bacterial endocarditis
- Cervical lymph node abscesses

History
- Mild to severe sore throat
- Young child that possibly stops eating
- Muscle and joint pain
- Chills, malaise, headache
- Pain, frequently referred to the ears
- Constant urge to swallow
- Constricted feeling in the back of the throat

Physical findings
- Fever
- Swollen, tender submandibular lymph nodes
- Generalized inflammation of pharyngeal wall
- Swollen tonsils projecting from between the pillars of the fauces and exuding white or yellow follicles
- Purulent drainage with application of pressure to tonsillar pillars
- Uvula possibly edematous and inflamed

Test results
LABORATORY
- Throat culture reveals the infecting organism.
- Serum white blood cell count usually reveals leukocytosis.

General
- Symptom relief

Diet
- Adequate fluid intake

Activity
- Rest, as needed

Medication
- Aspirin or acetaminophen
- Antibiotics

Surgery
- Possible tonsillectomy

✤ NURSING CONSIDERATIONS

Nursing diagnoses
- Acute pain
- Anxiety
- Impaired swallowing
- Ineffective breathing pattern
- Risk for aspiration
- Risk for deficient fluid volume

Key outcomes
The patient will:
- express feelings of increased comfort and decreased pain
- verbalize a decrease in anxiety
- swallow without pain or aspiration
- maintain effective breathing pattern
- show no signs of aspiration
- demonstrate adequate fluid intake and balanced intake and output.

Nursing interventions
- Encourage oral fluids.
- Offer a child ice cream and flavored drinks and ices.
- Provide humidification.
- Encourage gargling to soothe the throat and remove debris from tonsillar crypts.

AFTER SURGERY
- Maintain a patent airway.
- Prevent aspiration by side positioning.
- Keep suction equipment readily available.
- Provide water after gag reflex returns.
- Later, encourage nonirritating oral fluids.
- Avoid milk products and salty or irritating foods.
- Provide prescribed analgesics for pain relief.
- Encourage deep-breathing exercises.

Monitoring
- Hydration status
- Effect of pain medication

BEFORE SURGERY
- Bleeding abnormalities

AFTER SURGERY
- Vital signs
- Signs and symptoms of bleeding
- Respiratory status

◆ **NURSING ALERT** Immediately report excessive bleeding, increased pulse rate, or decreasing blood pressure.

▶ PATIENT TEACHING

Be sure to cover:
- disorder, diagnostic tests, and treatment
- importance of completing the entire course of antibiotics
- avoidance of irritants
- the need for soft foods for approximately 3 weeks after surgery to decrease risk of rebleeding
- medication administration, dosage, and possible adverse effects
- possibility of throat discomfort and some bleeding postoperatively
- expectation of a white scab to form in the throat 5 to 10 days postoperatively
- need to report bleeding, ear discomfort, or a fever for 3 days or more.

◆ **NURSING ALERT** The greatest risk of bleeding is 7 to 10 days postoperatively.

✱ RESOURCES

Organizations
American Academy of Allergy, Asthma and Immunology: *www.aaaai.org*
Mayo Clinic: *www.mayoclinic.com*
National Institute of Allergy and Infectious Disease: *www.niaid.nih.gov*

Selected references
Deason, J., and Hope, B. "A 23-year-old Man with Chest Pressure, Pallor, Tachypnea, and Tonsillitis," *Journal of Emergency Nursing* 31(2):199-202, April 2005.

Giger, R., et al. "Hemorrhage risk after Quinsy Tonsillectomy," *Otolaryngology—Head and Neck Surgery* 133(5):729-34, November 2005.

Ohashi, M., et al. "Severe Acute Tonsillitis Caused by Rothia Dentocariosa in a Healthy Child," *Pediatric Infectious Disease Journal* 24(5):466-67, May 2005.

Webb, C.J., et al. "Tonsillar Size is an Important Indicator of Recurrent Acute Tonsillitis," *Clinical Otolaryngology & Allied Sciences* 29(4):369-71, August 2004.

Toxic shock syndrome

● OVERVIEW

Description
- Inflammatory response syndrome linked to bacterial infections
- Acute and life-threatening condition
- Also called *TSS*

Pathophysiology
- Exoproteins are produced by infecting organisms that are toxic in nature.
- TSST-1 is the most common toxin; staphylococcal enterotoxin B is the second most common.
- For illness to develop, the patient must be infected with a toxigenic strain of *Staphylococcus aureus* and lack antibodies to that strain.

Causes
- Penicillin-resistant *S. aureus*

Risk factors
- Tampon use
- Varicella infection
- Streptococcal pharyngitis
- Childbirth
- Abortion

Incidence
- Affects 1 in 100,000, primarily affecting young individuals
- Half of all cases in settings other than menstruation
- Affects both sexes and all ages

Common characteristics
- In the early convalescent period: fever, hypotension, rash, multiorgan dysfunction, and desquamation.
- Menstruation (most common setting for TSS occurrence)
- Bacteremia (in about 60% of patients)

Complications
- Septic abortion
- Musculoskeletal and respiratory infections
- Staphylococcal bacteremia
- Renal and myocardial dysfunction
- Adult respiratory distress syndrome
- Desquamation of the skin
- Peripheral gangrene
- Muscle weakness
- Neuropsychiatric dysfunction

✳ ASSESSMENT

History
- Possible recent streptococcal infection
- Possible tampon usage or menstruation
- Intense myalgia, headache
- Nausea, vomiting, diarrhea
- Sore throat
- Dizziness

Physical findings
- Fever (104° F [40° C] or higher)
- Pharyngeal infection, strawberry tongue
- Hypotension
- Altered mental status
- Macular erythroderma (generalized or local)
- Peripheral edema
- Vaginal hyperemia, purulent vaginal discharge

Test results
LABORATORY
- Isolation of *S. aureus* from vaginal discharge or infection site supports the diagnosis. (See *Guidelines for diagnosing toxic shock syndrome.*)
- Blood urea nitrogen level shows azotemia.
- Urinalysis shows pyuria.
- Serum albumin shows hypoalbuminemia.
- Serum calcium shows hypocalcemia.
- Serum phosphorus shows hypophosphatemia.
- Complete blood count shows leukocytosis or leukopenia.
- Platelet count shows thrombocytopenia.
- Serum creatinine level is elevated.

◆ TREATMENT

General
- Aggressive fluid resuscitation
- Correction of electrolyte imbalances
- Supportive treatment such as possible ventilatory support
- Identification and decontamination of toxin production site

Diet
- No restrictions

Activity
- Bed rest until acute phase resolved

Medication
- Antibiotics
- Inotropics
- Vasopressors
- I.V. immunoglobulin

Surgery
- Examination and irrigation of recent surgical wounds

GUIDELINES FOR DIAGNOSING TOXIC SHOCK SYNDROME

Toxic shock syndrome is typically diagnosed when the following have occurred:
- fever 102° F (38.9° C) or higher
- diffuse macular erythrodermal rash (sunburn rash)
- hypotension (systolic blood pressure 90 mm Hg or less in adults or under the 5th percentile for age)
- involvement of at least three organ systems:
  - GI (vomiting, diarrhea)
  - muscular (myalgias, or liver function test results of at least twice the normal upper limit)
  - mucous membrane hyperemia (conjunctiva, vagina, oropharyngeal)
  - renal (blood urea nitrogen or creatinine level at least two times upper limit of normal, or pyuria)
  - hepatic (total serum bilirubin or aminotransferase level two times normal level)
  - hematologic (thrombocytopenia)
  - central nervous system (disorientation or change in level of consciousness)
- desquamation 1 or 2 weeks after onset of illness, especially of palms and soles
- other conditions ruled out.

❖ NURSING CONSIDERATIONS

Nursing diagnoses
- Acute pain
- Decreased cardiac output
- Deficient fluid volume
- Hyperthermia
- Impaired tissue integrity
- Ineffective tissue perfusion: Cardiopulmonary, cerebral, GI, peripheral, or renal

Key outcomes
The patient will:
- express feelings of increased comfort and decreased pain
- maintain adequate cardiac output
- maintain adequate fluid volume
- remain afebrile
- maintain collateral circulation
- maintain tissue perfusion and cellular oxygenation.

Nursing interventions
- Administer medications, as ordered.
- Assess fluid balance and replace fluids I.V. as ordered.
- Reorient, as needed.
- Use appropriate safety measures to prevent injury.
- Use standard precautions for any vaginal discharge and lesion drainage.

Monitoring
- Cardiovascular status
- Fluid and electrolyte status
- Neurologic status
- Vital signs
- Pulmonary status
- Response to treatment
- Complications

▶ PATIENT TEACHING

Be sure to cover:
- disorder, diagnostic tests, and treatment
- need to avoid using tampons, especially superabsorbent ones, because of the risk of recurrence
- TSS prevention.

✹ RESOURCES

Organizations
Mayo Clinic: *www.mayoclinic.com*
National Center for Infectious Diseases—Division of Bacterial and Mycotic Diseases: *www.cdc.gov/ncidod/dbmd*
Toxic Shock Syndrome Information Service: *www.toxicshock.com*
U.S. Food and Drug Administration: *www.fda.gov*

Selected references
Arora, S. "A Case of Non-Menstrual Staphylococcal Toxic Shock Syndrome," *Journal of General Internal Medicine* 19(Suppl 1):24-25, April 2004.
Chuang, Yu-Yu, et al. "Toxic Shock Syndrome in Children: Epidemiology, Pathogenesis, and Management," *Pediatric Drugs* 7(1):11-25, 2005.
Hidalgo-Carballal, A., and Suarez-Mier, M.P. "Sudden Unexpected Death in a Child with Varicella Caused by Necrotizing Fasciitis and Streptococcal Toxic Shock Syndrome," *American Journal of Forensic Medicine & Pathology* 27(1):93-96, March 2006.
Kasper, D.L., et al., eds. *Harrison's Principles of Internal Medicine*, 16th ed. New York: McGraw-Hill Book Co., 2005.

Toxoplasmosis

● OVERVIEW

Description
- One of the most common infectious diseases
- Usually causes localized infection
- May produce significant generalized infection, especially in an immunodeficient patient
- Once infected, organism carried for life and with possibility of reactivation of acute infection
- Congenital type characterized by lesions in the central nervous system (CNS); may result in stillbirth or serious birth defects

Pathophysiology
- Upon ingestion, the causative parasites are released from latent cysts by the digestive process, then invade and multiply in the GI tract.
- Parasites disseminate to a variety of organs, especially lymphatic tissue, skeletal muscle, myocardium, retina, placenta, and the CNS (most commonly).
- The parasite infects host cells and replicates, then invades adjoining cells, resulting in cell death and focal necrosis surrounded by an acute inflammatory response.

Causes
- The protozoan *Toxoplasma gondii*, which exists in trophozoite forms in the acute stages of infection and in cystic forms (tissue cysts and oocysts) in latent stages
- Transmitted by ingestion of tissue cysts in raw or undercooked meat or by fecal-oral contamination from infected cats
- Congenital toxoplasmosis due to transplacental transmission

Incidence
- Infects up to 70% of people in United States
- Occurs worldwide; less common in cold or hot, arid climates and at high elevations

Common characteristics
- Fever
- Rash
- Constitutional symptoms

Complications
- Seizure disorder
- Vision loss (see *Ocular toxoplasmosis*)
- Mental retardation
- Deafness
- Generalized infection
- Stillbirth
- Congenital toxoplasmosis

✳ ASSESSMENT

History
- Possible immunocompromised state, exposure to cat feces, or ingestion of poorly cooked meat
- Malaise, fatigue
- Myalgia, headache, sore throat
- Vomiting

Physical findings
- Fever (if generalized, possibly 106° F [41.1° C])
- Cough, dyspnea, cyanosis, coarse crackles
- Delirium, seizures
- Diffuse maculopapular rash (except on the palms, soles, and scalp)
- In infant with congenital toxoplasmosis:
  - Hydrocephalus or microcephalus
  - Jaundice, purpura, rash
  - Strabismus, blindness
  - Epilepsy, mental retardation
  - Lymphadenopathy, splenomegaly, and hepatomegaly

Test results
LABORATORY
- Specimens (such as bronchoalveolar lavage material from immunocompromised patients or lymph node biopsy) show parasites.
- Intraperitoneal inoculation with blood or other body fluids into mice or tissue cultures show isolation of parasites.
- Polymerase chain reaction detects parasite's genetic material (especially in detecting congenital infections in utero).

◆ TREATMENT

General
- No treatment in otherwise healthy patient who isn't pregnant
- Seizure precautions

Diet
- No restrictions

Activity
- Rest periods when fatigued

Medication
- Pyrimethamine plus sulfadiazine with Leucovorin

OCULAR TOXOPLASMOSIS

Ocular toxoplasmosis (active chorioretinitis) is characterized by focal necrotizing retinitis. It accounts for about 25% of all cases of granulomatous uveitis. Although usually the result of a congenital infection, it may not appear until adolescence or young adulthood, when infection is reactivated.

Symptoms include blurred vision, scotoma, pain, photophobia, and impairment or loss of central vision. Vision improves as inflammation subsides but usually without recovery of lost visual acuity. Ocular toxoplasmosis may subside after treatment with prednisone.

❖ NURSING CONSIDERATIONS

Nursing diagnoses
- Activity intolerance
- Acute pain
- Deficient fluid volume
- Fatigue
- Hyperthermia
- Impaired skin integrity
- Ineffective breathing pattern
- Risk for injury

Key outcomes
The patient will:
- return to previous activity level
- express feelings of increased comfort and decreased pain
- have an adequate fluid volume
- report having an increased energy level
- remain afebrile
- maintain skin integrity
- maintain respiratory rate within 5 breaths/minute of baseline
- remain free from injury.

Nursing interventions
- Give tepid sponge baths to decrease fever.
- Administer medications, as ordered.
- Provide chest physiotherapy and administer oxygen, as needed. Assist ventilations, if needed.

  ⬡ NURSING ALERT Don't palpate the patient's abdomen vigorously; this could lead to a ruptured spleen. For the same reason, discourage vigorous activity.
- Report all cases of toxoplasmosis to the local public health department.

Monitoring
- Neurologic status
- Response to treatment
- Complications

▶ PATIENT TEACHING

Be sure to cover:
- disorder, diagnostic tests, and treatment
- necessary medication, including the need for frequent blood tests
- importance of regularly scheduled follow-up care
- prevention of the spread of toxoplasmosis (the need to wash hands after working with soil, cook meat thoroughly and freeze promptly, cover children's sandboxes, and keep flies away from food because flies transport oocysts)
- need for pregnant woman to avoid cleaning and handling cat litter boxes, or to wear gloves.

Discharge planning
- Refer the patient for follow-up with a neurologist or infectious diseases specialist, if needed.

✹ RESOURCES

Organizations
National Center for Infectious Diseases: *www.cdc.gov/ncidod*
National Institute of Allergy and Infectious Diseases: *www.niaid.nih.gov*

Selected references
Dzitko, K., et al. "Toxoplasma Gondii: Serological Recognition of Reinfection," *Experimental Parasitology* 112(2):134-37, February 2006.

Kasper, D.L., et al., eds. *Harrison's Principles of Internal Medicine*, 16th ed. New York: McGraw-Hill Book Co., 2005.

Many, A., and Koren, G. "Toxoplasmosis during Pregnancy," *Canadian Family Physician* 52:29-30, 32, January 2006.

Sukthana, Y. "Toxoplasmosis: Beyond Animal to Humans," *Trends in Parasitology* 22(3):137-42, March 2006.

Trigeminal neuralgia

● OVERVIEW

Description
- Painful disorder of the 5th cranial (trigeminal) nerve, which affects chewing movements and sensations of the face, scalp, and teeth (see *Trigeminal nerve function and distribution*)
- Can subside spontaneously
- Remissions lasting from several months to years
- Also known as *tic douloureux*

Pathophysiology
- A trigger zone is stimulated, and interaction or short-circuiting of touch and pain fibers occurs.
- Paroxysmal attacks of excruciating facial pain result.

Causes
- Exact cause unknown
- Afferent reflex phenomenon
- Compression of the nerve root by:
  - Posterior fossa tumors
  - Middle fossa tumors
  - Vascular lesions
- Multiple sclerosis
- Herpes zoster

Incidence
- Affects those over age 40 and about 25% more women than men
- Right side of face affected more commonly than left

Common characteristics
- Sudden onset of severe, throbbing pain
- Contortion of affected side of face

Complications
- Excessive weight loss
- Depression
- Social isolation

✳ ASSESSMENT

History
- Searing or burning pain that occurs in lightning-like jabs
  - Pain that lasts from 1 to 15 minutes (usually 1 or 2 minutes)
  - Pain that's localized in an area innervated by the trigeminal nerve
  - Pain that's initiated by a light touch to a hypersensitive area
- Attacks possibly following:
  - Draft of air
  - Exposure to heat or cold
  - Eating, smiling, and talking
  - Drinking hot or cold beverages
  - Period that's free from pain

Physical findings
- Favoring (splinting) of affected area
- Affected side of face unwashed and unshaven
- Patient never touching affected area
- No impairment of sensory or motor function

Test results
IMAGING
- Skull X-ray, computed tomography scan, and magnetic resonance imaging results rule out sinus or tooth infections and tumors.

◆ TREATMENT

General
- Clinical trials investigating use of transmitter-receptor or ion channel-specific drugs

Diet
- No restrictions

Activity
- As tolerated

Medication
- Anticonvulsants
- Analgesics

Surgery
- Microsurgery
- Radiosurgery with stereotactic technique
- Gamma radiosurgery to trigeminal root (noninvasive)

TRIGEMINAL NERVE FUNCTION AND DISTRIBUTION

Function
- Motor: chewing movements
- Sensory: sensations of face, scalp, and teeth (mouth and nasal chamber)

Distribution
I ophthalmic
II maxillary
III mandibular

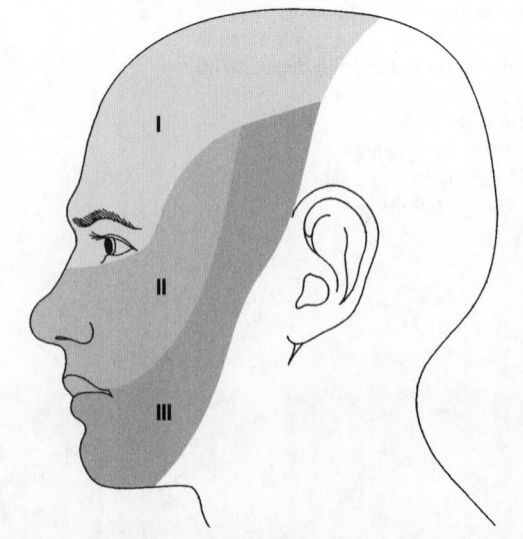

✤ NURSING CONSIDERATIONS

Nursing diagnoses
- Activity intolerance
- Acute pain
- Anxiety
- Fatigue
- Imbalanced nutrition: Less than body requirements
- Ineffective coping
- Ineffective role performance

Key outcomes
The patient will:
- perform activities of daily living within confines of the disorder
- express feelings of increased comfort and decreased pain
- express feelings of decreased anxiety
- express feelings of increased energy
- consume required caloric intake daily
- demonstrate adaptive coping behaviors
- perform routine roles within the confines of the disorder.

Nursing interventions
- Provide emotional support.
- Provide nutritional management.
- Administer medications, as ordered.
- After microsurgery, provide postcraniotomy care.

Monitoring
- Characteristics of each attack
- Precipitating factors of each attack
- Response to medications
- Postoperatively, neurologic function and vital signs

▶ PATIENT TEACHING

Be sure to cover:
- preoperative teaching, if indicated
- disorder, diagnostic tests, and treatment
- medication administration, dosage, and possible adverse effects
- nutritional management
- prevention of neuralgia attacks.

✱ RESOURCES

Organizations
American Chronic Pain Association: *www.theacpa.org*
American Pain Foundation: *www.painfoundation.org*
Trigeminal Neuralgia Association: *www.tna-support.org.*

Selected references
Aryan, H.E., et al. "Multimodality Treatment of Trigeminal Neuralgia: Impact of Radiosugery and High Resolution Magnetic Resonance Imaging," *Journal of Clinical Neuroscience* 13(2):239-44, February 2006.

Cox, C.L., et al. "Cranial Nerve Damage," *Emergency Nurse* 12(2):14-21, May 2004.

Crucci, G., et al. "Diagnostic Accuracy of Trigeminal Reflex Testing in Trigeminal Neuralgia," *Neurology* 66(1):139-41, January 2006.

Diseases, 4th ed. Philadelphia: Lippincott Williams & Wilkins, 2006.

Handbook of Pathophysiology, Philadelphia: Lippincott Williams & Wilkins, 2005.

Lin, Y.W., et al. "Fatal Paranasal Sinusitis Presenting as Trigeminal Neuralgia," *Headache* 46(1):174-78, January 2006.

Truini, A., et al. "New Insight into Trigeminal Neuralgia," *Journal of Headache and Pain* 6(4):237-39, September 2005.

Tuberculosis

● OVERVIEW

Description
- Acute or chronic infection characterized by pulmonary infiltrates and the formation of granulomas with caseation, fibrosis, and cavitation
- Prognosis excellent with proper treatment
- Also known as *TB*

Pathophysiology
- Multiplication of the bacillus *Mycobacterium tuberculosis* causes an inflammatory process where deposited.
- A cell-mediated immune response follows, usually containing the infection within 4 to 6 weeks.
- The T-cell response results in the formation of granulomas around the bacilli, making them dormant. This confers immunity to subsequent infection.
- Bacilli within granulomas may remain viable for many years, resulting in a positive purified protein derivative or other skin test for TB.
- Active disease develops in 5% to 15% of those infected.
- Transmission occurs when an infected person coughs or sneezes, spreading infected droplets.

Causes
- Exposure to *M. tuberculosis*
- Occasionally, exposure to other strains of mycobacteria

Risk factors
- Close contact with newly diagnosed tuberculosis patient
- History of prior TB
- Multiple sexual partners
- Recent immigration from Africa, Asia, Mexico, or South America
- Gastrectomy
- History of silicosis, diabetes, malnutrition, cancer, Hodgkin's disease, or leukemia
- Drug and alcohol abuse
- Residence in mental health facility
- Nursing home residence
- Immunosuppression and use of corticosteroids
- Prison residence
- Homelessness

Incidence
- Decrease in cases from 25,787 (1993) to 14,874 (2003)
- More prevalent in individuals ages 25 to 44
- Twice as common in men as in women
- Four times as common in nonwhites as in whites
- Higher in Black and Hispanic men between ages 25 and 44
- Highest in people who live in crowded, poorly ventilated, unsanitary conditions
- Medication-resistant strains continuing to be troublesome

Common characteristics
- Weakness and fatigue
- Anorexia, weight loss
- Low-grade fever
- Night sweats

Complications
- Massive pulmonary tissue damage
- Respiratory failure
- Bronchopleural fistulas
- Pneumothorax
- Pleural effusion
- Pneumonia
- Infection of other body organs by small mycobacterial foci
- Liver involvement disease secondary to drug therapy

✳ ASSESSMENT

History
PRIMARY INFECTION
- May be asymptomatic after a 4- to 8-week incubation period
- Weakness and fatigue
- Anorexia
- Weight loss
- Low-grade fever
- Night sweats
REACTIVATED INFECTION
- Chest pain
- Productive cough for blood, or mucopurulent or blood-tinged sputum
- Low-grade fever

Physical findings
- Dullness over the affected area
- Crepitant crackles
- Bronchial breath sounds
- Wheezes
- Whispered pectoriloquy

Test results
LABORATORY
- Tuberculin skin test reaction is positive in both active and inactive tuberculosis.
- Stains and cultures of sputum, cerebrospinal fluid, urine, drainage from abscess, or pleural fluid show heat-sensitive, nonmotile, aerobic, and acid-fast bacilli.
IMAGING
- Chest X-rays show nodular lesions, patchy infiltrates, cavity formation, scar tissue, and calcium deposits.
- Computed tomography or magnetic resonance imaging scans show presence and extent of lung damage or support the diagnosis.
DIAGNOSTIC PROCEDURES
- Bronchoscopy specimens show heat-sensitive, nonmotile, aerobic, acid-fast bacilli.

◆ TREATMENT

General
- After 2 to 4 weeks, disease is no longer infectious; patient can resume normal activities while continuing to take medication.

Diet
- Well-balanced, high-calorie

Activity
- Rest, initially

Medication
- Antitubercular therapy for at least 6 months with daily oral doses of:
  - isoniazid
  - rifampin
  - pyrazinamide
  - ethambutol, added in some cases
- Second-line drugs including:
  - capreomycin
  - streptomycin
  - aminosalicylic acid (para-aminosalicylic acid)
  - pyrazinamide
  - cycloserine

Surgery

- For some complications

❖ NURSING CONSIDERATIONS

Nursing diagnoses

- Fatigue
- Imbalanced nutrition: Less than body requirements
- Impaired gas exchange
- Ineffective airway clearance
- Ineffective coping
- Ineffective therapeutic regimen management
- Risk for injury

Key outcomes

The patient will:

- identify measures to prevent or reduce fatigue
- consume required daily caloric intake
- maintain adequate ventilation and oxygenation
- maintain a patent airway
- use support systems to assist with coping
- express an understanding of the illness and comply with treatment modalities
- remain free from injury.

Nursing interventions

- Administer medications as ordered.
- Isolate the infectious patient in a quiet, properly ventilated room, as per guidelines from the Centers for Disease Control and Prevention, and maintain tuberculosis precautions.
- Provide diversional activities.
- Properly dispose of secretions.
- Provide adequate rest periods.
- Provide well-balanced, high-calorie foods.
- Provide small frequent meals.
- Consult with dietitian if oral supplements are needed.
- Perform chest physiotherapy.
- Provide supportive care.
- Include the patient in care decisions.

Monitoring

- Vital signs
- Intake and output
- Daily weight
- Complications
- Adverse reactions

- Visual acuity if taking ethambutol
- Liver and kidney function tests

▶ PATIENT TEACHING

Be sure to cover:

- disorder, diagnostic tests, and treatment
- medication administration, dosage, and possible adverse effects
- when to notify the physician
- isolation
- postural drainage and chest percussion
- coughing and deep-breathing exercises
- regular follow-up examinations
- signs and symptoms of recurring tuberculosis
- possible decreased oral contraceptive effectiveness while taking rifampin
- need to consume a high-calorie, high-protein, balanced diet
- TB prevention (see *Preventing tuberculosis*).

Discharge planning

- Refer anyone exposed to an infected patient for tuberculin skin tests and appropriate follow-up.
- Refer the patient to local support groups such as the American Lung Association.
- Refer the patient to a smoking cessation program, if indicated.

✴ RESOURCES

Organizations

American Lung Association: *www.lungusa.org*
Centers for Disease Control and Prevention: *www.cdc.gov*
National Institute of Allergy and Infectious Diseases: *www.niaid.nih.gov*
U.S. Department of Labor Occupational Safety & Health Administration: *www.osha.gov*
World Health Organization: *www.who.int*

Selected references

Forget, E.J., and Menzies, D. "Adverse Reactions to First-Line Antituberculosis Drugs," *Expert Opinion on Drug Safety* 5(2):232-49, March 2006.

Glickman, S.W., et al. "Medicine. A Portfolio of Drug Development for Tuberculosis," *Science* 311(5765):1246-247, March 2006.

Jereb, J.A., et al. "Commentary on the Risk of Active Tuberculosis," *Archives of Pediatrics & Adolescent Medicine* 160(3):317-18, March 2006.

Kaufmann, S.H. "Robert Koch, the Noel Prize, and the Ongoing Threat of Tuberculosis," *New England Journal of Medicine* 353(23):2423-426, December, 2005.

Rubin, E.J. "Toward a New Therapy for Tuberculosis," *New England Journal of Medicine* 352(9):933-34, March 2005.

Williams, V.G. "Tuberculosis: Clinical Features, Diagnosis, and Management," *Nursing Standard* 29(22):49-53, February 2006.

PREVENTING TUBERCULOSIS

Explain respiratory and standard precautions to a hospitalized patient with tuberculosis. Before discharge, tell him that he must take precautions to prevent spreading the disease, such as wearing a mask around others, until his practitioner tells him he's no longer contagious. He should tell all health care providers he sees, including his dentist and eye doctor, that he has tuberculosis so that they can institute infection-control precautions.

Teach the patient other specific precautions to avoid spreading the infection. Tell him to cough and sneeze into tissues and to dispose of the tissues properly. Stress the importance of washing his hands thoroughly in hot, soapy water after handling his own secretions. Also instruct him to wash his eating utensils separately in hot, soapy water.

Tularemia

● OVERVIEW

Description
- *Francisella tularensis* (gram-negative pleomorphic bacterium) causing disease in humans and animals
- As few as 10 organisms able to cause disease
- Incubation period 3 to 4 days
- Six forms:
  - Ulceroglandular form
  - Glandular form
  - Oculoglandular form
  - Oropharyngeal form
  - Pneumonic form
  - Septicemic form

Pathophysiology
- *F. tularensis* gains access to the host by skin or mucous membrane inoculation, inhalation, or ingestion.
- After inoculation, a papule (that eventually evolves into an ulcer) and high fever develop.

Causes
- Bites of ticks and deerflies
- Eating or drinking contaminated food or water
- Contact with the blood of an infected animal, especially rabbits
- Breathing in the bacteria *F. tularensis*

Incidence
- About 200 cases in humans annually
- Occurs more commonly in the south-central and western United States

Common characteristics
- Swollen lymph nodes
- Fever

Complications
- Pneumonia
- Lung abscess
- Respiratory failure
- Rhabdomyolysis
- Meningitis
- Pericarditis
- Osteomyelitis

✳ ASSESSMENT

History
- Tick bite
- Exposure to contaminated food or water
- Exposure to contaminated blood
- Abrupt onset of fever, chills, headache, and malaise

Physical findings
ULCEROGLANDULAR
- Ulcers at the site of inoculation
- Swollen regional lymph nodes
GLANDULAR
- Swollen regional lymph nodes
OCULOGLANDULAR
- Painful
- Red eye
- Purulent exudates
- Swollen submandibular, preauricular, or cervical lymph nodes
OROPHARYNGEAL
- Sore throat
- Abdominal pain
- Nausea
- Vomiting
- Diarrhea
- Occasionally, GI bleeding
PNEUMONIC
- Dry cough
- Dyspnea
- Pleuritic chest pain
SEPTICEMIC
- Fever, chills, myalgia, malaise, and weight loss
- Absence of ulcer

Test results
LABORATORY
- White blood cell count is normal or elevated.
- Blood or sputum cultures are positive for *F. tularensis*.
- Serology may detect antibodies against *F. tularensis*.
IMAGING
- Chest X-ray may reveal pneumonia.

◆ TREATMENT

General
- Proper skin care

Diet
- Increased fluid intake

Activity
- As tolerated

Medication
- IV., I.M., or oral antibiotics
- Antipyretics

✤ NURSING CONSIDERATIONS

Nursing diagnoses
- Acute pain
- Diarrhea
- Hyperthermia
- Imbalanced nutrition: Less than body requirements
- Impaired gas exchange
- Impaired skin integrity
- Ineffective breathing pattern
- Risk for deficient fluid volume

Key outcomes
The patient will:
- express feelings of increased comfort and decreased pain
- return to a normal elimination pattern
- remain afebrile
- maintain adequate nutritional intake
- maintain adequate ventilation and oxygenation
- have warm, dry, and intact skin
- maintain normal breathing pattern
- regain or maintain normal fluid balance.

Nursing interventions
- Give prescribed drugs.
- Replace lost fluids through diet or I.V. fluids.

Monitoring
- Intake and output
- Vital signs
- Signs of dehydration

▶ PATIENT TEACHING

Be sure to cover:
- disorder, diagnostic tests, and treatment
- medication administration, dosage, and possible adverse effects
- complications and when to notify the physician
- preventive measures, such as using insect repellent containing DEET on skin, or treating clothing with repellent containing permethrin.

✹ RESOURCES

Organizations
National Center for Infectious Diseases – Division of Bacterial and Mycotic Diseases: *www.cdc.gov/ncidod/dbmd*
National Institute of Allergy and Infectious Diseases: *www.niaid.nih.gov*
U.S. Department of Labor Occupational Safety & Health Administration: *www.osha.gov*

Selected references
Buckingham, S.C. "Tick-borne Infections in Children: Epidemiology, Clinical Manifestations, and Optimal Management Strategies," *Paediatric Drugs* 7(3):163-76, 2005.
Daya, M., and Nakamura, Y. "Pulmonary Disease from Biological Agents: Anthrax, Plague, Q Fever, and Tularemia," *Critical Care Clinics* 21(4):747-63, vii, October 2005.
Farlow, J., et al. "*Francisella tularensis* in the United States," *Emerging Infectious Diseases* 11(12):1835-841, December 2005.
Isherwood, K.E., et al. "Vaccination Strategies for *Francisella tularensis*," *Advanced Drug Delivery Reviews* 57(9):1403-14, June 2005.
Schmitt, P., et al. "A Novel Screening ELISA and a Confirmatory Western blot Useful for Diagnosis and Epidemiological Studies of Tularemia," *Epidemiology and Infection* 133(4):759-66, August 2005.

Upper respiratory infection

● OVERVIEW

Description
- Acute, usually afebrile viral infection that causes inflammation of the upper respiratory tract
- Transmission through airborne respiratory droplets or through contact with contaminated objects, including hands
- Accounts for 30% to 50% of time lost from work by adults and 60% to 80% of time lost from school by children, more than any other illness
- Communicable for 2 to 3 days after onset of symptoms
- Usually benign and self-limiting

Pathophysiology
- Rhinoviruses infect cells by attaching to specific receptors.
- Infiltration with neutrophils, lymphocytes, plasma cells, and eosinophils occurs.
- Mucus-secreting glands become hyperactive and nasal turbinates become engorged. (See *What happens in an upper respiratory infection.*)

Causes
- More than 200 viruses, including rhinoviruses, coronaviruses, myxoviruses, adenoviruses, coxsackieviruses, and echoviruses
- Mycoplasma
- Viral infection of the upper respiratory tract passages and consequent mucous membrane inflammation responsible for 90% of cases

Incidence
- Most common infectious disease
- More prevalent in children, adolescent boys, and women
- Occurs more often in the colder months in temperate climates; occurs more often during rainy season in tropics

Common characteristics
- Nasal discharge
- Malaise
- Erythematous nasal and pharyngeal mucosa

Complications
- Secondary bacterial infection, causing sinusitis, otitis media, pharyngitis, or lower respiratory tract infection

✳ ASSESSMENT

History
- Exposure to persons with upper respiratory infection
- Sore throat
- Fatigue
- Malaise
- Myalgia
- Fever

Physical findings
- Copious nasal discharge that often irritates the nose
- Increased erythema of nasal and pharyngeal mucous membranes
- Nasal quality to voice
- Excoriated skin around nose

Test results
- There are no diagnostic tests for this disorder.

◆ TREATMENT

General
- Use of humidified inspired air
- Prevention of chilling

Diet
- Increased fluid intake

Activity
- Rest periods, as needed

Medication
- Acetylsalicylate acid
- Ibuprofen
- Acetaminophen
- Throat lozenges
- Antitussives
- In infants, saline nose drops and mucus aspiration with a bulb syringe

---

WHAT HAPPENS IN AN UPPER RESPIRATORY INFECTION

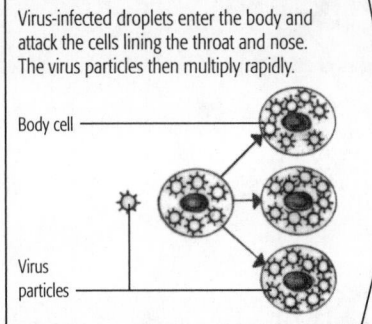

Virus-infected droplets enter the body and attack the cells lining the throat and nose. The virus particles then multiply rapidly.

Body cell

Virus particles

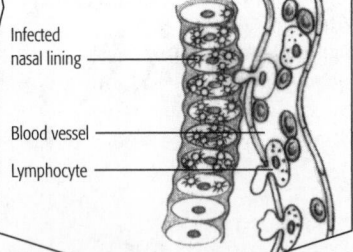

The immune system responds by sending lymphocytes to the infected mucosa, causing blood vessels in the nasal mucosa to swell. This swelling causes secretion of excess fluid—the classic symptom of a runny nose.

Infected nasal lining

Blood vessel

Lymphocyte

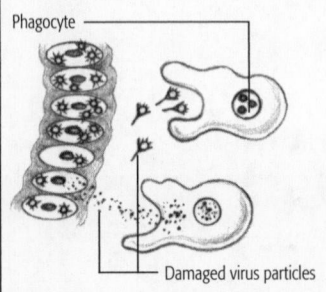

Phagocytes engulf and destroy dead virus particles and damaged cells. Soon the symptoms disappear.

Phagocyte

Damaged virus particles

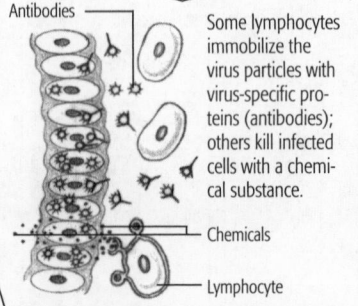

Antibodies

Some lymphocytes immobilize the virus particles with virus-specific proteins (antibodies); others kill infected cells with a chemical substance.

Chemicals

Lymphocyte

- Vitamin therapy, interferon administration, and experimental vaccines (under investigation)

♣ NURSING CONSIDERATIONS

Nursing diagnoses
- Acute pain
- Fatigue
- Hyperthermia
- Ineffective airway clearance
- Ineffective breathing pattern
- Risk for infection

Key outcomes
The patient will:
- express feeling of increased comfort and decreased pain
- report increased energy
- remain afebrile
- expectorate sputum effectively and maintain a patent airway
- maintain effective breathing pattern and express feelings of comfort in maintaining air exchange
- remain free from further signs or symptoms of infection.

Nursing interventions
- Give prescribed drugs.
- Encourage use of a lubricant on nostrils to decrease irritation.
- Assist with relieving throat irritation with sugarless hard candy or cough drops.
- Suggest use of a warm bath or heating pad to reduce aches and pains.
- Suggest a hot or cold steam vaporizer to relieve nasal congestion.

Monitoring
- Body temperature
- Respiratory status
- Response to treatment
- Adverse effects of medication

▶ PATIENT TEACHING

Be sure to cover:
- avoidance of overuse of nose drops or sprays
- how to avoid spreading colds
- proper hand-washing technique.

Discharge planning
- Refer the patient for medical care if a high fever persists, level of consciousness changes, or significant respiratory symptoms develop.

✷ RESOURCES

Organizations
Centers for Disease Control and Prevention: *www.cdc.gov*
Harvard University Consumer Health Information: *www.intelihealth.com*
National Health Information Center: *www.health.gov/nhic/*
National Library of Medicine: *www.nlm.nih.gov*

Selected references
Arroll, B. "Non-Antibiologic Treatments for Upper-Respiratory Tract Infections (Common Cold)," *Respiratory Medicine* 99(12):1477-484, December 2005.
Diseases, 4th ed. Philadelphia: Lippincott Williams & Wilkins, 2006.
Eccles, R. "Understanding the Symptoms of the Common Cold and Influenza," *The Lancet Infectious Diseases* 5(11):718-25, November 2005.
Kasper, D.L., et al., eds. *Harrison's Principles of Internal Medicine,* 16th ed. New York: McGraw-Hill Book Co., 2005.
Sitzman, K. "Managing the Common Cold," *AAOHN Journal* 53(2):96, February 2005.

Urinary tract infection, lower

● OVERVIEW

Description
- Two forms:
  - Cystitis (infection of the bladder)
  - Urethritis (infection of the urethra)
- Most urinary tract infections (UTIs) responding readily to treatment
- Possible recurring and resistant bacterial flare-ups during therapy

  ✴ **AGE-RELATED CONCERN** In adult males and children, lower UTIs are typically associated with anatomic or physiologic abnormalities and require close evaluation.

Pathophysiology
- Local defense mechanisms in the bladder break down.
- Bacteria invade the bladder mucosa and multiply.
- Bacteria can't be readily eliminated by normal urination.
- The pathogen's resistance to prescribed antimicrobial therapy usually causes bacterial flare-up during treatment.
- Recurrent lower UTIs result from reinfection by the same organism or a new pathogen.

Causes
- Ascending infection by a single gram-negative, enteric bacterium, such as *Escherichia coli, Klebsiella, Proteus, Enterobacter, Pseudomonas,* and *Serratia*
- Simultaneous infection with multiple pathogens

Risk factors
- Natural anatomical variations
- Trauma or invasive procedures
- Urinary tract obstructions
- Vesicourethral reflux
- Urinary stasis
- Diabetes
- Immobility
- Inadequate fluid consumption

Incidence
- Nearly 10 times more common in females than in males (except elderly males)
- Affects 10% to 20% of all females at least once

Common characteristics
- Urinary urgency and frequency
- Dysuria

Complications
- Damage to the urinary tract lining
- Infection of adjacent organs and structures

✳ ASSESSMENT

History
- Urinary urgency and frequency
- Bladder cramps or spasms
- Pruritus
- Feeling of warmth during urination
- Nocturia or dysuria
- Urethral discharge (in men)
- Low back or flank pain
- Malaise and chills
- Nausea and vomiting

Physical findings
- Pain or tenderness over the bladder
- Hematuria
- Fever
- Cloudy, foul-smelling urine

Test results
LABORATORY
- Microscopic urinalysis shows red blood cell and white blood cell counts greater than 10 per high-power field suggests lower UTI.
- Clean-catch urinalysis showing bacterial count of more than 100,000/ml confirms UTI.
- Sensitivity testing determines appropriate antimicrobial therapy.
- If the patient history and physical examination warrant, a blood test or a stained smear of urethral discharge rules out venereal disease.

IMAGING
- Voiding cystourethrography or excretory urography may demonstrate congenital anomalies that predispose the patient to recurrent UTIs.

◆ TREATMENT

General
- Sitz baths or warm compresses

Diet
- Increased fluid and fruit juice intake, especially cranberry

Activity
- No restrictions

Medication
- Antimicrobials

Surgery
- Warranted for recurrent infections from infected renal calculi, chronic prostatitis, or structural abnormalities

❖ NURSING CONSIDERATIONS

Nursing diagnoses
- Acute pain
- Disturbed sleep pattern
- Impaired urinary elimination
- Risk for infection
- Risk for injury
- Sexual dysfunction

Key outcomes
The patient will:
- report increased comfort and decreased pain
- verbalize feeling well rested after undisturbed periods of sleep
- demonstrate skill in managing the urinary elimination pattern
- remain free from further signs or symptoms of infection
- remain free from injury
- reestablish sexual activity at the pre-illness level.

Nursing interventions
- Collect all urine specimens appropriately.
- Administer medications, as ordered.
- Encourage oral fluid intake, unless contraindicated.
- Use sitz baths or warm compresses, as needed.

Monitoring
- Intake and output
- Urine characteristics
- Voiding patterns
- Vital signs
- Adverse effects of antimicrobial therapy

▶ PATIENT TEACHING

Be sure to cover:
- disorder, diagnostic tests, and treatment
- importance of completing the prescribed course of antibiotic therapy
- medication administration, dosage and possible adverse effects
- warm sitz baths to relieve perineal discomfort
- proper cleaning after toileting.

✷ RESOURCES

Organizations
American Association of Kidney Patients: *www.aakp.org*
National Institute of Diabetes & Digestive & Kidney Diseases: *www.niddk.nih.gov*

Selected references
Diseases, 4th ed. Philadelphia: Lippincott Williams & Wilkins, 2006.
Falagas, M.E., and Vergidis, P.I. "Urinary Tract Infections in Patients with Urinary Diversion," *American Journal of Kidney Diseases* 46(6):1030-1037, December 2005.
Schaeffer, A.J., et al. "The Natural Course of Uncomplicated Lower Urinary Tract Infection in Women Illustrated by a Randomized Placebo-Controlled Study," *Journal of Urology* 173(2):467-68, February 2005.
Schroeder, A.R., et al. "Choice of Urine Collection Methods for the Diagnosis of Urinary Tract Infection in Young Febrile Infants," *Archives of Pediatrics & Adolescent Medicine* 159(10)915-22, October 2005.
van Merode, T., et al. "Acute Uncomplicated Lower Urinary Tract Infections in General Practice: Clinical and Microbiological Cure Rates after Three- versus Five-Day Treatment with Trimethoprim," *European Journal of General Practice* 11(2):55-58, June 2005.

Urticaria and angioedema

● OVERVIEW

Description
- Common allergic reactions
- Occur separately or simultaneously
- Acute (present for less than 6 weeks) or chronic (present for at least 6 weeks)
- Urticaria also known as *hives*

Pathophysiology
- Urticaria is an episodic, rapidly occurring, usually self-limiting skin reaction. It involves only the superficial portion of the dermis, which erupts with local wheals surrounded by an erythematous flare.
- Angioedema involves additional skin layers and produces deeper, larger wheals (usually on the hands, feet, lips, genitalia, and eyelids). It causes diffuse swelling of loose subcutaneous tissue and may affect the upper respiratory and GI tracts.
- Several mechanisms and disorders may provoke urticaria and angioedema. They include immunoglobulin (Ig) E–induced release of mediators from cutaneous mast cells and binding of IgG or IgM to antigen, resulting in complement activation.

Causes
- Exact cause unknown
- Cholinergic trigger (heat, exercise, stress)
- Drug allergy
- Food allergy
- Hormones
- Inhalant allergens (animal dander, cosmetics)
- Insect bite
- Occupational skin exposure
- Rheumatological disease
- Thyroid abnormality
- Viral infection

Incidence
- Affect about 20% of general population at any given time
- More common after adolescence, with highest incidence in the 30s
- More common in females than males

Common characteristics
- Raised, red wheals
- Diffuse edema

Complications
- Skin abrasion and secondary infection
- Laryngeal edema
- Respiratory arrest
- Severe abdominal colic

✳ ASSESSMENT

History
- Drug history including nonprescription preparations, such as vitamins, aspirin, and antacids
- Reported frequently troublesome foods and environmental factors
- Exposure to physical factors, such as cold, sunlight, exercise, and trauma (dermatographism)
- Adverse reaction to iodinated contrast media used for diagnostic radiological studies

Physical findings
- Distinct, raised, evanescent dermal wheals surrounded by a reddened flare
- Nonpitting swelling of deep subcutaneous tissue on the eyelids, lips, genitalia, and mucous membranes that doesn't itch but may burn and tingle
- Respiratory stridor and hoarseness
- Anxiety, gasping for breath, and difficulty speaking
- Abdominal colic with or without nausea and vomiting
- Signs of anaphylaxis, such as hypotension, respiratory distress, stridor

Test results
LABORATORY
- Decreased serum levels of C1, C4, and C2 inhibitors confirm the diagnosis.
DIAGNOSTIC PROCEDURES
- Diagnosis can be confirmed through careful skin testing with the suspected offending substance to see if a local wheal and flare result.

◆ TREATMENT

General
- Emergency treatment for signs of anaphylaxis
- Limited contact with triggering factors
- Desensitization to the triggering antigen

Diet
- Avoidance of food allergens

Activity
- As tolerated

Medication
- Antihistamines
- Systemic glucocorticoids

NURSING CONSIDERATIONS

Nursing diagnoses
- Acute pain
- Anxiety
- Disturbed body image
- Impaired gas exchange
- Impaired oral mucous membrane
- Impaired skin integrity
- Ineffective airway clearance
- Ineffective breathing pattern
- Powerlessness
- Risk for infection

Key outcomes
The patient will:
- express feelings of increased comfort and decreased pain
- expressed a reduced level of anxiety
- verbalize feelings about a changed body image
- maintain adequate ventilation and oxygenation
- maintain intact oral mucous membranes
- exhibit improved or healed lesions or wounds
- maintain a patent airway
- maintain respiratory rate within 5 breaths/minute of baseline
- express feelings of control over well-being
- remain free from signs or symptoms of infection.

Nursing interventions
- Maintain a patent airway.
- Reduce or minimize environmental exposure to offending allergens and irritants, such as wools and harsh detergents.
- If food is a suspected cause, gradually eliminate suspected foods from the diet, and watch for improvement of signs and symptoms.
- Administer medications, as ordered.

Monitoring
- Vital signs, with attention to respiratory status
- Skin, for signs of secondary infection caused by scratching
- Response to treatment

PATIENT TEACHING

Be sure to cover:
- disorder, diagnostic tests, and treatment
- how to identify the cause of urticaria and angioedema by keeping a diary to record exposure to suspected offending substances and signs and symptoms that appear after exposure
- how to monitor nutritional status and food replacements for nutrients lost by excluding allergy-provoking foods and beverages
- need to keep fingernails short to avoid abrading the skin when scratching
- signs and symptoms that indicate a skin infection.

RESOURCES

Organizations
Allergic Diseases Resource Center: *www.worldallergy.org*
American Academy of Dermatology: *www.aad.org*
American College of Allergy, Asthma and Immunology: *www.allergy.mcg.edu*

Selected references

Baxi, S., and Dinakar, C. "Urticaria and Angioedema," *Immunology and Allergy Clnics of North America* 25(2):353-67, vii, May 2005.

Bork, K., et al. "Hereditary Angioedema: New Findings Concerning Symptoms, Affected Organs, and Course," *American Journal of Medicine* 119(3):267-74, March 2006.

Kaplan, A.P., and Greaves, M.W. "Angioedema," *Journal of the American Academy of Dermatology* 53(3):373-88, September 2005.

Kasper, D.L., et al., eds. *Harrison's Principles of Internal Medicine*, 16th ed. New York: McGraw-Hill Book Co., 2005.

The Merck Manual of Diagnosis & Therapy, 18th ed. Whitehouse Station, N.J.: Merck and Co., Inc., 2006.

Picado, C. "Non-steroidal Anti-Inflammatory Drug-Induced Urticaria and Angioedema: More Research on Mechanisms Needed," *Clinical and Experimental Allergy* 35(6):698-99, June 2005.

Uterine cancer

● OVERVIEW

Description
- Prolferation of cancer cells in the endometrium
- Most common gynecologic cancer

Pathophysiology
- Uterine cancer is usually an adenocarcinoma.
- Metastasis occurs late (usually from the endometrium to the cervix, ovaries, fallopian tubes, and other peritoneal structures; it may spread to distant organs, such as the lungs and the brain, by way of the blood or the lymphatic system; lymph node involvement can also occur).
- Less common uterine tumors include adenoacanthoma, endometrial stromal sarcoma, lymphosarcoma, mixed mesodermal tumors (including carcinosarcoma), and leiomyosarcoma.

Causes
- Exact cause unknown

Risk factors
- Low fertility index and anovulation
- History of infertility or failure of ovulation
- Abnormal uterine bleeding
- Obesity, hypertension, diabetes, or nulliparity
- Familial tendency
- History of uterine polyps or endometrial hyperplasia
- Estrogen replacement therapy

Common characteristics
- Abnormal vaginal bleeding

Incidence
- Most common in postmenopausal women between ages 50 and 60 (uncommon between ages 30 and 40 and rare before age 30)
- Most premenopausal patients having history of anovulatory menstrual cycles or other hormonal imbalances
- About 33,000 new cases reported annually; about 5,500 resulting in death

Complications
- Anemia
- Intestinal obstruction
- Ascites
- Increasing pain
- Hemorrhage

✳ ASSESSMENT

History
- Presence of risk factors
- Spotting and protracted, heavy menses (in younger patient)
- Possible bleeding beginning 12 or more months after menses stopped (in postmenopausal woman)
- Vaginal discharge, initially watery, then increasingly blood streaked

Physical findings
- Palpable enlarged uterus (advanced disease)
- Abdominal tenderness

Test results
DIAGNOSTIC PROCEDURES
- Endometrial, cervical, or endocervical biopsy confirms the presence of cancer cells.
- Fractional dilatation and curettage are used to identify the problem when the disease is suspected but the endometrial biopsy is negative.
- Multiple cervical biopsies and endocervical curettage pinpoint cervical involvement.
- Schiller's test involves staining the cervix and vagina with an iodine solution that turns healthy tissues brown (cancerous tissues resist the stain).

◆ TREATMENT

General
- Radiation therapy

Diet
- Well-balanced; no restrictions

Activity
- As tolerated

Medication
- Hormonal therapy
- Chemotherapy

Surgery
- Total abdominal hysterectomy, bilateral salpingo-oophorectomy or, possibly, omentectomy with or without pelvic or para-aortic lymphadenectomy
- Total pelvic exenteration

Nursing diagnoses

- Acute pain
- Anxiety
- Disturbed body image
- Fear
- Impaired urinary elimination
- Ineffective coping
- Risk for infection
- Sexual dysfunction

Key outcomes

The patient will:

- express feelings of increased comfort and decreased pain
- express feelings of decreased anxiety
- express positive feelings about self
- discuss fears and concerns
- maintain adequate urine output
- demonstrate positive coping behaviors
- remain free from signs and symptoms of infection
- express feelings and perceptions about change in sexual performance with partner.

Nursing interventions

- Encourage verbalization and provide support.
- Administer medications, as ordered.
- Encourage the patient to breathe deeply and cough.

Monitoring

AFTER SURGERY

- Wound site and drainage system
- Vital signs
- Postoperative complications
- Pain control

INTERNAL RADIATION THERAPY

- Safety precautions (time, distance, and shielding)
- Movement (limited while source is in place)
- Vital signs
- Complications from radiation therapy, such as skin reaction, vaginal bleeding, abdominal discomfort, and dehydration

Be sure to cover:

- disorder, diagnostic tests, and treatment
- preoperative and postoperative care
- (if the patient is premenopausal) that removal of her ovaries will induce menopause
- safety measures involved in internal radiation therapy
- dietary modifications
- medication administration, dosage, and possible adverse effects.

Discharge planning

- Refer the patient to resource and support services.

Organizations

American Cancer Society: *www.cancer.org*
Guide to Internet Resources for Cancer: *www.cancerindex.org*
National Cancer Institute: *www.nci.org*

Selected references

Ackermann, S., et al. "Awareness of General and Personal Risk Factors for Uterine Cancer Among Healthy Women," *European Journal of Cancer Prevention* 14(6):519-24, December 2005.

Ahlberg, K., et al. "Fatigue, Psychological Distress, Coping Resources, and Functional Status during Radiotherapy for Uterine Cancer," *Oncology Nursing Forum* 32(3):633-40, May 2005.

Atlas of Pathophysiology, 2nd ed. Philadelphia: Lippincott Williams & Wilkins, 2005.

Gold, M.A., et al. "Effects of Tubal Occlusion on Dissemination of Uterine Cancer," *International Journal of Gynecological Cancer* 14(Suppl 1):6, September-October 2004.

Loizzi, V., et al. "Hormone Replacement Therapy on Ovarian and Uterine Cancer Risk and Cancer Survivors: How Shall We Do No Harm?" *International Journal of Gynecological Cancer* 15(3):420-25, May-June 2005.

Vancomycin intermediate-resistant *Staphylococcus aureus*

● OVERVIEW

Description
- Common infection in chronically ill patients; most likely developing in health care setting; apparently not spread to family members, household contacts, other patients, or health care workers
- *Staphylococcus aureus* (MRSA) normally most reliably and effectively treated with vancomycin; MRSA with decreased susceptibility to vancomycin possibly a sign that vancomycin-resistant strains are emerging
- Also called *VISA* and *glycopeptide intermediate-resistant* Staphylococcus aureus

Pathophysiology
- Genes encode resistance and are carried on plasmids that transfer themselves from cell to cell.
- Resistance is mediated by enzymes that substitute a different molecule for the terminal amino acid so that vancomycin can't bind.

Causes
- Direct contact with infected or colonized patient or colonized health care worker or contact with contaminated surface such as overbed table

Incidence
- First discovered in mid-1996; four cases detected in the United States
- Noted in patients receiving multiple courses of vancomycin for MSRA infections
- Colonized patient more than 10 times as likely to become infected with the organism such as through a breach in the immune system

Common characteristics
- Causative organism able to live for weeks on such surfaces as patient gowns, bed linens, and handrails
- No specific symptoms; cultures found incidentally

Complications
- Sepsis
- Multisystem organ involvement
- Death in the immunocompromised patient

✳ ASSESSMENT

History
- Possible breach in the immune system or surgery or condition predisposing the patient to the infection
- Multiple antibiotic use

Physical findings
- Carrier patient commonly asymptomatic but may exhibit signs and symptoms related to the primary diagnosis
- Possible evidence of cardiac, respiratory, or other major symptoms

Test results
LABORATORY
- Culture may show staphylococci with decreased susceptibility to vancomycin after 24-hour incubation.

◆ TREATMENT

General
- With an infection, possibly no treatment (stop all antibiotics and simply wait for normal bacteria to repopulate and replace the strain)
- Colonized patient placed in contact isolation until culture-negative or discharged

Diet
- No restrictions

Activity
- Rest periods when fatigued

Medication
- Antimicrobials

✤ NURSING CONSIDERATIONS

Nursing diagnoses
- Acute pain
- Decreased cardiac output
- Deficient fluid volume
- Hyperthermia
- Impaired tissue integrity
- Ineffective tissue perfusion: Cardio-pulmonary

Key outcomes
The patient will:
- express feelings of increased comfort and decreased pain
- maintain adequate cardiac output
- have an adequate fluid volume
- remain febrile
- maintain adequate circulation to impaired tissues
- attain and maintain hemodyamic stability.

Nursing interventions
- Consider grouping infected patients together and having the same nursing staff care for them.
- Institute contact isolation precautions.
- Ensure judicious and careful use of antibiotics. Encourage physicians to limit the use of antibiotics.
- Use infection-control practices, such as wearing gloves before and after contact with infectious body tissues and proper hand washing, to reduce the spread of VISA.

Monitoring
- Vital signs
- Response to treatment
- Complications

▶ PATIENT TEACHING

Be sure to cover:
- disorder, diagnostic tests, and treatment
- need for family and friends to wear personal protective equipment when they visit the patient and how to dispose of it
- medication administration, dosage, and possible adverse effects.

✳ RESOURCES

Organizations
National Center for Infectious Diseases
www.cdc.gov/ncidod
National Institute of Allergy and Infectious Diseases: *www.niaid.nih.gov*
National Library of Medicine:
www.nlm.nih.gov

Selected references
Appelbaum., R.C. "The Emergence of Vancomycin-Intermediate and Vancomycin-Resistant *Staphylococcus aureus*," *Clinical Microbiology and Infection* 12(Suppl 1):16-23, March 2006.

Bhateja, P., et al. "Characterization of Laboratory-Generated Vancomycin Intermediate Resistant *Staphylococcus aureus* Strains," *International Journal of Antimicrobial Agents* 27(3):201-11, March 2006.

Cui, L., et al. "Correlation between Reduced Daptomycin Susceptibility and Vancomycin Resistance in Vancomycin-Intermediate *Staphylococcus aureus*," *Antimicrobial Agents and Chemotherapy* 50(3):1079-82, March 2006.

Howden, B.P. "Recognition and Management of Infections Caused by Vancomycin-Intermediate *Staphylococcus aureus* (VISA) and Heterogenous VISA (hVISA)," *Internal Medicine Journal* 35(Suppl 2):S136-40, December 2005.

Kasper, D.L., et al., eds. *Harrison's Principles of Internal Medicine*, 16th ed. New York: McGraw-Hill Book Co., 2005.

Varicella

● OVERVIEW

Description
- Acute, highly contagious infection that can occur at any age
- Same virus that causes chickenpox, thought to become latent until the sixth decade of life, or later, causing herpes zoster (shingles)
- Transmission through direct contact (primarily with respiratory secretions, less often with skin lesions) and indirect contact (through airwaves)
- Possible congenital varicella in infants whose mothers had acute infections in first or early second trimester
- Commonly known as *chickenpox*

Pathophysiology
- Localized replication of the virus occurs (probably in the nasopharynx), leading to seeding of the reticuloendothelial system and development of viremia.
- Diffuse and scattered skin lesions result with vesicles involving the corium and dermis with degenerative changes (ballooning) and infection of localized blood vessels.
- Necrosis and epidermal hemorrhage result; vesicles eventually rupture and release fluid or are reabsorbed.

Causes
- Varicella-zoster herpesvirus

Incidence
- Most common in children ages 5 to 9 but can occur at any age
- Neonatal infection rare, probably because of transient maternal immunity
- Occurs worldwide; endemic in large cities with outbreaks occurring sporadically
- Equally affects all races and both sexes
- Seasonal distribution variable; in temperate areas, incidence higher during late winter and spring

Common characteristics
- Incubation period lasting from 13 to 17 days
- Communicable from 48 hours before lesions erupt until after vesicles are crusted over

Complications
- With scratching due to severe pruritus, infection, scarring, impetigo, furuncles, and cellulitis
- Reye's syndrome
- Pneumonia
- Myocarditis
- Bleeding disorders
- Arthritis
- Nephritis
- Hepatitis
- Acute myositis
- Congenital varicella-caused hypoplastic deformity, limb scarring, retarded growth, and central nervous system and eye problems

✱ ASSESSMENT

History
- Recent exposure to someone with chickenpox
- Malaise, headache, and anorexia

Physical findings
- Temperature 101° to 103° F (38.3° to 39.4° C)
- Crops of small, erythematous macules on the trunk or scalp
- Macules progressing to papules and then clear vesicles on an erythematous base (so-called dewdrops on rose petals)
- Vesicles becoming cloudy and breaking easily; then scabs forming
- Rash that spreads to face and, rarely, to extremities
- Rash containing a combination of red papules, vesicles, and scabs in various stages
- Ulcers on mucous membranes of the mouth, conjunctivae, and genitalia

Test results
LABORATORY
- Isolation of virus from vesicular fluid occurs within the first 3 to 4 days of the rash.
- Giemsa stain distinguishes the varicella-zoster virus from the vaccinia-variola virus.
- Serum samples contain antibodies 7 days after onset of symptoms.
- Serologic testing differentiates rickettsial pox from varicella.

◆ TREATMENT

General
- Strict isolation until all the vesicles have crusted over; for congenital chickenpox, no isolation

Diet
- Increased fluid intake

Activity
- Rest periods when fatigued

Medication
- Antipruritics
- Antibiotics
- Analgesic and antipyretic
- Acyclovir (Zovirax)
- Varicella-zoster immune globulin

♣ NURSING CONSIDERATIONS

Nursing diagnoses
- Disturbed body image
- Fatigue
- Hyperthermia
- Impaired skin integrity
- Readiness for enhanced management of therapeutic regimen
- Risk for imbalanced fluid volume
- Risk for infection
- Social isolation

Key outcomes
The patient will:
- verabalize feelings about changed body image
- report or demonstrate an increased energy level
- remain afebrile
- exhibit improved or healed lesions or wounds
- demonstrate the skin care regimen
- maintain adequate fluid balance
- remain free from signs of secondary infection
- interact with family and peers to decrease feelings of isolation.

Nursing interventions
- Observe an immunocompromised patient for manifestations of complications, such as pneumonitis and meningitis, and report them immediately.
- Provide skin care comfort measures (calamine lotion, cornstarch, sponge baths, or showers).
- Administer varicella-zoster immune globulin, if ordered, to lessen the severity of the disease.
- Institute strict isolation measures until all skin lesions have crusted.
- Prevent exposure to pregnant women.

Monitoring
- Response to treatment
- Complications
- Skin integrity
- Signs and symptoms of dehydration
- Signs and symptoms of infection
- Adverse drug reactions

▶ PATIENT TEACHING

Be sure to cover:
- disorder, diagnostic tests, and treatment
- how to correctly apply topical antipruritic medications.
- importance of good hygiene and keeping the child's fingernails trimmed
- need for the child to avoid scratching the lesions
- need for parents to watch for and immediately report signs of complications (severe skin pain and burning may indicate a serious secondary infection and require prompt medical attention)
- need for parents to refrain from giving the child aspirin because of its association with Reye's syndrome
- signs and symptoms of Reye's syndrome and the need to immediately report them to the physician.

✹ RESOURCES

Organizations
Centers for Disease Control and Prevention: *www.cdc.gov*
World Health Organization: *www.who.int*

Selected references
Breuer, J. "Varicella Vaccination for Healthcare Workers," *British Medical Journal* 330(7489):433-34, February 2005.

Kasper, D.L., et al., eds. *Harrison's Principles of Internal Medicine*, 16th ed. New York: McGraw-Hill Book Co., 2005.

Neu, A.M. "Indications for Varicella Vaccination Post-Transplant," *Pediatric Transplantation* 9(2):141-44, April 2005.

Plourd, D.M., and Austin, K. "Correlation of a Reported History of Chickenpox with Seropositive Immunity in Pregnant Women," *Journal of Reproductive Medicine* 50(10):779-83, October 2005.

Sandy, M.C. "Herpes Zoster: Medical and Nursing Management," *Clinical Journal of Oncology Nursing* 9(4):443-46, August 2005.

Seward, J.F., and Orenstein, W.A. "Commentary: The Case for Universal Varicella Immunization," *Pediatric Infectious Disease Journal* 25(1):45-46, January 2006.

Vasculitis

● OVERVIEW

Description
- Autoimmune condition that includes a broad spectrum of disorders characterized by blood vessel inflammation and necrosis
- Clinical effects dependent on the vessels involved and reflective of tissue ischemia caused by blood flow obstruction

Pathophysiology
- The process is initiated by excessive circulating antigen, which triggers the formation of soluble antigen-antibody complexes. The reticuloendothelial system can't effectively clear these complexes, which are deposited in blood vessel walls.
- Increased vascular permeability (associated with the release of vasoactive amines by platelets and basophils) enhances this deposition. The deposited complexes activate the complement cascade and result in chemotaxis of neutrophils, which release lysosomal enzymes.
- Vessel damage and necrosis result.

Causes
- Several theories:
  – Follows serious infectious disease and may be related to high doses of antibiotics
  – Formation of autoantibodies directed at the body's own cellular and extracellular proteins, which can lead to the activation of inflammatory cells or cytotoxicity
  – Cell-mediated (T-cell) immune response
  – In atopic individuals, exposure to allergens

Incidence
- Can affect a person at any age (except mucocutaneous lymph node syndrome, which affects only children)

Common characteristics
- Any blood vessel can be affected

Complications
- Renal failure, renal hypertension, glomerulitis
- Fibrous scarring of the lung tissue
- Stroke
- GI bleeding, intestinal obstruction
- Myocardial infarction and pericarditis
- Rupture of mesenteric aneurysms

✳ ASSESSMENT

History
- Varied findings, depending on blood vessels involved

POLYARTERITIS NODOSA
- Fever
- Weight loss
- Malaise
- Headache
- Abdominal pain
- Myalgias

Physical findings
POLYARTERITIS NODOSA
(DEPENDS ON BODY SYSTEM)
- Hypertension (renal)
- Arthritic changes (musculoskeletal)
- Rash, purpura, nodules, and cutaneous infarcts (skin)
- Altered mental status and seizures (central nervous system)
- Respiratory distress, peripheral edema, hepatomegaly, peripheral vasoconstriction (cardiovascular)

Test results
DIAGNOSTIC PROCEDURES
- Not all vasculitis disorders can be diagnosed definitively through specific tests. The most useful general diagnostic procedure is biopsy of the affected vessel.

◆ TREATMENT

General
- Avoidance of antigenic drugs

Diet
- Avoidance of antigenic foods

Activity
- Avoidance of offending environmental substances

Medication
- Corticosteroids
- Antihypertensives
- Analgesics
- Immunosuppressives
- Antineoplastics

✿ NURSING CONSIDERATIONS

Nursing diagnoses
- Activity intolerance
- Chronic pain
- Decreased cardiac output
- Disturbed body image
- Disturbed sensory perception: Visual
- Hyperthermia
- Imbalanced nutrition: Less than body requirements
- Impaired gas exchange
- Impaired oral mucous membrane
- Impaired physical mobility
- Impaired skin integrity
- Ineffective breathing pattern
- Ineffective tissue perfusion: Cardiopulmonary
- Risk for infection
- Risk for injury

Key outcomes
The patient will:
- verbalize the importance of balancing activity, as tolerated, with rest
- express feelings of increased comfort and decreased pain
- maintain adequate cardiac output
- express positive feelings about self
- maintain optimal functioning within the confines of his visual impairment
- maintain a normal body temperature
- consume adequate daily caloric intake
- demonstrate adequate ventilation and oxygenation
- maintain intact oral mucuous membranes
- maintain joint range of motion and muscle strength to the fullest extent possible
- expereince healing of wounds and lesions without complications
- maintain a respiratory rate wthin 5 breaths/minute of baseline
- attain hemodynamic stability
- remain free from signs and symptoms of infection
- remain free from injury.

Nursing interventions
- Assess for dry nasal mucosa. Instill nose drops to lubricate the mucosa and minimize crusting; irrigate nasal passages with warm normal saline solution.
- Keep the patient well hydrated (about 3 L of fluid daily).

- Make sure that the patient with decreased visual acuity has a safe environment.
- Regulate environmental temperature to prevent additional vasoconstriction caused by cold.
- Provide emotional support to the patient and family members.

Monitoring
- Vital signs and neurologic status
- Signs and symptoms of organ involvement
- Laboratory values
- GI disturbances and renal function tests
- Intake and output and daily weight for edema

▶ PATIENT TEACHING

Be sure to cover:
- disorder, diagnostic tests, and treatment
- how to recognize adverse effects of drug therapy, watch for signs of bleeding, and report any of these findings to the physician
- importance of wearing warm clothes and gloves when going outside in cold weather.

Discharge planning
- Refer the patient to a smoking cessation program, if appropriate.

✹ RESOURCES

Organizations
Johns Hopkins Vasculitis Center: *www.vasculitis.med.jhu.edu*
Lupus Foundation of America: *www.lupus.org*
National Institute of Allergy and Infectious Diseases: *www.niaid.nih.gov*

Selected references
Kasper, D.L., et al., eds. *Harrison's Principles of Internal Medicine*, 16th ed. New York: McGraw-Hill Book Co., 2005.

Kim, S., and Dedeoglu, F. "Update on Pediatric Vasculitis," *Current Opinion in Pediatrics* 17(6):695-702, December 2005.

The Merck Manual of Diagnosis & Therapy, 18th ed. Whitehouse Station, N.J.: Merck and Co., Inc., 2006.

Rodriguez-Pla, A., and Stone, J.H. "Vasculitis and Systemic Infections," *Current Opinion in Rheumatology* 18(1):39-47, January 2006.

Russell, J.P., amd Gibson, L.E. "Primary Cutaneous Small Vessel Vasculitis: Approach to Diagnosis and Treatment," *International Journal of Dermatology* 45(1):3-13, January 2006.

Vitiligo

Description
- Hypopigmentation condition of the skin
- May cause a serious cosmetic problem
- Concurrent risk of other diseases, especially thyroid

Pathophysiology
- Destruction of melanocytes and circulating antibodies results in hypopigmented areas.

Causes
- Apparently, both genetic and environmental components
- About 30% of patients with a first-degree relative with the same disorder
- Precipitating factors:
  - Stressful physical or psychological events
  - Chemical agents, such as phenols and catechols
- Associated concurrent diseases:
  - Thyroid dysfunction
  - Pernicious anemia
  - Addison's disease
  - Aseptic meningitis
  - Diabetes mellitus

Incidence
- Affects about 1% of U.S. population
- Onset at any age
- About 50% of cases beginning between ages 10 and 30
- No racial predilection
- Affects males and females about equally; however, women tending to seek treatment more than men

Common characteristics
- Loss of pigment
- Locally increased sunburn

Complications
- Extreme photosensitivity in depigmented areas
- Hypersensitivity reactions to therapeutic agents and to dyes or cosmetics used to camouflage lesions

History
- Family history of vitiligo

Physical findings
- Depigmented or stark-white skin patches; almost imperceptible on fair-skinned whites
- Patches usually bilaterally symmetrical, with distinct borders that may be raised and hyperpigmented (see *Recognizing vitiligo*)
- Patches most likely over bony prominences, around orifices, within body folds, and at sites of traumatic injury
- Hair within lesions also possibly white
- Prematurely gray hair
- Ocular pigment changes

Test results
DIAGNOSTIC PROCEDURES
- Wood's light examination in a darkened room shows vitiliginous patches in fair-skinned patients.
- Skin biopsy confirms the diagnosis.

General
- Sunscreens
- Cosmetics and skin dyes as cover-ups
- Possibility of underlying thyroid disorder ruled out

Diet
- As tolerated

Activity
- As tolerated

Medication
- Repigmentation compounds
- Depigmentation creams

Surgery
- Skin grafting

RECOGNIZING VITILIGO

This illustration shows characteristic depigmented skin patches in vitiligo. These patches are usually bilaterally symmetrical, with distinct borders.

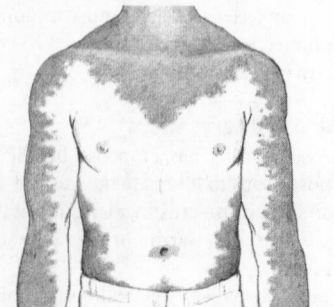

✤ NURSING CONSIDERATIONS

Nursing diagnoses
- Disturbed body image
- Risk for injury

Key outcomes
The patient will:
- verbalize feelings about changed body image
- remain free from injury.

Nursing interventions
- Encourage expression of feelings about the patient's appearance.
- Offer emotional support and reassurance.
- Reinforce treatment goals.

Monitoring
- Response to treatment
- Complications

▶ PATIENT TEACHING

Be sure to cover:
- disorder, diagnostic tests, and treatment
- that exposure to sunlight also darkens normal skin in patients undergoing repigmentation therapy
- use of sunscreen, sunglasses, and protective clothing
- that results of depigmentation are permanent
- adverse effects of sunlight.

Discharge planning
- Refer the patient to the National Vitiligo Foundation.

✸ RESOURCES

Organizations
American Academy of Dermatology:
www.aad.org
Dermatology Foundation:
www.dermfnd.org
National Vitiligo Foundation:
www.nvfi.org

Selected references

Don, P., et al. "Treatment of Vitiligo with Broadband Ultraviolet B and Vitamins," *International Journal of Dermatology* 45(1):63-65, January 2005.

Kostovic, K., and Pasic, A. "New Treatment Modalities for Vitiligo: Focus On Topical Immunomodulators," *Drugs* 65(4):447-59, 2005.

Leone, G., et al. "Tacalcitol and Narrow-Band Phototherapy in Patients with Vitiligo," *Clinical & Experimental Dermatology* 31(2):200-205, March 2006.

Ongenae, K., et al. "Psychosocial Effects of Vitiligo," *Journal of the European Academy of Dermatology and Venereology* 20(1):1-8, January 2006.

Tjioe, M., et al. "Topical Macrolide Immunomodulators: A Role in the Treatment of Vitiligo?" *American Journal of Clinical Dermatology* 7(1):7-12, 2006.

Volvulus

OVERVIEW

Description
- Twisting of the intestine at least 180 degrees on itself
- Marked by sudden onset of severe abdominal pain
- Results in blood vessel compression
- Causes obstruction both proximal and distal to the twisted loop
- Occurs in a bowel segment long enough to twist, most commonly the sigmoid colon (small bowel common site in children)
- Other common sites including the stomach and cecum

Pathophysiology
- The colon twists on its mesentery.
- A closed loop obstruction occurs, affecting venous drainage and arterial inflow.
- Cecal volvulus is a congenital defect in the peritoneum with inadequate fixation of the cecum. (See *What happens in volvulus.*)

Causes
- Anomaly of bowel rotation in utero
- Ingested foreign body
- Adhesions
- Meconium ileus (in patients with cystic fibrosis)

Risk factors
- Straining at stool
- Pregnancy
- Intestinal malignancy
- Hernia
- High-bulk diet
- History of previous attacks
- Use of chronic neuropsychotropic drugs
- Chronic constipation and laxative abuse

Incidence
- Varies worldwide in cases of volvulus of the large bowel
- Accounts for 1% to 5% of all large-bowel obstructions in advanced Western populations
- Most common sites: sigmoid colon (80%), cecum (15%), transverse colon (3%), and splenic flexure (2%)
- Common in regions of Africa, Southern Asia, and South America
- About 50% of large-bowel obstructions caused by volvulus occurring in the "volvulus belt" of Africa and the Middle East
- Affects men and women equally

Common characteristics
- Severe abdominal pain and distention
- Vomiting
- Constipation

Complications
- Strangulation of the twisted bowel loop
- Bowel ischemia and infarction
- Bowel perforation

ASSESSMENT

History
- Severe abdominal pain
- Bilious vomiting
- Constipation

Physical findings
- Abdominal distention
- Palpable abdominal mass

Test results
LABORATORY
- White blood cell count, in strangulation, is greater than 15,000/ml; in bowel infarction, it's greater than 20,000/ml.
IMAGING
- Abdominal X-rays may show multiple distended bowel loops and a large bowel without gas. In midgut volvulus, abdominal X-rays may be normal.
- In cecal volvulus, barium enema shows barium filling the colon distal to the affected section of cecum; in sigmoid volvulus, barium may twist to a point and, in adults, take on an "ace of spades" configuration.

TREATMENT

General
- For adults with sigmoid volvulus, nonsurgical treatment: proctoscopy to check for infarction and reduction by careful insertion of a flexible sigmoidoscope to deflate the bowel

Diet
- Nothing by mouth until condition resolves

Activity
- Bed rest until condition resolves

Medication
- I.V. therapy
- Antibiotics
- Analgesics

Surgery
- Warranted for children with midgut volvulus
- Detorsion (untwisting)
- Resection and anastomosis

NURSING CONSIDERATIONS

Nursing diagnoses
- Acute pain
- Deficient fluid volume
- Imbalanced nutrition: Less than body requirements
- Ineffective tissue perfusion: GI
- Risk for infection

Key outcomes
The patient will:
- express feelings of increased comfort and decreased pain
- maintain normal fluid balance
- achieve adequate caloric and nutritional intake
- regain normal bowel function
- remain free of signs and symptoms from infection

Nursing interventions
- Encourage verbalization and provide support.
- Administer mediations, as ordered.
- Administer I.V. fluids, as ordered.

Monitoring
- Pain control
- Bowel function
- Vital signs
- Fluid and electrolyte balance
- Nasogastric tube function and drainage
- Wound site

PATIENT TEACHING

Be sure to cover:
- disorder, diagnostic tests, and treatment
- preoperative teaching
- medication administration, dosage, and possible adverse effects
- signs and symptoms of infection
- importance of follow-up care.

RESOURCES

Organizations
Digestive Disease National Coalition: *www.ddnc.org*
National Digestive Diseases Information Clearinghouse: *www.niddk.nih.gov/health/digest/nddic.htm*

Selected references
Consorti, E.T., and Liu, T.H. "Diagnosis and Treatment of Caecal Volvulus," *Postgraduate Medical Journal* 81(962):772-76, December 2005.

McNally, P. *GI/Liver Secrets,* 3rd ed. Philadelphia: Hanley & Belfus, Inc. 2006.

Mourra, N., et al. "Chronic Schistosomiasis: An Incidental Finding in Sigmoid Volvulus," *Journal of Clinical Pathology* 59(1):111, January 2006.

Tiah, L., and Goh, S.H. "Sigmoid Volvulus: Diagnostic Twists and Turns," *European Journal of Emergency Medicine* 13(2):84-87, April 2006.

Tsang, T.K., et al. "Gastrointestinal: Sigmoid Volvulus," *Journal of Gastroenterology & Hepatology* 20(5):790, May 2005.

WHAT HAPPENS IN VOLVULUS

Although volvulus may occur anywhere in a bowel segment long enough to twist, the most common site, as this illustration depicts, is the sigmoid colon, causing edema within the closed loop and obstruction at its proximal and distal ends.

Normal bowel segment

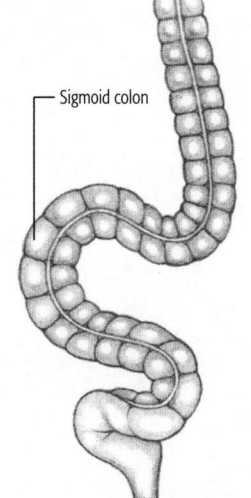

Sigmoid colon

Volvulus

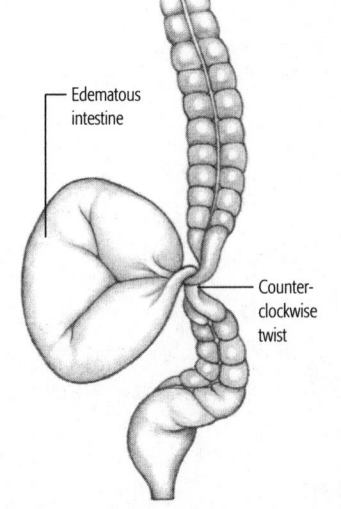

Edematous intestine

Counter-clockwise twist

Von Willebrand's disease

● OVERVIEW

Description
- Hereditary bleeding disorder characterized by prolonged bleeding time, moderate deficiency of clotting factor VIII (antihemophilic factor), and impaired platelet function
- Also known as *angiohemophilia, pseudohemophilia,* and *vascular hemophilia*

Pathophysiology
- Mild to moderate deficiency of factor VIII and defective platelet adhesion prolong coagulation time.
- This results from a deficiency of von Willebrand's factor (factor VIII_{VWF}), which appears to occupy the factor VIII molecule and may be necessary for the production of factor VIII and proper platelet function.
- Defective platelet function is characterized by decreased agglutination and adhesion at the bleeding site, reduced platelet retention when filtered through a column of packed glass beads, and diminished ristocetin-induced platelet aggregation.

Causes
- Inherited as an autosomal dominant trait
- Acquired form identified in patients with cancer and immune disorders

Incidence
- Affects both males and females; tends to be more common in males

Common characteristics
- Bleeding from the skin or mucosal surfaces
- In females, excessive uterine bleeding

Complications
- Hemorrhage

✳ ASSESSMENT

History
- Possible family history of the disease
- Easy bruising and frequent bleeding from the nose or gums (petechiae are rare)
- Menorrhagia
- Hemorrhage after a laceration or surgery
- Possible episodes of GI bleeding

Physical findings
- Bruises
- Clinical bleeding

Test results
LABORATORY
- Bleeding time is prolonged (more than 6 minutes).
- Partial thromboplastin time is slightly prolonged (more than 45 seconds).
- Factor VIII–related antigen levels are absent or reduced and factor VIII activity level is low.
- Platelet aggregation is defective in vitro (using the ristocetin coagulation factor assay test).
- Platelet count and clot retraction are normal.

◆ TREATMENT

General
- Dependent on the symptoms and underlying disease
- Decreasing bleeding time by local measures and replacing factor VIII and, consequently, factor VIII_{VWF}
- Avoidance of aspirin

Diet
- No restrictions

Activity
- Alternation of activities and rest periods if patient is fatigued after a bleeding episode

Medication
- Cryoprecipitate (cryoprecipitated antihemophilic factor)
- Plasma products or vasopressin analogue
- Factor VIII concentrates

✣ NURSING CONSIDERATIONS

Nursing diagnoses
- Activity intolerance
- Anxiety
- Disabled family coping
- Fatigue
- Ineffective coping
- Ineffective tissue perfusion: Cardiopulmonary
- Risk for deficient fluid volume
- Risk for injury

Key outcomes
The patient (or family) will:
- verbalize the importance of balancing activity, as tolerated, with rest
- verbalize strategies to reduce anxiety level
- seek support systems and exhibit adequate coping behaviors
- express feelings of energy and decreased fatigue
- exhibit adequate coping skills
- show evidence of hemodynamic stabillity
- maintain normal fluid volume
- remain free from injury.

Nursing interventions
- Focus on measures to control bleeding and on patient teaching to prevent bleeding, unnecessary trauma, and complications.
- Provide emotional support, as necessary.
- During a bleeding episode, elevate the area if possible, and apply cold compresses and gentle pressure to the bleeding site. (Pressure is often the only treatment necessary.)
- Give medications or transfusions, as ordered.
- If the patient is fatigued after a bleeding episode, alternate activities and rest periods.
- After bleeding episodes and surgery, be alert for signs of further bleeding.
- Prevent potential injury by using an electric razor, keeping the room free from clutter, and providing a cushioned sitting and sleeping surface (such as a convoluted foam mattress).

Monitoring
- Signs and symptoms of decreased tissue perfusion
- Vital signs
- Bleeding from the skin, mucous membranes, and wounds
- After surgery, bleeding time or other clotting procedure for 24 to 48 hours and for signs of new bleeding
- Adverse reactions to blood products

▶ PATIENT TEACHING

Be sure to cover:
- disorder, diagnostic tests, and treatment
- need to notify the physician after even minor trauma and before all surgery, including dental procedures, to determine whether replacement of blood components is necessary
- warnings against using aspirin and other drugs that impair platelet function (teach the patient and his parents how to recognize over-the-counter medications that contain aspirin)
- special precautions to prevent bleeding episodes
- importance of wearing a medical identification bracelet.

Discharge planning
- Refer parents of an affected child for genetic counseling.

✶ RESOURCES

Organizations
Centers for Disease Control and Prevention: *www.cdc.gov*
The Merck Manual Online Medical Library: *www.merck.com/mmhe*
National Hemophilia Foundation: *www.hemophilia.org*

Selected references
Franchini, M. "Thrombotic Complications to von Willebrand Disease," *Hematology* 11(1):49-52, February 2006.

Handbook of Pathophysiology, 2nd ed. Philadelphia: Lippincott Williams & Wilkins, 2005.

James, A.H. "von Willebrand Disease," *Obstetrical & Gynecological Survey* 61(2):136-45, February 2006.

Kasper, D.L., et al., eds. *Harrison's Principles of Internal Medicine,* 16th ed. New York: McGraw-Hill Book Co.

Michiels, J.J., et al. "Characterization, Classification, and Treatment of von Willebrand Diseases: A Critical Appraisal of the Literature and Personal Experiences," *Seminars in Thrombosis and Hemostasis* 31(5):577-601, November 2005.

Professional Guide to Diseases, 8th ed. Philadelphia: Lippincott Williams & Wilkins, 2005.

Tierney, L., et al. *Current Medical Diagnosis & Treatment 2006.* New York: McGraw-Hill Book Co., 2006.

Yoshida, K., et al. "Acquired von Willebrand Disease Type IIA in Patients with Aortic Valve Stenosis," *Annals of Thoracic Surgery* 81(3)1114-116, March 2006.

Vulvovaginitis

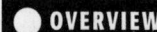

OVERVIEW

Description
- Inflammation of the vulva (vulvitis) and vagina (vaginitis)
- Good prognosis good with treatment

Pathophysiology
- Because of the proximity of the vulva and vagina, inflammation of one usually precipitates inflammation of the other.

Causes
VAGINITIS
- Protozoan infection (*Trichomonas vaginalis*)
- Fungal infection (*Candida albicans*)
- Bacterial infection (bacterial vaginosis)
- Venereal infection (*Neisseria gonorrhoeae)*
- Viral infection with venereal warts or herpes simplex virus type 2

VULVITIS
- Parasitic infection (*Phthirus pubis*, crab louse)
- Traumatic injury
- Poor personal hygiene
- Chemical irritations
- Allergic reactions, such as to douches or toilet paper
- Retention of a foreign body such as a tampon

Risk factors
- Pregnancy
- Hormonal contraceptives
- Diabetes mellitus
- Systemic broad-spectrum antibiotics
- Vaginal mucosa and vulval atrophy in menopausal women

Incidence
- Occurs at any age
- Affects most females at some time

Common characteristics
- Vaginal itching and discharge in most cases
- Vaginal discharge in many cases

Complications
- Inflammation of the perineum
- Skin breakdown
- Secondary infection

- Dyspareunia
- Dysuria

ASSESSMENT

History
TRICHOMONAL VAGINITIS
- Vaginal irritation and itching
- Urinary symptoms, such as burning and frequency

CANDIDAL VAGINITIS
- Intense vaginal itching

BACTERIAL VAGINOSIS
- Fishy-smelling discharge
- May be asymptomatic

GONORRHEA
- May be asymptomatic
- Dysuria

ACUTE VULVITIS
- Vulvar burning, pruritus
- Severe dysuria
- Dyspareunia

Physical findings
TRICHOMONAL VAGINITIS
- Thin, bubbly, green-tinged, and malodorous vaginal discharge

CANDIDAL VAGINITIS
- Thick, white, cottage cheese–like discharge
- Red, edematous mucous membranes with white flecks on vaginal wall

BACTERIAL VAGINOSIS
- Gray, foul, fishy-smelling discharge

GONORRHEA
- Profuse and purulent discharge

HERPESVIRUS INFECTION
- Ulceration or vesicle formation on the perineum (active phase)
- Severe edema that may involve entire perineum (chronic infection)

ACUTE VULVITIS
- Vulvar edema and erythema

Test results
LABORATORY
- Wet slide preparation and microscopic examination of vaginal exudates are used in obtaining various test results:
  - Vaginitis diagnosis requires identification of the infectious organism.
  - In trichomonal infections, the presence of motile, flagellated trichomonads confirms the diagnosis.

  - In monilial vaginitis, 10% potassium hydroxide is added to the slide; diagnosis requires identification of *C. albicans* fungus.
  - In bacterial vaginosis, saline wet mount shows the presence of clue cells, giving it a stippled appearance.
  - Gonorrhea requires a culture of vaginal exudate to confirm the diagnosis.
- Diagnosis of vulvitis or a suspected sexually transmitted disease (STD) may require a complete blood count, urinalysis, cytology screening, biopsy of chronic lesions to rule out cancer, and culture of exudate from acute lesions.

TREATMENT

General
- Cold compresses or cool sitz baths to relieve pruritus
- Warm compresses for severe inflammation
- Avoidance of drying soaps
- Loose clothing to promote air circulation
- For chronic vulvitis, changing problematic environmental factors

Diet
- No restrictions

Activity
- No restrictions

Medication
- Antibacterials
- Antiprotozoals
- Topical corticosteroids
- Antipruritics
- Topical estrogen ointments
- Antivirals

Nursing diagnoses
- Acute pain
- Disturbed body image
- Ineffective coping
- Ineffective sexuality patterns
- Risk for impaired skin integrity
- Risk for infection

Key outcomes
The patient will:
- express feelings of increased comfort and decreased pain
- express concerns about self-concept, self-esteem, and body image
- with her partner, use available counseling or support groups and develop effective coping mechanisms
- with her partner, verbalize feelings regarding the condition and how it affects their sexuality
- maintain intact skin integrity
- remain free from signs or symptoms of infection.

Nursing interventions
- Encourage expression of feelings.
- Help to develop effective coping strategies.
- Provide comfort measures.
- Use meticulous hand-washing technique.
- Report cases of STDs to the public health authorities.
- Administer medications, as ordered.

Monitoring
- Response to treatment
- Vaginal discharge
- Signs and symptoms of secondary infection

Be sure to cover:
- disorder, diagnostic tests, and treatment
- correlation between sexual contact and spread of vaginal infections
- use of condoms to prevent or decrease the spread of sexually transmitted infections
- notification of sexual partners of the need for treatment
- abstinence from sexual intercourse until the infection resolves
- completion of prescribed medication, even if symptoms subside
- proper application of vaginal ointments and suppositories
- need for meticulous hand washing before and after drug administration
- prevention of skin breakdown and secondary infections
- good hygiene practices
- wearing all-cotton white underpants and avoiding tight-fitting pants and panty hose
- abstinence from alcoholic beverages with metronidazole therapy
- that metronidazole therapy may turn the urine dark brown.

Organizations
American College of Obstetricians and Gynecologists: *www.acog.org*
American Society for Reproductive Medicine: *www.asrm.org*

Selected references
Kokotos. F., "Vulvovaginitis," *Pediatrics in Review/American Academy of Pediatrics* 27(3):116-17, March 2006.

Merkley, K. "Vulvovaginitis and Vaginal Discharge in the Pediatric Patient," *Journal of Emergency Nursing* 31(4):400-402, August 2005.

Say, P.J., and Jacyntho, C. "Difficult-to-Manage Vaginitis," *Clinical Obstetrics and Gynecology* 48(4):753-68, December 2005.

Theroux, R. "Factors Influencing Women's Decisions to Self-treat Vaginal Symptoms," *Journal of the American Academy of Nurse Practitioners* 17(4):156-62, April 2005.

West Nile encephalitis

OVERVIEW

Description
- An infectious disease, part of a family of vector-borne diseases that also includes malaria, yellow fever, and Lyme disease
- Mortality rate from 3% to 15%; higher in elderly population
- Ticks infected with the virus found in Africa and Asia only; role of ticks in transmission and maintenance of the virus uncertain
- Also called *West Nile virus (WNV)*

Pathophysiology
- Mosquitoes become infected by feeding on birds contaminated with the virus.
- The virus is transmitted to a human by the bite of an infected mosquito (mostly the Culex species).
- The incubation period is 5 to 15 days after exposure.
- Disease primarily causes inflammation or encephalitis of the brain.

Causes
- A flavivirus commonly found in humans, birds, and other vertebrates in Africa, West Asia, and the Middle East

Risk factors
- Recent chemotherapy
- Recent organ transplantation
- Immunocompromised state
- Pregnancy
- Advanced age
- Breast-feeding

Incidence
- In temperate areas, occurs mainly in late summer or early fall
- In milder climates, can occur year-round
- Risk greater in areas with active cases
- Greatest risk in those over age 50 and those with compromised immune systems
- No documented evidence that human fetus is at risk due to a woman's infection with WNV

Common characteristics
- Mostly asymptomatic; only 1 in 300 get sick
- Generalized malaise

Complications
- Neurologic impairment
- Seizures
- Death

ASSESSMENT

History
- Headache
- Body aches
- Neck stiffness
- Possible recent exposure to bodies of water, dead birds, or recent mosquito bites

Physical findings
- Fever
- Skin rash
- Swollen lymph glands
- Stupor and disorientation

Test results
LABORATORY
- White blood cell (WBC) count is normal or increased.
- The enzyme-linked immunosorbent assay (ELISA) and the IgM Antibody Capture (MAC)-ELISA allow a rapid and definitive diagnosis.
- Accurate diagnosis is possible only when serum or cerebrospinal fluid specimens are obtained while the patient is still hospitalized with acute illness and they show an elevated WBC cell count and protein levels.

IMAGING
- Magnetic resonance imaging may show inflammation.

TREATMENT

General
- No specific treatment
- Respiratory support

Diet
- Increased fluid intake

Activity
- Rest periods when fatigued

Medication
- Antipyretics

Nursing diagnoses
- Acute pain
- Decreased cardiac output
- Deficient fluid volume
- Hyperthermia
- Impaired tissue integrity
- Ineffective tissue perfusion: Cardiopulmonary

Key outcomes
The patient will:
- express feelings of increased comfort and decreased pain
- exhibit adequate cardiac output
- exhibit an adequate fluid volume
- remain afebrile
- maintain collateral circulation
- maintain hemodynamic stability.

Nursing interventions
- Maintain adequate hydration with I.V. fluids.
- Administer medications, as ordered.
- Provide respiratory support measures, when applicable.
- Use standard precautions when handling blood or other body fluids.
- Report any suspected cases of West Nile encephalitis to the state department of health.

Monitoring
- Fluid and electrolyte status
- Neurologic status
- Vital signs

Be sure to cover:
- disorder, diagnostic tests, and treatment
- proper use of insect repellants, which can irritate the eyes and mouth, and to avoid applying repellant to the hands of children (repellant shouldn't be applied to children under age 3)
- expected course and outcomes of the illness
- need to drink fluids to avoid dehydration
- how to control mosquitoes from breeding by:
  - cleaning out birdbaths and wading pools at least once per week
  - cleaning roof gutters and downspout screens regularly
  - eliminating any standing water
  - not allowing water to collect in trash cans
  - turning over or removing containers in yards where rainwater collects, such as in toys and old tires.

Discharge planning
- Refer the patient to an infectious disease specialist. (See *Preventing West Nile virus.*)

Organizations
National Center for Infectious Diseases: *www.cdc.gov/ncidod*
National Institute of Allergy and Infectious Disease: *www.niaid.nih.gov*
World Health Organization: *www.who.int*

Selected references
Abroug, F., et al. "A Cluster Study of Predictors of Severe West Nile Virus Infection," *Mayo Clinic Proceedings* 81(1):12-16, January 2006.
Avalos-Bock, S.A. "West Nile Virus and the U.S. Blood Supply: New Tests Substantially Reduce the Risk of Transmission via Donated Blood Products," *AJN* 105(12):34, 36-37, December 2005.
Civen, R., et al. "West Nile Virus Infection in the Pediatric Population," *Pediatric Infectious Disease Journal* 25(1):75-78, January 2006.

PREVENTING WEST NILE VIRUS

To reduce the risk of infection with West Nile encephalitis, advise patients to:
- stay indoors at dawn, dusk, and early evening when mosquitoes are biting
- wear long-sleeved shirts and long pants when outdoors
- apply insect repellent sparingly to exposed skin (Effective repellents contain 20% to 30% DEET [N,N-diethyltoluamide]. DEET in concentrations greater than 30% can cause adverse effects, particularly in children, and should be avoided; adults should apply repellent on children with no more than 10% DEET.)
- not use repellent under clothing
- not apply repellent over cuts, wounds, sunburn, or irritated skin
- wash repellent off daily and reapply, as needed.

Whooping cough

● OVERVIEW

Description
- Highly contagious respiratory infection
- Typically causes an irritating cough that becomes paroxysmal and ends in a high-pitched, inspiratory whoop
- Follows a 6- to 8-week course that includes three 2-week stages with varying symptoms
- Also called *pertussis*

Pathophysiology
- The infecting organism adheres to ciliated epithelial cells and multiplies.
- The resulting local mucosal damage induces paroxysmal coughing, which enhances disease transmission.
- Various toxins produced during the infection impair local defenses and cause local tissue damage. Toxins may also cause direct central nervous system injury.

Causes
- Nonmotile, gram-negative coccobacillus *Bordetella pertussis;* occasionally, *B. parapertussis* or *B. bronchiseptica* (see Bordetella pertussis)
- Spreads indirectly through soiled linen and other articles contaminated by respiratory secretions
- Typically transmitted by direct inhalation of contaminated droplets from someone in the acute disease stage

Incidence
- Fifty percent of cases seen in under-immunized children younger than age 1
- Commonly occurs in schools, nursing homes, and residential facilities
- Epidemics occurring every 3 to 5 years without seasonal variation

Common characteristics
CATARRHAL (INITIAL) STAGE
- Hacking nocturnal cough
- Anorexia
- Sneezing, lacrimation, and rhinnorhea
PAROXYSMAL (SECOND) STAGE
- Spasmodic, recurrent coughing with tenacious mucus; cough typically ending in a loud, crowing, inspiratory whoop
- Vomiting (if patient chokes on mucus)
CONVALESCENT (THIRD) STAGE
- Gradual subsidence of paroxysmal coughing and vomiting

Complications
- Increased venous pressure
- Anterior eye chamber hemorrhage
- Detached retina and blindness
- Rectal prolapse
- Inguinal or umbilical hernia
- Encephalopathy, seizures
- Atelectasis or pneumonitis
- Apnea, anoxia (in infants)
- Otitis media
- Pneumonia
- Cerebral hemorrhage

✳ ASSESSMENT

History
- Possible lack of immunization coupled with exposure to pertussis during previous 3 weeks

Physical findings
- Low or normal body temperature
- Mild conjunctivitis
- Listlessness
- Engorged neck veins
- Epistaxis during paroxysmal coughing
- Exhaustion and cyanosis after coughing spell
- Diminished breath sounds, upper airway wheezing
- Cough that produces a high-pitched "whooping" sound
- Vomiting from repeated coughing
- Choking spells (in infants)

Test results
LABORATORY
- White blood cell count and differential show lymphocytosis.
- Nasopharyngeal swabs and sputum culture find *B. pertussis* in early disease stages.
- Direct immunofluorescence shows antigen.

◆ TREATMENT

General
- For infants and elderly patients, hospitalization with vigorous supportive therapy and fluid and electrolyte replacement

Diet
- Adequate nutrition with small, frequent meals
- Increased fluid intake

Activity
- Rest periods when fatigued

Medication
- Oxygen
- Antibiotics

BORDETELLA PERTUSSIS

This microscopic enlargement shows *Bordetella pertussis,* the nonmotile, gram-negative coccobacillus that commonly causes whooping cough. After entering the tracheobronchial tree, pertussis causes mucus to become increasingly tenacious. The classic 6-week course of whooping cough follows.

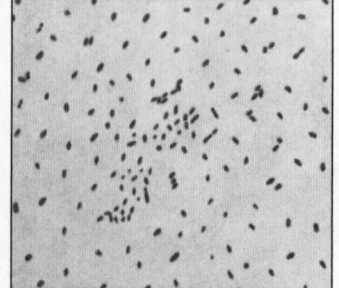

♣ NURSING CONSIDERATIONS

Nursing Diagnoses
- Activity intolerance
- Acute pain
- Anxiety
- Deficient fluid volume
- Impaired gas exchange
- Ineffective airway clearance
- Ineffective breathing pattern
- Risk for infection
- Risk for injury

Key Outcomes
The patient will:
- return to a normal activity level
- express feelings of increased comfort and decreased pain
- identify strategies to reduce anxiety
- attain and maintain normal fluid and electrolyte balance
- maintain adequate ventilation and oxygenation
- maintain a patent airway
- remain free from adventitious breath sounds
- remain free from infection
- remain free from injury.

Nursing interventions
- Maintain infection control precautioins (mask only) for 5 to 7 days after antibiotic therapy begins.
- Provide oxygen and moist air, as ordered; if needed, assist respiration.
- Suction secretions, as necessary.
- Elevate the head of the bed to ease breathing.
- Create a quiet environment to decrease coughing stimulation.
- Assess for complications caused by excessive coughing.
- Provide emotional support to the patient and parents, as appropriate.
- Report cases to local public health authorities.

Monitoring
- Respiratory status
- Acid-base balance
- Fluid and electrolyte balance

▶ PATIENT TEACHING

Be sure to cover:
- disorder, diagnostic tests, and treatment
- need for the patient's close contacts to get medical care
- when to notify the practitioner
- importance of immunization and vaccinations and the need to notify the practitioner of adverse reactions to the vaccine.

Discharge planning
- Refer the patient to a pulmonologist for follow-up care, as indicated.

✳ RESOURCES

Organizations
American Lung Association: *www.lungusa.org*
Centers for Disease Control and Prevention: *www.cdc.gov*
Harvard Medical School's Consumer Health Information: *www.intelihealth.com*
National Health Information Center: *www.health.gov/nhic/*
National Institute of Allergy and Infectious Diseases: *www.niaid.nih.gov*
National Library of Medicine: *www.nlm.nih.gov*

Selected references
Casey, I.R., and Pichichero, M.E. "Acellular Pertussis Vaccine Safety and Efficacy in Children, Adolescents and Adults," *Drugs* 65(10):1367-389, 2005.

Edwards, K., and Freeman, D.M. "Adolescent and Adult Pertussis: Disease Burden and Prevention," *Current Opinion in Pediatrics* 18(1):77-80, February 2006.

Hu, J.J., et al. "Survey of Pertussis in Patients with Prolonged Cough," *Journal of Microbiology, Immunology, and Infection* 39(1):54-58, February 2006.

Kasper, D.L., et al, eds. *Harrison's Principles of Internal Medicine,* 16th ed. New York: McGraw-Hill Book Co., 2005.

Part II > TREATMENTS

Ablation therapy for arrhythmias

● OVERVIEW

- Destroys heart tissue that's creating a heart beat originating outside the sinoatrial node or permitting conduction of such foci.
- Type of ablation performed dependent on the type of arrhythmia and the presence of other heart disease:
  - Surgical ablation
  - Minimally invasive ablation
  - The Maze or Cox-Maze III procedure (gold standard for arrhythmia treatment)
  - Radiofrequency ablation
  - Microwave, ultrasound, laser ablation, and cryoablation

Indications
- Atrial fibrillation
- Atrial flutter
- Supraventricular tachycardia, including atrioventricular (AV) nodal reentry and Wolff-Parkinson-White syndrome, and ventricular tachycardias

▶ PROCEDURE

- The procedure is typically performed under conscious sedation with an I.V. tranquilizer and opioid. General anesthesia is used in children and selected adults undergoing surgical ablation.
- A nonsurgical procedure generally takes place in the electrophysiology laboratory. The patient's groin area is shaved and his neck, upper chest, arm, and groin are cleaned with antiseptic.
- A local anesthetic is used.
- Two to five map and ablating electrode catheters are inserted via the femoral or internal jugular vein into the left, right or both sides of the heart. The coronary sinus may also be evaluated
- Anticoagulation with I.V. heparin is used to reduce the risk of embolism.
- The patient is connected to monitors for electrocardiography, heart rate, blood pressure, pulse oximetry and, possibly, hemodynamic monitoring.
- After the catheters are in place, the heart's conduction system is assessed and present rhythm confirmed.

- The physician then uses a pacemaker to initiate the arrhythmia. Then the physician steers the catheters to determine the arrhythmia area of origin. Energy is applied to ablate the source.
- To help facilitate the ablation process, three-dimensional electroanatomical mapping systems are projected on monitors. Intracardiac echocardiography may also be used.
- When the ablation is complete, the physician monitors the electrocardiogram (ECG) to verify correction of the arrhythmic trigger.
- The physician removes the catheters from the groin and pressure is applied to the site.

◆ **NURSING ALERT** The patient may feel some discomfort or a burning sensation in the chest when the tissue is being destroyed. Determine his analgesic needs if the patient would like extra pain medication. Also remind him that the discomfort is normal and that he should try to lie quietly and avoid taking deep breaths.

Complications
- Death (rare)
- Cardiac complications: high-grade AV block, cardiac tamponade, coronary artery spasm or thrombosis, pericarditis, arrhythmias, hypotension
- Retroperitoneal bleeding
- Hematoma and infection at access site
- Thromboembolism, vascular injury
- Hypotension
- Transient ischemic attack or stroke
- Pulmonary vein stenosis
- Pneumothorax
- Left atrial-esophageal fistula
- Acute pyloric spasm or gastric hypomotility
- Phrenic nerve paralysis

✳ NURSING INTERVENTIONS

Pretreatment care
- Explain the treatment and preparation to the patient and his family.
- Verify that the patient has signed an appropriate consent form.
- Obtain a 12-lead ECG and laboratory tests, as ordered.
- Confirm that cardiac drugs with electrophysiologic effects, such as beta-adrenergic blockers, calcium-channel blockers, digoxin, and class I and III antiarrhythmics, were reduced or discontinued, as instructed. Verify that warfarin (Coumadin) therapy has also been stopped as ordered, and obtain serum coagulation testing.
- Ask the woman of childbearing age if it's possible that she could be pregnant, and notify the physician of results because exposure to radiation should be avoided.
- Confirm that the patient has had no food or fluids since 12 a.m. the day of the procedure.

◆ **NURSING ALERT** Left atrial ablation a flutter is contraindicated if an atrial thrombus is present. Left ventricular ablation is contraindicated if a left ventricular thrombus is present. Ablation catheters usually aren't inserted through a mechanical prosthetic heart valve.

Posttreatment care
- Enforce bed rest for 1 to 6 hours, as ordered, with the operative leg extended during this time to prevent bleeding.
- Initiate anticoagulant therapy to prevent thromboembolic events.

MONITORING
- Cardiac rhythm for arrhythmias
- Vital signs
- Insertion site

Patient teaching
Be sure to cover:
- insertion site care, emphasizing keeping the area clean and dry and reporting any redness, swelling, or drainage
- reporting of signs and symptoms indicating that his arrhythmia is recurring
- healing possibly taking up to 6 to 8 weeks
- medication administration, dosage, and possible adverse effects
- pulse monitoring and recording
- (for ablation along the triscuspid or mitral valve annulus) need for antibiotics to prevent endocarditis that may be recommended for up to 12 weeks postablation.

Adrenalectomy

- Surgical resection or removal of one or both of the adrenal glands
- May be performed laparascopically or through abdominal incision.

Indications
- Adrenal hyperfunction
- Hyperaldosteronism
- Benign or malignant adrenal tumor
- Secondary treatment of neoplasms or corticotropin oversecretion
- Pheochromcytoma

▶ PROCEDURE

- After the patient is anesthetized, an anterior (transperitoneal) or a posterior (lumbar) approach is used.
- The adrenal gland is identified and dissected free from the upper pole of the kidney.
- Wound closure follows.
- If adrenalectomy is done because of a tumor, the glands are explored first; then the tumor is resected or one or both of the glands is removed.
- In pheochromocytoma, the affected adrenal gland is excised, and the abdominal organs are palpated for other tumors.

Complications
- Acute life-threatening adrenal crisis
- Hemorrhage
- Poor wound healing
- Hypoglycemia
- Electrolyte disturbances
- Pancreatic injury
- Hypotension (with gland removal)
- Hypertension (with gland manipulation)

✴ NURSING INTERVENTIONS

Pretreatment care
- Explain the treatment and preparation to the patient and family.
- Make sure the patient has signed an appropriate consent form.
- Administer medications to control hypertension, edema, diabetes, cardiovascular symptoms, and increased infection risk, as needed and ordered.
- Administer aldosterone antagonists for blood pressure control, as ordered.
- Give glucocorticoids on the morning of surgery, as ordered.
- Draw blood samples for laboratory test, as ordered.

FOR PATIENT WITH PHEOCHROMOCYTOMA
- One to 2 weeks before surgery, administer:
  - catecholamine-synthesis blockers as ordered
  - medications to control hypertension and tachycardia as ordered.
- Monitor patient for the following:
  - Arrhythmias
  - Palpitations
  - Severe headache
  - Hypertension
  - Hyperglycemia
  - Nausea, vomiting
  - Diaphoresis
  - Vision disturbances

Posttreatment care
TO COUNTERACT SHOCK
- Administer I.V. vasopressors; titrate the dosage to the patient's blood pressure response, as ordered.
- Increase the I.V. fluid rate, as ordered.
- Administer glucocorticoids I.V., as ordered.
- Administer analgesics, as ordered.
- Keep the room cool.

MONITORING
- Vital signs
- Intake and output
- Hemorrhage and shock
- Invasive arterial pressure
- Adrenal hypofunction
- Acute adrenal crisis
- Hypoglycemia
- Serum electrolyte levels
- Surgical wound and dressings
- Abdominal distention and return of bowel sounds

Patient teaching
Be sure to cover:
- medication administration, dosage, and possible adverse effects
- avoidance of sudden steroid withdrawal
- complications
- when to notify the physician
- follow-up medical care
- adjustment of steroid dosage during stress or illness
- signs and symptoms of adrenal insufficiency
- reversal of physical disease signs within a few months (with adrenal hyperfunction)
- wound care instructions
- signs and symptoms of infection
- stress-reduction techniques, if appropriate
- importance of wearing medical identification.

Amputation

● OVERVIEW

- Surgical removal of an extremity (see *Common levels of amputation*)
- Closed technique: skin flaps used to cover the bone stump
- Open (guillotine) amputation: tissue and bone are cut flush; wound is left open to be repaired in a second operation

Indications

- To preserve function in a remaining part
- To prevent death
- Severe trauma
- Gangrene
- Cancer
- Vascular disease
- Congenital deformity
- Thermal injury

▶ PROCEDURE

- The patient receives general or local anesthesia.

CLOSED TECHNIQUE

- Tissue is incised to the bone, leaving sufficient skin to cover the limb end.
- Bleeding is controlled by tying off the bleeding vessels above the site.
- The bone (or joint) is sawed and filed, with the periosteum removed about ¼″ (0.5 cm) from the bone end.
- All vessels are ligated and nerves are divided.
- Opposing muscles are sutured over the bone end and periosteum.
- Skin flaps are closed and an incisional drain is placed.
- Soft dressings are applied; rigid dressings may be used in below-the-knee amputation.

OPEN OR GUILLOTINE AMPUTATION

- A perpendicular incision is made through the bone and all tissue.
- The wound isn't sutured closed.
- A large, bulky dressing is applied.

Complications

- Infection
- Contractures
- Skin breakdown, necrosis
- Phantom pain

✳ NURSING INTERVENTIONS

Pretreatment care

- Explain the treatment and preparation to the patient and family.
- Make sure the patient has signed an appropriate consent form.
- Provide emotional support.
- Arrange for the patient to meet with a well-adjusted amputee, if possible.
- Demonstrate prescribed exercises.
- Administer broad-spectrum antibiotics, as ordered.

Posttreatment care

- Elevate the affected limb, as ordered.
- Provide analgesics, as ordered.
- Keep the stump wrapped properly with elastic compression bandages or a stump shrinker, as ordered.
- Provide cast care if a rigid plaster dressing has been applied.
- Maintain the patient in proper body alignment.
- Provide regular physical therapy.
- Encourage frequent ambulation.
- Encourage active or passive range-of-motion exercises.
- Help the patient with turning and positioning without propping the limb on a pillow.
- Provide emotional support.

MONITORING

- Vital signs
- Intake and output
- Surgical wound and dressings
- Bleeding
- Drain patency and drainage
- Pain

Patient teaching

Be sure to cover:

- medication administration, dosage, and possible adverse effects
- postoperative care and rehabilitation
- prosthesis and its care
- phantom limb sensation
- daily examination of the distal limb
- daily limb care and dressings
- signs and symptoms of infection
- complications
- when to notify the physician
- use of elastic bandages or a stump shrinker
- proper crutch use, as appropriate
- activities to toughen the residual limb
- follow-up care
- referral for psychological counseling or social services, as indicated
- referral to a local support group.

COMMON LEVELS OF AMPUTATION

Amputation may be performed at a wide range of sites. Review this list for common types and levels of amputation.

- *Partial foot:* removal of one or more toes and part of the foot
- *Total foot:* removal of the foot below the ankle joint
- *Ankle (Syme's amputation):* removal of the foot at the ankle joint
- *Below-the-knee:* removal of the leg 5″ to 7″ (12.5 to 17.5 cm) below the knee
- *Knee disarticulation:* removal of the patella, with the quadriceps brought over the end of the femur, or fixation of the patella to a cut surface between the condyles (Gritti-Stokes amputation)
- *Above-the-knee:* removal of the leg from 3″ (7.5 cm) above the knee
- *Hip disarticulation:* removal of the leg and hip or the leg and pelvis
- *Hemipelvectomy:* removal of a leg and half of the pelvis
- *Fingers:* removal of one or more fingers at the hinge or condyloid joints
- *Wrist disarticulation:* removal of the hand at the wrist
- *Below-the-elbow:* removal of the lower arm about 7″ below the elbow
- *Elbow disarticulation:* removal of the lower arm at the elbow
- *Above-the-elbow:* removal of the arm from 3″ above the elbow

Angioplasty, percutaneous transluminal coronary

● OVERVIEW

- Nonsurgical alternative to coronary artery bypass surgery; commonly called *PTCA*
- Uses a tiny balloon catheter to dilate a coronary artery narrowed by atherosclerotic plaque
- May include placement of a regular or drug-eluting stent

Indications
- Documented myocardial ischemia
- Proximal lesion in a single coronary artery
- Multivessel disease
- Acute myocardial infarction (MI)
- Totally occluded coronary arteries
- Post-thrombolytic therapy with high-grade stenosis
- Previous coronary artery bypass surgery
- High risk for complications associated with coronary artery bypass surgery
- Stenosis that narrows the arterial lumen by 70% or greater

▶ PROCEDURE

- The catheter insertion site, usually femoral, is prepared and anesthetized.
- A guide wire is inserted into the femoral artery using a percutaneous or cutdown approach.
- The catheter is guided fluoroscopically to the target coronary artery.
- The lesion is confirmed by angiography.
- A small, double-lumen, balloon-tipped catheter is inserted over the guide wire and positioned properly.
- The balloon is inflated repeatedly with normal saline solution and contrast medium for about 15 to 30 seconds, to a pressure of 6 atmospheres.
- The expanding balloon compresses the plaque, expanding the arterial lumen and pressure gradients across the stenotic area.
- The balloon is inflated repeatedly until the residual gradient decreases to about 20% or until the pressure gradient measures less than 16 mm Hg. The stent is fixed to a vessel during the procedure

- Angiography is repeated.
- The catheter and sheath are removed and pressure is applied to the insertion site.
- Depending on facility policy, a pressure device may be applied to the insertion site.

Complications
- Arterial dissection
- Coronary artery rupture
- Cardiac tamponade
- Myocardial ischemia or infarction
- Abrupt reclosure of the affected artery (occurs within a few hours)
- Restenosis (occurs within 30 days to 6 months)
- Coronary artery spasm
- Arrhythmias
- Bleeding
- Hematoma
- Thromboembolism
- Adverse reactions to contrast medium

✳ NURSING INTERVENTIONS

Pretreatment care
- Explain the treatment and preparation to the patient and family.
- Make sure the patient has signed an appropriate consent form.
- Tell the patient that contrast medium injection may cause a flushing sensation or transient nausea.
- Check for and report a history of allergies or adverse reactions to shellfish, iodine, or contrast medium.
- Restrict food and fluid intake for at least 6 hours before the procedure.
- Obtain results of coagulation studies, complete blood count, serum electrolyte studies, and blood typing and crossmatching, as ordered.
- Weigh the patient.
- Insert I.V. line and arterial line, if ordered; apply electrocardiogram leads, automatic blood pressure cuff, and pulse oximeter.
- Locate and mark bilateral distal pulses.
- Administer a sedative, as ordered.

Posttreatment care
- Administer anticoagulants and I.V. nitroglycerin, as ordered.
- Administer I.V. fluids, as ordered.

- Keep the affected extremity straight, as ordered.
- Elevate the head of the bed no more than 15 degrees, as ordered.
- If an expanding ecchymosis appears, mark the area, and obtain hemoglobin and hematocrit samples, as ordered.
- Report bleeding sites to the physician, and apply direct pressure to them.
- After sheath removal, apply direct pressure to the insertion site until hemostasis occurs.
- Apply a pressure dressing, as ordered.

MONITORING
- Vital signs
- Intake and output
- Heart rate and rhythm
- Electrocardiogram results
- Invasive arterial pressures
- Peripheral pulses
- Neurovascular status of extremities
- Hematoma formation, ecchymosis, or bleeding at the catheter insertion site
- Chest pain or other angina symptoms
- Signs and symptoms of infection
- Fluid overload
- Abrupt arterial reclosure

Patient teaching
Be sure to cover:
- medication administration, dosage, and possible adverse effects
- puncture site care
- activity restrictions, if applicable
- follow-up care and testing
- signs and symptoms of bleeding, infection, and restenosis
- complications
- when to notify the physician.

Appendectomy

● OVERVIEW

- Surgical removal of an inflamed vermiform appendix
- Prevents imminent rupture or perforation of the appendix
- May involve laparoscopy for diagnosis and appendix removal

Indications
- Acute appendicitis

▶ PROCEDURE

- The patient receives general anesthesia.
- The surgeon makes an incision in the right lower abdominal quadrant to expose the appendix.
- In laparoscopic appendectomy, three to four small abdominal incisions are made.
- The base of the appendix is ligated.
- A purse-string suture is placed in the cecum.
- Excessive fluid or tissue debris is removed from the abdominal cavity.
- The incision is closed.
- If perforation occurs, one or more Penrose drains or abdominal sump tubes, or both, are placed before the incision is closed.

Complications
- Infection
- Paralytic ileus

WITH PERFORATION
- Local or general peritonitis
- Paralytic ileus
- Intestinal obstruction
- Abscess

✳ NURSING INTERVENTIONS

Pretreatment care
- Explain the treatment and preparation to the patient and family.
- Make sure the patient has signed an appropriate consent form.
- Administer prophylactic antibiotics, as ordered.
- Administer I.V. fluids, as ordered.
- Insert a nasogastric (NG) tube, as ordered.
- Place the patient in Fowler's position.
- Avoid giving analgesics, cathartics, or enemas or applying heat to the abdomen.
- Provide reassurance.

Posttreatment care
- Place the patient in Fowler's position after anesthesia wears off.
- Ensure the patency of drainage catheters and tubes.
- Encourage the patient to ambulate as soon as possible.
- Encourage coughing, deep breathing, and frequent position changes.
- Gradually resume oral intake after NG tube removal and return of bowel sounds.
- Assist with emergency treatment of peritonitis if needed.

MONITORING
- Vital signs
- Intake and output
- Bowel sounds
- Surgical wounds and dressings
- Signs and symptoms of peritonitis
- Drainage
- Complications

Patient teaching
Be sure to cover:
- medication administration, dosage, and possible adverse effects
- signs and symptoms of infection
- signs and symptoms of intestinal obstruction
- complications
- when to notify the physician
- wound care
- activity restrictions
- follow-up care.

Biliopancreatic diversion

● OVERVIEW

- Procedure that restricts both food intake and the amount of calories and nutrients the body absorbs to achieve long-term, major weight loss in individuals weighing more than 100 lb (45 kg) over their ideal body weight
- Stomach capacity: 4 to 5 oz after biliopancreatic diversion (BPD), compared with 1 oz after standard gastric bypass operation, making it a less restrictive option
- Two types of BPD surgery:
  - BPD: stomach removed just below the esophagus forming a small pouch; remaining pouch connected to the ileum, freed duodenal and jejunal limbs of the small intestine then connected to the lower end of the ileum.
  - BPD with duodenal switch (BPD/DS): smaller part of stomach removed; pyloric valve and small segment of the duodenum retained, duodenal area then connected to the ileum; remaining portion of stomach, duodenum, and jejunum then reconnected to lower end of the ileum.

Indications

- Obesity for at least 5 years without a history of alcohol abuse, untreated depression, or other psychiatric disorder
- Body mass index (BMI) 40 or higher despite repeated attempts to lose weight
- BMI 35 to 40 and presence of a life-threatening or disabling condition related to weight

▶ PROCEDURE

- The patient is placed under general anesthesia. With an open procedure, a large incision is made in the abdomen. With the laparoscopic approach, several small incisions are made, carbon dioxide gas is insufflated into the abdomen to separate the organs, and smaller instruments and a camera are used to guide the surgery.

BPD

- All but a portion of the stomach is removed.
- The stomach pouch is connected directly to the ileum, through an opening made in the mesothelium.
- The bypassed portions of the intestine are anastomosed to the final 2′ to 4′ (1.2 m) of ileum, forming a common channel before entering the colon.
- The newly anastomosed sites are checked for leakage by filling with sterile saline solution.

BPD/DS

- The pyloric valve and about 2″ (5 cm) of the proximal duodenum is preserved, as a large portion of the stomach is excised, parallel to the greater curvature.
- An opening in the mesothelium is created and the ileum is attached to the residual duodenum.
- The detached stomach, duodenum, and jejunum are connected to the final 2′ to 4′ (0.6 to 1.2 m) of the distal ileum, as in BPD.

Complications

- Loose stools or dumping syndrome
- Malodorous gas
- Serious deficiencies in protein, fat, calcium, iron, or vitamins B_{12}, A, D, E, and K due to malabsorption
- Paralytic ileus
- Stomal ulcers (rare with BPD/DS)
- Anemia
- Infection or poor wound healing at the incision site
- Peritonitis
- Embolization of the large bowel or lungs
- Gallstones due to rapid weight loss
- Death (rare)

✳ NURSING INTERVENTIONS

Pretreatment care

- Verify that the patient has signed an informed consent form, that preoperative testing results are available, and that patient has completed preoperative bowel cleansing and not had anything to eat or drink after midnight.
- Insert an I.V. access device
- Administer an antibiotic, as ordered.

- Explain the treatment, preparation, and postoperative care to the patient and his family, including I.V. therapy, need for a nasogastric (NG) tube for a few days after surgery, and possible insertion of abdominal drains.
- Prepare the patient for early postoperative ambulation.

Posttreatment care

- Maintain I.V. replacement therapy, as ordered.
- Keep the NG tube patent, but don't reposition it.
- Provide care of incisions and skin folds, as indicated.
- Encourage regular coughing and deep-breathing exercises.
- Teach splinting the incision site.
- Administer medications, as ordered.
- Provide comfort measures.

MONITORING

- Incision and drainage
- Vital signs, intake and output, and daily weight

◈ **NURSING ALERT** Immediately report signs and symptoms of anastomotic leakage, including low-grade fever, malaise, slight leukocytosis, abdominal distention, tenderness, hemorrhage, hypovolemic shock, blood in stool, and wound drainage.

- Abdominal pain or cramps and shoulder pain

Patient teaching

Be sure to cover:
- avoidance of abdominal straining and lifting until the practitioner approves
- return to activities, as directed
- follow-up appointments
- dumping syndrome and relief measures
- lifestyle changes and changes in taste and tolerance for different foods
- need for lifelong fat-soluble (A, D, E, K) vitamin supplementation
- follow-up laboratory studies
- medication administration, dosage, and adverse effects
- incision site care
- signs and symptoms of infection
- complications
- when to notify the practitioner.

Bone marrow transplantation

● OVERVIEW

- Infusion of fresh or stored bone marrow into bloodstream
- Autologous donation: bone marrow harvested from the patient (before chemotherapy or radiation, or during remission) and frozen for later use
- Syngeneic donation: bone marrow donated by the patient's identical twin
- Allogeneic donation: bone marrow donated by a histocompatible individual

Indications
- Aplastic anemia
- Severe combined immunodeficiency disease
- Acute leukemia
- Chronic leukemia
- Lymphoma
- Multiple myeloma
- Certain solid tumors
- Sickle cell anemia

▶ PROCEDURE

- With autologous donation, the patient's bone marrow is harvested and frozen 2 weeks before transplantation, and then thawed before infusion.
- With syngeneic or allogeneic donation, donor marrow is obtained in the operating room the same day as transplantation and is brought to the patient's room immediately; transplantation takes place at the bedside.
- An antihistamine or analgesic is administered, as ordered.
- The physician infuses the marrow through a central venous catheter over 2 to 4 hours.

Complications
DURING INFUSION
- Fluid volume overload
- Anaphylaxis
- Pulmonary fat embolism
AFTER INFUSION
- Infection
- Abnormal bleeding
- Renal insufficiency
- Venous occlusive disease
- With allogeneic donation: graft-versus-host disease (GVHD)

✳ NURSING INTERVENTIONS

Pretreatment care
- Explain the treatment and patient preparation.
- Make sure the patient has signed an appropriate consent form.
- Keep diphenhydramine and epinephrine readily available to manage transfusion reactions.
- Start an I.V. line., and administer I.V. fluids, as ordered.
- Obtain an administration set without a filter for bone marrow infusion.
- Administer medications, as ordered.

◆ **NURSING ALERT** Be alert for signs and symptoms of bronchospasm, urticaria, erythema, chest pain, and back pain.

Posttreatment care
- Maintain asepsis.
- Institute safety measures.
- Administer ordered transfusions.
- Obtain blood samples for laboratory analysis, as ordered.
MONITORING
- Vital signs
- Infection
- Hemorrhage
- Laboratory results
- GVHD

Patient teaching
Be sure to cover:
- medication administration, dosage, and possible adverse effects
- infection control measures
- bleeding precautions
- central venous catheter care
- signs and symptoms of transplant failure
- complications
- when to notify the physician
- emergency telephone numbers
- follow-up care.

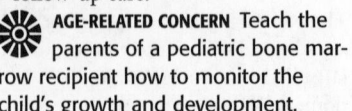 **AGE-RELATED CONCERN** Teach the parents of a pediatric bone marrow recipient how to monitor the child's growth and development.

Bowel resection

- Bowel resection with ostomy: diseased bowel excised and stoma created on the outer abdominal wall for feces elimination; laparoscopic approach possible for standard colostomy and end-ileostomy
- Bowel resection with anastomosis: diseased intestinal tissue surgically resected and remaining segments connected or anastomosed (preferred surgical technique for treating localized bowel cancer)

Indications
BOWEL RESECTION WITH OSTOMY
- Inflammatory bowel disease
- Familial adenomatous polyposis
- Diverticulitis
- Advanced colorectal cancer

BOWEL RESECTION WITH ANASTOMOSIS
- Localized obstructive disorders secondary to diverticulitis, intestinal polyps, adhesions, or malignant or benign intestinal lesions

- All procedures are performed under general anesthesia

Bowel resection with ostomy
- The surgeon makes an incision in the abdominal wall. (The location depends on the bowel area to be resected and type of ostomy required.)
- The diseased bowel segment is resected, possibly along with several more inches of bowel.
- The surgeon creates a stoma.

ABDOMINOPERINEAL RESECTION
- A low abdominal incision is made and the sigmoid colon is divided.
- The proximal end of the colon is brought out through another, smaller abdominal incision to create an end stoma.
- A wide perineal incision is made and the anus, rectum, and distal portion of the sigmoid colon are resected.
- The abdominal wound is closed and abdominal drains are placed.
- The perineal wound may be left open, packed with gauze, or closed; several Penrose drains are placed.

ILEOSTOMY
- The surgeon resects all or part of the colon and rectum (proctocolectomy).
- A permanent ileostomy is created by bringing the end of the ileum out through a small abdominal incision in the right lower quadrant to create a stoma.

ILEOANAL RESERVOIR
- A colectomy is performed and an ileal loop or the distal ileum is used to create a stoma for a temporary ileostomy.
- The rectal mucosal layer is removed and an internal pouch is made with a portion of the ileum.
- A pouch-anal anastomosis is performed.
- The temporary ileostomy is usually closed after 3 to 4 months.

KOCK ILEOSTOMY
- The surgeon removes the colon, rectum, and anus, and closes the anus.
- A reservoir is constructed from a loop of the terminal ileum.
- A portion of the ileum is intussuscepted to form a nipple valve.
- The upper part of the sutured and cut ileum is pulled down and sutured to form a pouch.
- The nipple valve is used to create a stoma by pulling it through the abdominal wall and suturing it flush with the skin. A catheter is placed in the stoma.

Bowel resection with anastomosis
- An abdominal incision is made, depending on location of the lesion.
- The diseased area is resected, along with a wide margin of surrounding normal tissue.
- Remaining bowel segments are anastomosed end-to-end or side-to-side.
- The incision is closed, and a sterile dressing is applied.

Complications
- Hemorrhage
- Sepsis
- Ileus
- Fluid and electrolyte imbalance
- Skin excoriation
- Pelvic abscess
- Incompetent nipple valve (with a Kock ileostomy)
- Bleeding or leakage from the anastomosis site
- Peritonitis, postresection obstruction, wound infection, or atelectasis
- Psychological problems

(continued)

☼ NURSING INTERVENTIONS

Pretreatment care
- Explain preoperative and postoperative procedures and equipment to the patient and his family.
- Discuss postoperative analgesia.
- Verify that the patient has signed the appropriate consent form.
- Tell the patient what to expect for fecal drainage and bowel movement control for the type of ostomy performed.
- Provide total parenteral nutrition, as ordered.
- Administer an antibiotic and other medications, as ordered.

Posttreatment care
- Provide meticulous wound care.
- Administer an analgesic, as ordered.
- Maintain I.V. replacement therapy, as ordered.
- Keep the nasogastric tube patent, but don't reposition it.
- After an abdominoperineal resection, irrigate the perineal area, as ordered.
- Maintain catheter patency and connect to low intermittent suction or straight drainage if the patient has a Kock pouch with a catheter inserted in the stoma; irrigate, as ordered:
- Encourage deep-breathing and coughing exercises; encourage splinting of the incision site, as necessary.
- For anastomosis patients, encourage oral fluid intake and give stool softeners and laxatives, as ordered.
- Encourage the patient to express feelings and concerns.
- Arrange for a consultation with an enterostomal therapist, as appropriate.

MONITORING
- Vital signs and intake and output
- Fluid and electrolyte balance
- Stoma appearance and drainage; skin appearance around stoma
- Drainage from catheter inserted into Kock pouch
- Signs of infection, peritonitis, and sepsis

◈ **NURSING ALERT** Immediately report excessive blood or mucus draining from the stoma, which could indicate hemorrhage or infection. Immediately report signs and symptoms of anastomotic leakage, including low-grade fever, malaise, slight leukocytosis, abdominal distention, tenderness, hemorrhage, hypovolemic shock, and bloody stool or wound drainage.

Patient teaching
Be sure to cover:
- medication administration, dosage, and possible adverse effects
- stoma and skin care; ostomy type, function, and care
- resumption of sexual intercourse
- dietary restrictions with emphasis on high fluid intake
- avoidance of alcohol, laxatives, and diuretics (unless approved by the physician)
- bowel retraining for appropriate ostomy patients; use of sitz baths (after abdominoperineal resection)
- signs and symptoms of inflammation and infection
- follow-up care.

Carpal tunnel release

● OVERVIEW

- Surgery to decompress the median nerve
- Relieves pain and restores function in the wrist and hand
- May be performed as outpatient surgery with local anesthesia
- Contraindicated in rheumatoid arthritis, mass lesions, and repeat surgery

Indications

- Carpal tunnel syndrome unrelieved by splinting or medication

▶ PROCEDURE

- Surgeon can choose from several approaches, but entire transverse carpal tunnel ligament must be transected to achieve adequate compression of median nerve.
- The surgeon makes an incision around the thenar eminence.
- The flexor retinaculum is exposed and transected to relieve pressure on the median nerve.
- Neurolysis (stretching of the nerve) may be performed to free flattened nerve fibers.
- A small incision may be made in a puncture site to decompress the median nerve. (See *Endoscopic carpal tunnel release.*)

Complications

- Hematoma
- Infection
- Painful scar formation
- Tenosynovitis
- Nerve damage

☀ NURSING INTERVENTIONS

Pretreatment care

- Explain the treatment and preparation to the patient and family.
- Make sure the patient has signed an appropriate consent form.
- Explain that the patient will have a dressing wrapped around the hand and lower arm after surgery and that this will remain in place for 1 to 2 days.
- Tell the patient he may experience pain once the anesthetic wears off but that analgesics will be available.
- Demonstrate rehabilitative exercises, and have the patient perform a return demonstration.

Posttreatment care

- Keep the affected hand elevated to reduce swelling and discomfort.
- Administer analgesics, as ordered.
- ◆ **NURSING ALERT** Report severe, persistent pain or tenderness, which may indicate tenosynovitis or formation of hematoma.
- Encourage the patient to perform wrist and finger exercises.
- Assess the need for home care and follow-up.

MONITORING

- Vital signs
- Circulation in the affected arm and hand
- Sensory and motor function in the affected arm and hand
- Surgical dressings
- Drainage or bleeding
- Pain
- Complications
- Response to treatment

Patient teaching

Be sure to cover:

- medication administration, dosage, and possible adverse effects
- elevation of hand
- surgical incision care
- dressing changes
- daily wrist and finger exercises
- avoidance of overusing the affected wrist or lifting objects heavier than a thin magazine
- signs and symptoms of infection
- complications
- when to notify the physician
- follow-up care
- referral to occupational therapy, especially if the disorder is work-related.

ENDOSCOPIC CARPAL TUNNEL RELEASE

Endoscopic carpal tunnel release is an alternative to open carpal tunnel release. Its advantages include less scar tenderness, earlier return to work and activities of daily living, and earlier return of pinch and grip strength. Complications are comparable to those seen with the open technique, but patient satisfaction is greater with this method.

The procedure may use the single-portal or double-portal technique. In either, the carpal tunnel is approached through small incisions that allow endoscope passage along the ulnar border of the transverse carpal ligament. The ligament is sharply divided after transverse fibers are well visualized. The antebrachial fascia proximally is divided under direct vision.

Contraindications to the procedure include rheumatoid arthritis, mass lesions, and repeat surgery.

Cataract removal

● OVERVIEW

- Removal of a cataract, or lens opacity
- May involve intracapsular cataract extraction (ICCE) or extracapsular cataract extraction (ECCE)
- May be followed by immediate placement of an intraocular lens implant

AGE-RELATED CONCERN ECCE is the primary treatment for congenital and traumatic cataracts. It's characterically used to treat children and young adults because the posterior capsule adheres to the vitreous until about age 20. By leaving the posterior capsule undisturbed, ECCE avoids disruption and loss of vitreous.

Indications

- Congenital cataract
- Traumatic cataract

▶ PROCEDURE

- The patient may receive a local or general anesthetic.

AGE-RELATED CONCERN Children are typically given general anesthesia to keep them in a deep sleep and pain-free; adults usually are awake but sedated and pain-free with local anesthesia.

- In ICCE, the entire lens is removed, most commonly with a cryoprobe.
- In ECCE, the anterior capsule, cortex, and nucleus are removed, leaving the posterior capsule intact; manual extraction, irrigation and aspiration, or phacoemulsification may be used.
- After the incision is enlarged, a lens may be implanted into the capsular sac.
- If the lens is implanted without sutures, miotic agents are administered.
- In ICCE and ECCE, a peripheral iridectomy may be done and alpha-chymotrypsin may be instilled in the anterior chamber.
- The surgeon closes the sutures and instills antibiotic drops or ointment.
- Miotics may be administered.
- A patch and shield are applied to the eye.

Complications

- Pupillary block
- Corneal decompensation
- Vitreous loss
- Hemorrhage
- Cystoid macular edema
- Lens dislocation
- Secondary membrane opacification
- Retinal detachment

❊ NURSING INTERVENTIONS

Pretreatment care

- Explain the treatment and preparation to the patient including eye drops and their purpose.
- Make sure the patient has signed an appropriate consent form.
- Explain that patient will wear an eye patch temporarily after surgery.
- Perform an antiseptic facial scrub, as ordered.

Posttreatment care

- Institute safety precautions.
- Assist the patient with ambulation.
- Have the patient wear an eye shield, especially when sleeping.
- Maintain the eye patch.
- Approach the patient from the unaffected side.

MONITORING
- Vital signs
- Pain
- Bleeding
- Drainage
- Intraocular pressure
- Complications

Patient teaching

Be sure to cover:
- medication administration, dosage, and possible adverse effects
- importance of sleeping on the unaffected side
- temporary loss of depth perception and decrease in peripheral vision on the operative side
- avoidance of activities that increase intraocular pressure
- avoidance of strenuous exercise for 6 to 10 weeks postoperatively
- when to change the eye patch
- use of eye shield, especially during sleep
- importance of wearing dark glasses to relieve glare
- contact lens care, if applicable
- likelihood of visual instability for several weeks after surgery
- increase in visual acuity as the affected eye heals
- follow-up care
- when to notify the physician (especially for sudden eye pain, red or watery eyes, photophobia, or sudden vision changes).

Cerebellar stimulator implantation

● OVERVIEW

- Suppresses tremors by delivering mild electrical stimulation to block signals (that cause tremors) from the thalamus, subthalamic nucleus, or globus pallidus without destroying brain tissue
- Target areas identified by a computed tomography scan or magnetic resonance imaging of the brain; microelectrode recording technique of choice to map brain
- Components: implantable lead with four electrodes at the end; neurostimulator with an external programming system to change stimulation settings; extension wire to connect the lead to the neurostimulator
- Can be performed on one or both sides of the brain (majority of patients with Parkinson's disease requiring stimulators placed on both sides of the brain)
- Procedure usually staged with each side of the brain done on separate days
- Stimulation adjustable and can be changed as symptoms change

Indications
- Essential tremor
- Parkinson's disease

▶ PROCEDURE

Lead placement
- The patient's scalp is anesthetized with local anesthetic.
- I.V. sedation may also used for patient comfort, but generally the patient remains awake during the lead placement.
- An incision is made on the top of the head behind the hairline and a small opening (burr hole) is made.
- The neurologist and neurosurgeon identify the target sites using microelectrode mapping.
- Once the target site has been confirmed, a permanent stimulator lead is inserted through the burr hole.
- The patient is asked to answer questions and perform some tasks during the procedure to test the stimulation and maximize symptom control.
- I.V. sedation is administered and the lead is anchored to the skull with a plastic cap and the scalp incision is sutured shut.

Neurostimulator placement
- The neurostimulator is generally placed at a later time, usually under general anesthesia.
- A small incision is made in the upper chest near the collar bone. A subcutaneous pocket is formed and the neurostimulator is implanted under the skin.
- The lead is attached to an extension cable which is passed under the skin of the scalp, neck, and shoulder and connected to the neurostimulator.
- Programming of the neurostimulator usually takes place 3 to 4 weeks after implantation.

Complications
- Infection
- Paresthesia
- Paralysis
- Ataxia
- Intracerebral hemorrhage
- Seizures
- Stroke
- Confusion

✳ NURSING INTERVENTIONS

Pretreatment care
- Perform a complete neurologic assessment.
- Explain the treatment and preparation to the patient and his family.
- Verify that the patient has signed an appropriate consent form.
- Tell the patient that his head may be shaved in the operating room.

Posttreatment care
- Administer medications, as ordered.
- Assist with activities of daily living, as appropriate.
- Make sure dressings stay clean, dry, and intact.

MONITORING
- Vital signs
- Dressing and incision
- Neurologic status

◈ **NURSING ALERT** Notify the surgeon immediately if you detect a worsening of mental status, pupillary changes, or focal signs, such as increasing weakness in an arm or leg.

- Fluid and electrolyte balance
- Signs and symptoms of infection

Patient teaching
Be sure to cover:
- medication administration, dosage, and possible adverse effects
- wound care
- occurrence of headache and facial swelling for 2 or 3 days after surgery
- postoperative leg and deep breathing exercises and use of antiembolism stockings or a pneumatic compression device
- signs and symptoms of infection, complications, and when to notify the practitioner
- follow-up care
- such activity restrictions as light activities for the first 2 weeks after surgery gradually leading to moderate to heavy activities at 4 to 6 weeks after surgery
- use of magnet to activate and deactivate the neurostimulator.

Cerebral aneurysm repair

● OVERVIEW

- Surgical repair: clipping the aneurysm neck with at least one titanium clip
- Endovascular repair: use of electrically detachable platinum coils that promote electrothrombosis within the aneurysm
- Decision to obliterate an aneurysm surgically through a craniotomy and clipping or to use endovascular methods based on the patient's condition

  ✳ **AGE-RELATED CONCERN** Treatment depends on the patient's age and the location of the aneurysm. Younger patients commonly undergo surgical clipping because coiling has a high recurrence rate. However, posterior fossa aneurysms (especially the basilar artery tip) tend to be treated using the coil procedure. In most major aneurysm centers, many cases are still obliterated by surgical clipping, although coiling is being used more frequently.

  ✳ **AGE-RELATED CONCERN** The prognosis is always guarded, but is affected by the patient's age and neurologic condition, the presence of other diseases, and the extent and location of the aneurysm.

Indications
- Cerebral aneurysm (usually arise at arterial junction in the circle of Willis)

▶ PROCEDURE

Clipping
- General anesthesia is used and the area of the skull where the craniotomy will occur is shaved. The exact position of the opening depends on the approach that the neurosurgeon will use to reach the aneurysm.
- The bone flap is removed and the various layers of tissue are cut away to expose the brain.
- Brain tissue is gently retracted back to expose the area containing the aneurysm.
- Surgical techniques performed through a microscope are then used to dissect the aneurysm away from the vessels feeding the aneurysm and expose the neck to receive the clip.

- The clip is placed on the neck of the aneurysm to stop the flow of blood into the aneurysm, causing it to deflate or obliterate.
- The brain tissue is carefully lowered back into place, the various layers sutured closed, and the bone flap is reseated for healing.
- The skin and other outer layers are also sutured closed.

Coiling
- A specially trained radiologist called a neurointerventionist performs the procedure using fluoroscopic angiography. A microcatheter is threaded from the patient's femoral artery to the aneurysm. The catheter is used to place small platinum coils within the aneurysm using a delivery wire.
- Once the coil has been maneuvered into place, an electrical charge is sent through the delivery wire that disintegrates the stainless steel of the coil, separating it from the delivery wire, which is then removed from the body.
- Several coils may be necessary to block the neck of the aneurysm from the normal circulation and obliterate it, as with the clip procedure.
- The coils act as a thrombogenic agent, causing blood to coagulate in the aneurysm, decreasing the risk of rupture.

  ◈ **NURSING ALERT** Coil treatment is contraindicated if the patient has a cerebral hematoma (which precludes anticoagulation during the procedure) or an aneurysm with a wide opening. The coil mass could lapse into the parent artery, partially or completely occluding it and causing a stroke.

Complications
- Infection
- Rebleeding
- Vasospasm
- Neurologic damage
- Hypothermia

✳ NURSING INTERVENTIONS

Pretreatment care
- Check laboratory values, electrocardiogram, and chest X-rays, as ordered; notify the surgeon or radiologist of any abnormalities.
- Explain all tests, neurologic examinations, treatments, and procedures to the patient and his family and reinforce surgeon's explanations, as necessary.
- Perform a neurologic examination.
- Verify that the patient has signed a consent form.

Posttreatment care
- Assist with obtaining a postoperative magnetic resonance angiogram, which may be performed to confirm good clip placement, total obliteration of the aneurysm, and continued blood flow through the neighboring vessels.
- Administer I.V. fluids, as ordered.
- Administer treatments for vasospasm, as ordered.
- Administer oxygen, as indicated; suction and turn the patient.
- Administer heparin infusion and then aspirin for patients who received a coil.
- Apply elastic stockings or compression boots to reduce the risk of deep vein thrombosis.
- Arrange for home health care or rehabilitation services, as needed.

MONITORING
- Vital signs, including blood pressure
- Neurologic status; signs and symptoms of increased intracranial pressure
- Laboratory values
- Intake and output
- Femoral puncture site for bleeding or hematoma; leg for signs of ischemia

  ◈ **NURSING ALERT** Notify the surgeon immediately if you notice pain, pallor, pulselessness, poikilothermia (cool to touch), or paresthesia.

Patient teaching
Be sure to cover:
- signs of rebleeding to report, such as headache, nausea, vomiting, and changes in level of consciousness
- follow-up skull X-ray or magnetic resonance angiography.

Chemoembolization of liver

● OVERVIEW

- Primary liver cancer (also known as *hepatoma* or *hepatocellular carcinoma*): derives its blood exclusively from the hepatic artery; extremely vascular tumor
- Arterial chemotherapy infusion of the liver and chemoembolization of the liver (transarterial chemoembolization, or TACE): involve chemotherapy injected into the hepatic artery supplying the liver tumor; however, with chemoembolization, additional injected material blocks small branches of hepatic artery
- Provides relief or lessens the severity of disease; however, not curative and produces less than 50% decrease in tumor size
- Can be used only in patients with relatively preserved liver function

Indications
- Hepatoma or hepatocellular carcinoma

▶ PROCEDURE

- An interventional radiologist works closely with an oncologist, who determines the amount of chemotherapy that the patient receives at each session. Some patients may undergo repeat sessions at 6- to 12-week intervals.
- Under fluoroscopy imaging, a catheter is inserted into the femoral artery in the groin, threaded into the aorta, and advanced into the hepatic artery.
- When the branches of the hepatic artery that feed the liver cancer are identified, the chemotherapy is infused.
- Different types of compounds, such as gelfoam or small metal coils, are used as an additional step of embolizing the small blood vessels.
- The procedure takes 1 to 2 hours, and then the catheter is removed and a compression device is placed over the puncture site.

Complications
- Systemic chemotherapeutic adverse effects
- Inflammation of the gallbladder (cholecystitis)
- Intestinal and stomach ulcers
- Pancreatitis
- Liver failure
- Blocking of the feeding vessels to the tumor with chemoembolization possibly making future attempts at intra-arterial infusions impossible

✳ NURSING INTERVENTIONS

Pretreatment care
- Review the procedure with the patient and emphasize the importance of remaining still during the procedure. Also review possible adverse reactions of the treatment.
- Review laboratory results, as ordered, and notify the practitioner of results.
- Provide pretreatment medications, as ordered.
- Check for patient allergies.
- Verify that the patient has signed an informed consent form.

Posttreatment care
- Maintain sandbag or other compression device over the puncture site.
- Administer analgesics, as ordered.
- Provide emotional support.
- Refer the patient and his family to support services available in the community.

MONITORING
- Signs of bleeding from the femoral artery puncture
- Pulses in the affected extremity
- Laboratory test results

◈ **NURSING ALERT** Generally, liver test results get worse during the 2 or 3 days after the procedure. This worsening reflects the death of the tumor (and some nontumor) cells.

- Puncture site inspection
- Abdominal pain and low-grade fever
- Adverse effects

Patient teaching
Be sure to cover:
- medication administration, dosage, and possible adverse effects
- signs and symptoms to report to the physician
- need for follow-up care, including repeat of liver imaging studies in 6 to 12 weeks to assess the size of the tumor in response to the treatment.

Cholecystectomy

OVERVIEW

- Surgical removal of the gallbladder
- May be performed as an open abdominal surgical procedure or as a laparoscopic procedure

Indications
- Gallbladder or biliary duct disease refractory to drug therapy, dietary changes, and other supportive treatments

PROCEDURE

- The open abdominal and laparoscopic approaches require general anesthesia.

ABDOMINAL CHOLECYSTECTOMY
- A right subcostal or paramedial incision is made.
- The surgeon surveys the abdomen.
- Laparotomy packs are used to isolate the gallbladder from the surrounding organs.
- After biliary tract structures are identified, cholangiography or ultrasonography may be used to identify gallstones.
- The bile ducts are visualized using a choledoscope.
- The ducts are cleared of stones after insertion of a Fogarty balloon-tipped catheter.
- The surgeon ligates and divides the cystic duct and artery and removes the entire gallbladder.
- A choledochotomy may be performed, with a T tube inserted into the common bile duct.
- A Penrose drain may be placed into the ducts.
- The incision is closed and a dressing is applied.

LAPAROSCOPIC CHOLECYSTECTOMY
- A small incision is made just above the umbilicus.
- Carbon dioxide or nitrous oxide is injected into the abdominal cavity.
- A trocar, connected to an insufflator, is inserted through the incision.
- A laparoscope is passed through the trocar to view the intra-abdominal contents.

- The patient is placed in a 30-degree, reverse Trendelenburg's position and tilted slightly to the left.
- With laparoscopic guidance, the surgeon makes three incisions in the right upper quadrant: one below the xiphoid process in the midline; one below the right costal margin in the midclavicular line; and one in the anterior axillary line at the umbilical level.
- Using the laparoscope, the surgeon passes instruments through the three incisions to clamp and tie off the cystic duct and excise the gallbladder.
- The gallbladder is removed through the umbilical opening.
- The surgeon sutures all four incisions and places a dressing over each.

Complications
- Peritonitis
- Postcholecystectomy syndrome
- Atelectasis
- Bile duct injury
- Small bowel injury
- Wound infection
- Ileus
- Urinary retention
- Retained gallstones

NURSING INTERVENTIONS

Pretreatment care
- Explain the treatment and preparation to the patient and family.
- Make sure the patient has signed an appropriate consent form.
- Withhold oral intake, as ordered.
- Administer preoperative medications, as ordered.

ABDOMINAL APPROACH
- Tell the patient that:
  - a nasogastric (NG) tube will be in place for 1 to 2 days and an abdominal drain will be in place for 3 to 5 days after surgery
  - a T tube may remain in place for up to 2 weeks
  - he may be discharged with the T tube in place.

LAPAROSCOPIC APPROACH
- Tell the patient that:
  - an indwelling urinary catheter will be inserted into the bladder

  - a NG tube will be placed in the stomach
  - tubes are usually removed in the postanesthesia room
  - three small incisions will be covered with a small sterile dressing
  - discharge may occur on the day of surgery or 1 day after.

Posttreatment care
- Administer medications, as ordered.
- Place the patient in low Fowler's position.
- Attach the NG tube to low intermittent suction, as ordered.
- Report drainage greater than 500 ml after 48 hours.
- Provide meticulous skin care, especially around drainage tube insertion sites.
- After NG tube removal, introduce foods, as ordered.
- Clamp the T tube before and after each meal, as ordered.
- After laparoscopic cholecystectomy, start clear liquids, as ordered, when the patient has fully recovered from anesthesia.
- Assist with early ambulation.
- Encourage coughing and deep-breathing exercises.
- Encourage incentive spirometry use.
- Provide analgesics, as ordered.

MONITORING
- Vital signs
- Intake and output
- Complications
- Postcholecystectomy syndrome
- Respiratory status
- Amount and characteristics of drainage
- Surgical dressings
- Position and patency of drainage tubes

Patient teaching
Be sure to cover:
- medication administration, dosage, and possible adverse effects
- coughing and deep-breathing exercises
- T tube home care, if applicable
- signs and symptoms of biliary obstruction
- signs and symptoms of infection
- complications
- when to notify the physician
- follow-up care.

Cochlear implant

● OVERVIEW

- Auditory prosthetic device that improves auditory awareness; may improve hearing enough so the patient can understand conversation
- Works by directly stimulating the auditory nerve that transmits impulses to the brain's hearing center (see *Cochlear implant: A closer look*)

Indications
- Deafness secondary to sensorineural hearing loss

▶ PROCEDURE

- The surgeon implants the internal component of the device, complete with one or more electrodes, into the cochlea.
- A receiver is implanted behind the top of the auricle.
- On postoperative day 10 to 15, when wound healing is complete, the patient wears an external component consisting of a small microphone with an ear hook over the ear.
- The external component is connected to a speech processor and a transmitter coil with a magnet that keeps it in place over the receiver stimulator.
- The device picks up sound through the microphone and sends it to the processor, where it is broken down and stored.
- The converted sound information is transferred to the external device, further processed, and sent through any surviving nerve cells to the brain's hearing center, allowing the patient to hear.

Complications
- Infection
- Feelings of depression

✳ NURSING INTERVENTIONS

Pretreatment care
- Explain the treatment and preparation to the patient and family.
- Make sure the patient has signed an appropriate consent form.
- When addressing the patient, speak slowly in a clear, loud voice. Give the patient time to process the information and respond.
- Develop alternative communication methods, as indicated.

Posttreatment care
- Report incisional redness, swelling, or drainage.
- Administer analgesics, as ordered.

MONITORING
- Vital signs
- Incision site
- Drainage
- Infection

Patient teaching
Be sure to cover:
- medication administration, dosage, and possible adverse effects
- information about sensorineural hearing loss
- fact that hearing won't return to preloss level
- importance of learning how to interpret sounds produced by the device
- complications
- when to notify the physician
- follow-up care.

COCHLEAR IMPLANT: A CLOSER LOOK

The illustration below shows a patient with a cochlear implant in place.

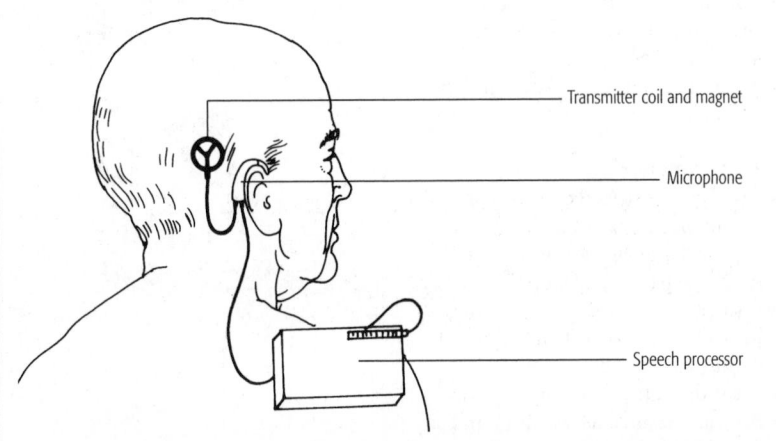

Transmitter coil and magnet

Microphone

Speech processor

Corneal transplantation

OVERVIEW

- Replacement of a damaged part of the cornea with healthy corneal tissue from a donor
- Most common type of transplant surgery; has highest success rate
- Indicated when corneal damage is too severe for treatment with corrective lenses; may be combine with other eye procedures (such as cataract surgery) to resolve multple eye problems
- Vision not completely functional until healing is complete, which may take up to 1 year, during which time the sutures remain in place
- Also called *keratoplasty*

Indications

- Keratoconus
- Fuchs' dystrophy
- Pseudophakic button keratopathy
- Chemical burns to cornea
- Mechanical trauma
- Infection by viruses, bacteria, fungi, or protozoa

NURSING ALERT Although the cornea isn't normally vascular, some corneal diseases cause vascularization into the cornea. In such patients, careful testing of both donor and recipient is done, and repeated surgery may be needed for a successful transplant.

PROCEDURE

- The patient may receive a local or general anesthetic.
- A disc of tissue is removed from the center of the eye and replaced with a disc from the donor eye. The circular incision is made using a trepone.
- In penetrating keratoplasty—the most common type of corneal transplant—the disc removed and the replacement disc are the entire thickness of the cornea.
- In lamellar keratoplasty, only the outer layer of the cornea is removed and replaced.
- The donor cornea is attached with fine sutures and an eye patch and shield applied.

Complications

- Infection
- Glaucoma
- Retinal detachment
- Cataract formation
- Rejection of donor cornea
- Photophobia

NURSING INTERVENTIONS

Pretreatment care

- Explain the treatment and preparation to the patient and family.
- Make sure the patient has signed an appropriate consent form.
- Explain that a bandage and protective shield will be placed over the eye postoperatively.
- Administer a sedative or an osmotic agent, as ordered, to reduce intraocular pressure.
- Perform an antiseptic facial scrub, if ordered.

Posttreatment care

- Instill corticosteroid eyedrops or topical antibiotics, as ordered.
- Administer analgesics, as ordered.
- Assist the patient to lie on his back or the unaffected side.
- Keep the head of the bed flat or slightly elevated, as ordered.
- Assist the patient with ambulation.
- Keep all personal items within the patient's field of vision.

MONITORING

- Vital signs
- Dressings
- Drainage
- Pain

NURSING ALERT Immediately report sudden, sharp, or excessive pain; bloody, purulent, or clear viscous drainage; and fever.

Patient teaching

Be sure to cover:

- medication administration, dosage, and possible adverse effects
- signs and symptoms of graft rejection
- importance of assessing the graft *daily* for the rest of the patient's life
- fact that healing will be slow and vision may not be completely restored until sutures are removed
- follow-up care
- avoidance of activities that increase intraocular pressure
- photophobia precautions
- importance of using an eye shield when sleeping
- avoidance of driving or participating in physical activities until the physician approves
- complications
- when to notify the physician.

Coronary artery bypass grafting

● OVERVIEW

- Grafting of a blood vessel segment from another part of the body to create an alternate circulatory route that bypasses an occluded area of a coronary artery, thus restoring normal blood flow to the myocardium
- Usually the saphenous vein or internal mammary artery used for grafting
- Can relieve anginal pain and improve cardiac function, and may enhance the quality of life
- Sometimes involves a minimally invasive surgical procedure
- Commonly called *CABG*

Indications

- Medically uncontrolled angina that adversely affects quality of life
- Left main coronary artery disease (CAD)
- Severe proximal left anterior descending coronary artery stenosis
- Three-vessel CAD with proximal stenoses or left ventricular dysfunction
- Three-vessel CAD with normal left ventricular function at rest, but with inducible ischemia and poor exercise capacity

▶ PROCEDURE

- The patient receives general anesthesia.
- The surgeon makes a series of incisions in the patient's thigh or calf and removes a saphenous vein segment for grafting; internal mammarian artery segments also may be removed.
- A medial sternotomy is done and the heart is exposed.
- Cardiopulmonary bypass is initiated.
- Cardiac hypothermia and standstill are induced.
- The surgeon sutures one end of the venous graft to the ascending aorta and the other end to a patent coronary artery distal to the occlusion.
- This procedure is repeated for each artery that will be bypassed.
- Once the grafts are in place, the surgeon flushes the cardioplegic solution from the heart.

- Cardiopulmonary bypass is discontinued.
- Epicardial pacing electrodes are implanted.
- A chest tube is inserted.
- The incision is closed and a sterile dressing is applied.

Complications

- Cardiac arrhythmias
- Hypertension or hypotension
- Cardiac tamponade
- Thromboembolism
- Hemorrhage
- Postpericardiotomy syndrome
- Myocardial infarction
- Stroke
- Postoperative depression or emotional instability
- Pulmonary embolism
- Decreased renal function
- Infection

✳ NURSING INTERVENTIONS

Pretreatment care

- Explain the treatment and preparation to the patient and family.
- Make sure the patient has signed an appropriate consent form.
- Explain what to expect during the immediate postoperative period including:
  - endotracheal tube and mechanical ventilator
  - cardiac monitor
  - nasogastric tube, chest tube, indwelling urinary catheter, and arterial line
  - epicardial pacing wires
  - pulmonary artery catheter.
- Institute cardiac monitoring.
- The evening before surgery, have the patient shower with antiseptic soap as ordered.
- Restrict food and fluids after midnight, as ordered.
- Provide sedation, as ordered.
- Assist with pulmonary artery catheterization and insertion of arterial lines.

Posttreatment care

- Keep emergency resuscitative equipment immediately available.

- Maintain arterial pressure within the limits set by the physician.
- Adjust ordered I.V. medications according to facility protocol.
- Maintain chest tube patency.
- Administer medications, as ordered.
- Assist with weaning the patient from the ventilator, as appropriate.
- Promote chest physiotherapy.
- Encourage coughing, deep breathing, and incentive spirometry use.
- Assist the patient with range-of-motion (ROM) exercises.

MONITORING

- Vital signs
- Intake and output
- Heart rate, rhythm, and heart sounds
- Hemodynamic values
- Complications
- Nutritional status
- Electrocardiogram
- Arterial blood gas analysis
- Breath sounds
- Peripheral vascular status
- Respiratory status, breath sounds
- Neurologic status
- Renal function
- Chest tube patency and drainage
- Surgical wounds and dressings
- Drainage
- Electrolyte imbalances

Patient teaching

Be sure to cover:
- medication administration, dosage, and possible adverse effects
- incentive spirometry
- ROM exercises
- incision care
- signs and symptoms of infection, arterial reocclusion, and postpericardiotomy syndrome
- how to identify and cope with postoperative depression
- complications
- when to notify the physician
- dietary restrictions
- activity restrictions; adequate rest periods
- prescribed exercise program
- smoking cessation
- follow-up care
- referral to the Mended Hearts Club and American Heart Association for information and support.

Craniotomy

● OVERVIEW

- A surgical opening into the skull, exposing the brain for treatment
- May involve supratentorial or infratentorial approach

Indications
- Ventricular shunt placement
- Tumor excision
- Abscess drainage
- Hematoma aspiration
- Aneurysm clipping

▶ PROCEDURE

- The anesthetist starts a peripheral I.V. line, a central venous pressure line, and an arterial line.
- The patient receives a general or local anesthetic.
- For a supratentorial craniotomy, the surgical approach may be frontal, parietal, temporal, occipital, or a combination.
- For an infratentorial craniotomy, the surgeon makes an incision slightly above the neck, in the back of the skull.
- The surgeon marks an incision line and cuts through the scalp to the cranium, forming a scalp flap that is folded to one side.
- The surgeon then bores four or five holes through the skull in the corners of the cranial incision and cuts out a bone flap.
- After pulling aside or removing the bone flap, the surgeon incises and retracts the dura, exposing the brain.
- The surgeon then proceeds with the required surgery.
- The dura mater is closed, and a drain may be used.
- If swelling is expected, the bone flap may not be replaced to prevent undue pressure.
- Periosteum and muscle are approximated. Skin closure is performed and dressings are applied.

Complications
- Infection
- Vasospasm
- Hemorrhage
- Increased intracranial pressure (ICP)
- Diabetes insipidus
- Syndrome of inappropriate antidiuretic hormone secretion
- Seizures
- Cranial nerve damage

✳ NURSING INTERVENTIONS

Pretreatment care
- Explain the treatment and preparation to the patient and family.
- Make sure the patient has signed an appropriate consent form.
- Tell the patient that his head will be shaved in the operating room.
- Explain the intensive care unit and equipment the patient will see postoperatively.
- Perform a complete neurologic assessment.

Posttreatment care
- Maintain a patent airway.
- Administer oxygen and medications, as ordered.
- Position the patient on his side with the head of the bed elevated 15 to 30 degrees.
- Turn the patient carefully every 2 hours.
- Encourage careful deep breathing and coughing.
- Suction gently, as needed.
- Make sure the dressings stay clean, dry, and intact.
- Ensure a quiet, calm environment.
- Maintain seizure precautions.

Monitoring
- Vital signs
- Intake and output
- Level of consciousness
- Respiratory status
- ICP
- Heart rate and rhythm
- Hemodynamic values
- Fluid and electrolyte balance
- Urine specific gravity
- Daily weight
- Drain patency
- Surgical wound and dressings
- Drainage
- Complications

 NURSING ALERT Notify the physician immediately if you detect a worsening mental status, pupillary changes, or focal signs, such as increasing weakness in an arm or leg. These findings may indicate increased ICP.

Patient teaching
Be sure to cover:
- medication administration, dosage, and possible adverse effect
- surgical wound care
- probability of headache and facial swelling for 2 to 3 days after surgery
- postoperative leg exercises and deep breathing
- use of antiembolism stockings or a pneumatic compression device
- signs and symptoms of infection and complications
- when to notify the physician
- use of a wig, hat, or scarf until hair grows back
- avoidance of alcohol and smoking
- follow-up care.

Cryosurgery

● OVERVIEW

- Tissue destruction by application of extreme cold
- Most commonly involves liquid nitrogen or nitrous oxide
- Success of procedure dependent on lesion type, extent and depth of freezing, and duration between freezing and thawing

Indications

- Actinic and seborrheic keratoses
- Leukoplakia
- Molluscum contagiosum
- Verrucae
- Early basal cell epithelioma and squamous cell carcinoma
- Cervicitis
- Chronic cervical erosion
- Cervical polyps
- Condyloma acuminata
- Cataracts
- Retinal tears or holes

▶ PROCEDURE

- The procedure varies with the area being treated.

DERMATOLOGIC CRYOSURGERY

- The patient may receive a local anesthetic.
- The correct temperature and depth for freezing are determined.
- A superficial lesion may simply be palpated and inspected to determine the correct temperature and depth for freezing; skin cancer requires use of thermocouple needles and a tissue temperature monitor to ensure adequate freezing of the deepest tissue in the lesion.
- If thermocouple needles are used, they are inserted and secured into the base of the lesion.
- The operative site is cleaned with povidone-iodine solution.
- A cotton-tipped applicator dipped in liquid nitrogen or the complex cryosurgical unit is used to freeze the lesion.
- The lesion may be refrozen several times to ensure its destruction.
- For each cycle of refreezing the tumor to ensure its destruction, monitor and record the number of seconds that elapse until the tissue reaches –4° F (–20° C) and the number of seconds it takes for the tissue to thaw.
- After cryosurgery, the area is left uncovered.

GYNECOLOGIC CRYOSURGERY

- The surgery is performed 1 week after the patient's menstrual cycle ends.
- The patient is placed in the lithotomy position.
- A speculum is inserted into the vagina.
- After locating and inspecting the cervix, the physician slides the cryoprobe through the speculum and places it against the cervix to freeze the tissue, which later becomes necrotic and sloughs off.

OPHTHALMIC CRYOSURGERY

- The physician instills mydriatic and anesthetic eyedrops into the affected eye.
- After the eye dilates and becomes numb, the cryoprobe is placed on the conjunctiva, directly over the anterior retinal break.
- To treat the posterior retinal area, the physician cuts an opening in the conjunctiva and rotates the eye to expose a large portion of the sclera.
- After the procedure, a patch is applied to the affected eye.

Complications

Variable but may include:
- hypopigmentation
- secondary infection
- damage to blood vessels, nerves, and tear ducts
- cervical stenosis.

✳ NURSING INTERVENTIONS

Pretreatment care

- Explain the treatment and preparation to the patient and family.
- Make sure the patient has signed an appropriate consent form.
- Check the patient's history for allergies and hypersensitivities.
- Tell the patient to expect to feel a cold sensation and then a burning sensation during the procedure.
- Ask the patient to stay as still as possible.
- Before gynecologic cryosurgery, tell the patient she may experience transient headache, dizziness, flushing, or cramping during the procedure.

Posttreatment care

- Apply an ice bag to relieve swelling.
- Administer analgesics, as ordered.

DERMATOLOGIC CRYOSURGERY

- Clean the area gently with a cotton-tipped applicator soaked in hydrogen peroxide.

GYNECOLOGIC CRYOSURGERY

- Provide perineal care, as necessary.
- Have the patient wear a perineal pad.

OPHTHALMIC CRYOSURGERY

- Remove the eye patch after the anesthesia wears off.

MONITORING

- Vital signs
- Type and amount of vaginal drainage (for gynecologic cryosurgery)

Patient teaching

Be sure to cover:
- medication administration, dosage, and possible adverse effects
- when to notify the physician
- complications
- follow-up care.

DERMATOLOGIC PATIENT

Be sure to cover:
- expectation of pain, redness, swelling, and blister formation within 6 hours of treatment
- flattening and possible bleeding of the blister within a few days, and sloughing off of the blister in 2 to 3 weeks
- warnings against breaking the blister
- expectation of serous exudation during the first postoperative week, accompanied by development of a crust or eschar
- skin site care
- ways to prevent hypopigmentation
- signs and symptoms of infection.

GYNECOLOGIC PATIENT

Be sure to cover:
- expectation of a heavy, watery vaginal discharge for several weeks
- avoidance of tampons
- avoidance of sexual intercourse while discharge is present
- signs and symptoms of infection.

OPHTHALMIC PATIENT

Be sure to cover:
- importance of notifying the physician immediately of sudden vision changes or increased eye pain.

Cystectomy

- Partial or total removal of the urinary bladder and surrounding structures (see *Types of cystectomy*)
- Total cystectomy: necessitates permanent urinary diversion into an ileal or colonic conduit

Indications
- Advanced bladder cancer
- Bladder disorders such as interstitial cystitis
- Frequent recurrence of widespread papillary tumors not responding to endoscopic or chemotherapeutic management

▶ PROCEDURE

PARTIAL CYSTECTOMY
- The surgeon makes a midline low or transverse incision from the umbilicus to the symphysis pubis.
- The bladder is opened and the tumor removed, along with a small portion of healthy tissue.
- The wound is closed, leaving a Penrose drain and suprapubic catheter in place

TOTAL (SIMPLE) CYSTECTOMY
- The surgeon makes a midline abdominal incision.
- The entire bladder is removed, leaving only a portion of the urethra.

RADICAL CYSTECTOMY
- In addition to the bladder, the seminal vesicles and prostate in male patients and the uterus, ovaries, fallopian tubes, and anterior vagina in female patients are removed.
- Depending on the extent of cancer, the urethra and surrounding lymph nodes also may be removed.

TO COMPLETE A TOTAL OR RADICAL CYSTECTOMY
- Urinary diversion is done by attaching the ureters to an external collection device, such as a cutaneous ureterostomy, conduit of the large or small bowel, or continent urinary neobladder.

Complications
- Bleeding

- Hypotension
- Nerve injury, such as to the genitofemoral or peroneal nerve
- Anuria
- Stoma stenosis
- Urinary tract infection
- Pouch leakage
- Electrolyte imbalances
- Ureteroileal junction stenosis
- Vascular compromise
- Loss of sexual or reproductive function
- Psychological problems relating to changes in body image

✻ NURSING INTERVENTIONS

Pretreatment care
- Explain the treatment and preparation to the patient and family.
- Make sure the patient has signed an appropriate consent form.
- Arrange for a visit by an enterostomal therapist.
- Address the patient's concerns about inevitable loss of sexual or reproductive function.
- Explain the equipment the patient will see immediately after surgery.
- If possible, arrange for the patient to visit the intensive care unit.
- Perform standard bowel preparation, as ordered.
- Administer enemas or oral polyethylene glycol-electrolyte solution, as ordered.
- Administer antibiotics, as ordered.

Posttreatment care
- Administer medications, as ordered.
- Report urine output of less than 30 ml/hour.

- Maintain patency of the indwelling urinary catheter or stoma as appropriate, and irrigate, as ordered.
- Test all drainage from the nasogastric tube, abdominal drains, indwelling urinary catheter, and urine collection appliance for blood; notify the physician of positive findings.
- Change abdominal dressings, maintaining asepsis.
- Encourage frequent position changes, coughing, deep breathing, and early ambulation.
- Offer emotional support.

MONITORING
- Vital signs
- Intake and output
- Surgical wound and dressings
- Drainage
- Hypovolemic shock
- Stoma (if present)
- Frank hematuria and clots
- Respiratory status
- Infection

Patient teaching
Be sure to cover:
- medication administration, dosage, and possible adverse effects
- signs and symptoms of infection
- abnormal bleeding, including persistent hematuria
- complications
- when to notify the physician
- urinary diversion care
- home care nursing visits, if appropriate
- possibility of cancer recurrence
- follow-up care
- referral to a support group such as the United Ostomy Association if appropriate
- referral for psychological and sexual counseling as appropriate.

TYPES OF CYSTECTOMY

In cystectomy, surgery may be partial, simple, or radical.
- *Partial cystectomy* involves resection of a portion of the bladder wall. Commonly preserving bladder function, this surgery is most often indicated for a single, easily accessible bladder tumor.
- *Total* or *simple cystectomy* involves resection of the entire bladder. It's indicated for benign conditions limited to the bladder. It may also be performed as a palliative measure, such as to stop bleeding, when cancer isn't curable.
- *Radical cystectomy* is generally indicated for muscle-invasive primary bladder carcinoma. Besides removing the bladder, this procedure removes several surrounding structures. This extensive surgery typically causes impotence in men and sterility in women.
  After removal of the entire bladder, the patient requires a permanent urinary diversion, such as an ileal conduit or a continent urinary pouch.

Electroconvulsive therapy

● OVERVIEW

- Electric current delivered to the patient's brain by electrodes placed (bilaterally or unilaterally) on his temples
- Produces seizure lasting from 30 seconds to 1 minute
- Requires a multidisciplinary approach

Indications
- Affective disorders
- Selective schizophrenias
- Severe depression when other therapies are ineffective

◆ NURSING ALERT Contraindications to electroconvulsive therapy (ECT) include brain tumors, space-occupying lesions, and other brain diseases that cause increased intracranial pressure. The severity of any physical illness, such as heart, liver, or kidney disease as well as the psychiatric disorder, should be weighed against each other before ECT is initiated.

▷ PROCEDURE

- Attach the patient to an electronic blood pressure monitor and check his baseline vital signs. Attach a pulse oximeter, insert an I.V. catheter, and attach him to the electrocardiogram (ECG) monitor.
- Attach the EEG electrodes and stimulus electrodes to the rubber headband. Coat the electrodes with conduction gel and place the band around the patient's head. Place the large, silver-colored stimulus electrodes on each temple at about eye level. Space the small, brown EEG electrodes across the forehead.
- Connect the stimulus electrodes to the stimulus output receptacle on the machine.
- Run the EEG/ECG machine in the self-test mode to print the date, time, treatment parameters, a brief ECG strip, and EEG monitors.
- The physician administers glycopyrrolate (Robinul) or atropine, followed by methohexital (Brevital). Methohexital acts very rapidly. Expect an

abrupt loss of consciousness when the appropriate dose is infused.
- After the patient is unconscious, succinylcholine (Anectine) is administered. A tremor or fasciculation of various muscle groups occurs due to the depolarizing effect of this drug. Because succinylcholine also causes complete facial paralysis, mechanical ventilation is started at this time. A rubber mouthpiece is inserted and positive-pressure oxygen is given.
- The physician initiates the stimulus, and mild seizurelike activity occurs for about 30 seconds. The patient's jaw and extremities must be supported while avoiding contact with metal. The patient's vital signs as well as ECG and EEG rhythm strips are monitored and skin is assessed for burns.

Complications
- Respiratory distress
- Malignant hyperthermia
- Persistent memory loss

☆ NURSING INTERVENTIONS

Pretreatment care
- Review the procedure with the patient and what to expect before, during, and after the procedure.
- Verify that the patient has signed an appropriate consent form.
- If the patient is taking benzodiazepines before the procedure, obtain an order to begin tapering and discontinue the drugs 3 to 4 days preprocedure. Benzodiazepines and anticonvulsants (such as razepam [Ativan] and phenytoin [Dilantin]) negatively affect the patient's response to treatment.
- Make sure all equipment, drugs, and emergency equipment are available.
- Attach the ECG and EEG monitors.
- Complete a preprocedure assessment and set treatment parameters, as ordered, for pulse width (ms), frequency (Hz), duration (sec), and current (amp), based on patient's age, medication use, seizure threshold, and other factors.
- Plug in the electronic blood pressure monitor. Make sure that the crash cart, with emergency drug kit, defib-

rillator, suction equipment, endotracheal intubation tray, and oxygen is readily available and that needed medications are properly prepared.
- Verify the orders and gather the appropriate equipment.
- After arrival in the ECT room, identify the patient and check his nothing-by-mouth status.
- Make sure that the patient's history, physical examination, and dental evaluation and necessary test results are documented in his chart.
- Help the patient remove dentures, partial plates, or other foreign objects from his mouth to prevent choking. Make sure that the patient removes all jewelry, metal objects, and prosthetic devices before the procedure.
- Have the patient wear a hospital gown and ask him to void to prevent incontinence during the procedure. Assist the patient onto the stretcher.

Posttreatment care
- When spontaneous ventilation returns, usually in 3 to 5 minutes, discontinue mechanical ventilation.
- As the patient becomes more alert, speak quietly and explain what's happening. Remove the rubber mouthpiece.
- Place the patient on his side to maintain a patent airway.
- Discharge the patient from the recovery area when he can move all four extremities, can breathe and cough adequately, is roused and oriented when called, has an Aldrete score of 7 or greater, has stable vital signs and temperature within 1° F (0.6° C) of the pretreatment value, and has a normal swallowing reflex.
- Obtain a physician's order for patient release from the recovery area.

MONITORING
- Vital signs
- Temperature to assess for malignant hyperthermia
- Respiratory status
- Neurologic status

Patient teaching
Be sure to cover:
- Signs and symptoms to report to the practitioner
- follow-up care

Endarterectomy, carotid

● OVERVIEW

- Surgical removal of atheromatous plaque from the inner lining of the carotid artery
- Improves intracranial perfusion by increasing blood flow through the carotid artery

Indications
- Reversible ischemic neurologic deficit
- Completed stroke
- Transient ischemic attack
- High-grade asymptomatic or ulcerative lesions

▶ PROCEDURE

- Cervical block anesthesia, sedatives, or light general anesthesia may be used.
- A longitudinal incision is made over the area of the carotid bifurcation.
- The soft tissue is dissected for exposure of the carotid artery and its bifurcation.
- The external, common, and internal carotid arteries are clamped to evaluate perfusion.
- If perfusion is inadequate, the surgeon inserts a shunt to permit blood flow past the obstruction and to ensure adequate cerebral perfusion during surgery.
- After the artery is stabilized, a heparin infusion is started to prevent thrombosis.
- An arteriotomy is made over the stenotic area. The incision is lengthened to expose the full extent of the occluding plaque.
- The plaque or plaques are dissected free from the arterial wall. The intima is cleaned with heparin solution.
- The arteriotomy is closed and a synthetic or autogenous patch may be used to restore the arterial lumen if it's small.
- Before complete closure, blood flow is temporarily restored through the arteries to wash any free plaques, air, or thrombi away from the internal carotid artery.
- The occluding clamps are removed from the external and common carotid arteries. The internal carotid artery clamp is removed last to ensure that any minor debris missed will be flushed harmlessly into the external rather than the internal carotid artery.
- A drain is inserted through a separate stab incision.
- The wound is closed and a dressing is applied.

Complications
- Blood pressure lability
- Preoperative stroke
- Temporary or permanent loss of carotid body function
- Thrombosis
- Respiratory distress
- Wound infection
- Ipsilateral vascular headache
- Seizures
- Intracerebral hemorrhage
- Vocal cord paralysis
- Transient or permanent neurologic deficit

✳ NURSING INTERVENTIONS

Pretreatment care
- Explain the treatment and preparation to the patient and family.
- Make sure the patient has signed an appropriate consent form.
- Explain postoperative care and equipment.
- Perform a complete neurologic assessment.
- Assist with any invasive procedures, as appropriate.
- Obtain a baseline electroencephalogram before the patient is anesthetized, as ordered.

Posttreatment care
- Perform a neurologic assessment every hour for the first 24 hours; check extremity strength, fine hand movements, speech, orientation, and level of consciousness.
- Obtain an electrocardiogram if the patient experiences chest pain or arrhythmias.
- Administer medications, as ordered.

MONITORING
- Vital signs
- Intake and output
- Heart rate and rhythm
- Neurologic status
- Respiratory status
- Surgical wound and dressings
- Drainage
- Cervical edema
- Infection
- Seizures
- Pain

Patient teaching
Be sure to cover:
- medication administration, dosage, and possible adverse effects
- surgical wound care
- signs and symptoms of infection and complications
- when to notify the physician
- risk factor modification, including:
  – smoking cessation
  – lipid-lowering therapy
  – weight reduction
  – control of hypertension and diabetes mellitus
  – regular exercise regimen
- follow-up care
- management of neurologic, sensory, or motor deficits
- referral to a home health care agency, as indicated.

External enhanced coronary perfusion

● OVERVIEW

- Noninvasive procedure that can reduce the symptoms of angina pectoris by increasing coronary blood flow in ischemic areas of the heart
- Involves the use of the external enhanced coronary perfusion (EECP) device to inflate and deflate a series of compressive cuffs wrapped around the patient's calves, lower thighs, and upper thighs; inflation and deflation of cuffs modulated by events in the cardiac cycle via computer-interpreted electrocardiogram (ECG) signals
- Concept of counterpulsation: based on a favorable response of the left ventricle to reduce arterial pressure during the systolic period; heart can be rested and its demand for oxygen reduced, if left ventricular pressure can be reduced; increases stroke volume per unit work and efficiency of the left ventricle; coronary flow and collateral flow to ischemic regions of myocardium increased

Indications

- Stable or unstable angina pectoris
- Patients considered at high risk for revascularization procedures or in whom revascularization isn't technically possible
- Heart failure
- Cardiogenic shock

◆ **NURSING ALERT** EECP shouldn't be used to treat patients with uncontrolled heart failure, severe valvular disease, uncontrolled arrhythmias, hemorrhage, coagulopathy, thrombophlebitis, and peripheral vascular diseases involving iliofemoral arterial obstruction.

▶ PROCEDURE

- The EECP device is placed on the patient's legs and set to inflate and deflate a series of compression cuffs wrapped around the patient's calves, lower thighs, and upper thighs.
- At the start of treatment, external compression is progressively increased, as needed, to raise diastolic pressures gradually. Finger plethysmography is used to monitor correct timings.
- Inflation and deflation of the cuffs are modulated by events in the cardiac cycle via computer-interpreted ECG signals.
- During diastole, the cuffs inflate sequentially from the calves proximally, resulting in augmented diastolic central aortic pressure and increased coronary perfusion pressure. Rapid and simultaneous decompression of the cuffs at the onset of systole permits systolic unloading and decreased cardiac workload.
- Patients are treated with EECP 1 or 2 hours per day for a total of 35 hours. The first week of treatment is limited to 1 hour daily to facilitate familiarization and monitor patient tolerance before increasing the daily treatment time. Two hours of treatment on the same day is usually separated by a rest period.

Complications

- Discomfort from the pulsatile movement and pressure on legs and buttocks

✻ NURSING INTERVENTIONS

Pretreatment care

- At each visit and before treatment begins, take and record the patient's resting blood pressure readings. Also measure and record the sitting pulse and respiratory rates.

◆ **NURSING ALERT** Patients with blood pressure over 180/110 mm Hg or a heart rate more than 120 beats/minute should have these conditions treated before beginning EECP.

- The patient's legs are examined for areas of redness, ecchymosis, and signs of other vascular problems.
- Advise the patient to urinate immediately before treatment.
- Ask the patient about symptoms of angina and review the patient's record.

Posttreatment care

- Place the patient in a comfortable position and give supplemental oxygen, as indicated.
- Administer medications.
- Provide support for the patient's family.

MONITORING

- Cardiac status; continuous cardiac monitoring
- Vital signs
- Intake and output
- Effect of medications

Patient teaching

Be sure to cover:

- signs and symptoms of heart failure
- measures to eliminate or minimize discomfort from the pulsatile movement and pressure on legs and need to notify the practitioner if the pulsating sensation becomes uncomfortable
- recording of each anginal attack; its time of occurrence, duration, and severity; its relationship to precipitating factors; and the number of nitroglycerin tablets used to ease the attack
- follow-up care.

Extracorporeal membrane oxygenation

● OVERVIEW

- Group of supportive therapies that oxygenizes blood outside the body
- Exposes a patient's lungs to low pressures, allowing them to rest and providing a means for oxygen delivery and carbon dioxide removal
- Lowers fraction of inspired oxygen (FIO_2) concentrations and volumes via mechanical ventilation, thereby reducing the risk of oxygen toxicity and barotrauma
- Also called *ECMO* or *extracorporeal life support*

Indications

- Severe acute respiratory failure
- Acute respiratory distress syndrome
- Perioperative cardiac failure
- Primary myocardial failure
- Bridge to transplantation

▶ PROCEDURE

- The physician uses strict aseptic technique to insert a cannula percutaneously into the appropriate vessel.
- The patient receives a loading dose of heparin I.V.
- The catheter is connected to the ECMO circuit and therapy is initiated; a continuous heparin infusion is maintained throughout therapy. An ECMO specialist remains at the patient's bedside.
- As blood leaves the patient's body, it's pumped through a membrane oxygenator, which acts as an artificial lung, supplying oxygen to the blood.
- A roller pump regulates the blood flow to the oxygenator, turning off whenever the pump flow is greater than blood return to the patient; excessive pressure on the right atrium or major vessels is averted. The pump automatically restarts when the flow rate balances.

AGE-RELATED CONCERN Typical blood flow rates for adults range from 70 to 90 ml/kg/minute; for children, 80 to 100 ml/kg/minute; and for neonates, 120 to 170 ml/kg/minute.

- An in-line fiber-optic catheter is used to monitor venous oxygen levels.
- Before returning to the patient, the blood passes through a heat exchanger where it's warmed to prevent hypothermia.

Complications

- Mechanical: clots in the circuit, vessel damage, air in circuit, oxygenator failure, pump or heat exchanger malfunction, failure of the circuit or circuit monitoring equipment
- Patient: seizures, intracranial bleeding, hemorrhage, thrombocytopenia, myocardial stun, hypertension, pericardial tamponade, pneumothorax, pulmonary hemorrhage, acute tubular necrosis, hyperbilirubinemia, infection, sepsis, metabolic acidosis or alkalosis, electrolyte imbalances involving potassium, sodium, and calcium, hyperglycemia or hypoglycemia

✳ NURSING INTERVENTIONS

Pretreatment care

- Reinforce the practitioner's explanation of the procedure, equipment, and follow-up care.
- Verify that an appropriate consent form is signed.
- As appropriate, inform the patient that he'll have an endotracheal (ET) tube in place and will be connected to a mechanical ventilator.
- Review other equipment that may be used and provide emotional support.
- Administer sedation, as ordered, to reduce pain and restrict movement during catheter insertion and treatment.

Posttreatment care

- After ECMO is initiated and the patient's gas exchange shows signs of improvement, expect to lower ventilator settings. Stay alert for changes in tidal volumes, which should increase as the lungs improve.
- If the patient becomes hemodynamically unstable, expect to administer dopamine (Intropin) to raise blood pressure and dobutamine (Dobutrex) to improve cardiac output; titrate dosages to desired response.
- Maintain a patent airway and ventilator function, as appropriate.

- Administer supplemental oxygen and suction, as necessary.
- Inspect catheter insertion sites for oozing or hematoma; change dressings, as needed. If necessary, weigh saturated dressings to determine fluid volume loss.
- If hematoma develops, palpate and mark borders to monitor for size increase.
- Perform chest physiotherapy and change the patient's position frequently. Make sure that the ECMO circuit is unimpaired.
- Administer sedatives and analgesia and apply soft restraints, as ordered.
- Expect to administer blood transfusions, including packed red blood cells to increase the oxygen-carrying capacity of the blood and to help stabilize the patient's intravascular volume.
- Anticipate platelet transfusion if the patient's platelet count drops below 100,000/mm³.
- Offer emotional support to the patient's family.

MONITORING

- ET tube patency, position, and function, and mechanical ventilation
- Oxygen saturation levels and arterial blood gas levels
- Cardiac and hemodynamic status (central venous pressure, pulmonary artery pressure, and cardiac output)
- Intake and output, weight, blood urea nitrogen, and serum creatinine levels
- Signs and symptoms of acute renal failure
- Activated clotting times
- Affected extremity distal to the ECMO catheter insertion site for pulses, color, and temperature at least every 2 hours

⊡ NURSING ALERT A thready or absent pulse; a pale, cyanotic, or cool extremity; and a decrease in sensation indicate that the extremity isn't receiving adequate blood flow. This is an emergency that must be reported to the practitioner immediately.

Patient teaching

Be sure to cover:
- monitoring techniques and devices
- signs and symptoms indicating improvement in condition
- care measures necessary.

Femoral popliteal bypass

● OVERVIEW

- Used to restore blood flow to the leg with a femoral artery occlusion
- Also called *femoral-popliteal* or *fem-pop bypass*

Indications

- Vessel damaged by an arteriosclerotic or thromboembolic disorder
- Arterial occlusive disease
- Limb-threatening acute arterial occlusion unresponsive to thrombolytic drug therapy
- Vessel trauma, infection, or congenital defect
- Vascular disease unresponsive to drug therapy or nonsurgical revascularization

▶ PROCEDURE

- The procedure may be done under local or general anesthesia.
- I.V. antibiotics may be administered prophylactically during or just after the procedure; blood pressure drugs may be titrated to maintain the desired range.
- The surgical area is thoroughly cleaned with an antiseptic solution.
- If the saphenous vein will be used, an incision is made in the thigh and the other tissues are retracted until the vein can be seen. An appropriate length of the vein is excised for grafting and prepared (the vein is reversed so that the end that was originally located in the groin is now connected to the popliteal artery to eliminate hindrance of the valves).
- If the saphenous vein is inadequate, a synthetic vein graft is used.
- The saphenous access incision is closed and smaller incisions are made in the groin area to access the femoral artery and behind the knee for the popliteal artery.
- One end of the vein graft is attached above the blockage femorally, and the free end of the graft is tunneled next to the artery to the popliteal site, where it's sutured in place.

- Blood flow is initiated through the graft and the connections are assessed for leakage.
- A repeat arteriogram is performed to confirm that blood flow has been restored.
- The incisions are closed and dressings are applied.

Complications

- Vessel or nerve injury
- Thrombus or emboli formation
- Myocardial infarction
- Cardiac arrhythmias
- Hemorrhage
- Infection
- Edema
- Pulmonary edema
- Graft occlusion, narrowing, dilation, or rupture

✳ NURSING INTERVENTIONS

Pretreatment care

- Explain the treatment and preparation to the patient and his family.
- Verify that the patient has signed an appropriate consent form.
- Explain postoperative care.
- Perform a complete neurovascular assessment; mark the location of distal peripheral pulses bilaterally (if present) for ease of monitoring during and after the procedure (may require Doppler ultrasound localization in affected extremity).
- Obtain baseline vital signs and blood pressure.
- Obtain or verify the completion of the baseline 12-lead electrocardiogram and laboratory studies.
- Restrict food and fluids, as ordered.
- Give the patient an aspirin before the procedure, as ordered.
- Notify the surgeon if the patient is sensitive or allergic to any medications, latex, iodine, tape, contrast dyes, or anesthetic agents.
- Notify the surgeon if there's a history of bleeding disorders or if the patient is taking anticoagulants, aspirin, or other medications that affect blood clotting. It may be necessary to stop these medications before the procedure.

- Make sure the surgeon marks the site where the procedure is to be performed.
- Shave the areas around the surgical sites, as ordered.
- Initiate peripheral I.V. access; inform the patient that his heart rhythm will be monitored during the procedure.
- Insert a urinary catheter after preparing the patient for the procedure.
- Administer sedation, as ordered.

Posttreatment care

- Administer medications, as ordered.
- Position the patient, as ordered, and encourage frequent turning, keeping pressure off the graft site.
- Provide comfort measures and analgesics, as needed.
- Perform incision site care and dressing changes, as ordered.
- Assist with initial transfers and ambulation when cleared by the practitioner, and explain recommended activity levels to the patient.
- Encourage frequent incentive spirometer use, coughing, and deep breathing.
- Assist with and teach the patient range-of-motion exercises.

MONITORING

- Vital signs, heart rate and rhythm, and neurovascular status (per facility policy)
- Incision site
- Signs and symptoms of infection
- Intake and output
- Complications, including abnormal bleeding, graft occlusion, chest pain, and breathing difficulty with embolism or pulmonary edema

Patient teaching

Be sure to cover:
- medication administration, dosage, and possible adverse effects
- monitoring of lower extremities for changes in temperature, color, and sensation, and any return of preoperative symptoms, warranting notification of the surgeon
- incision site care
- signs and symptoms of infection and possible complications
- lifestyle changes including need for low-cholesterol diet, smoking cessation, and regular exercise
- follow-up care for monitoring of blood pressure and cholesterol levels.

Gastric bypass

● OVERVIEW

- Malabsorption and restriction procedure in which a small stomach pouch is created using sutures and is attached to a portion of the jejunum; reduces the body's intake of calories, thus achieving potentially significant weight loss
- Postoperatively, because stomach is smaller, allows patient to feel fuller faster
- Also referred to as a *Roux-en-Y bypass*

Indications

- Body mass index (BMI) of 40 or more and at least 100 lb (45 kg) over recommended weight (normal BMI, 18.5 to 25)
- BMI of 35 or more plus a life-threatening illness that can be improved with weight loss, such as sleep apnea, type 2 diabetes, and heart disease

▶ PROCEDURE

- The surgery is performed under general anesthesia.
- The surgeon divides the stomach into a small upper section and a larger bottom section using staples similar to stitches.
- After the stomach has been divided, the surgeon connects a section of the small intestine (commonly the jejunum) to the pouch.
- The surgeon then reconnects the base of the Roux limb with the remaining portion of the small intestines from the bottom of the stomach, forming a V-shape.
- Gastric bypass can also be performed using a laparoscope.
- With laparoscopy, small incisions are made in the abdomen. Carbon dioxide is insufflated to separate the organs from one another. The surgeon the passes slender surgical instruments through these incisions with a laparoscope to perform the procedure and video monitoring during the surgery.

◆ **NURSING ALERT** If the patient weighs more than 350 lb (159 kg) or if he has had previous ab-

dominal surgery, laparoscopy may be contraindicated.

Complications

- Bleeding
- Infections
- Gallstones
- Vomiting
- Iron or vitamin B_{12} deficiencies leading to anemia
- Calcium deficiency leading to osteoporosis
- Dumping syndrome (nausea, vomiting' diarrhea, dizziness, and sweating)

✳ NURSING INTERVENTIONS

Pretreatment care

- Perform a complete physical examination to evaluate the patient's overall health. Also complete a psychological evaluation to determine if he'll be adhering to the new lifestyle.
- Explain the treatment and preparation to the patient and his family.
- Verify that the patient has signed an appropriate consent form.
- Obtain blood samples for hematologic and chemistry studies, as ordered.
- Withhold food and fluids, as ordered.
- Begin I.V. fluid replacement and total parenteral nutrition (TPN), as ordered.
- Prepare the patient for abdominal X-rays, as ordered.
- Explain postoperative care and equipment.
- Monitor the patient's vital signs, intake and output, nutritional status, and laboratory test results.
- Complete the preoperative verification process.

Posttreatment care

- Maintain I.V. replacement therapy, as ordered.
- Keep the nasogastric tube patent, but don't reposition it.
- Encourage regular turning, coughing, deep-breathing exercises, and use of incentive spirometry.
- Encourage splinting of the incision site with coughing and movement.
- Administer medications, as ordered.

- Place the patient in low or semi-Fowler's position.
- Provide wound care, as necessary.
- After bowel sounds return, begin oral intake, providing six small feedings per day. Encourage fluids to prevent dehydration.
- Provide comfort measures.

MONITORING

- Vital signs
- Intake and output and daily weight
- Signs of dehydration, peritonitis, sepsis, infection, or postresection obstruction

◆ **NURSING ALERT** Monitor for and immediately report signs and symptoms of anastomotic leakage, including low-grade fever, malaise, slight leukocytosis, abdominal distention, tenderness, hemorrhage, hypovolemic shock, and bloody stool or wound drainage.

- Abdominal pain, cramping, or shoulder pain
- Bowel sounds
- Laboratory test results
- Incision site
- Drainage
- Complications of morbid obesity, such as pneumonia, thromboembolism, skin breakdown, and delayed wound healing

Patient teaching

Be sure to cover:
- medication administration, dosage, and possible adverse effects
- excessive bleeding from surgical sites
- signs and symptoms of infection
- signs and symptoms of obstruction or perforation
- surgical wound care
- dumping syndrome and measures to prevent it
- nutritional counseling (including liquid and pureed foods initially, small meals, reduction of fat intake), weight loss patterns, and need for adherence to dietary plan
- follow-up visits
- possible need for replacement of iron, calcium, vitamin B_{12}, or other nutrients.

Heart valve replacement

● OVERVIEW

- Excision of a diseased heart valve and replacement with a mechanical or biological valve prosthesis
- Usually involves a medial sternotomy approach
- Alternatively, may involve a minimally invasive-port access approach

Indications

- Severe aortic valvular stenosis or insufficiency
- Severe mitral valvular stenosis or insufficiency
- Damage or disease from bacterial endocarditis, rheumatic fever, calcific degeneration, or congenital abnormalities

▶ PROCEDURE

- After the patient is anesthetized, a medial sternotomy is performed, and cardiopulmonary bypass is initiated.
- The coronary arteries are cannulated and perfused with a cold cardioplegic solution.
- For aortic valve replacement, the aorta is clamped above the right coronary artery.
- For mitral valve replacement, the left atrium is incised to expose the mitral valve.
- The diseased valve is excised.
- The surgeon sutures around the margin of the valve annulus.
- The suture is threaded through the sewing ring of the prosthetic valve.
- Using a valve holder, the prosthesis is positioned, and the sutures are secured.
- The patient is removed from the bypass machine.
- As the heart fills with blood, the surgeon vents the aorta and ventricle for air.
- Epicardial pacemaker leads and a chest tube are inserted.
- The incision is closed, and a sterile dressing is applied.

Complications

- Postpericardiomotomy syndrome
- Cardiac arrhythmias
- Hemorrhage
- Coagulopathy
- Stroke
- Prosthetic valve endocarditis
- Valve dysfunction or failure
- Renal failure
- Pulmonary embolism
- Thromboembolism
- Infection

✳ NURSING INTERVENTIONS

Pretreatment care

- Explain the treatment and preparation to the patient and family.
- Make sure the patient has signed an appropriate consent form.
- Explain postoperative care and equipment.
- Obtain results of laboratory studies, including blood typing and cross-matching, chest X-ray, and 12-lead electrocardiogram.

Posttreatment care

- Administer medications, as ordered.
- Assist with temporary epicardial pacing, as indicated.
- Maintain mean arterial pressure within prescribed guidelines.
- Maintain the chest tube system as ordered.
- Administer I.V. fluids and blood products, as ordered.
- Perform chest physiotherapy.
- Assist with weaning from the mechanical ventilator, as indicated.
- Encourage coughing, turning, deep breathing, and use of incentive spirometry.
- Assist with early ambulation.

MONITORING

- Vital signs
- Intake and output
- Daily weight
- Complications
- Cardiovascular status
- Heart rate and rhythm
- Heart sounds, including prosthetic valve sounds
- Hemodynamic values
- Respiratory status
- Arterial blood gas analysis
- Laboratory test results
- Surgical wound and dressings
- Abnormal bleeding
- Drainage
- Sternal stability

Patient teaching

Be sure to cover:

- medication administration, dosage, and possible adverse effects
- surgical wound care
- signs and symptoms of infection
- signs and symptoms of postpericardiotomy syndrome
- complications
- when to notify the physician
- anticoagulant therapy
- infective endocarditis prophylaxis
- abnormal bleeding
- balancing activity with rest
- prescribed dietary and activity restrictions
- prescribed exercise program
- follow-up care
- importance of informing all health care providers of the prosthetic valve
- importance of wearing medical identification.

Heart valvuloplasty, percutaneous balloon

● OVERVIEW

- Insertion of a balloon-tipped catheter through the femoral vein or artery and into the heart, followed by repeated balloon inflation against the leaflets of a diseased heart valve
- Helps expand the constricted valve, promoting more adequate cardiac output and heart functioning

Indications

- Congenital valve defects
- Valve calcifications
- Valvular stenosis
- Poor candidate for invasive valve surgery

▶ PROCEDURE

- After the patient is sedated, the catheter site is cleaned and draped. A local anesthetic is then injected into the tissue surrounding the catheter insertion site.
- The physician inserts a catheter into the femoral artery (for left heart valve) or the femoral vein (for a right heart valve).
- The balloon-tipped catheter is passed through this catheter and guided by fluoroscopy into the heart.
- The deflated balloon is inserted in the valve opening and repeatedly inflated with a solution containing normal saline solution and a contrast media.
- As the balloon inflates, the valve leaflets split free from one another, permitting them to open and close properly and increase the valvular orifice.
- The surgeon removes the balloon-tipped catheter.
- The femoral catheter may be left in place in case the patient needs to return to the laboratory for a repeat procedure

Complications

- Valvular insufficiency
- Embolism
- Valve leaflet damage
- Infection
- Bleeding and hematoma at the arterial or venous puncture site

- Arrhythmias
- Myocardial ischemia and infarction
- Circulatory insufficiency distal to the catheter entry site
- Restenosis
- Guidewire perforation of the ventricle, leading to tamponade

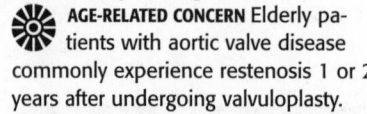 **AGE-RELATED CONCERN** Elderly patients with aortic valve disease commonly experience restenosis 1 or 2 years after undergoing valvuloplasty.

※ NURSING INTERVENTIONS

Pretreatment care

- Review the purpose of the procedure and what nursing measures to expect after insertion of the device.
- Initiate I.V. therapy, as prescribed.
- Prepare the patient's groin area.
- Verify that an appropriate consent form has been signed.
- Provide emotional support.
- Monitor electrocardiogram (ECG) and pulmonary artery and hemodynamic status; if a central catheter is already in place, monitor vital signs and intake and output.
- Restrict food and fluid intake, as ordered.
- Obtain routine laboratory studies, report abnormal results, and verify that blood typing and crossmatching are complete.
- Palpate bilateral distal pulses and complete a vascular assessment of the extremities, mark the pulse points with a skin marker, and record the assessment findings. Use Doppler ultrasonography, if needed, to locate all pulses.
- Administer a sedative and withhold other medications, as ordered.
- Complete the preoperative verification process.

Posttreatment care

- Maintain sandbag or other compression device over cannulation site to minimize bleeding, as ordered.
- Prevent excessive hip flexion by keeping affected leg straight and elevating the head of the bed no more than 15 degrees.
- If needed, prepare for catheter removal in 6 to 12 hours after valvuloplasty. Afterward, apply a pressure dressing and assess vital signs.
- Admininster I.V. fluids and medications, as ordered.
- If an expanding ecchymotic area appears, mark the area to help determine the pace of expansion. If bleeding occurs, apply direct pressure and notify the physician.
- Auscultate for murmurs, which may indicate worsening valvular insufficiency. Report changes to the physician immediately.

MONITORING

- Vital signs, intake and output
- Catheter insertion site for hematoma formation, ecchymosis, or hemorrhage
- ECG and hemodynamic status (if central catheter in place)
- Peripheral pulses distal to insertion site, and color, temperature, and capillary refill of extremities

 NURSING ALERT Notify the physician immediately if pulses are absent.

Patient teaching

Be sure to cover:

- signs to report to the physician, including bleeding or increased bruising at the puncture site, or recurrence of symptoms of valvular insufficiency, such as breathlessness or decreased exercise tolerance
- diet and activity restrictions
- medication administration, dosage, and possible adverse effects
- need for prophylactic antibiotics during dental surgery or other invasive procedures
- follow-up care.

Hernia repair, inguinal

● OVERVIEW

- Surgical repair of a hernia
- May involve herniorrhaphy (which returns the protruding intestine to the abdominal cavity and repairs an abdominal wall defect) or hernioplasty (which reinforces the weakened area around the repair with plastic, steel or tantalum mesh, or wire)
- Laparoscopic repair typical for uncomplicated hernias
- Usually done on an elective basis, but emergency surgery necessary for a strangulated or incarcerated hernia (may necessitate hospitalization for several days with a nasogastric tube in place)

Indications
- Groin hernias
- Hernias of the anterior abdominal wall

▶ PROCEDURE

- General or spinal anesthesia is used.
- The surgeon makes an incision over the herniated area or views area laparoscopically.
- The herniated tissue is manipulated back to its proper position.
- The defect in the muscle or fascia is repaired.
- If necessary, the defect is reinforced with wire, mesh, or another material.
- The incision is closed and a dressing is applied.

Complications
- Infection
- Bleeding
- Hernia recurrence
- Bowel or bladder injury.

✳ NURSING INTERVENTIONS

Pretreatment care
- Explain the treatment and preparation to the patient and family.
- Make sure the patient has signed an appropriate consent form.
- Explain postoperative care.
- Shave the surgical site, as ordered.
- Administer an enema, as ordered.
- Administer a sedative, as ordered.

Posttreatment care
- Administer medications, as ordered.
- Reduce pressure on the incision site.
- Take measures to prevent constipation.
- Encourage early ambulation.
- Make sure the patient voids within 12 hours after surgery; if necessary, insert a urinary catheter or assist with insertion.
- Provide comfort measures.
- Apply an ice bag to the scrotum, if appropriate.
- Apply a scrotal bridge or truss, if appropriate.

MONITORING
- Vital signs
- Intake and output
- Complications
- Surgical wound and dressings
- Drainage
- Infection

Patient teaching
Be sure to cover:
- medication administration, dosage, and possible adverse effects
- activity restrictions
- incision care
- signs and symptoms of infection
- complications
- when to notify the physician
- follow-up care
- possible need for a job change if the patient regularly does heavy lifting or other strenuous activities
- signs and symptoms of hernia recurrence
- hernia prevention
- use of scrotal support or ice packs (in males)
- high-fiber diet
- adequate oral fluid intake
- referral to a weight reduction program, if indicated
- referral to a smoking cessation program, if indicated.

Hyperbaric oxygenation

● OVERVIEW

- Medical treatment that delivers 100% oxygen to a patient in a special pressurized chamber
- Increases oxygen in the plasma and its availability to hypoxic cells and tissues
- Increases white blood cells and stimulates the formation of new capillaries and nerve endings around wound sites; pushes other dissolved harmful gases out of the circulatory system and causes vasoconstriction without decrease in oxygenation
- Involves specialized chambers that deliver oxygen at atmospheric pressures 1½ to 3 times that at sea level
- Oxygen delivered in special masks or acrylic hoods that provide for a continuous flow of air across the face and venting of carbon dioxide outside the chamber
- Regular air pressurized within most chambers, although some are pressurized with 100% oxygen
- Treatment protocols variable in length, frequency, and inpatient or outpatient location by type of disorder

Indications
- Carbon monoxide or cyanide poisoning
- Gas or air embolism
- Decompression sickness
- Osteoradionecrosis
- Drug overdose
- Clostridial gas gangrene
- Combined with other treatments for:
  – Anemia from severe blood loss
  – Crush injuries or wounds with severe tissue ischemia
  – Compartment syndrome
  – Graft and flap salvage
  – Injury from radiation, thermal burns
  – Necrotizing soft tissue infections
- Neurologic disease

▶ PROCEDURE

- The patient enters the hyperbaric chamber on a stretcher (monoplace— one patient) or may be treated while in a chair, recliner, or stretcher (multiplace—holding from 2 to 16 patients).
- Oxygen delivery devices are applied to the patient, often with a transcutaneous oxygen monitor on the arm.
- The chamber is sealed and pressurized to the ordered air pressure, for the prescribed amount of time. Patients are monitored visually and staff speak directly to the patient to assess adjustment and difficulties via special communication lines. An attendant monitors the chamber during treatment.
- The pressure is gradually decompressed at the end of the treatment phase, and the oxygen delivery device is removed.

Complications
- Oxygen toxicity syndrome
- Painful, bloody discharge from sinuses
- Edema, rupture, or retraction of tympanic membrane
- Temporary deterioration of visual acuity; accelerated maturation of cataracts
- Ataxia
- Vertigo
- Tinnitus; hearing loss
- Hypoglycemia in patients with type 1 diabetes
- Nausea or vomiting
- Flatulence; colicky abdominal pain
- Tooth pain, implosion, or explosion
- Sudden decreased level of consciousness
- Hemiplegia

✳ NURSING INTERVENTIONS

Pretreatment care
- Obtain baseline vital signs, and assess heart and lung sounds. If wounds are involved, perform an assessment.
- Explain how therapy is delivered, and what safety measures are in place and communication devices are used.
- Verify that an informed consent form has been signed.
- Determine if the patient has a history of claustrophobia; if so, notify the physician and administer a mild sedative, as ordered.

- Explain to the patient and family that an electrocardiogram, arterial line, hemodynamic monitoring lines, I.V. lines, or mechanical ventilation may be used within the chambers as needed.
- Teach the patient that cigarettes and fire risk materials; hand warmers; watches, jewelry, and metal objects; hair spray, make-up, perfume, deodorant, shaving lotion, skin lotions, and any other alcohol or petroleum-based product; newspapers; battery-operated equipment; and hearing aids, hard contact lenses, and dental plates aren't permitted in the chamber for safety reasons.
- Inform the patient that some ear discomfort or popping, an increase in temperature of the chamber, and a motorlike noise are to be expected as the chamber is pressurized. Once pressurized fully, the ambient temperature will decrease to comfortable levels and the noise will stop.
- Teach the patient methods to clear pressure in the eustachian tubes and to notify the attendant promptly if the discomfort doesn't improve.
- Tell the patient he may experience transient light-headedness, fatigue, headache, or vomiting after the treatment.
- Assist the patient, as needed, into all-cotton clothes and shoe covers.

Posttreatment care
- Provide comfort measures.
- Offer emotional support.
- Administer medications, as ordered.
MONITORING
- Vital signs
- Hemodynamic values
- Heart rate and rhythm
- Intake and output
- Pulse oximetry
- Neurologic, pulmonary, skin, sensory, and mental status for complications

Patient teaching
Be sure to cover:
- signs of oxygen toxicity and other complications to report to the physician immediately
- medication administration, dosage, and possible adverse effects
- safety guidelines for each treatment
- follow-up care.

Hysterectomy

● OVERVIEW

- Surgical removal of the uterus
- May be performed abdominally, vaginally, or through a laparoscope
- When done laparoscopically, allows the surgeon to perform preparatory steps before removing the uterus through the vagina
- Subtotal hysterectomy: removal of the entire uterus except the cervix
- Total hysterectomy: removal of both the uterus and cervix
- Panhysterectomy: removal of the entire uterus, ovaries, and fallopian tubes
- Radical hysterectomy: removal of the uterus, ovaries, fallopian tubes, adjoining ligaments and lymph nodes, upper one-third of the vagina, and surrounding tissues

Indications

- Malignant or benign tumor of the uterus, cervix, or adnexa
- Uterine bleeding and hemorrhage
- Uterine rupture or perforation
- Life-threatening pelvic infection
- Endometriosis unresponsive to conservative treatment
- Pelvic floor relaxation or prolapse

▶ PROCEDURE

- The patient receives general anesthesia.

ABDOMINAL APPROACH

- The surgeon makes a midline vertical incision from the umbilicus to the symphysis pubis, or makes a horizontal incision in the lower abdomen.
- The uterus and accompanying structures are excised and removed.
- The incision is closed, and a dressing and perineal pad are applied.

VAGINAL APPROACH

- An incision is made above the vagina near the cervix.
- The uterus is excised and removed through the vaginal canal.
- The opening is closed to the peritoneal cavity with sutures.
- A perineal pad is applied.

LAPAROSCOPIC APPROACH

- An incision is made in the umbilicus.

- Nitrous oxide or carbon dioxide is infused into the abdominal cavity.
- The patient is placed in Trendelenburg's position.
- The laparoscope is inserted. (If an operative laparoscope is used, no other incision is required.)
- Several other small abdominal incisions are made to pass instruments.
- The uterus is excised vaginally, along with other accompanying structures, as necessary.
- The incision is closed, and a dressing and perineal pad are applied.

Complications

- Wound infection
- Urinary retention
- Abdominal distention
- Thromboembolism
- Pneumonia
- Hemorrhage
- Ureteral or bowel injury
- Wound dehiscence
- Pulmonary embolism
- Paralytic ileus
- Psychological problems

✳ NURSING INTERVENTIONS

Pretreatment care

- Explain the treatment and preparation to the patient and family.
- Make sure the patient has signed an appropriate consent form.
- Administer an enema the evening before surgery.
- Administer prophylactic antibiotics, as ordered.
- Make sure laboratory tests have been performed, including a pregnancy test, if indicated; report abnormal results.
- Explain postoperative care, including expected abdominal cramping and moderate amounts of drainage. If the patient will have an abdominal hysterectomy, explain that an indwelling urinary catheter or suprapubic tube, as well as a nasogastric or rectal tube, may be inserted.
- Institute deep vein thrombosis prophylaxis, as ordered.
- Provide information regarding estrogen replacement therapy, if appropriate.

Posttreatment care

- Administer medications, as ordered.
- Provide indwelling urinary catheter or suprapubic catheter care, if appropriate.
- Provide perineal care.

  ◈ **NURSING ALERT** Notify the physician if the patient saturates more than one pad every 4 hours.

- Encourage the patient to cough, breathe deeply, and turn at least every 2 hours.
- Administer I.V. fluids, as ordered.
- Withhold oral intake status until peristalsis returns.
- Keep the patient in a supine position, low Fowler's, or semi-Fowler's position, as ordered.
- Assist with early ambulation.
- Encourage the patient to perform prescribed exercises.
- Assist with suture or staple removal (usually on fifth postoperative day).

MONITORING

- Vital signs
- Intake and output
- Complications
- Surgical wound and dressings
- Vaginal drainage (color, odor, and amount)
- Abnormal bleeding
- Infection
- Bowel sounds
- Respiratory status
- Pain management

Patient teaching

Be sure to cover:

- medication administration, dosage, and possible adverse effects
- coughing and deep-breathing exercises and use of incentive spirometry
- signs and symptoms of infection
- complications
- when to notify the physician
- activity restrictions, including sexual activity
- early ambulation
- avoidance of tub baths, douching, and sexual activity until after the 6-week checkup
- importance of a high-protein, high-residue diet
- increased oral fluid intake (3,000 ml/day), as ordered
- follow-up care
- wound care
- pain management.

Implantable cardioverter-defibrillator

● OVERVIEW

- Monitors the heart for bradycardia, ventricular tachycardia, and fibrillation and delivers shocks or paced beats when indicated
- Stores information and electrocardiograms (ECGs) and tracks treatments and their outcome
- Allows information retrieval to evaluate the device's function and battery status and to adjust the settings
- Depending on the model, may deliver bradycardia pacing (both single- and dual-chamber), antitachycardia pacing, cardioversion, and defibrillation
- Also called *ICD*

Indications
- Cardiac arrhythmias refractory to drug therapy, surgery, or catheter ablation
- Therapy for atrial arrhythmias such as atrial fibrillation
- Ventricular defibrillation for automated treatment of life-threatening ventricular arrhythmias.

 NURSING ALERT ICDs are contraindicated for patients with transient or reversible ventricular tachyarrhythmia or as the sole treatment of atrial arrhythmia.

▶ PROCEDURE

- The transvenous route with fluoroscopy is the most commonly used operative procedure. The thoracotomy approach may be used for patients who have mediastinal adhesions from previous sternal surgery. The subxiphoid approach may also be used. A median sternotomy may be used if the patient requires other cardiac surgery such as revascularization.
- One or more lead wires are attached to the epicardium.
- A programmable pulse generator is inserted into a pocket made under the right or left clavicle.
- The device is programmed and checked for proper functioning.

Complications
- Infection

- Venous thrombosis and embolism
- Pneumothorax
- Pectoral or diaphragmatic muscle stimulation
- Arrhythmias
- Cardiac tamponade
- Heart failure
- Lead dislodgment
- ICD malfunction, resulting in untreated ventricular fibrillation and cardiac arrest

✖ NURSING INTERVENTIONS

Pretreatment care
- Explain the treatment and patient preparation.
- Make sure the patient has signed an appropriate consent form.
- Obtain baseline vital signs and a 12-lead ECG.
- Evaluate the patient's radial and pedal pulses.
- Assess the patient's mental status.
- Restrict food and fluids before the procedure, as ordered.
- Explain postoperative care.
- If the patient is monitored, document and report any arrhythmias.
- Administer medications, as ordered, and prepare to assist with medical procedures (such as defibrillation), if indicated.

Posttreatment care
- Obtain a printed status report verifying the ICD type and model, status (on or off), detection rates, and therapies to be delivered (such as pacing, antitachycardia pacing, cardioversion, and defibrillation).
- Don't remove the occlusive dressing for the first 24 hours without a physician's order.
- After the first 24 hours, begin passive range-of-motion exercises, if ordered, and progress, as tolerated.
- If the patient experiences cardiac arrest, initiate cardiopulmonary resuscitation (CPR) and advanced cardiac life support (wearing latex gloves to avoid experiencing an ICD shock).

 NURSING ALERT For external defibrillation, use anteroposterior paddle placement; don't place paddles directly over the pulse generator.

MONITORING
- Vital signs
- Intake and output
- Heart rate and rhythm
- Complications
- Surgical incision and dressings
- Drainage
- Infection

 NURSING ALERT Monitor for signs and symptoms of a perforated ventricle with resultant cardiac tamponade. Findings may include persistent hiccups, distant heart sounds, pulsus paradoxus, hypotension accompanied by narrow pulse pressure, increased venous pressure, bulging neck veins, cyanosis, decreased urine output, restlessness, and complaints of fullness in the chest. Notify the physician immediately, and prepare the patient for emergency surgery.

Patient teaching
Be sure to cover:
- medication administration, dosage, and possible adverse effects
- signs and symptoms of infection
- complications
- when to notify the physician
- importance of wearing medical alert identification that indicates ICD placement and of carrying ICD information at all times
- what to do in an emergency, such as calling 911 and having a family member perform CPR if the ICD fails
- avoidance of placing excessive pressure over the insertion site or moving or jerking the area, until the physician approves
- prescribed activity restrictions
- what to expect when the ICD discharges
- notifying the physician when the ICD discharges
- importance of informing airline personnel and health care workers who perform diagnostic tests (such as computed tomography scans and magnetic resonance imaging) of ICD presence
- possible disruption of the ICD by electrical or electronic devices
- follow-up care.

Intra-aortic balloon counterpulsation

● OVERVIEW

- Temporarily supports the heart's left ventricle by mechanically displacing blood by an intra-aortic balloon attached to an external pump console
- Increases the supply of oxygen-rich blood to the myocardium and decreases myocardial oxygen demand
- Also used to monitor myocardial perfusion and the effects of drugs on myocardial function and perfusion
- Usually inserted through the common femoral artery and positioned with its tip just distal to the left subclavian artery
- Also called *IABP*

Indications
- Low cardiac output disorders
  - Refractory angina
  - Ventricular arrhythmias
  - Cardiogenic shock
- Cardiac instability
  - Myocardial infarction
  - High-grade lesions
- Support measures
  - Bypass surgery
  - Angioplasty
  - Cardiac catheterization

▶ PROCEDURE

Before the physician inserts the balloon, he puts on sterile gloves, a gown, and a mask, cleans the site with povidone-iodine solution, and covers the area with a sterile drape.

PERCUTANEOUS INSERTION
- The physician may insert the balloon percutaneously through the femoral artery into the descending thoracic aorta, using a modified Seldinger technique.
- He accesses the vessel with an 18G angiography needle, removes the inner stylet, passes the guide wire through the needle, and then removes the needle.
- An introducer (dilator and sheath assembly) is passed over the guide wire into the vessel until 1″ (2.5 cm) remains above the insertion site.
- The inner dilator is removed, leaving the introducer sheath and guide wire in place.
- After passing the balloon over the guide wire into the introducer sheath, the physician advances the catheter into position—⅜″ to ⅘″ (1 to 2 cm) distal to the left subclavian artery under fluoroscopic guidance.
- The balloon is then attached to the control system to start counterpulsation.

SURGICAL INSERTION
- The surgeon may decide to insert the catheter through a femoral arteriotomy.
- After making an incision and isolating the femoral artery, the surgeon attaches a Dacron graft to a small opening in the arterial wall and passes the catheter through this graft.
- Using fluoroscopic guidance, he advances the catheter up the descending thoracic aorta and positions the catheter tip between the left subclavian and renal arteries.
- The Dacron graft is sewn around the catheter at the insertion point and the other end is connected to the pump console.

- If the balloon can't be inserted through the femoral artery, the surgeon may use the transthoracic method and insert it in an antegrade direction through the anterior wall of the ascending aorta.
- He positions it ⅜″ to ⅕″ beyond the left subclavian artery and brings the catheter out through the chest wall.

Complications
- Arterial embolism
- Extension or rupture of an aortic aneurysm
- Femoral or iliac artery perforation
- Femoral artery occlusion
- Sepsis
- Bleeding at the insertion site

✳ NURSING INTERVENTIONS

Pretreatment care
- Depending on facility policy, you or a perfusionist must balance the pressure transducer in the external pump console and calibrate the oscilloscope monitor to ensure accuracy.
- Tell the patient that the physician will place a special balloon catheter in his aorta to help his heart pump more easily.
- Let the patient know that the balloon will be removed after his heart can resume an adequate workload.
- Explain the insertion procedure; mention that the catheter will be connected to a large console next to the patient's bed.
- Verify that the patient has signed an appropriate consent form.
- Record the patient's baseline vital signs and hemodynamic results, if available.
- Monitor the electrocardiogram (ECG) continuously in lead II; obtain a baseline 12-lead ECG.
- Provide oxygen, as needed.
- Maintain and monitor arterial line and pulmonary artery catheter.
- Insert an indwelling urinary catheter; monitor intake and output.

(continued)

- Assess the patient's left arm and peripheral leg pulses and document sensation, movement, color, and temperature of the arm and legs.
- Give the patient a sedative, as ordered.

NURSING ALERT Have a defibrillator, suction, temporary pacemaker, and emergency drugs readily available in case the patient develops complications, such as an arrhythmia, during insertion.

Posttreatment care

- Obtain chest X-ray, as ordered, to verify correct balloon placement
- Adjust heparin drip according to protocol to maintain partial thromboplastin time (PTT) at 1 to 2 times the normal value; monitor PTT according to facility policy.

NURSING ALERT If the control system malfunctions or becomes inoperable, don't let the balloon catheter remain dormant for more than 30 minutes. Inflate the balloon manually until another control system becomes available.

WEANING THE PATIENT FROM INTRA-AORTIC BALLOON COUNTERPULSATION

- To begin weaning, gradually decrease the frequency of balloon augmentation to 1:2 and 1:4, as ordered.
- Assist frequency is usually maintained for 1 hour or longer, depending on facility policy. If the patient's hemodynamic status remain stable during this time, weaning may continue.

NURSING ALERT Don't leave the patient on a low augmentation setting for more than 2 hours to prevent embolus formation.

- Assess the patient's tolerance of weaning and notify the physician if the patient shows signs of hemodynamic instability .

REMOVING THE INTRA-AORTIC BALLOON

- If the balloon was inserted percutaneously, the cardiologist usually removes the catheter. If the balloon was inserted surgically, the surgeon closes the Dacron graft and sutures the insertion site.
- Make sure PTT is within normal limits before the balloon is removed to prevent hemorrhage at insertion site.
- Turn off the control system and disconnect the connective tubing from the catheter to ensure balloon deflation.
- The practitioner withdraws the balloon until the proximal end of the catheter contacts the distal end of the introducer sheath.
- The practitioner then applies pressure below the puncture site and removes the balloon and introducer sheath as a unit, allowing a few seconds of free bleeding to prevent thrombus formation.
- To promote distal bleed-back, apply pressure above the puncture site for 30 minutes or until bleeding stops, if facility policy permits. (Sometimes this is the practitioner's responsibility.)
- After balloon removal, provide wound care according to facility policy.
- Enforce bedrest with the head of the bed elevated no more than 30 degrees.
- Change dressing at insertion site every 24 hours, or as needed, using sterile technique.

MONITORING

- Vital signs
- Arm pulses, sensation and movement, and arm color and temperature; pedal and posterior tibial pulses; as well as color, sensation, and temperature in the affected limb

NURSING ALERT Loss of left arm pulses may indicate upward balloon displacement. Notify the practitioner of changes in left-arm pulse.

- Intake and output
- Laboratory test results
- Signs of of bleeding, especially at the insertion site
- Pulmonary artery pressure and pulmonary artery wedge pressure (PAWP) every 1 or 2 hours

NURSING ALERT A rising PAWP reflects preload, signaling increased ventricular pressure and workload; notify the practitioner if this occurs. Some patients require I.V. nitroprusside (Nipride) during intra-aortic balloon counterpulsation to reduce preload and afterload.

Patient teaching

Be sure to cover:
- positionig and movement restrictions
- rationale for pump
- signs and symptoms of complications and need to report to the physician immediately.

Joint replacement

● OVERVIEW

- Total or partial replacement of a joint with a synthetic prosthesis
- Restores joint mobility and stability and relieves pain
- May involve any joint except a spinal joint
- Most commonly involves the hip and knee (see *Arthroplasty variations*)
- Also called *arthroplasty*

Indications
- Severe chronic arthritis
- Degenerative joint disorders
- Extensive joint trauma

▶ PROCEDURE

- The procedure varies slightly depending on the joint and its condition.

TOTAL HIP REPLACEMENT
- The patient is placed in a lateral decubitus position and receives a regional or general anesthetic.
- An incision is made to expose the hip joint.
- The hip capsule is incised or excised as indicated.

ARTHROPLASTY VARIATIONS

Arthroplasty, the surgical reconstruction or replacement of a joint, is done to restore mobility of the joint and function to the muscles and ligaments. Other than total joint replacement, two types of arthroplastic surgery include joint resection and interpositional reconstruction.

Joint resection involves removing a portion of the bone from a stiffened joint, creating a gap between the bone and the socket, to improve the range of motion. Scar tissue eventually fills this gap. Although pain is relieved and motion is restored, the joint is less stable.

Interpositional reconstruction involves reshaping the joint and placing a prosthetic disk between the reshaped bony ends forming the joint. The prosthesis may be made of metal, plastic, or from body tissue, such as fascia, or skin. However, with repeated injury and surgical reshaping, the patient eventually may need total joint replacement.

In recent years, joint replacement has become the operation of choice for most knee and hip problems. Elbow, shoulder, ankle, and finger joints are more likely to be treated with joint resection or interpositional reconstruction.

- The joint is dislocated to expose the acetabulum and head of the femur.
- The acetabulum is shaped and reamed to accept the socket of the ball-and-socket hip prosthesis.
- The device is secured in place.
- Polymethylmethacrylate adhesive is used to secure the device in place if the prosthesis is cemented.
- The process is repeated for the other side of the hip.
- After the prosthesis parts are in place, the surgeon fits them together to restore the joint.
- The incision is closed in layers and a dressing is applied.

Complications
- Infection
- Hypovolemic shock
- Fat embolism
- Thromboembolism
- Pulmonary embolism (PE)
- Nerve compromise
- Prosthesis dislocation or loosening
- Heterotrophic ossification
- Avascular necrosis
- Atelectasis
- Pneumonia
- Deep vein thrombosis (DVT)

✳ NURSING INTERVENTIONS

Pretreatment care
- Explain the treatment and patient preparation.
- Make sure the patient has signed an appropriate consent form.
- Explain postoperative care.
- Reassure the patient that analgesics will be available as needed.
- Provide emotional support.

Posttreatment care
- Administer medications, as ordered.
- Maintain bed rest for the prescribed period.
- Maintain the affected joint in proper alignment.
- Assess the patient's pain level and provide analgesics, as ordered.
- Change dressings, as ordered.
- Reposition the patient frequently.
- Encourage frequent coughing and deep breathing.
- Encourage adequate fluid intake.

- Exercise the affected joint, as ordered.
- If joint displacement occurs, notify the physician.
- If traction is used to correct joint displacement, periodically check weights and other equipment.

MONITORING
- Vital signs
- Intake and output
- Complications
- Surgical wound and dressings
- Drainage
- Abnormal bleeding
- Respiratory status
- Neurovascular status of the affected extremity
- Infection

Patient teaching
Be sure to cover:
- medication administration, dosage, and and possible adverse effects
- signs and symptoms of infection
- signs and symptoms of joint dislodgment
- complications
- when to notify the physician
- incision care
- follow-up care
- signs and symptoms of DVT and PE
- prescribed exercise regimen
- prescribed activity restrictions
- physical therapy
- range-of-motion exercises and use of a continuous passive motion device, as appropriate
- infective endocarditis prophylaxis.

AFTER HIP REPLACEMENT
Be sure to cover:
- importance of maintaining hip abduction
- avoidance of crossing his legs when sitting
- avoidance of flexing his hips more than 90 degrees when rising from a bed or chair
- using a chair with high arms and a firm seat
- importance of sleeping on a firm mattress
- proper use of crutches or a cane.

Laryngectomy

● OVERVIEW

- Partial or complete surgical removal of the larynx
- May be performed with other treatments for cancer, such as radiation therapy or chemotherapy
- Total laryngectomy: entire larynx removed, along with any affected surrounding structures such as the lymph nodes
- Partial laryngectomy: performed if small tumor; usually, one vocal chord removed

Indications
- Cancer
- Relief of symptoms associated with cancer

▶ PROCEDURE

- General anesthetic is administered.

Endoscopic resection
- The surgeon places an endoscope into the patient's throat.
- He inserts surgical instruments through the endoscope to remove the cancer or laser the affected tissues away. The laser, similar to a scalpel, can cut through tissue, but causes less bleeding.

Partial laryngectomy
- In this procedure, part of the larynx is removed and at least part of one vocal cord is kept so that the patient's retains the ability to speak, but his voice may be hoarse or weak.
- There are several different types of partial laryngectomy, depending on the location of the cancer:
  - Cordectomy removes the vocal cords only
  - Supraglottic laryngectomy removes the supraglottis only
  - Hemilaryngectomy removes half of the larynx; retaining the patient's voice
  - Partial laryngectomy removes portion of the larynx; helping retain the patient's ability to speak.

Total laryngectomy
- This procedure involves the removal of the entire larynx with the formation of a permanent stoma.
- If the patient has nodes larger than 1 cm, a neck dissection may be done in which all the lymph nodes on the affected side are removed. The sternocleidomastoid, internal jugular vein, and accessory nerve may also be removed if the lymph nodes adjacent to them are cancerous. Because the accessory nerve controls shoulder movement, the shoulder may be stiff and difficult to move after surgery. If the muscle is removed, the patient's neck might appear thinner and sunken on the affected side over time.

Complications
- Infection
- Hemorrhage (ruptured carotid artery)
- Edema
- Aspiration
- Fistula
- Tracheostomy stenosis
- Neurovascular injury
- Complications from anesthesia

❊ NURSING INTERVENTIONS

Pretreatment care
- Make sure that diagnostic testing has been completed and documented and any abnormal findings reported to the practitioner
- Tell the patient what to expect postoperatively, such as a feeding tube, neck edema, drains to help reduce the swelling, attachment to a ventilator, and the inability to speak.
- Arrange a visit with a patient who has undergone a laryngectomy.
- Arrange for the speech language pathologist to meet the patient and his family before surgery.
- Help the patient choose a temporary way to communicate, such as writing, alphabet board, or sign language.
- Verify that a consent form has been signed.

Posttreatment care
- Maintain ventilation as ordered; assist with weaning as indicated

- Make sure there's a spare tracheotomy tube at the bedside that's the same size as the patient's tube.
- Keep the head of bed elevated as ordered.
- Provide tracheostomy care; suction as indicated.
- Maintain patency of. tubes; administer fluids as ordered.
- Help the patient turn and perform deep-breathing exercises to help mobilize secretions in the lungs. Suction the patient as indicated.
- Maintain patency of nasogastric (NG) tube; begin tube feedings or parenteral therapy as ordered.
- Provide mouth care.
- Administer medications as ordered.
- Provide emotional support; keep call bell within reach and provide a means of communication for the patient.
- Arrange for home care nursing and speech therapy referrals.

MONITORING
- Vital signs and intake and output
- Respiratory status including breath sounds and pulse oximetry
- Response to ventilator settings
- Wound site for drainage, bleeding, edema, and wound dehiscence
- Pain
- Laboratory test results

Patient teaching
Be sure to cover:
- Restrictions such as inability to smell aromas, blow his nose, whistle, gargle, or sip or suck on a straw.
- Care of permanent tracheostomy as indicated, care and cleaning of the stoma, and ways to provide humidification and oxygenation.
- Alternative speech methods

Laser eye surgery

● OVERVIEW

- Laser-assisted in-situ keratomileusis (LASIK): corrects vision by changing the curvature of the cornea
  - Recovery normally quick with fewer adverse effects and complications than other methods of vision correction
  - Significant improvement in vision common soon after surgery
  - Newer technique: wavefront-guided LASIK, involving special mapping of small irregularities in the patient's cornea and customizing of the laser shaping procedure to correct these defects
- Photorefractive keratectomy (PRK): uses the Excimer laser to correct vision by reshaping the cornea without creating a corneal flap
- Phototherapeutic keratectomy (PTK): removes roughness or cloudiness from corneas, use alone or with traditional corneal surgical techniques

Indications
LASIK AND PRK
- Low to high levels of nearsightedness, farsightedness, and astigmatism
PTK
- Corneal degeneration and dystrophy
- Corneal irregularities
- Superficial scars

▶ PROCEDURE

The area around the eyes is draped and anesthetic eye drops are applied. When the eye is completely numb, an eyelid holder is placed between the eyelids to keep the patient from blinking.
- With LASIK: A special ring is applied to the eye and suction pressure is applied. Then a micro keratome is used to create a hinged flap of thin corneal tissue, which is suctioned open with the ring and then removed.
- With PRK, the surgeon removes the epithelium of the cornea. The patient looks directly at a target light while the laser reshapes the cornea. The laser is programmed with the information gathered in the preoperative examination. The laser treatment is completed in less than 2 minutes usually.

- The protective layer is folded back into place.
- For the patient who's nearsighted, the surgeon makes the steep cornea flatter by removing tissue from the cornea's center. Similarly, for the patient who's farsighted, the surgeon makes the flat cornea steeper by removing tissue outside of the central optical zone.
- For the patient with astigmatism, the cornea is made more spherical, thus eliminating multiple focusing points within the eye.
- PTK treatments vary depending on the corneal disorder, and goals vary based on the patient's symptoms. The laser allows corneas to be treated with a cool beam of light that evaporates tissue, producing a smoother surface.
- After LASIK procedure, the patient's eyes are examined with a slit lamp microscope and an eye shield is applied; after PRK and PTK, the patient's eyes are examined with a slit lamp microscope and a bandage contact lens and eye shield is applied. Anti-inflammatory and antibiotic medications may be administered after PRK.

Complications
- Infection
- Failure of treatment
- Double vision or night vision problems (PRK)
- New astigmatism (PRK)

✳ NURSING INTERVENTIONS

Pretreatment care
- Explain the treatment and preparation to the patient and his family.
- Verify that the patient had a baseline visual evaluation and refraction before the procedure and, if he's a contact lens wearer, hasn't worn his lenses for at least 2 weeks before the baseline examination for soft lenses, 3 weeks for rigid gas permeable or toric soft lenses, or 4 weeks for hard lenses; nor worn them since the examination.
- Make sure the patient has signed an appropriate consent form.
- Verify that the patient isn't wearing eye makeup, lotions, perfume, or creams, and the eyelids and lashes have been washed.

- Explain that a protective shield may be placed over the eye postoperatively.
- Explain that, immediately after surgery, his eye may feel itchy, burning, watery, or as if a foreign body is in it; however, he must avoid rubbing the eye because rubbing can result in injuring the surgical area.
- Inform the patient that his vision may be blurry with halos or starbursts around lights and a sensitivity to glare for a few days.
- Make sure the patient has someone to drive him home after the procedure.
- Administer a sedative or an osmotic agent, as ordered, to reduce intraocular pressure.

Posttreatment care
- Instill corticosteroid eyedrops or topical antibiotics as ordered.
- Administer analgesics as ordered.
- Help the patient lie on his back or the unaffected side.
- Keep the head of the bed flat or slightly elevated as ordered.
- Assist the patient with ambulation.
- Assess for pain and administer analgesics as ordered.
MONITORING
- Operative site
- Pain

⬥ **NURSING ALERT** Immediately report sudden, sharp, or excessive pain; bloody, purulent, or clear viscous drainage; and fever.
- Vital signs

Patient teaching
- Medications
- Follow-up care, including postsurgical follow-up appointment in 24 to 48 hours.
- Avoidance of: eye makeup for 1 to 2 weeks; sports for about 3 days; strenuous or contact sports for about 1 month; swimming, whirlpools, and hot tubs for about 8 weeks
- Precautions for photophobia
- Use of eye shield for about 1 month when sleeping
- Avoidance of driving until approved by the practitioner
- Signs and symptoms to report: sudden, sharp, or excessive pain; bloody, purulent, or clear viscous drainage; and fever.

Lithotripsy

OVERVIEW

- Noninvasive procedure for removing obstructive renal calculi or gallstones
- Extracorporeal shock-wave lithotripsy (ESWL): use of high-energy shock waves to break up calculi and allow their normal passage
- Percutaneous ultasonic lithotripsy (PUL): invasive procedure using ultrasonic shock waves at close range
- Common replacements for surgical removal of renal calculi (except when kidney is nonfunctional and must be removed)
- Now commonly replaced by laparoscopic cholecystectomy for gallstones
- Contraindicated in urinary or biliary tract obstruction distal to the calculi; in renal or gallbladder cancer; in calculi that are fixed to the kidney, ureter, or gallbladder or located below the iliac crest level; in patients with pacemakers; and during pregnancy

Indications

- Potentially obstructive calculi
- Emergency treatment for acute renal obstruction

PROCEDURE

- The patient receives I.V. or oral sedation, or the use of a transcutaenous electrical nerve stimulator.

ESWL

- The patient is placed in a semireclining or supine position on the hydraulic stretcher of the ESWL machine on a water-filled cushion (or submerged in lukewarm water for gallstones) through which the shock waves are directed from the lithotriptor.
- The generator is focused on the calculi using biplane fluoroscopy confirmation.
- The generator is activated to direct high-energy shock waves through the cushion or water at the calculi.
- Shock waves are synchronized to the patient's R waves on the electrocardiogram (ECG) and fired during diastole.
- The number of waves fired depends on the size, number, and composition of the calculi (500 to 2,000 shocks delivered during a treatment).

PUL

- The patient receives local anesthesia or oral sedation.
- Gallstones can be broken up by several percutaneous fragmentation devices besides ultrasound, such as laser pulses and electrohydraulics, utilizing electric sparks.
- Overall procedures for gallstones and renal calculi are similar, except for placement of the percutaneous devices into the gallbladder or common bile duct versus the renal pelvis.

Complications

- Hemorrhage
- Hematomas
- Obstruction (biliary or ureteral)

NURSING INTERVENTIONS

Pretreatment care

- Explain the treatment and preparation to the patient and family.
- Make sure the patient has signed an appropriate consent form.
- Explain postprocedure care. If ESWL will be done for gallstones, explain that the patient may have mild pain afterward.
- Arrange for the patient to see the ESWL device before treatment if possible.

Posttreatment care

- Administer medications, as ordered.
- Maintain a patent indwelling urinary catheter and I.V. line.
- Strain urine for calculi fragments, and send the specimen to the laboratory.
- Report frank or persistent bleeding.
- Encourage ambulation as early as possible.
- Increase the patient's fluid intake, as ordered.
- Provide comfort measures.
- Report severe pain.

NURSING ALERT Immediately report severe unremitting pain, persistent hematuria, inability to void, fever and chills, or recurrent nausea and vomiting.

MONITORING

- Vital signs
- Intake and output
- Complications
- Urine color and pH
- Pain

Patient teaching

Be sure to cover:
- medication administration, dosage, and possible adverse effects
- complications
- when to notify the physician
- importance of daily oral fluid intake of 3 to 4 qt (3 to 4 L) for about 1 month after treatment
- straining of all urine for the first week after treatment, saving fragments in the container provided, and bringing the container to first follow-up visit
- likelihood of pain occurring as fragments pass, slight redness or bruising, blood-tinged urine for several days, and mild GI upset after the procedure
- prescribed activity restrictions
- prescribed dietary recommendations
- ways to prevent new calculi formation
- follow-up care.

Loop electrosurgical excision

⬤ OVERVIEW

- Loop electrosurgical excision procedure (LEEP): performed with a thin, low-voltage electrified wire loop to remove abnormal cervical tissue
- Performed after abnormal Papanicolaou (Pap) test results have been confirmed by colposcopy and cervical biopsy
- After LEEP: specimen examined again for cancerous cells
- Can be as effective as cryotherapy or laser treatment
- Also known as large loop excision of the transformation zone

Indications

- Removal of abnormal cervical tissue
- Removal of abnormal tissue high in the cervical canal that can't be seen during colposcopy; may be done instead of a cone biopsy
- Microinvasive cervical cancer
- Abnormal Pap test

▶ PROCEDURE

- LEEP is usually performed as an outpatient procedure.
- A cervical block is injected to anesthetized the cervix; in addition an oral or I.V. pain medication may also be used.
- An acetic acid or iodine solution, which makes abnormal cells more visible, may be applied to the cervix before the procedure.
- The patient is placed in the lithotomy position and the practitioner inserts a speculum to examine the vagina and cervix.

Complications

- Uterine perforation
- Bleeding
- Infection
- Cervical stenosis
- Infertility
- Decreased cervical mucus
- Cervical incompetence

✳ NURSING INTERVENTIONS

Pretreatment care

- Explain the treatment and preparation to the patient.
- Verify that the patient has signed an appropriate consent form.
- Provide emotional support.
- Obtain and document results of diagnostic studies, medical history, and physical examination; notify the practitioner of abnormalities.
- Make sure the patient has fasted and used an enema preoperatively as ordered.
- Administer I.V. fluids as ordered.

Posttreatment care

- Administer analgesics as ordered.
- Institute safety precautions.

MONITORING

- Vital signs
- Intake and output
- Type and amount of vaginal drainage
- Pain

NURSING ALERT Be sure to report continuous, sharp abdominal pain that doesn't respond to analgesics; this indicates possible uterine perforation, a potentially life-threatening complication.

- Signs and symptoms of infection

Patient teaching

Be sure to cover:

- Medications and possible adverse reactions
- Possibility of postoperative abdominal cramping and pain in the pelvis and lower back.
- Appearance of postoperative vaginal drainage—dark brown during the first week; discharge or spotting may occur for approximately 3 weeks
- Possibility of heavier-than-normal for the first two or three menstrual cycles after the procedure.
- Use of sanitary napkins instead of tampons for 3 weeks.
- Avoidance of doucing and sexual intercourse for 3 weeks.
- Signs to report: increased bleeding, infection
- Return to activities in 1 to 3 days
- Follow-up care

Lung volume reduction surgery

● OVERVIEW

- Removal of diseased portion of the lung increasing chest cavity space
- Can alter flattened diaphragm of a patient with emphysema to assume a more normal shape, making the diaphragm function better
- Results in diminished shortness of breath, greater exercise tolerance, and better quality of life

Indications
- Severe chronic obstructive pulmonary disease (COPD)

▶ PROCEDURE

- The patient receives general anesthesia.
- Portions of one or both of the patient's lungs are removed surgically by opening the chest wall or by thoracoscopy.
- One or more chest tubes are placed during surgery to prevent lung tissue collapse.

Thoracoscopy (unilateral or bilateral)
- Thoracoscopy is a minimally invasive technique (sometimes called *VATS* or *video-assisted thoracic surgery*).
- The patient is positioned supine but is slightly raised on the affected side, with the arm held above his head.
- Three small (about 1″ [2.5-cm]) J incisions are made between the ribs.
- A videoscope is placed through one of the incisions. A stapler and grasper are inserted in the other incisions to remove damaged areas and to reseal the remaining lung.
- Sutures are used to close the incisions.
- The patient may be repositioned and the procedure performed on the other side.

Sternotomy (bilateral)
- An incision is made through the breastbone to expose both lungs.
- Both lungs are reduced at the same time.
- The chest bone is wired together and the skin is closed.

- This is the most invasive technique and is used when thoracoscopy isn't appropriate.
- It's used only for patients with upper lobe disease.

Thoracotomy (unilateral)
- For the thoracotomy technique, an incision is made between the ribs and the ribs are separated with retractors. The incision is about 5″ to 12″ (13 to 30 cm) long.
- The lung is reduced as required.
- The muscle and skin are closed by sutures.
- Thoracotomy is commonly used when the surgeon can't visualize the lung clearly through the thoracoscope or when dense scar tissue exists.

Complications
- Subcutaneous crepitus, which may indicate tracheal or bronchial perforation or pneumothorax
- Hypoxemia
- Cardiac arrhythmias
- Bleeding
- Infection
- Bronchospasm
- Air leakage
- Pneumonia
- Stroke
- Myocardial infarction

✳ NURSING INTERVENTIONS

Pretreatment care
- Review with the patient the surgeon's description of the technique to be used, and explain pretreatment and posttreatment nursing care.
- Verify that an appropriate consent form has been signed.
- Note and document patient allergies.
- Instruct the patient to fast for 6 to 12 hours before the test.
- Obtain vital signs and results of preprocedure studies; report abnormal findings.
- An I.V. sedative may be given.
- Remove the patient's dentures.

Posttreatment care
- Maintain a patent airway and adequate oxygenation.

- Position the patient to promote chest expansion postoperatively.
- Provide pulmonary rehabilitation; suctioning, deep breathing, percussion, incentive spirometry, and respiratory treatments as ordered.
- Provide chest tube care.
- Provide measures for pain control.
- Check the follow-up chest X-ray for pneumothorax.

◆ **NURSING ALERT** Immediately report subcutaneous crepitus around the patient's face, neck, or chest because these may indicate tracheal or bronchial perforation or pneumothorax.

MONITORING
- Vital signs, pulse oximetry, and intake and output
- Respiratory status
- Sputum characteristics
- Chest tube function, patency and drainage
- Incisional site
- Signs and symptoms of bleeding

Patient teaching
Be sure to cover:
- Respiratory care measures such as coughing, use of an incentive spirometer, and other pulmonary rehabilitation measures
- Signs and symptoms of infection or complications, such as increased shortness of breath, hemoptysis, or chest pain.
- Medications and possible adverse reactions
- Incision site care.
- Activity restrictions

Mastectomy

● OVERVIEW

- Breast excision done primarily to remove malignant breast tissue and regional lymphatic metastases
- May involve one of various procedures (see *Types of mastectomy*)
- May be combined with radiation and chemotherapy

Indications
- Breast cancer
- Female history of breast cancer (prophylactic)

▶ PROCEDURE

TOTAL MASTECTOMY
- The entire breast is removed without dissecting the lymph nodes.
- A skin graft may be applied if necessary.

MODIFIED RADICAL MASTECTOMY
- Axillary lymph nodes are resected while the pectoralis major is left intact.
- The pectoralis minor may be removed.
- If the patient has small lesions and no metastasis, breast reconstruction may follow immediately or a few days later.

RADICAL MASTECTOMY
- The entire breast, axillary lymph nodes, underlying pectoral muscles, and adjacent tissues are removed.
- Skin flaps and exposed tissue are covered with moist packs.
- The chest wall and axilla are irrigated before closure.

EXTENDED RADICAL MASTECTOMY
- The breast, underlying pectoral muscles, axillary contents, and upper internal mammary (mediastinal) lymph node chain are removed.
- After closure of the mastectomy site, a drain or catheter may be inserted.
- Large pressure dressings may be applied if a drain isn't inserted.

Complications
- Infection
- Delayed healing
- Lymphedema
- Change in self-concept

✳ NURSING INTERVENTIONS

Pretreatment care
- Explain the treatment and preparation to the patient and family.
- Make sure the patient has signed an appropriate consent form.
- Explain postoperative care.
- Take baseline arm measurements on both sides.
- Restrict food and fluids, as ordered.
- If the patient will have a radical mastectomy, explain that skin on the anterior surface of one thigh may be shaved and prepared in case she needs a graft.
- Provide emotional support.

Posttreatment care
- Administer medications, as ordered.
- Elevate the patient's arm on a pillow.
- Regularly check the suction tubing to ensure proper functioning.
- Initiate flexion and extension arm exercises, as ordered.

- Place a sign in the patient's room indicating that no blood pressure readings, injections, or venipunctures should be performed on the affected arm.
- Gently encourage the patient to look at the operative site.
- Encourage her to express her feelings.
- Arrange a fitting for a temporary breast pad after 2 to 3 days.

MONITORING
- Vital signs
- Intake and output
- Complications
- Surgical wound and dressings
- Drainage
- Abnormal bleeding
- Infection
- Emotional response

Patient teaching
Be sure to cover:
- medication administration, dosage, and possible adverse effects
- signs and symptoms of infection
- complications
- when to notify the physician
- ways to prevent infection
- importance of using the affected arm as much as possible
- range-of-motion exercises and other postoperative exercises
- temporary breast prosthesis, as needed
- avoidance of blood pressure readings, injections, and venipunctures on the affected arm
- avoidance of keeping the affected arm in a dependent position for a prolonged period
- protecting the affected arm from injury
- adequate rest periods
- monthly breast self-examinations
- follow-up care
- permanent prosthesis, which can be fitted 3 to 4 weeks after surgery
- referrals to the American Cancer Society and Reach to Recovery.

TYPES OF MASTECTOMY

The type of mastectomy performed depends on the extent of tissue and lymph node involvement.
- A *lumpectomy* (partial mastectomy) or a *total (simple) mastectomy* may be done if the tumor is confined to breast tissue and no lymph node involvement is detected. A total mastectomy also may be used palliatively for advanced, ulcerative cancer and to treat extensive benign disease.
- *Modified radical mastectomy* – the standard surgery for stage I and II breast cancer – removes small, localized tumors. It has replaced radical mastectomy as the most widely used breast cancer surgery. Besides causing less disfigurement than radical mastectomy, it reduces postoperative arm edema and shoulder problems.
- *Radical mastectomy* controls the spread of larger, metastatic lesions. Later, breast reconstruction may be performed using a portion of the latissimus dorsi.
- *Extended radical mastectomy* is used to treat cancer in the medial quadrant of the breast or in subareolar tissue. This rare procedure may prevent possible metastasis to the internal mammary lymph nodes.

Mohs' microsurgery

● OVERVIEW

- Highly specialized treatment for total removal of skin cancers
- Also called *Mohs' surgery* or, formerly, *chemosurgery*

Indications
- Basal cell carcinoma

▶ PROCEDURE

- A local anesthetic is applied and the tumor is scraped using a curette. A thin piece of tissue is then surgically removed around the scraped skin and carefully divided into pieces that fit on a microscope slide. The edges are marked with colored dyes; a careful map or diagram of the removed tissue is made; and the tissue is frozen by the technician.
- Most bleeding is controlled using pressure; occasionally, a small blood vessel needs to be tied using suture material. A pressure dressing is then applied, and the patient is asked to wait while the slides are being processed.
- The surgeon studies the slides microscopically to tell if any tumor is still present. If cancer cells exist, they can be located by referring to the map. Another layer of tissue is then removed, and the procedure is repeated until the surgeon is satisfied that the entire base and sides of the wound have no cancer cells. It usually takes removal of two or three layers of tissue (called stages) to complete the surgery.

Complications
- Bleeding
- Infection
- Temporary or permanent numbness
- Scarring of the area
- Return of skin cancer

❉ NURSING INTERVENTIONS

Pretreatment care
- Review the procedure with the patient and answer questions.
- Verify that a consent form has been signed.
- A biopsy may be done before the procedure to confirm skin cancer.
- The patient may need to stop taking aspirin or aspirin-containing products at least 1 week before the surgery because it may interfere with the normal blood clotting mechanism.

Posttreatment care
- Provide skin care, as ordered.
- If stitches are present, provide care, as ordered.
- Administer pain medication, as ordered.
- Apply ice to the area.

MONITORING
- Vital signs
- Operative site
- Wound drainage
- Vital signs
- Sensation in the operative area

Patient teaching
Be sure to cover:
- skin care with the patient
- signs of complications, such as persistent bleeding or signs of infection, and when to notify the physician
- use of ice packs
- medication administration, dosage, and possible adverse effects
- skin cancer prevention measures
- follow-up care and possible plastic surgery.

Nephrectomy

● OVERVIEW

- Surgical removal of a kidney
- May be unilateral or bilateral
- Partial nephrectomy: resection of a portion of the kidney
- Simple nephrectomy: removal of the entire kidney
- Radical nephrectomy: resection of the entire kidney and surrounding fat tissue
- Nephroureterectomy: removal of the entire kidney, entire ureter, and perinephric fat
- Laparaoscopic nephrectomy: used with simple and partial nephrectomies to procure a donor kidney for transplantation

INDICATIONS
- Renal cell carcinoma
- Harvest of a healthy kidney for transplantation
- Renal trauma or infection
- Hypertension
- Hydronephrosis
- Inoperable renal calculi

▶ PROCEDURE

- The patient receives general anesthesia.

TRADITIONAL NEPHRECTOMY
- The surgeon makes a flank incision (thoracicoabdominal or transthoracic) to expose the kidney.
- The kidney is freed of fat and adhesions.
- The lower pole of the kidney is released.
- The upper third of the ureter is freed, double-clamped, cut between the clamps, and ligated on both ends.
- The vascular pedicle is freed and double-clamped.
- The renal artery and the renal vein are clamped.
- The kidney is removed distal to the clamps.
- The surrounding perinephric fat and ureter are resected.
- A flank catheter and Penrose drain may be inserted.
- The wound is sutured closed.

LAPAROSCOPIC NEPHRECTOMY
- The surgeon makes four or five ½″ incisions.
- Narrow surgical instruments are inserted into the abdomen through the previously made incisions.
- The surgeon uses a small camera to help visualize inside the abdomen to clamp the vasculature.
- The surgeon makes a 2½″ incision and removes the kidney.
- The incisions are closed with sutures.

Complications
- Infection
- Hemorrhage
- Atelectasis
- Pneumonia
- Deep vein thrombosis
- Pulmonary embolism

✳ NURSING INTERVENTIONS

Pretreatment care
- Explain the treatment and preparation to the patient and family.
- Make sure the patient has signed an appropriate consent form.
- Explain postoperative care.
- Restrict oral intake, as ordered.
- Administer I.V. fluids, as ordered.

Posttreatment care
- Administer medications, as ordered.
- Provide care for the I.V. line, nasogastric tube, and indwelling urinary catheter.
- Notify the physician if urine output falls below 50 ml/hour.
- Maintain drain patency.
- Change dressings, as ordered.
- Resume oral feedings, as ordered.
- Encourage coughing, deep breathing, incentive spirometry, and position changes.
- Encourage early and regular ambulation.
- Apply antiembolism stockings, as ordered.

MONITORING
- Vital signs
- Intake and output
- Daily weight
- Complications
- Surgical wound and dressings
- Abnormal bleeding
- Drainage
- Bowel sounds
- Respiratory status
- Hemorrhage and shock
- Infection

Patient teaching
Be sure to cover:
- medication administration, dosage, and possible adverse effects
- coughing and deep-breathing exercises
- signs and symptoms of infection
- complications
- when to notify the physician
- intake and output monitoring
- prescribed fluid intake and dietary restrictions
- prescribed activity restrictions
- follow-up care
- importance of wearing medical identification.

Pacemaker insertion

⬤ OVERVIEW

- Pacemaker: battery-operated generator that controls heart rate by emitting timed electrical signals that trigger contraction of the heart muscle; may be temporary or permanent

Indications
TEMPORARY PACEMAKER
- Emergency treatment of symptomatic bradycardia
- Bridge to permanent pacemaker implantation or to determine the effect of pacing on cardiac function
- Open-heart surgery

PERMANENT PACEMAKER
- Symptomatic bradycardia
- Advanced symptomatic atrioventricular block
- Sick sinus syndrome
- Sinus arrest
- Sinoatrial block
- Stokes-Adams syndrome
- Tachyarrhythmias
- Arrhythmias caused by antiarrhythmics

▶ PROCEDURE

- Insertion or application of a *temporary pacemaker* varies, depending on the device. (See *Types of temporary pacemakers.*)

PERMANENT PACEMAKER
- The pacemaker is implanted using a transvenous endocardial approach.
- The patient is sedated and the chest or abdomen is prepared.
- A 3″ to 4″ (7.5 to 10 cm) incision is made in the selected site.
- The electrode catheter is inserted through a vein and guided by fluoroscopy to the heart chamber appropriate for the pacemaker type.
- Pacemaker leads are inserted.
- A pacing system analyzer is used to set the pulse generator to the proper stimulating and sensing thresholds.
- The pulse generator is attached to the leads and implanted into a pocket of muscle in the chest wall.
- The incision is closed, and a tight occlusive dressing is applied.

Complications
- Infection
- Venous thrombosis, embolism
- Pneumothorax
- Pectoral or diaphragmatic muscle stimulation from the pacemaker
- Arrhythmias
- Cardiac tamponade
- Heart failure
- Pacemaker malfunction

✳ NURSING INTERVENTIONS

Pretreatment care
- Explain the treatment and preparation to the patient and family.
- Make sure the patient has signed an appropriate consent form.
- Explain postoperative care.
- Obtain baseline vital signs and a 12-lead electrocardiogram (ECG)
- Restrict food and fluids, as ordered.
- Establish I.V. access.

Posttreatment care
- Administer medications, as ordered.
- Maintain continuous cardiac monitoring.
- Document the type of pacemaker inserted, lead system, pacemaker mode, and pacing guidelines.
- If the patient requires defibrillation, place paddles at least 4″ (10 cm) from the pulse generator; avoid anteroposterior paddle placement.
- After first 24 hours, begin passive range-of-motion exercises on the affected arm, if ordered.

MONITORING
- Vital signs
- Intake and output
- Complications
- Surgical wound and dressing
- Drainage
- Abnormal bleeding
- Infection
- Cardiac rate and rhythm; ECG
- Pacemaker function

Patient teaching
Be sure to cover:
- medication administration, dosage, and possible adverse effects
- complications and when to notify the physician
- incision care
- prescribed activity restrictions
- how to monitor the heart rate and rhythm and pacemaker function
- prescribed diet and exercises
- pacemaker identification
- importance of informing medical personnel of the implanted pacemaker before certain diagnostic tests
- follow-up care.

TYPES OF TEMPORARY PACEMAKERS

Temporary pacemakers come in three types: transcutaneous, transvenous, and epicardial.

Transcutaneous pacemaker
Completely noninvasive and easily applied, a transcutaneous pacemaker proves especially useful in an emergency. To perform pacing with the device, the physician places electrodes on the skin directly over the heart and connects them to a pulse generator.

Transvenous pacemaker
This balloon-tipped pacing catheter is inserted via the subclavian or jugular vein into the right ventricle. The procedure can be done at the bedside or in the cardiac catheterization laboratory. A transvenous pacemaker offers better control of the heartbeat than a transcutaneous pacemaker. However, electrode insertion takes longer, limiting its usefulness in emergencies.

Epicardial pacemaker
Implanted during open-heart surgery, an epicardial pacemaker permits rapid treatment of postoperative complications. During surgery, the physician attaches the leads to the heart and runs them out through the chest incision. Afterward, the leads are coiled on the patient's chest, insulated, and covered with a dressing. If pacing is needed, the leads are simply uncovered and attached to a pulse generator. When pacing is no longer needed, the leads can be removed under local anesthesia.

Pancreatectomy and pancreaticoduodenectomy

● OVERVIEW

- Surgical removal of part or all of the pancreas
- May involve various types of resections, drainage procedures, and anastomoses to treat pancreatic diseases when more conservative techniques have failed
- Common resections: pancreatoduodenectomy or Whipple procedure

Indications
- Pancreatic cancer
- Chronic pancreatitis
- Islet cell tumor or insulinoma

▶ PROCEDURE

- The patient is anesthetized.
- The surgeon makes an abdominal incision.
- The remainder of the procedure is based on evaluation of the pancreas, liver, gallbladder, and common bile duct.
- If the disease is localized, portions of the pancreas and surrounding organs are resected.
- For metastatic disease in the liver or lymph nodes or tumor invasion of the aorta or superior mesenteric artery, the obstruction may be bypassed to lessen pain.
- With pancreacticoduodenectomy, the surgeon removes the head of the pancreas, the entire duodenum, a portion of the jejunum, the distal third of the stomach, and the lower half of the common bile duct, with the reestablishment of continuity of the billiary, pancreatic, and GI tract systems; the surgeon inserts two drains into the abdomen and closes the wound.

Complications
- Hemorrhage
- Fistula formation
- Abscess
- Common bile duct obstruction
- Pseudocyst
- Insulin dependence
- Paralytic ileus

✳ NURSING INTERVENTIONS

Pretreatment care
- Explain the treatment and preparation to the patient and family.
- Make sure the patient has signed an appropriate consent form.
- Explain postoperative care.
- Provide emotional support.
- Administer analgesics, as ordered.
- Arrange for required diagnostic studies, as ordered.
- Provide enteral or parenteral nutrition before surgery, if ordered.
- Provide low-fat, high-calorie feedings, as ordered.
- Administer oral hypoglycemic agents or insulin, as ordered.
- Administer mechanical and antibiotic bowel preparation as well as prophylactic systemic antibiotics, as ordered.
- Assist with nasogastric tube and indwelling urinary catheter insertion.

Posttreatment care
- Administer medications, as ordered.
- Administer plasma expanders and I.V. fluids, as ordered.
- Administer oxygen, as ordered.
- Encourage deep breathing, coughing, and incentive spirometry use.
- Maintain the patency of drainage tubes.
- Change dressings, and provide incision care, as ordered.
- Use a wound pouching system to contain drainage, as needed.

◈ **NURSING ALERT** Monitor for and report absent bowel sounds, severe abdominal pain, vomiting, or fever. These findings may indicate a fistula or paralytic ileus.

MONITORING
- Vital signs
- Hemodynamic values
- Intake and output
- Nutritional status
- Pulmonary status
- Complications
- Infection
- Surgical wound and dressing
- Abnormal bleeding
- Drainage
- Metabolic alkalosis or acidosis
- Serum glucose and calcium levels
- Bowel sounds

Patient teaching
Be sure to cover:
- medication administration, dosage, and possible adverse effects
- incision care
- signs and symptoms of infection
- complications
- when to notify the physician
- home blood glucose monitoring
- how to recognize and manage hypoglycemia and hyperglycemia
- prescribed dietary and activity restrictions
- pancreatic enzyme replacement, if necessary
- follow-up care.

Parathyroidectomy

OVERVIEW

- Surgical removal of one or more of the four parathyroid glands; number of glands removed dependent on the underlying cause of excessive parathyroid hormone secretion

Indications
- Primary hyperparathyroidism
- Adenoma
- Glandular hyperplasia
- Cancer

PROCEDURE

- The patient is anesthetized.
- The surgeon makes a cervical neck incision and exposes the thyroid gland.
- The four parathyroid glands are located and tagged.
- If a gland can't be located, a cervical thymectomy and thyroid lobectomy are done on the side where the gland is missing, and a specimen is sent for an immediate frozen section.
- If the missing gland isn't found in the removed tissue, the procedure may be stopped and localization studies done before a second surgery.
- Alternatively, the sternum may be opened and the mediastinum explored for the missing gland.
- When all four parathyroids are found, they are examined for hyperplasia.
- Affected glands are removed.
- The surgeon tags the remaining glands or any remnant of a gland that wasn't removed.
- A Penrose drain or closed wound drainage device is inserted, and the wound is sutured.

Complications
- Hemorrhage
- Infection
- Recurrent laryngeal nerve damage
- Hypoparathyroidism

NURSING INTERVENTIONS

Pretreatment care
- Explain the treatment and preparation to the patient and family.
- Make sure the patient has signed an appropriate consent form.
- Explain postoperative care, including the likelihood that talking and swallowing will be painful for the first few days after surgery.
- Administer I.V. fluids and medications, such as diuretics and antihypercalcemic agents, as ordered.

Posttreatment care
- Administer medications, as ordered.
- Keep the patient in high Fowler's position.
- Encourage coughing, deep breathing, and incentive spirometry use.
- Provide surgical wound care, as ordered.
- Keep a tracheotomy tray at the bedside for the first 24 hours after surgery.

MONITORING
- Vital signs
- Intake and output
- Complications
- Surgical wound and dressings
- Drainage
- Abnormal bleeding
- Infection
- Respiratory status
- Voice quality and speaking ability
- Serum calcium levels

NURSING ALERT Watch for and report signs and symptoms of increased neuromuscular excitability, including positive Chvostek's and Trousseau's signs, numbness and tingling of the fingers and toes or around the mouth, muscle cramps, and tetany.

Patient teaching
Be sure to cover:
- medication administration, dosage, and possible adverse effects
- incision site care
- signs and symptoms of infection
- complications
- when to notify the physician
- coughing and deep-breathing exercises
- incentive spirometry use
- importance of consulting the physician before taking nonprescription drugs, especially magnesium-containing laxatives and antacids, mineral oil, and vitamins A and D
- maintaining a high-calcium, low-phosphorus diet, as ordered, after total parathyroidectomy
- signs and symptoms of hypercalcemia and hypocalcemia
- prescribed activity restrictions
- follow-up care.

Pericardiocentesis

⬤ OVERVIEW

- Needle aspiration of pericardial fluid for analysis
- Therapeutic and diagnostic; most useful as an emergency measure to relieve cardiac tamponade
- Fluid specimen used to confirm and identify cause of pericardial effusion and determine therapy
- Excess pericardial fluid: may accumulate after inflammation, cardiac surgery, rupture, or penetrating trauma to the pericardium
- Rapidly forming effusions: may induce cardiac tamponade, a potentially lethal syndrome marked by increased intrapericardial pressure that prevents complete ventricular filling and reduces cardiac output
- Slowly forming effusions: pose less immediate danger and allow the pericardium more time to adapt to accumulating fluid
- Pericardial effusions classified as transudates (from mechanical factors) or exudates (from inflammation)

Indications
- Cardiac tamponade
- Pericardial effusion

▷ PROCEDURE

- The physician cleans the skin with sterile gauze pads soaked in povidone-iodine solution and injects an anesthetic is injected.
- The physician attaches a 50-ml syringe to one end of a three-way stopcock and the cardiac needle to the other.
- The V_1 lead (precordial leadwire) of the electrocardiogram (ECG) may be attached to the hub of the aspirating needle using the alligator clips to help determine if the needle is in contact with the epicardium during the procedure.
- An echocardiogram may also be used to help guide needle placement.
- The physician inserts the needle through the chest wall into the pericardial sac, maintaining aspiration until fluid appears in the syringe.

- The needle should be angled 35 to 45 degrees toward the tip of the right scapula between the left costal margin and the xiphoid process; this minimizes the risk of lacerating the coronary vessels or the pleura.
- Observe the ECG tracing when the cardiac needle is being inserted; ST-segment elevation indicates that the needle has reached the epicardial surface and should be retracted slightly.

◈ **NURSING ALERT** An abnormally shaped QRS complex may indicate perforation of the myocardium. Premature ventricular contractions usually indicate that the needle has touched the ventricular wall. Watch for grossly bloody fluid aspirate, which may indicate inadvertent puncture of a cardiac chamber.

- After the needle is positioned, the physician attaches a clamp to the skin surface so it won't advance further.
- Assist the physician by labeling and numbering the specimen tubes and cleaning the top of the tube used for culture and sensitivity with povidone-iodin solution.
- A pericardial catheter may be connected to a drainage bag or to low suction drainage.
- The insertion site is cleaned and dressed.

Complications
- Laceration of a coronary artery or the myocardium (potentially fatal)
- Vasovagal arrest
- Infection
- Cardiac arrhythmias
- Myocardial perforation
- Respiratory distress

✳ NURSING INTERVENTIONS

Pretreatment care
- Explain the procedure to the patient and answer questions.
- Tell the patient that the anesthetic may cause brief burning and local pain.
- Verify that a consent form has been signed.
- Tell the patient that he may feel pressure when the needle is inserted into the pericardial sac.

- Inform the patient that he'll be monitored closely during and after the procedure.
- Instruct the patient to be still during the procedure; tell him that a sedative may be given to help him relax.
- Connect the patient to the bedside monitor set to read lead V_1.
- Make sure that a defibrillator and emergency drugs are readily available.
- Provide adequate lighting at the puncture site.
- Put the patient in the supine position with his thorax elevated 60 degrees.

◈ **NURSING ALERT** To minimize the risk of complications, echocardiography should precede pericardiocentesis to determine the effusion site.

Posttreatment care
- If bacterial culture and sensitivity tests are scheduled, record on the laboratory request any antimicrobials the patient is receiving.
- If anaerobic organisms are suspected, consult the laboratory about proper collection technique to avoid exposing the aspirate to air.
- Send specimens to the laboratory immediately.
- Provide care to aspiration site, as indicated.
- Provide continuous cardiac monitoring and document rhythm strips.
- Dispose of equipment according to facility policy.

MONITORING
- Vital signs
- Oxygen saturation
- Cardiac status including rate, rhythm, and heart sounds
- Aspiration site
- Signs and symptoms of respiratory and cardiac distress

◈ **NURSING ALERT** Watch especially for signs of cardiac tamponade: muffled and distant heartbeat, jugular vein distention, paradoxical pulse, and shock.

Patient teaching
Be sure to cover:
- medication administration, dosage, and possible adverse effects
- signs and symptoms of recurrent effusion, infection, and cardiac arrhythmia to report to the physician.

Prostatectomy

● OVERVIEW

- Surgical removal of the prostate
- Transurethral resection of the prostate (TURP): prostate removal via insertion of a resectoscope into the urethra
- May be performed by an open surgical approach, such as suprapubic prostatectomy, retropubic prostatectomy (which allows pelvic lymph node dissection for prostate cancer staging), or perineal prostatectomy (safer for obese patients and those who have had lower abdominal or pelvic surgery)

Indications

- Prostate cancer
- Obstructive benign prostatic hyperplasia

▶ PROCEDURE

TURP

- The patient is placed in a lithotomy position and anesthetized.
- The surgeon introduces a resectoscope into the urethra and advances it to the prostate.
- A clear irrigating solution is instilled, and the obstruction is visualized.
- The resectoscope's cutting loop is used to resect prostatic tissue and restore the urethral opening.

SUPRAPUBIC PROSTATECTOMY

- The patient receives a general anesthetic and placed in a supine position.
- A horizontal incision is made just above the pubic symphysis.
- Fluid is instilled into the bladder.
- A small incision is made in the bladder wall to expose the prostate.
- The surgeon shells out prostatic tissue with a finger.
- The obstruction is cleared and bleeding points are ligated.
- A suprapubic drainage tube and Penrose drain are inserted.

RETROPUBIC PROSTATECTOMY

- The patient is anesthetized and placed in a supine position.
- A horizontal suprapubic incision is made.
- The prostate is approached from between the bladder and pubic arch.

- Another incision is made in the prostatic capsule, and the obstructing tissue is removed.
- Bleeding is controlled.
- A suprapubic tube and Penrose drain are inserted.

PERINEAL PROSTATECTOMY

- The patient is anesthetized and placed in an exaggerated lithotomy position.
- The surgeon makes an inverted U-shaped incision in the perineum.
- The entire prostate is removed, along with the seminal vesicles.
- The urethra is anastomosed to the bladder.
- The incision is closed, leaving a Penrose drain in place.

Complications

- Hemorrhage
- Infection
- Urine retention and incontinence
- Impotence

✳ NURSING INTERVENTIONS

Pretreatment care

- Explain the treatment and preparation to the patient and family.
- Make sure the patient has signed an appropriate consent form.
- Explain postoperative care.
- Administer an enema, as ordered.
- Restrict foods and fluids, as ordered.
- Provide emotional support.

Posttreatment care

- Administer medications, as ordered.
- Maintain urinary catheter and suprapubic tube patency, as ordered.
- Keep the urinary collection container below the bladder level.
- Administer antispasmodics and analgesics, as ordered.
- Offer sitz baths.
- Arrange for psychological and sexual counseling, as needed.

 NURSING ALERT Never administer medication rectally in a patient who has had a total prostatectomy.

MONITORING

- Vital signs
- Intake and output
- Urine characteristics
- Complications

 NURSING ALERT Monitor for and report signs and symptoms of dilutional hyponatremia, such as altered mental status, muscle twitching, and seizures.

- Surgical wound and dressings
- Drainage
- Abnormal bleeding
- Infection

 NURSING ALERT Monitor for and report signs and symptoms of epididymitis, including fever, chills, groin pain, and a swollen, tender epididymis.

- Fluid and electrolyte status

Patient teaching

Be sure to cover:

- medication administration, dosage, and possible adverse effects
- incision care
- signs and symptoms of infection and abnormal bleeding
- complications
- when to notify the physician
- importance of drinking ten 8-oz glasses of water daily and urinating at least every 2 hours
- likelihood of experiencing transient urinary frequency and dribbling after catheter removal
- how to perform Kegel exercises
- avoidance of caffeine-containing beverages
- prescribed activity restrictions
- sitz baths
- follow-up care, including annual prostate-specific antigen testing.

Radiation therapy

● OVERVIEW

- Destroys ability of cancer cells to grow and multiply by either decreasing the mitosis rate or impairing synthesis of deoxyribonucleic or ribonucleic acid

EXTERNAL THERAPY
- Delivery of high levels of radiation (externally) to a specific body area
- Also called *external beam radiation* or *teletherapy*

INTERNAL THERAPY
- Placement of a radiation source in a specific body area or onto a body surface; also called *brachytherapy*
- May be administered locally or systemically, using various approaches:
  - Interstitial approach: direct implantation of a radioactive substance sealed in an applicator in the tumor or surrounding tissue, or applicator placement on top of a body surface
  - Intracavitary approach: use of an unsealed radioactive substance for temporary delivery into a hollow body cavity; may involve use of a remote afterloader, with radiation delivered at very high doses to a specific area daily for 3 to 5 days (in-patient or out-patient)
  - Intraoperative approach: delivery of a large dose of external radiation to the tumor and surrounding tissue during surgery
  - Hyperthermic approach: exposure of body tissues to high temperatures
  - Radiolabeled antibody approach: delivery of radiation directly to the cancer site; antibodies actively seek out and destroy the cancer cells, which may help lessen the risk of damage to healthy cells
  - Systemic approach: systemic delivery of radiation using radioactive material in a solution or colloidal suspension given orally or I.V. that's used for primary and metastatic thyroid cancer

Indications
- Primary cancer
- Metastatic cancer

▶ PROCEDURE

EXTERNAL THERAPY
- The radiation oncologist may mark precise treatment areas on the patient's skin with tiny tattoo dots of semipermanent ink.
- The patient is placed on the treatment table and is instructed to lie immobile.
- A large machine directs radiation at the target site for the prescribed period, usually 1 or 2 minutes.

INTERSTITIAL OR INTRACAVITARY APPROACH
- The surgeon usually inserts the applicator for the radioactive source in the operating room, with the patient under anesthesia.
- The radioactive source is placed in the applicator after the patient returns to his room.
- If the radioactive source isn't permanent, it's left in place for 24 to 72 hours and then removed in the patient's room.

I.V., ORAL, OR INTRACAVITARY APPROACH
- After intracavitary instillation of a suspension, the patient lies on a flat surface and is rotated every 15 minutes for 2 to 3 hours.

Complications
- Dehydration
- Localized skin burns
- Hemorrhage
- Neurologic dysfunction
- Leukemia and other cancers
- Cataracts
- Alopecia
- Xerostomia
- Thrombocytopenia
- Genetic mutation
- Sterility
- Bone marrow suppresion (external)
- Dysfunction or structural change in body parts within irradiated area (external)

✣ NURSING INTERVENTIONS

Pretreatment care
- Explain the treatment and preparation to the patient and family.

- Make sure the patient has signed an appropriate consent form.
- Obtain a thorough patient history.
- Obtain baseline white blood cell and platelet counts.
- Evaluate the patient for possible problems in positioning, range of motion, and comfort.
- Prepare the patient for a temporary appearance change if the implant is placed in a visible area.

Posttreatment care
EXTERNAL THERAPY
- Implement measures to control bleeding and prevent infection.
- Provide meticulous skin care.
- Provide comfort measures and supportive care.
- Monitor the patient's vital signs.
- Monitor WBC and platelet counts.

INTERNAL THERAPY
- Reassure the patient that normal activities can be resumed after the temporary radiation source has been removed or the permanent source has decayed.
- Report and properly store a dislodged radioactive implant, according to facility policy.
- Follow facility policy regarding radiation precautions.

MONITORING
- Vital signs
- Intake and output
- Complications
- Abnormal bleeding
- Infection

Patient teaching
Be sure to cover:
- radiation therapy and potential adverse effects
- avoidance of applying lotions, medications, and such to area receiving external therapy
- use of sunblock
- activity restrictions, as appropritae
- restriction of children and pregnant visitors
- follow-up care
- home management of adverse effects
- complications
- when to notify the physician
- need for temporary isolation after ingestion or instillation of a radioactive source
- referral to support groups such as the American Cancer Society.

Radioactive iodine therapy

● OVERVIEW

- Therapeutic administration of the radioisotope iodine 131 (^{131}I)
- Causes acute radiation thyroiditis and gradual thyroid atrophy
- Eventually reduces thyroid hormone levels
- Rarely requires an inpatient stay after administration, unless the patient received a large radioiodine dose (30 mCi or greater)

Indications
- Hyperthyroidism
- Thyroid cancer

▶ PROCEDURE

- In the nuclear medicine or radiation therapy department, the patient receives an oral dose of ^{131}I or ^{123}I.
- A larger dose is given for thyroid cancer than for hyperthyroidism.
- To treat hyperthyroidism, the dose depends on thyroid size and the gland's degree of radiosensitivity.

Complications
- Hypothyroidism
- Radiation thyroiditis
- Dysphagia
- Salivary gland inflammation
- Thyroid crisis
- Thyroid storm

❈ NURSING INTERVENTIONS

Pretreatment care
- Explain the treatment and preparation to the patient and family.
- Make sure the patient has signed an appropriate consent form.
- Discontinue thyroid hormone antagonists 4 to 7 days before ^{131}I administration, as ordered.
- Make sure the patient isn't taking the antiarrhythmic drug amiodarone.

Posttreatment care
- Institute radiation precautions until the facility's radiation safety officer determines the radiation level has fallen to within a safe zone.
- Encourage increased oral fluid intake for the first 48 hours after treatment.
- Instruct the patient to flush the toilet twice after each use for the first 48 hours.
- Provide disposable eating utensils.
- Caution the patient against close contact with young children and pregnant women for 7 days after treatment.

MONITORING
- Vital signs
- Intake and output
- Complications

Patient teaching
Be sure to cover:
- adverse effects and complications
- the fact that urine and saliva will be slightly radioactive for 24 hours and that vomitus will be highly radioactive for 6 to 8 hours after treatment
- proper excrement disposal
- likelihood that maximum effects may not occur for 3 months
- prescribed thyroid hormone antagonists
- periodic laboratory tests (serum thyroid hormone)
- signs and symptoms of hypothyroidism and hyperthyroidism
- signs and symptoms of radiation thyroiditis
- when to notify the physician
- avoidance of salicylates
- importance for a female of childbearing age to avoid conception for several months after therapy
- follow-up care.

Radiofrequency ablation of tumors

● OVERVIEW

- Insertion of radiofrequency ablation (RFA) energy through needle to destory tumor
- Highly successful, less expensive, and preferred treatment
- Minimally invasive procedure; most patients can return home on same day of procedure
- May also be performed with laparoscopy or during open surgery; percutaneous approach preferred by most radiologists because it's less invasive and produces fewer complications
- Able to destroy a tumor and a small rim of normal tissue around the liver's edges without affecting most of the normal liver; however, not used to treat liver tumors if there's active metastasis
- Can destroy small liver tumors (less than 5 cm in diameter) but it can't eliminate microscopic tumors
- Used when surgery isn't possible or if the patient is a poor surgical risk

Indications
- Liver tumors
- Kidney tumors
- Pain management for small bone cancer

▶ PROCEDURE

- A local anesthetic is injected into the site and the patient is sedated by I.V. injection.
- The physician guides a special needle through the skin and into the tumor by images from ultrasound or computed tomography (CT) scanning.
- When properly positioned, a plunger is advanced so that the electrodes extend from the needle tip. When fully extended, the electrodes resemble an open umbrella.
- Insulated wires to the needle electrodes and to grounding pads are placed on the patient's back or thigh, to connect the radiofrequency generator. It produces alternating electric current in the range of radiofrequency waves.
- The needle sends RFA current from the hollow core of the needle to penetrate and destroy the tumor. In addition, heat from radiofrequency energy closes up small blood vessels, reducing the risk of bleeding.

Complications
- Injury to adjacent organs and tissues (such as gallbladder, bile ducts, diaphragm, and bowel loops) requiring surgical correction
- Shoulder pain
- Gallbladder inflammation
- Thermal damage to the bowel or adjacent tissues
- Postablation syndrome
- Bleeding

�֍ NURSING INTERVENTIONS

Pretreatment care
- Explain the procedure to the patient.
- Verify that an appropriate consent form has been signed.
- Make sure that the patient has taken nothing by mouth from midnight the evening before treatment.
- Know that medications may need to be restricted before treatment, such as aspirin (usually stopped 10 days before) or blood thinners (such as warfarin [Coumadin]).
- Have the patient void before the procedure.
- Identify and record baseline laboratory values.

Posttreatment care
- Help the patient assume a comfortable position.
- Note color, amount, and character of drainage.
- Remove and dispose of all equipment properly.
- Make sure the patient has a computed tomography (CT) scan or magnetic resonance imaging (MRI) of the liver scheduled within a few hours to 1 week after RFA to ensure that all tumor tissue has been destroyed and to detect complications.

MONITORING
- Vital signs
- Dressing and drainage
- Complications
- Pain
- Nausea

Patient teaching
Be sure to cover:
- interpretation of follow-up CT scan or MRI to determine if the entire liver tumor appears to have been eliminated
- repeat CT scanning possible every 3 months to check for new tumors
- postablation syndrome: flulike symptoms that appear 3 to 5 days after the procedure and usually last 5 days, but can last a few weeks
- complications and when to notify the practitioner
- follow up care.

Restrictive gastric surgeries

● OVERVIEW

- Combination of procedures that use both restriction and malabsorption methods to produce weight loss
- Types include adjustable gastric banding and vertical banded gastroplasty
- Results in a smaller stomach so the patient feels fuller faster, thus significantly reduces caloric intake
- Not as successful as other types of gastric surgeries

Indications
- Body mass index (BMI) of 40 or more and at least 100lb (45 kg) over his recommended weight (normal BMI, 18.5 to 25)
- A BMI of 35 or more with a life-threatening illness that can be improved with weight loss, such as sleep apnea, type 2 diabetes, and heart disease

▶ PROCEDURE

- The surgery is performed with the patient under anesthesia.
- The small stomach pouch is created using bands (gastric banding), staples (stomach stapling), or a combination. The surgeon leaves a narrow passage in the newly created pouch so that food can still go through the remainder of the stomach and small intestines. except it does so more slowly.

Complications
- Bleeding
- Infections
- Bowel obstruction
- Peritonitis
- Gallstones
- Gastritis
- Vomiting
- Dumping syndrome

✳ NURSING INTERVENTIONS

Pretreatment care
- A complete medical examination is done to evaluate overall health. A psychological evaluation is also done to determine if the patient will be adhering to the new lifestyle. Extensive nutritional counseling is done with the patient.
- Explain the treatment and preparation to the patient and his family.
- Verify that the patient has signed an appropriate consent form.
- Obtain serum samples for hematologic studies as ordered.
- Begin I.V. fluid replacement and total parenteral nutrition (TPN) as ordered.
- Prepare the patient for abdominal X-rays as ordered.
- Explain postoperative care and equipment.
- Monitor the patient's vital signs, intake and output, nutritional status, and laboratory test results.

Posttreatment care
- Maintain I.V. replacement therapy as ordered.
- Keep the nasogastric tube patent, but don't reposition it.
- Provide wound care as indicated
- Encourage regular coughing and deep breathing exercises and splinting of the incision site as needed.
- Administer medications as ordered.
- Provide pain relief measures.
- Place the patient in low or semi-Fowler's position.
- Administer tube feedings or TPN as ordered.

MONITORING
- Vital signs
- Respiratory status

NURSING ALERT Watch for hypotension, bradycardia, and respiratory changes; these may signal hemorrhage and shock.

- Intake and output, daily weights
- Signs of dehydration, peritonitis, sepsis, infection, or postresection obstruction

NURSING ALERT Monitor for and immediately report signs and symptoms of anastomotic leakage, including low-grade fever, malaise, slight leukocytosis, abdominal distention, tenderness, hemorrhage, hypovolemic shock, and bloody stools or wound drainage.

- Abdominal pain, abdominal cramps or shoulder pain
- Complications
- Laboratory test results
- Dumping syndrome: weakness, nausea, flatulence, and palpitations occurring within 30 minutes after a meal

Patient Teaching
Be sure to cover:
- Importance of reporting abnormal bleeding
- Signs and symptoms of infection, obstruction, perforation or abnormal bleeding
- Coughing and deep-breathing exercises, splinting of incision
- Wound care
- Dumping syndrome and how to prevent it
- Anticipated pattern of weight loss: average of 10 lb (4.5 kg) per month usually lost; stable weight 18 to 24 months after surgery with greatest rate of weight loss at the very beginning
- Follow-up care to address his physical and mental health status, change in weight, and nutritional needs
- Exercise and dietary patterns; need to chew food slowly and eat small frequent meals
- Dietary restrictions, including reduced intake of fat and foods high in sugar; separation of fluid and food intake by at least 30 minutes
- Vitamin and mineral supplementation.

Spinal surgery

OVERVIEW

- Laminectomy: removes one or more of the bony laminae that cover the vertebrae; typically done to relieve pressure on the spinal cord or spinal nerve roots
- Arthrodesis: grafting of bone chips between vertebral space to stabilize spine
- Kyphoplasty: uses cement-like substances injected into vertebrae under fluoroscopy
- Laminoplasty: involves reconstruction of the lamina to increase amount of space available for neural tissue
- Microdiskectomy: alternative to laminectomy for decompressing and repairing damaged lumbar disks
- Rod implantation: attachment of hooks, rods, and wires to redistribute stress to the spine and keep the bone in proper alignment
- Vertebroplasty: picks up the pieces of a fracture and supports the vertebral body by cementing it back into a solid unit

Indications
- Herniated disk
- Compression fracture
- Vertebral dislocation
- Spinal cord tumor
- Vertebrae seriously weakened by trauma or disease
- Spinal stenosis (laminoplasty)

ROD IMPLANTATION
- Scoliosis
- Birth defects
- Fractures
- Marfan syndrome
- Neurofibromatosis
- Neuromuscular diseases
- Severe injuries
- Tumors

PROCEDURE

LAMINECTOMY
- The patient receives a general anesthetic and is placed in a prone or side-lying position.
- A midline vertical incision is made.
- The fascia and muscles are stripped off the bony laminae.
- One or more sections of laminae are removed to expose the spinal defect (herniated disk, bone spur, disk fragment).

ARTHRODESIS
- The patient receives a general anesthetic.
- For cervical fusion, the anterior approach is usually used; for lumbar and thoracic fusion, the posterior approach is used.
- The surgeon exposes the affected vertebrae.
- If a bone graft is used, an incision is made in the donor's hip and pieces or chips of the bone are removed, usually from the iliac crest.
- Bone chips, bone bank, or both are shaped and inserted into the defect.
- Wire, spinal plates, rods, or screws are used to secure bone grafts into several vertebrae surrounding the unstable area.
- The incision is closed and a dressing, splint, or cast is applied.
- External traction, such as a halo device, may be applied if surgery involves the cervical spine.

KYPHOPLASTY
- The patient receives general or local anesthesia and is placed in a prone position. The procedure is performed with fluoroscopy.
- After a small incision is made in the back, a narrow tube is inserted into the affected area, and a balloon inserted and inflated.
- This inflation creates a cavity inside the vertebrae as well as elevates the fracture to return the vertebrae to a normal position.
- After the balloon is removed, the cavity is filled with a cementlike material that hardens quickly to stabilize the bone.
- This procedure is repeated for all involved vertebrae.

- A dressing is then applied to the incision site when the procedure is complete.

LAMINOPLASTY
- The patient receives a general anesthetic and is placed in a prone position.
- A midline vertical incision is made.
- One side of the vertebrae is cut to form a "hinge" and the other side is cut all the way through.
- Small titanium mini-plates and pieces of bone are then inserted and the vertebrae are put back in place with an increased spinal space.
- This increased space allows for decompression of spinal cord and nerve roots.

MICRODISKECTOMY
- The procedure may be performed on an outpatient basis; the patient receives local anesthesia.
- Under guided X-ray visualization, the surgeon locates the damaged disk and removes the nerve root and injured disk tissues.
- The incision is stapled and may be covered with a dressing.

ROD IMPLANTATION
- The procedure is performed by a neurology or orthopedic surgical team usually under general anesthesia.
- The surgery is usually done at the same time as spinal fusion.
- The surgeon can use a posterior or anterior approach.
- The surgeon strips the muscles away from the surgical site and the bone surface is peeled away. This helps the bone graft to fuse better.
- In some cases, the vertebral disk is removed to provide a larger area for the spinal fusion.
- Rods, hooks, and wires are inserted and secured to stabilize the area and the incision is closed.

VERTEBROPLASTY
- The patient receives a local anesthetic and is placed in the prone position.
- A small incision is made in the back through which the surgeon threads a narrow tube.
- Using fluoroscopy to guide it to the correct position, the tube creates a path through the back into the fractured vertebrae.

(continued)

- The cavity is filled with cement-like material that hardens quickly, stabilizing the bone.
- The incision is closed, and a dressing is applied.

Complications
- Infection
- Bleeding
- Spinal fluid leakage
- Nerve or muscle damage
- Paralysis (rod implantation)

✻ NURSING INTERVENTIONS

Pretreatment care
- Explain the treatment and preparation to the patient and his family.
- Verify that the patient has signed an appropriate consent form.
- Discuss postoperative recovery and rehabilitation. Reassure the patient that analgesics and muscle relaxants will be available during recovery.
- Tell the patient that he'll return from surgery with a dressing over the incision and that there may be activity restrictions.
- Just before surgery, perform a baseline assessment of motor function and sensation in the patient's lower trunk, legs, and feet as well as upper extremities and fingers for cervical involvement. Carefully document results for comparison with postoperative findings.

Posttreatment care
- Administer medications, as ordered.
- Maintain activity restrictions, as ordered.
- Log roll the patient after laminectomy and keep the head of the bed flat or elevated no more than 45 degrees for at least 24 hours after surgery.
- Perform wound care and dressing changes, as ordered.
- After rod implantation, change patient's position frequently and have a physical therapist help the patient to learn self-care activities and how to perform range-of-motion and strengthening exercises.

MONITORING
- Vital signs
- Intake and output
- Surgical wound and dressings
- Drainage and bleeding
- Possible cerebrospinal fluid leakage
- Motor, sensory, and overall neurologic function

Patient teaching
Be sure to cover:
- medication administration, dosage, and possible adverse effects
- incision site care
- signs and symptoms of infection
- showering with back facing away from the stream of water
- activity restrictions
- exercise regimen
- proper body mechanics and body alignment
- follow-up care.

Splenectomy

● OVERVIEW

- Surgical removal of the spleen
- Performed based on severity of condition suggseting spleen removal; may be performed by open surgery or laparascopically
- May require long-term treatment with antibiotics following surgery

Indications
- Hematologic disorders
- Traumatic splenic rupture
- Hypersplenism
- Hereditary spherocytosis
- Chronic idiopathic thrombocytopenic purpura
- Hodgkin's disease

▶ PROCEDURE

- The patient is placed under general anesthesia.
- The peritoneal cavity is exposed through a left rectus paramedial or subcostal incision.
- The splenic artery, vein, and ligaments are ligated.
- The spleen is removed.
- After carefully checking for bleeding, the abdomen is closed.
- A drain may be placed in the left sub-diaphragmatic space.
- The incision site is sutured and dressed.

Complications
- Bleeding
- Infection
- Pneumonia
- Atelectasis

※ AGE-RELATED CONCERN Children have an increased risk of death due to infection after a splenectomy, especially in the 2 years following surgery.

✳ NURSING INTERVENTIONS

Pretreatment care
- Explain the treatment and preparation to the patient and family.
- Make sure the patient has signed an appropriate consent form.
- Report abnormal results of blood studies.
- Administer blood products, vitamin K, or fresh frozen plasma, as ordered.
- Obtain vital signs, and perform a baseline respiratory assessment.
- Notify the physician if you suspect respiratory infection; surgery may be delayed.
- Explain postoperative care.
- Administer antibiotics, as ordered.

Posttreatment care
- Administer medications and I.V. fluids, as ordered.
- Assist with early ambulation.
- Encourage coughing, deep breathing, and incentive spirometry use.
- Administer analgesics, as needed and ordered.
- Provide comfort measures.
- Provide incision care, as ordered.
- Change dressings, as ordered.
- Maintain patency of drains.

MONITORING
- Vital signs
- Intake and output
- Complications
- Surgical wound and dressings
- Drainage
- Abnormal bleeding
- Hematologic studies
- Infection

Patient teaching
Be sure to cover:
- medication administration, dosage, and potential adverse effects
- coughing and deep-breathing techniques
- signs and symptoms of infection and bleeding
- complications
- when to notify the physician
- ways to prevent infection, including possible long-term antibiotic therapy
- incision care
- adherence to therapy
- follow-up care.

Stereotactic radiosurgery

● OVERVIEW

- Stereotactic radiosurgery (SRS): noninvasive delivery of single high dose of radiation (l-day session) to an area of the brain to treat abnormalities, tumors, or other functional disorders
- May be the primary treatment used with inaccessible tumors, or as an adjunct to other treatments with recurring or malignant tumor
- Forms of SRS:
  – particle beam (proton) and cobalt 60-based (gamma knife)—used for small tumors
  – linear accelerator based—used for larger tumors (greater than 3.5 cm)
- Fractionated stereotactic radiotherapy: radiation administered over several days or weeks by the same procedure; larger total radiation dose
- Three-dimensional computer-aided planning and high degree of immobilization allowing for minimal amount of radiation to healthy brain tissue

Indications
- Brain tumors (benign and malignant)
- Trigeminal neuralgia
- Essential tremor
- Parkinson's tremor or rigidity
- Arteriovenous malformations

▶ PROCEDURE

- Before performing SRS, the patient is fitted with a stereotactic frame that allows for precise delivery of radiation to the required area. For fractionated radiotherapy, the frame is attached to a rigid plastic mask that contours to the patient's skeletal frame and is reused. The frame for single use is bolted to the patient's head with metal bolts.
- The patient doesn't require anesthesia, although local anesthesia may be used to attach the frame to the patient's head.
- Radiation is then aimed at the tumor from various directions. The amount of radiation required directly correlates to the exact size and location of the tumor, as determined by magnetic resonance imaging and computed tomography scanning.
- The frame is detached when the procedure is complete.

Complications
- Headache
- Recurrence of tumor
- Nausea and vomiting
- Fatigue

✳ NURSING INTERVENTIONS

Pretreatment care
- Explain the treatment and preparation to the patient and his family.
- Verify that the patient has signed an appropriate consent form.
- Answer questions about pretreatment studies or these procedures and remind the patient that the frame will be applied for the procedure, but removed when the procedure is complete.
- Obtain baseline vital signs.
- Provide reassurance.

Posttreatment care
- Administer medications, as ordered.
- Provide comfort measures and supportive care.

MONITORING
- Vital signs
- Mental status

Patient teaching
Be sure to cover:
- medication administration, dosage, and possible adverse effects
- complications and when to notify the physician
- follow-up care
- support groups such as American Cancer Society.

Thoracotomy

● OVERVIEW

- Surgical incision into the thoracic cavity, most commonly performed to remove part or all of a lung and thus spare healthy lung tissue from disease
- May involve pneumonectomy, lobectomy, segmental resection, or wedge resection
- Exploratory thoracotomy: done to evaluate the chest and pleural space for chest trauma and tumors
- Decortication: removal or stripping of the fibrous membrane covering the visceral pleura; helps reexpand the lung in empyema
- Thoracoplasty: removes part or all of one rib to reduce chest cavity size, decreasing the risk of mediastinal shift; may be done when tuberculosis has reduced lung volume

Indications
- Diseased lung tissue requiring removal

▶ PROCEDURE

- The patient is anesthetized.
- In a posterolateral thoracotomy, the incision starts in the submammary fold of the anterior chest, is drawn below the scapular tip and along the ribs, and then curves posteriorly and up to the scapular spine.
- In an anterolateral thoracotomy, the incision begins below the breast and above the costal margins, extending from the anterior axillary line and then turning downward to avoid the axillary apex.
- In a median sternotomy, a straight incision is made from the suprasternal notch to below the xiphoid process; the sternum must be transected with an electric or air-driven saw.
- Once the incision is made, the surgeon removes tissue for a biopsy.
- Bleeding sources are tied off.
- Injuries within the thoracic cavity are located and repaired.
- The ribs may be spread and the lung exposed for excision.

PNEUMONECTOMY
- The surgeon ligates and severs the pulmonary arteries.
- The mainstem bronchus leading to the affected lung is clamped.
- The bronchus is divided and closed with nonabsorbable sutures or staples.
- The lung is removed.
- To ensure airtight closure, a pleural flap is placed over the bronchus and closed.
- The phrenic nerve is severed on the affected side.
- After air pressure in the pleural cavity stabilizes, the chest is closed.

LOBECTOMY
- The surgeon resects the affected lobe.
- Appropriate arteries, veins, and bronchial passages are ligated and severed.
- One or two chest tubes are inserted for drainage and lung reexpansion.

SEGMENTAL RESECTION
- The surgeon removes the affected lung segment.
- The appropriate artery, vein, and bronchus are ligated and severed.
- Two chest tubes are inserted to aid lung reexpansion.

WEDGE RESECTION
- The affected area is clamped, excised, and sutured.
- The surgeon inserts two chest tubes to aid lung reexpansion.
- After completing the procedure requiring the thoracotomy, the surgeon closes the chest cavity and applies a dressing.

Complications
- Hemorrhage
- Infection
- Tension pneumothorax
- Bronchopleural fistula
- Empyema
- Persistent air space that the remaining lung tissue doesn't expand to fill

✳ NURSING INTERVENTIONS

Pretreatment care
- Explain the treatment and preparation to the patient and family.
- Make sure the patient has signed an appropriate consent form.
- Explain postoperative care.
- Arrange for laboratory studies and tests; report abnormal results.
- Withhold food and fluids, as ordered.

Posttreatment care
- Administer medications, as ordered.
- After pneumonectomy, make sure the patient lies only on the operative side or his back until stabilized.
- Make sure chest tubes are patent and functioning.
- Provide comfort measures.
- Encourage coughing, deep breathing, and incentive spirometry use.
- Have the patient splint the incision, as needed.
- Perform passive range-of-motion (ROM) exercises, progressing to active ROM exercises.
- Perform incision care and dressing changes, as ordered.

MONITORING
- Vital signs
- Intake and output
- Complications
- Respiratory status
- Lung sounds
- Surgical wound and dressings
- Drainage
- Abnormal bleeding

◉ **NURSING ALERT** Monitor for and immediately report dyspnea, chest pain, hypotension, irritating cough, vertigo, syncope, anxiety, subcutaneous emphysema, or tracheal deviation from the midline. These findings indicate tension pneumothorax.

Patient teaching
Be sure to cover:
- medication administration, dosage, and possible adverse effects
- coughing and deep-breathing techniques
- incentive spirometry
- incision care and dressing changes
- signs and symptoms of infection
- complications and when to notify the physician
- monitoring of sputum characteristics
- ROM exercises and prescribed physical activity restrictions
- ways to prevent infection
- smoking cessation
- wound care and dressing change care
- home health care, as needed
- follow-up care.

Thyroidectomy

● OVERVIEW

- Surgical removal of all or part of the thyroid gland

Indications
- Hyperthyroidism
- Respiratory obstruction caused by goiter
- Thyroid cancer

▶ PROCEDURE

- The patient is anesthetized.
- The surgeon extends the patient's neck fully and determines the incision line by measuring bilaterally from each clavicle.
- The surgeon cuts through the skin, fascia, and muscle and raises skin flaps from the strap muscles.
- The muscles are separated at midline, revealing the isthmus of the thyroid.
- The thyroid artery and veins are ligated to help prevent bleeding.
- The surgeon locates and visualizes the laryngeal nerves and parathyroid glands.
- Thyroid tissue is dissected and removed.
- A Penrose drain or a closed wound drainage device is inserted, and the wound is closed.

Complications
- Hemorrhage
- Parathyroid damage
- Hypocalcemia
- Tetany
- Laryngeal nerve damage
- Vocal cord paralysis
- Thyroid storm

✳ NURSING INTERVENTIONS

Pretreatment care
- Explain the treatment and preparation to the patient and family.
- Make sure the patient has signed an appropriate consent form.
- Explain postoperative care.
- Inform the patient that some hoarseness and a sore throat will occur after surgery.
- Make sure the patient has followed the preoperative drug regimen as ordered.
- Collect blood samples for serum thyroid hormone measurement.
- Obtain a 12-lead electrocardiogram.

Posttreatment care
- Administer medications, as ordered.
- Keep the patient in high Fowler's position.
- Evaluate the patient's speech for signs of laryngeal nerve damage.
- Keep a tracheotomy tray at the bedside for 24 hours after surgery.
- Provide surgical wound care and dressing changes, as ordered.
- Provide comfort measures.
- Maintain patency of drains.

MONITORING
- Vital signs
- Intake and output
- Surgical wound and dressings
- Drainage
- Abnormal bleeding
- Respiratory status
- Hypocalcemia (Chvostek's and Trousseau's signs)
- Thyroid storm

Patient teaching
Be sure to cover:
- medication administration, dosage, and possible adverse effects
- signs and symptoms of respiratory distress
- signs and symptoms of hypothyroidism and hyperthyroidism
- signs and symptoms of infection
- signs and symptoms of hypocalcemia
- abnormal bleeding
- complications and when to notify the physician
- prescribed thyroid hormone replacement therapy
- calcium supplements, as indicated
- incision care and dressing changes
- follow-up care.

Tracheotomy

- Surgical creation of an opening into the trachea through the neck
- May be permanent or temporary

Indications
- Prolonged mechanical ventilation
- To prevent aspiration in an unconscious or paralyzed patient
- Upper airway obstruction caused by trauma, burns, epiglottitis, or a tumor
- To remove lower tracheobronchial secretions in a patient who can't clear them

- The technique varies with the type of tube used.
- If an endotracheal (ET) tube isn't already in place, it's inserted with the patient under general anesthesia.
- A horizontal incision is made in the skin below the cricoid cartilage, and vertical incisions are made in the trachea.
- A tracheostomy tube is placed between the second and third tracheal rings.
- Retraction sutures may be placed in the stomal margins.
- The tube cuff (if present) is inflated.
- Ventilation and suction are performed.
- Oxygen is administered.
- The ET tube is removed.

Complications
- Hemorrhage
- Edema
- Aspiration of secretions
- Pneumothorax
- Subcutaneous emphysema
- Infection
- Airway obstruction
- Hypoxia
- Arrhythmias

Pretreatment care
- Explain the treatment and preparation to the patient and family.
- Make sure the patient has signed an appropriate consent form.
- Obtain appropriate supplies or a tracheotomy tray.
- Devise an appropriate communication system.
- Obtain samples for arterial blood gas (ABG) analysis and other required diagnostic tests; report abnormal results.

Posttreatment care
- Administer medications, as ordered.
- Turn the patient every 2 hours and provide chest physiotherapy.
- Provide oxygen and humidification, as ordered.
- Suction the airway, as indicated.
- Monitor cuff pressures, as ordered (usually should measure less than 25 cm H_2O [18 mm Hg]).
- Provide comfort measures.
- Perform incision care and dressing changes, as ordered.
- Keep a sterile tracheostomy tube with obturator (including a tube one size smaller) at the bedside.

MONITORING
- Vital signs
- Intake and output
- Respiratory status
- Lung sounds
- Pulmonary secretions
- Surgical wound and dressings
- Drainage
- Abnormal bleeding
- Complications
- ABG values
- Pulse oximetry values
- Tracheostomy tube cuff pressures
- Peritracheal edema

Patient teaching
Be sure to cover:
- medication administration, dosage, and possible adverse effects
- tracheostomy and tube care and reinsertion of tube, if appropriate
- protection of the stoma from water
- use of a foam filter over the stoma in winter
- signs and symptoms of infection
- complications
- when to notify the physician
- proper disposal of expelled secretions
- follow-up care.

Traction

● OVERVIEW

- Treatment that exerts a pulling force on a part of the body, usually the spine, pelvis, or a long bone of the arm or leg
- Type of mechanical traction used (skin or skeletal) dependent on the patient's condition, age, weight, and skin condition as well as the purpose and expected duration of traction
- Skin traction: applied directly to the skin (indirectly to the bone); used when a light, temporary, or noncontinuous pulling force is required
- Skeletal traction: device inserted through the bone and attached to traction equipment to exert a direct, constant, longitudinal pulling force; applied by an orthopedist

Indications
- Fracture
- Dislocation
- Deformity
- Contracture
- Muscle spasm

⬡ **NURSING ALERT** Skin traction is contraindicated in patients with severe injury with open wounds, allergy to tape, thrombophlebitis, circulatory disturbances, dermatitis, and varicose veins. Skeletal traction is contraindicated in patients with infections such as osteomyelitis.

▶ PROCEDURE

SKIN TRACTION
- Mechanical traction is applied at the patient's bedside.
- Adhesive or nonadhesive traction tape (or another skin traction device) is used to exert a pulling force (5 to 8 lb [2.25 to 3.5 kg]) on the skin.
- Types of skin traction include Buck's extension, pelvic (with a pelvic belt), and cervical (with a cervical halter).

SKELETAL TRACTION
- Skeletal traction is applied under local, general, or spinal anesthesia in aseptic surroundings.
- The physician inserts pins, wires, or tongs into or through the affected bone.
- Weights are attached to the pins, wires, or tongs; the usual weight is 25 to 40 lb (11.5 to 18 kg).
- Types of skeletal traction include balanced skeletal, overhead arm, and cervical with tongs.
- Pads, slings, or pushers may be used along with traction.

Complications
- Pressure ulcers
- Muscle atrophy
- Weakness
- Contractures
- Osteoporosis
- Urinary stasis and calculi
- Pneumonia
- Thrombophlebitis
- Osteomyelitis
- Nonunion or delayed union of the bone
- Complications of immobility
- Feelings of depression

✳ NURSING INTERVENTIONS

Pretreatment care
- Explain the treatment and preparation to the patient and family.
- Make sure the patient has signed an appropriate consent form.
- Set up appropriate traction equipment and a frame according to established facility policy.

Posttreatment care
- Administer medications, as ordered.
- Show the patient how much movement is permitted.
- Provide comfort measures.
- Unwrap skin traction every shift and assess the skin for redness, warmth, blisters, and other signs of breakdown.
- Maintain the patient in proper body alignment; reposition as necessary.
- Provide meticulous skin care.
- Administer pin care, as ordered.
- Encourage coughing and deep-breathing exercises.
- Assist with ordered range-of-motion exercises for unaffected extremities.
- Apply elastic support stockings, as ordered.
- Provide dietary fiber and sufficient fluids.
- Administer stool softeners, laxatives, or enemas, as needed and ordered.
- Inspect traction equipment for kinks, knots, or frays in ropes; make sure the weights hang freely and don't touch the floor.

MONITORING
- Vital signs
- Intake and output
- Skin condition
- Infection
- Complications of immobility
- Neurovascular status of extremities

Patient teaching
Be sure to cover:
- medication administration, dosage, and possible adverse effects
- set-up and care of traction equipment
- use of an overhead trapeze
- pin care
- signs and symptoms of infection
- complications and when to notify the physician
- preventing and managing complications of immobility
- dietary recommendations
- follow-up care.

Transjugular intrahepatic portosystemic shunt

● OVERVIEW

- Insertion of small, flexible tube made of medical grade plastic or wire mesh to create a new passageway from the portal vein to the hepatic vein, diverting blood flow away from the liver
- Diverts blood that's returning to the heart from the spleen and intestines, thereby reducing pressure in the portal system within the liver
- Also known as *TIPS*

Indications
- End-stage portal hypertension
- Active, or recurrent, varices despite treatment
- Ascites unresponsive to other treatments

▶ PROCEDURE

- The patient receives general anesthesia or conscious sedation.
- The procedure is done in a specially equipped suite with emergency equipment and staffing. The patient's electrocardiogram and oxygen status are monitored during the procedure.
- The interventional radiologist threads a catheter through a small incision in the skin near the jugular vein in the neck and guides it through the vena cava to the hepatic vein, using fluoroscopy or ultrasonography.
- With X-ray guidance, the radiologist directs a special needle through the wall of the hepatic vein, across a gap, and into the portal vein.
- Dye is injected to verify catheter placement.
- A balloon is used to dilate the new tract, then one to three stents are inserted and opened to maintain the flow.
- Dye is reinjected to verify correct flow from hepatic vein to portal vein to inferior vena cava.
- The catheter is removed and the incision sutured and bandaged.

Complications
- Bleeding or bruising at the catheter site
- Hematoma of the neck or liver area
- Cardiac arrhythmias
- Liver capsule rupture
- Septicemia
- Hepatic failure
- Encephalopathy
- Shunt failure
- Exsanguination and death

✳ NURSING INTERVENTIONS

Pretreatment care
- Make sure that preliminary evaluation and diagnostic testing has been completed, as ordered.
- Review the procedure with the patient and answer questions.
- Verify that a consent form has been signed.
- Review with the patient what to expect postoperatively.
- Perform a baseline cardiopulmonary and abdominal assessment, including height and weight.
- Make sure that the patient doesn't take anything by mouth after midnight before the procedure.
- Make sure that pre-existing treatments have been performed, as ordered.
- Note allergies and medications the patient is taking.

Posttreatment care
- Maintain continuous cardiac and hemodynamic monitoring, as ordered.
- Provide catheter site care and dressing changes.
- Measure abdominal girth; when bowel sounds return, expect to begin oral feedings.
- Maintain nothing-by-mouth status until the gag reflex returns.
- Maintain patency of I.V. tubes and provide hydration, as ordered.
- Administer medications, as ordered, including analgesics, as needed.
- Reorient the patient, as necessary.
- Encourage the patient to breathe deeply and cough, as indicated; assist with using an incentive spirometer.
- Assist with ambulation, as ordered.

MONITORING
- Vital signs
- Cardiopulmonary and hemodynamic status
- Mental status
- Intake and output; daily weight
- Catheter site for signs and symptoms of bleeding and infection

◆ **NURSING ALERT** Because of the patient's underlying liver disease, coagulation may be altered. Monitor the dressing at least every 30 minutes initially, and then every 1 or 2 hours. Immediately report bright red drainage on the dressing.

- Abdomen for bowel sounds and distention

◆ **NURSING ALERT** Insertion should cause the patient's abdominal girth to gradually decrease. However, because of the underlying liver disease, bleeding can occur at the catheter insertion site. Be alert to increases in abdominal girth, and notify the physician immediately. An increase may indicate bleeding or that the stent isn't functioning.

Patient teaching
Be sure to cover:
- exercise and driving restrictions
- signs and symptoms of complications and what to report to the physician
- medication administration, dosage, and possible adverse effects
- dietary restrictions
- need for rest and drinking plenty of fluids, except alcoholic beverages
- avoidance of lifting heavy objects or performing strenuous exercises
- smoking cessation
- follow-up care and testing.

Transmyocardial laser revascularization

OVERVIEW

- Used to treat inoperable cardiac ischemia in patients with persistent angina, that's unrelieved by other methods (angioplasty, coronary artery surgery), by improving blood flow to those areas of the heart
- Employs a special carbon dioxide (CO_2) laser that creates small channels in poorly perfused but nonnecrotic ventricular heart tissue, stimulating reperfusion of the muscle through new collateral circulation
- New channels thought to promote angiogenesis (growth of new capillaries)
- Also known as *TMR*

Indications

- Angina
- Inoperable heart disease

NURSING ALERT TMR is contraindicated if the heart muscle is severely damaged or necrotic from a myocardial infarction or if the heart muscle has too much scar tissue.

PROCEDURE

- The patient is given general anesthesia but doesn't require cardiopulmonary bypass or heart stoppage.
- A small incision is made in the left or middle of the chest.
- The underlying tissues are separated and retracted to expose the heart muscle.
- The laser hand piece is positioned over the poorly perfused ventricular muscle. The CO_2 laser creates 20 to 40 1-mm wide channels in the left ventricle. The channels penetrate all layers of the heart but the pericardial holes quickly close. The channels through the myocardium and endocardium remain open.
- The laser is guided by a computer that monitors the patient's electrocardiogram so that the laser cuts only between heartbeats—when the ventricle is filled with blood and the heart is relatively still. This helps to prevent arrhythmias.

Complications

- Cardiac tamponade
- Hypovolemic shock
- Arrhythmias

NURSING INTERVENTIONS

Pretreatment care

- Tests required before TMR include cardiac catheterization, echocardiogram, positron emission tomography, dobutamine echocardiography, and cardiac magnetic resonance imaging.
- Review the disorder and the procedure with the patient and answer questions.
- Verify that a consent form has been signed.
- Review with the patient what to expect postoperatively.
- Perform a baseline assessment and verify pulse quality.
- Make sure the patient doesn't take anything by mouth after midnight before the procedure.
- Check that treatments have been performed, as ordered.

- Note allergies and medications the patient is taking.

Posttreatment care

- Maintain patency of I.V. tubes and provide hydration, as ordered.
- Administer medications, as ordered.
- Encourage coughing and deep-breathing exercises, as indicated; assist with incentive spirometry.
- Assist with ambulation, as ordered.
- Provide wound care, as indicated

MONITORING

- Vital signs
- Cardiopulmonary status including heart rate and rhythm, heart and lung sounds, hemodynamic status, pulse oximetry
- Intake and output
- Peripheral pulses
- Abdominal sounds
- Signs and symptoms of infection

Patient teaching

Be sure to cover:

- exercise and driving restrictions
- supervised cardiac rehabilitation program, as ordered
- complications and when to notify physician
- medication administration, dosage, and possible adverse effects
- dietary restrictions
- how effects of therapy may be immediate or gradual; or how symptoms may not completely resolve, but activity tolerance will improve
- follow-up care.

Ventricular assist device

● OVERVIEW

- Provides support to a failing heart and provides systemic and pulmonary support
- Implanted to divert blood from an impaired ventricle to an artificial pump; pump synchronizes to the patient's electrocardiogram (ECG) and functions as the ventricle
- Also called *VAD*
- Right VAD (RVAD): diverts blood from the failing right ventricle to the VAD, which then pumps blood to the pulmonary circulation via the VAD connection to the pulmonary artery
- Left VAD (LVAD): diverts blood from the failing left ventricle to the VAD, which then pumps blood back to the body via the VAD connection to the aorta
- When RVAD and LVAD are used, biventricular (BiVAD) support provided

Indications
- Ventricular failure
- Cardiac transplantation
- Refractory cardiogenic shock
- Cardiopulmonary bypass

▶ PROCEDURE

- The patient is given general anesthesia.
- An incision is made through the breastbone to expose the heart; heparin is administered to keep the blood from clotting.
- Cardiopulmonary bypass is initiated.
- An incision is made to form a pocket for the LVAD in the abdominal wall.
- Small incisions are placed through the diaphragm to allow placement of the tubes, which are used to channel blood from the ventricle to the LVAD and connect the pump to the aorta.
- An incision is also made through the abdominal wall to connect the VAD to an external power source.
- The surgeon cannulates the left ventricle with the inflow tube and the aorta with the outflow tube.
- When the pump is adequately supporting the heart, the patient is removed from the heart-lung machine.
- All incisions are sutured and dressings are applied.

Complications
- Hemorrhage
- Air embolus
- Thrombus
- Infection
- Lethal arrhythmias

✷ NURSING INTERVENTIONS

Pretreatment care
- Review the purpose of the VAD and what to expect after its insertion.
- Verify that an appropriate consent form has been signed.
- Provide emotional support.
- Monitor ECG, pulmonary artery and hemodynamic status, and intake and output.
- Administer ongoing medications, as ordered.
- Before surgery, restrict food and fluid intake, and monitor cardiac function.

Posttreatment care
- Maintain I.V. fluid therapy, as ordered.
- Keep the patient immobile to prevent accidental extubation, contamination, or disconnection of the VAD.
- Maintain cardiac output at 5 to 8 L/minute, central venous pressure at 8 to 16 mm Hg, pulmonary artery wedge pressure at 10 to 20 mm Hg, mean arterial pressure at greater than 60 mm Hg, and left atrial pressure between 4 and 12 mm Hg.

◈ **NURSING ALERT** Monitor the patient for signs and symptoms of poor perfusion and ineffective pumping, including arrhythmias, hypotension, low capillary refill, cool skin, oliguria or anuria, confusion, anxiety, and restlessness.

- Use sterile technique in dressing changes. Change the dressing site over the cannula sites daily or according to facility policy.
- Maintain chest tube patency and function. Notify the practitioner if drainage is greater than 150 ml/hour over 2 hours.
- Obtain laboratory test results; assess for bleeding.
- When stable, turn the patient every 2 hours and begin range-of-motion (ROM) exercises.
- Administer antibiotics prophylactically, if ordered.
- Give heparin, as ordered, to prevent clotting in the pump head and formation of thrombus.
- Provide comfort measures and supportive care

◈ **NURSING ALERT** If ventricular function fails to improve within 4 days, the patient may need a transplant. Provide psychological support for the patient and his family as they endure referral.

MONITORING
- Cardiopulmonary status: breath sounds, oxygen saturation or mixed venous oxygen saturation, vital signs, hemodynamic parameters, cardiac output, ECG, peripheral pulses
- Peripheral pulses
- Incisions, cannula insertion sites, and dressings
- Fluid and electrolyte balance
- Signs and symptoms of bleeding and infection

Patient teaching
Be sure to cover:
- medication administration, dosage, and possible adverse effects
- coughing and deep-breathing exercises and incentive spirometery
- activity restrictions
- wound care
- signs and symptoms of infection
- signs and symptoms of increasing heart failure, bleeding, pulmonary embolism, or cerebral embolism, with instructions to noticy the physician promptly
- care for the exit port and battery pack
- referral for home care
- follow-up care.

Part III > PROCEDURES

Arterial pressure monitoring

● OVERVIEW

- Permits direct continuous measurement of systolic, diastolic, and mean pressures; also allows arterial blood sampling
- Indicated when highly accurate or frequent blood pressure measurements are required, for example, in patient with low cardiac output and high systemic vascular resistance
- Also indicated for patients receiving titrated doses of vasoactive drugs or needing frequent blood sampling
- Generally more accurate than indirect methods based on blood flow alone (such as palpation and auscultation of blood pressure) because systemic vascular resistance is also reflected
- Also known as *intra-arterial pressure monitoring*

Contraindications
ABSOLUTE
- Severe injury to the extremity
- Positive Allen's test
- Injury proximal to the vessel
- Local skin compromise
RELATIVE
- Atherosclerotic arterial disease
- Vasospastic arterial disease
- Hypercoagulable state
- Artery site that's prone to infection

❖ EQUIPMENT

CATHETER INSERTION
Gloves • sterile gown • mask • protective eyewear • sterile gloves • 16G to 20G catheter (type and length dependent on the insertion site, patient's size, and other anticipated uses of the line) • preassembled preparation kit (if available) • sterile drapes • sheet protector • prepared pressure transducer system • ordered local anesthetic • sutures • syringe and needle (21G to 25G, 1") • I.V. pole • tubing and medication labels • site care kit • arm board and soft wrist restraint (for a femoral site, an ankle restraint) • optional: shaving kit (for femoral artery insertion)

BLOOD SAMPLE COLLECTION
If an *open system* is in place: Gloves • gown • mask • protective eyewear • sterile 4" × 4" gauze pads • sheet protector • 500-ml I.V. bag • 5- to 10-ml syringe for discard sample • syringes of appropriate size and number for ordered laboratory tests • laboratory request forms and labels • needleless device (depending on your facility's policy) • specimen tubes

If a *closed system* is in place: Gloves • gown • mask • protective eyewear • syringes of appropriate size and number for ordered laboratory tests • laboratory request forms and labels • alcohol pads • blood transfer unit • specimen tubes

ARTERIAL LINE TUBING CHANGES
Gloves • gown • mask • protective eyewear • sheet protector • preassembled arterial pressure tubing with flush device and disposable pressure transducer • sterile gloves • 500-ml bag of I.V. flush solution (such as D_5W or normal saline solution) • 500 or 1,000 units of heparin • syringe and needle (21G to 25G, 1") • medication label • pressure bag • site care kit • tubing labels

ARTERIAL CATHETER REMOVAL
Gloves • mask • gown • protective eyewear • two sterile 4" × 4" gauze pads • sheet protector • sterile suture removal set • dressing • hypoallergenic tape

FEMORAL LINE REMOVAL
Additional sterile 4" × 4" gauze pads • small sandbag • adhesive bandage

CATHETER-TIP CULTURE
Sterile scissors • sterile container • sterile gloves

Equipment preparation
- Wash your hands thoroughly.
- Maintain asepsis throughout all procedures.
- Set up and prime the monitoring system.
- Assemble equipment, maintaining sterile technique.
- Set the alarms on the bedside monitor according to your facility's policy.

▮▮ ESSENTIAL STEPS

- Explain the procedure to the patient and family members.
- Make sure the patient has signed an appropriate consent form.
- Wear appropriate personal protective equipment throughout all procedures.
- Check the patient's history for an allergy or a hypersensitivity to iodine or the ordered local anesthetic.
- Position the patient for easy access to the catheter insertion site.
- Place a sheet protector under the site.
- If the catheter will be inserted into the radial artery, perform Allen's test to assess collateral circulation in the hand.

◈ **NURSING ALERT** Even though thrombosis of the radial artery at the catheter site is common, ischemic injury of the hand is rare if there is adequate ulnar collateral flow.

INSERTING AN ARTERIAL CATHETER
- The physician prepares and anesthetizes the insertion site and covers the surrounding area with sterile drapes.

◈ **NURSING ALERT** Cannulation of the brachial artery isn't recommended because of the potential for thrombosis and ischemia of the lower arm and hand.

- The physician then inserts the catheter into the artery and attaches it to the fluid-filled pressure tubing.
- While the physician holds the catheter in place, activate the fast-flush release to flush blood from the catheter.

- After each fast-flush, observe the drip chamber to verify the correct continuous flush rate.
- Observe for a waveform on the bedside monitor.
- The physician may suture the catheter in place, or you may secure it with hypoallergenic tape.
- Cover the insertion site with a sterile dressing.
- With a radial or brachial site, immobilize the insertion site according to your facility's policy.
- With a femoral site, assess the need for immobilization of the lower extremity and maintain the patient on bed rest, with the head of the bed raised no more than 15 to 30 degrees, to prevent the catheter from kinking.
- Level the zeroing stopcock of the transducer with the phlebostatic axis, then zero the transducer system to atmospheric pressure.
- Activate monitor alarms, as appropriate.

OBTAINING BLOOD SAMPLE FROM AN OPEN SYSTEM
- Turn off or temporarily silence the monitor alarms, according to facility policy.
- Open a sterile 4″ × 4″ gauze pad.
- Remove the dead-end cap from the stopcock nearest the patient and place it on the gauze pad.
- Insert the syringe for the discard sample into the stopcock, turn off the stopcock to the flush solution, and withdraw 5 to 10 ml, according to facility policy.

⬥ **NURSING ALERT** Don't use the discarded sample for laboratory studies because it's diluted with flushing solution.

- If you feel resistance, reposition the affected extremity and check the insertion site for obvious problems and resume blood withdrawal.
- Turn the stopcock halfway back to the open position to close the system in all directions.
- Remove the discard syringe, and dispose of the blood in the syringe, observing universal precautions.
- Place the syringe for the laboratory sample in the stopcock, turn off the stopcock to the flush solution, and

slowly withdraw the required amount of blood.
- For each additional sample required, repeat this procedure.

⬥ **NURSING ALERT** Obtain blood for coagulation tests from the final syringe to prevent dilution from the flush device.

- After you've obtained the blood samples, turn off the stopcock to the syringe and remove it.
- Activate the fast-flush release to clear the tubing, turn off the stopcock to the patient, and repeat the fast flush to clear the stopcock port.
- Turn off the stopcock to the stopcock port, and replace the dead-end cap.
- Reactivate the monitor alarms.
- Attach the needleless device to the filled syringes, and transfer the blood samples to the appropriate specimen tubes.
- Label the tubes and send them to the laboratory.
- Check the monitor for return of the arterial waveform and pressure reading. (See *Understanding the arterial waveform.*)

OBTAINING BLOOD SAMPLE FROM A CLOSED SYSTEM
- Locate the closed-system reservoir and blood sampling site.
- Deactivate or temporarily silence monitor alarms, according to facility policy.
- Clean the sampling site with an alcohol pad.
- Holding the reservoir upright, grasp the flexures and slowly fill the reservoir with blood to be discarded over 3 to 5 seconds.
- If you feel resistance, reposition the affected extremity, and check the catheter site for obvious problems and resume blood withdrawal.
- Turn off the one-way valve to the reservoir by turning the handle perpendicular to the tubing.
- Using a syringe with attached cannula, insert the cannula into the sampling site, making sure the plunger is depressed to the bottom of the syringe barrel.
- Slowly fill the syringe, then grasp the cannula near the sampling site, and remove the syringe and cannula as one unit.
- Repeat the procedure, as needed.
- After filling the syringes, turn the one-way valve parallel to the tubing.

(continued)

UNDERSTANDING THE ARTERIAL WAVEFORM

Normal arterial blood pressure produces a characteristic waveform, representing ventricular systole and diastole. The waveform has five distinct components: the anacrotic limb, systolic peak, dicrotic limb, dicrotic notch, and end diastole.

The *anacrotic limb* marks the waveform's initial upstroke, which results as blood is rapidly ejected from the ventricle through the open aortic valve into the aorta. The rapid ejection causes a sharp rise in arterial pressure, which appears as the waveform's highest point. This is called the *systolic peak.*

As blood continues into the peripheral vessels, arterial pressure falls, and the waveform begins a downward trend. This part is called *the dicrotic limb.* Arterial pressure usually will continue to fall until pressure in the ventricle is less than pressure in the aortic root. When this occurs, the aortic valve closes. This event appears as a small notch (the *dicrotic notch*) on the waveform's downside.

When the aortic valve closes, diastole begins, progressing until the aortic root pressure gradually descends to its lowest point. On the waveform, this is known as *end diastole.*

Normal arterial waveform

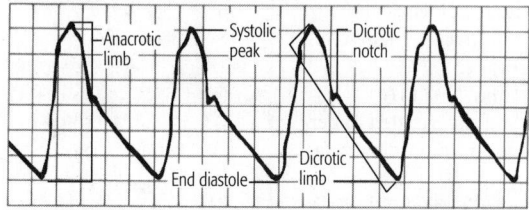

- Smoothly push down on the plunger until the flexures lock in place in the fully closed position and all fluid has been reinfused over a 3- to 5-second period.
- Activate the fast-flush release to clear blood from the tubing and reservoir.
- Clean the sampling site with an alcohol pad.
- Reactivate the monitor alarms.
- Using the blood transfer unit, transfer blood samples to the specimen tubes.
- Send all labeled samples to the laboratory.

CHANGING ARTERIAL LINE TUBING
- Determine how much tubing length to change, according to facility policy.
- Inflate the pressure bag to 300 mm Hg, check it for air leaks, and release the pressure.
- Prepare the I.V. flush solution, prime the pressure tubing and transducer system, and add medication and tubing labels.

◆ **NURSING ALERT** Priming tubing under pressure may cause microbubble formation.

- Apply 300 mm Hg of pressure to the system and hang the I.V. bag on a pole.
- Place the sheet protector under the affected extremity.
- Carefully remove the dressing from the catheter insertion site.
- Turn off or temporarily silence the monitor alarms, according to facility policy.
- Turn off the flow clamp of the tubing segment that you'll change.
- Carefully disconnect the tubing from the catheter hub.
- Immediately insert new tubing into the catheter hub, secure the tubing, and activate the fast-flush release to clear it.
- Reactivate the monitor alarms.
- Apply an appropriate dressing.
- Level the zeroing stopcock of the transducer with the phlebostatic axis, and zero the transducer system to atmospheric pressure.

REMOVING ARTERIAL CATHETER
- Determine if you're permitted to perform this procedure, according to facility policy.
- Record the patient's systolic, diastolic, and mean blood pressures.

- Obtain a manual blood pressure reading to establish a new baseline.
- Turn off the monitor alarms and turn off the flow clamp to the flush solution.
- Carefully remove the dressing over the insertion site.
- Remove any sutures, using the suture removal kit.
- Withdraw the catheter using a gentle, steady motion, keeping the catheter parallel to the artery during withdrawal.
- Immediately apply pressure to the site with a sterile 4″ × 4″ gauze pad for at least 10 minutes (longer if bleeding or oozing persists) until hemostasis is obtained.
- Apply additional pressure to a femoral site or if the patient has coagulopathy or is receiving anticoagulants.
- Cover the site with an appropriate dressing and secure the dressing with tape.
- According to facility policy, make a pressure dressing for a femoral site by folding in half four sterile 4″ × 4″ gauze pads, place the dressing over the femoral site, and cover it with a tight adhesive bandage; then cover the bandage with a sandbag.
- Maintain the patient on bed rest for 6 hours with the sandbag in place.
- Observe the site for bleeding.
- Assess the extremity distal to the site by evaluating color, pulses, and sensation every 15 minutes for the first 4 hours, every 30 minutes for the next 2 hours, then hourly for the next 6 hours.

OBTAINING A CATHETER-TIP CULTURE
- If infection is suspected, obtain a culture of the catheter by cutting the tip so it falls into the sterile container, label the specimen, and send it to the laboratory.

♦ **SPECIAL CONSIDERATIONS**

- Observe the pressure waveform on the monitor for abnormalities that may reflect arrhythmias (such as atrial fibrillation), aortic stenosis, aortic insufficiency, pulsus alternans, or pulsus paradoxus. (See *Recognizing abnormal waveforms.*)
- Change the pressure tubing every 2 to 3 days, according to facility policy.
- Change the catheter site dressing, according to facility policy.
- Regularly assess the site for signs of infection, such as redness and swelling.

◆ **NURSING ALERT** Be aware that erroneous pressure readings may result from a catheter that's clotted or positional, loose connections, addition of extra stopcocks or extension tubing, inadvertent entry of air into the system, or improper calibration, leveling, or zeroing of the monitoring system.

◆ **NURSING ALERT** A disparity of 5 to 20 mm Hg between direct and indirect arterial pressure measurements is a generally accepted range.

- If the catheter lumen clots, check the flush system for proper pressure.
- Regularly assess the amount of flush solution in the I.V. bag, and maintain 300 mm Hg pressure in the pressure bag.

Complications
- Nerve compression and injury, especially with axillary arteries
- Hemorrhage
- Infection
- Aneurysm
- Embolism
- Arterial spasm
- Necrosis of overlying skin
- Thrombosis
- Vasovagal reactions
- Hematoma
- Arteriovenous fistula
- Pseudoaneurysm

▶ PATIENT TEACHING

Be sure to cover:
- why the procedure is performed
- how the arterial catheter is inserted
- keeping the affected limb still
- anticipated duration of catheter placement
- discomfort at the insertion site
- monitoring and care performed while the arterial catheter is in place
- when to notify the nurse, such as for bleeding.

◆ DOCUMENTATION

- Date and time of system setup, tubing or flush change, dressing change, and site care
- Systolic, diastolic, and mean pressure
- Neurovascular status of extremity distal to the site
- Amount of flush solution infused
- Patient position when blood pressure reading is obtained
- Appearance of the waveform
- Comparison with auscultated blood pressure
- Appearance of the insertion site, noting evidence of bleeding or infection
- Patient teaching

Selected references

Bourgoin, A., et al. "Increasing Mean Arterial Pressure in Patients with Septic Shock: Effects on Oxygen Variables and Renal Function," *Critical Care Medicine* 33(4):780-86, April 2005.

Eggen, M.A., and Brock-Utne, J.G. "Arthritis Increase in Arterial Pressure Waveform: Remember the Stopcock," *Anesthesia & Analgesia* 101(1):298-99, July 1005.

Garretson, S. "Haemodynamic Monitoring Arterial Catheters," *Nursing Standard* 19(31):55-64, April 2005.

Michard, F. "Changes in Arterial Pressure during Mechanical Ventilation," *Anesthesiology* 103(2):419-28, August 2005.

Mukkamala, R., et al. "Continuous Cardiac Output Monitoring by Peripheral Blood Pressure Waveform Analysis," *IEEE Transactions on Bio-Medical Engineering*, 53(3):459-67, March 2006.

Rose, J.C., et al. "Continuous Monitoring of the Microcirculation in Neurocritical Care: An Update on Brain Tissue Oxygenation," *Current Opinions in Critical Care* 12(2):97-102, April 2006.

RECOGNIZING ABNORMAL WAVEFORMS

Understanding a normal arterial waveform is relatively straightforward. But an abnormal waveform is more difficult to decipher. Abnormal patterns and markings, however, may provide important diagnostic clues to the patient's cardiovascular status, or they may simply signal trouble in the monitor. Use this table to help you recognize and resolve waveform abnormalities.

Abnormality	Possible causes	Nursing interventions
ALTERNATING HIGH AND LOW WAVES IN A REGULAR PATTERN 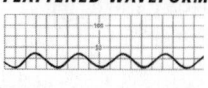	• Ventricular bigeminy	• Check the patient's electrocardiogram to confirm ventricular bigeminy. The tracing should reflect premature ventricular contractions every second beat.
FLATTENED WAVEFORM 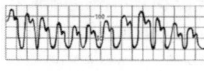	• Overdamped waveform or hypotensive patient	• Check the patient's blood pressure with a sphygmomanometer. If you obtain a reading, suspect overdamping. Correct the problem by trying to aspirate the arterial line. If you succeed, flush the line. If the reading is very low or absent, suspect hypotension.
SLIGHTLY ROUNDED WAVEFORM WITH CONSISTENT VARIATIONS IN SYSTOLIC HEIGHT 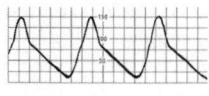	• Patient on ventilator with positive end-expiratory pressure	• Check the patient's systolic blood pressure regularly. The difference between the highest and lowest systolic pressure reading should be less than 10 mm Hg. If the difference exceeds that amount, suspect pulsus paradoxus, possibly from cardiac tamponade.
SLOW UPSTROKE 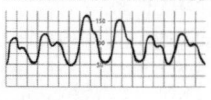	• Aortic stenosis	• Check the patient's heart sounds for signs of aortic stenosis. Also, notify the physician, who will document suspected aortic stenosis in his notes.
DIMINISHED AMPLITUDE ON INSPIRATION	• Pulsus paradoxus, possibly from cardiac tamponade, constrictive pericarditis, or lung disease	• Note systolic pressure during inspiration and expiration. If inspiratory pressure is at least 10 mm Hg less than expiratory pressure, call the physician. • If you're also monitoring pulmonary artery pressure, observe for a diastolic plateau. This occurs when the mean central venous pressure (right atrial pressure), mean pulmonary artery pressure, and mean pulmonary artery wedge pressure are within 5 mm Hg of one another.

Bedside blood glucose and hemoglobin testing

● OVERVIEW

- For monitoring at bedside; also convenient for patient's home use
- Provides fast and accurate results, allowing immediate intervention
- Performed to detect hyperglycemia, such as from diabetes mellitus or use of steroid drugs; or hypoglycemia, such as from overly rapid glucose use, which may occur with strenuous exercise or infection
- Also performed to detect low hemoglobin values—such as from anemia, recent hemorrhage, or fluid retention—causing hemodilution; or elevated hemoglobin values, such as from hemoconcentration from polycythemia or dehydration

Contraindications
- None known

❖ EQUIPMENT

Lancet • microcuvette • photometer • gloves • alcohol pads • gauze pads

Equipment preparation
- Wash your hands thoroughly.
- Take the equipment to the patient's bedside.
- Before using a microcuvette, note its expiration date.
- Plug the AC adapter into the photometer power inlet. Then plug the other end of the adapter into the wall outlet.
- Turn on the photometer.
- If the photometer hasn't been used recently, insert the control cuvette to make sure the photometer is working properly.

▌▍▋ ESSENTIAL STEPS

- Confirm the patient's identity using two patient identifiers according to facility policy.
- Explain the procedure to the patient.
- Put on clean gloves.
- Select an appropriate puncture site, such as the fingertip or earlobe of an adult.

◈ **NURSING ALERT** In an adult, avoid using the second finger as a puncture site because it's usually the most sensitive; the thumb, which may have thickened skin or calluses; and a ring-bearing finger because blood must circulate freely.

✸ **AGE-RELATED CONCERN** In an infant, use the heel or great toe as a puncture site for this procedure.

- Keep the patient's finger straight and ask him to relax it.
- To promote blood flow to the sampling point, hold the finger between the thumb and index finger of your nondominant hand.
- Gently rock the patient's finger as you move your fingers from the top knuckle to the fingertip.
- Use an alcohol pad to clean the puncture site, wiping in a circular motion from the center of the site outward.
- Dry the site thoroughly with a gauze pad.
- Pierce the skin quickly and sharply with the lancet and apply the microcuvette, which automatically draws a precise amount of blood (approximately 5 µl).
- Place the microcuvette into the photometer.
- Watch for results to appear on the photometer screen within 40 seconds to 4 minutes. (See *How to use a bedside blood glucose and hemoglobin monitor.*)
- Place a gauze pad over the puncture site until the bleeding stops.
- Dispose of the lancet and microcuvette according to your facility's policy.
- Remove your gloves and wash your hands.
- Notify the physician if the test result is outside the expected parameters.

NURSING ALERT When using glucose levels to monitor drug or diet therapy in a patient with diabetes mellitus, results may require immediate action.

✦ SPECIAL CONSIDERATIONS

- A microcuvette can be stored for up to 2 years; however, after the microcuvette vial is opened, the shelf life is 90 days.
- Before taking a blood sample, operate the photometer with the control cuvette to check for proper function.
- Avoid using a cold, cyanotic, or swollen area as the puncture site to ensure an adequate blood sample.

Complications
- Pain
- Bleeding

▶ PATIENT TEACHING

Be sure to cover:
- purpose of the test and how it will be performed
- that a pinprick sensation may be felt in the finger during blood sampling
- that the finger must be held still during the procedure
- test result and its implications for further treatment.

●◇ DOCUMENTATION

- Date and time of the test
- Values obtained from the photometer
- Any interventions performed
- Name of the physician and time notified of abnormal results as well as any orders given
- Patient teaching and patient's response to the procedure

Selected references

"Be Aware of False Glucose Results with Point-of-Care Testing," *ISMP Medication Safety Alert,* 10(18). Institute for Safe Medication Practices, 2005.

Blake, D.R., and Nathan, D.M. "Point-of-Care Testing for Diabetes," *Critical Care Nursing Quarterly* 27(2):150-61, April-June 2004.

Hudson, K. "Tech Update: Get Bedside Results with Point-of-Care Testing," *Nursing Management* 36(1):45-46, January 2005.

Rodis, J.L., and Thomas, R.A. "Stepwise Approach to Developing Point-of-Care Testing Services in the Community/Ambulatory Pharmacy Setting," *Journal of the American Pharmacists Association* 46(5):594-604, 2006.

HOW TO USE A BEDSIDE BLOOD GLUCOSE AND HEMOGLOBIN MONITOR

Monitoring blood glucose and hemoglobin levels at the patient's bedside is a straightforward procedure. A photometer, such as the HemoCue analyzer featured here, relies on capillary action to draw blood into a disposable microcuvette.

HemoCue gives accurate results without having to pipette, dispense, or mix blood and reagents to obtain readings. This method of obtaining blood minimizes a health care worker's exposure to the patient's blood and decreases the risk of cross-contamination. It also eliminates the risk of leakage, broken tubes, and splattered blood.

A plastic, disposable microcuvette functions as a combination pipette, test tube, and measuring vessel. It contains a reagent that produces a precise chemical reaction as soon as it contacts blood. The photometer is powered by a battery or an AC adapter. One model is calibrated at the factory and seldom needs to be recalibrated, returning to zero between tests. Use the cuvette included with each system to test photometer function.

Follow the three steps depicted here when using the HemoCue system.

After you pierce the skin, the microcuvette draws blood automatically.	Next, place the microcuvette into the photometer.	The photometer screen displays the blood glucose or hemoglobin levels.

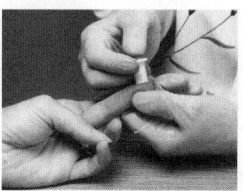 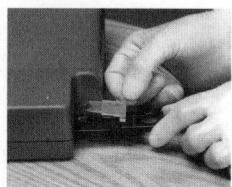 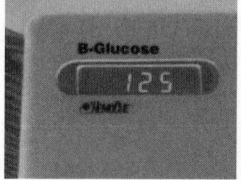

Bladder and bowel retraining

- Indicated for loss or impairment of urinary or anal sphincter control; age- or disease-related changes in genitourinary (GU) or GI system function or, less commonly, in other body systems, such as the musculoskeletal and nervous systems; and fecal stasis and impaction
- May be needed to treat such elimination problems as bladder and fecal incontinence (especially in elderly patients), which can have serious psychosocial effects and threaten a patient's ability to live independently

Contraindications
- None known

Readily accessible toilet or commode • intake and output record or retraining schedule • personal hygiene supplies (soap, water, washcloth, towel)

Equipment preparation
- Wash hands thoroughly.
- Ensure clear pathway to toilet or commode.

- Explain the treatment and preparation to the patient and his family.

BLADDER RETRAINING
- Make sure that the patient maintains adequate daily fluid intake.
- Frequently assess the patient's mental and functional status.
- Encourage or assist the patient to void every 2 hours (or more frequently to maintain dryness between voidings).
- Respond to patient calls promptly, and help him get to the bathroom as quickly as possible.
- Implement an exercise program for strengthening pelvic floor muscles such as Kegel exercises.
- Suggest biofeedback to reinforce pelvic muscle contraction, as needed.
- When the patient can stay dry for 2 hours, increase the time between voidings by 30 minutes each day until a 3- to 4-hour voiding schedule is achieved.
- Have the patient empty his bladder completely before bedtime.

BOWEL RETRAINING
- Remind or help the patient to get to the toilet or commode 15 to 20 minutes before his usual bowel movement time.
- Ask the patient if the bowel movement felt complete, allowing more time if needed and tolerated.
- Encourage the patient to alternately contract and release his abdominal muscles, sway back and forth on the toilet, or take a large breath, hold briefly while bearing down, and then release it to stimulate peristalsis .

⚙ **AGE-RELATED CONCERN** Stay with a patient who has dementia, and reinforce the need to remain on the toilet.
- Encourage a fiber-rich diet that includes raw, leafy vegetables, unpeeled fruits, and whole grains, such as bran cereals.
- Encourage adequate daily fluid intake.
- Promote regular exercise.

- Perform a careful assessment of diet, fluid status, dentition and swallowing, usual bowel and bladder patterns in the past, laxative use and ability to comprehend and follow instructions.
- Regularly reassess food and fluid intake, character and patterns of voiding, and mental capacity to respond to the treatment program.
- Monitor the patient's vital signs, fluid intake and output, and diet patterns to determine baseline values.
- Assess the patient for signs and symptoms of urinary tract infection (UTI) or incomplete elimination.
- Provide support and help the patient deal with feelings of shame, embarrassment, or powerlessness caused by loss of control.
- Praise the patient's successful efforts. Encourage persistence, tolerance, and a positive attitude.
- Maximize the patient's independence while minimizing risks to his self-esteem.
- Refer the patient for dental, GU, physical, and speech therapy (for swallowing), as needed, to improve contributing factors and proper intake before initiating an individualized therapy program.

Complications
- Skin breakdown
- Infection

Be sure to cover:
- how to manage the steps of retraining
- need for gradual elimination of laxative use, if necessary, and how to transition to the use of natural laxatives, such as prunes or prune juice
- possible episodes of periodic incontinence, with emphasis that occurrence doesn't mean program failure
- signs and symptoms of infection and when to notify the physician.

- Document the bowel or bladder training steps provided to the patient and his understanding of this information.
- Document the patient's progress.
- Document any medications, including laxatives, and the patient's response to them.

Selected references
Bharucha, A.E. "Update of Tests of Colon and Rectal Structure and Function," *Journal of Clinical Gastroenterology* 40(2):96-103, February 2006.

Jumadilova, Z., et al. "Urinary Incontinence in the Nursing Home: Resident Characteristics and Prevalence of Drug Treatment," *American Journal of Managed Care* 11(Suppl 4):S112-120, July 2005.

Karon, S. "A Team Approach to Bladder Retraining: A Pilot Study," *Urological Nursing* 25(4):269-76, August 2005.

Bladder irrigation, continuous

● OVERVIEW

- Helps prevent urinary tract obstruction by flushing out small blood clots that form after prostate or bladder surgery; may also be used for a nonsurgical patient
- Used to treat an irritated, inflamed, or infected bladder lining
- Creates a mild tamponade with continuous flow of irrigating solution through the bladder that may help prevent venous hemorrhage

Contraindications
- None known

❖ EQUIPMENT

One 4,000-ml container or two 2,000-ml containers of solution (usually normal saline solution) or prescribed amount of medicated solution • Y-type tubing made specifically for bladder irrigation • alcohol or chlorhexidine pad

Equipment preparation
- Use Y-type tubing to allow immediate irrigation with reserve solution.
- Large volumes of irrigating solution are usually required during the first 24 to 48 hours after surgery.
- Before starting, double-check the irrigating solution against the practitioner's order.
- If the solution contains an antibiotic, check the patient's chart to make sure that he isn't allergic to the drug.
- Make sure that the patient remains on bed rest throughout continuous bladder irrigation, unless specified otherwise.
- Assemble all equipment at the patient's bedside (see *Setup for continuous bladder irrigation*).

▌▌▌ ESSENTIAL STEPS

- Confirm the patient's identity using two patient identifiers according to facility policy.
- Wash your hands and put on gloves.
- Explain the procedure and provide privacy.
- Insert the spike of the Y-type tubing into the container of irrigating solution.
- If you have a two-container system, insert one spike into each container.
- Squeeze the drip chamber on the spike of the tubing.
- Open the flow clamp and flush the tubing to remove air that could cause bladder distention.
- Close the clamp.
- Hang the bag of irrigating solution on the I.V. pole.
- Clean the opening to the inflow lumen of the catheter with the alcohol or chlorhexidine pad.

- Insert the distal end of the Y-type tubing securely into the inflow lumen (third port) of the catheter using sterile technique.
- Make sure that the catheter's outflow lumen is securely attached to the drainage bag tubing.
- Open the flow clamp under the container of the irrigating solution and set the drip rate, as ordered.
- To prevent air from entering the system, don't allow the primary container to empty completely before replacing it.
- If you have a two-container system, simultaneously close the flow clamp under the nearly empty container and open the flow clamp under the reserve container. This prevents reflux of irrigating solution from the reserve container into the nearly empty one.
- Hang a new reserve container on the I.V. pole and insert the tubing, maintaining asepsis.
- Empty the drainage bag about every 4 hours, or as needed.

SETUP FOR CONTINUOUS BLADDER IRRIGATION

In continuous bladder irrigation, a triple-lumen catheter allows irrigating solution to flow into the bladder through one lumen and flow out through another, as shown in the inset. The third lumen is used to inflate the balloon that holds the catheter in place.

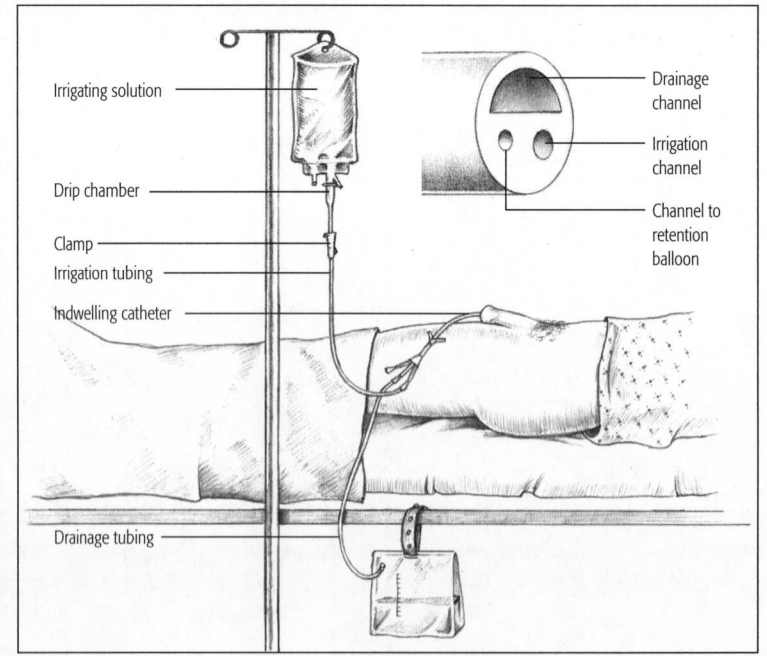

- Use sterile technique to avoid the risk of contamination.
- Monitor the patient's vital signs at least every 4 hours during irrigation, increasing the frequency if the patient becomes unstable.

◆ SPECIAL CONSIDERATIONS

- Check inflow and outflow lines periodically for kinks to make sure that the solution is running freely.
- If the solution flows rapidly, check the lines frequently.
- Measure the outflow volume accurately. The outflow should be the same or slightly more than the inflow volume, allowing for urine production.

NURSING ALERT Postoperative inflow volume exceeding outflow volume may indicate bladder rupture at the suture lines or renal damage; notify the practitioner immediately.

- Assess outflow for changes in appearance and for blood clots, especially if irrigation is being done postoperatively to control bleeding.

NURSING ALERT If drainage is bright red, irrigating solution should be infused rapidly with the clamp wide open until drainage clears. Notify the practitioner immediately if you suspect hemorrhage.

- If the drainage is clear, the solution is usually given at a rate of 40 to 60 drops/minute. The practitioner usually specifies the rate for antibiotics.
- Encourage oral fluid intake of 2 to 3 qt (2 to 3 L)/day, unless contraindicated.

Complications
- Infection that's caused by interruptions in a continuous irrigation system
- Bladder distention that's caused by obstruction in the catheter's outflow lumen

▶ PATIENT TEACHING

Be sure to cover:
- notifying the nurse if the patient experiences abdominal discomfort
- remaining on bed rest (unless otherwise specified).

●◆ DOCUMENTATION

- Completion of each container of solution, including date, time, and amount of fluids on the intake and output record
- Time and amount of fluid each time you empty the drainage bag
- Type of solution infused
- Appearance of the drainage and patient complaints
- Date, time, and name of physician notified of abnormal findings and orders given
- Patient tolerance of procedure

Selected references
Braasch, M., et al. "Irrigation and Drainage Properties of Three-way Urethral Catheters," *Urology* 67(1):40-44, January 2006.

Chan, P.T., et al. "A Modified Bladder Irrigation System after Transurethral Resection of Prostate," *International Journal of Urology* 11(Suppl 11):A72, October 2004.

Cutts, B. "Developing and Implementing a New Bladder Irrigation Chart," *Nursing Standard* 20(8):48-52, November 2005.

Burn wound care

● OVERVIEW

- Aims to maintain the patient's physiologic stability, repair skin integrity, prevent infection, and maximize functionality and psychosocial health
- Dramatic improvement in success of overall treatment with competent care immediately after a burn
- Burn severity determined by the depth and extent of the burn and the presence of other factors, such as age, complications, and coexisting illnesses; with burns involving more than 20% of total body surface, fluid resuscitation to support body's compensatory mechanisms without overwhelming them
- Requires careful positioning and regular exercise for burned extremities to help maintain joint function, prevent contractures, and minimize deformity

Contraindications
None known

❖ EQUIPMENT

Normal saline solution • sterile bowl • scissors • tissue forceps • ordered topical medication • burn gauze • roller gauze • elastic netting or tape • fine mesh gauze • elastic gauze • cotton-tipped applicators or sterile tongue depressor • ordered pain medication • three pairs of sterile gloves • sterile gown, mask, surgical cap • heat lamps • impervious plastic trash bag • cotton bath blanket • 4″ × 4″ gauze pad

Equipment preparation
- A sterile field is required and all equipment and supplies used in the dressing should be sterile.
- Open equipment packages using aseptic technique.
- Arrange supplies on a sterile field in the order of their use.

  ◆ **NURSING ALERT** Dress the cleanest areas first and the most contaminated areas last to prevent cross-contamination. Be aware that you may need to dress in stages to avoid exposing all wounds at the same time to help prevent excessive pain or cross-contamination.

▮▮ ESSENTIAL STEPS

- Give the ordered analgesic about 20 minutes before beginning wound care to maximize patient comfort and cooperation.
- Explain the procedure and provide privacy.
- Turn on overhead heat lamps to keep the patient warm. Make sure that they don't overheat him.
- Pour warmed normal saline solution into the sterile bowl in the sterile field.
- Wash your hands.

REMOVING A DRESSING WITHOUT HYDROTHERAPY
- Put on a gown, a mask, and sterile gloves.
- Remove dressing layers down to the innermost layer by cutting the outer dressings with sterile blunt scissors.
- Lay open these dressings.
- If the inner layer appears dry, soak it with warm normal saline solution to ease removal.
- Remove the inner dressing with sterile tissue forceps or your gloved hand.
- Dispose of soiled dressings carefully in an impervious plastic trash bag according to facility policy.
- Dispose of your gloves and wash your hands.
- Put on a new pair of sterile gloves.
- Using gauze pads moistened with normal saline solution, gently remove exudate and old topical drug.
- Carefully remove all loose eschar with sterile forceps and scissors, if ordered.
- Assess the wound's condition. It should appear clean, with no debris, loose tissue, purulence, inflammation, or darkened margins.
- Before applying a new dressing, remove your gown, gloves, and mask.
- Discard them properly; put on a clean mask, surgical cap, gown, and sterile gloves.

APPLYING A WET DRESSING

- Soak fine-mesh gauze and the elastic gauze dressing in a large sterile basin containing the ordered solution.
- Wring out the fine-mesh gauze until it's moist but not dripping, and apply it to the wound.
- Warn the patient that he may feel transient pain when you apply the dressing.
- Wring out the elastic gauze dressing and position it to hold the fine-mesh gauze in place.
- Roll elastic gauze dressing over the fine-mesh dressing to keep it intact.
- Cover the patient with a cotton bath blanket to prevent chills.
- Change the blanket if it becomes damp and use an overhead heat lamp, if necessary.
- Change the dressings frequently, as ordered, to keep the wound moist, especially if you're using silver nitrate. If the dressings become dry, silver nitrate becomes ineffective and the silver ions may damage tissue.
- To maintain moist dressings, some protocols call for irrigating the dressing with solution at least every 4 hours through small slits cut into the outer dressing.

APPLYING A DRY DRESSING WITH A TOPICAL DRUG

- Remove old dressings and clean the wound (as described previously).
- Apply the drug to the wound in a thin layer—about 2 to 4 mm thick—with your sterile gloved hand or a sterile tongue blade.
- Apply several layers of burn gauze over the wound to contain the drug but allow exudate to escape.
- Cut the dressing to fit only the wound areas.
- Don't cover unburned areas.
- Cover the entire dressing with roller gauze and secure it with elastic netting or tape.

PROVIDING ARM AND LEG CARE

- Apply the dressings from the distal to the proximal area to stimulate circulation and prevent constriction.
- Wrap the burn gauze once around the arm or leg so the edges overlap slightly.
- Continue wrapping until the gauze covers the wound.
- Apply a dry roller gauze dressing to hold bottom layers in place.
- Secure with elastic netting or tape.

PROVIDING HAND AND FOOT CARE

- Wrap each finger separately with a single $4'' \times 4''$ gauze pad to allow the patient to use his hands and to prevent webbing contractures.
- Place the hand in a functional position and secure using a dressing.
- Apply splints, if ordered.
- Put gauze between each toe, as appropriate, to prevent webbing contractures.

PROVIDING CHEST, ABDOMEN, AND BACK CARE

- Apply the ordered drug to the wound in a thin layer.
- Cover the entire burned area with sheets of burn gauze.
- Wrap with roller gauze or apply a specialty vest dressing to hold the burn gauze in place.
- Secure the dressing with elastic netting or tape.
- Make sure that the dressing doesn't restrict respiratory motion, especially in very young or elderly patients, or in those with circumferential injuries.

PROVIDING SCALP AND FACIAL CARE

- If the patient has scalp burns, clip or shave the hair around the burn, as ordered.
- Clip other hair until it's about 2″ (5 cm) long to prevent contamination of burned scalp areas.
- Shave facial hair if it comes in contact with burned areas. Typically, facial burns are managed with milder topical agents (such as triple antibiotic ointment) and are left open to air.
- If dressings are required, make sure that they don't cover the eyes, nostrils, or mouth.

PROVIDING EAR CARE

- Clip hair around the affected ear.
- Remove exudate and crusts with cotton-tipped applicators dipped in normal saline solution.
- Place a layer of $4'' \times 4''$ gauze behind the auricle to prevent webbing.
- Apply the ordered topical drug to $4'' \times 4''$ gauze pads and place them over the burned area.
- Before securing the dressing with a roller bandage, position the patient's ears normally to avoid damaging the auricular cartilage.
- Assess the patient's hearing ability.

PROVIDING EYE CARE

- Clean the area around his eyes and eyelids with a cotton-tipped applicator and normal saline solution every 4 to 6 hours, or as needed, to remove crust and drainage.
- Give ordered eye ointments or drops.
- If his eyes can't be closed, apply lubricating ointments or drops, as ordered.
- Be sure to close his eyes before applying eye pads to prevent corneal abrasion.
- Don't apply topical ointments near his eyes without a practitioner's order.

(continued)

PROVIDING NASAL CARE

- Check the patient's nostrils for inhalation injury, such as the presence of inflamed mucosa, singed vibrissae, and soot.
- Clean his nostrils with cotton-tipped applicators dipped in normal saline solution.
- Remove crust.
- Apply the ordered ointments.
- If he has a nasogastric tube, use tracheostomy ties to secure the tube.
- Be sure to check tracheostomy ties frequently for tightness caused by swelling facial tissue.
- Clean the area around the tube every 4 to 6 hours.

◆ SPECIAL CONSIDERATIONS

- Thorough assessment and documentation of the wound's appearance are essential to detect infection and other complications.

  NURSING ALERT Healthy granulation tissue appears clean, pinkish, faintly shiny, and free from exudate. A purulent wound or green-gray exudate indicates infection, an overly dry wound suggests dehydration, and a wound with a swollen, red edge suggests cellulitis. Suspect a fungal infection if the wound is white and powdery.

- Blisters protect underlying tissue; leave them intact unless they impede joint motion, become infected, or cause discomfort.
- Be sure to meet the increased nutritional needs of the patient with healing burns; extra protein and carbohydrates are required to accommodate an almost doubled basal metabolism.
- If you must manage a burn with topical drugs, exposure to air, and no dressing, watch for such problems as wound adherence to bed linens, poor drainage control, and partial loss of topical drugs.
- Skin integrity is repaired through aggressive wound debridement, followed by maintenance of a clean wound bed until the wound heals or is covered with a skin graft.
- Full-thickness burns and some deep partial-thickness burns must be debrided and grafted in the operating room, taking place as soon as possible after fluid resuscitation.
- Most wounds are managed with twice-daily dressing changes using topical antibiotics.
- Burn dressings encourage healing by barring germ entry and removing exudate, eschar, and other debris that host infection.

- After thorough wound cleaning, topical antibacterial agents are applied, and the wound is covered with absorptive, coarse mesh gauze.
- Roller gauze typically tops the dressing and is secured with elastic netting or tape.

Complications

- Infection (most common)
- Sepsis
- Allergic reaction to ointments or dressings
- Renal failure
- Multisystem organ dysfunction
- Hypothermia
- Hypovolemia

PATIENT TEACHING

Be sure to cover:
- what to expect, including preparing the patient for scarring, but advising him that proper therapy can minimize scarring
- wound management and pain control
- prescribed exercises and activity
- encouragement and emotional support, including referrals to burn survivor support groups
- home-care follow-up including discharge planning.

DOCUMENTATION

- Dates and times for all care provided
- Wound's appearance and condition
- Special dressing-change techniques
- Topical drugs given
- Positioning of the burned area
- Patient's tolerance of the procedure

Selected references

Gilbride, J. "Not Just Skin Deep: A History of Pediatric Burn Trauma," *Pediatric Nursing* 31(5):412-13, September-October 2005.

Hall, B. "Wound Care for Burn Patients in Acute Rehabilitation Settings," *Rehabilitation Nursing* 30(3):114-19, May-June 2005.

Kavanagh, S., et al. "Care of Burn Patients in the Hospital," *Burns* 30(8):A2-6, December 2004.

Laskowski-Jones, L. "First Aid for Burns," *Nursing* 36(1):41-43, January 2006.

Mendez-Eastman, S. "Burn Injuries," *Plastic Surgical Nursing* 25(3):133-39, July-September 2005.

Nowlin, A. "The Delicate Business of Burn Care," *RN* 69(l):52, 56-57, January 2006.

Supple, K.G. "Handle with Care. An Overview of Burn Injury," *Advance for Nurse Practitioners* 13(7):24-29, July 2005.

Cardiac monitoring

- Allows continuous observation of heart's electrical activity
- Uses electrodes placed on the patient's chest to transmit electrical signals that are converted into a tracing of cardiac rhythm on an oscilloscope
- Displays heart rate and rhythm, which may be printed out; sounds alarm if heart rate rises above or falls below specified limits; and recognizes and counts abnormal heartbeats and changes.
- May use hardwire monitoring in which a patient is connected to a monitor at his bedside or the rhythm is transmitted to a remote location
- May use telemetry in which a small, battery-powered, portable transmitter connected to ambulatory patients sends electrical signals to another location, where they're displayed on a monitor screen, allowing patients to be mobile and safely isolated from electrical hazards; especially useful for monitoring arrhythmias during sleep, rest, exercise, or stressful situations

Contraindications
- None known

EQUIPMENT

Cardiac monitor • patient cable with leadwires • disposable pregelled electrodes (number of electrodes varies from three to five, depending on patient's needs) • alcohol pads • 4″ × 4″ gauze pads • optional: clippers, washcloth

TELEMETRY MONITORING
Transmitter • transmitter pouch • telemetry battery pack, leads, electrodes

Equipment preparation
- Wash your hands thoroughly.
- Turn the cardiac monitor on to warm up the unit while you prepare other equipment and the patient.
- Insert the cable into the appropriate socket in the monitor.
- Check each leadwire for the location of attachment to the patient: right

arm (RA), left arm (LA), right leg (RL), left leg (LL), and chest (C).
- Connect an electrode to each of the leadwires.
- For telemetry monitoring, insert a new battery into the transmitter.
- Test the battery's charge by pressing the button at the top of the telemetry unit and test the unit to make sure that the battery is operational.
- If the leadwires aren't permanently affixed to the telemetry unit, attach them securely to the correct outlet.

ESSENTIAL STEPS

- Confirm the patient's identity using two patient identifiers according to facility policy.
- Explain the procedure to the patient.
- Provide for patient privacy.

HARDWIRE MONITORING
- Determine electrode positions on the patient's chest, based on the system and lead you're using. (See *Positioning monitoring leads.*)
- If the leadwires and patient cable aren't permanently attached, verify that the electrode placement corresponds to the label on the patient cable.
- If necessary, clip the hair from an area about 4″ (10 cm) in diameter around each electrode site and clean the area with soap and water and dry completely to remove skin secretions that might interfere with electrode function; use an alcohol pad to clean area if skin is diaphoretic or oily.
- Gently abrade the dried area by rubbing it briskly until it reddens to remove dead skin cells and to promote better electrical contact with living cells.
- Remove the backing from the pregelled electrode.
- Apply the electrode to the site and press firmly to ensure a tight seal.
- Repeat the above procedure with the remaining electrodes.
- When all the electrodes are in place, check for a tracing on the cardiac monitor and assess the quality of the electrocardiogram (ECG).

NURSING ALERT To avoid electric shock, make sure all electrical equipment is grounded.

- To verify that the monitor detects each beat, compare the digital heart rate display with your count of the patient's pulse.
- If necessary, use the gain control to adjust the size of the rhythm tracing and the position control to adjust the waveform position on the recording paper.
- Set the upper and lower limits of the heart rate alarm, based on unit policy, and turn on the alarm.

TELEMETRY MONITORING
- Expose the patient's chest, and select the lead arrangement.
- Remove the backing from one of the gelled electrodes.
- Apply the electrode to the appropriate site by pressing one side of the electrode against the patient's skin, pulling the skin taut, and then pressing the remainder of the electrode against the taut skin.
- Press your fingers in a circular motion around the electrode to fix the gel and stabilize the electrode.
- Repeat the above procedure for each electrode.
- Attach an electrode to the end of each leadwire.
- Place the transmitter in the pouch and tie the pouch strings around the patient's neck and waist, making sure that the pouch fits snugly without causing discomfort.
- If a pouch isn't available, place the transmitter in the patient's pocket.
- Check the patient's waveform for clarity, position, and size, adjusting the gain and baseline, as needed.

SPECIAL CONSIDERATIONS

- Make sure all electrical equipment and outlets are grounded, and keep the patient clean and dry to avoid electric shock and interference.
- Open the electrode packages before use to prevent the gel from drying.
- Avoid placing the electrodes on bony prominences, hairy areas, areas where defibrillator pads will be placed, or areas for chest compression.
- If the patient's skin is exceptionally oily, scaly, or diaphoretic, rub the electrode site with a dry 4″ × 4″ gauze

pad before applying the electrode to help reduce interference in the tracing.

- If the patient's respirations distort the recording, ask him to hold his breath briefly to reduce baseline wander in the tracing.
- Assess skin integrity, and reposition the electrodes every 24 hours or as necessary.

Complications

- Skin excoriation or breakdown
- Allergic reaction
- Electric shock

▶ PATIENT TEACHING

Be sure to cover:
- purpose of the procedure
- how the telemetry monitor works
- importance of pressing a button when symptoms occur (to produce an ECG recording at the central station)
- removal of the transmitter before taking a shower or bath.

✦ DOCUMENTATION

- Date and time monitoring began
- Monitoring lead used
- Rhythm strip at least every 8 hours with changes in patient's condition, labeling rhythm strip with patient's name, room number, medical record number, date, and time
- Patient teaching; patient's understanding of the procedure

Selected references

Lapensky, J. "Integrated Technologies Transform Telemetry," *Nursing Management* 36(12):23-26, December 2005.

Schneck, M.J., et al. "Utility of Routine Telemetry in Patients with Acute Stroke or Transient Ischemic Attacks," *Stroke* 37(2):702, February 2006.

Singer, A.J., et al. "Telemetry Monitoring During Transport of Low-Risk Chest Pain Patients From The Emergency Department: Is It Necessary?" *Academic Emergency Medicine* 12(10):965-69, October 2005.

POSITIONING MONITORING LEADS

This chart shows the correct electrode positions for some of the monitoring leads you'll use most often. For each lead, you'll see electrode placement for a five-leadwire system, a three-leadwire system, and a telemetry system.

In the two-hardwire systems, the electrode positions for one lead may be identical to the electrode positions for another lead. In this case, you simply change the lead selector switch to the setting that corresponds to the lead you want. In some cases, you'll need to reposition the electrodes.

In the telemetry system, you can create the same lead with two electrodes that you do with three, simply by eliminating the ground electrode.

The illustrations below use these abbreviations: RA, right arm; LA, left arm; RL, right leg; LL, left leg; C, chest; and G, ground.

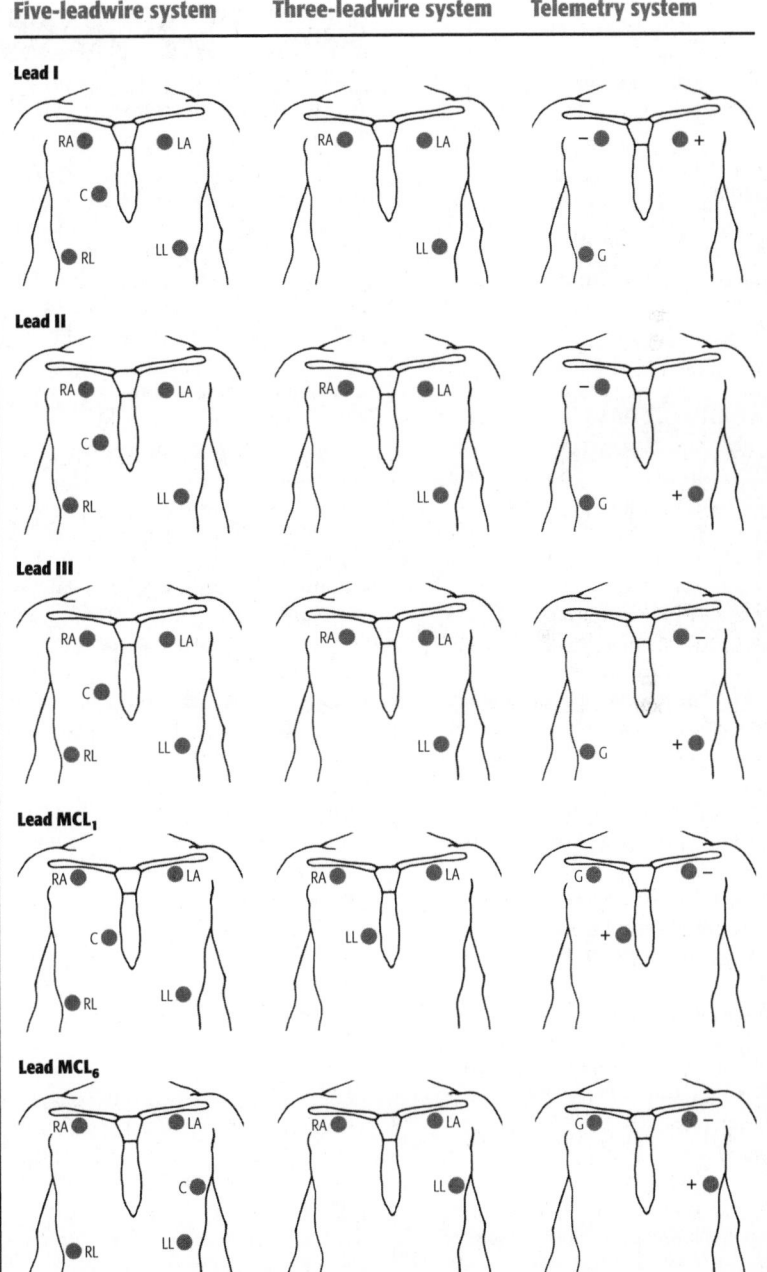

Five-leadwire system   **Three-leadwire system**   **Telemetry system**

Lead I

Lead II

Lead III

Lead MCL₁

Lead MCL₆

Cardiac output measurement

● OVERVIEW

- Used for evaluating cardiac function by showing amount of blood ejected by the heart
- Has a normal range of 4 to 8 L/ minute
- May be determined by bolus thermodilution technique (most common method) done at bedside (see *Understanding the thermodilution method*)
- May also be determined using Fick method and dye dilution test (see *Other methods for measuring cardiac output*)

Contraindications

ABSOLUTE

- Trauma at the access site or to adjacent structures
- Full-thickness burn, infection, or cellulitis over the insertion site
- Uncooperative or agitated patient
- Distorted local anatomy or landmarks at insertion site (as a result of surgery, irradiation, trauma, or congenital malformations)
- Previous use of the vessel for a sclerosing agent (such as from chemotherapeutic agents)
- Suspected or actual injury to the superior vena cava
- Significant carotid artery disease in the internal jugular vein
- Recent unsuccessful contralateral cannulation (because of the possibility of bilateral hematomas and the threat to airway patency) in the internal jugular vein

RELATIVE

- Coagulopathy or anticoagulant therapy

UNDERSTANDING THE THERMODILUTION METHOD

To measure cardiac output by the thermodilution method, a specific quantity of solution colder than the patient's blood is injected into the right atrium through a port on a pulmonary artery catheter. This indicator solution mixes with the blood as it travels through the right ventricle into the pulmonary artery. A thermistor on the catheter registers the change in temperature of the flowing blood. A computer then plots the temperature change over time, which produces a curve that indicates the measurement of blood flow (cardiac output).

- Hemothorax or pneumothorax on contralateral side (ipsilateral side preferred)
- Suspected or known prior injury to the vein
- Anticipated mastectomy on the side of central access
- Vasculitis
- Previous recent long-term cannulation of the vessel

❖ EQUIPMENT

THERMODILUTION METHOD

Thermodilution pulmonary artery (PA) catheter in position • output computer and cables (or a module for the bedside cardiac monitor) • closed or open injectant delivery system • 10-ml syringe • 500-ml bag of dextrose 5% in water or normal saline solution • crushed ice and water (if iced injectant is used)

Equipment preparation

- Wash your hands thoroughly.
- Assemble the equipment at the patient's bedside.
- Insert the closed injectant system tubing into the 500-ml bag of I.V. solution.
- Connect the 10-ml syringe to the system tubing and prime the tubing with I.V. solution until it's free of air, then clamp the tubing.
- After clamping the tubing, connect the primed system to the stopcock of the proximal injectant lumen of the PA catheter.
- Connect the temperature probe from the cardiac output computer to the closed injectant system's flow-through housing device.
- Connect the cardiac output computer cable to the thermistor connector on the PA catheter and verify the blood temperature reading.

- Turn on the cardiac output computer and enter the correct computation constant (determined by the volume and temperature of the injectant and the size and type of catheter), as provided by the catheter's manufacturer.
  ✸ **AGE-RELATED CONCERN** For a child, adjust the computation constant to reflect a smaller volume and catheter size.

▌▌▌ ESSENTIAL STEPS

- Confirm the patient's identity using two patient identifiers according to facility policy.
- Explain that the procedure will help to determine how well the patient's heart is pumping and causes no discomfort.
- Place your patient in a comfortable position and tell him not to move during the procedure.
- Maintain asepsis throughout the procedure.
- Verify the presence of a pulmonary artery waveform on the cardiac monitor.
- Unclamp the I.V. tubing, withdraw exactly 10 ml of solution, and reclamp the tubing.
- Turn the stopcock at the catheter injectant hub to open a fluid path between the injectant lumen of the PA catheter and the syringe.
- Press the START button on the cardiac output computer or wait for an "Inject" message to flash.
- Inject the solution smoothly within 4 seconds, making sure it doesn't leak at the connectors.
- If available, analyze the contour of the thermodilution washout curve on a strip chart recorder for a rapid upstroke and a gradual, smooth return to the baseline.
- Repeat these steps until three values are within 10% to 15% of the median value.

- Compute the average, and record the patient's cardiac output.
- Return the stopcock to its original position, and make sure the injectant delivery system tubing is clamped.
- Again verify the presence of a pulmonary artery waveform on the cardiac monitor.
- Discontinue cardiac output measurements when patient is hemodynamically stable and weaned from vasoactive and inotropic drugs.
- Disconnect and discard the injectant delivery system and the I.V. bag.
- Cover any exposed stopcocks with air-occlusive caps.

◆ SPECIAL CONSIDERATIONS

- The adequacy of a patient's cardiac output is better assessed by calculating his cardiac index (CI), adjusted for his body size.
- To calculate the patient's CI, divide his cardiac output by his body surface area (BSA), a function of height and weight (normal CI for adults ranges from 2.5 to 4.2 L/minute/m^2).

AGE-RELATED CONCERN Normal CI for infants and children is 3.5 to 4 L/minute/m^2; for elderly adults, 2 to 2.5 L/minute/m^2; and for pregnant women, 3.5 to 6.5 L/minute/m^2.

- Add the amount of fluid injected for cardiac output measurement to the patient's total intake.
- After cardiac output measurement, make sure the clamp on the injectant bag is secured to prevent inadvertent delivery of the injectant to the patient.

Complications
- Fluid volume overload
- Pulmonary artery perforation
- Pulmonary infarction
- Catheter knotting
- Local or systemic infection
- Cardiac arrhythmias

▶ PATIENT TEACHING

Be sure to cover:
- need for cardiac output measurements and what to expect during the procedure
- importance of remaining still during the procedure
- implications of cardiac output results.

●◆ DOCUMENTATION

- Date, time, and results of cardiac output, CI, and other hemodynamic values and vital signs at the time of measurement
- Patient's position during measurement and any unusual occurrences such as bradycardia
- Explanations given to the patient and the patient's response to the procedure

Selected references

Baulig, W., et al. "Cardiac Output Measurement by Pulse Dye Densitometry in Cardiac Surgery," *Anaesthesia* 60(10):968-73, October 2005.

Pittman, J., et al. "Continuous Cardiac Output: Monitoring With Pulse Contour Analysis: A Comparison With Lithium Indicator Dilution Cardiac Output Measurement," *Critical Care Medicine* 33(9):2015-2021, September 2005.

Taguchi, N., et al. "Cardiac Output Measurement by Pulse Dye Densitometry Using Three Wavelengths," *Pediatric Critical Care Medicine* 5(4):343-50, July 2004.

OTHER METHODS FOR MEASURING CARDIAC OUTPUT

In the *Fick method* (especially useful in detecting low cardiac output [CO] levels), the blood's oxygen content is measured before and after it passes through the lungs. First, blood is removed from the pulmonary and the brachial arteries and analyzed for oxygen content. Second, a spirometer measures oxygen consumption (the amount of air entering the lungs each minute). Third, CO is calculated using this formula:

$$CO \text{ (L/minute)} = \frac{\text{oxygen consumption (ml/minute)}}{\text{arterial oxygen content - venous oxygen content (ml/minute)}}$$

In the *dye dilution test,* a known volume and concentration of dye is injected into the pulmonary artery and measured by simultaneously sampling the amount of dye in the brachial artery. To calculate CO, these values are entered into a formula or plotted into a time and dilution-concentration curve. A computer, similar to the one used for the thermodilution test, performs the computation. Dye dilution measurements are particularly helpful in detecting intracardiac shunts and valvular regurgitation.

Cardioversion, synchronized

● OVERVIEW

- Indicated for stable paroxysmal atrial tachycardia, unstable paroxysmal supraventricular tachycardia, atrial fibrillation, atrial flutter, and ventricular tachycardia
- Delivery of an electric charge to the myocardium synchronized with the R wave so current won't be given on a vulnerable T wave and disrupt repolarization
- Results in immediate depolarization, interrupting reentry circuits and allowing the sinoatrial node to resume control
- Treatment of choice for arrhythmias that don't respond to vagal massage or drug therapy, such as unstable supraventricular tachycardia, unstable atrial fibrillation, unstable atrial flutter, and monomorphic ventricular tachycardia
- Elective or urgent procedure, depending on how well the patient tolerates the arrhythmia
- Immediate defibrillation possibly necessary when preparing for cardioversion because patient's condition can deteriorate quickly

Contraindications
- None known

❖ EQUIPMENT

Cardioverter-defibrillator • conductive gel pads • anterior, posterior, or transverse paddles electrocardiogram (ECG) monitor with recorder • sedative • oxygen therapy equipment • airway • handheld resuscitation bag • emergency pacing equipment • emergency cardiac drugs • automatic blood pressure cuff (if available) • pulse oximeter

Equipment preparation
- Make sure all equipment is at the bedside.
- Check to make sure that the battery is charged or that the unit is plugged into an electrical source.

▮▮ ESSENTIAL STEPS

- Confirm the patient's identify using two patient identifiers according to facility policy.
- Explain the procedure to the patient and make sure he has signed a consent form.
- Check his recent serum potassium and magnesium levels and arterial blood gas results.
- Check recent digoxin levels. Digitalized patients may undergo cardioversion, but tend to require lower energy levels to convert.

◈ **NURSING ALERT** If the patient takes digoxin, withhold the dose on the day of the procedure.

- Withhold food and fluids for 6 to 12 hours before the procedure.
- Obtain a 12-lead ECG to serve as a baseline.
- Check to see if the physician has ordered cardiac drugs before the procedure.
- Verify that the patient has a patent I.V. site in case drugs become necessary.
- Connect the patient to a pulse oximeter and automatic blood pressure cuff, if available.
- Consider giving oxygen for 5 to 10 minutes before cardioversion to promote myocardial oxygenation.
- If the patient wears dentures, evaluate whether they support his airway or may cause airway obstruction. If they may cause an obstruction, remove them.
- Place the patient in the supine position and assess vital signs, level of consciousness (LOC), cardiac rhythm, and peripheral pulses.
- Remove the oxygen delivery device before cardioversion to prevent combustion.
- Have epinephrine (Adrenalin), lidocaine (Xylocaine), and atropine at the patient's bedside.
- Make sure the resuscitation bag is at the bedside.
- Give a sedative, as ordered. Sedation is considered moderate to deep with reflexes intact and with the patient still able to breathe adequately.
- Carefully monitor blood pressure and respiratory rate until he recovers.

- Press the POWER button to turn on the defibrillator.
- Push the SYNC button to synchronize the machine with the patient's QRS complexes. Make sure the SYNC button flashes with each of the patient's QRS complexes. You should see a bright green flag flash on the monitor.
- Turn the ENERGY SELECT dial to the ordered amount of energy.

⬕ **NURSING ALERT** Advanced cardiac life support protocols call for a monophasic energy dose of 50 to 100 joules for a patient with unstable supraventricular tachycardia, 100 to 200 joules for a patient with atrial fibrillation, 50 to 100 joules for a patient with atrial flutter, and 100 joules for a patient who has monomorphic ventricular tachycardia with a pulse. If there's no response with the first shock, the health care provider should increase the joules in a step-wise manner.

- Remove paddles from machine and prepare them as if you were defibrillating the patient.
- Place conductive gel pads or paddles in the same positions you would to defibrillate.
- Make sure everyone stands away from the bed; push the discharge buttons.
- Hold the paddles in place and wait for energy to be discharged—the machine has to synchronize the discharge with the QRS complex.
- Check the waveform on the monitor.
- If the arrhythmia fails to convert, repeat the procedure two or three more times at 3-minute intervals.
- Gradually increase the energy level with each additional countershock.
- After cardioversion, frequently assess the patient's LOC and respiratory status, including airway patency, respiratory rate and depth, and need for supplemental oxygen.

⬕ **NURSING ALERT** The patient may require airway support because he's heavily sedated.

- Record a postcardioversion 12-lead ECG, and monitor the patient's ECG rhythm for 2 hours or per facility sedation protocol.
- Check for electrical burns and treat as needed.

✦ SPECIAL CONSIDERATIONS

- Improper synchronization may result if the patient's ECG tracing contains artifact-like spikes, such as peaked T waves or bundle-branch heart blocks when the R' wave may be taller than the R wave.

Complications

- Transient, harmless arrhythmias (common), such as atrial, ventricular, and junctional premature beats
- Serious ventricular arrhythmias, such as ventricular fibrillation resulting from high amounts of electrical energy, digoxin toxicity, severe heart disease, electrolyte imbalance, or improper synchronization with the R wave

▶ PATIENT TEACHING

Be sure to cover:
- procedure and what to expect
- how to monitor and record pulse, as indicated
- signs and symptoms of recurrent arrhythmia.

◆ DOCUMENTATION

- Date and time of procedure
- Voltage given with each attempt
- Rhythm strips before and after the procedure
- Patient's tolerance of procedure

Selected references

American Heart Association. "2005 AHA Guidelines for Cardiopulmonary Care: Interventional Consensus on Science," *Circulation* 112(22 Suppl): IV-I-IV-221, November 2005.

Jacoby, J.L., et al. "Synchronized Emergency Department Cardioversion of Atrial Dysrhythmias Saves Time, Money and Resources," *Journal of Emergency Medicine* 28(1):27-30, January 2005.

Stellbrink, C., and Schimpf, T. "Anticoagulation During Cardioversion in Patients With Atrial Fibrillation: Current Clinical Practice," *American Journal of Cardiovascular Drugs* 5(3):155-62, 2005.

Wazni, O., et al. "C Reactive Protein Concentration and Recurrence of Atrial Fibrillation After Electrical Cardioversion," *Heart* 91(10):1303-305, October 2005.

Xavier, L.C., and Memon, A. "Synchronized Cardioversion of Unstable Supraventricular Tachycardia Resulting in Ventricular Fibrillation," *Annals of Emergency Medicine* 44(2):178-80, August 2004.

Catheter, urinary (indwelling), insertion, care, and removal

● OVERVIEW

- Remains in bladder to provide continuous urine drainage
- Has an inflated balloon at its distal end to prevent it from slipping out of the bladder after insertion
- Relieves bladder distention caused by urine retention and allows continuous urine drainage when the urinary meatus is swollen from childbirth, surgery, or local trauma
- Also indicated for urinary tract obstruction (by a tumor or enlarged prostate), urine retention or infection from neurogenic bladder paralysis caused by spinal cord injury or disease, and any illness in which the patient's urine output must be monitored closely
- Requires keeping catheter site clean to prevent infection and other complications
- Removed when bladder decompression is no longer necessary, when patient can resume voiding, or when catheter is obstructed
- May require bladder retraining before catheter removal, depending on duration of catheterization
- Also known as *Foley* or *urinary retention catheter*

Contraindications
- Urethral trauma
- Urethral obstruction

❖ EQUIPMENT

CATHETER INSERTION
Prepackaged sterile disposable kit that contains all the equipment usually available; if not available then sterile indwelling catheter (latex or silicone #10 to #22 French [average adult sizes are #16 to #18 French]) • syringe filled with 5 to 8 ml of sterile water • washcloth • towel • soap and water • two linen-saver pads • sterile gloves • sterile drape • sterile fenestrated drape • sterile cotton-tipped applicators (or cotton balls and plastic forceps) • povidone-iodine or other antiseptic cleaning agent • urine receptacle • sterile water-soluble lubricant in syringe • sterile drainage collection bag • intake and output sheet • adhesive tape • optional: urine-specimen container and laboratory request form, leg band with Velcro closure, gooseneck lamp, or pillows or rolled blankets or towels

CATHETER CARE
Soap and water • basin • sterile gloves • washcloth • leg bag • adhesive tape or leg band • optional: safety pin, gooseneck lamp or flashlight, adhesive remover, and specimen container

CATHETER REMOVAL
Gloves • alcohol pad • 10-ml syringe with a luer-lock • bedpan • linen-saver pad • optional: clamp for bladder retraining

Equipment preparation
CATHETER INSERTION
- Check the order for insertion on the patient's chart to determine if a catheter size or type has been specified.
- Wash your hands thoroughly.
- Select the appropriate equipment, and assemble it at the patient's bedside.
- Bring all equipment to the patient's bedside.

┃┃■ ESSENTIAL STEPS

- Confirm the patient's identify using two patient identifiers according to facility policy.
- Explain the procedure to the patient and provide privacy.
- Maintain asepsis throughout procedure.

CATHETER INSERTION
- Check the patient's chart and ask when he voided last.
- Percuss and palpate the bladder and ask if he feels the urge to void.
- Place a female patient in the supine position with her knees flexed and separated and her feet flat on the bed, about 2′ (61 cm) apart.

✸ **AGE-RELATED CONCERN** Some elderly female patients or those with severe contractures may find it more comfortable to lie on the side with the knees drawn up to the chest during the insertion. Additionally, an elderly patient may need pillows or towels or blankets to provide support with positioning.

- Place the male patient in the supine positioning with his legs extended and flat on the bed.
- Ask the patient to hold the position to give you a clear view of the urinary meatus and to prevent contamination of the sterile field.
- Use the washcloth to clean the patient's genital area and perineum thoroughly with soap and water and dry the area with the towel.
- Wash your hands again.
- Place the linen-saver pads on the bed between the patient's legs and under the hips.
- To create the sterile field, open the prepackaged kit or equipment tray and place it between the female patient's legs or next to the male patient's hip.
- If the sterile gloves are the first item on the top of the tray, put them on.
- Without contaminating your gloves, place the sterile drape under the patient's hips and drape the lower abdomen with the sterile fenestrated drape so that only the genital area remains exposed.

- Open the rest of the kit, putting on the sterile gloves if you haven't already done so.
- Open the packet of povidone-iodine and use it to saturate the sterile cotton balls or applicators, taking care not to spill the solution on the equipment.
- Open the water-soluble lubricant and apply it to the catheter tip

NURSING ALERT A syringe prefilled with water-soluble lubricant may be used, if policy allows, to instill lubricant directly into the male urethra instead of on the catheter tip. This prevents trauma to the urethral lining and possible urinary tract infection.

- Attach the drainage bag to the other end of the catheter. (In a commercial kit, the drainage bag may be attached.)
- Make sure all tubing ends remain sterile and close the clamp at the emptying port of the drainage bag.
- Check the balloon for leaks by inflating it with the prefilled syringe of sterile water or normal saline solution and inspect it for leaks, then aspirate the solution to deflate the balloon.
- For a female patient, separate the labia majora and labia minora as widely as possible with the thumb, middle, and index fingers of your nondominant hand to visualize the urinary meatus.
  - Keep the labia well separated throughout the procedure, so they don't contaminate the urinary meatus once it's cleaned.
  - With your dominant hand, use a sterile, cotton-tipped applicator (or sterile cotton ball with the plastic forceps) and wipe one side of the urinary meatus with a single downward motion.
  - Wipe the other side with another sterile applicator or cotton ball in the same way and then wipe directly over the meatus with still another sterile applicator or cotton ball.
- For a male patient, hold the penis with your nondominant hand, retracting the foreskin if the man isn't circumcised.

- Gently lift and stretch the penis to a 60-degree to 90-degree angle and hold the penis this way throughout the procedure, to straighten the urethra.
- Use your dominant hand to clean the glans with a sterile cotton-tipped applicator or a sterile cotton ball held in forceps, working in a circular motion, from the urinary meatus outward.
- Repeat the procedure using another sterile applicator or cotton ball. If the lubricant syringe is being used, gently insert the tip of the syringe into the urethra and instill the 10 ml of lubricant as per facility policy.
- Pick up the catheter with your dominant hand, holding it close to the tip, and insert it into the urinary meatus.
- To facilitate insertion by relaxing the sphincter, ask the patient to cough as you insert the catheter.
- Tell the patient to breathe deeply and slowly to further relax the sphincter.

NURSING ALERT Never force a catheter during insertion. Maneuver it gently as the patient bears down or coughs. If you still meet resistance, stop and notify the physician. Sphincter spasms, strictures, misplacement in the vagina (in females), or an enlarged prostate (in males) may cause resistance.

- For the female patient, advance the catheter about 2″ to 3″ (5 to 7.5 cm) until urine begins to flow.
  - If the catheter is inadvertently inserted into the vagina, leave it there as a landmark and begin the procedure again using new supplies.
- For the male patient, advance the catheter to the bifurcation 5″ to 7½″ (12.5 to 19 cm) and check for urine flow.
  - If the foreskin was retracted, replace it to prevent compromised circulation and painful swelling.
- When urine stops flowing, attach the prefilled syringe to the luer-lock and inflate the balloon to keep the catheter in place in the bladder.

NURSING ALERT Never inflate a balloon without first establishing urine flow, which assures you that the catheter is in the bladder.

- Attach the drainage bag to the catheter and hang it below bladder level to prevent urine reflux into the bladder, which can cause infection, and to facilitate gravity drainage of the bladder.
- Some drainage systems have an air-lock chamber to prevent bacteria from traveling to the bladder from urine in the drainage bag.
- Secure the catheter to the female patient's thigh to prevent possible tension on the urogenital trigone.
- Secure the catheter to the male patient's anterior thigh to prevent pressure on the urethra at the penoscrotal junction, which can lead to formation of urethrocutaneous fistulas; traction on the bladder; and alteration in the normal direction of urine flow. As an alternative, secure the catheter to the patient's thigh using a leg band with a Velcro closure to decrease skin irritation.

CATHETER CARE
- Explain the procedure to the patient.
- Provide privacy.
- Make sure that the lighting is adequate so that you can see the perineum and catheter tubing clearly (use a gooseneck lamp or flashlight, if needed).
- Inspect the catheter for any problems.
- Check the urine drainage for mucus, blood clots, sediment, and turbidity. If present, obtain a urine specimen (collect at least 3 ml of urine, but don't fill the specimen cup more than halfway) and notify the physician.
- Inspect the outside of the catheter where it enters the urinary meatus for encrusted material and suppurative drainage and inspect the tissue around the meatus for irritation or swelling.

(continued)

- Remove the leg band, or if adhesive tape was used to secure the catheter, remove the adhesive tape, inspecting the area for signs and symptoms of adhesive burns (redness, tenderness, or blisters).
- Put on gloves.
- Clean the outside of the catheter and the tissue around the meatus, using soap and water.

NURSING ALERT To avoid contaminating the urinary tract, always clean by wiping away from—never toward—the urinary meatus. Avoid pulling on the catheter while you're cleaning it. This can injure the urethra and the bladder wall. It can also expose a section of the catheter that was inside the urethra, so that when you release the catheter, the newly contaminated section will reenter the urethra, introducing potentially infectious organisms.

- Use a dry gauze pad to remove encrusted material.
- Remove your gloves, reapply the leg band, and reattach the catheter to the leg band. Alternatively, if a leg band isn't available, tape the catheter on the opposite side to prevent skin hypersensitivity or irritation.
- If necessary, clean residue from the previous tape site with adhesive remover.

NURSING ALERT Provide enough slack before securing the catheter to prevent tension on the tubing, which could injure the urethral lumen or bladder wall.

- Attach the drainage tubing to the sheet using a plastic clamp on the tubing or, if there's no clamp, wrap a rubber band around the drainage tubing, insert the safety pin through a loop of the rubber band, and pin the tubing to the sheet below bladder level.
- Attach the collection bag (below bladder level) to the bed frame.

CATHETER REMOVAL
- Provide privacy.
- Explain the procedure and tell the patient that he may feel slight discomfort.
- Tell the patient that you'll check on him periodically during the first 6 to 24 hours (after catheter removal) to make sure voiding resumes.
- Put on gloves.
- Place a linen-saver pad under the patient's buttocks.
- Attach the syringe to the luer-lock mechanism on the catheter.
- Pull back on the plunger of the syringe to deflate the balloon by aspirating the injected fluid (amount of fluid injected is usually indicated on the tip of the catheter's balloon lumen).
- Because urine may leak as the catheter is removed, offer the patient a bedpan.
- Grasp the catheter, and pinch it with your thumb and index finger to prevent urine from flowing back into the urethra.
- Gently pull the catheter from the urethra.
- If you meet resistance, notify the physician.
- Remove the bedpan.
- For the first 24 hours after catheter removal, note the time and amount of each voiding.

◆ SPECIAL CONSIDERATIONS

CATHETER INSERTION
- Several types of catheters are available with balloons of various sizes; each type has its own method of inflation and closure.
- The balloon size determines the amount of solution needed for inflation, and the exact amount is printed on the distal extension catheter used for inflating the balloon.

NURSING ALERT Injecting a catheter with air makes identification difficult and doesn't guarantee deflation of the balloon for removal.

- If the physician orders a urine specimen for laboratory analysis, obtain it at the time of catheterization, and send it to the laboratory with the appropriate request form.
- Inspect the catheter and tubing periodically to detect compression kinking that could obstruct urine flow.
- Empty the collection bag at least every 8 hours or more frequently, if needed.
- Some hospitals encourage changing catheters at regular intervals, such as every 30 days, if the patient will have long-term continuous drainage.
- Check facility policy before catheterization to determine the maximum amount of urine that may be drained at one time (although this practice is controversial, some facilities limit the amount to 700 to 1,000 ml).

NURSING ALERT Observe the patient carefully for adverse reactions, such as hypovolemic shock, caused by removing excessive volumes of residual urine. Clamp the catheter at the first sign of an adverse reaction, and notify the physician.

CATHETER CARE AND REMOVAL

- Follow your facility's policy on the use of specific cleaning agents for catheter care.
- A physician's order is needed to apply antibiotic ointments to the urinary meatus after cleaning.
- To avoid damaging the urethral lumen or bladder wall, always disconnect the drainage bag and tubing from the bed linen and bed frame before helping the patient out of bed.
- When possible, attach a leg bag to allow the patient greater mobility.
- If the patient will be discharged with an indwelling catheter, teach him how to use a leg bag.
- Encourage patients with unrestricted fluid intake to increase intake to at least 3 qt (3 L)/day to flush the urinary system and reduce sediment formation.
- To prevent urinary sediment and calculi from obstructing the drainage tube, some patients are placed on an acid-ash diet to acidify the urine.
- After catheter removal, assess the patient for incontinence (or dribbling), urgency, persistent dysuria or bladder spasms, fever, chills, or palpable bladder distention and report their occurrence to the physician.
- When changing catheters after long-term use (usually 30 days), you may need a larger size catheter because the meatus enlarges, causing urine to leak around the catheter.
- Regardless of the catheter care policy, the equipment and the patient's genitalia require inspection twice daily.

Complications

- Urinary tract infection
- Traumatic injury to the urethral and bladder mucosa
- Bladder atony or spasms
- Sediment build-up in the catheterization system
- Acute renal failure
- Urine retention

▶ PATIENT TEACHING

Be sure to cover:
- why catheterization is needed
- what to expect during the procedure and what the patient can do to help
- importance of deep-breathing exercises to promote relaxation during insertion
- care of the catheter and equipment
- importance of not pulling on the catheter and keeping the drainage bag below the level of the bladder
- need to increase fluid intake
- what to expect during catheter removal
- home care including daily catheter maintenance, signs and symptoms of urinary tract infection or obstruction to report, catheter irrigation (if appropriate), fluid intake, follow-up for catheter changes, and clean intermittent self-catheterization, as appropriate.

◆ DOCUMENTATION

- Date, time, and size and type of indwelling catheter insertion
- Amount, color, and other characteristics of urine emptied from the bladder and in drainage bag
- Intake and output
- Patient's tolerance for the procedure
- Urine specimens sent for laboratory analysis
- Date and time of catheter care and type of care performed
- Condition of the perineum and urinary meatus
- Date and time catheter was removed
- Time and volume of voiding after catheter removal

Selected references

Abadi, S., et al. "Misleading Positioning of a Foley Catheter Balloon," *British Journal of Radiology* 79(938):175-76, February 2006.

Addison, R. "Choosing a Urinary Catheter for Short and Long-Term Use," *Professional Nurse* 19(12):41-44, August 2004.

Bardsley, A. "Use of Lubricant Gels in Urinary Catheterization," *Nursing Standard* 20(8):41-46, November 2005.

Morey, A.F. "Consensus Statement on Urethral Trauma," *Journal of Urology* 174(3):968-69, September 2005.

Ribby, K.J. "Decreasing Urinary Tract Infections Through Staff Development, Outcomes, and Nursing Process," *Journal of Nursing Care Quality* 21(2):194-98, April-June 2006.

Central venous pressure monitoring

⬤ OVERVIEW

- Permits assessment of cardiac function and evaluation of venous return; indirectly gauges how well the heart is pumping
- Tracks central venous pressure (CVP) (an index of right ventricular function), which increases with increasing circulating blood volume (due to enhanced venous return, for example) and decreases with reduced circulating blood volume (due to reduced venous return, for example)
- Achieved by means of a catheter that's connected to a manometer or pressure monitor and advanced through a vein until its tip lies near the right atrium
- Done intermittently or continuously (see *Understanding CVP monitoring*)
- Also provides access with central venous (CV) line to a large vessel for rapid, high-volume fluid administration and allows frequent blood withdrawal for laboratory samples

Contraindications

ABSOLUTE

- Trauma at the access site or to adjacent structures
- Full-thickness burn, infection, or cellulitis over the insertion site
- Uncooperative or agitated patient

UNDERSTANDING CVP MONITORING

In central venous pressure monitoring, a catheter is inserted percutaneously (or, using a cutdown method) into a vein and advanced until its tip lies in or near the right atrium. Because no major valves lie at the junction of the vena cava and right atrium, pressure at end diastole reflects back to the catheter. When connected to a manometer, the catheter measures central venous pressure (CVP), an indicator of right ventricular function.

To measure the patient's volume status, a disposable plastic water manometer may be attached between the I.V. line and the central catheter with a three- or four-way stopcock. CVP may also be monitored continuously through a CV catheter attached to a pressure transducer. CVP is recorded in centimeters of water (cm H_2O) or millimeters of mercury (mm Hg). Normal CVP ranges from 2 to 8 cm H_2O (2 to 6 mm Hg).

- Distorted local anatomy or landmarks at insertion site (as a result of surgery, irradiation, trauma, or congenital malformations)
- Previous use of the vessel for a sclerosing agent (such as from chemotherapeutic agents)
- Suspected or actual injury to the superior vena cava
- Significant carotid artery disease in the internal jugular vein
- Recent unsuccessful contralateral cannulation (because of the possibility of bilateral hematomas and the threat to airway patency) in the internal jugular vein

RELATIVE

- Coagulopathy or anticoagulant therapy
- Hemothorax or pneumothorax on contralateral side (ipsilateral side preferred)
- Suspected or known prior injury to the vein
- Anticipated mastectomy on the side of central access
- Vasculitis
- Previous recent long-term cannulation of the vessel

❖ EQUIPMENT

INTERMITTENT CVP MONITORING
Disposable CVP manometer set • leveling device (such as a rod from a reusable CVP pole holder) • additional stopcock • extension tubing (if needed) • I.V. pole • I.V. solution • I.V. drip chamber and tubing

CONTINUOUS CVP MONITORING
Pressure monitoring kit with disposable pressure transducer • leveling device • bedside pressure module • continuous I.V. flush solution • pressure bag

WITHDRAWING BLOOD SAMPLES THROUGH THE CV LINE
Appropriate number of syringes for the ordered tests • 5- or 10-ml syringe for the discard sample

USING AN INTERMITTENT CV LINE
Syringe with normal saline solution • syringe with heparin flush solution

▌▌▌ ESSENTIAL STEPS

- Confirm the patient's identity using two patient identifiers according to facility policy.
- Explain all procedures to the patient and his family.
- Make sure the patient has signed an appropriate consent form.
- Wash your hands thoroughly.
- Gather the necessary equipment at the bedside.
- Maintain asepsis and wear appropriate personal protective equipment.
- Assist the physician as he inserts the CV catheter in a procedure similar to that used for pulmonary artery pressure monitoring.

INTERMITTENT MONITORING WITH WATER MANOMETER

- Place the patient in a supine position in bed.
- Align the base of the manometer with the zero reference point (at the level of the right atrium) by using a leveling device, typically at the fourth intercostal space at the midaxillary line.
- Mark the appropriate place on the patient's chest so that all subsequent recordings will be made using the same location.

⬡ **NURSING ALERT** If the patient can't tolerate a supine position, place him in semi-Fowler's position and use the same degree of elevation for all subsequent measurements.

- Attach the water manometer to an I.V. pole or place it next to the patient's chest with the zero reference point level with the right atrium. (See *Measuring CVP with a water manometer.*)
- Verify that the water manometer is connected to the I.V. tubing.
- Turn off the stopcock to the patient, and slowly fill the manometer with I.V. solution until the fluid level is 10 to 20 cm H_2O higher than the patient's expected CVP value.
- Turn off the stopcock to the I.V. solution and open the stopcock to the patient, watching the fluid level in the manometer drop.
- Record CVP at the end of expiration, noting the value either at the bottom of the meniscus or at the midline of the small floating ball, depending on the type of water manometer used.

- After you've obtained the CVP value, turn on the stopcock to resume the I.V. infusion and adjust the I.V. drip rate as required.
- Make the patient comfortable.

CONTINUOUS MONITORING WITH WATER MANOMETER
- Make sure the stopcock is turned on so that the ports to I.V. solution, CVP column, and patient are open.

NURSING ALERT When the stopcock is turned "on" to the patient, manometer, and I.V. solution, I.V. solution infusion increases CVP readings.

- Assess the patient closely for changes.

CONTINUOUS MONITORING WITH PRESSURE MONITORING SYSTEM
- Make sure the CV line or the proximal lumen of a multilumen pulmonary artery catheter is attached to the system.
- Set up a pressure transducer system connecting the pressure tubing from the CVP catheter hub to the transducer.
- Connect the flush solution container to a flush device.
- To obtain values, lie the patient flat.
- Zero the transducer, leveling the transducer air-fluid interface stopcock with the right atrium.
- Read the CVP value from the digital display on the monitor, and note the waveform.

NURSING ALERT Make sure the patient is still when taking a CVP reading with a continuous pressure monitoring system to prevent artifact.

✦ SPECIAL CONSIDERATIONS

- Arrange for daily chest X-rays to check catheter placement, as ordered.
- Care for insertion site and change the dressing every 24 to 48 hours, according to facility policy.

NURSING ALERT Watch for signs of air embolism, including sudden onset of pallor, cyanosis, hypoxia, dyspnea, coughing, tachycardia, and cardiovascular collapse.

- Wash your hands before changing dressing and use sterile gloves and technique when redressing.

- When removing the old dressing, observe for signs of infection and note complaints of tenderness.
- Apply ointment to the insertion site during dressing changes, if directed by facility policy, and cover the site with a sterile gauze dressing or a clear occlusive dressing.
- After the initial CVP reading, reevaluate readings frequently to establish a baseline for the patient, and report a fluctuation in CVP of more than 2 cm H_2O to the physician.
- Change the I.V. solution and tubing, according to facility policy.
- Label I.V. solution, tubing, and dressing with date, time, and your initials.

Complications
- Pneumothorax
- Local or systemic infection
- Hemorrhage or hematoma
- Thrombus
- Vessel or adjacent organ puncture
- Air embolism
- Arrhythmias

▶ PATIENT TEACHING

Be sure to cover:
- purpose of the procedure

- implications of CVP values
- need to lie flat and still during measurements
- signs and symptoms of complications
- what to expect during catheter removal.

●◆ DOCUMENTATION

- Date and time of dressing, tubing, solution changes, and CVP reading
- Condition and care of insertion site
- Patient's tolerance of the procedure
- Date, time, and name of physician notified of abnormal results, complications and orders given

Selected references
Craig, J., and Mathieu, S. "Is Central Venous Pressure Monitoring Appropriate for Assessment of Perioperative Fluid Balance?" *British Journal of Hospital Medicine* 67(2):108, February 2006.

Ho, A.M., et al. "Accuracy of Central Venous Pressure Monitoring During Simultaneous Continuous Infusion Through the Same Catheter," *Anaesthesia* 60(10):1027-1030, October 2005.

MEASURING CVP WITH A WATER MANOMETER

To ensure accurate central venous pressure (CVP) readings, make sure the manometer base is aligned with the patient's right atrium (the zero reference point). The manometer set usually contains a leveling rod to allow you to determine this quickly.

After adjusting the manometer's position, examine the typical three-way stopcock, as shown here. By turning it to any position shown, you can control the direction of fluid flow. Four-way stopcocks are also available.

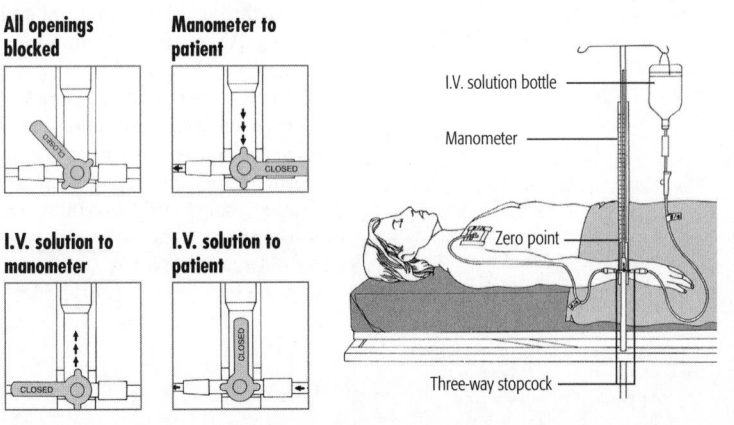

All openings blocked

Manometer to patient

I.V. solution to manometer

I.V. solution to patient

I.V. solution bottle

Manometer

Zero point

Three-way stopcock

Chemotherapy administration

OVERVIEW

- Requires specific skills in addition to those used when giving other drugs
- May require specialized equipment or administration through an unusual route
- Exact dosage necessary to avoid potentially fatal complications
- Although I.V. (using peripheral or central veins) used most commonly, may also be given orally; subcutaneously; I.M.; intra-arterially, into a body cavity or pleural space, through a central venous catheter; or through an Ommaya reservoir into the spinal canal
- Route dependent on drug pharmacodynamics and tumor characteristics
- If malignant tumor confined to one area, use of a localized or regional method, which allows delivery of a high dose directly to the tumor
- Regional chemotherapy: advantageous because many solid tumors don't respond to drug levels that are safe for systemic administration
- Adjuvant chemotherapy: used to be sure no undetectable metastasis exists in patients who have had surgery or radiation therapy
- Induction chemotherapy (or neoadjuvant or synchronous chemotherapy) before surgery or radiation therapy: improves survival rates by shrinking a tumor before surgical excision or radiation therapy

Contraindications
- None known

EQUIPMENT

Prescribed drug • aluminum foil or brown paper bag (if drug is photosensitive) • normal saline solution • syringes and needleless adapters • infusion pump or controller • gloves • impervious containers labeled CAUTION: BIOHAZARD

Equipment preparation
- Verify the drug, dosage, and administration route.
- Make sure you know the immediate and delayed adverse effects.
- Follow administration guidelines.

ESSENTIAL STEPS

- Confirm the patient's identity using two patient identifiers according to facility policy.
- Explain the procedure to the patient.
- Assess the patient's physical condition and medical history.
- Make sure you understand what drug needs to be given and by what route. Determine the best site to give the drug.
- When selecting the site, consider drug compatibilities, frequency of administration, and the vesicant potential of the drug.
- Continuous infusion of a vesicant drug should be done through a central venous line or a vascular access device.
- Nonvesicant agents (including irritants) may be given by direct I.V push, through the side port of an infusing I.V. line, or as a continuous infusion.
- Because vein integrity decreases with time, some facilities require that vesicants be given before other drugs. Also, because vesicants increase vein fragility, some facilities require vesicants be given after other drugs (check facility policy).

- Evaluate the patient, paying attention to recent laboratory studies, including complete blood cell count, blood urea nitrogen level, platelet count, urine creatinine level, and liver function studies.
- Determine if the patient has received chemotherapy previously, and note severity of adverse effects.
- Check his history for drugs that might interact with chemotherapy.

⬥ **NURSING ALERT** Don't mix chemotherapeutic drugs with other drugs. If you have questions or concerns, talk with the physician or pharmacist before giving the drug.

- Double-check the chart for the complete chemotherapy protocol order, including the patient's name, drug's name, dosage, route, rate, and frequency of administration.
- Check if the drug's dosage depends on certain laboratory values.
- Some facilities require two nurses to read the dosage order and check the drug and amount given.
- Check to see if an antiemetic, fluids, a diuretic, or electrolyte supplements are to be given before, during, or after chemotherapy.
- Evaluate the patient's understanding and make sure a consent form has been signed.
- Wear gloves through all stages of handling the drug.
- Before giving the drug, perform a new venipuncture proximal to the old site.

⬥ **NURSING ALERT** Avoid using an existing peripheral I.V. line and never test vein patency with a chemotherapeutic drug.

- To identify an administration site, examine the patient's veins, starting with his hand then his forearm.
- After an appropriate line is in place, infuse 10 to 20 ml of normal saline solution to test vein patency.
- Give the drug as appropriate: nonvesicants by I.V. push or admixed in a bag of I.V.fluid; vesicants by I.V. push through a piggyback set connected to a rapidly infusing I.V. line.
- During I.V. administration, closely monitor for signs of hypersensitivity or extravasation.

- Check for adequate blood return after 5 ml of drug has been infused or according to facility policy.
- Infuse 20 ml of normal saline solution after infusion of the drug, between administration of different chemotherapeutic drugs, and before discontinuing the I.V. line.
- Dispose of used needles and syringes carefully in a sharps container.
- To prevent aerosol dispersion of chemotherapeutic drugs, don't clip needles. Place the needles intact in an impervious container for incineration.
- Dispose of I.V. bags, bottles, gloves, and tubing in a properly labeled, covered trash container.
- Wash your hands thoroughly after giving chemotherapeutic drugs.

◆ SPECIAL CONSIDERATIONS

- Check frequently for signs of extravasation and allergic reaction (swelling, redness, and urticaria).

NURSING ALERT If you suspect extravasation, stop infusion immediately. Leave I.V. catheter in place and notify the physician. A conservative method for treating extravasation involves aspirating residual drug from the tubing and I.V. catheter, instilling an I.V. antidote, and then removing the I.V. catheter. Afterward, apply heat or cold to the site and elevate the limb.

- To avoid breakdown, some drugs shouldn't be exposed to direct sunlight. To protect from sunlight, cover vial with a brown paper bag or aluminum foil.
- When giving vesicants, avoid sites where damage to underlying tendons or nerves may occur (veins in the antecubital fossa, near the wrist, or the dorsal surface of the hand).
- If you're unable to stay with the patient, use an infusion pump or controller to ensure drug delivery within the prescribed time and rate.
- Observe him regularly during and after treatment for adverse reactions.
- Monitor vital signs throughout infusion.

- Record the types and amounts of drugs the patient received.
- Maintaining a list is especially important if he has received drugs that have a cumulative effect and that can be toxic to such organs as the heart or kidneys.

Complications

- Nausea and vomiting, ranging from mild to debilitating
- Bone marrow suppression, leading to neutropenia and thrombocytopenia
- Intestinal irritation
- Stomatitis
- Pulmonary fibrosis
- Cardiotoxicity
- Nephrotoxicity
- Neurotoxicity
- Anemia
- Alopecia
- Urticaria
- Radiation recall (if drugs are given with, or soon after, radiation therapy)
- Anorexia
- Esophagitis
- Diarrhea
- I.V. administration that may also cause extravasation, inflammation, ulceration, necrosis, loss of vein patency

▶ PATIENT TEACHING

Be sure to cover
- drugs being given, including route and frequency
- possible adverse reactions to chemotherapy
- possible drugs that can be given to treat some of the adverse reactions
- measures to alleviate adverse effects
- importance of follow-up care.

●❖ DOCUMENTATION

- Location and description of the I.V. site before treatment and presence of blood return during bolus administration
- Drugs and dosages given
- Sequence of drug administration
- Needle type and size
- Amount and type of flushing solution
- Site's condition after treatment
- Adverse reactions and measures to treat
- Patient's tolerance of the procedure
- Topics discussed with patient and his family

Selected references

Hendershot, E., et al. "Outpatient Chemotherapy Administration: Decreasing Wait Times for Patients and Families," *Journal of Pediatric Oncology Nursing* 22(1):31-37, January-February 2005.

Schulmeister, L. "Look-alike, Sound-alike Oncology Medications," *Clinical Journal of Oncology Nursing* 100(1):35-41, February 2006.

Treleaven, J., et al. "Obtaining Consent for Chemotherapy," *British Journal of Haematology* 132(5):552-59, March 2006.

Wyatt, A., et al. "Cutaneous Reactions to Chemotherapy and Their Management," *American Journal of Clinical Dermatology* 7(1):45-63, 2006.

Chest tube insertion

● OVERVIEW

- Allows drainage of air (in pneumothorax), fluid (in hemothorax or pleural effusion), or both from the pleural space, for the patient with partial or complete lung collapse, thus promoting lung reexpansion
- For pneumothorax: second intercostal space usual insertion site because air rises to the top of the intrapleural space (see *Performing needle thoracentesis*)
- For hemothorax or pleural effusion: sixth to eighth intercostal spaces common insertion sites because fluid settles to the lower levels of the intrapleural space
- For removal of air and fluid: both high and low insertion sites used

Contraindications
RELATIVE
- Systemic anticoagulation or coagulopathy
- Small (less than 20%), stable pneumothorax

❖ EQUIPMENT

Two pairs sterile gloves • sterile drape • facility-approved skin preparation solution such as povidone-iodine solution • vial of 1% lidocaine • 10-ml syringe • alcohol pad • 22G 1″ needle • 25G ⅜″ needle • sterile scalpel (usually with #11 blade) • sterile forceps • two rubber-tipped clamps for each chest tube inserted • sterile 4″ × 4″ gauze pads • two sterile 4″ × 4″ drain dressings (gauze pads with slit) • 3″ or 4″ (7.5 to 10 cm) sturdy, elastic tape • 1″ adhesive tape for connections • appropriate size chest tube (#16 to #20 French catheter for air or serous fluid; #28 to #40 French catheter for blood, pus, or thick fluid), with or without a trocar • sterile Kelly clamp • suture material (usually 2-0 silk with cutting needle) • thoracic drainage system • sterile drainage tubing (6′ [1.8 m]) and connector • sterile Y-connector (for two chest tubes on the same side) • optional: petroleum gauze

Equipment preparation
- Thoroughly wash your hands before setting up equipment and before all procedures.
- Check the expiration date on the sterile packages, and inspect for tears.
- Assemble all equipment in the patient's room and set up the thoracic drainage system, placing it next to the patient's bed below the chest level to facilitate drainage.

▐▮ ESSENTIAL STEPS

- Explain the procedure to the patient and his family.
- In a nonemergency situation, make sure the patient has signed an appropriate consent form.
- Maintain asepsis throughout the procedure.
- Wear appropriate personal protective equipment throughout the procedure.
- Provide for the patient's privacy.
- Record baseline vital signs and respiratory assessment.
- Position the patient in high Fowler's, semi-Fowler's, or the supine position if he has a pneumothorax; leaning over the overbed table or straddling a chair with his arms dangling over the back if he has hemothorax; or lying on his unaffected side with arms extended over his head for either pneumothorax or hemothorax.
- Open the chest tube tray using sterile technique.
- Assist the physician with cleaning the area with povidone-iodine solution.
- Wipe the rubber stopper of the lidocaine vial with an alcohol pad, invert the bottle, and hold it for the doctor to withdraw the anesthetic.
- After the physician anesthetizes the site, he makes a small incision and inserts the chest tube.
- Reassure the patient, as necessary.
- Connect the chest tube to the thoracic drainage system.
- Open the packages containing the 4″ × 4″ drain dressings and gauze pads, and put on sterile gloves.
- Place two 4″ × 4″ drain dressings around the insertion site, one from the top and the other from the bottom.
- Place several 4″ × 4″ gauze pads on top of the drain dressings and tape the dressings, covering them completely.
- Tape the chest tube to the patient's chest distal to the insertion site to help prevent accidental tube dislodgment.
- Tape the junction of the chest tube and the drainage tube to prevent separation.
- Make sure that the tubing remains level with the patient and there are no dependent loops.

PERFORMING NEEDLE THORACENTESIS

For a patient with life-threatening tension pneumothorax, needle thoracentesis temporarily relieves pleural pressure until a practitioner can insert a chest tube.

How needle thoracentesis works
A needle attached to a flutter valve is inserted into the affected pleural space. (If no flutter valve is available, one can be made from a perforated finger cot or glove attached with a rubber band.) When the patient exhales, trapped air escapes by way of the flutter valve instead of being retained under pressure. The flutter valve also prevents air from entering the patient's involved lung during inhalation.

How to perform needle thoracentesis
If a practitioner isn't available, you may need to perform the procedure (depending on your state's Nurse Practice Act as well as your facility's policy). Here's how to proceed:
- Clean the skin around the second intercostal space at the midclavicular line with povidone-iodine solution, using a circular motion, starting at the center and working outward.
- Insert a sterile 16G (or larger) needle over the superior portion of the rib and through the tissue covering the pleural cavity. The vein, artery, and nerve lie behind the rib's inferior border.
- Listen for a hissing sound signaling the needle's entry into the pleural cavity.
- If you're using a flutter valve, secure it to the needle. The arrow on the valve indicates the direction of airflow.
- Place a sterile glove on the distal end of the valve to collect drainage.
- Leave the needle in place until a chest tube can be inserted.

- Immediately after the drainage system is connected, instruct the patient to take a deep breath, hold it momentarily, and slowly exhale to assist drainage of the pleural space and lung reexpansion.
- Call for a portable chest X-ray to check tube position.
- Take the patient's vital signs every 15 minutes for 1 hour, then as his condition indicates.
- Auscultate the patient's lungs at least every 4 hours following the procedure to assess air exchange in the affected lung.

NURSING ALERT Diminished or absent breath sounds indicate that the lung hasn't reexpanded.

✦ SPECIAL CONSIDERATIONS

- Clamping the chest tube isn't recommended because of the risk of tension pneumothorax.
- During patient transport, keep the thoracic drainage system below chest level.

NURSING ALERT If the chest tube comes out, cover the site immediately with 4″ × 4″ gauze pads and tape in place. Stay with the patient, and monitor vital signs every 10 minutes. Look for signs and symptoms of tension pneumothorax (hypotension, distended jugular veins, absent breath sounds, tracheal shift, hypoxemia, weak and rapid pulse, dyspnea, tachypnea, diaphoresis, chest pain). Have another staff member notify the physician and gather equipment needed to reinsert tube.

- Place the rubber-tipped clamps at bedside.

NURSING ALERT If the drainage system cracks, or a tube disconnects, clamp the chest tube as close to the insertion site as possible.

NURSING ALERT No air or liquid can escape from the pleural space while the tube is clamped; observe the patient closely for signs and symptoms of tension pneumothorax while clamp is in place.

- The tube may be clamped with the large, smooth, rubber-tipped clamps for several hours before removal.

- As an alternative to clamping the tube, submerge the distal end in a container of normal saline solution to create a temporary water seal while you replace the drainage system. Follow facility policy.
- Look for signs and symptoms of respiratory distress, an indication that air or fluid remains trapped in the pleural space.
- Chest tubes are usually removed within 7 days to prevent infection. (See *Removing a chest tube.*)

Complications
- Injury to the heart, great vessels, or lungs, liver, spleen, or diaphragm
- Bleeding from the chest wall
- Occlusion of the chest tube
- Subcutaneous air pocketing
- Local or systemic infection
- Contralateral tension pneumothorax

▶ PATIENT TEACHING

Be sure to cover:
- why a chest tube is needed and what to expect during insertion, care, and removal of the chest tube
- coughing, deep breathing exercises, and using an incentive spirometer to expand the lung and prevent complications
- need for pain control and the options available

- need to report a sudden onset of shortness of breath or chest pain.

✦⊃ DOCUMENTATION

- Date and time of chest tube insertion
- Location of insertion site and appearance
- Drainage system and suction used
- Name of the physician performing the procedure
- Patient's tolerance of the procedure
- Use of analgesics
- Patient teaching performed
- Presence of drainage and bubbling

NURSING ALERT Be sure to include drainage on the patient's intake and output record.

- Type, amount, and consistency of drainage
- Vital signs, auscultation findings, complications, and nursing actions taken

Selected references
Coughlin, A.M., and Parchinsky, C. "Go With the Flow of Chest Tube Therapy," *Nursing* 36(3):36-41, March 2006.

Giacomini, M., et al. "How to Avoid and Manage Pneumothorax," *Journal of Vascular Access* 7(1):7-14, January-March 2006.

Roman, M., and Mercado, D. "Review of Chest Tube Use," *Medsurg Nursing* 15(1):41-43, February 2006.

REMOVING A CHEST TUBE

After the patient's lung has reexpanded, you may assist the practitioner in removing the chest tube. First, obtain the patient's vital signs and perform a respiratory assessment. After explaining the procedure to the patient, administer an analgesic, as ordered, 30 minutes before tube removal. Then follow the steps listed below:
- Place the patient in semi-Fowler's position or on his unaffected side.
- Place a linen-saver pad under the affected side to protect the linen from drainage and to provide a place to put the chest tube after removal.
- Put on clean gloves and remove the chest tube dressings, being careful not to dislodge the chest tube. Discard soiled dressings.
- The practitioner puts on sterile gloves, holds the chest tube in place with sterile forceps, and cuts the suture anchoring the tube.
- Make sure the chest tube is securely clamped, and then instruct the patient to perform Valsalva's maneuver by exhaling fully and bearing down. *Valsalva's maneuver effectively increases intrathoracic pressure.*
- The doctor holds an airtight dressing, usually petroleum gauze, *so that he can cover the insertion site with it immediately after removing the tube.* After he removes the tube and covers the insertion site, secure the dressing with tape. Be sure to cover the dressing completely with tape *to make it as airtight as possible.*
- Dispose of the chest tube, soiled gloves, and equipment according to your facility's policy.
- Take vital signs as ordered, and assess the depth and quality of the patient's respirations. Assess the patient carefully for signs and symptoms of pneumothorax, subcutaneous emphysema, or infection.

Closed-wound drain management

● OVERVIEW

- Promotes healing and prevents swelling by suctioning serosanguineous fluid that accumulates around a wound site
- Typically inserted during surgery in anticipation of substantial postoperative drainage
- Reduces risk of infection and skin breakdown and the number of dressing changes
- Common types include Hemovac and Jackson-Pratt closed drainage systems, which consist of perforated tubing connected to portable vacuum unit with distal end of the tubing lying in the wound, and usually leaving the body from a site other than the primary suture line
- Calls for drainage to be emptied and measured frequently to maintain maximum suction and prevent strain on the suture line

Contraindications
- None known

❖ EQUIPMENT

Graduated biohazard cylinder • sterile laboratory container, if needed • alcohol pads • gloves • gown • face shield • trash bag • sterile gauze pads • antiseptic cleaning agent • prepackaged povidone-iodine swabs • optional: label

❚❚❚ ESSENTIAL STEPS

- Explain the procedure to the patient and provide privacy.
- Wash your hands thoroughly.
- Maintain asepsis throughout the procedure.
- Wear appropriate personal protective equipment throughout the procedure.
- Unclip the vacuum unit from the patient's bed or gown.
- Release the vacuum by removing the spout plug on the collection chamber, allowing the container to expand completely as it draws in air.
- Empty the unit's contents into a graduated biohazard cylinder, and note the amount and appearance of the drainage.
- If diagnostic tests will be performed on the fluid specimen, pour the drainage directly into a sterile laboratory container, note the amount and appearance, label the specimen, and send it to the laboratory.
- Use an alcohol pad to clean the unit's spout and plug.
- To reestablish the vacuum, fully compress the vacuum unit.

- With one hand holding the unit compressed, replace the spout plug with your other hand. (See *Using a closed-wound drainage system.*)
- Check the patency of the equipment, and make sure the tubing is free from twists, kinks, and leaks.

◈ **NURSING ALERT** The vacuum unit should remain compressed when you release manual pressure; rapid reinflation indicates an air leak (such as an insecure spout plug).

- Secure the vacuum unit to the patient's gown, below wound level to promote drainage.
- Observe the sutures that secure the drain to the patient's skin; look for signs of pulling or tearing and for swelling or infection of the surrounding skin.
- Gently clean the sutures with sterile gauze pads soaked in an antiseptic cleaning agent or with a povidone-iodine swab.
- Properly dispose of drainage, solutions, and trash bag, and clean or dispose of soiled equipment and supplies according to facility policy.
- Remove and discard your gloves and personal protective equipment and wash your hands thoroughly.

USING A CLOSED-WOUND DRAINAGE SYSTEM

The portable closed-wound drainage system draws drainage from a wound site, such as the chest wall postmastectomy shown at left, by means of a Y-tube. To empty the drainage, remove the plug and empty it into a graduated cylinder. To reestablish suction, compress the drainage unit against a firm surface to expel air and, while holding it down, replace the plug with your other hand, as shown below middle. The same principle is used for the Jackson-Pratt bulb drain, as shown below right.

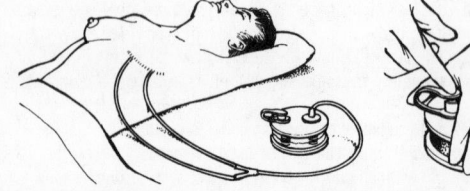 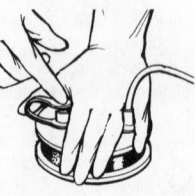 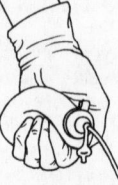

- Empty the drain and measure its contents once during each shift if drainage has accumulated; more often if drainage is excessive to maintain maximum suction and avoid straining the drain's suture line.
- Empty the drain and measure its contents before the patient ambulates to prevent the weight of drainage from pulling on the drain as the patient ambulates.
- If the patient has more than one closed drain, number the drains so you can record drainage from each site.

⬥ **NURSING ALERT** Be careful not to mistake chest tubes for closed-wound drains because the vacuum of a chest tube should never be released.

Complications
- Occlusion of the tubing by fibrin, clots, or other particles that reduce or obstruct drainage
- Local infection

Be sure to cover:
- purpose of closed-wound drainage system
- importance of not pulling on drains and of having the drain emptied before ambulation
- signs and symptoms to report, such as redness or pain at insertion site
- how to empty drains and provide site care, if patient is to go home before drains are removed.

- Date and time of drain emptying and location of drain
- Appearance of the drain site and presence of swelling or signs of infection
- Equipment malfunction and consequent nursing action
- Patient's tolerance of the treatment
- Patient teaching
- Color, consistency, type, and amount of drainage on the intake and output record (if patient has more than one drain, number the drains, and record the information separately for each drainage site)

Selected references
Parker, M.J., et al. "Closed Suction Drainage for Hip and Knee Arthroplasty: A Meta-analysis," *Journal of Bone and Joint Surgery* 86-A(6):1145-152, June 2004.

Colostomy and ileostomy care

● OVERVIEW

- Indicated for patient with ascending or transverse colostomy or ileostomy who wears an external pouch to collect watery or pasty fecal matter, control odor, and protect the stoma and peristomal skin
- Requires knowledge of disposable pouching systems that can be used for 2 to 7 days; some models last longer
- Requires all pouching systems to be changed immediately if a leak develops, or emptied when one-third to one-half full
- May require that pouches for patients with ileostomy be emptied 4 to 5 times daily
- May use pouching system that provides the best adhesive seal and skin protection for individual patient; also depends on stoma location and structure, availability of supplies, wearing time, consistency of effluent, personal preference, and finances

Contraindications
- None known

❖ EQUIPMENT

Pouching system • stoma measuring guide • stoma paste • plastic bag • water • washcloth • towel • closure clamp • toilet or bedpan • water or pouch cleaning solution • gloves • facial tissues • optional: ostomy belt, paper tape, mild nonmoisturizing soap, skin shaving equipment, liquid skin sealant, and pouch deodorant

Pouching systems may be drainable or closed-bottomed, disposable or reusable, adhesive-backed, and one-piece or two-piece.

║▌ ESSENTIAL STEPS

- Confirm patient's identity using two patient identifiers according to facility policy.
- Explain the procedure to the patient.
- Wash your hands thoroughly.

- Wear appropriate personal protective equipment, when necessary, throughout all procedures.
- Provide for patient privacy.

FITTING THE POUCH AND SKIN BARRIER
- Measure the stoma using the stoma measuring guide.
- For a pouch with an attached skin barrier, select the pouch system with an appropriate opening size.
- For an adhesive-backed pouch with a separate skin barrier, trace the selected size opening onto the adhesive backing and cut out the opening.
- If the adhesive-backed pouch has pre-cut openings, select an opening that's ⅛″ larger than the stoma; if the pouch comes without an opening, cut the hole ⅛″ wider than the measured tracing.

◆ **NURSING ALERT** A cut-to-fit system works best for an irregularly shaped stoma.

- A two-piece pouching system with flanges may be used. (See *Applying a skin barrier and pouch.*)
- Avoid a pouch that's too tight to avoid trauma to the stoma or too big to avoid skin exposure to fecal matter and moisture.

◆ **NURSING ALERT** Because the stoma has no pain receptors, a constrictive opening could injure the stoma or skin tissue without the patient feeling any warning discomfort.

- The patient with a descending or sigmoid colostomy who has formed stools and whose ostomy doesn't secrete much mucus may wear only a pouch whose opening closely matches stoma size.

APPLYING OR CHANGING THE POUCH
- Put on gloves, and remove and discard the old pouch.
- Wipe the stoma and peristomal skin gently with a facial tissue.
- Wash the peristomal skin with mild soap and water and gently pat it dry.
- Allow the skin to dry thoroughly.
- Inspect the peristomal skin and stoma.
- If necessary, shave the hair away from the stoma to promote a better seal and avoid skin irritation from hair pulling against the adhesive.
- If applying a separate skin barrier, peel off the paper backing of the prepared skin barrier, center the barrier

over the stoma, and press gently to ensure adhesion.
- Outline the stoma on the back of the skin barrier, if desired, with a thin ring of stoma paste to provide extra skin protection.
- Remove the paper backing from the adhesive side of the pouching system, center the pouch opening over the stoma, and press gently to secure.
- For a pouching system with flanges, align the lip of the pouch flange with the bottom edge of the skin barrier flange and gently press around the circumference of the pouch flange until the pouch clicks into its secured position. Holding the barrier against the skin, gently pull on the pouch to confirm the seal between flanges.
- Encourage the patient to stay in position for about 5 minutes as his body warmth improves adherence and softens a rigid skin barrier.
- Attach an ostomy belt to further secure the pouch, if desired. (Some pouches have belt loops, and others have plastic adapters for belts.)
- Leave a bit of air in the pouch to allow drainage to fall to the bottom.
- Apply the closure clamp, if necessary.
- If desired, apply paper tape in a picture-frame fashion to the pouch edges for additional security.

EMPTYING THE POUCH
- Put on gloves.
- Tilt the bottom of the pouch upward and remove the closure clamp.
- Turn up a cuff on the lower end of the pouch and allow it to drain into the toilet or bedpan.
- Wipe the bottom of the pouch and reapply the closure clamp.
- Rinse the bottom portion of the pouch with cool tap water, if desired.

◆ **NURSING ALERT** Don't aim water up near the top of the pouch when rinsing because this may loosen the seal on the skin.

- A two-piece flanged system can also be emptied by unsnapping the pouch and letting the drainage flow into the toilet.
- Release flatus through the gas release valve, if present, or by tilting the pouch bottom upward, releasing the clamp, and expelling the flatus.

◆ **NURSING ALERT** Never make a pinhole in a pouch to release gas because this destroys the odor-proof seal.

- Remove gloves.

♦ SPECIAL CONSIDERATIONS

- Demonstrate and explain the procedure to the patient and encourage self-care.
- Use adhesive solvents and removers only after patch-testing the patient's skin to detect skin irritation or hypersensitivity reactions.
- Use a liquid skin sealant, if necessary, to give additional protection from drainage and adhesive irritants.
- Between 6 weeks and 1 year after surgery, the stoma will shrink to its permanent size and pattern-making preparations will be unnecessary un-

less the patient gains weight, has additional surgery, or injures the stoma.

- Remove the pouching system if the patient reports burning or itching beneath it or purulent drainage around the stoma.
- Notify the physician or therapist of any skin irritation, breakdown, rash, or unusual appearance of the stoma or peristomal area.
- Use commercial pouch deodorants, if desired.
- If the patient wears a reusable pouching system, suggest that he obtain two or more systems so he can wear one while the other dries after cleaning.
- Change the pouching system, if possible, when the bowel is least active, usually between 2 and 4 hours after meals.

Complications
- Stoma injury
- Allergic reaction
- Skin irritation and breakdown

▶ PATIENT TEACHING

Be sure to cover:
- how to perform ostomy self-care
- care of equipment
- signs and symptoms of adverse effects and appropriate interventions
- importance of avoiding odor-causing foods, such as fish, eggs, onions, and garlic
- need for follow-up care
- strategies for emotional adjustment
- availability of ostomy support groups.

● DOCUMENTATION

- Date and time of ostomy care
- Location of the stoma
- Condition of the stoma, including size, shape, and color
- Character of drainage, including color, amount, type, and consistency
- Condition of the peristomal skin, including redness, irritation, breakdown, bleeding, or other conditions
- Type of appliance used, appliance size, and type of adhesive used
- Patient teaching and the patient's response to self-care

Selected references

Berg, K., and Seidler, H. "Randomized Crossover Comparison of Adversely Coupled Colostomy Pouching Systems," *Ostomy/Wound Management* 51(3):30-32, 34, 36, March 2005.

Cronin, E. "Best Practice in Discharging Patients With a Stoma," *Nursing Times* 101(47):67-68, November 2005.

Notter, J. and Burnard, P. "Preparing for Loop Ileostomy Surgery: Women's Accounts from a Qualitative Study," *International Journal of Nursing Studies* 43(2):147-59, February 2006.

Ratliff, C.R., et al. "Descriptive Study of Peristomal Complications," *Journal of Wound, Ostomy, and Continence Nursing* 32(1):33-37, January-February 2005.

APPLYING A SKIN BARRIER AND POUCH

Fitting a skin barrier and ostomy pouch properly can be done in a few steps. A commonly used, two-piece pouching system with flanges is depicted below.

Measure the stoma using a measuring guide.

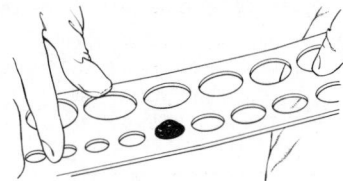

Trace the appropriate circle carefully on the back of the skin barrier.

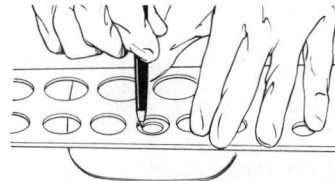

Cut the circular opening in the skin barrier. Bevel the edges to keep them from irritating the patient.

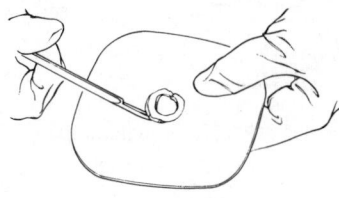

Remove the backing from the skin barrier and moisten it or apply barrier paste, as needed, along the edge of the circular opening.

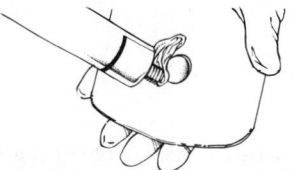

Center the skin barrier over the stoma, adhesive side down, and gently press it to the skin.

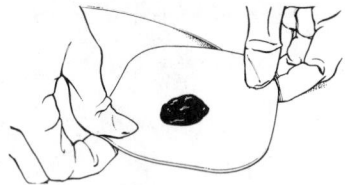

Gently press the pouch opening onto the ring until it snaps into place.

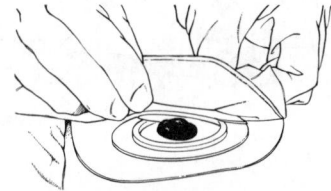

Continuous passive motion therapy

● OVERVIEW

- Postoperative treatment that moves patient's joint through full range of motion (ROM), without using muscles, aiding in recovery after joint surgery
- Improves or maintains joint mobility and helps prevent contractures
- Indicated for temporary or permanent loss of mobility; total knee replacement; anterior cruciate ligament reconstruction; tendon repair; joint manipulation under anesthesia; arthroscopic debridement of adhesions; open reduction and internal fixation (stabilization) of intra-articular fractures; rotator cuff repair; or articular cartilage micro fracture or transplantation
- Continuous passive motion (CPM) devices available for the knee, ankle, shoulder, elbow, wrist, and hand (see *Continuous passive motion machine*)
- Gradually moves the joint resulting in accelerated recovery time by decreasing soft-tissue stiffness, increasing ROM, promoting healing of joint surfaces and soft tissue, and preventing the development of motion-limiting adhesions (scar tissue)

Contraindications

- Unhealed or unstable fracture
- Septic joints
- Acute thrombophlebitis

❖ EQUIPMENT

Passive motion device ● optional: pillow, adhesive tape, gauze for padding bone prominences

Equipment preparation

- Review manufacturer's instructions and facility policy about using the device.
- Make sure the settings on the device are as ordered by the practitioner and physical therapist and that it's in working order.
- Wash hands thoroughly.
- Specialty CPM machines entail a more involved setup, and a therapist is usually needed for calibration and setup.

❚❚❚ ESSENTIAL STEPS

- The practitioner determines how the CPM unit should be used by the patient (such as speed, duration of usage, amount of motion, and rate of increase of motion); the calibrations are set by the manufacturer or physical therapist.
- Review the procedure with the patient.
- Inform the patient about the purpose of the device and that the joint will be moved through a ROM for an extended period. Tell him that the CPM machine can significantly reduce recovery time, promote healing, reduce the development of adhesions and scar tissue, and decrease stiffness.
- Apply the device, as indicated, using the prescribed settings.

CONTINUOUS PASSIVE MOTION MACHINE

Postoperatively, a continuous passive motion machine may be used to aid in exercising the patient's affected joint. This is an illustration of one such device used for the lower leg.

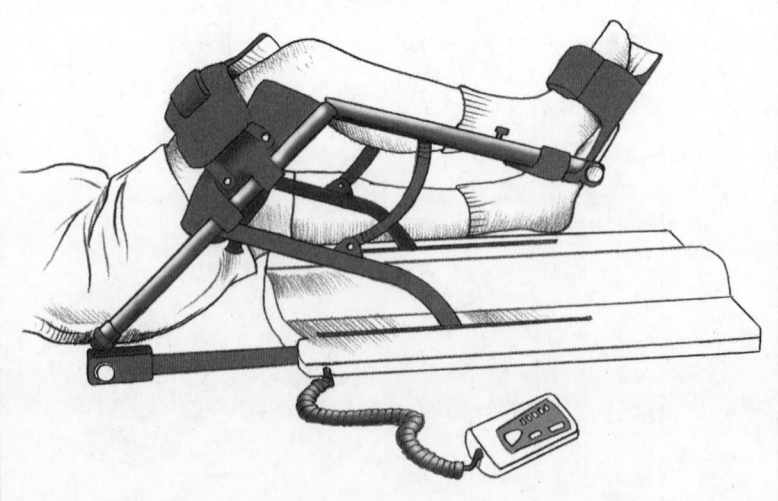

- Keep the patient as comfortable as possible.
- Give analgesics, as ordered, and monitor for adverse effects.
- Maintain proper body alignment.
- Use splints or braces, as ordered.
- Elevate the affected area and apply ice, as tolerated, when the patient's joint isn't in motion.
- Monitor the patient's vital signs.
- Monitor laboratory test results.
- Assess mobility and ROM; inspect skin area where device is attached for any changes.
- Monitor the patient for complications.

Complications
- Increased pain
- Intolerance of the procedure

Be sure to cover:
- use of device and intended effect, including how to apply the device and what settings should be used
- activity restrictions and lifestyle changes, as appropriate
- how to use the device at home, if ordered
- instructions for physical and occupational therapy, as indicated
- importance of follow-up care.

- Time and date of procedure
- Settings ordered, length of time patient tolerated setting, any changes in settings and reason for changes
- Patient's tolerance of procedure
- Patient teaching and return demonstration, as appropriate

Selected references
Friemert, B., et al. "Benefits of Active Motion for Joint Position Sense," *Knee Surgery, Sports Traumatology, and Arthroscopy* 23:1-7, November 2005.

Lynch, D., et al. "Continuous Passive Motion Improves Shoulder Joint Integrity Following Stroke," *Clinical Rehabilitation* 19(6):594-99, September 2005.

Zeifang, E., et al. "Continuous Passive Motion Versus Immobilisation in a Cast after Surgical Treatment of Idiopathic Club Foot in Infants: A Prospective, Blinded, Randomized, Clinical Study," *The Journal of Bone and Joint Surgery* 87(12):1663-65, December 2005.

Continuous renal replacement therapy

● OVERVIEW

- Indicated for patients with acute renal failure and those unable to tolerate traditional hemodialysis such as patients with hypotension
- Given round the clock, providing patients with continuous therapy and sparing them the destabilizing hemodynamic and electrolyte changes characteristic of intermittent hemodialysis (IHD)
- Slow continuous ultrafiltration: uses arteriovenous access and the patient's blood pressure to circulate blood through a hemofilter; patient doesn't receive any fluids
- Continuous arteriovenous hemofiltration (CAVH): uses the patient's blood pressure and arteriovenous access to circulate blood through a flow resistance hemofilter; patient receives replacement fluids to maintain filter patency and systemic blood pressure
- Continuous arteriovenous hemodialysis (CAVH-D): combines hemodialysis with hemofiltration; infusion pump moves dialysate solution concurrent to blood flow, adding the ability to continuously remove solute while removing fluid; like CAVH, may also be performed in patients with hypotension and fluid overload
- Continuous venovenous hemofiltration (CVVH): similar to CAVH except that a vein provides access that's channeled through the "arterial" lumen of a dual-lumen catheter and then mechanically pumped to the hemofilter
- Continuous venovenous hemodialysis: similar to CAVH-D, except that a vein provides access while a pump is used to move dialysate solution concurrent with blood flow

Contraindications
- None known

❖ EQUIPMENT

Hemofiltration device • catheter-access • hemodynamic monitoring devices • pump • collection device • pressure monitors, as appropriate • replacement fluid or solution • gauze pads • povidone-iodine solution • syringes with needles • heparin solution • gloves (clean and sterile) • personal protective equipment

Equipment preparation
- Wash your hands thoroughly
- Ensure that solutions are readily available for use
- Assemble the equipment at the patient's bedside according to the manufacturer's recommendations and your facility's policy, and explain the procedure to the patient. (See *Setup for CAVH and CVVH*.)

▐▐ ESSENTIAL STEPS

- Confirm the patient's identify using two patient identifiers according to facility policy.
- Weigh the patient, take baseline vital signs, and make sure that all necessary laboratory studies have been done (such as electrolyte levels, coagulation factors, complete blood count, blood urea nitrogen, and creatinine studies).
- Ensure that the patient has signed a consent form if catheter is to be inserted. If necessary, assist with inserting the catheters into the femoral artery and vein, using strict sterile technique. An internal arteriovenous fistula or external arteriovenous shunt may sometimes be used instead of the femoral route. If ordered, flush both catheters with the heparin flush solution to prevent clotting.
- Apply occlusive dressings to the insertion sites, and mark the dressings with the date and time. Secure the tubing and connections with tape.
- Put on sterile gloves and mask.
- Prepare the connection sites by cleaning them with gauze pads soaked in povidone-iodine solution, and then connect them to the exit port of each catheter.
- Turn on the hemofilter and monitor the blood-flow rate through the circuit. The flow rate is typically 500 to 900 ml/hour.
- Inspect the ultrafiltrate during the procedure. It should remain clear yellow, with no gross blood. Pink-tinged or blood ultrafiltrate may signal a membrane leak in the hemofilter, which permits bacterial contamination. If a leak occurs, notify the practitioner so that the hemofilter can be replaced.
- If the ultrafiltrate flow rate decreases, raise the bed to increase the distance between the collection device and the hemofilter. Lower the bed to decrease the flow rate.

(continued)

SETUP FOR CAVH AND CVVH

Continuous renal replacement therapy is frequently performed using one of the two systems described here.

Continuous arteriovenous hemofiltration

In continuous arteriovenous hemofiltration (CAVH), the physician inserts two large-bore, single-lumen catheters. One catheter is inserted into an artery—most commonly, the femoral artery. The other catheter is inserted into a vein, usually the femoral, subclavian, or internal jugular vein. During CAVH, the patient's arterial blood pressure serves as a natural pump, driving blood through the arterial line. A hemofilter removes water and toxic solutes (ultrafiltrate) from the blood. Replacement fluid is infused into a port on the arterial side. The same port can be used to infuse heparin. The venous line carries the replacement fluid and purified blood to the patient.

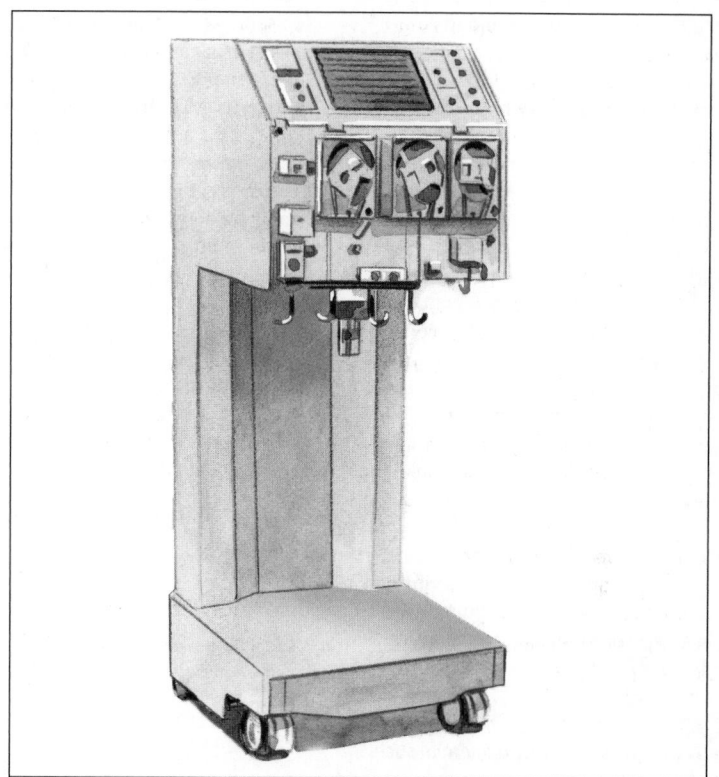

Continuous venovenous hemofiltration

In continuous venovenous hemofiltration (CVVH), the physician inserts a special double-lumen catheter into a large vein, commonly the subclavian, femoral, or internal jugular vein (as shown at right). Because the catheter is in a vein, an external pump is used to move blood through the system. The patient's venous blood moves through the "arterial" lumen to the pump, which then pushes the blood through the catheter to the hemofilter. Here, water and toxic solutes (ultrafiltrate) are removed from the patient's blood and drain into a collection device. Blood cells aren't removed because they're too large to pass through the filter. As the blood exits the hemofilter, it's then pumped through the "venous" lumen back to the patient.

Several components of the pump provide safety mechanisms. Pressure monitors on the pump maintain the flow of blood through the circuit at a constant rate. An air detector traps air bubbles before the blood returns to the patient. A venous trap collects blood clots that may be in the blood. A blood leak detector signals when blood is found in the ultrafiltrate; a venous clamp operates if air is detected in the circuit or if there's a disconnection in the blood line.

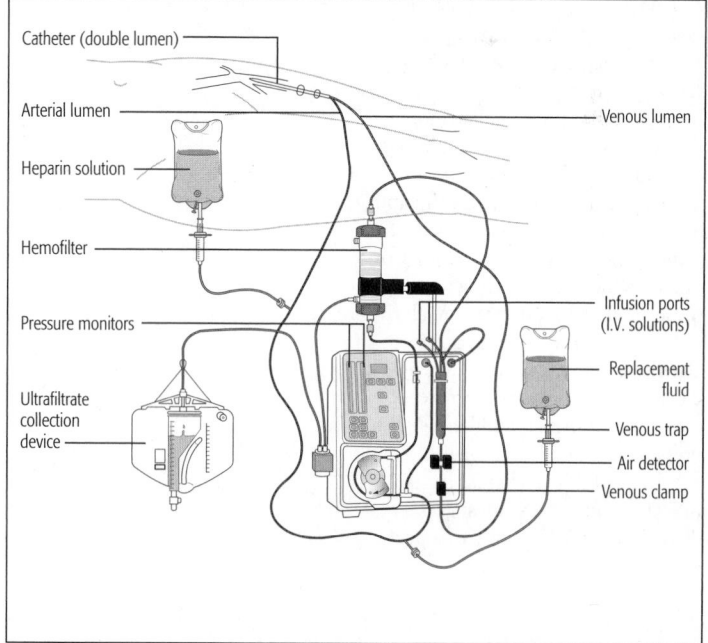

NURSING ALERT Clamping the ultrafiltrate line is contraindicated with some types of hemofilters because pressure may build up in the filter, clotting it and collapsing the blood compartment.

- Calculate the amount of filtration replacement fluid every hour, as ordered, or according to your facility's policy. Infuse the prescribed amount and type of replacement fluid through the infusion pump into the arterial side of the circuit.

NURSING ALERT When calculating the amount of replacement fluid, total the amount of fluid in the collection device from the previous hour with other fluid losses the patient may have (such as blood loss, emesis, or nasogastric tube drainage). From this total, subtract the patient's fluid intake for the past hour and the net fluid loss prescribed by the practitioner.

- Assess hemodynamic parameters, including pulmonary artery pressure, central venous pressure, pulmonary artery wedge pressure, and blood pressure hourly, or more frequently, if indicated.

NURSING ALERT Stay alert for indications of hypovolemia, such as falling blood pressure and a decrease in hemodynamic pressures, from too rapid removal of ultrafiltrate, or of hypervolemia due to excessive fluid replacement with a decrease in ultrafiltrate.

- Institute continuous cardiac monitoring, as indicated, for arrhythmias (may indicate electrolyte imbalance).
- If the patient is receiving CVVH and the pressure alarm sounds, check the catheter for kinks, disconnections, or other problems. Determine whether the arterial or venous pressure alarm sounded; if it's the arterial pressure alarm, check the arterial lumen and if it's the venous pressure alarm, check the venous lumen. A sudden rise in pressure indicates blockage in the catheter or tubing, whereas a significant drop in pressure suggests a disconnection or opening of a port.

- Because blood flows through an extracorporeal circuit during CAVH and CVVH, the blood in the hemofilter may need to be anticoagulated. To do this, infuse heparin in low doses (usually starting at 500 units/hour) into an infusion port on the arterial side of the setup. Measure thrombin clotting time or the activated clotting time. This ensures that the circuit, not the patient, is anticoagulated. A normal value for activated clotting time is 100 seconds; during continuous renal replacement therapy it's kept between 100 and 300 seconds, depending on the patient's clotting times. If the value is too high or low, the practitioner adjusts the heparin dose accordingly.

- Monitor the patient's vital signs and weight hourly, or as indicated.
- Assess the leg for signs of obstructed blood flow, such as coolness, pallor, and weak pulse. Check the groin area on the affected side for signs of hematoma. Ask the patient whether he has pain at the insertion sites.
- If possible, infuse medications or blood through another line rather than the venous line to prevent clotting in the hemofilter.
- Assess all pulses (dorsalis pedis, posterior tibial, popliteal, and femoral) in the affected leg every hour for the first 4 hours, then every 2 hours.
- To help prevent clots in the hemofilter and prevent kinks in the catheter, make sure the patient doesn't bend the affected leg more than 30 degrees at the hip.
- Obtain serum electrolyte levels every 4 to 6 hours, or as ordered; anticipate adjustments in replacement fluid or dialysate based on the results.
- Inspect the site dressing every 4 to 8 hours for infection and bleeding. To prevent infection, perform skin care at the catheter insertion sites every 48 hours, using sterile technique. Cover the sites with an occlusive dressing.

Complications
- Bleeding, hemorrhage
- Hemofilter occlusion
- Infection
- Hypotension
- Thrombosis
- Hypothermia
- Air embolism

Be sure to cover:
- care of the equipment and catheter sites
- signs and symptoms to report
- importance of keeping the extremity still.

- Time treatment began
- Type of therapy and solutions used, including amounts
- Hemodynamic parameters
- Weights
- Pulses including location and character
- Care to access site
- Medications infused including date and time of administration
- Patient's tolerance of procedure

Selected references

American Nephrology Nurses Association. "Standards and Guidelines of Practice for Continuous Renal Replacement Therapy (Revised 2005 edition)," Pitman, N.J., 2005.

Niu, S.E, and Li, I.C. "Quality of Life of Patients Having Renal Replacement Therapy," *Journal of Advanced Nursing* 51(1):15-21, July 2005.

Schatell, D. "Home Dialysis, Home Dialysis Central, and What You Can Do Today," *Nephrology Nursing Journal* 32(2):235-38, March-April 2005.

Debridement

● OVERVIEW

- Removes necrotic tissue by mechanical, chemical, or surgical means
- Includes wet-to-dry dressings, irrigation, hydrotherapy, and excision of dead tissue with forceps and scissors
- May be performed at the bedside or a specially prepared area such as a hydrotherapy tub
- May involve combination of debridement techniques
- Conservative sharp debridement: removes necrotic tissue by using a scalpel, scissors, or laser
- Wet-to-dry dressings: used for wounds with extensive necrotic tissue and minimal drainage
- Irrigation of a wound with a pressurized antiseptic solution: cleans tissue and removes wound debris and excess tissue
- Hydrotherapy: involves immersing the patient in a tank of warm water, with intermittent agitation of the water
- Daily debridement: prevents hemorrhage and the need for surgical interventions
- Other debridement techniques: chemical debridement (with wound cleaning beads or topical agents that remove exudate and debris) or surgical excision and skin grafting (usually reserved for deep burns or ulcers)

Contraindications

- Closed blisters over partial-thickness burns

❖ EQUIPMENT

CONSERVATIVE SHARP DEBRIDEMENT
Ordered pain medication • two pairs of sterile gloves • two gowns or aprons • mask • cap • sterile scissors • sterile forceps • sterile gauze pads • sterile solutions and medications, as ordered • hemostatic agents, as ordered
WET-TO-DRY DRESSINGS
Sterile saline solution • waterproof trash bag • sterile gauze pads • clean gloves • tape or adhesive bandage
IRRIGATION
Prescribed irrigating solution • irrigation syringe or catheter • clean gloves
HYDROTHERAPY
Hydrotherapy tub • sterile dressings • waterproof trash bag • clean gloves
DAILY DEBRIDEMENT (FOR HEMORRHAGE CONTROL)
Needle holder • gut suture with needle • silver nitrate sticks

Equipment preparation

- Review the order for debridement, including prescribed solutions and type of debridement
- Ensure that solutions are at the proper temperature
- Administer medication for pain
- Assemble equipment at the bedside, as appropriate
- Check the expiration date on each sterile package and inspect for tears
- Place waterproof trash bag near patient to avoid reaching over the sterile field or wound

▮▮ ESSENTIAL STEPS

- Confirm the patient's identify using two patient identifiers according to facility policy.
- Explain the procedure to the patient and family
- Assist the patient in using distraction and relaxation techniques, as appropriate
- Provide privacy
- Wash hands thoroughly
- Maintain asepsis through the procedure
- Wear personal protective equipment

CONSERVATIVE SHARP DEBRIDEMENT
- Expose only the area to be debrided to prevent chilling and fluid and electrolyte loss.
- Remove the dressings and clean the wound.
- Remove your soiled gloves, and put on sterile gloves.
- Lift loosened edges of eschar with forceps.
- Use the blunt edge of scissors or forceps to probe the eschar.
- Cut the dead tissue from the wound with scissors.
- Leave a ¼″ (0.6-cm) edge on remaining eschar to avoid cutting into viable tissue.
- Irrigate the wound to remove debris.
- Because debridement removes only dead tissue, bleeding should be minimal. If bleeding occurs, apply gentle pressure on the wound with sterile gauze pads and apply a hemostatic drug.
- If bleeding persists, notify the practitioner; maintain pressure on the wound until he arrives.
- Excessive bleeding or spurting vessels may require ligation.
- Perform additional procedures, such as an applying topical drugs and replacing dressings, as ordered.

WET-TO-DRY DRESSING
- Put on clean gloves.
- Slowly remove the old dressings, using saline solution to moisten parts of the dressing that don't easily pull away. Discard old dressing and gloves in a waterproof trash bag.
- Put on sterile gloves.

- Using sterile technique, moisten a gauze pad with saline solution and loosely pack it into the wound. Make sure that the entire wound surface is lightly covered.
- Apply an outer dressing and secure it with tape or an adhesive bandage.
- Remove the dressing after it completely dries and becomes adherent to the necrotic tissue (4 to 6 hours).

IRRIGATION
- Using sterile technique, instill a slow, steady stream of solution into the wound with an irrigating syringe or catheter.

HYDROTHERAPY
- Prepare the tub and check the patient's vital signs.
- Assist the patient into the tub.
- After the affected area has been in the water for the prescribed time, put on clean gloves, remove old dressings, and discard items in a waterproof trash bag.
- Spray rinse and pat dry the patient before reapplying sterile dressings.

✦ SPECIAL CONSIDERATIONS

- If possible, work with an assistant to complete the procedure quickly, thus limiting the patient's pain
- Monitor the patient's vital signs, peripheral pulses, and pulse oximetry.
- Monitor the patient for signs of bleeding.
- Assess the patient for complications.
- Assess the patient's pain level and response to analgesics.
- Assess the patient for signs and symptoms of infection.
- Monitor laboratory test results.

Complications
- Infection
- Bleeding or hemorrhage
- Fluid and electrolyte imbalance

▶ PATIENT TEACHING

Be sure to cover:
- why the procedure is needed
- that the procedure is painful but that pain medication will be readily available
- distraction and relaxation techniques.

⚫◇ DOCUMENTATION

- Date and time of debridement
- Area debrided
- Solutions and drugs used
- Wound condition, including signs of infection or skin breakdown
- Patient's tolerance of procedure
- Indications for additional therapy

Selected references

Andersen, I. "Debridement Methods in Wound Care," *Nursing Standard* 20(24):65-66, 67, 70, February 2006.

Beitz, J.M. "Wound Debridement: Therapeutic Options and Care Considerations," *Nursing Clinics of North America* 40(2):233-49, June 2005.

Davies, C.E., et al. "Exploring Debridement Options for Chronic Venous Leg Ulcers," *British Journal of Nursing* 14(7):393-97, April 2005.

Ichioka, S., et al. "Benefits of Surgical Reconstruction in Pressure Ulcers with a Non-advancing Edge and Scar Formation," *Journal of Wound Care* 14(7):301-305, July 2005.

Mosti, G., et.al. "The Debridement of Hard to Heal Leg Ulcers by Means of a New Device Based on Fluid-jet Technology," *International Wound Journal* 2(4):310-14, December 2005.

Defibrillation

● OVERVIEW

- Performed as the definitive treatment for the patient with ventricular fibrillation
- Involves using electrode paddles to direct an electric current through the patient's heart causing the myocardium to depolarize which, in turn, encourages the sinoatrial node to resume control of the heart's electrical activity
- May be monophasic (delivery of a single current of electricity [high amount] that travels in one direction between the two pods on the patient's chest) or biphasic (delivery of electrical current that travels in a positive direction for a specified time and then reverses to a negative direction [usually less energy required])
- When performed, electrode paddles delivering current placed on patient's chest or, during cardiac surgery, directly on the myocardium
- Also used to treat the patient with pulseless ventricular tachycardia

Contraindications
- None known

❖ EQUIPMENT

Defibrillator • external paddles • internal paddles (sterilized for cardiac surgery) • conductive medium pads • electrocardiogram (ECG) monitor with recorder • oxygen therapy equipment • handheld resuscitation bag • airway equipment • emergency pacing equipment • emergency cardiac medications

▐▐▌ ESSENTIAL STEPS

- Assess the patient to determine unresponsiveness and absence of respirations and pulse.

  NURSING ALERT In an infant, use the brachial artery to assess for a pulse.

- Call for help and perform cardiopulmonary resuscitation (CPR) until the defibrillator and emergency equipment arrives.

  NURSING ALERT Use personal protective equipment during resuscitation.

- Expose the patient's chest.
- If the defibrillator has "quick-look" capability, place the paddles on the patient's chest to quickly view the cardiac rhythm. Otherwise, connect the monitoring leads of the defibrillator to the patient, and assess his cardiac rhythm.

  NURSING ALERT Because ventricular fibrillation leads to death if not corrected, the success of defibrillation depends on your early recognition and quick treatment of this arrhythmia.

- Apply conductive pads at the paddle placement positions.
- For anterolateral placement, position one paddle to the right of the upper sternum, just below the right clavicle, and the other over the fifth or sixth intercostal space at the left anterior axillary line.
- For anteroposterior placement, position the anterior paddle directly over the heart at the precordium, to the left of the lower sternal border and the flat posterior paddle under the patient's body beneath the heart and immediately below the scapulae (but not under the vertebral column).
- Turn on the defibrillator.
- Set the energy level for 200 joules for an adult patient when using a monophasic defibrillator or 120 joules (commonly) when using a biphasic defibrillator.
- Charge the paddles by pressing the charge buttons, located either on the machine or on the paddles themselves.
- Place the paddles over the conductive pads and press firmly against the patient's chest using 25 lb of pressure.

- Reassess the patient's cardiac rhythm.
- If the patient remains in ventricular fibrillation or pulseless ventricular tachycardia, instruct all personnel to stand clear of the patient and the bed.
- Discharge the current by pressing both paddle charge buttons simultaneously.
- Perform 5 cycles (2 minutes) of CPR and then check the patient's rhythm.
- Tell someone to reset the energy level on the defibrillator (or on the paddles) to 360 joules, or the biphasic energy equivalent, if necessary.
- Announce that you're preparing to defibrillate, and repeat the procedure.
- Perform five cycles (2 minutes) of CPR, and then check the patient's rhythm.
- If debfibrillation is again necessary, tell someone to reset the energy level to 360 joules, or the biphasic energy equivalent.
- Follow the same procedure.
- When possible, secure an airway and confirm placement. Always minimize the amount of time chest compressions must be stopped.
- When available, give epinephrine or vasopressin.
- Consider possible causes for failure of the patient's rhythm to convert, such as acidosis or hypoxia.
- If defibrillation restores a normal rhythm, check the patient's central and peripheral pulses and obtain a blood pressure reading, heart rate, and respiratory rate.
- Assess the patient's level of consciousness, cardiac rhythm, breath sounds, skin color, and urine output.
- Obtain baseline arterial blood gas levels and a 12-lead ECG.
- Provide supplemental oxygen, ventilation, and drugs, as needed.
- Check the patient's chest for electrical burns, and treat them, as ordered, with corticosteroid or lanolin-based creams.
- Prepare defibrillator for immediate reuse.

- Defibrillators vary from one manufacturer to the next, so familiarize yourself with your facility's equipment.
- Defibrillator operation should be checked at least every 8 hours and after each use.
- Defibrillation can be affected by several factors, including paddle size and placement, condition of the patient's myocardium, duration of the arrhythmia, transthoracic impedance, and the number of countershocks.
- Familiarize yourself with the automatic and semiautomatic external defibrillators used in your facility to assure early and effective defibrillation. (See *Using an automated external defibrillator.*)

Complications
- Accidental electric shock to those providing care
- Skin burns

▶ PATIENT TEACHING

Be sure to cover:
- events leading to defibrillation
- what treatment (such as medications and oxygen) the patient can now expect
- that the patient is being closely monitored
- how equipment being used (such as continuous cardiac monitor) works.

●◆ DOCUMENTATION

- Date and time of event, location, and person who found patient
- Events leading up to defibrillation
- Assessment findings indicating the need for defibrillation
- Person performing defibrillation
- Number of times defibrillation was performed and voltage used with each attempt
- Paddle placement
- Success of defibrillation (return of pulse)

- Dosage, route, and time of any medications administered
- Other interventions performed and patient response
- Postdefibrillation patient assessment, including ECG
- Time and name of physician notified
- Names of staff who assisted
- Family notification of defibrillation Documentation may be recorded on a code record for a precise, quick, and chronological recording.

Selected references
Bubien, R.S., et al. "Cardiac Defibrillation and Resynchronization Therapies: Principles, Therapies, and Management Implications," *AACN Clinical Issues* 15(3):340-61, July-September 2004.

Germano, J.J., et al. "Frequency and Causes of Implantable Cardioverter-Defibrillator Therapies: Is Device Therapy Proarrhythmic?" *American Journal of Cardiology* 97(8):1255-261, April 2006.

Gullick, J. "A Study into Safe and Efficient Use of Defibrillators by Nurses," *Nursing Times* 100(44):42-44, November 2004.

Gura, M.T. "Implantable Cardioverter Defibrillator Therapy," *Journal of Cardiovascular Nursing* 20(4):276-87, July-August 2005.

Marett, B.E. "American Heart Association Releases New Guidelines," *Journal of Emergency Nursing* 32(1):63-64, February 2006.

USING AN AUTOMATED EXTERNAL DEFIBRILLATOR

It's estimated that 70% of sudden cardiac arrests are due to ventricular fibrillation (VF). An automated external defibrillator, or AED, is a defibrillator that can detect VF and rapid ventricular tachycardia (VT). After these rhythms are detected, the fully automated AED charges itself and delivers a shock. This reduces the time required for defibrillation.

Speedy defibrillation is the most important determinant of survival in a patient with VF. The longer it takes for defibrillation to occur, the less likely it becomes for defibrillation to be able to convert VF to a rhythm with a pulse. Defibrillation should occur before CPR is started in an unresponsive and pulseless patient, unless a defibrillator isn't immediately available or if the AED indicates that the heart rhythm detected, such as asystole, shouldn't be shocked.

Types of AEDs
There are two basic types of AEDs: semiautomated (or shock-advisory) and fully automated. A semiautomated AED signals that the patient has a shockable arrhythmia (VF or pulseless VT with a rate greater than a rate preset by the manufacturer), but the nurse must push the button for defibrillation to occur. The fully automated AED assesses the heart rhythm and automatically defibrillates if it detects VF or rapid VT – it requires only that the operator attach the defibrillatory pads and turn on the device.

Using a semiautomated AED
Until the Advanced Cardiac Life Support (ACLS) team arrives, follow this procedure if your patient is unresponsive.
- First, assess your patient. If he's unresponsive, not breathing, and pulseless, call for help as you get an AED and attach it to the patient. Start CPR if there is a delay in obtaining or attaching the AED.
- Turn on the power to the AED. Place one electrode pad on the chest, just below the right clavicle. Place the other pad at the cardiac apex to the left of the nipple line with the center of the electrode in the midaxillary line. The standard anterior-posterior positions may also be used as an acceptable alternative approach.
- Press the button to analyze the patient's heart rhythm. If the AED indicates that the patient has a shockable rhythm, make sure everyone is clear of the bed, and push the shock button.
- Defibrillate up to three times, if indicated. If the AED indicates that no further shocks are required, check for spontaneous pulse and respirations. Otherwise, check for pulse and breathing after the third defibrillation.
- If there is no pulse, perform CPR for 1 minute, then check the pulse. If it's still absent, press the AED button to analyze the rhythm. If the AED indicates that the patient has a shockable rhythm, defibrillate up to three times, if indicated.
- Continue this sequence until either shock is no longer advised (in which case, continue CPR), the pulse returns (in which case, assess vital signs, support airway and breathing, and provide appropriated medications for blood pressure and heart rate and rhythm), or the ACLS team arrives.

Doppler blood flow detector use

- Allows determination of arterial blood flow when flow may be compromised, such as in a cool, edematous, pale, cyanotic, or apparently pulseless extremity
- Shows placement of an arterial insertion or puncture
- More sensitive than palpation for determining pulse rate; especially useful when pulse is faint or weak
- Detects motion of red blood cells, as opposed to palpation, which detects arterial wall expansion and retraction

Contraindications
- Use over an open or draining lesion

Doppler ultrasound blood flow detector • coupling or transmission gel • soft cloth • antiseptic solution or soapy water

- Confirm the patient's identity using two patient identifiers according to facility policy.
- Explain the procedure to the patient.
- Wash your hands thoroughly.
- Apply a small amount of coupling gel or transmission gel (not water-soluble lubricant) to the ultrasound probe.
- Position the probe on the skin directly over the selected artery.
- Set the volume control to the lowest setting.
- If your model doesn't have a speaker, plug in the earphones and slowly raise the volume.
- To obtain the best signal, tilt the probe 45 degrees from the artery, making sure to put gel between the skin and the probe.
- Slowly move the probe in a circular motion to locate the center of the artery and the Doppler signal (a hissing noise at the heartbeat).
- Avoid moving the probe rapidly because it distorts the signal.
- Count the signals for 60 seconds to determine the pulse rate.
- After you've measured the pulse rate, clean the probe with a soft cloth soaked in antiseptic solution or soapy water, according to the manufacturer's recommendations.

- Doppler ultrasound is helpful in measuring the ankle-brachial index (ABI; the difference in systolic blood pressure in the ankle and arm) and in detecting peripheral arterial disease.

◈ **NURSING ALERT** An ABI less than 0.5 indicates critical leg ischemia.

- Failure to position the transducer properly can interfere with results.
- If the patient has a threat to vascular integrity, such as recent orthopedic surgery or an indwelling arterial catheter above the affected site, frequently check pulses for any changes in circulation.
- If you don't hear any noise when you turn on the Doppler ultrasound, replace the battery.
- To avoid a loud static noise, turn the volume all the way down and hold the probe against the skin before turning on the Doppler ultrasound.

Complications
- None known

Be sure to cover:
- how the procedure is performed
- need to lie still and not to move the involved body part during assessment
- that the procedure doesn't involve pain but the gel may feel cold
- that loud noises may be heard, but that this is normal
- further teaching based on the test results, diagnosis, and prognosis.

- Indication for the procedure
- Time, date, location, and quality of the pulse as well as the pulse rate
- Instructions given to the patient

Selected references

Blaivas, M. "Ultrasound-Guided Peripheral I.V. Insertion in the ED," *American Journal of Nursing* 105(10):54-57, October 2005.

French, L. "Community Nurse Use of Doppler Ultrasound in Leg Ulcer Assessment," *British Journal of Community Nursing* 10(9):S6-S10, passim, September 2005.

Ozbudak, O., et al. "Doppler Ultrasonography in the Detection of Deep Vein Thrombosis in Patients with Pulmonary Embolism," *Journal of Thrombosis and Thrombolysis* 21(2):159-62, April 2006.

Patel, U. "The Potential Value of Power Doppler Ultrasound Imaging Compared With Gray-Scale Ultrasound Findings in the Diagnosis of Local Recurrence After Prostatectomy," *Clinical Radiology* 61(4):323-24, April 2006.

Ear irrigation

● OVERVIEW

- Involves washing the external auditory canal with a stream of solution to clean the canal of discharges, soften and remove impacted cerumen, or dislodge a foreign body
- Relieves localized inflammation and discomfort
- Must be performed carefully to avoid causing patient discomfort or vertigo and to avoid increasing the risk of otitis media

⬥ NURSING ALERT Because irrigation can contaminate the middle ear if the tympanic membrane is ruptured, an otoscopic examination always precedes ear irrigation.

Contraindications
ABSOLUTE
- Suspected tympanic membrane perforation
- Infectious process present

RELATIVE
- Recent ear or head trauma
- Large foreign body present
- Tympanic membrane or ear canal deformities present

❖ EQUIPMENT

Ear irrigation syringe (rubber bulb) • otoscope with aural speculum • prescribed irrigant • large basin • linen-saver pad and bath towel • cotton balls or cotton-tipped applicators • 4″ × 4″ gauze pad • optional: adjustable light (such as a gooseneck lamp), container for irrigant, tubing, clamp, and syringe with ear tip, normal saline solution, gloves, cotton

Equipment preparation
- Wash your hands thoroughly.
- Select the appropriate syringe, and obtain the prescribed irrigant.
- Put the container of irrigant into the large basin filled with hot water to warm the solution to body temperature 98.6° F (37° C) because extreme temperature changes may produce nausea and dizziness.
- Test the temperature of the solution by sprinkling a few drops on your inner wrist.

⬥ NURSING ALERT Avoid extreme temperature changes of the irrigant, which can affect inner ear fluids, causing nausea and dizziness.

- Inspect equipment (syringe or catheter tips) for breaks or cracks; inspect all metal tips for roughness.

▌▌▌ ESSENTIAL STEPS

- Confirm the patient's identity using two patient identifiers according to facility policy.
- Explain the procedure to the patient and provide privacy.
- Put on gloves if you expect contact with drainage.
- Inspect the auditory canal of the ear that will be irrigated using an otoscope.

⬥ NURSING ALERT Ear irrigation is contraindicated when a vegetable (such as a pea) obstructs the auditory canal because it can swell in contact with an irrigant, causing intense pain and complicating removal of the object.

Don't irrigate the ear if a battery (or a battery part) is lodged in the ear because battery acid could leak and irrigation would spread caustic material throughout the canal.

- Help the patient to a sitting position with his head tilted slightly forward and toward the affected side.
- If the patient can't sit, have him lie on his back and tilt his head slightly forward and toward the affected ear.
- Make sure you have adequate lighting.
- If the patient is sitting, place the linen-saver pad (covered with the bath towel) on his shoulder and upper arm, under the affected ear (if he's lying down, cover his pillow and the area under the affected ear).
- Have the patient hold the emesis basin close to his head under the affected ear.
- Clean the auricle and the meatus of the auditory canal with a cotton-tipped applicator moistened with normal saline or the prescribed irrigating solution.
- Draw the irrigant into the syringe and expel any air.
- Straighten the auditory canal; then insert the syringe tip and start the flow. (See *How to irrigate the ear canal.*)

✳ AGE-RELATED CONCERN To examine the ear canal of an older child or adult, gently pull the pinna up and back; in a child under age 3, pull the pinna down and back.

- If the patient reports pain or dizziness during irrigation, stop the procedure, recheck the temperature of the irrigant, inspect the patient's ear with the otoscope, and resume irrigation, as indicated.
- When the syringe is empty, remove it and inspect the return flow.
- Refill the syringe, and continue the irrigation until the return flow is clear.

⬥ NURSING ALERT Never use more than 500 ml of irrigant during the procedure.

- Remove the syringe, and inspect the ear canal for cleanliness with the otoscope.
- Dry the patient's auricle and neck.
- Remove the bath towel and linen-saver pad.
- Help the seated patient lie on his affected side with the 4″ × 4″ gauze pad under his ear to promote drainage of residual debris and solution.

- Avoid dropping or squirting irrigant on the tympanic membrane because this can startle the patient and cause discomfort.
- If you're using an irrigating catheter instead of a syringe, adjust the flow of solution to a steady, comfortable rate with a flow clamp.

◈ **NURSING ALERT** Don't raise the container more than 6″ (15 cm) above the ear because the resulting

pressure can damage the tympanic membrane.

- If the physician directs you to place a cotton pledget in the ear canal to retain some of the solution, pack the cotton loosely and instruct the patient not to remove it.
- If irrigation doesn't dislodge impacted cerumen, the physician may order you to instill several drops of glycerin, carbamide peroxide (Debrox), or a similar preparation two to three times daily for 2 to 3 days, and then to irrigate the ear again.

Complications
- Trauma to the mucous membranes
- Pain
- Vertigo
- Infection
- Nausea and vomiting
- Tinnitus
- Ruptured tympanic membrane
- Otitis media

HOW TO IRRIGATE THE EAR CANAL

Follow these guidelines for irrigating the ear canal.
- Gently pull the auricle up and back to straighten the ear canal. (For a child, pull the ear down and back.)
- Have the patient hold an emesis basin beneath the ear to catch returning irrigant. Position the tip of the irrigating syringe at the meatus of the auditory canal. Don't block the meatus because you'll impede backflow and raise pressure in the canal.

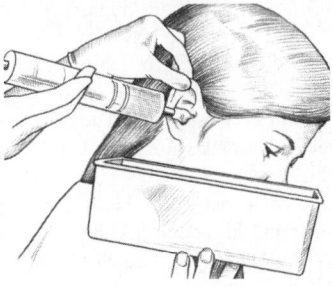

- Tilt the patient's head toward the opposite ear, and point the syringe tip upward and toward the posterior ear canal. This angle prevents damage to the tympanic membrane and guards against pushing debris farther into the canal.

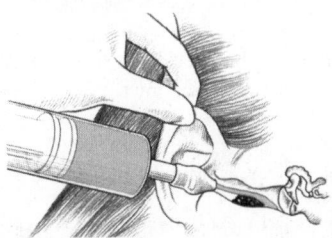

- Direct a steady stream of irrigant against the upper wall of the ear canal, and inspect return fluid for cloudiness, cerumen, blood, or foreign matter.

Be sure to cover:
- why the procedure is needed and how it's performed
- signs and symptoms to report, such as abnormal discharge, pain, vertigo, or hearing problems
- proper ear care at home, such as preventing cerumen impaction and preventing insertion of foreign bodies.

- Date and time of irrigation and which ear was irrigated
- Volume and type of solution used
- Appearance of the canal before and after irrigation
- Appearance of the return flow
- Patient's tolerance of the procedure and any comments he made about his condition, especially related to his hearing acuity

Selected references

Baer, S. "Knowing When to Treat Ear Wax," *Practitioner* 249(1670):328, 330, 332, May 2005.

Dimmit, P. "Cerumen Removal Products," *Journal of Pediatric Health Care* 19(3):332-36, September-October 2005.

Shefelbine, S.E., et al. "Mitigation of Hearing Loss from Semi-Circular Canal Transection in Pseudomonas Otitis Media with Ciprofloxacin-Dexamethasone Irrigation," *Otology & Neurology* 27(2):265-69, February 2006.

Williams, D. "Does Irrigation of the Ear to Remove Impacted Wax Improve Hearing?" *British Journal of Community Nursing* 10(5):228-32, May 2005.

Electrocardiography

⬤ OVERVIEW

- Measures the heart's electrical activity as waveforms
- Identifies myocardial ischemia and infarction, rhythm and conduction disturbances, chamber enlargement, electrolyte imbalances, and drug toxicity
- Uses electrodes attached to the skin to detect electric currents in the heart and transmit them to electrocardiogram (ECG) machine that produces a record of cardiac activity
- Requires knowledge of standard 12-lead ECG; uses 10 electrodes to measure electrical potential from 12 different leads: the standard bipolar limb leads (I, II, III), three unipolar augmented leads (aV_R, aV_L, aV_F), and six unipolar precordial or chest leads (V_1 to V_6)
- Measures and averages the difference between the electrical potential of electrode sites for each lead and graphs them over time creating the standard electrocardiography complex, called PQRST (see *Reviewing ECG waveforms and components*)
- Used during exercise (stress ECG) to monitor heart rate, blood pressure, and ECG waveforms as the patient walks on a treadmill or pedals a stationary bicycle
- May be used at home where ambulatory patient wears a portable Holter monitor to record heart activity continually over 24 hours

Contraindications
- None known

❖ EQUIPMENT

ECG machine • recording paper • disposable pregelled electrodes • 4″ × 4″ gauze pads • optional: clippers, marking pen

Equipment preparation
- Place the ECG machine close to the patient's bed.
- Plug the cord into the wall outlet.
- If the patient is already connected to a cardiac monitor, remove the electrodes to accommodate the precordial leads and minimize electrical interference on the ECG tracing.
- Keep the patient away from electrical fixtures and power cords.

▮▮ ESSENTIAL STEPS

- Confirm the patient's identity using two patient identifiers according to facility policy.
- Explain the procedure to the patient.
- Wash your hands thoroughly.
- Provide for patient privacy.
- Have the patient lie in a supine position in the center of the bed with his arms at his sides, raising the head of the bed to make him more comfortable.
- Expose the patient's arms and legs, and cover him appropriately.

◈ **NURSING ALERT** The patient's arms and legs should be relaxed to minimize muscle trembling, which can cause electrical interference.

- If the bed is too narrow for the patient to relax or the patient is trembling and is nonresponsive to common measures, such as a blanket for warmth, ask him to place his hands under his buttocks to reduce muscle tension, which can interfere with the ECG tracing.
- Select flat, fleshy areas to place the electrodes, avoiding muscular and bony areas.

◈ **NURSING ALERT** If the patient has an amputated limb, choose a site on the stump.

- If an area is excessively hairy, clip it.

REVIEWING ECG WAVEFORMS AND COMPONENTS

An electrocardiogram (ECG) waveform has three basic components: P wave, QRS complex, and T wave. These elements can be further divided into PR interval, J point, ST segment, U wave, and QT interval.

P wave and PR interval
The P wave represents atrial depolarization. The PR interval represents the time it takes an impulse to travel from the atria through the AV nodes and bundle of His. The PR interval measures from the beginning of the P wave to the beginning of the QRS complex.

QRS complex
The QRS complex represents ventricular depolarization (the time it takes for the impulse to travel through the bundle branches to the Purkinje fibers). The Q wave appears as the first negative deflection in the QRS complex; the R wave as the first positive deflection. The S wave appears as the second negative deflection or the first negative deflection after the R wave.

J point and ST segment
Marking the end of the QRS complex, the J point also indicates the beginning of the ST segment. The ST segment represents part of ventricular repolarization.

T wave and U wave
Usually following the same deflection pattern as the P wave, the T wave represents ventricular repolarization. The U wave follows the T wave but isn't always seen. The U wave represents delayed repolarization of the ventricular conduction system.

QT interval
The QT interval represents ventricular depolarization and repolarization. It extends from the beginning of the QRS complex to the end of the T wave.

- Clean excess oil or other substances from the skin to enhance electrode contact and allow it to dry.
- Peel off the contact paper from disposable electrodes and apply them directly to the prepared site, as recommended by the manufacturer, with the lead connection pointing superiorly.
- Connect the limb leadwires to the electrodes as follows: the white or RA leadwire goes to the right arm; the green or RL leadwire to the right leg; the red or LL leadwire to the left leg; the black or LA leadwire to the left arm; and the brown or V_1 to V_6 leadwire to the chest.
- Expose the patient's chest and put a small amount of electrode gel or paste or a disposable electrode at each electrode position. (See *Positioning chest electrodes.*)
- If your patient is a woman, be sure to place the chest electrodes below the breast tissue and displace the breast tissue of a large-breasted woman laterally.
- Check to see that the paper speed selector is set to the standard 25 mm/second and that the machine is set to full voltage.
- Enter the appropriate patient identification data.
- If any part of the waveform extends beyond the paper when you record the ECG, adjust the normal standardization to half-standardization and note this adjustment on the ECG strip because it will affect results.
- Ask the patient to relax, lie still, breathe normally, and not talk when you record the ECG.
- Press the AUTO button and observe the tracing quality as the machine records all 12 leads automatically, recording three consecutive leads simultaneously. (Some machines have a display screen so you can preview waveforms before the machine records them on paper.)
- When the machine finishes recording the 12-lead ECG, remove the electrodes and clean the patient's skin.
- After disconnecting the leadwires from the electrodes, dispose of or clean the electrodes, as indicated.

✦ SPECIAL CONSIDERATIONS

- If the patient's respirations distort the recording, ask him to hold his breath briefly while you record the ECG.
- If the patient has a pacemaker, you can perform an ECG with or without a magnet, according to the physician's orders, noting the presence of a pacemaker and the use of the magnet (to turn off the pacemaker) on the strip.

Complications
- Skin sensitivity to electrodes
- Allergic symptoms (ranging from mild to severe) when patients with latex sensitivity are exposed to any latex materials found in electrodes, cables, or leadwires

▶ PATIENT TEACHING

Be sure to cover:
- why the procedure is needed and how it's performed
- that the test doesn't hurt and won't cause an electrical shock
- that the test takes up to 10 minutes to perform
- that electrodes will be attached to the arms, legs, and chest and that the gel may feel cold
- need to lie still, relax, not talk, and breathe normally during the procedure.

◆◇ DOCUMENTATION

- Indications for the ECG
- Patient's name, age, gender, and date on the ECG tracing
- Date and time of the ECG and significant responses by the patient in nurse's notes
- Patient's tolerance of the procedure

Selected references
Alinier, G., et al, "12-Lead ECG Training: The Way Forward," *Nurse Education Today* 26(1):87-92, January 2006.

Colyar, M. "Interpreting a 12-Lead ECG," *Advance for Nurse Practitioners* 12(4):18, 21-23, April 2004.

Gregory, J. "Using the 12-Lead ECG to Assess Acute Coronary Patients," *British Journal of Nursing* 14(2):1135-140, November-December 2005.

Jahrsdoerfer, M., et al. "Clinical Usefulness of the EASI 12-Lead Continous Electrocardiographic Monitoring System," *Critical Care Nurse* 25(5):28-30, 32-37, October 2005.

Pyne, C.C. "Classification of Acute Coronary Syndromes Using the 12-Lead Electrocardiogram as a Guide," *AACN Clinical Issues* 15(4):558-67, October-December 2004.

POSITIONING CHEST ELECTRODES

To ensure accurate test results, position chest electrodes as follows:

V_1: Fourth intercostal space at right border of sternum
V_2: Fourth intercostal space at left border of sternum
V_3: Halfway between V_2 and V_4
V_4: Fifth intercostal space at midclavicular line
V_5: Fifth intercostal space at anterior axillary line (halfway between V_4 and V_6)
V_6: Fifth intercostal space at midaxillary line, level with V_4

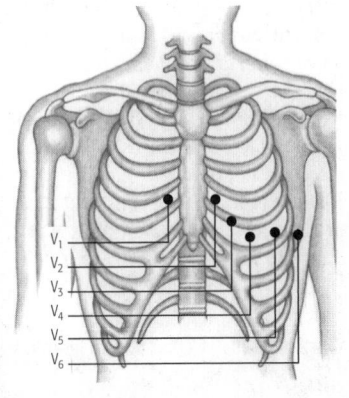

Electrocardiography, posterior and right chest lead placement

POSTERIOR LEAD PLACEMENT
- Used to identify electrocardiographic (ECG) changes associated with the heart's posterior surface
- May provide clues to posterior wall infarction so that appropriate treatment can begin
- Typically performed with a standard ECG and involves recording only the additional posterior leads: V_7, V_8, and V_9

RIGHT CHEST LEAD PLACEMENT
- Obtains information from the right side of the heart to assess interior and right ventricular ischemia or infarction
- Determines inferior wall myocardial infarction (MI) and suspected right ventricular involvement: 25% to 50% of MI patients having right ventricular involvement; many also having high creatinine kinase levels
- Early identification of a right ventricular MI essential because it requires different treatment

Contraindications
- None known

❖ EQUIPMENT

Multichannel or single-channel ECG machine with recording paper • disposable pregelled electrodes • 4″ × 4″ gauze pads • optional: clippers

Equipment preparation
- Place the ECG machine close to the patient.
- Plug the power cord into the wall outlet or confirm that the battery is charged.
- Keep the patient away from electrical fixtures and power cords to minimize electrical interference.
- Make sure that the paper speed is set at 25 mm/second and amplitude at 1 mV/10 mm.

▌▌▌ ESSENTIAL STEPS

- Confirm the patient's identity using two patient identifiers according to facility policy.
- Explain the procedure to the patient and his family.
- Wash your hands thoroughly.
- Provide privacy and expose his arms, chest, and legs.
- Prepare the electrode sites according to the manufacturer's instructions.
- When the ECG is complete, remove the electrodes and clean the patient's skin.

POSTERIOR LEAD PLACEMENT
- To ensure good skin contact, clip the site if the patient has considerable back hair.
- If you're using a multichannel ECG machine, begin by attaching a disposable electrode to the V_7 position on the left posterior axillary line, fifth intercostal space. Then attach the V_4 leadwire to the V_7 electrode.

◈ **NURSING ALERT** Because of the location of the heart's posterior surface, changes associated with myocardial damage aren't apparent on a standard 12-lead ECG.

- Next, attach a disposable electrode to the patient's back at the V_8 position on the left midscapular line, fifth intercostal space, and attach the V_5 leadwire to this electrode.
- Finally, attach a disposable electrode to the patient's back at the V_9 position, just left of the spinal column at the fifth intercostal space (as shown below), and attach the V_6 leadwire to the V_9 electrode.

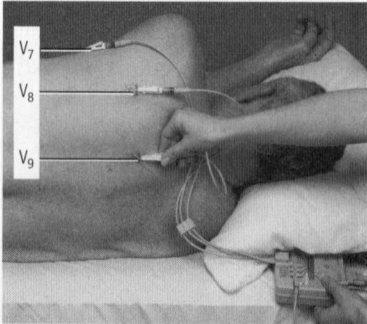

- If you're using a single-channel ECG machine, put electrode gel at locations for electrodes V_7, V_8, and V_9 and con-

nect the brown leadwire to the V_7 electrode.
- Turn on the machine and make sure the paper speed is set for 25 mm/second, standardizing the machine if necessary.
- Press AUTO and the machine will record.
- If you're using a multichannel ECG machine, all leads will print out as a straight line except the leads labeled V_4, V_5, and V_6, which should be relabeled leads V_7, V_8, and V_9, respectively.
- If you're using a single-channel ECG machine, turn the selector knob to "V" to record the V_7 lead, stop the machine, and reposition the electrode to the V_8 position and record that lead, repeating the procedure for the V_9 position.
- If you think you may need more than one posterior lead ECG, use a marking pen to mark the electrode sites on his skin to permit accurate comparison for future tracings.

RIGHT CHEST LEAD PLACEMENT
- Place the patient in a supine position or, if he has difficulty lying flat, in semi-Fowler's position.
- Choose flat, fleshy (not bony or muscular), hairless areas, such as the inner aspects of the wrist and ankles, for placement of the extremity electrodes.
- Clean the sites with the gauze pads to promote good skin contact.
- Connect the leadwires to the electrodes. The leadwires are color-coated and lettered.
- Attach the electrodes to the appropriate extremities: white (RA) to the right arm, black (LA) to the left arm, green (RL) to the right leg, and red (LL) to the left leg.
- If there's excessive hair in the area, clip it.
- Locate the correct sites for chest lead placement (as shown top of next page).
- For a female patient, place the electrodes under the breast tissue.
- Feel between the patient's ribs for the second intercostal space on the left (the notch at the top of the sternum, where the manubrium joins the body of the sternum), count down two spaces to the fourth intercostal space, and apply an electrode to the site and attach leadwire V_{1R}.

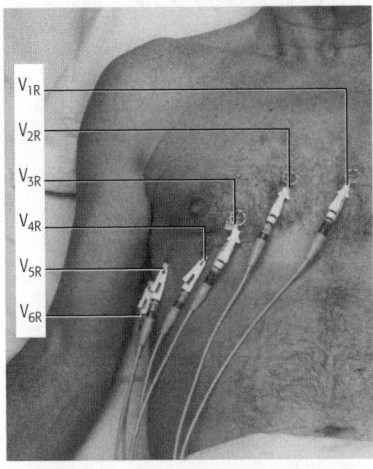

- Move your fingers across the sternum to the fourth intercostal space on the right side of the sternum and apply an electrode to that site and attach lead V_{2R}.
- Move your finger down to the fifth intercostal space and over to the midclavicular line and place an electrode here and attach lead V_{4R}.
- Visualize a line between V_{2R} and V_{4R}. Apply an electrode midway on this line and attach lead V_{3R}.
- Move your finger horizontally from V_{4R} to the right midaxillary line and apply a disposable electrode to this site and attach lead V_{6R}.
- Move your fingers along the same horizontal line to the midpoint between V_{4R} and V_{6R} (the right anterior midaxillary line) and apply an electrode to this site and attach lead V_{5R}.
- Turn on the electrocardiography machine.
- Ask the patient to breathe normally but not to talk during the recording so that muscle movement won't distort the tracing.
- Enter any appropriate patient information required by the machine you're using.
- If necessary, standardize the machine, causing a square tracing of 10 mm (two large squares) to appear on the ECG paper when the machine is set for 1 mV (1 mV = 10 mm).
- Press the AUTO key to record all 12 leads automatically.
- Check your facility's policy for the number of readings to obtain. Some facilities rquire at least two ECGs so one can be sent for interpretation

while the other stays in the patient's chart. If the ECG is to be put in the chart, it may need to be labeled "preliminary."
- After recording the ECG, turn off the machine.
- Clearly label the ECG with the patient's name, the date, and the time.
- Label the tracing as "right chest ECG" to distinguish it from a standard 12-lead ECG.

✦ SPECIAL CONSIDERATIONS

POSTERIOR LEAD PLACEMENT

- The number of leads may vary according to the cardiologist's preference.
- If right posterior leads are requested, position the patient on his left side, and identify the same landmarks on the right side of the patient's back for leads V_{7R}, V_{8R}, and V_{9R}.
- If the ECG machine won't operate unless all leadwires are connected, you may need to connect the limb leadwires and the leadwires for V_1, V_2, and V_3.

RIGHT CHEST LEAD PLACEMENT

- For best results, place the electrodes symmetrically on the limbs.
- If the patient's wrist or ankle is covered by a dressing, or if the patient is an amputee, choose an area that's available on both sides.

Complications
- Skin sensitivity reactions

▶ PATIENT TEACHING

Be sure to cover:
- why the procedure is needed and how it's performed
- that the test doesn't hurt and won't cause an electrical shock
- that the test takes up to 10 minutes to perform
- that electrodes will be attached to the arms, legs, and chest and that the gel may feel cold
- need to lie still, relax, not talk, and breathe normally during the procedure.

◆◇ DOCUMENTATION

- Indications for the posterior or right chest lead ECG
- Date and time the ECG was performed
- Copy of the ECG, if available
- Patient's tolerance to the procedure
- Patient's name, age, gender, date, and time on the ECG tracing

Selected references
Brown, D.F., and Nadel, E.S. "Posterior Wall Myocardial Infarction," *Journal of Emergency Medicine* 27(1):75-78, July 2004.
Chockalingam, A., et al. "Right Ventricular Myocardial Infarction: Presentation and Acute Outcomes," *Angiology* 56(4):371-76, July-August 2005.
Hosino, Y., et al. "Electrocardiographic Abnormality of Pure Posterior Myocardial Infarction," *Internal Medicine* 43(9):883-85, September 2004.
Khan, S., et al. "Prevalence of Right Ventricular Myocardial Infarction in Patient with Acute Inferior Wall Myocardial Infarction," *International Journal of Clinical Practice* 58(4):354-57, April 2004.
Moye, S., et al. "The Electrocardiogram in Right Ventricular Myocardial Infarction," *American Journal of Emergency Medicine* 23(6):793-99, October 2005.
Rotondo, N., et al. "Electrocardiographic Manifestations: Acute Inferior Wall Myocardial Infarction," *Journal of Emergency Medicine* 26(4):433-40, May 2004.

Electrocardiography, signal-averaged

● OVERVIEW

- Identifies risk for sustained ventricular tachycardia in patients with malignant ventricular tachycardia, a history of myocardial infarction (MI), unexplained syncope, nonischemic congestive cardiomyopathy, or nonsustained ventricular tachycardia
- Helps the physician determine if the patient needs an invasive procedure, such as electrophysiologic testing or angiography
- Detects low-amplitude signals or late electrical potentials that reflect slow conduction or disorganized ventricular activity through abnormal or infarcted regions of the ventricles (on standard 12-lead ECG, noise from muscle tissue, electronic artifacts, and electrodes masking late potentials that have low amplitude)
- Performed by recording noise-free surface ECG in three specialized leads for several hundred beats

Contraindications

- None known

❖ EQUIPMENT

Signal-averaged electrocardiography machine • signal-averaged computer • record of patient's surface ECG for 200 to 300 QRS complexes • three bipolar electrodes or leads • alcohol pads • optional: clippers

Equipment preparation

- Check to ensure that the machine is in working order.
- Review manufacturer's instructions and facility policy for use.
- Explain the procedure to the patient.

▌▌▆ ESSENTIAL STEPS

- Confirm the patient's identify using two patient identifiers according to facility policy.
- Place the patient in a supine position; have him lie as still as possible.
- Tell the patient to breathe normally but not to speak during the procedure.
- If the patient has hair on his chest, clip the area, rub it with alcohol, and dry it before placing electrodes.

PLACING ELECTRODES FOR SIGNAL-AVERAGED ELECTROCARDIOGRAPHY

To prepare for signal-averaged electrocardiography, place the electrodes in the X, Y, and Z orthogonal positions shown here. These positions bisect one another to provide a three-dimensional, composite view of ventricular activation.

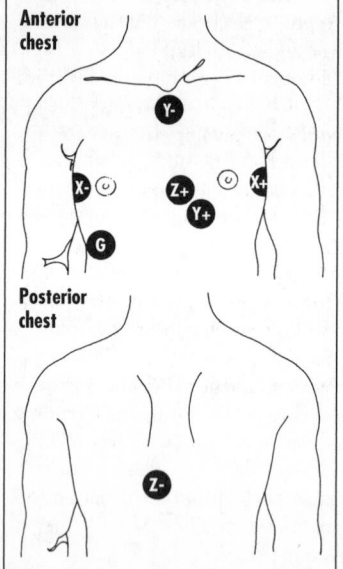

KEY

X+ Fourth intercostal space, midaxillary line, left side
X- Fourth intercostal space, midaxillary line, right side
Y+ Standard V_3 position (or proximal left leg)
Y- Superior aspect of manubrium
Z+ Standard V_2 position
Z- V_2 position, posterior
G Ground; eighth rib on right side

- Place the leads in the X, Y, and Z positions. (See *Placing electrodes for signal-averaged electrocardiography.*)
- The ECG machine gathers input from the leads and amplifies, filters, and samples the signals; the computer collects and stores data for analysis.
- Crucial values are those showing QRS complex duration, duration of the portion of the QRS complex with an amplitude under 40 uV, and the root mean square voltage of the last 40 msec.

◆ SPECIAL CONSIDERATIONS

- Muscle movement may cause a false-positive result. Patients who are restless or in respiratory distress are poor candidates for signal-averaged electrocardiography.
- Proper electrode placement and skin preparation are essential.

  NURSING ALERT Low-amplitude signals are indicated by a QRS complex duration greater than 110 msec; a duration of more than 40 msec for the amplitude portion under 40 uV; and a root mean square voltage of less than 25 uV during the last 40 msec of the QRS complex. All three factors aren't needed to consider the result positive or negative. Final interpretation depends on individual patient factors.

- Validity of signal-averaged electrocardiography in patients with bundle-branch heart block is unknown because myocardial activation doesn't follow the usual sequence in these patients.

Complications
- Skin sensitivity reactions

▶ PATIENT TEACHING

Be sure to cover:
- why the procedure is needed
- that the procedure usually 10 to 30 minutes
- that the results will help the physician determine the risk for a certain type of arrhythmia
- performance of procedure along with other tests, such as echocardiography, Holter monitoring, electrophysiology studies, and stress testing.

●◆ DOCUMENTATION

- Time of the procedure
- Reason for procedure
- Patient's tolerance of the procedure
- Results of the procedure

Selected references
Bennhagen, R.G., et aL. "Serial Signal-Averaged Electrocardiography in Children After Cardiac Transplantation," *Pediatric Transplantation* 9(6):773-79, December 2005.

Budeus, M., et al. "Prediction of Atrial Fibrillation After Coronary Artery Bypass Grafting: The Role of Chemoreflex-Sensitivity and P Wave Signal-Averaged ECG," *International Journal of Cardiology* 106(1):67-74, January 2006.

Haghjoo, M., et al. "Does the Abnormal Signal-Averaged Electrocardiogram Predict Future Appropriate Therapy in Patients with Implantable Cardioverter-Defibrillators?" *Journal of Electrocardiology* 39(2):50-55, April 2006.

Lee, K.L., and Lau, C.P. "The Use of Signal-Averaged Electrocardiogram in Risk Stratification after Acute Myocardial Infarction in the Modern Era," *European Heart Journal* 26(8):747-48, April 2005.

End-of-life care

● OVERVIEW

- Provides physical comfort and emotional support as patient approaches death and helps patient and family through the stages of dying (see *Five stages of dying*)
- Requires recognition of signs and symptoms of impending death, including reduced respiratory rate and depth, decreased or absent blood pressure, weak or erratic pulse rate, lowered skin temperature, decreased level of consciousness (LOC), diminished sensorium and neuromuscular control, diaphoresis, pallor, cyanosis, and mottling
- May require following the directives of living wills stating desire for death unimpeded by artificial support, such as from defibrillators, mechanical ventilators, life-sustaining drugs, and ventricular assist devices

Contraindications
- None known

❖ EQUIPMENT

Clean bed linens • clean gowns • gloves • water-filled basin • soap • washcloth • towels • lotion • linen-saver pads • petroleum jelly • suction equipment, as necessary • personal protective equipment, as necessary • optional: indwelling urinary catheter

Equipment preparation
- Assemble necessary equipment at the patient's bedside.
- Wash hands thoroughly.
- Provide for comfort and support to the patient and family.

▮▮▮ ESSENTIAL STEPS

- Explain all care to the patient, even if he's unconscious, and his family.
- Provide for privacy.
- Wear appropriate personal protective equipment, when necessary.

PROVIDING PHYSICAL COMFORT
- Take vital signs and observe for pallor, diaphoresis, and decreased LOC.
- Reposition the patient at least every 2 hours.
- Make sure the bed sheets cover the patient loosely to reduce discomfort caused by pressure on arms and legs.
- When the patient's vision and hearing start to fail, turn his head toward the light and speak to him from near the head of the bed.

⬥ **NURSING ALERT** Because hearing may be acute despite loss of consciousness, avoid whispering or speak-

---

FIVE STAGES OF DYING

According to Elisabeth Kübler-Ross, author of *On Death and Dying,* the dying patient may progress through five psychological stages in preparation for death. Although each patient experiences these stages differently, and not necessarily in this order, understanding them will help you meet your patient's needs.

Denial
When the patient first learns of his terminal illness, he refuses to accept the diagnosis. He may experience physical symptoms similar to a stress reaction (shock, fainting, pallor, sweating, tachycardia, nausea, and GI disorders). During this stage, be honest with the patient but not blunt or callous. Maintain communication with him so he can discuss his feelings when he accepts the reality of death. Don't force the patient to confront this reality.

Anger
Once the patient stops denying his impending death, he may show deep resentment toward those who will live on after he dies (you, other staff, and his own family members). Although you may instinctively draw back from the patient or even resent this behavior, remember that he's dying and has a right to be angry. After you accept his anger, you can help him find different ways to express it and can help his family members to understand it.

Bargaining
Although the patient acknowledges his impending death, he attempts to bargain with God or fate for more time. He will probably strike this bargain secretly. If he does confide in you, don't urge him to keep his promises.

Depression
In this stage, the patient may first experience regrets about his past and then grieve about his current condition. He may withdraw from his friends, family, doctor, and you. He may suffer from anorexia, increased fatigue, or self-neglect. You may find him sitting alone, in tears. Accept the patient's sorrow, and if he talks to you, listen. Provide comfort by touch, as appropriate. Resist the temptation to make optimistic remarks or cheerful small talk.

Acceptance
In this last stage, the patient accepts without emotion the inevitability and imminence of his death. The patient may simply desire the quiet company of a family member or friend. If a family member or friend can't be present, stay with the patient to satisfy his final needs. Remember that many patients die before reaching this stage.

ing inappropriately about the patient in his presence.

- Change the bed linens and the patient's gown, as needed.
- Provide skin care and adjust the room temperature for the patient's comfort.
- If the patient is incontinent, provide frequent perineal care, use linen-saver pads beneath his buttocks, or obtain an order to insert a catheter, if appropriate.
- Gently suction the patient's mouth and upper airway to remove secretions, as indicated.
- Elevate the head of the bed to facilitate breathing.
- Offer fluids frequently, and lubricate the patient's lips and mouth with petroleum jelly to counteract dryness caused by breathing through the mouth.
- If the comatose patient's eyes are open, provide appropriate eye care to prevent corneal ulceration.

NURSING ALERT Corneal ulceration can cause blindness and prevent the use of these tissues for transplantation after death.

- Provide ordered pain medication I.V. to keep the patient comfortable.

PROVIDING EMOTIONAL SUPPORT
- Fully explain all care and treatments to the patient.
- Answer any questions as candidly as possible, without sounding callous.
- Allow the patient to express his feelings, which may range from anger to loneliness.
- Take time to talk with the patient by sitting near the head of the bed and avoiding looking rushed or unconcerned.
- Notify his family, if they're absent, when the patient wishes to see them.
- Let the patient and his family discuss death at their own pace.
- Offer to contact a member of the clergy or social services, if desired.

✦ SPECIAL CONSIDERATIONS

- If the patient has signed a living will and the physician has written a "no code" order on the progress notes and order sheets, be sure to communicate this to all staff involved in the patient's care. Be aware of state and facility policies regarding advance directives and living wills.
- Orient his family to the unit and facility; explain the patient's needs, treatments, and care plan; offer to teach them specific skills so they can take part in care; and provide emotional support.
- At an appropriate time, ask the patient's family if they have considered organ and tissue donation and check the patient's records to determine whether he completed an organ donor card.

▶ PATIENT TEACHING

Be sure to cover:
- all procedures and care
- advanced directives
- pain relief and comfort care measures
- services and supports available
- what to expect as death approaches
- organ donation, as appropriate
- emotional responses to dying, as appropriate.

●✦ DOCUMENTATION

- Changes in the patient's vital signs, intake and output, and LOC
- Physical and emotional care given
- Advance directives
- Times of cardiac arrest and the end of respiration
- Time and name of physician notified
- Family or staff members present at time of death

Selected references

Holmberg, L. "Communication in Action Between Family Caregivers and a Palliative Home Care Team," *Journal of Hospice and Palliative Nursing* 8(5):276-87, September 2006.

Jones, R.W. "SHARING: Diamond in the Rough," *Nursing* 35(11):53, November 2005.

Mazanec, P., and Tyler, M.K. "Cultural Considerations in End-of-Life Care," *AJN* 103(3):50-58, March 2003.

Ufema, J. "Insights On Death & Dying: Missing the Moment," *Nursing* 35(10):20, October 2005.

Ufema, J. "Insights On Death & Dying: Taking the Mask Off," *Nursing* 35(2):66-67, February 2005.

Endotracheal tube care

- Performed to ensure airway patency and prevent complications until the patient can maintain independent ventilation
- Includes frequent assessment of airway status, maintenance of proper cuff pressure to prevent tissue ischemia and necrosis, repositioning of the tube to avoid traumatic manipulation, and constant monitoring for complications

Contraindications

- None known

❖ EQUIPMENT

MAINTAINING THE AIRWAY
Stethoscope • suction equipment • gloves

REPOSITIONING THE ET TUBE
10-ml syringe • compound benzoin tincture • stethoscope • adhesive or hypoallergenic tape or Velcro tube holder • suction equipment • sedative or 2% lidocaine • gloves • handheld resuscitation bag with mask in case of accidental extubation

REMOVING THE ET TUBE
10-ml syringe • suction equipment • supplemental oxygen source with mask • cool-mist, large-volume nebulizer • handheld resuscitation bag with mask • gloves • equipment for reintubation

Equipment preparation

- Wash hands thoroughly before all procedures.
- Assemble all equipment at the patient's bedside.
- When repositioning the endotracheal (ET) tube, using sterile technique, set up the suction equipment.
- When removing the ET tube, set up the suction and supplemental oxygen equipment and have all equipment for emergency reintubation ready.

❚❚❚ ESSENTIAL STEPS

- Confirm the patient's identity using two patient identifiers according to facility policy.
- Explain the procedure to the patient even if he doesn't appear to be alert.
- Provide for patient privacy.
- Wear appropriate personal protective equipment, when necessary, throughout all procedures.
- Put on clean gloves.

MAINTAINING THE AIRWAY

- Auscultate the patient's lungs at any sign of respiratory distress.
- If you detect an obstructed airway, determine the cause and treat it accordingly.
- If secretions are obstructing the lumen of the tube, suction the secretions from the tube. (See "Tracheal suction," page 836.)
- If the ET tube has slipped from the trachea into the right or left mainstem bronchus, indicated by absent breath sounds over one lung, obtain a chest X-ray, as ordered, to verify tube placement and, if necessary, reposition the tube.

REPOSITIONING THE ET TUBE

- Get help from another nurse to prevent accidental extubation during the procedure if the patient coughs.

◈ **NURSING ALERT** To prevent traumatic manipulation of the tube, instruct the assisting nurse to hold it as you carefully untape the tube or unfasten the Velcro tube holder.

- Hyperoxygenate the patient and then suction the patient's trachea through the ET tube to remove any secretions, which can cause the patient to cough during the procedure.
- Suction the patient's pharynx to remove any secretions that may have accumulated above the tube cuff to prevent aspiration of secretions during cuff deflation.
- When freeing the tube, locate a landmark, such as a number on the tube, or measure the distance from the patient's mouth to the top of the tube so that you have a reference point when moving the tube.
- Deflate the cuff by attaching a 10-ml syringe to the pilot balloon port and

aspirating air until you meet resistance and the pilot balloon deflates.

◈ **NURSING ALERT** Deflate the cuff before moving the ET tube because the cuff forms a seal within the trachea and movement of an inflated cuff can damage the tracheal wall and vocal cords.

- Reposition the tube as necessary, noting new landmarks or measuring the length.
- To reinflate the cuff, instruct the patient to inhale, and slowly inflate the cuff using a 10-ml syringe attached to the pilot balloon port.
- As you do this, use your stethoscope to auscultate the patient's neck to determine the presence of an air leak.
- When air leakage ceases, stop cuff inflation and, while still auscultating the patient's neck, aspirate a small amount of air until you detect a minimal air leak, indicating that the cuff is inflated at the lowest pressure possible to create an adequate seal.
- If the patient is being mechanically ventilated, aspirate to create a minimal air leak during the inspiratory phase of respiration because the positive pressure of the ventilator during inspiration will create a larger leak around the cuff.
- Note the amount of air required to achieve a minimal air leak.
- Measure cuff pressure, and compare the reading with previous pressure readings to prevent overinflation.
- Verify placement of the ET tube by auscultating both lung fields to verify breath sounds; listen over the epigastric area to confirm that the ET tube wasn't positioned in the stomach. Carbon dioxide levels may also be monitored to verify placement, and a chest X-ray may be required.
- Use benzoin and tape to secure the tube in place, or refasten the Velcro tube holder.
- Make sure the patient is comfortable and the airway patent.
- When the cuff is inflated, measure its pressure at least every 8 hours to avoid overinflation.

REMOVING THE ET TUBE

- Check the physician's order to remove the ET tube.
- Obtain another nurse's assistance to prevent traumatic manipulation of

the tube when it's untaped or unfastened.

- Elevate the head of the patient's bed to approximately 90 degrees.
- Suction the patient's oropharynx and nasopharynx to remove any accumulated secretions and to help prevent aspiration of secretions when the cuff is deflated.
- Using a handheld resuscitation bag or the mechanical ventilator, give the patient several deep breaths through the ET tube to hyperinflate his lungs and increase his oxygen reserve.
- Attach a 10-ml syringe to the pilot balloon port, and aspirate air until you meet resistance and the pilot balloon deflates.

NURSING ALERT If you fail to detect an air leak around the deflated cuff, notify the physician immediately and don't proceed with extubation. Absence of an air leak may indicate marked tracheal edema, which can result in total airway obstruction if the ET tube is removed.

- If you detect the proper air leak, untape or unfasten the ET tube while the assisting nurse stabilizes the tube.
- Insert a sterile suction catheter through the ET tube.
- Apply suction, and to reduce the risk of laryngeal trauma, ask the patient to take a deep breath, open his mouth fully, and pretend to cry out.
- Simultaneously, remove the ET tube and the suction catheter in one smooth, outward and downward motion, following the natural curve of the patient's mouth.

NURSING ALERT Suctioning during extubation removes secretions retained at the end of the tube and prevents aspiration.

- Give the patient supplemental oxygen.
- For maximum humidity, use a cool-mist, large-volume nebulizer to help decrease airway irritation, patient discomfort, and laryngeal edema.
- Encourage the patient to cough and deep-breathe.
- Remind him that a sore throat and hoarseness are to be expected and will gradually subside.
- Make sure the patient is comfortable and the airway is patent.
- After extubation, auscultate the patient's lungs frequently and be alert

for stridor or other evidence of upper airway obstruction.
- If ordered, draw an arterial sample for blood gas analysis.

◆ SPECIAL CONSIDERATIONS

- Use sedation or direct instillation of 2% lidocaine (if ordered) to numb the airway when repositioning an ET tube in patients with highly sensitive airways.
- After extubation of a patient who has been intubated for an extended time, keep reintubation supplies readily available for at least 12 hours or until you're sure he can tolerate extubation.
- Never extubate a patient unless someone skilled at intubation is readily available.
- If you inadvertently cut the pilot balloon on the cuff, leave the tube in place, and immediately call the physician to remove the damaged ET tube and replace it with one that's intact.

Complications

- Traumatic injury to the larynx or trachea
- Ventilatory failure
- Airway obstruction
- Laryngospasm
- Tracheal edema

▶ PATIENT TEACHING

Be sure to cover:
- why the ET tube is being repositioned
- how the procedure will be done
- need to lie still and keep head still during repositioning
- how the ET tube will be removed and what the patient can do to help
- that the patient will be monitored closely after intubation
- that patient's throat will be sore and his voice may be hoarse, but this is temporary
- need for coughing and deep breathing
- possible need for supplemental oxygen therapy.

●◆ DOCUMENTATION

- Date and time of tube repositioning
- Reason for repositioning (such as malposition shown by chest X-ray)
- New tube position
- Total amount of air in the cuff after the procedure
- Any complications and interventions
- Patient's tolerance of the procedure
- Date and time of extubation
- Presence or absence of stridor or other signs of upper airway edema
- Type of supplemental oxygen administered
- Complications and required subsequent therapy
- Patient teaching

Selected references

Birkett, K.M., et al. "Reporting Unplanned Extubation," *Intensive & Critical Care Nursing* 21(2):65-75, April 2005.

O'Donnell, J.M. "A Comparison of Endotracheal Tube Cuff Pressures Using Estimation Techniques and Direct Intracuff Measurement," *AANA Journal* 72(4):250-51, August 2004.

Yeh, S.H., et al. "Implications of Nursing Care in the Occurrence and Consequences of Unplanned Extubation in Adult Intensive Care Units," *International Journal of Nursing Studies* 41(3):255-62, March 2004.

End-tidal carbon dioxide monitoring

- Shows carbon dioxide (CO_2) concentration in exhaled gas
- May indicate a range or simply whether CO_2 is present during exhalation
- Measures amount of infrared light absorbed by airway gas during inspiration and expiration with photodetector and shows data converted to a CO_2 value and a corresponding waveform, or capnogram, if capnography is used (see *Understanding ETCO$_2$ monitoring*)
- Provides information about patient's pulmonary, cardiac, and metabolic status that aids patient management and helps prevent clinical compromise
- Helps wean a patient with a stable acid-base balance from mechanical ventilation
- Confirms correct endotracheal (ET) tube placement during ET intubation and detects accidental esophageal intubation because CO_2 isn't normally produced by the stomach
- Detects accidental ET tube displacement or extubation when used throughout intubation
- Reduces need for frequent arterial blood gas (ABG) measurements, especially when combined with pulse oximetry
- Assesses resuscitation efforts and identifies the return of spontaneous circulation
- Detects apnea (no CO_2 is exhaled when breathing stops)
- Used as standard procedure during anesthesia administration and mechanical ventilation

Gloves • mainstream or sidestream CO_2 monitor • CO_2 sensor • airway adapter, as recommended by the manufacturer (neonatal adapter may have a much smaller dead space, making it appropriate for a smaller patient)

Equipment preparation

- If the monitor you're using isn't self-calibrating, calibrate it as the manufacturer directs.
- If you're using a sidestream CO_2 monitor (the airway adapter is positioned at the airway), be sure to replace the water trap between patients, if directed.
- Newer sidestream models don't require water traps.

UNDERSTANDING ETco$_2$ MONITORING

The optical portion of an end-tidal carbon dioxide (ETco$_2$) monitor contains an infrared light source, a sample chamber, a special carbon dioxide (CO_2) filter, and a photodetector. The infrared light passes through the sample chamber and is absorbed in varying amounts, depending on the amount of CO_2 the patient has just exhaled. The photodetector measures CO_2 content and relays this information to the microprocessor in the monitor, which displays the CO_2 value and waveform.

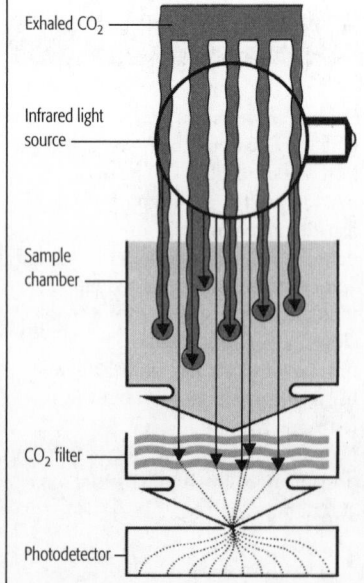

Exhaled CO_2

Infrared light source

Sample chamber

CO_2 filter

Photodetector

- Confirm the patient's identity using two patient identifiers according to facility policy.
- Wash your hands thoroughly.
- Explain the purpose of end-tidal carbon dioxide (ETCO$_2$) monitoring and its expected duration to the patient and his family.

◆ **NURSING ALERT** The effects of manual resuscitation or ingestion of alcohol or carbonated beverages can alter the detector's findings.

- Apply the ETCO$_2$ detector or monitor immediately after ET intubation and position the airway adapter directly on the ET tube.
- For a nonintubated patient, place the adapter at or near the patient's airway. (An oxygen-delivery cannula may have a sample port through which gas can be aspirated for monitoring.)
- Turn on all alarms to settings appropriate for your patient and adjust the alarm volume so it can be heard.

◆ **NURSING ALERT** Color changes detected after fewer than six ventilations can be misleading.

- Wear gloves when handling the airway adapter to prevent cross-contamination.
- Change the airway adapter with every breathing circuit and ET tube change.
- Place the adapter on the ET tube to avoid contaminating exhaled gases with fresh gas flow from the ventilator.
- If you're using a heat and moisture exchanger, you may be able to position the airway adapter between the exchanger and breathing circuit.
- If your patient's $ETCO_2$ values differ from his partial pressure of arterial carbon dioxide, assess him for factors that can influence $ETCO_2$ — especially when the differential between arterial and $ETCO_2$ values (the arterial absolute difference of carbon dioxide) is above normal.
- Because $ETCO_2$ monitoring doesn't assess oxygenation, concurrent use with pulse oximetry may provide more complete information.
- If the CO_2 waveform is available, assess it for height, frequency, rhythm, baseline, and shape to help evaluate gas exchange.

⬢ NURSING ALERT In a nonintubated patient, exhaled gas is more likely to mix with ambient air, and exhaled CO_2 may be diluted by fresh gas flow from the nasal cannula.

- $ETCO_2$ monitoring commonly is discontinued when the patient has been weaned effectively from mechanical ventilation or when he's no longer at risk for respiratory compromise.

⬢ NURSING ALERT After extubation, continuous $ETCO_2$ monitoring may indicate a need for reintubation.

- When using a disposable $ETCO_2$ detector, always check its color under fluorescent or natural light because the dome looks pink under incandescent light.

Complications
- Inaccurate measurements, such as from poor sampling technique, calibration drift, contamination of optics with moisture or secretions, or equipment malfunction, possibly leading to misdiagnosis and improper treatment

Be sure to cover:
- why $ETCO_2$ monitoring is needed
- how long the monitoring will continue.

- Date and time $ETCO_2$ monitoring was initiated
- Indications for monitoring
- Initial $ETCO_2$ value and ventilator settings
- Description of the waveform, if one appears on the monitor
- Print out of waveform if the monitor has a printer
- $ETCO_2$ values with vital signs
- $ETCO_2$ values whenever significant changes in waveform or patient status occur, and before and after weaning, respiratory, and other interventions
- ABG analysis with corresponding $ETCO_2$ values
- Patient teaching

Selected references

Hillier, S.C., and Schamberger, M.S. "Transcutaneous and End-Tidal Carbon Dioxide Analysis: Complimentary Monitoring Strategies," *Journal of Intensive Care Medicine* 20(5):307-309, September-October 2005.

Sullivan, K.J., et al. "End-Tidal Carbon Dioxide Monitoring in Pediatric Emergencies," *Pediatric Emergency Care* 21(5):326-32, May 2005.

Yosefy, C., et al. "End-Tidal Carbon Dioxide as a Predictor of the Arterial PCO_2 in the Emergency Department Setting," *Emergency Medicine Journal* 21(5):557-59, September 2004.

Fecal occult blood testing

- Detects presence of occult blood in feces and distinguishes between true melena and melena-like stools
- Performed for early detection of colorectal cancer (80% of patients with this disorder testing positive)
- Confirmed positive test result possibly indicating other conditions, such as ulcers and diverticula
- Two common occult blood screening tests: Hematest (an orthotolidin reagent tablet) and the Hemoccult slide (filter paper impregnated with guaiac); produces blue reaction in fecal smear if occult blood loss exceeds 5 ml in 24 hours
- Newer test: ColoCARE; requires no fecal smear

Contraindications
RELATIVE
- Actively bleeding hemorrhoids
- Menses

EQUIPMENT

Test kit • glass or porcelain plate • tongue blade or other wooden applicator • gloves

Equipment preparation
- Ensure that kit and wooden applicator are readily available.
- Check patient's history for drugs that may affect test.

ESSENTIAL STEPS

- Confirm the patient's identity using two patient identifiers according to facility policy.
- Explain the procedure to the patient and why it's being performed.
- Put on gloves and collect a stool specimen.

HEMATEST
- Use a wooden applicator to smear a bit of stool on the filter paper supplied with the test kit.
- If you've performed a digital rectal examination, wipe the finger you used for examination on a square of the filter paper.
- Place the filter paper with the stool smear on a glass plate.
- Remove a reagent tablet from the bottle, and immediately replace the cap tightly.
- Place the tablet in the center of the stool smear on the filter paper.
- Add one drop of water to the tablet, and allow it to soak in for 5 to 10 seconds.
- Add a second drop, letting it run from the tablet onto the specimen and filter paper.
- If necessary, tap the plate gently to dislodge any water from the top of the tablet.

> **NURSING ALERT** Certain medications, such as iron supplements and bismuth compounds, can darken stools so that they resemble melena.

- After 2 minutes, the filter paper will turn blue if the test result is positive. Don't read the color that appears on the tablet itself or develops on the filter paper after the 2-minute period.

- Note the results, and discard the filter paper.

> **NURSING ALERT** Reassure the patient that a single positive test result doesn't necessarily confirm GI bleeding or indicate colorectal cancer.

- Remove and discard your gloves, and wash your hands thoroughly.

HEMOCCULT TEST
- Open the flap on the slide packet.
- Use a wooden applicator to apply a thin smear of the stool specimen to the guaiac-impregnated filter paper exposed in box A.
- If you've performed a digital rectal examination, wipe the finger you used on a square of the filter paper.
- Apply a second smear from another part of the specimen to the filter paper exposed in box B.
- Allow the specimen to dry for 3 to 5 minutes.
- Open the flap on the reverse side of the slide package, and place 2 drops of Hemoccult-developing solution on the paper over each smear.
- A blue reaction will appear in 30 to 60 seconds if the test result is positive.
- Record the results and discard the slide package.
- Remove and discard your gloves, and wash your hands thoroughly.

- Make sure stool specimens aren't contaminated with urine, soap solution, or toilet tissue, and test them as soon as possible after collection.
- Test samples from several different portions of the same specimen because occult blood from the upper GI tract isn't always evenly dispersed throughout the formed stool; likewise, blood from colorectal bleeding may occur mostly on the outer stool surface.
- Use only fresh reagent tablets and discard expired ones.
- Protect Hematest tablets from moisture, heat, and light.
- To confirm a positive result, the test must be repeated at least three times while the patient follows a high-fiber diet and refrains from eating red meat, poultry, fish, turnips, and horseradish for 48 to 72 hours before and during the test.
- As ordered, have the patient discontinue use of iron preparations, bromides, iodides, rauwolfia derivatives, indomethacin, colchicine, salicylates, potassium, phenylbutazone, oxyphenbutazone, bismuth compounds, steroids, and ascorbic acid for 48 to 72 hours before and during the test to ensure accurate test results.

Be sure to cover:
- indications for fecal occult blood testing
- using the Hemoccult slide packet at home
- using a ColoCARE test packet at home (see *Home tests for fecal occult blood*)
- dietary restrictions before and during testing
- withholding certain medications before and during testing, test results, and any follow-up care.

- Date and time of the test
- Type of test and result
- Any unusual characteristics of the stool tested
- Date, time, and name of physician notified of positive test results

Selected references

Evans-Smith, P. *Taylor's Clinical Nursing Skills.* Philadelphia: Lippincott Williams & Wilkins, 2005.

O'Leary, B.A., et al. "Cost-Effectiveness of Colorectal Cancer Screening: Comparison of Community-Based Flexible Sigmoidoscopy With Fecal Occult Blood Testing and Colonoscopy," *Journal of Gastroenterology and Hepatology* 19(1):38-47, January 2004.

Ouyang, D.L., et al. "Noninvasive Testing for Colorectal Cancer: A Review," *American Journal of Gastroenterology* 100(6):1393-403, June 2005.

HOME TESTS FOR FECAL OCCULT BLOOD

A new fecal occult blood test, ColoCARE, doesn't require the patient to handle stool, making the procedure safer, simpler, and more acceptable to patients.

To perform the ColoCARE test at home, tell the patient to avoid red meat and vitamin C supplements for 2 days before the test. He should check with his practitioner about discontinuing any medications before the test.

Tell the patient to flush the toilet twice just before performing the test to remove any toilet-cleaning chemicals from the tank. Tell him to defecate into the toilet but to throw no toilet paper into the bowl. Within 5 minutes, he should remove the test pad from its pouch and float it printed side up on the surface of the water. Tell him to watch the pad for 15 to 30 seconds for any evidence of blue or green color changes, and have him record the result on the reply card.

Tell him to perform this test with three consecutive bowel movements and then send the completed card to his practitioner. However, he should call his practitioner immediately if he notes a positive color change in the first test.

Gastric lavage

- Flushes the stomach and removes ingested substances through a tube after poisoning or drug overdose; useful in patients who have central nervous system depression or an inadequate gag reflex
- Also used to empty the stomach before an endoscopic examination
- Continuous or intermittent; usually done in the emergency room or intensive care unit by a physician, gastroenterologist, or nurse

Contraindications

- Already compromised esophagus (after ingestion of corrosive substances , such as lye, petroleum distillates, ammonia, alkalis, or mineral acids), which may become perforated by lavage tube

Lavage setup (two graduated containers for drainage, three pieces of large lumen rubber tubing, Y-connector, and clamp or hemostat) • 2 to 3 L of normal saline solution, tap water, or appropriate antidote, as ordered • Ewald tube or any large-lumen gastric tube, typically #36 to #40 French • I.V. pole • water-soluble lubricant or anesthetic ointment • stethoscope • hypoallergenic tape • 50-ml bulb or catheter-tip syringe • gloves • face shield • linen-saver pad or towel • Yankauer or tonsiltip suction device • suction apparatus • labeled specimen container • laboratory request form • norepinephrine • basin of ice, if ordered • optional: patient restraints, charcoal tablets

Equipment preparation

NURSING ALERT A prepackaged, syringe-type irrigation kit may be used for intermittent lavage. For poisoning or drug overdose, the continuous lavage setup is faster and more effective for diluting and removing the harmful substance.

- Connect one of the three pieces of large-lumen tubing to the irrigant container.
- Insert the Y-connector stem in the other end of the tubing.
- Connect the remaining two pieces of tubing to the free ends of the Y-connector.
- Place the unattached end of one of the tubes into one of the drainage containers. (Later, you'll connect the other piece of tubing to the patient's gastric tube.)
- Clamp the tube leading to the irrigant.
- Suspend the entire setup from the I.V. pole, hanging the irrigant container at the highest level.
- If iced lavage is ordered, chill the ordered irrigant in a basin of ice.
- Lubricate the end of the lavage tube with water-soluble lubricant or anesthetic ointment.

- Provide privacy.
- Wash your hands and put on gloves and a face shield.
- Drape the towel or linen-saver pad over the patient's chest to protect from spills.
- The physician inserts the lavage tube nasally and advances it slowly; forceful insertion may injure tissues and cause epistaxis. Tube placement is checked by injecting about 30 cc of air with the bulb syringe, then auscultating the patient's abdomen with a stethoscope.

NURSING ALERT The patient may vomit when the lavage tube reaches the posterior pharynx; be prepared to suction the airway immediately.

- After the tube passes the posterior pharynx, put the patient in Trendelenburg's position and turn him to his left in a three-quarter prone posture to minimize passage of gastric contents into the duodenum and prevent the patient from aspirating vomitus.
- After securing the tube with tape and making sure the irrigant inflow tube on the lavage setup is clamped, connect the unattached end of the irrigant inflow tube to the lavage tube.
- Allow stomach contents to empty into the drainage container before instilling irrigant. This confirms proper tube placement and decreases risk of overfilling the stomach with irrigant and inducing vomiting.
- If using a syringe irrigation set, aspirate stomach contents with a 50-ml bulb or catheter-tip syringe before instilling irrigant.
- After you confirm proper tube placement, begin gastric lavage by instilling about 250 ml of irrigant to assess patient's tolerance and prevent vomiting.
- If using a syringe, instill about 50 ml of solution at a time until you've instilled between 250 and 500 ml. Clamp the inflow tube and unclamp the outflow tube to allow irrigant to flow out.
- If using the syringe irrigation kit, aspirate the irrigant with the syringe and empty into a calibrated container. Measure outflow to make sure it at least equals the amount of irrigant in-

stilled. This prevents stomach distention and vomiting.
- If drainage amount is significantly less than instilled amount, reposition the tube until sufficient solution flows out. Gently massage the abdomen over the stomach to promote outflow.
- Repeat the inflow-outflow cycle until returned fluids appear clear, signaling that the stomach no longer contains harmful substances or bleeding has stopped.
- Assess vital signs, urine output, and level of consciousness (LOC) every 15 minutes. Notify the physician of changes.
- If ordered, remove the lavage tube.

✦ SPECIAL CONSIDERATIONS

- To control GI bleeding, the physician may order continuous stomach irrigation including a vasoconstrictor. The drug is delivered directly to the liver via the portal septum, thus preventing systemic circulation that can cause a hypertensive response.
- Alternatively, the outflow tube can be clamped for a prescribed period after instilling irrigant and vasoconstrictive drug and before withdrawing it. This allows the mucosa time to absorb the drug.
- Never leave a patient alone during gastric lavage. Watch for changes in LOC and monitor vital signs frequently; the vagal response to intubation can depress the patient's heart rate.
- If you need to restrain the patient, secure restraints on one side of the bed or stretcher so you can free them quickly.
- Keep tracheal suctioning equipment nearby; watch closely for airway obstruction caused by vomiting or excess oral secretions.
- Suction the oral cavity often to ensure an open airway and prevent aspiration.
- If the patient doesn't have an adequate gag reflex, he may need an endotracheal tube before the procedure.
- When aspirating the stomach for ingested poisons or drugs, save the contents in a labeled container for laboratory analysis.
- After lavage to remove poisons or drugs, mix charcoal tablets with the irrigant and administer the mixture through the tube, if ordered.
- When lavage is done to stop bleeding, keep precise intake and output records to determine amount of bleeding. When large volumes of fluid are instilled and withdrawn, serum electrolyte and arterial blood gas levels may be measured during or after lavage.

Complications
- Vomiting and aspiration
- Bradyarrhythmias
- After iced lavage, possible lowered body temperature, triggering cardiac arrhythmias

▶ PATIENT TEACHING

Be sure to cover
- why the procedure is needed
- what to expect during the procedure.

●◆ DOCUMENTATION

- Date and time of lavage
- Size and type of NG tube used
- Volume and type of irrigant
- Amount of drained gastric contents
- Color and consistency of drainage
- Intake and output
- Vital signs and LOC
- Drugs instilled through the tube
- Time the tube was removed
- Patient's tolerance of the procedure

Selected references
Bartlett, D. "Acetaminophen Toxicity," *Journal of Emergency Nursing* 30(3):281-83, June 2004.
Heard, K. "Gastrointestinal Decontamination," *Medical Clinics of North America* 89(6):1067-1078, November 2005.
Madden, M.A. "Pediatric Poisonings: Recognition, Assessment, and Management," *Critical Care Nursing Clinics of North America* 17(4):395-404, xi, December 2005.

Gastrostomy feeding button care

● **OVERVIEW**

- Used as an alternative feeding device for an ambulatory patient receiving long-term enteral feedings
- Approved by the Food and Drug Administration for 6-month implantation; can be used to replace gastrostomy tubes, if necessary
- Inserted into established stoma (15-minute procedure); lies almost flush with skin; only top of safety plug is visible
- Advantages: cosmetic appeal, ease of maintenance, reduced skin irritation and breakdown, and less likelihood of becoming dislodged or migrating (compared with ordinary feeding tube)
- Has one-way antireflux valve inside mushroom dome that prevents accidental leakage of gastric contents; usually replaced after 3 to 4 months because antireflux valve wears out

Contraindications

ABSOLUTE
- Intestinal obstruction that prohibits use of the bowel
- Diffuse peritonitis
- Intractable vomiting
- Paralytic ileus
- Severe diarrhea that makes metabolic management difficult

RELATIVE
- Severe pancreatis
- Enterocutaneous fistulae
- GI ischemia

❖ **EQUIPMENT**

Gastrostomy feeding button of the correct size (all three sizes, if the correct one isn't known) • obturator • water-soluble lubricant • gloves • feeding accessories, including adapter, feeding catheter, food syringe or bag, and formula • catheter clamp • cleaning equipment, including water, syringe, cotton-tipped applicator, pipe cleaner, and mild soap or povidone-iodine solution • optional: I.V. pole, pump to provide continuous infusion over several hours

❚❙❚ **ESSENTIAL STEPS**

- Explain the insertion, reinsertion, and feeding procedure to the patient.
- Tell the patient that the physician will perform the initial insertion.
- Make sure the patient has signed the appropriate consent form.
- Wash your hands and put on gloves. (See *How to reinsert a gastrostomy feeding button.*)
- Attach the adapter and feeding catheter to the syringe or feeding bag.
- Clamp the catheter and fill the syringe or bag and catheter with formula.

HOW TO REINSERT A GASTROSTOMY FEEDING BUTTON

If your patient's gastrostomy feeding button pops out (with coughing, for example), it needs to be reinserted. Here are some steps to follow.

Prepare the equipment
Collect the feeding button, an obturator, and water-soluble lubricant. If the button is to be reinserted, wash it with soap and water and rinse it thoroughly.

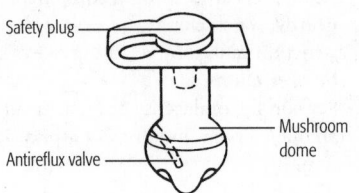

Safety plug

Mushroom dome

Antireflux valve

Insert the button
- Check the depth of the patient's stoma to make sure you have a feeding button of the correct size.
- Clean around the stoma.
- Lubricate the obturator with a water-soluble lubricant, and distend the button several times to ensure patency of the antireflux valve within the button.
- Lubricate the mushroom dome and the stoma.
- Gently push the button through the stoma into the stomach.

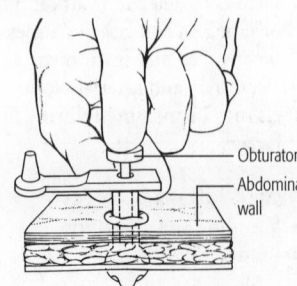

Obturator

Abdominal wall

- Remove the obturator by gently rotating it as you withdraw it, to keep the antireflux valve from adhering to it.
- If the valve sticks nonetheless, gently push the obturator back into the button until the valve closes.
- After removing the obturator, make sure the valve is closed.
- Next, close the flexible safety plug, which should be relatively flush with the skin surface.

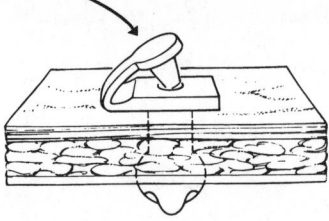

- If you need to administer a feeding right away, open the safety plug and attach the feeding adapter and feeding tube.
- Deliver the feeding, as ordered.

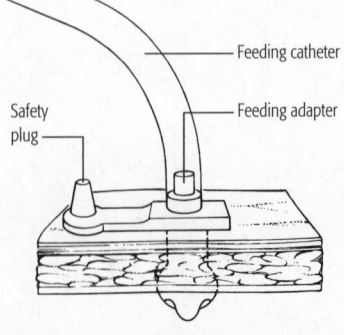

Feeding catheter

Feeding adapter

Safety plug

- Open the safety plug and attach the adapter and feeding catheter to the button.
- Elevate the syringe or feeding bag above stomach level, and gravity-feed the formula for 15 to 30 minutes, varying the height, as needed, to alter the flow rate.
- Use a pump for continuous infusion or for feedings lasting several hours.
- Refill the syringe before it's empty to prevent air from entering the stomach and distending the abdomen.
- After the feeding, flush the button with 10 ml of water.
- Lower the syringe or bag below stomach level to allow burping.
- Remove the adapter and feeding catheter; the antireflux valve should prevent gastric reflux.
- Snap the safety plug in place to keep the lumen clean and prevent leakage if the antireflux valve fails.
- If the patient feels nauseated or vomits after the feeding, vent the button with the adapter and feeding catheter to control emesis.
- Wash the catheter and syringe or feeding bag in warm, soapy water and rinse thoroughly.
- Clean the catheter and adapter with a pipe cleaner.
- Rinse well before using for the next feeding.
- Soak the equipment once a week according to manufacturer's recommendations.

- If the button pops out while feeding, reinsert it, estimate the formula already delivered, and resume feeding.
- Once daily, clean the peristomal skin with mild soap and water or povidone-iodine solution, and let the skin air-dry for 20 minutes, to avoid skin irritation.
- Clean the peristomal site whenever spillage from the feeding bag occurs.

Complications
- Nausea and vomiting
- Abdominal distention
- Exit-site infection
- Exit-site leakage
- Peritonitis

Be sure to cover:
- how the gastrostomy feeding button is inserted and cared for
- how to use the button for feedings
- how to clean the equipment
- peristomal skin care
- when and who to call for questions.

- Date, time, and duration of feeding
- Amount and type of feeding formula used
- Patient's tolerance of the procedure
- Intake and output
- Appearance of the stoma and surrounding skin
- Skin care

Selected references
Goldberg, E., et al. "Gastrostomy Tube: Facts, Fallacies, Fistulas and False Tracts," *Gastroenterology Nursing* 28(6):485-93, November/December 2005.

Michaud, L., et al. "Longevity of Balloon-Sized Skin-Level Gastrostomy Device," *Journal of Pediatric Gastroenterology and Nutrition* 38(4):426-29, April 2004.

O'Dowd, M., et al. "New Approaches to Percutaneous Gastrostomy," *Seminars in Interventional Radiology. Interventional Radiology in the GI Tract* 21(3):191-97, September 2004.

Usuba, T., et al., "Analysis of Buried Bumper Syndrome after Percutaneous Endoscopic Gastrostomy Due to Use of a Button-type Kit," *Digestive Endoscopy* 19(1):18-21, January 2007.

Hemodialysis

● **OVERVIEW**

- Indicated for patients in renal failure
- Removes blood from the body, circulates it through a purifying dialyzer, and then returns the blood to the body
- For long-term treatment, typically used with arteriovenous (AV) fistula as the access device; various other access sites can be used (see *Hemodialysis access sites*)
- Works on the principle of differential diffusion across a semipermeable membrane, which extracts by-products of protein metabolism, such as urea and uric acid as well as creatinine and excess body water
- Restores or maintains balance of the body's buffer system and electrolyte level, promoting rapid return to normal serum values and preventing complications associated with uremia
- Used for regular long-term treatment of patients with chronic end-stage renal disease, temporary support for patients with acute reversible renal failure and, less commonly, for acute poisoning

❖ EQUIPMENT

PREPARING THE HEMODIALYSIS MACHINE
Hemodialysis machine with appropriate dialyzer • I.V. solution, administration sets, lines, and related equipment • dialysate • optional: heparin, 3-ml syringe with needle, medication label, hemostats

HEMODIALYSIS WITH A DOUBLE-LUMEN CATHETER
Povidone-iodine pads • two sterile 4″ × 4″ gauze pads • two 3-ml and two 5-ml syringes • tape • heparin bolus syringe • clean gloves • sterile labels • sterile markers

HEMODIALYSIS WITH AN AV FISTULA
Two winged fistula needles (each attached to a 10-ml syringe filled with heparin flush solution) • linen-saver pad • povidone-iodine pads • sterile 4″ × 4″ gauze pads • tourniquet • clean gloves • adhesive tape • sterile labels • sterile markers

HEMODIALYSIS WITH AN AV GRAFT
Alcohol pads • povidone-iodine pads • sterile pads • two sterile shunt adapters • sterile Teflon connector • two bulldog clamps • two 10-ml syringes • normal saline solution • four short strips of adheisve tape • sterile shunt spreader, sterile label, sterile marker (optional)

DISCONTINUING HEMODIALYSIS WITH A DOUBLE-LUMEN CATHETER
Sterile 4″ × 4″ gauze pads • povidone-iodine pads • precut gauze dressing • clean gloves • sterile gloves • normal saline solution • alcohol pads • heparin flush solution • luer-lock injection caps • optional: transparent occlusive dressing, skin barrier preparation, tape, materials for culturing drainage

DISCONTINUING HEMODIALYSIS WITH AN AV FISTULA
Clean gloves • sterile 4″ × 4″ gauze pads • two adhesive bandages • hemostats • optional: sterile absorbable gelatin sponges (Gelfoam), topical thrombin solution

DISCONTINUING HEMODIALYSIS WITH AN AV GRAFT
Sterile gloves • bulldog clamps • hemostats • Teflon connector • tap • sterile gauze pads • povidone-iodine solution • alcohol pads

Equipment preparation

- Prepare the hemodialysis equipment following the manufacturer's instructions and hospital protocol.
- Be sure to test the dialyzer and dialysis machine for residual disinfectant after rinsing, and test all the alarms.

▌▌▌ ESSENTIAL STEPS

- Wash your hands thoroughly before all procedures.
- Confirm the patient's identity using two patient identifiers according to facility policy.
- If the patient is undergoing hemodialysis for the first time, explain the procedure in detail.
- Maintain strict sterile technique to prevent introducing pathogens into the patient's bloodstream during dialysis.

- Wear appropriate personal protective equipment, as necessary, throughout all procedures.
- Weigh the patient and compare his present weight to his weight after the last dialysis and his target weight to determine ultrafiltration requirements.
- Record baseline vital signs, taking blood pressure while the patient's sitting and standing; auscultate the heart for rate, rhythm, and abnormalities; assess for edema; observe respiratory rate, rhythm, and quality; and check the patient's mental status.
- Assess the condition and patency of the access site.
- Check for problems since the last dialysis, and evaluate previous laboratory data.
- Help the patient into a comfortable position (supine or sitting in recliner chair with feet elevated).
- Support the access site and rest it on a clean drape.
- Label all medications, medication containers, and other solutions on and off the sterile field.

BEGINNING HEMODIALYSIS WITH A DOUBLE-LUMEN CATHETER
- If extension tubing isn't already clamped, clamp it to prevent air from entering the catheter.
- Clean each catheter extension tube, clamp, and luer-lock injection cap with povidone-iodine pads to remove contaminants.
- Place a sterile 4″ × 4″ gauze pad under the extension tubing, and place two 5-ml syringes and two sterile gauze pads on the drape.
- Prepare the anticoagulant regimen, as ordered.
- Identify arterial and venous blood lines, and place them near the drape.
- To remove clots and ensure catheter patency, remove catheter caps, attach syringes to each catheter port, open the clamp, aspirate 1.5 to 3 ml of blood, close the clamp, and flush each port with 5 ml of heparin flush solution.
- To gain patient access, remove the syringe from the arterial port, attach the line to the arterial port, and administer the heparin according to protocol to prevent clotting in the extracorporeal circuit.

- Grasp the venous blood line and attach it to the venous port, open the clamps on the extension tubing, and secure the tubing to the patient's extremity with tape to reduce tension on the tube and minimize trauma to the insertion site.
- Begin hemodialysis according to facility policy.

BEGINNING HEMODIALYSIS WITH AN AV FISTULA
- Flush the fistula needles, using attached syringes containing heparinized saline solution, and set them aside.
- Place a linen-saver pad under the patient's arm.
- Using sterile technique, clean a 3″ × 10″ (8 × 25 cm) area of skin over the fistula with povidone-iodine pads. (If the patient is sensitive to iodine, use chlorhexidine gluconate [Hibiclens] or alcohol instead.)
- Discard each pad after one wipe.
- Apply a tourniquet above the fistula to distend the veins and facilitate venipuncture, making sure you avoid occluding the fistula.
- Put on clean gloves.
- Remove the fistula needle guard and squeeze the wing tips firmly together.

- Insert the arterial needle at least 1″ (2.5 cm) above the anastomosis, being careful not to puncture the fistula.
- Release the tourniquet and flush the needle with heparin flush solution to prevent clotting.
- Clamp the arterial needle tubing with a hemostat, and secure the wing tips of the needle to the skin with adhesive tape to prevent it from dislodging within the vein.
- Perform another venipuncture with the venous needle a few inches above the arterial needle.
- Flush the venous needle with heparin flush solution.
- Clamp the venous needle tubing, and secure the wing tips of the venous needle as you did the arterial needle.
- Remove the syringe from the end of the arterial tubing, uncap the arterial line from the hemodialysis machine, and connect the two lines.
- Tape the connection securely to prevent it from separating during the procedure.
- Remove the syringe from the end of the venous tubing, uncap the venous line from the hemodialysis machine, and connect the two lines.

- Tape the connection securely to prevent it from separating during the procedure.
- Release the hemostats and start hemodialysis.

BEGINNING HEMODIALYSIS WITH AN AV GRAFT
- Remove the bulldog clamps and place them within easy reach of the sterile field.
- Remove the graft dressing, and use sterile technique to clean the shunt.
- Assemble the graft adapters according to the manufacturer's instructions.
- Clean the artierial and venous graft connection with povidone-iodine pads. Use a separate pad for each tube, and wipe in one direction only, from the insertion site to the connection site.
- Allow the tubing to air dry.
- Put on sterile gloves.
- Clamp the arterial and venous sides with bulldog clamps.
- Open the shunt by separating its sides with your fingers or with a sterile shunt spreader, if available. Both sides of the shunt should be exposed.
- Inspect the Teflon connector on one side of the shunt to see if it's damaged

(continued)

HEMODIALYSIS ACCESS SITES

Hemodialysis requires vascular access. The site and type of access depends on expected duration of dialysis, surgeon's preference, and patient's condition.

Subclavian vein catheterization
Using the Seldinger technique, the surgeon inserts an introducer needle into the subclavian vein. He then inserts a guide wire through the introducer needle and removes the needle. Using the guide wire, he threads a 5″ to 12″ (12.5- to 30.5-cm) plastic or Teflon catheter (with a Y-hub) into the patient's vein.

vein. He then inserts a guide wire through the introducer needle and removes the needle. Using the guide wire, he threads a 5″ to 12″ plastic or Teflon catheter with a Y-hub or two catheters, one for inflow and the other placed about ½″ (1.3 cm) distal to the first for outflow.

to make a common opening ⅛″ to ¼″ (3 to 6 mm) long.

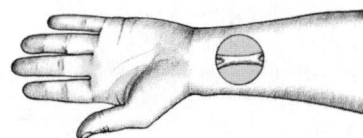

Arteriovenous graft
To create a graft, the surgeon makes an incision in the patient's forearm, upper arm, or thigh. He then tunnels a natural or synthetic graft under the skin and sutures the distal end to an artery and the proximal end to a vein.

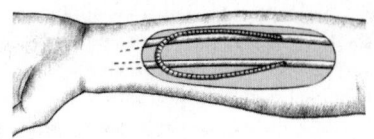

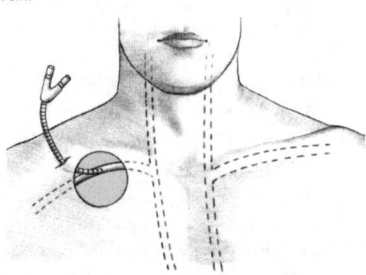

Femoral vein catheterization
Using the Seldinger technique, the surgeon inserts an introducer needle into the left or right femoral

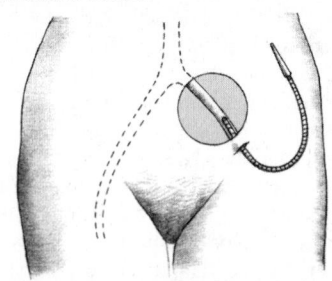

Arteriovenous fistula
To create a fistula, the surgeon makes an incision in the patient's lower forearm, then a small incision in the side of an artery, and another in the side of a vein. He sutures the edges of the incisions together

or bent. If necessary, replace it before proceeding. Note which side contains the connector so you can use the new one to close the shunt after treatment.

- Attach a shunt adapter and 10-ml syringe filled with about 8 ml of normal saline solution to the side of the shunt containing the Teflon connector.
- Attach the new Teflon connector to the side of the shunt with the second adapter. Attach the second 10-ml syringe filled with about 8 ml of normal saline solution to the same side.
- Flush the shunt's arterial tubing by releasing its clamp and gently aspirating it with the normal saline solution–filled syringe.
- Flush the tubing slowly while observing it for signs of fibrin buildup; repeat the procedure on the venous side of the shunt.
- Secure the shunt to the adapter connection with adhesive tape.
- Connect the arterial and venous lines to the adapters and secure the connections with tape. Tape each line to the patient's arm.
- Begin hemodialysis according to facility policy.

DISCONTINUING HEMODIALYSIS WITH A DOUBLE-LUMEN CATHETER

- Clamp the extension tubing to prevent air from entering the catheter.
- Clean all connection points on the catheter and blood lines as well as the clamps to reduce the risk of systemic or local infections.
- Place a clean drape under the catheter, and place two sterile 4″ × 4″ gauze pads on the drape beneath the catheter lines.
- Soak the pads with povidone-iodine solution.
- Prepare the catheter flush solution with normal saline or heparin flush solution, as ordered.
- Put on clean gloves.
- Grasp each blood line with a gauze pad and disconnect each line from the catheter.
- Flush each port with normal saline solution to clean the extension tubing and catheter of blood.
- Administer additional heparin flush solution, as ordered, to ensure catheter patency. Then attach luer-lock injection caps to prevent entry of air or loss of blood.

- Clamp the extension tubing.
- Re-dress the catheter insertion site; also re-dress it if it's occluded, soiled, or wet.
- During the dressing change, position the patient in a supine position with his face turned away from the insertion site so that he doesn't contaminate the site by breathing on it.
- Change gloves after washing your hands, and remove the outer occlusive dressing.
- Put on sterile gloves, remove the old inner dressing, and discard the gloves and the inner dressing.
- Set up a sterile field, and observe the site for drainage, obtaining a drainage sample for culture if necessary.
- Notify the physician if the suture appears to be missing.
- Put on sterile gloves and clean the insertion site with an alcohol pad to remove skin oils.
- Clean the site with a povidone-iodine pad and allow it to air-dry.
- Place a precut gauze dressing under the catheter, and place another gauze dressing over the catheter.
- Apply a skin barrier preparation to the skin surrounding the gauze dressing, and cover the gauze and catheter with a transparent occlusive dressing.
- Apply a 4″ to 5″ (10 to 12.5 cm) piece of 2″ tape over the cut edge of the dressing to reinforce the lower edge.

DISCONTINUING HEMODIALYSIS WITH AN AV FISTULA

- Turn the blood pump on the hemodialysis machine to 50 to 100 ml/ minute.
- Put on clean gloves and remove the tape from the connection site of the arterial lines.
- Clamp the needle tubing with the hemostat and disconnect the lines. The blood in the machine's arterial line will continue to flow toward the dialyzer, followed by a column of air. Just before the blood reaches the point where the normal saline solution enters the line, clamp the blood line with another hemostat.
- Unclamp the normal saline solution to allow a small amount to flow through the line.
- Unclamp the hemostat on the machine line to allow all blood to flow into the dialyzer where it passes

through the filter and back to the patient through the venous line.
- After the blood is retransfused, clamp the venous needle tubing and the machine's venous line with hemostats and turn off the blood pump.
- Remove the tape from the connection site of the venous lines and disconnect the lines.
- Remove the venipuncture needle and apply pressure to the site with a folded 4″ × 4″ gauze pad until all bleeding stops, usually within 10 minutes.
- Apply an adhesive bandage.
- Repeat the procedure on the arterial line.
- Disinfect and rinse the delivery system according to the manufacturer's instructions.

DISCONTINUING HEMODIALYSIS WITH AN AV GRAFT

- Wash your hands.
- Turn the blood pump on the hemodialysis machine to 50 to 100 ml/ minute.
- Put on sterile gloves.
- Remove the tape from the connection site of the arterial line.
- Clamp the arterial cannula with a bulldog clamp, and then disconnect the lines. Just before the blood reaches the point where the normal saline solution enters the line, clamp the blood line with a hemostat.
- Unclamp the normal saline solution to allow a small amount to flow through the line.
- Reclamp the normal saline solution line and unclamp the hemostat on the machine line.
- Just before the last volume of blood enters the patient, clamp the venous cannula with a bulldog clamp and the machine's venous line with a hemostat.
- Remove the tape from the connection site of the venous lines.
- Turn off the blood pump and disconnect the lines.
- Reconnect the graft cannula. Remove the older of the two Teflon connectors and discard it. Connect the graft, positioning the Teflon connector equally between the two cannulas.
- Remove the bulldog clamp.
- Secure the graft connection with plasticized or hypoallergenic tape.

- Clean the graft and its site with the gauze pads soaked with povidone-iodine solution.
- When the cleaning procedure is finished, remove the povidone-iodine with alcohol pads.
- Make sure that blood flows through the graft adequately.
- Apply a dressing to the graft site and wrap it securely (but not too tightly) with elastic gauze bandages.
- Attach the bulldog clamps to the outside dressing.
- When hemodialysis is complete, assess the patient's weight, vital signs, and mental status. Compare your findings with your predialysis assessment data.
- Document your findings.
- Disinfect and rinse the delivery system according to the manufacturer's instructions.

✦ SPECIAL CONSIDERATIONS

- Obtain blood samples from the patient, as ordered, usually before beginning hemodialysis.

> ◈ **NURSING ALERT** To avoid pyrogenic reactions and bacteremia with septicemia resulting from contamination, use strict sterile technique while preparing the machine.

- Immediately report any machine malfunction or equipment defect.
- Avoid unnecessary handling of hemodialysis tubing.

- Assess the catheter insertion site for signs of infection, such as purulent drainage, inflammation, and tenderness.

> ◈ **NURSING ALERT** Complete each step of dialysis correctly to avoid unnecessary blood loss or inefficient treatment from poor clearances or inadequate fluid removal. Failure to perform accurate hemodialysis therapy can lead to patient injury and even death.

- If bleeding continues after you remove an AV fistula needle, apply just enough pressure with a sterile, absorbable gelatin sponge or topical thrombin solution to stop bleeding.
- Monitor vital signs throughout hemodialysis at least hourly or as often as every 15 minutes, if necessary.
- After dialysis is complete, assess the patient's weight, vital signs, and mental status, and compare the findings with your predialysis assessment.
- Perform periodic tests for clotting time on the patient's blood samples and samples from the dialyzer.
- If the patient receives meals during treatment, make sure they're light.
- Continue necessary drug administration during dialysis unless the drug would be removed in the dialysate; if so, administer the drug after dialysis.

Complications
- Fever
- Dialysis disequilibrium syndrome
- Hypovolemia
- Hypotension
- Hyperglycemia

- Hypernatremia
- Hyperosmolarity
- Cardiac arrhythmias
- Angina
- Exsanguination
- Thrombosis or stenosis of AV fistula

▶ PATIENT TEACHING

Be sure to cover:
- how to care for the vascular access site at home (see *Caring for an arteriovenous fistula at home*)
- how to perform hemodialysis at home—usually a complex process requiring 2 to 3 months to feel comfortable and be competent
- telephone number of the dialysis center.

◆◇ DOCUMENTATION

- Time treatment began
- Any problems with treatment
- Vital signs and weight before and during treatment
- Time blood specimens were taken for testing, the test results, and treatment for complications
- Time the treatment was completed
- Patient's response to treatment
- Condition of vascular access site and site care

Selected references
Cleary, J., and Drennan, J. "Quality of Life of Patients on Haemodialysis for End-Stage Renal Disease," *Journal of Advanced Nursing* 51(6):577-86, September 2005.

Desmet, C., et al. "Falls in Hemodialysis Patient: Prospective Study of Incidence, Risk Factors, and Complications," *American Journal of Kidney Diseases* 45(1):148-52, January 2005.

Harwood, L., et al. "Preparing for Hemodiaylsis: Patient Stressors and Responses," *Nephrology Nursing Journal* 32(3):295-302, May-June 2005.

Holley, J.L., et al. "Managing Homeless Dialysis Patient," *Nephrology News & Issues* 20(1):49-50, 52-53, January 2006.

CARING FOR AN ARTERIOVENOUS FISTULA AT HOME

Before the patient leaves the hospital, teach him how to care for his arteriovenous (AV) fistula. Be sure to cover:
- the need to keep the incision clean and dry to prevent infection
- the need to clean the site daily until it heals completely and the sutures are removed (usually 10 to 14 days after surgery)
- the need to notify the practitioner of pain, swelling, redness, or drainage at the site
- using a stethoscope to auscultate for bruits and how to palpate a thrill
- using the arm freely after the site heals
- the need to allow no treatments or procedures on the arm with the AV fistula, including blood pressure monitoring or needle punctures
- the need to avoid putting excessive pressure on the arm
- the need to avoid sleeping on the arm with the AV fistula, wearing constricting clothing on it, or lifting heavy objects or straining with it
- the need to avoid getting the hemodialysis access site wet for several hours after dialysis
- exercises for the affected arm with a native AV fistula to promote vascular dilation and enhance blood flow, starting by squeezing a small rubber ball or other soft object for 15 minutes, when advised by the practitioner.

Hyperthermia-hypothermia therapy

● OVERVIEW

- Raises, lowers, or maintains body temperature through conductive heat or cold transfer between the blanket and the patient
- For manual use: temperature on unit and blanket reaches and maintains this temperature regardless of patient's temperature
- For automatic use: patient's temperature is monitored by thermistor probe (rectal, skin, or esophageal) and unit alternates heating and cooling cycles, as necessary, to achieve and maintain desired body temperature
- Used most commonly to reduce high fever when more conservative measures—such as baths, ice packs, and antipyretics—are unsuccessful
- Also used in maintaining normal temperature during surgery or shock; inducing hypothermia during surgery to decrease metabolic activity and thereby reduce oxygen requirements; reducing intracranial pressure; controlling bleeding and intractable pain in patients with amputations, burns, or cancer; and providing warmth in cases of severe hypothermia

Contraindications
ABSOLUTE
- None known

RELATIVE
- Impaired circulation
- Advanced age
- Impaired skin integrity

❖ EQUIPMENT

Hyperthermia-hypothermia control unit • operation manual • fluid for the control unit (distilled water or distilled water and 20% ethyl alcohol) • thermistor probe (rectal, skin, or esophageal) • patient thermometer • one or two hyperthermia-hypothermia blankets • one or two disposable blanket covers (or one or two sheets or bath blankets) • lanolin or a mixture of lanolin and cold cream • adhesive tape • towel • sphygmomanometer • gloves and gowns, if necessary • optional: protective wraps for the patient's hands and feet

Disposable hyperthermia-hypothermia blankets are available for single-patient use.

Equipment preparation
- Read the operation manual.
- Wash your hands thoroughly.
- Inspect the control unit and each blanket for leaks and the plugs and connecting wires for broken prongs, kinks, and fraying.

◆ **NURSING ALERT** If you detect or suspect malfunction, don't use the equipment.

- Prepare one or two blankets by covering them with disposable covers (or use a sheet or bath blanket when positioning the blanket on the patient) to absorb perspiration and condensation, which could cause tissue breakdown if left on the skin.
- Connect the blanket to the control unit, and set the controls for manual or automatic operation and for the desired blanket or body temperature, as ordered.
- Make sure the machine is properly grounded before plugging it in.
- Turn on the machine and add liquid to the unit reservoir, if necessary, as fluid fills the blanket.
- Allow the blanket to preheat or precool so that the patient receives immediate thermal benefit.

❙❙❚ ESSENTIAL STEPS

- Confirm the patient's identity using two patient identifiers according to facility policy.
- Explain the procedure to the patient and his family.
- Make sure the patient or responsible family member has signed the appropriate consent form, per facility policy.
- Assess the patient's condition.
- Make sure the room is warm and free from drafts.
- Help the patient into a hospital gown with cloth ties rather than metal snaps or pins to prevent heat or cold injury.
- Take the patient's vital signs, and assess level of consciousness, pupil reaction, limb strength, and skin condition.
- Keeping the bottom sheet in place and the patient recumbent, roll the patient to one side and slide the blanket halfway underneath him, so its top edge aligns with his neck.
- Roll the patient back, and pull and flatten the blanket across the bed.
- Place a pillow under the patient's head.
- Make sure the patient's head doesn't lie directly on the blanket because the blanket's rigid surface may be uncomfortable and the heat or cold may lead to tissue breakdown.
- If necessary, use a sheet or bath blanket as insulation between the patient and the blanket.
- Apply lanolin or a mixture of lanolin and cold cream to the patient's skin where it touches the blanket to help protect the skin from heat or cold sensation.
- In automatic operation, insert the thermistor probe in the patient's rectum and tape it in place to prevent accidental dislodgment.
- If rectal insertion is contraindicated, tuck a skin probe deep into the axilla, and secure it with tape.
- If the patient is comatose or anesthetized, an esophageal probe may be inserted.
- Plug the other end of the probe into the correct jack on the unit's control panel.
- Place a sheet or, if ordered, the second hyperthermia-hypothermia blanket over the patient, increasing thermal benefit by trapping cooled or heated air.
- Wrap the patient's hands and feet if he wishes, to minimize chilling and promote comfort.
- Monitor vital signs and perform a neurologic assessment every 5 minutes until the desired body temperature is reached and then every 15 minutes until temperature is stable, or as ordered.
- Check fluid intake and output hourly, or as ordered.
- Observe the patient for color changes in skin, lips, and nail beds, and for edema, induration, inflammation, pain, or sensory impairment; if these

occur, discontinue the procedure and notify the physician.
- Reposition the patient every 30 minutes to 1 hour, unless contraindicated, to prevent skin breakdown.
- Keep the patient's skin, bedclothes, and blanket cover free from perspiration and condensation, and reapply cream to exposed body parts, as needed.
- Some units must remain plugged in for at least 30 minutes after use to allow the condenser fan to remove water vapor from the mechanism; follow the manufacturer's directions.
- Continue to monitor the patient's temperature until it stabilizes because body temperature can fall as much as 5° F (2.8° C) after this procedure.
- Remove all equipment from the bed.
- Dry the patient and make him comfortable.
- Supply a fresh gown, if necessary, and cover the patient lightly.
- Continue to perform neurologic checks and monitor vital signs, fluid intake and output, and general condition every 30 minutes for 2 hours and then hourly, or as ordered.
- Return the equipment to the central supply department for cleaning, servicing, and storage.

✦ SPECIAL CONSIDERATIONS

- If the patient shivers excessively during hypothermia treatment, discontinue the procedure and notify the physician immediately.

▣ **NURSING ALERT** Shivering increases tissue oxygen demand and may lead to mixed venous desaturation, lactic acidosis, and ischemia of vital organs.

✸ **AGE-RELATED CONCERN** Elderly patients who have diminished cardiopulmonary reserves are particularly at risk for complications related to shivering.

- Avoid lowering the temperature more than 1° every 15 minutes to prevent premature ventricular contractions.
- Don't use pins to secure catheters, tubes, or blanket covers because an accidental puncture can result in fluid leakage and burns.

- With hyperthermia or hypothermia therapy, the patient may experience a secondary defense reaction (vasoconstriction or vasodilation) that causes body temperature to rebound and thus defeat the treatment's purpose.
- If the patient requires isolation, use a disposable blanket or place the nondisposable blanket, blanket cover, and probe in a plastic bag clearly marked with the type of isolation so that the central supply department can give it special handling.
- To avoid bacterial growth in the reservoir or blankets, always use sterile distilled water and change it monthly.
- Check to see if facility policy calls for adding a bacteriostatic agent to the water.
- Avoid using deionized water because it can corrode the system.
- To gradually increase body temperature, especially in postoperative patients, the physician may order a disposable blanket warming system. (See *Using a warming system*.)
- The control unit is equipped with an alarm to warn of abnormal temperature fluctuations and a circuit breaker that protects against current overload.

Complications
- Shivering
- Marked changes in vital signs
- Increased intracranial pressure
- Respiratory distress or arrest
- Cardiac arrest
- Oliguria; anuria
- Increased tissue oxygen demand

▶ PATIENT TEACHING

Be sure to cover:
- reason for procedure and what to expect during it
- signs and symptoms to report
- need for frequent monitoring and position changes
- when the unit will be removed.

●✛ DOCUMENTATION

- Date, time, and duration of treatment
- Type of hyperthermia-hypothermia unit used
- Control settings (manual or automatic and temperature settings)
- Patient's tolerance of treatment
- Signs of and measures for treating complications
- Pulse, respirations, blood pressure, neurologic signs, fluid intake and output, and skin condition
- Frequency of position changes
- Patient's temperature and that of the blanket (every 30 minutes)
- Patient teaching

Selected references

Basoglu, O.K., et al. "The Efficacy of Incentive Spirometry in Patients with COPD," *Respirology* 10(3):349-53, June 2005.

Hsu, L.L., et al. "Positive Expiratory Pressure Device Acceptance by Hospitalized Children with Sickle Cell Disease is Comparable to Incentive Spirometry," *Respiratory Care* 50(5):624-27, May 2005.

Ong, G.L. "Incentive Spirometry for Children with Sickle Cell Disorder," *Nursing Times* 101(42):55-57, October 2005.

USING A WARMING SYSTEM

Shivering, the compensatory response to falling body temperature, may use more oxygen than the body can supply, especially in a surgical patient. A warming system such as the Bair Hugger patient-warming system helps to gradually increase body temperature. Like a large hair dryer, the warming unit draws air through a filter, warms the air to the desired temperature, and circulates it through a hose to a warming blanket placed over the patient.

When using the warming system, be sure to:
- use a bath blanket in a single layer over the warming blanket to minimize heat loss
- place the warming blanket directly over the patient with the paper side facing down and the clear tubular side facing up
- make sure the connection hose is at the foot of the bed
- take the patient's temperature during the first 15 to 30 minutes and at least every 30 minutes while the warming blanket is in use
- obtain guidelines from the patient's physician for discontinuing use of the warming blanket.

Incentive spirometry

● OVERVIEW

- Encourages deep breathing by providing visual feedback to the patient such as the balls rising in response to respirations
- Increases lung volume, boosts alveolar inflation, and promotes venous return
- Hyperinflates the alveoli for a longer time than a normal deep breath, preventing and reversing the alveolar collapse that causes atelectasis and pneumonitis
- May be used by patients at low risk for developing atelectasis; those at high risk possibly needing a volume incentive spirometer, which measures lung inflation more precisely
- Benefits patient on prolonged bed rest, especially a postoperative patient who may regain normal respiratory pattern slowly due to predisposing factors such as abdominal or thoracic surgery, advanced age, inactivity, obesity, smoking, and decreased ability to cough effectively and expel lung secretions
- Use of spirometer requiring adaptation in presence of an open tracheal stoma

Contraindications

- Patients who are unable to cooperate or demonstrate the proper use of the device
- Patients who are unable to deep-breathe effectively

❖ EQUIPMENT

Flow or volume incentive spirometer, as indicated, with sterile disposable tube and mouthpiece (the tube and mouthpiece are sterile on first use and clean on subsequent uses) • stethoscope • watch • pencil • paper

Equipment preparation

- Wash your hands thoroughly.
- Assemble the equipment at the patient's bedside.
- Remove the sterile flow tube and mouthpiece from the package, and attach them to the device.
- Set the flow rate or volume goal as determined by the physician or respiratory therapist and based on the patient's preoperative performance.

▐▐▌ ESSENTIAL STEPS

- Confirm the patient's identity using two patient identifiers according to facility policy.
- Assess the patient's condition.
- Explain the procedure to the patient.
- Help the patient into a comfortable sitting or semi-Fowler's position to promote optimal lung expansion.

  ◆ **NURSING ALERT** Tilting a flow incentive spirometer decreases the required patient effort and reduces the exercise's effectiveness.

- Auscultate the patient's lungs to provide a baseline for comparison with posttreatment auscultation.
- Instruct the patient to insert the mouthpiece and close his lips tightly around it.
- Tell him to exhale normally and then inhale as slowly and as deeply as possible.
- Ask the patient to retain the entire volume of air he inhaled for 3 seconds or, if you're using a device with a light indicator, until the light turns off.
- Note the tidal volume.
- Tell the patient to remove the mouthpiece and exhale normally.
- Allow him to relax and take several normal breaths before attempting another breath with the spirometer.
- Repeat this sequence 5 to 10 times during every waking hour.
- Encourage him to cough after each effort because deep lung inflation may loosen secretions and facilitate their removal and observe any expectorated secretions.
- Auscultate the patient's lungs, and compare findings with the first auscultation.
- Instruct the patient to remove the mouthpiece, wash it in warm water, and shake it dry.
- Place the mouthpiece in a plastic storage bag between exercises, and label it and the spirometer, if applicable, with the patient's name.

- If the patient is scheduled for surgery, make a preoperative assessment of his respiratory pattern and capability to ensure the development of appropriate postoperative goals.
- Teach the patient how to use the spirometer preoperatively so that he can concentrate on your instructions and practice the exercise.
- Tell the patient to avoid exercising at mealtime to prevent nausea.
- Provide paper and pencil so the patient can note exercise times and volumes.
- Immediately after surgery, encourage the patient to use the exercise frequently to ensure compliance and enable assessment of his achievement.

Complications
- Hyperventilation
- Increased surgical pain
- Nausea
- Barotrauma (emphysematous lungs)
- Hypoxemia secondary to interruption of prescribed oxygen therapy
- Exacerbation of bronchospasm
- Fatigue

Be sure to cover:
- purpose of incentive spirometry and how to use the device
- importance of recording exercise times and volumes, so the patient can see improvement
- importance of performing this exercise regularly to maintain alveolar inflation.

- Preoperative teaching
- Preoperative flow or volume levels
- Date and time of the procedure, type of spirometer, flow or volume levels achieved, and number of breaths taken
- Patient's condition before and after the procedure, his tolerance of the procedure, and the results of both auscultations (see *Documenting flow and volume levels*)

Selected references

Basoglu, O.K., et al. "The Efficacy of Incentive Spirometry in Patients with COPD," *Respirology* 10(3):349-53, June 2005.

Hsu, L.L., et al. "Positive Expiratory Pressure Device Acceptance by Hospitalized Children with Sickle Cell Disease is Comparable to Incentive Spirometry," *Respiratory Care* 50(5):624-27, May 2005.

Ong, G.L. "Incentive Spirometry for Children with Sickle Cell Disorder," *Nursing Times* 101(42):55-57, October 2005.

Reardon, C.C., et al. "Intrapulmonary Percussive Ventilation vs. Incentive Spirometry for Children with Neuromuscular Disease," *Archives of Pediatrics & Adolescent Medicine* 159(6):526-31, June 2005.

DOCUMENTING FLOW AND VOLUME LEVELS

When using a flow incentive spirometer, compute the volume by multiplying the setting by the duration that the patient keeps the ball (or balls) suspended. For example, if the patient suspends the ball for 3 seconds at a setting of 500 cc during each of 10 breaths, multiply 500 cc by 3 seconds and record this total (1,500 cc) and the number of breaths, as follows: 1,500 cc × 10 breaths.

When using a volume-incentive spirometer, take the volume reading directly from the spirometer. For example, record 1,000 cc × 5 breaths.

Insulin pump therapy

- External device that delivers insulin continuously under the surface of the skin
- Keeps blood glucose levels as close to normal as possible
- Provides lifestyle flexibility for traveling, exercising, working, or eating without worry of injections and when the insulin will take effect
- Also called *continuous subcutaneous insulin infusion*

Contraindications

- None known

Insulin pump • infusion set • reservoir containing insulin • alcohol pads • occlusive dressing • clean gloves

Equipment preparation

- Check the order for insulin prescribed.
- Attach insulin reservoir to pump and program pump according to manufacturer's instructions.
- Assess patient's blood glucose level as a baseline value.

- Confirm the patient's identity using two patient identifiers according to facility policy.
- Review information about the procedure and the functioning of the pump with the patient.
- Verify that an appropriate consent form has been signed.
- Wear gloves and clean the area around the intended insertion site and allow the area to dry. A small, soft cannula (called an infusion set) is inserted under the skin of the patient's abdomen, thigh, or leg. (Usually the patient requires 12 insertions per month.)
- Insert the infusion device and apply a sterile occlusive dressing over the site. Attach the pump to the infusion set.
- The pump is programmed according to the patient's needs. The basal rate (a continuous preprogrammed rate) is usually 40% to 50% of the total daily dose of insulin. There may be several different basal rates throughout a 24-hour period based on activity patterns, hormonal changes, and other factors that affect insulin needs. (See *How an insulin pump works.*)
- Bolus rates are programmed by the user to compensate for eating. This is usually a pre-meal bolus dose given around the time of a meal or snack.
- The pump is clipped to the patient's clothing for easy access.

✦ SPECIAL CONSIDERATIONS

- Monitor vital signs.
- Monitor blood glucose levels.
- Make sure the pump is functioning properly and assess the patency of the infusion set.
- Watch for complications.

Complications

- Pump malfunction, resulting in hypoglycemia or hyperglycemia
- Skin site infection

▶ PATIENT TEACHING

Be sure to cover:
- operation of the pump, manuals, and available resources
- vendor contact information
- delivery of a precise dose of insulin based on his current needs, as established by his practitioner
- need to follow set guidelines for safety purposes
- importance of good nutrition and exercise habits
- blood glucose testing and how to make decisions about how much insulin to take for food intake
- diabetes education, as indicated
- signs and symptoms of hypoglycemia and hyperglycemia and emergency measures to take if such complications occur
- signs and symptoms of infection at the infusion insertion sites
- change of infusion sites, as ordered
- insulin needs during illness or stress
- importance of follow-up care

•✦ DOCUMENTATION

- Pre- and postprocedure vital signs
- Time and date of cannula insertion and condition and location of the site
- Make and model of pump used
- Time, date the infusion instituted with the delivery, and bolus rates noted
- Patient teaching performed
- Patient's condition before and after the insulin pump was instituted, his tolerance of the procedure, any complications noted and the nursing actions taken

Selected references

Fisher, L.K., and Halvorson, M. "Future Developments in Insulin Pump Therapy: Progression from Continuous Subcutaneous Insulin Infusion to a Sensor-Pump System," *Diabetes Educator* 32(1):47S-52S, January-February 2006.

Low, K.G., et al. "Insulin Pump Use in Young Adolescents with Type 1 Diabetes: A Descriptive Study," *Pediatric Diabetes* 6(1):22-31, March 2005.

Wittlin, S.D. "Treating the Spectrum of Type 2 Diabetes: Emphasis on Insulin Pump Therapy," *Diabetes Educator* 32(1):39S-46S, January-February 2006.

HOW AN INSULIN PUMP WORKS

The insulin pump delivers a continuous preprogrammed basal rate of insulin to the patient via a catheter that's inserted through the skin into the subcutaneous tissue.

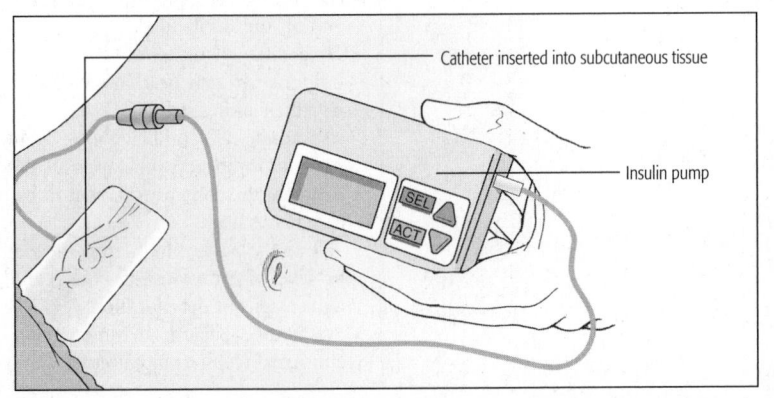

Catheter inserted into subcutaneous tissue

Insulin pump

Intracranial pressure monitoring

● OVERVIEW

- Indicated for head trauma with bleeding or edema, overproduction or insufficient absorption of cerebrospinal fluid (CSF), cerebral hemorrhage, and space-occupying brain lesions
- Used to measure pressure exerted by the brain, blood, and CSF against the inside of the skull
- Detects elevated intracranial pressure (ICP) early, allowing prompt intervention to avert or diminish neurologic damage caused by cerebral hypoxia and shifts of brain mass
- May use four basic ICP monitoring systems, including intraventricular catheter, subarachnoid bolt, epidural sensor, and intraparenchymal pressure monitoring
- Typically performed by a neurosurgeon in the operating room, emergency department, or intensive care unit (ICU)

Contraindications
INTRAVENTRICULAR CATHETER MONITORING
- Stenotic cerebral ventricles
- Cerebral aneurysms in path of catheter placement
- Suspected vascular lesions

❖ EQUIPMENT

Monitoring unit and transducers as ordered • 16 to 20 sterile 4″ × 4″ gauze pads • linen-saver pads • hair clippers • sterile drapes • chlorhexidine solution • sterile gown • surgical mask • sterile gloves • head-dressing supplies (two rolls of 4″ elastic gauze dressing, one roll of 4″ roller gauze, adhesive tape) • optional: suction apparatus, I.V. pole, and yardstick

Equipment preparation
- Set up monitoring units according to your facility's guidelines for your unit.
- Various types of preassembled ICP monitoring units are available, each with its own setup protocols designed to reduce the risk of infection by eliminating the need for multiple stopcocks, manometers, and transducer dome assemblies.

  NURSING ALERT Insertion of an ICP monitoring device and setting up equipment for the monitoring system requires strict asepsis to reduce the risk of central nervous system (CNS) infection.

▌▌▮ ESSENTIAL STEPS

- Confirm the patient's identity using two patient identifiers according to facility policy.
- Explain the procedure to the patient or his family.
- Make sure the patient or a responsible family member has signed an appropriate consent form.
- Provide privacy if the procedure is being done in an open emergency department or ICU.
- Wash your hands thoroughly.
- Wear appropriate personal protection equipment, when necessary, throughout all procedures.
- Obtain baseline routine and neurologic vital signs to aid in prompt detection of decompensation during the procedure.
- Place the patient in the supine position and elevate the head of the bed 30 degrees (or as ordered).
- Document the number of bed crank rotations, or hang a yardstick on an I.V. pole and mark the exact elevation.
- Place linen-saver pads under the patient's head.
- Clip his hair at the insertion site, as indicated by the physician, to decrease the risk of infection.
- Drape the patient with sterile drapes.
- Scrub the insertion site for 2 minutes with chlorhexidine solution.
- The physician puts on the sterile gown, mask, and sterile gloves and opens the interior wrap of the sterile supply tray and proceeds with insertion of the catheter or bolt.
- Label all medications, medication containers, and other solutions on and off the sterile field.
- To facilitate placement of the device, hold the patient's head in your hands or attach a long strip of 4″ roller gauze to one side rail, and bring it across the patient's forehead to the opposite rail.
- Reassure the conscious patient to help ease his anxiety.
- Talk to the patient frequently to assess his level of consciousness (LOC) and detect signs of deterioration.
- Watch for cardiac arrhythmias and abnormal respiratory patterns.

- After insertion, put on sterile gloves and apply chlorhexidine solution and a sterile dressing to the site.
- If not done by the physician, connect the catheter to the appropriate monitoring device, depending on the system used.

- If the physician has set up a ventriculostomy drainage system, attach the drip chamber to the headboard or bedside I.V. pole, as ordered.

  ◈ **NURSING ALERT** Positioning the drip chamber too high can increase ICP; positioning it too low can cause excessive CSF drainage.

- Inspect the insertion site at least every 24 hours (or according to your facility's policy) for redness, swelling, and drainage.
- Clean the insertion site, apply chlorhexidine solution, and apply a fresh sterile dressing.

(continued)

INTERPRETING ICP WAVEFORMS

Three waveforms—A, B, and C—are used to monitor intracranial pressure (ICP). A waves are an ominous sign of intracranial decompensation and poor compliance. B waves correlate with changes in respiration, and C waves correlate with changes in arterial pressure.

Normal waveform
A normal ICP waveform typically shows a steep upward systolic slope followed by a downward diastolic slope with a dicrotic notch. In most cases, this waveform occurs continuously and indicates an ICP between 0 and 15 mm Hg—normal pressure.

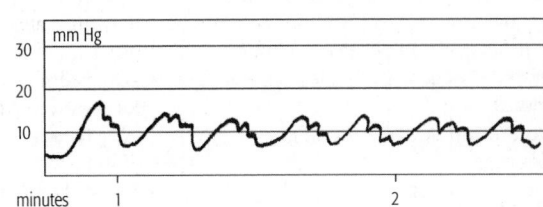

A waves
The most clinically significant ICP waveforms are A waves, which may reach elevations of 50 to 100 mm Hg, persist for 5 to 20 minutes, then drop sharply—signaling exhaustion of the brain's compliance mechanisms. A waves may come and go, spiking from temporary rises in thoracic pressure or from any condition that increases ICP beyond the brain's compliance limits. Activities, such as sustained coughing or straining during defecation can cause temporary elevations in thoracic pressure.

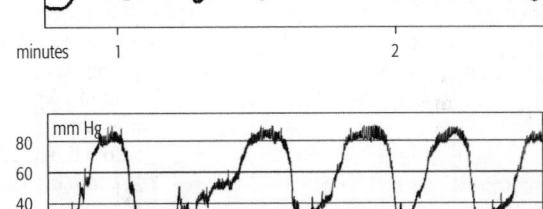

B waves
B waves, which appear sharp and rhythmic with a sawtooth pattern, occur every 1½ to 2 minutes and may reach elevations of 50 mm Hg. The clinical significance of B waves isn't clear, but the waves correlate with respiratory changes and may occur more frequently with decreasing compensation. Because B waves sometimes precede A waves, notify the physician if B waves occur frequently.

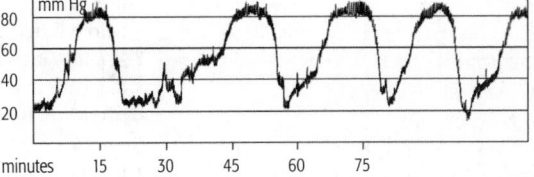

C waves
Like B waves, C waves are rapid and rhythmic, but they aren't as sharp. Clinically insignificant, they may fluctuate with respirations or systemic blood pressure changes.

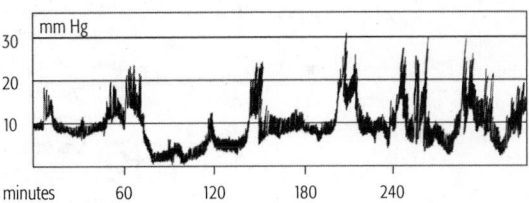

Waveform showing equipment problem
A waveform that looks like the one shown at right signals a problem with the transducer or monitor. Check for line obstruction, and determine if the transducer needs rebalancing.

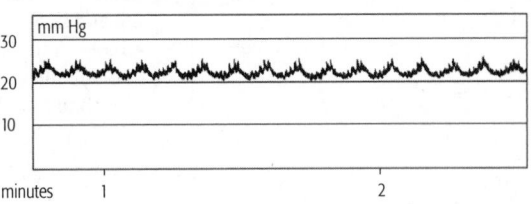
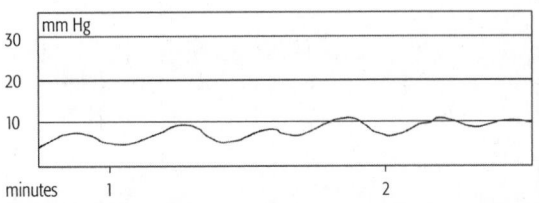

- Assess the patient's clinical status, and take routine and neurologic vital signs every hour, or as ordered.
- Obtain orders for waveforms and pressure parameters.
- Calculate cerebral perfusion pressure (CPP) hourly; use the equation:
  CPP = MAP − ICP
  (MAP refers to mean arterial pressure).
- Observe digital ICP readings and waves. (See *Interpreting ICP waveforms,* page 767.)

NURSING ALERT The pattern of ICP readings is more significant than any single reading. Notify the physician immediately if you observe continually elevated ICP readings that last several minutes.

- Record and describe any CSF drainage.

◆ SPECIAL CONSIDERATIONS

AGE-RELATED CONCERN In infants, ICP monitoring can be performed without penetrating the scalp using a photoelectric transducer with a pressure-sensitive membrane taped to the anterior fontanel. The external method is restricted to infants because pressure readings can be obtained only at fontanels.

- Osmotic diuretics, such as I. V. mannitol, reduce cerebral edema by shrinking intracranial contents by drawing water from tissues into plasma.
- When administering mannitol, monitor serum electrolyte levels and osmolality readings closely to avoid dehydration.
- To avoid rebound increased ICP when giving mannitol, administer 50 ml of albumin with the mannitol bolus, monitoring for a residual rise in ICP before it decreases.

NURSING ALERT Monitor the patient with heart failure or severe renal dysfunction for problems adapting to the increased intravascular volumes.

- Fluid restriction, usually 1,200 to 1,500 ml/day, prevents cerebral edema from developing or worsening.
- Steroid therapy, although controversial, may be used to lower elevated ICP by reducing sodium and water concentration in the brain.

NURSING ALERT Administer steroids with antacids and histamine-2 receptor antagonists to reduce the risk of peptic ulcers and monitor for GI bleeding and hyperglycemia.

- Barbiturate-induced coma reduces the brain's metabolic demand, reducing cerebral blood flow, thereby lowering ICP.
- Hyperventilation with oxygen from a handheld resuscitation bag or ventilator eliminates excess carbon dioxide, constricting cerebral vessels and reducing cerebral blood volume and ICP.

NURSING ALERT Hyperventilation with a handheld resuscitation bag or a ventilator should be performed with care because there's increasing evidence that hyperventilation can lead to frank ischemia in areas of marginally perfused brain.

- Before tracheal suctioning, hyperventilate the patient with 100% oxygen and suction for no more than 15 seconds to avoid inducing hypoxia and increasing cerebral blood flow.
- Because fever raises brain metabolism, which increases cerebral blood flow and ICP, reduce fever by administering acetaminophen, sponge baths, or a hypothermia blanket.

NURSING ALERT Rebound increases in ICP and brain edema may occur if rapid rewarming takes place after hypothermia or if cooling measures induce shivering.

- Withdrawal of CSF through the drainage system reduces CSF volume and thus reduces ICP.
- If a skull-bone flap is surgically removed to provide room for the swollen brain to expand, keep the site clean and dry to prevent infection and maintain sterile technique when changing the dressing.
- Watch for signs of decompensation: pupillary dilation (unilateral or bilateral); decreased pupillary response to light; decreasing LOC; rising systolic blood pressure and widening pulse pressure; bradycardia; slowed, irregular respirations; and, in late decompensation, decerebrate posturing.

Complications
- Hemorrhage
- CNS infection
- Seizure activity

⬥ **NURSING ALERT** Excessive loss of CSF can result from faulty stopcock placement or a drip chamber that's positioned too low. Such loss can rapidly decompress the cranial contents and damage bridging cortical veins, leading to hematoma formation, rupture of existing hematomas or aneurysms, and hemorrhage.

▶ PATIENT TEACHING

Be sure to cover:
- why the procedure is needed and how it will be performed
- monitoring and nursing care involved with ICP monitoring
- importance of proper body positioning to reduce ICP
- importance of avoiding Valsalva's maneuver and isometric muscle contractions
- need to remain calm and quiet
- indications for removing the monitor and how it will be performed.

●◆ DOCUMENTATION

- Time and date of the insertion procedure
- Name of physician performing the procedure
- Patient's response to the procedure
- Insertion site and the type of monitoring system used
- Hourly ICP digital readings, waveforms, and CPP (in your notes, on a flowchart, or directly on readout strips, depending on your facility's policy)
- Factors that affect ICP (for example, drug therapy, stressful procedures, or sleep)
- Routine and neurologic vital signs hourly
- Neurologic assessment findings
- Amount, character, and frequency of any CSF drainage and ICP reading in response to drainage
- Patient teaching and emotional support given

Selected references

Cremer, O.L., et al. "Need for Intracranial Pressure Monitoring Following Severe Traumatic Brain Injury," *Critical Care Medicine* 34(5):1583-84, May 2006.

Kuo, J.R., et al. "Intraoperative Applications of Intracranial Pressure Monitoring in Patients with Severe Head Injury," *Journal of Clinical Neuroscience* 13(2):218-223, February 2006.

March, K. "Intracranial Pressure Monitoring: Why Monitor?" *AACN Clinical Issues* 16(4):456-75, October-December 2005.

Marcoux, K.K. "Management of Increased Intracranial Pressure in the Critically Ill Child with an Acute Neurological Injury," *AACN Clinical Issues* 16(2):212-31, April-June 2005.

Iontophoresis

- Delivers dermal analgesia quickly (in 10 to 20 minutes) with minimal discomfort and without distorting the tissue
- May be performed with an iontophoretic drug-delivery system, a handheld battery-powered device with two electrodes that uses a mild electric current to deliver charged ions of lidocaine 2% and epinephrine 1:100,000 solution into the skin
- Acts quickly and is an excellent choice for numbing an I.V. injection site, especially in children

Contraindications

- Implanted pacemaker or other implanted device sensitive to electricity
- Allergy or sensitivity to lidocaine or epinephrine
- Use over scarred skin

Dose-control device with battery • drug-delivery electrode kit • lidocaine 2% with epinephrine 1:100,000 solution • alcohol pads • syringe with needle • gloves • tongue blade

Equipment preparation

- Thoroughly wash your hands before preparing the equipment.
- Gather the equipment at the bedside.
- Turn on the dose-control device and check that the battery has a charge.

- Confirm the patient's identity using two patient identifiers according to facility policy.
- Ask the patient if he has any allergies or sensitivity to medications.

AGE-RELATED CONCERN If the patient is a child, ask the parents if he has any allergies or sensitivities to lidocaine or epinephrine.

- Explain the procedure to the patient and tell him that he may feel tingling or warmth under the electrode pads while they're on the skin.
- Examine the patient's skin and select intact electrode placement sites, avoiding areas with pimples, unhealed wounds, or ingrown hairs.

NURSING ALERT Avoid placing electrodes over bony prominences and damaged, denuded, or recently scarred skin, which could impede electrical conduction.

- With alcohol pads, briskly rub an area slightly larger than the electrode at each site.
- Remove the paper flap from the back of the drug-delivery electrode.
- Draw up the lidocaine with epinephrine in a syringe according to the amount indicated on the electrode pad (about 1 ml for a standard-sized pad and about 2.5 ml for a large pad).
- Remove the needle from the syringe and saturate the medication pad with the lidocaine and epinephrine solution. (See photo below.)

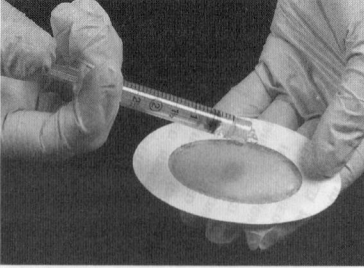

- Remove the remaining backing from the drug-delivery pad and apply the pad to the selected I.V. site.
- Remove the backing from the grounding electrode, and apply it to the second prepared site about 4″ to 6″ (10 to 15 cm) away.

- Connect the lead clips: red (positive charge) to the drug-delivery electrode and black (negative charge) to the grounding electrode.
- Turn on the device. (See *Using an iontophoresis delivery device.*)
- After the dose has been delivered, remove the electrodes.
- Assess the skin at the drug-delivery site for numbness by touching it with a blunt object such as a tongue blade.
- Promptly prepare the site and perform the venipuncture because the numbness may last only a few minutes.
- Discard gloves and wash your hands.

◆ SPECIAL CONSIDERATIONS

- To avoid interfering with energy emission, don't tape or compress the electrodes.
- If you need to stop the treatment for any reason, press the OFF button and hold it until the device beeps and turns off.

■ **NURSING ALERT** When turning the device off, don't disconnect the lead clips or the electrodes until all signals have stopped because the device is still transmitting energy until it turns off.

Complications
- Allergic reaction
- Prolonged redness at site

▶ PATIENT TEACHING

Be sure to cover:
- purpose of the procedure
- equipment to be used
- feelings and sensations experienced during the procedure
- length of time it takes for analgesia to occur (approximately 10 to 20 minutes)
- need to report a bothersome tingling sensation during the procedure.

●◆ DOCUMENTATION

- Date and time of treatment, sites used, and whether analgesia was achieved
- Whether an allergic response occurred and the resulting treatment, if necessary

Selected references

Brown, M.B., et al. "Dermal and Transdermal Drug Delivery Systems: Current and Future Prospects," *Drug Delivery* 13(3):175-87, May-June 2006.

Pasero, C. "Lidocaine Iontophoresis for Dermal Procedure Analgesia," *Journal of Perianesthesia Nursing* 21(1):48-52, February 2006.

Strout, T., et al. "Reducing Pain in ED Patients During Lumbar Puncture: The Efficacy and Feasibility of Iontophoresis, Collaborative Approach," *Journal of Emergency Nursing* 30(5):423-30, October 2004.

USING AN IONTOPHORESIS DELIVERY DEVICE

An iontophoresis delivery device automatically operates at the lowest current, 2 milliamperes (mA) — as indicated by a green light — unless you increase the level to 3 or 4 mA by pressing the ON button. If your patient has discomfort at a higher setting, reduce the current by pushing the ON button until the appropriate light indicates the desired level. The device is calibrated to deliver a dose of 40 mA-minutes, after which it will automatically stop. If the setting remains at 4 mA, treatment is completed in 10 minutes. However, if you decrease the setting because the patient has discomfort, the device automatically adjusts to a longer treatment time to deliver the entire dose.

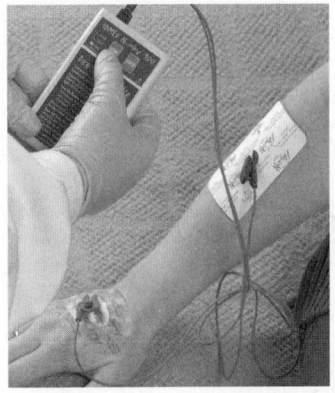

Latex allergy protocol

OVERVIEW

- Increasing use of latex (natural rubber) in health care products and medical equipment associated with hypersensitivity among health care workers and patients
- Product hazardous when protein in latex comes in direct contact with mucous membranes or is inhaled such as when powdered latex surgical gloves are used
- People at increased risk for developing latex allergy: those who undergo multiple surgical procedures (especially with spina bifida), health care workers (especially in emergency department and operating room), latex product manufacturers, and those with genetic predisposition to latex allergy
- Symptoms of latex allergy: generalized itching; itchy, watery, or burning eyes; sneezing and coughing (hay fever–type symptoms); rash; hives; bronchial asthma, scratchy throat, or difficulty breathing; edema of the face, hands, or neck; and anaphylaxis
- Diagnosis of latex allergy based on patient's history and physical examination; results of skin testing and blood tests (Alastat test, Hycor assay, the Pharmacia Cap test, and enzyme-linked immunosorbent assay) confirming diagnosis
- Identification of patient at risk for latex allergy based on asking latex allergy-specific questions during health history (see *Latex allergy screening*)
- Three categories of latex sensitivity based on the extent of sensitization:
  – Group 1: history of anaphylaxis or systemic reaction when exposed to a natural latex product
  – Group 2: history of nonsystemic allergic reaction
  – Group 3: no history of latex hypersensitivity but high risk because of associated medical condition, occupation, or allergy

NURSING ALERT Due to the risk of a life-threatening hypersensitivity reaction, a patient with sensitivity to latex should have no contact with latex. Keep a cart with latex-free equipment in the patient's room.

EQUIPMENT

Latex allergy patient identification wristband • latex-free equipment, including room contents • anaphylaxis kit • optional: latex allergy sign

Equipment preparation

- After you've determined that the patient is sensitive to latex, place him in a private room.
- If a private room isn't possible, make the room latex-free to prevent the spread of airborne particles from latex products used on the other patient.

ESSENTIAL STEPS

- Assess for latex allergy in all patients, including those admitted to the delivery room or short-procedure unit or those having a surgical procedure.
- If the patient has a confirmed latex allergy, bring a cart with latex-free supplies into his room.
- Document on the patient's chart (according to facility policy) that the patient has a latex allergy.
- Place a latex allergy identification bracelet on the patient, if required by facility policy.
- If the patient will be receiving anesthesia, make sure that "latex allergy" is clearly visible on the front of his chart.
- Notify the circulating nurse in the surgical unit, the postanesthesia care unit nurses, and any other team members that the patient has a latex allergy. (See *Anesthesia induction and latex allergy.*)
- If the patient is transported to another area, make sure that the latex-free cart accompanies him and that all staff who come in contact with him wear latex-free gloves.
- Place a mask with cloth ties on the patient when he leaves his room to protect him from inhaling airborne latex particles.
- Make sure I.V. access is accomplished using all latex-free products.

LATEX ALLERGY SCREENING

To determine if your patient has a latex sensitivity or allergy, ask these screening questions:
- What is your occupation?
- Have you experienced an allergic reaction, local sensitivity, or itching following exposure to any latex products, such as balloons or condoms?
- Do you have shortness of breath or wheezing after blowing up balloons or after a dental visit? Do you have itching in or around your mouth after eating a banana?
  If your patient answers yes to any of these questions, proceed with the following questions:
- Do you have a history of allergies, dermatitis, or asthma? If so, what type of reaction do you have?
- Do you have any congenital abnormalities? If yes, explain.
- Do you have any food allergies? If so, what specific allergies do you have? Describe your reaction.
- If you experience shortness of breath or wheezing when blowing up latex balloons, describe your reaction.
- Have you had any previous surgical procedures? Did you experience associated complications? If so, describe them.
- Have you had previous dental procedures? Did complications result? If so, describe them.
- Are you exposed to latex in your occupation? Do you experience a reaction to latex products at work? If so, describe your reaction.

- Post a LATEX ALLERGY sign on the I.V. tubing to prevent access of the line using latex products.
- Flush I.V. tubing with 50 ml of I.V. solution to rinse the tubing out because of latex ports in the I.V. tubing.
- Place a warning label on I.V. bags that says, DO NOT USE LATEX INJECTION PORTS.
- Use a latex-free tourniquet or a latex tourniquet over clothing, if none are available.
- Remove the vial stopper to mix and draw up medications.
- Use latex-free oxygen administration equipment; remove the elastic and tie equipment on with gauze.
- Wrap your stethoscope with a latex-free product to protect the patient.
- Wrap Tegaderm over the patient's finger before using pulse oximetry.
- Use latex-free syringes when administering medication.
- Have an anaphylaxis kit readily available.
- If your patient has an allergic reaction to latex, you must act immediately.

◆ **NURSING ALERT** Be prepared to treat life-threatening hypersensitivity with antihistamines, epinephrine, corticosteroids, I.V. fluids, oxygen, intubation, and mechanical ventilation, if necessary.

◆ SPECIAL CONSIDERATIONS

- Signs and symptoms of latex allergy usually occur within 30 minutes of anesthesia induction, but can occur up to 5 hours later.
- If you suspect that you're sensitive to latex, contact employee health services concerning facility protocol for latex-sensitive employees.
- Use latex-free products as often as possible to reduce your exposure to latex.
- Remember that people allergic to certain "cross-reactive" foods (apricots, cherries, grapes, kiwis, passion fruit, bananas, avocados, chestnuts, tomatoes, and peaches) may be allergic to latex.

◆ **NURSING ALERT** Don't assume that because something doesn't look like rubber, it isn't latex. Latex is found in a wide variety of equipment, including electrocardiograph leads, oral and nasal airway tubing, tourniquets, nerve stimulation pads, temperature strips, and blood pressure cuffs.

▶ PATIENT TEACHING

Be sure to cover:
- explanation of latex allergy
- signs and symptoms of latex allergy
- importance of wearing latex allergy identification
- importance of telling all health care workers of latex allergy
- what to do if hypersensitivity reaction occurs
- measures to reduce latex exposure.

●◆ DOCUMENTATION

- Patient history of allergies, including reactions to latex
- Signs and symptoms observed or reported by patient
- Notification of other departments of latex allergy
- Allergy identification placed on wrist
- Latex allergy alert placed on medical record and in patient's room
- Cart with latex-free items placed in room
- Measures taken to prevent latex exposure
- Patient teaching

Selected references

Beckford-Ball, J. "Tackling Latex Allergies in Patients and Nursing Staff," *Nursing Times* 10(24):26-27, June 2005.

Chiu, A.M., and Kelly, K.J. "Anaphylaxis: Drug Allergy, Insect Stings, and Latex," *Immunology and Allergy Clinics of North America* 25(2):389-405, vii, May 2005.

Kimata, H. "Latex Allergy in Infants Younger than 1 Year," *Clinical and Experimental Allergy* 34(12):1910-915, December 2004.

Noble, K.A. "The Patient with Latex Allergy," *Journal of Perianesthesia Nursing* 20(4):285-88, August 2005.

ANESTHESIA INDUCTION AND LATEX ALLERGY

Latex allergy can cause signs and symptoms in conscious and anesthetized patients.

Causes of intraoperative reaction	Signs and symptoms in conscious patient	Signs and symptoms in anesthetized patient
• Latex contact with mucous membrane	• Abnormal cramping	• Bronchospasm
• Latex contact with intraperitoneal serosal lining	• Anxiety	• Cardiopulmonary arrest
• Inhalation of airborne latex particles during anesthesia	• Bronchoconstriction	• Facial edema
• Injection of antibiotics and anesthetic agents through latex ports	• Diarrhea	• Flushing
	• Feeling of faintness	• Hypotension
	• Generalized pruritus	• Laryngeal edema
	• Itchy eyes	• Tachycardia
	• Nausea	• Urticaria
	• Shortness of breath	• Wheezing
	• Swelling of soft tissue (hands, face, tongue)	
	• Vomiting	
	• Wheezing	

Manual ventilation

- Device that consists of a bag and a nonrebreathing valve that can be attached to face mask or directly to endotracheal or tracheostomy tube to allow manual delivery of oxygen or room air to lungs of patient who can't breathe independently; oxygen administration with resuscitation bag also used to improve compromised cardiorespiratory system
- Usually an emergency measure; also used when patient is disconnected temporarily from mechanical ventilator, such as during a tubing change, during transport, or before suctioning
- Also known as *hand-held resuscitation bag* or *bag-mask ventilation*

Contraindications
- None known

USING A PEEP VALVE

Add positive end-expiratory pressure (PEEP) to manual ventilation by attaching a PEEP valve to the resuscitation bag. This may improve oxygenation if the patient hasn't responded to increased fraction of inspired oxygen levels. Always use a PEEP valve to manually ventilate a patient who has been receiving PEEP on the ventilator.

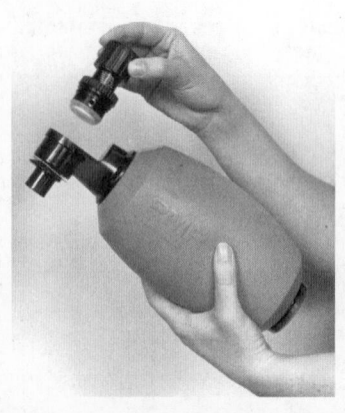

Hand-held resuscitation device ● oxygen source (wall unit or tank) ● oxygen tubing ● nipple adapter attached to oxygen flowmeter ● optional: oxygen accumulator, positive end-expiratory pressure (PEEP) valve (see *Using a PEEP valve*)

Equipment preparation
- Unless the patient is intubated or has a tracheostomy, select a mask that fits snugly over the mouth and nose and attach the mask to the resuscitation bag.
- Connect the bag-mask device to oxygen, if available, by attaching one end of the tubing to the bottom of the bag and the other end to the nipple adapter on the flowmeter of the oxygen source.
- Turn on the oxygen, and adjust the flow rate according to the patient's condition.
- To increase the concentration of inspired oxygen, you can add an oxygen accumulator (also called an *oxygen reservoir*), which attaches to an adapter on the bottom of the bag, permitting a fraction of inspired oxygen of up to 100%.
- If time allows, set up suction equipment.

- Wash your hands thoroughly.
- Confirm the patient's identity using two patient identifiers according to facility policy.
- Explain the procedure to the patient.
- Wear personal protective equipment throughout the procedure.
- Check the patient's upper airway for foreign objects and remove them, if present.
- Suction the patient to remove any secretions that may obstruct the airway.
- If necessary, insert an oropharyngeal or nasopharyngeal airway to maintain airway patency.
- If appropriate, remove the bed's headboard and stand at the head of the bed to help keep the patient's neck extended and to free space at the side of the bed for other activities such as cardiopulmonary resuscitation.
- Tilt the patient's head backward, if not contraindicated, and pull his jaw forward to move the tongue away from the base of the pharynx and prevent obstruction of the airway. (See *How to use a bag-mask device.*)
- Keeping your nondominant hand on the patient's mask, exert downward pressure to seal the mask against his face.
- For an adult patient, use your dominant hand to compress the bag every 6 to 7 seconds to deliver approximately 1 L of air.
- Deliver breaths with the patient's own inspiratory effort, if any is present.
- Observe the patient's chest to ensure that it rises and falls with each compression.
- If ventilation fails to occur, check the fit of the mask and the patency of the patient's airway; if necessary, reposition the patient's head and ensure patency with an oral airway.
- Provide emotional support.

- Avoid neck hyperextension if the patient has a possible cervical injury; instead, use the jaw-thrust technique to open the airway.
- If you need both hands to keep the patient's mask in place and maintain hyperextension, use the lower part of your arm to compress the bag against your side.
- Observe for vomiting through the clear part of the mask. If vomiting occurs, stop the procedure immediately, lift the mask, wipe and suction vomitus, and resume resuscitation.

HOW TO USE A BAG-MASK DEVICE

Place the mask over the patient's face so that the apex of the triangle covers the bridge of the nose and the base lies between the lower lip and chin.

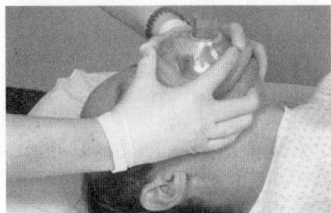

Make sure that the patient's mouth remains open underneath the mask. Attach the bag to the mask and to the tubing leading to the oxygen source.

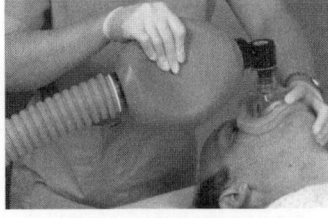

Or, if the patient has a tracheostomy or endotracheal tube in place, remove the mask from the bag and attach the device directly to the tube.

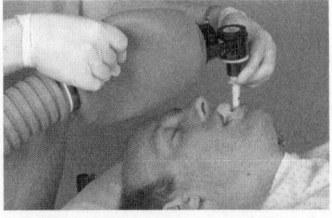

- Underventilation commonly occurs because the handheld resuscitation bag is difficult to keep positioned tightly on the patient's face while ensuring an open airway. Provision of effective ventilation is more likely when two rescuers use the bag-mask system: one rescuer holds the mask while the other rescuer squeezes the bag.
- The volume of air delivered to the patient varies with the type of bag used and the hand size of the person compressing the bag. Because the actual tidal volume delivered is impossible to determine in the clinical setting, the volume of air delivered to the patient should be titrated to produce visible chest expansion and maintenance of oxygen saturation (confirmed by pulse oximetry) in the patient with effective systemic perfusion.

Complications
- Aspiration of vomitus (can result in pneumonia)
- Gastric distention
- Underventilation

▶ PATIENT TEACHING

Be sure to cover:
- reasons for manual ventilation
- step-by-step actions to lessen anxiety

◗ DOCUMENTATION

- Date and time of the procedure
- Reason for manual ventilation
- Manual ventilation efforts
- Oxygen flow rate
- Breath sounds during ventilation
- Chest rising with ventilation
- Length of time receiving manual ventilation
- Vital signs
- Complications and the actions taken
- Patient's response to treatment
- Patient teaching and emotional support given
- Oxygen saturation in the patient with effective systemic perfusion

Selected references
Bennett, S., et al. "A Comparison of Three Neonatal Resuscitation Devices," *Resuscitation* 67(1):113-18, October 2005.
O'Donnell, C.P., et al. "Neonatal Resuscitation 2: An Evaluation of Manual Ventilation Devices and Face Masks," *Archives of Disease in Childhood: Fetal and Neonatal Edition* 90(5): F392-96, September 2005.
Pruitt, W.C. "Manual Ventilation by One or Two Rescuers," *Nursing* 34(11):43-45, November 2004.
Turki, M., et al. "Peak Pressures During Manual Ventilation," *Respiratory Care* 50(3):340-44, March 2005.

Mechanical ventilation

● OVERVIEW

- Method of supporting intubated patients during illness; supports the failing respiratory system until improvement in its function can occur
- Also indicated for central nervous system disorders, such as cerebral hemorrhage and spinal cord transection, acute respiratory distress syndrome, pulmonary edema, chronic obstructive pulmonary disease, flail chest, and acute hypoventilation
- Used with either positive or negative pressure
- When performed with positive-pressure ventilator, exerts positive pressure on patient's airway, causing inspiration while increasing tidal volume (V_T) with inspiratory cycles that may vary in volume, pressure, or time
- When performed with negative-pressure ventilator, creates negative pressure, which pulls the thorax outward and allows air to flow into the lungs; includes iron lung, cuirass (chest shell), and body wrap
- Performed with negative-pressure ventilators mainly to treat neuromuscular disorders, such as Guillain-Barré syndrome, myasthenia gravis, and poliomyelitis

Contraindications
- Living will or advance directive documenting patient's refusal to utilize mechanical ventilation

❖ EQUIPMENT

Positive pressure ventilator • negative pressure ventilator

Equipment preparation
- In most facilities, respiratory therapists assume responsibility for setting up the ventilator. If necessary, check the manufacturer's instructions for setting up the ventilator.
- Wash your hands thoroughly.
- Add sterile distilled water to the humidifier and connect the ventilator to the appropriate gas source.

▌▌▌ ESSENTIAL STEPS

- Confirm the patient's identity using two patient identifiers according to facility policy.
- Put on gloves and personal protective equipment.
- Connect the endotracheal tube to the ventilator.
- Observe for chest expansion and auscultate for bilateral breath sounds.
- Monitor the patient's arterial blood gas (ABG) values after initial ventilation setup (usually 20 to 30 minutes), after any changes in ventilator settings, and as the patient's clinical condition warrants.
- Adjust ventilator settings depending on ABG analysis.
- Check the ventilator tubing for condensation.
- Drain the condensate into a collection trap and empty.
- Don't drain the condensate into the humidifier.
- Monitor the in-line thermometer to ensure air is close to body temperature.
- When monitoring vital signs, count spontaneous and ventilator-delivered breaths.
- Change, clean, or dispose of ventilator tubing and equipment over 48 to 72 hours to reduce risk of bacterial contamination.
- When ordered, begin to wean patient from the ventilator.

◆ SPECIAL CONSIDERATIONS

- Make sure ventilator alarms are on at all times. (See *Responding to ventilator alarms.*)
- If the problem can't be identified, disconnect patient from the ventilator and use a handheld resuscitation bag to ventilate him.
- Provide emotional support to reduce anxiety, even if the patient is unresponsive.
- Unless contraindicated, turn the patient from side to side every 1 to 2 hours.
- Perform active or passive range-of-motion exercises.

- If permitted, position the patient upright at regular intervals.
- Prevent condensation in the tubing from flowing into the lungs.
- Provide care for the patient's artificial airway, as needed.
- Assess peripheral circulation and monitor urine output.
- Watch for fluid volume excess or dehydration.
- Place the call button within reach.
- Establish a method of communication, such as communication board.
- Give a sedative or neuromuscular-blocking drug, as ordered, to relax the patient and prevent spontaneous breathing efforts that interfere with the ventilator's action.
- Closely observe the patient with inability to breathe or talk.
- Reassure the patient and his family that the paralysis is temporary.
- Make sure that emergency equipment is readily available.
- Explain all procedures to ensure patient safety.
- Make sure that the patient gets adequate rest and sleep.
- Provide subdued lighting, low noise, and restricted staff.
- Observe for signs of hypoxia when weaning the patient.
- With the patient's input, schedule weaning around his daily regimen.
- As weaning progresses, encourge the patient to get out of bed.
- Suggest diversionary activities to take his mind off breathing.

Complications
- Tension pneumothorax
- Decreased cardiac output
- Reduced cerebral perfusion
- Oxygen toxicity
- Fluid volume excess
- Infection
- Barotrauma

Be sure to cover:
- what to expect during procedures
- reason for mechanical ventilation
- how weaning progresses
- coping strategies
- alternative methods of communication
- home use of ventilator, including:
  - ventilator care and settings
  - artificial airway care
- suctioning
- respiratory therapy
- communication
- nutrition
- therapeutic exercise
- signs and symptoms of infection and other complications
- troubleshooting equipment malfunction
- community resources.

RESPONDING TO VENTILATOR ALARMS

Signal	Possible cause	Nursing interventions
Low-pressure alarm	• Tube disconnected from ventilator	• Reconnect tube to ventilator.
	• Endotracheal (ET) tube displaced above vocal cords or tracheostomy tube extubated	• Check tube placement and reposition if needed. If extubation or displacement has occurred, ventilate patient manually and call physician immediately.
	• Leaking tidal volume from low cuff pressure (from an underinflated or ruptured cuff or a leak in the cuff or one-way valve)	• Listen for a whooshing sound around tube, indicating an air leak. If you hear one, check cuff pressure. If you can't maintain pressure, call the physician; he may need to insert a new tube.
	• Ventilator malfunction	• Disconnect the patient from the ventilator and ventilate him manually if necessary. Obtain another ventilator.
	• Leak in ventilator circuitry (from loose connection or hole in tubing, loss of temperature-sensitive device, or cracked humidification jar)	• Make sure all connections are intact. Check for holes or leaks in tubing and replace if necessary. Check the humidification jar and replace if cracked.
High-pressure alarm	• Increased airway pressure or decreased lung compliance caused by worsening disease	• Auscultate the lungs for evidence of increasing lung consolidation, barotrauma, or wheezing. Call physician if indicated.
	• Patient biting on oral ET tube	• Insert a bite block if needed. • Consider an analgesic or sedation, if appropriate.
	• Secretions in airway	• Look for secretions in the airway. To remove them, suction the patient or have him cough.
	• Condensate in large-bore tubing	• Check tubing for condensate and remove any fluid.
	• Intubation of right mainstem bronchus	• Auscultate the lungs for evidence of diminished or absent breath sounds in the left lung fields. • Check tube position. If it has slipped, call the physician; he may need to reposition it.
	• Patient coughing, gagging, or attempting to talk	• If the patient fights the ventilator, the physician may order a sedative or neuromuscular-blocking agent.
	• Chest wall resistance	• Reposition the patient to improve chest expansion. If repositioning doesn't help, administer the prescribed analgesic.
	• Failure of high-pressure relief valve	• Have faulty equipment replaced.
	• Bronchospasm	• Assess the patient for the cause. Report to the physician, and treat as ordered.

- Date and time of initiation of mechanical ventilation
- Type of ventilator used, also noting the settings
- Assessment findings, such as vital signs, breath sounds, use of accessory muscles, intake and output, and weight
- Complications and actions taken
- ABG analysis results and oxygen saturation levels
- Date and time of weaning sessions; the weaning method; and baseline and subsequent vital signs, oxygen saturation levels, and ABG values
- Patient's response to weaning, including LOC, spontaneous respiratory effort and rate, arrhythmias, skin color, and need for suctioning
- Patient, family, and caregiver teaching
- Ability of family members or caregiver to use equipment and provide care

Selected references

Christine, N. "Caring for the Mechanically Ventilated Patient: Part One," *Nursing Standard* 20(17):55-64, January 2006.

Goodman, S. "Implementing a Protocol for Weaning Patients Off Mechanical Ventilation," *Nursing in Critical Care* 11(1):23-32, January-February 2006.

Hampton, D.C., et al. "Evidence-Based Clinical Improvement for Mechanically Ventilated Patients," *Rehabilitation Nursing* 30(4):160-65, July-August 2005.

Manno, M.S. "Managing Mechanical Ventilation," *Nursing* 35(12):36-41, December 2005.

Rose, L. , and Nelson, S. "Issues in Weaning from Mechanical Ventilation: Literature Review," *Journal of Advanced Nursing* 54(1):73-85, April 2006.

Mixed venous oxygen saturation

● OVERVIEW

- Used to evaluate the patient's response to drug therapy, endotracheal tube suctioning, ventilator setting changes, positive end-expiratory pressure, and fraction of inspired oxygen
- Uses a fiber-optic thermodilution pulmonary artery (PA) catheter to continuously monitor oxygen delivery to tissues and oxygen consumption by tissues
- Allows rapid detection of impaired oxygen delivery; normal value, 75%

Contraindications

- None known

❖ EQUIPMENT

Fiber-optic PA catheter co-oximeter (monitor) • optical module and cable • gloves

Equipment preparation

- Review manufacturer's instructions for assembly and use of the fiber-optic PA catheter.
- Connect the optical module and cable to the monitor.
- Peel back catheter wrapping just enough to uncover the fiber-optic connector.
- Attach the fiber-optic connector to the optical module; don't remove the rest of the catheter.
- Calibrate the fiber-optic catheter.

❚❙❚ ESSENTIAL STEPS

- Confirm the patient's identity using two patient identifiers according to facility policy.
- Wash your hands thoroughly and put on gloves.
- Explain the procedure to the patient.
- Assist with insertion of the fiber-optic catheter.
- After insertion, ensure correct positioning and function.
- Observe the digital readout and record the mixed venous oxygen saturation ($S\bar{v}o_2$) on graph paper. (See $S\bar{v}o_2$ *waveforms.*)
- Repeat readings at least hourly to monitor and document trends.

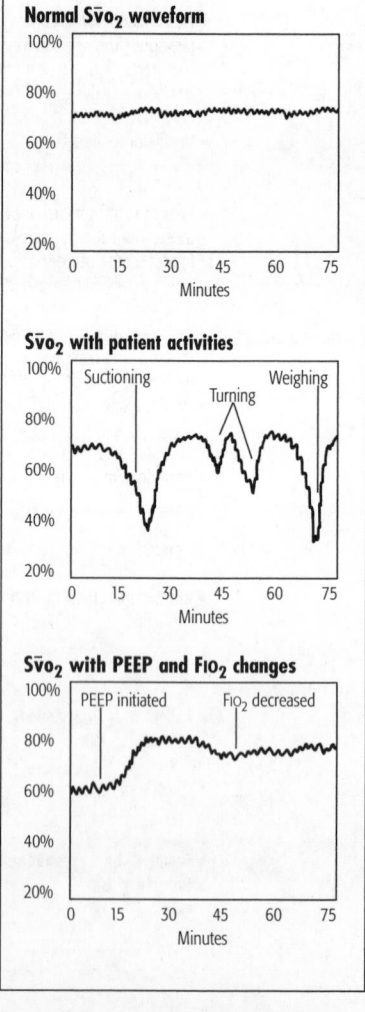

$S\bar{v}o_2$ WAVEFORMS

Normal $S\bar{v}o_2$ waveform

$S\bar{v}o_2$ with patient activities

$S\bar{v}o_2$ with PEEP and Fio_2 changes

- Set alarms 10% above and 10% below patient's current $S\bar{v}o_2$ reading.

RECALIBRATING THE MONITOR
- Draw a blood sample from the distal port of the PA catheter and send it for laboratory analysis.
- Compare the laboratory's $S\bar{v}o_2$ reading with that of the fiber-optic catheter.
- If the catheter values and monitor values differ by more than 4%, follow the manufacturer's instructions to enter the $S\bar{v}o_2$ value obtained by the laboratory into the oximeter.
- Recalibrate the monitor every 24 hours or whenever the catheter has been disconnected from the optical module.

✦ SPECIAL CONSIDERATIONS

NURSING ALERT If the patient's $S\bar{v}o_2$ drops below 60% or varies by more than 10% for 3 minutes or longer, reassess the patient. If the $S\bar{v}o_2$ doesn't return to the baseline value after nursing interventions, notify the physician. This could indicate hemorrhage, hypoxia, shock, or arrhythmias. $S\bar{v}o_2$ may also decrease as a result of increased oxygen demand from hyperthermia, shivering, or seizures.

- If the intensity of the tracing is low, make sure that all connections are secure and the catheter is patent and not kinked.
- If the tracing is damped or erratic, aspirate blood from the catheter to check for patency.
- If aspiration is unsuccessful, anticipate catheter replacement and notify the physician.
- Determine if the catheter is wedged by checking the PA waveform.
- If the catheter has wedged, turn the patient from side to side and instruct him to cough.
- If the catheter remains wedged, notify the physician immediately.
- Monitor for signs and symptoms of infection, such as redness or drainage at the catheter site.

Complications
- Thrombosis
- Thromboembolism
- Infection

▶ PATIENT TEACHING

Be sure to cover:
- reason for and steps of the procedure
- need for frequent monitoring.

⟡ DOCUMENTATION

- Date and time of procedure
- $S\bar{v}o_2$ value on a flowchart with tracing
- Significant changes in the patient's status and actions taken
- Condition of insertion site
- Measures for recalibrating, including date and time of recalibration
- $S\bar{v}o_2$ as measured by the fiber-optic catheter whenever a blood sample was obtained for laboratory analysis of $S\bar{v}o_2$ for comparison

Selected references
Kamijo, Y., et al. "Mixed Venous Oxygen Saturation Monitoring in Calcium Channel Blocker Poisoning: Tissue Hypoxia Avoidance Despite Hypotension," *American Journal of Emergency Medicine* 24(3):357-60, May 2006.

Rivers, E. "Mixed vs. Central Venous Oxygen Saturation May Not Be Numerically Equal, But Both Are Still Clinically Useful," *Chest* 129(3):507-508, March 2006.

Smartt, S. "The Pulmonary Artery Catheter: Gold Standard or Redundant Relic," *Journal of Perianesthesia Nursing* 20(6):373-79, December 2005.

Wang, X.R., et al. "A Preliminary Study on the Monitoring of Mixed Venous Oxygen Saturation through the Left Main Bronchus," *Critical Care* 10(1):R7, December 2005.

Moderate sedation

- Produces a minimally depressed level of consciousness (LOC) in patients undergoing tests and procedures such as minor bone fracture reduction, breast biopsy, vasectomy, dental or plastic reconstructive surgery, or endoscopy procedures
- Allows the patient to respond to verbal or tactile commands and maintain airway patency and protective reflexes while controlling anxiety and pain and producing amnesia
- Drugs used: propofol, benzodiazepines (midazolam and diazepam), and opioids (morphine, hydromorphone, and fentanyl), alone or in combination
- May be administered by specially trained physicians and nurses
- Also known as *conscious* or *procedural sedation*

■ **NURSING ALERT** Know whether your state board of nursing and your facility allow you to administer drugs that produce moderate sedation.

Contraindications
- Allergy to drug or its components
PROPOFOL SEDATION
- Patients with severe systemic disease that limits activities
- Difficult airways due to obstructive sleep apnea, marked obesity, inability to open mouth widely, or short neck with limited neck extension
- Increased risk of aspiration from upper GI bleeding, known gastric outlet obstructon, or known delayed gastric emptying
- Allergy to propofol or its components

I.V. access • I.V. solutions compatible with intended drugs • infusion pump • prescribed drugs • pulse oximetry • supplemental oxygen

Equipment preparation
- Ensure that ordered drugs are readily available and prepared.
- Assess patient's I.V. access to ensure patency; if access isn't available, initiate therapy using a large bore I.V. device.
- Wash hands thoroughly.

- Confirm the patient's identify using two patient identifiers according to facility policy.
- Explain the procedure to the patient and what to expect.
- Make sure that patient has maintained nothing-by-mouth (NPO) status in preparation for procedure.
- Obtain baseline vital signs and pulse oximetry readings.
- Monitor I.V. infusion.
- Assist with sedation administration, as appropriate.
- Monitor vital signs and oxygen saturation every 5 minutes during procedure.
- Titrate drug, as ordered, to achieve intended extent of sedation.
- Make sure that emergency equipment is readily available such as airway management, supplemental oxygen, suction equipment, and opioid reversal agents.

- Monitor vital signs every 15 minutes for the first hour or until patient is fully awake.
- Assess level of consciousness.

🔲 **NURSING ALERT** Administer analgesics for post-procedural pain carefully, especially if the patient received propofol. Propofol can increase the hypotensive effects of opioid analgesics.

- Evaluate for nausea, vomiting, dizziness

Complications
- Respiratory depression
- Cardiac irregularities

Be sure to cover:
- use of moderate sedation and what to expect
- need for frequent monitoring until patient is fully awake
- avoidance of decision-making until full effects of the drug have worn off
- need for a family member or friend to drive the patient home
- signs and symptoms to report
- follow-up care, as appropriate.

- Patient's status and proper preparation for intended procedure, including NPO status
- Baseline and ongoing vital signs and oxygen saturation levels
- Level of consciousness throughout sedation
- I.V. infusion, including solution and rate
- Drugs given for sedation (such as analgesics, antiemetics, or reversal agents), including name, dose, route, frequency, and patient's response
- Time and name of the physician notified of any changes in the patient's condition, such as somnolence, confusion, reduced reflexes, respiratory depression or obstruction, apnea, coma, hypotension, and nausea and vomiting
- Orders given, nursing actions, and the patient's response
- Patient's tolerance of procedure
- Discharge teaching, including name and telephone number for the patient to call with questions
- Person accompanying patient at discharge

Selected references
"Guidelines for Conscious Sedation and Monitoring during Gastrointestinal Endoscopy," National Guideline Clearinghouse. (February 2006) Available at: *http://www.guideline.gov/summary/summary.aspx?ss=15&doc_id=4141&nbr=31 77.* Accessed January 24, 2007.

Halliday, A.B. "Shades of Sedation," *Nursing* 36(4): 36-42, April 2006.

Nuccio, S.A., and Bean, K.B. "Moderate (Conscious) Sedation Update, Challenges, and Issues," *Gastroenterology Nursing* 28(2):173, March-April 2005.

Nasoenteric-decompression tube care

⬤ OVERVIEW

- Performed after a nasoenteric-decompression tube is inserted nasally and advanced beyond the stomach into the intestinal tract; also requires encouragement and support during insertion and removal of the tube and while the tube is in place
- Used to aspirate intestinal content for analysis and to treat intestinal obstruction; may also help to prevent abdominal distention after GI surgery
- Involves continuous monitoring to ensure tube patency, maintain suction and bowel decompression, and detect complications, such as skin breakdown and fluid-electrolyte imbalance

Contraindications
RELATIVE (TO TUBE INSERTION)
- Nasal polyps, deviated septum, or other obstruction

❖ EQUIPMENT

Suction apparatus with intermittent suction capability (stationary or portable unit) • container of water • intake and output record sheets • mouthwash and water mixture • sponge-tipped swabs • water-soluble lubricant or petroleum jelly • cotton-tipped applicators • safety pin • tape or rubber band • disposable irrigation set • irrigant • labels for tube lumens • optional: throat comfort measures, such as gargle, viscous lidocaine, throat lozenges, ice collar, sour hard candy, or gum

Equipment preparation
- Wash your hands thoroughly.
- Assemble the suction apparatus and set up the suction unit.
- Turn on the suction and occlude the end of the connecting tubing to check suction pressure.

❚❚❙ ESSENTIAL STEPS

- Confirm the patient's identity using two patient identifiers according to facility policy.
- Explain all procedures to the patient and his family.
- Wear appropriate personal protective equipment, when necessary, throughout all procedures.
- After tube insertion, have the patient lie quietly on his right side for about 2 hours to promote the tube's passage.
- After the tube advances past the pylorus, the tube can be advanced 2″ (5 cm) per hour as ordered.
- After the tube advances to the desired position, coil the excess external tubing and secure it to the patient's gown or bed linens with a safety pin attached to tape or a rubber band looped around it.
- When in the desired location, the tube may be taped to the patient's face.
- Maintain slack in the tubing so the patient can move comfortably and safely in bed.
- After securing the tube, connect it to the suction tubing to begin decompression.
- Check the suction machine at least every 2 hours to ensure proper functioning, tube patency, and bowel decompression.

🔷 **NURSING ALERT** Excessive negative pressure may draw the mucosa into the tube openings, impair the suction's effectiveness, and injure the mucosa.

- After decompression and before extubation provide a clear-to-full liquid diet, as ordered, to assess bowel function.
- Record intake and output accurately to monitor fluid balance.
- If you irrigate the tube, record the amount of instilled irrigant as INTAKE.

🔷 **NURSING ALERT** Normal saline solution is preferred over water for irrigation because normal saline is isotonic and helps to prevent electrolyte losses.

- Observe for signs and symptoms of fluid-electrolyte imbalance caused by suctioning, such as dry skin and mucous membranes, decreased urine output, lethargy, exhaustion, and fever.
- Watch for signs and symptoms of pneumonia related to the inability to cough effectively with a tube in place, such as fever, chest pain, tachypnea or labored breathing, and diminished breath sounds.
- Observe drainage for color, amount, consistency, odor, and any unusual changes.
- Check patency and placement at least every 4 hours.
- Empty the container every 8 hours and measure the contents.
- Provide mouth care frequently (at least every 4 hours) to increase the patient's comfort and promote a healthy oral cavity.

🔷 **NURSING ALERT** If the tube remains in place for several days, mouth breathing will leave the lips, tongue, and other tissues dry and cracked.

- Encourage the patient to brush his teeth or rinse his mouth with a mouthwash and water mixture.
- Lubricate the patient's lips with moistened swabs or petroleum jelly.
- Gently clean and lubricate the external nostrils at least every 4 hours with either petroleum jelly or water-soluble lubricant to prevent skin breakdown.
- Watch for signs of returned peristalsis, such as active bowel sounds, flatus, decreased abdominal distention and, possibly, a spontaneous bowel movement.

- For a Miller-Abbott tube, clamp the lumen leading to the mercury balloon and label it DO NOT TOUCH, label the other lumen SUCTION, to prevent accidentally instilling irrigant into the wrong lumen.
- If the suction machine works properly but no drainage accumulates in the collection container, suspect an obstruction in the tube.
- Use intermittent suction to reduce the risk of mucosal injury that may occur with continuous suction.
- To check the functioning of the suction unit, look for drainage in the connecting tube and dripping into the collecting container.
- As ordered, irrigate the tube with the irrigation set to clear the obstruction. (See *Clearing a nasoenteric-decompression tube obstruction.*)
- The patient may move short distances, if ambulatory, while connected to the unit or the tube can be disconnected, if ordered, and clamped briefly while he moves around.
- If the tubing irritates the patient's throat or makes him hoarse, offer mouthwash, gargles, viscous lidocaine, throat lozenges, an ice collar, sour hard candy, or gum as appropriate.

◈ NURSING ALERT If the tip of the balloon falls below the ileocecal valve (confirmed by X-ray), the tube can't be removed nasally and must be advanced and removed through the anus.

- If the balloon at the end of the tube protrudes from the anus, notify the physician. Most likely, the tube can be disconnected from suction, the proximal end severed, and the remaining tube removed gradually through the anus either manually or by peristalsis.

Complications

- Fluid and electrolyte imbalance
- Pneumonia
- Intussusception of the bowel
- Nasal or oral inflammation
- Nasal, laryngeal, or esophageal ulceration

Be sure to cover:
- purpose of the procedure
- how the tube is advanced
- what to expect during and after insertion
- signs and symptoms to report
- when the tube will be removed.

- Frequency and type of mouth and nose care provided
- Amount, color, consistency, and odor of the drainage in the collection container
- Amount of drainage on the intake and output sheet
- Amount and type of any irrigant or other fluid introduced through the tube or taken orally by the patient
- Amount and character of any vomitus
- Findings of abdominal assessment, such as bowel sounds, flatus, decreased abdominal distention, and passage of a bowel movement
- Patient's tolerance of the tube's insertion and removal
- Patient teaching

Selected references

Gallagher, J.J. "How to Recognize and Manage Abdominal Compartment Syndrome," *Nursing Management (Suppl)*:36-42, 2004.

McClave, S.A., and Ritchie, C.S. "The Role of Endoscopically Placed Feeding or Decompression Tubes," *Gastroenterology Clinics of North America* 35(1):83-100, March 2006.

Shayani, V., and Sarker, S. "Diagnosis and Management of Acute Gastric Distention Following Laparoscopic Adjustable Gastric Banding," *Obesity Surgery* 14(5):702-704, May 2004.

CLEARING A NASOENTERIC-DECOMPRESSION TUBE OBSTRUCTION

If your patient's nasoenteric-decompression tube appears to be obstructed, notify the physician right away. He may order measures such as those below to restore patency.

- First, disconnect the tube from suction and irrigate with normal saline solution. Use gravity flow to help clear the obstruction unless ordered otherwise.
- If irrigation doesn't reestablish patency, tug slightly on the tube to free it from the gastric mucosa because it may be against the intestinal wall.
- If gentle tugging doesn't restore patency, the tube may be kinked. Before manipulating the tube to try to clear the obstruction, take the following precautions:
  – Never reposition or irrigate a nasoenteric-decompression tube (without a physician's order) in a patient who has had GI surgery.
  – Avoid manipulating a tube in a patient who had the tube inserted during surgery as this may disturb new sutures.
  – Don't try to reposition a tube in a patient who was difficult to intubate (because of an esophageal stricture, for example).

Nasogastric tube insertion and removal

● OVERVIEW

- Nasogastric (NG) tube inserted for 48 to 78 hours after major surgery to decompress stomach and prevent vomiting until peristalsis resumes
- Used for other diagnostic and therapeutic applications, especially in assessing and treating upper GI bleeding, collecting gastric contents for analysis, performing gastric lavage, aspirating gastric secretions, and administering medications and nutrients
- Typically, have a radiopaque marker or strip at the distal end so that the tube's position can be verified by X-ray studies or fluoroscopy
- Most common types include the Levin tube, which has one lumen, and the Salem sump tube, which has two lumens, one for suction and drainage and a smaller one for ventilation, which prevents a vacuum from forming if the tube adheres to the stomach lining

Contraindications
ABSOLUTE
- Comatose patient
- Facial or basilar skull fracture with cribriform plate injury
- Hypothermic patients
RELATIVE
- History of known caustic ingestions
- Recent gastrectomy, esophagectomy, or oropharyngeal, gastric, or nasal surgery
- Known uncorrected coagulopathies or anticoagulant therapy

❖ EQUIPMENT

INSERTING AN NG TUBE
Tube (usually #12, #14, #16, or #18 French for a normal adult) • towel or linen-saver pad • facial tissues • emesis basin • penlight • 1″ or 2″ hypoallergenic tape • gloves • water-soluble lubricant • cup or glass of water with straw • pH test strip • tongue blade • catheter-tip or bulb syringe or irrigation set • safety pin • ordered suction equipment

REMOVING AN NG TUBE
Stethoscope • gloves • catheter-tip syringe • normal saline solution • towel or linen-saver pad • adhesive remover

Equipment preparation
- Thoroughly wash your hands.
- Check the physician's order to determine the type of tube to be inserted.
- Gather all necessary equipment.
- Inspect the NG tube for defects, such as rough edges or partially closed lumens.
- Check the tube's patency by flushing it with water.
- To ease insertion, increase a stiff tube's flexibility by coiling it around your gloved fingers for a few seconds.
- Stiffen a limp rubber tube by briefly chilling it in ice.

▌▌■ ESSENTIAL STEPS

- Confirm the patient's identity using two patient identifiers according to facility policy.
- Explain the procedure to the patient and his family.
- Provide for privacy.
- Wear personal protective equipment throughout all procedures.

INSERTING AN NG TUBE
- Inform the patient that he may experience nasal discomfort, that he may gag, and that his eyes may water.
- Emphasize that swallowing will ease the tube's advancement.
- Agree on a signal that the patient can use if he wants you to stop briefly during the procedure.
- Help the patient into high Fowler's position unless contraindicated.
- Drape the towel or linen-saver pad over the patient's chest.
- Have the patient gently blow his nose.
- Place the facial tissues and emesis basin within the patient's reach.
- Help the patient face forward with his neck in a neutral position.
- To determine how long the NG tube must be to reach the stomach, hold the end of the tube at the tip of the patient's nose, extend the tube to the patient's earlobe, and then down to the xiphoid process.

- Mark this distance on the tubing with the tape (average measurements for an adult range from 22″ to 26″ [56 to 66 cm]).

> **⊙ NURSING ALERT** Add 2″ (5 cm) to the measurement of NG insertion length for a tall patient, to ensure entry into the stomach.

- To determine which nostril will allow easier access, use a penlight and inspect for a deviated septum or other abnormalities, ask if he ever had nasal surgery or a nasal injury, assess airflow in both nostrils by occluding one nostril at a time while the patient breathes through his nose, then choose the nostril with the better airflow.
- Lubricate the first 3″ (7.6 cm) of the tube with a water-soluble gel.
- Instruct the patient to hold his head straight and upright.
- Grasp the tube with the end pointing downward, curve it if necessary, and carefully insert it into the more patent nostril.
- Aim the tube downward and toward the ear closer to the chosen nostril and advance it slowly to avoid pressure on the turbinates and resultant pain and bleeding.

> **⊙ NURSING ALERT** If the patient is coughing, choking, or otherwise showing signs of respiratory distress, withdraw the tube until symptoms subside.

- When the tube reaches the nasopharynx, you'll feel resistance.
- Instruct the patient to lower his head slightly to close the trachea and open the esophagus, then rotate the tube 180 degrees toward the opposite nostril to redirect it so that the tube won't enter the patient's mouth.

> **⊙ NURSING ALERT** If you can't pass the tube to the measured length, the tube is probably in the trachea and should be pulled back and reinserted.

- Unless contraindicated, to help pass the tube to the esophagus, offer the patient a cup of water with a straw or ice chips and direct him to sip and swallow as you slowly advance the tube.

ENSURING PROPER TUBE PLACEMENT
- Use a tongue blade and penlight to examine the patient's mouth and throat for signs of a coiled section of tubing indicating an obstruction.

NURSING ALERT Watch for respiratory distress signs, which can mean the tube is in the bronchus and must be removed immediately.

- Stop advancing the tube when tape mark reaches the patient's nostril.
- Attach a catheter-tip or bulb syringe to the tube and try to aspirate stomach contents. If you don't obtain stomach contents, position the patient on his left side to move the contents into the stomach's greater curvature, and aspirate again.

NURSING ALERT When confirming tube placement, never place the tube's end in a container of water. If the tube is in the trachea, the patient may aspirate water. Besides, water without bubbles doesn't confirm proper placement. Instead, the tube may be coiled in the trachea or the esophagus.

- Inspect the color of the aspirate and check the pH. Gastric fluid has a pH of 4 or less and is green, brown, clear, or straw-colored.
- Obtain an X-ray, as ordered.
- Secure the NG tube to the patient's nose with hypoallergenic tape.
- If the patient's skin is oily, wipe the bridge of his nose with an alcohol pad and allow it to dry.
- To reduce discomfort from the weight of the tube, wrap another piece of tape around the end of the tube and leave a tab. Next, fasten the tape tab to the patient's gown.
- Attach the tube to suction equipment, if ordered; set the suction pressure.
- Provide frequent nose and mouth care.

REMOVING AN NG TUBE

- Explain the procedure to the patient, informing him that it may cause nasal discomfort and sneezing or gagging.
- Assess bowel function by auscultating for peristalsis or flatus.
- Help the patient into semi-Fowler's position.
- Drape a towel or linen-saver pad across his chest.
- Wash your hands and put on gloves.
- Using a catheter-tip syringe, flush the tube with 10 ml of normal saline solution to ensure that the tube doesn't contain stomach contents that could irritate tissues during tube removal.
- Untape the tube from the patient's nose and unpin it from his gown.

- Clamp the tube by folding it in your hand.
- Ask the patient to hold his breath while you withdraw the tube.
- Immediately cover and remove the tube because its sight and odor may nauseate the patient.
- Assist the patient with thorough mouth care, and clean the tape residue from his nose.
- For the next 48 hours, monitor the patient for signs of GI dysfunction.

✦ SPECIAL CONSIDERATIONS

- If the patient has a deviated septum or other nasal condition that prevents nasal insertion, pass the tube orally after removing any dentures. Sliding the tube over the tongue, proceed as you would for nasal insertion.
- When using the oral route, remember to coil the end of the tube around your hand to curve and direct the tube downward at the pharynx.
- If your patient is unconscious, tilt his chin toward her chest to close the trachea and advance the tube between respirations to ensure that it doesn't enter the trachea.
- While advancing the tube in an unconscious patient (or one who can't swallow), stroke the patient's neck to encourage the swallowing reflex and to facilitate passage down the esophagus.
- While advancing the tube, observe for signs that it has entered the trachea, such as choking or breathing difficulties in a conscious patient and cyanosis in an unconscious patient or a patient without a cough reflex. If these signs occur, remove the tube.
- After tube placement, vomiting suggests tubal obstruction or incorrect position. Assess immediately to determine the cause.

▶ PATIENT TEACHING

Be sure to cover:
- reasons for NG tube insertion and what to expect during the procedure and removal

- how the patient can facilitate NG tube insertion, such as sipping water and swallowing
- discomfort in the nose and throat
- signs and symptoms to report, such as nausea, vomiting, abdominal distention, or increased pain after tube removal
- avoidance of food and drink for several hours after removal of NG tube.

Complications

- Skin erosion at the nostril
- Sinusitus
- Esophagitis
- Esophagotracheal fistula
- Gastric ulceration
- Pulmonary and oral infection
- Electrolyte imbalance and dehydration

●◆ DOCUMENTATION

- Date and time of insertion or removal
- Type and size of the NG tube
- Route of insertion
- Methods of confirming tube placement
- Length of tubing inserted
- Type and amount of suction, and describe the drainage, including the amount, color, consistency, and odor
- Periodic tube placement verification
- Patient's tolerance of NG tube insertion or removal
- Patient teaching

Selected references

Crisp, C.L. "Nasogastric Tube Insertion in a Child with Neurodevelopmental Disabilities: Size Does Matter: A Case Study," *Gastroenterology Nursing* 29(2):108-110. March -April 2006.

Higgins, D. "Nasogastric Tube Insertion," *Nursing Times* 101(37):28-29, September 2005.

Puttaswamy, R.K., et al. "A Novel Method for Replacement of a Blocked Fine-Bore Nasogastric Tube," *Journal of Laryngology and Otology* 118(8):659-60, August 2004.

Rushing, J., "Inserting a Nasogastric Tube," *Nursing* 35(5):22, May 2005.

Negative pressure wound therapy

● OVERVIEW

- Used to enhance delayed or impaired wound healing; also known as vacuum-assisted closure (VAC) therapy
- Applies localized subatmospheric pressure to draw the edges of the wound toward the center.
- A special dressing placed in the wound or over a graft or flap, which removes fluids from the wound and stimulates growth of healthy granulation tissue (See *Understanding VAC therapy*).
- Used for acute and traumatic wounds and pressure ulcers or chronic open wounds, such as diabetic ulcers, meshed grafts, and skin flaps

Contraindications
- Fistulas that involve organs or body cavities
- Necrotic tissue with eschar
- Untreated osteomyelitis
- Malignant wounds

❖ EQUIPMENT

Waterproof trash bag • goggles • gown, if indicated • emesis basin • normal saline solution • clean gloves • sterile gloves • sterile scissors • linen saver pad • 35-ml piston syringe with 19G catheter • reticulated foam • fenestrated tubing • evacuation tubing • skin protectant wipe • transparent occlusive air-permeable drape • evacuation canister • vacuum unit

Equipment preparation
- Assemble the device at the bedside.
- Set negative pressure according to the practitioner's order (25 to 200 mm Hg).

▮▮ ESSENTIAL STEPS

- Check the practitioner's order, and assess the patient's condition.
- Confirm the patient's identity using two patient identifiers according to facility policy.
- Explain the procedure, provide privacy, and wash your hands.
- If necessary, put on a gown and goggles to protect yourself from wound drainage and contamination.
- Place a linen-saver pad under the patient to catch spills.
- Position the patient to allow maximum wound exposure, and place the emesis basin under the wound to collect drainage.
- Put on clean gloves; remove the soiled dressing and discard.
- Attach the 19G catheter to the 35-ml piston syringe and irrigate the wound thoroughly using normal saline solution.
- Clean the area around the wound with normal saline solution; wipe intact skin with a skin protectant wipe and allow it to dry.
- Remove and discard your gloves and put on sterile gloves.
- Using sterile scissors, cut the foam to the shape and measurement of the wound. More than one piece may be

---

UNDERSTANDING VAC THERAPY

Vacuum-assisted closure (VAC) therapy may be used when a wound fails to heal in a timely manner through application of localized subatmospheric pressure at the wound site. This reduces edema and bacterial colonization and stimulates the formation of granulation tissue.

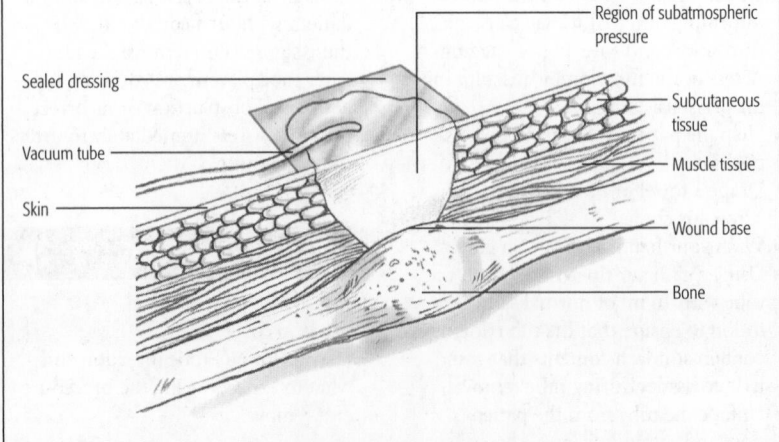

needed to make sure you get the right size.
- Carefully place the foam in the wound.
- Place the fenestrated tubing into the center of the foam; this delivers negative pressure to the wound.
- Place the transparent occlusive air permeable drape over the foam, enclosing the foam and the tubing together.
- Remove and discard your gloves.
- Connect the free end of the fenestrated tubing to the tubing that's connected to the evacuation canister.
- Turn on the vacuum unit and make sure the patient is comfortable.
- Dispose of drainage, solution, linen saver pad, and trash bag, and clean or dispose of soiled equipment and supplies according to guidelines.

◆ SPECIAL CONSIDERATIONS

- Change the dressing every 48 hours; try to coordinate dressing changes with the practitioner's visits so he can inspect the wound.
- Measure the amount of drainage every shift.
- Audible and visual alarms alert you if the unit is tipped greater than 45 degrees, the canister is full, the dressing has an air leak, or the canister becomes dislodged.

Complications
- Temporary increase in the patient's pain
- Risk of infection

▶ PATIENT TEACHING

Be sure to cover:
- reason for the procedure
- steps involved
- possible temporary increase in pain and use of analgesics as ordered.

◆◇ DOCUMENTATION

- Frequency and duration of therapy
- Amount of negative pressure applied
- Size and condition of the wound
- Drainage amount and appearance (if appropriate)
- Patient's tolerance of procedure

Selected references
Clubley, L., and Harper, L. "Using Negative Pressure Therapy for Healing of a Sternal Wound," *Nursing Times* 101(16):44-46, April 2005.
Gibson, K. "Vacuum-Assisted Closure," *AJN* 104(12):16, December 2004.
Malli, S. "Keep a Close Eye on Vacuum-Assisted Wound Closure," *Nursing* 35(7):25, July 2005.
Smith, N. "The Benefits of VAC Therapy in the Management of Pressure Ulcers," *British Journal of Nursing* 13(22): 1359-65, December 2004-January 2005.

Nephrostomy and cystostomy tube care

● OVERVIEW

- Two urinary diversion techniques—nephrostomy and cystostomy—ensure adequate drainage from kidneys or bladder and help prevent urinary tract infection or kidney failure (see *Urinary diversion techniques*)
- Nephrostomy: Performed for obstructive disease, such as calculi in the ureter or ureteropelvic junction, or an obstructing tumor; tube drains urine directly from a kidney when a disorder inhibits the normal flow of urine; tube usually placed percutaneously through renal cortex and medulla into renal pelvis from a lateral incision in the flank
- Cystostomy: Used after gynecologic procedures, bladder surgery, prostatectomy, and for severe urethral strictures or traumatic injury; tube drains urine from bladder, diverting it from urethra; tube inserted about 2″ (5 cm) above symphysis pubis; cystostomy tube may be used alone or with indwelling urethral catheter
- Care varies depending on type of tube used

Contraindications
- None known

❖ EQUIPMENT

Commercially prepared sterile dressing kits may be available.

DRESSING CHANGES
4″ × 4″ gauze pads • povidone-iodine solution or povidone-iodine pads or normal saline solution • sterile cup or emesis basin • paper bag • linen-saver pad • clean gloves • sterile gloves • precut 4″ × 4″ drain dressings or transparent semipermeable dressings • adhesive tape (preferably hypoallergenic)

NEPHROSTOMY-TUBE IRRIGATION
3-ml syringe • alcohol pad or povidone-iodine pad • normal saline solution • optional: hemostat

Equipment preparation
- Wash your hands thoroughly.
- Assemble all equipment at the patient's bedside.
- Open several packages of gauze pads, place them in the sterile cup or emesis basin, and pour the povidone-iodine solution over them (or open several packages of povidone-iodine pads).
- If you're using a commercially packaged dressing kit, open it using sterile technique.
- Fill the cup with antiseptic solution.
- Open the paper bag and place it away from the other equipment to avoid contaminating the sterile field with soiled supplies.

▌▌▌ ESSENTIAL STEPS

- Explain the procedure to the patient.
- Provide for privacy.
- Maintain asepsis throughout all procedures.
- Wear appropriate personal protective equipment, when necessary, throughout all procedures.

CHANGING A DRESSING
- Help the patient to lie on his back (for a cystostomy tube) or the side opposite the tube (for a nephrostomy tube).
- Place the linen-saver pad under the patient.
- Put on clean gloves.
- Carefully remove the tape around the tube, and then remove the wet or soiled dressing.
- Remove your soiled gloves and put on sterile gloves.
- Pick up a saturated pad or dip a dry one into the cup of antiseptic solution.
- Wipe around the wound only once with each pad or sponge, moving from the insertion site outward, discarding each used pad or sponge.
- Place sterile 4″ × 4″ drain dressings around the tube or apply a transparent semipermeable dressing over the site and tubing to allow observation of the site, depending on facility policy.
- Secure the dressing with hypoallergenic tape. Write the date on the dressing.
- Tape the tube to the patient's lateral abdomen to prevent tension on the tube.
- Dispose of all equipment appropriately.
- Clean the patient as necessary.

IRRIGATING A NEPHROSTOMY TUBE
- Fill the 3-ml syringe with the normal saline solution.
- Clean the junction of the nephrostomy tube and drainage tube with the alcohol pad or povidone-iodine pad, and disconnect the tubes.
- Insert the syringe into the nephrostomy tube opening, and instill 2 to 3 ml of saline solution into the tube.

URINARY DIVERSION TECHNIQUES

A cystostomy or a nephrostomy can be used to create permanent diversion, to relieve obstruction from an inoperable tumor, or to provide an outlet for urine after cystectomy. A temporary diversion can relieve obstruction from a calculus or ureteral edema.

In a *cystostomy*, a catheter is inserted percutaneously through the suprapubic area into the bladder. In a *nephrostomy*, a catheter is inserted percutaneously through the flank into the renal pelvis.

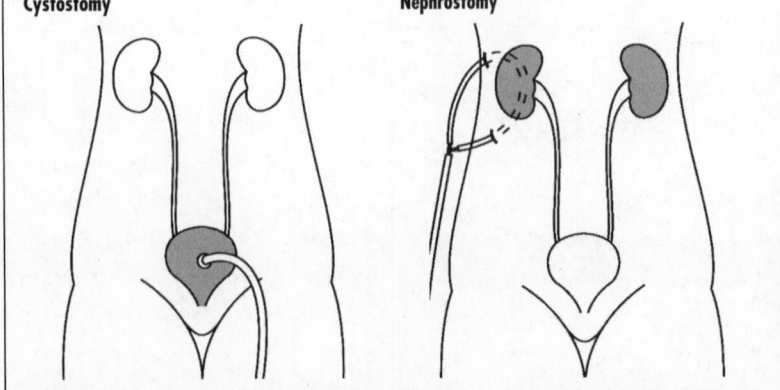

Cystostomy

Nephrostomy

- Gently and slowly aspirate the solution back into the syringe.

NURSING ALERT To avoid damaging the renal pelvis tissue when irrigating a nephrostomy tube, never pull back forcefully on the plunger of the syringe.

- If the solution doesn't return, remove the syringe from the tube and reattach it to the drainage tubing to allow the solution to drain by gravity.
- Dispose of all equipment appropriately.

✦ SPECIAL CONSIDERATIONS

- Change dressings once per day or more often if needed.

NURSING ALERT Never irrigate a nephrostomy tube with more than 5 ml of solution because the capacity of the renal pelvis is usually 4 to 8 ml.

- When necessary, gently irrigate a cystostomy tube as you would an indwelling urinary catheter.
- Check the nephrostomy tube frequently for kinks or obstructions because the pressure created by urine backing up in the tube can damage nephrons.
- Suspect an obstruction when the amount of urine in the drainage bag decreases or the amount of urine around the insertion site increases.
- If a blood clot or mucous plug obstructs a nephrostomy or cystostomy tube, try milking the tube gently to restore its patency, taking care not to dislodge the tube.
- Check the cystostomy tube for patency and the bladder for distention hourly for the first 24 hours after surgery.
- Keep the drainage bag below the level of the kidney at all times to prevent reflux of urine.
- If the tube becomes dislodged, cover the site with a sterile dressing and notify the physician immediately.
- If the physician orders the nephrostomy tube clamped before removal to determine readiness for removal, assess the patient for flank pain and fever, and monitor urine output while the tube is clamped.

Complications
- Urinary tract infection
- Nephron damage
- Perinephric abscess

▶ PATIENT TEACHING

Be sure to cover:
- how to clean the insertion site at home with soap and water, check for skin breakdown, and change the dressing daily
- how to increase fluid intake to 3 qt (3 L) per day, unless contraindicated
- how to change the leg bag (used during the day) or drainage bag (used at night)
- importance of reporting to the doctor signs and symptoms of infection or tube displacement
- how to wash the drainage container daily with a 1:3 vinegar and water solution, rinse it with plain water, and dry it on a clothes hanger or over the towel rack to prevent crystalline buildup.

●◆ DOCUMENTATION

- Color, character, and amount of drainage from the nephrostomy or cystostomy tube (if patient has more than one tube, describe each separately)
- Date and time of site care
- Condition of skin around site
- Amount and type of irrigant used and whether you obtained a complete return
- Patient teaching

Selected references

Jou, Y.C., et al., "Nephrostomy Tube-Free Percutaneous Nephrolithotomy for Patients with Large Stones and Staghorn Stones," *Urology* 56(1):30-34, January 2006.

Kim, S.C., et al. "Using and Choosing a Nephrostomy Tube after Percutaneous Nephrolithotomy for Large or Complex Stone Disease: A Treatment Streategy," *Journal of Endourology* 19(3):348-52, April 2005.

Modi, P., et al. "Laparascopic Ureteroneo-cystostomy for Distal Ureteral Injuries," *Urology* 66(4):751-53, October 2005.

Noninvasive positive airway pressure

● OVERVIEW

- Delivery of ventilatory support without need for an invasive artificial airway; may be given by a volume ventilator, a pressure-controlled ventilator, a bilevel positive airway pressure (Bi-PAP) device, or a continuous positive airway pressure (CPAP) device
- Noninvasive positive pressure ventilation (NPPV): used as an intermittent mode of assistance or as instantaneous and continuous support given to patients in acute respiratory distress
- CPAP: delivers continuous positive air pressure that improves breathing by counteracting intrinsic positive end-expiratory pressure decreasing preload and afterload, improving lung compliance, and decreasing the work of breathing
- CPAP devices: consist of a mask, tubes, and a fan that use air pressure to push the tongue forward and open the throat, which allows air to pass through the throat, and keeps the airways from being blocked, reducing snoring and preventing apnea
- BiPAP: delivers CPAP but also senses when an inspiratory effort is being made, thus delivers a higher pressure during inspiration; when flow stops, pressure returns to CPAP level; this positive pressure wave during inspiration unloads diaphragm, decreasing the work of breathing
- Indications: sleep apnea and sleep related breathing disorders, obstructive and mixed apnea, hypoxia, hypercapnia, acute or chronic respiratory failure, heart failure, acute pulmonary edema or asthma, cystic fibrosis, and restrictive thoracic disorders

Contraindications

⬙ **NURSING ALERT** If the patient has a decreased level of consciousness, has copious secretions, can't protect his airway, or is hemodynamically unstable, an intubation is needed.

❖ EQUIPMENT

Ventilatory device • mask and tubing appropriate for device • skin protectant dressing • oxygen supplementation if indicated

Equipment preparation

- Review manufacturer's instructions and facility policy for use and setup.
- Make sure that the correct-sized mask is available.
- Make sure the patient meets the criteria for the device.
- Wash your hands thoroughly.

▮▮ ESSENTIAL STEPS

- Explain the procedure and the intended effect to the patient.
- Verify that a consent form has been signed.
- Confirm the patient's identity using two patient identifiers according to facility policy.
- Choose the correct size of mask and initiate ventilator at CPAP of 0 cm water with a pressure support of 10 cm water.
- Hold the mask gently on the patient's face until the patient is comfortable and in full synchrony with the ventilator.
- Apply wound care dressing on the patient's nasal bridge and other pressure points, as appropriate.
- Secure the mask with head straps, but avoid a tight fit.
- Slowly increase CPAP to more than 5 cm water.
- Increase pressure support (that is, inspired positive airway pressure, 10 to 20 cm water) to achieve maximal exhaled tidal volume (10 to 15 ml/kg).
- Evaluate that ventilatory support is adequate, which is indicated by an improvement in dyspnea, a decreased respiratory rate, achievement of desired tidal volume, and good comfort for the patient.
- Oxygen supplementation is achieved through NPPV machine-to-machine oxygen saturation of greater than 90%.
- A backup rate may be provided in case the patient becomes apneic.
- In patients with hypoxemia, increase CPAP in increments of 2 or 3 cm water until the fraction of inspired oxygen is less than 0.6.
- Set the ventilator alarms and backup apnea parameters.

- Ask the patient to call for needs, and provide reassurance and encouragement.
- Monitor the patient with oximetry, and adjust ventilator settings after obtaining arterial blood gas results.
- Monitor vital signs and hemodynamics; assess cardiac rate and rhythm.
- Assess intake and output.
- Suction patient, as indicated, and assist with deep-breathing and coughing exercises.
- Monitor laboratory test results.

Complications
- Skin irritation
- Nose dryness and stuffiness
- Eye irritation
- Sinus pain or congestion
- Barotrauma
- Adverse hemodynamic effects, such as preload reduction and hypotension

Be sure to cover:
- importance of follow-up care
- use and care of the airway device
- need to try several masks to provide effective ventilation that's comfortable to him
- mask removal in case of panic or vomiting
- need for the mask to fit firmly over the nose and cheeks
- possible skin irritation necessitating a different size or kind of mask
- skin moisturizers specially made for users of CPAP devices (some petroleum-based products can damage the mask, so tell the patient to check with the manufacturer or supplier)
- use of nasal pillows that fit into the nostrils and relieve pressure on the bridge of the nose as appropriate; possible alternative use of a CPAP mask one night and nasal pillows the next night to increase comfort
- use of chin strap to help hold up the jaw to prevent air escape
- possible difficulty in wearing mask all night long, every night, from the beginning; suggestions to keep trying, even if he can only use the mask for 1 hour per night at first, then gradually increase it.

- Date and time of device application
- Length of device use
- Pressure settings
- Mask size and type
- Vitals signs, hemodynamic values, and pulse oximetry
- Skin protectant measures and skin appearance around mask area
- Patient's tolerance of procedure

Selected references
Dickerson, S.S., and Kennedy, M.C. "CPAP Devices: Encouraging Patients with Sleep Apnea," *Rehabilitation Nursing* 31(3):114-22, May-June 2006.

Loredo, J.S., et al. "Effect of Continuous Positive Airway Pressure versus Supplemental Oxygen on Sleep Quality in Obstructive Sleep Apnea: A Placebo CPAP-controlled Study," *Sleep* 29(4): 564-71, April 2006.

Pirret, A.M., et al. "Local Experience with the Use of Nasal Bubble CPAP in Infants with Bronchiolitis Admitted to a Combined Adult/Paediatric Intensive Care Unit," *Intensive and Critical Care Nursing: The Official Journal of the British Society of Critical Care Nurses* 21(5):314-19, October 2005.

Oronasopharyngeal suctioning

● OVERVIEW

- Suction catheter inserted through mouth or nostril removes secretions from pharynx
- Used to maintain patent airway in patient who can't clear airway effectively with coughing and expectoration (such as one who is unconscious or severely debilitated)
- Requires sterile equipment and sterile technique; clean technique may be used for tonsil tip suction device

Contraindications
- Deviated septum
- Nasal polyps
- Nasal obstruction
- Traumatic injury
- Epistaxis
- Mucosal swelling
- Used with caution in patients with nasopharyngeal bleeding or spinal fluid leakage into the nasopharyngeal area, trauma patients, patients receiving anticoagulant therapy, and those with blood dyscrasias

❖ EQUIPMENT

Wall suction or portable suction apparatus • collection bottle • connecting tubing • water-soluble lubricant • normal saline solution • disposable sterile container • sterile suction catheter (a #12 or #14 French for an adult, #8 or #10 French for a child, or pediatric feeding tube for an infant) • sterile gloves • clean gloves • nasopharyngeal or oropharyngeal airway (optional for frequent suctioning) • overbed table • waterproof trash bag • soap, water, and 70% alcohol for cleaning catheters • optional: tongue blade, tonsil tip suction device

Commercially prepared kits are available.

Equipment preparation
- Gather and place the suction equipment on the patient's overbed table or bedside stand.
- Position the table or stand on your preferred side of the bed to facilitate suctioning.
- Attach the collection bottle to the suctioning unit, and attach the connecting tubing to it.

- Date and then open the bottle of normal saline solution.
- Open the waterproof trash bag.

▌▌▌ ESSENTIAL STEPS

- Check your facility's policy to determine whether a physician's order is required for oropharyngeal suctioning.
- Review the patient's blood gas or oxygen saturation values, and check vital signs.
- Evaluate the patient's ability to cough and deep-breathe to determine his ability to move secretions up the tracheobronchial tree.
- Wash your hands thoroughly.
- Confirm the patient's identity using two patient identifiers according to facility policy.
- Explain the procedure to the patient, even if he's unresponsive.
- Ask the patient which nostril is more patent.
- Maintain asepsis throughout all procedures.
- Wear appropriate personal protective equipment throughout all procedures.
- Place the patient in semi-Fowler's or high Fowler's position, if tolerated, to promote lung expansion and effective coughing.
- Turn on the suction and set the pressure according to your facility's policy, usually between 80 and 120 mm Hg.

◆ **NURSING ALERT** Suctioning with excessively higher pressures cause undue trauma without enhancing secretion removal.

- Occlude the end of the connecting tubing to check suction pressure.
- Open the suction catheter kit or the packages containing the sterile catheter, container, and gloves.
- Put on the gloves; consider your dominant hand sterile and your nondominant hand nonsterile.
- Using your nondominant hand, pour the saline solution into the sterile container.
- With your nondominant hand, place a small amount of water-soluble lubricant on the sterile area.
- Pick up the catheter with your dominant (sterile) hand and attach it to the connecting tubing.

TIPS ON AIRWAY CLEARANCE

Deep-breathing and coughing are vital for removing secretions from the lungs. Other techniques used to help clear the airways include diaphragmatic breathing and forced expiration. Here's how to teach these techniques to your patients.

Diaphragmatic breathing
First, tell the patient to lie supine, with his head elevated 15 to 20 degrees on a pillow. Tell him to place one hand on his abdomen and then inhale so that he can feel his abdomen rise. Explain that this is known as "breathing with the diaphragm."

Next, instruct the patient to exhale slowly through his nose—or, even better, through pursed lips—while letting his abdomen collapse. Explain that this action decreases his respiratory rate and increases his tidal volume.

Suggest that the patient perform this exercise for 30 minutes several times a day. After he becomes accustomed to the position and has learned to breathe using his diaphragm, he may apply abdominal weights of 8.8 to 11 lb (4 to 5 kg). The weights enhance the movement of the diaphragm toward the head during expiration.

To enhance the effectiveness of exercise, the patient may also manually compress the lower costal margins, perform straight-leg lifts, and coordinate the breathing technique with a physical activity such as walking.

Forced expiration
Explain to the patient that forced expiration helps clear secretions while causing less traumatic injury than does a cough. To perform the technique, tell the patient to forcefully expire without closing his glottis, starting with a middle to low lung volume. Tell him to follow this expiration with a period of diaphragmatic breathing and relaxation.

Inform the patient that if his secretions are in the central airways, he may have to use a more forceful expiration or a cough to clear them.

- Use your nondominant hand to control the suction valve while your dominant hand manipulates the catheter.
- Instruct the patient to cough and breathe slowly and deeply several times before beginning suction to loosen secretions and minimize or prevent hypoxia. (See *Tips on airway clearance.*)

NASAL INSERTION
- Raise the tip of the patient's nose with your nondominant hand to straighten the passageway and facilitate insertion of the catheter.
- Without applying suction, gently insert the suction catheter into the patient's nares.
- Roll the catheter between your fingers to help it advance through the turbinates.
- Continue to advance the catheter approximately 5″ to 6″ (12.5 to 15 cm) until you reach the pool of secretions or the patient begins to cough.

ORAL INSERTION
- Without applying suction, gently insert the catheter into the patient's mouth.
- Advance the catheter 3″ to 4″ (7.5 to 10 cm) along the side of the patient's mouth until you reach the pool of secretions or the patient begins to cough.
- Suction both sides of the patient's mouth and pharyngeal area.

REMOVAL OF SECRETIONS
- Using intermittent suction, withdraw the catheter from either the mouth or the nose with a continuous rotating motion to minimize invagination of the mucosa into the catheter's tip and side ports.
- Apply suction for only 10 to 15 seconds at a time to minimize tissue trauma and hypoxia.
- Between passes, wrap the catheter around your dominant hand to prevent contamination.
- Clear the lumen of the catheter by dipping it in water and applying suction.
- Repeat the procedure until gurgling or bubbling sounds stop and respirations are quiet.
- After completing suctioning, pull off your sterile glove over the coiled catheter and discard it and the non-sterile glove along with the container of water.
- Flush the connecting tubing with normal saline solution.
- Wash your hands.

◆ SPECIAL CONSIDERATIONS

- If the patient has no history of nasal problems, alternate suctioning between nostrils to minimize traumatic injury.
- If repeated oronasopharyngeal suctioning is required, using a nasopharyngeal or oropharyngeal airway aids catheter insertion, reduces traumatic injury, and promotes a patent airway.
- Depressing the patient's tongue with a tongue blade during oropharyngeal suctioning helps you visualize the back of the throat and prevents the patient from biting the catheter.
- If the patient has excessive oral secretions, consider using a tonsil tip catheter because this allows the patient to remove oral secretions.
- Let the patient rest after suctioning while you continue to observe him. Monitor oxygen saturation levels closely.
- The frequency and duration of suctioning depend on the patient's tolerance for the procedure and on any complications.

Complications
- Increased dyspnea
- Hypoxia
- Bloody aspirate
- Nasal trauma

▶ PATIENT TEACHING

Be sure to cover:
- why suctioning is necessary
- what to expect during the procedure
- coughing and deep-breathing technique and why it's important.

Home care
Be sure to cover:
- oronasopharyngeal suctioning technique (include the patient's family and caregiver)
- how to use and care for suction equipment and catheters
- indications for calling the physician
- follow-up care.

●◆ DOCUMENTATION

- Date and time of suctioning
- Reason for suctioning
- Technique used
- Amount, color, consistency, and odor (if any) of the secretions
- Patient's respiratory status before and after the procedure
- Any complications and the nursing action taken
- Patient's tolerance for the procedure
- Patient teaching

Selected references

Castledine, G. "Nurse Negligence in Oral/Nasal Suctioning Caused Patients Distress and Put Them at Risk," *British Journal of Nursing* 15(2):67, January-February 2006.

Gungor, S., et al. "Oronasopharyngeal Suction Versus No Suction in Normal, Term, and Vaginally Born Infants: A Prospective Randomised Controlled Trial," *Australian and New Zealand Journal of Obstetrics and Gynaecology* 45(5):453-56, October 2005.

Vain, N.E., et al. "Oropharyngeal and Nasopharyngeal Suctioning of Meconium-Stained Neonates before Delivery of their Shoulders: Multicentre, Randomised Controlled Trial," *Lancet* 36(9434):597-602, August 2004.

Oropharyngeal handheld inhalers

● OVERVIEW

- Includes metered-dose inhalers or nebulizers, turbo-inhalers, and nasal inhalers
- Deliver topical medications to respiratory tract, enabling immediate absorption through the mucosal lining and producing local and systemic effects
- Used with inhalants, including bronchodilators, to improve airway patency and facilitate mucous drainage; mucolytics, which attain a high local concentration to liquefy tenacious bronchial secretions; and corticosteroids, to decrease inflammation

Contraindications
- Inability to form airtight seal around device
- Lack of coordination or clear vision needed to assemble turbo-inhaler
- Specific drug contraindications (for example, bronchodilator contraindicated if patient has tachycardia or history of cardiac arrhythmias associated with tachycardia)

❖ EQUIPMENT

Patient's medication record and chart • metered-dose inhaler, turbo-inhaler, or nasal inhaler • prescribed medication • normal saline solution (or another appropriate solution) for gargling • optional: emesis basin (see *Types of handheld inhalers*)

Equipment preparation
- Verify the order on the patient's medication record by checking it against the physician's order.
- Wash your hands thoroughly.
- Check the label on the inhaler against the order on the medication record.
- Verify the expiration date on the inhaler.

▌▌▌ ESSENTIAL STEPS

- Confirm the patient's identity using two patient identifiers according to facility policy.
- Explain the procedure to the patient.

USING A METERED-DOSE INHALER
- Shake the inhaler bottle to mix the medication and aerosol propellant.
- Remove the mouthpiece and cap.
- Insert the metal stem on the bottle into the small hole on the flattened portion of the mouthpiece and turn the bottle upside down.
- If the metered-dose inhaler has a spacer built into the inhaler, pull the spacer away from the section holding the medication canister until it clicks into place.
- Have the patient exhale; then place the mouthpiece in his mouth and close his lips around it.
- As you firmly push the bottle down against the mouthpiece, ask the patient to inhale slowly and to continue inhaling until his lungs feel full.

✺ AGE-RELATED CONCERN
An elderly patient may have difficulty depressing the medication canister due to weakness or arthritic pain.

- Remove the mouthpiece from the patient's mouth, and tell him to hold his breath for several seconds to allow the medication to reach the alveoli.
- Next, instruct him to exhale slowly through pursed lips, to keep the distal bronchioles open, allowing increased absorption and diffusion of the drug and better gas exchange.
- Have the patient gargle with normal saline solution or other appropriate solution, if desired, to remove medication from the mouth and the back of the throat.
- Rinse the mouthpiece thoroughly with warm water to prevent accumulation of residue.

USING A TURBO-INHALER
- Hold the mouthpiece in one hand, and with the other hand, slide the sleeve away from the mouthpiece as far as possible.
- Unscrew the tip of the mouthpiece by turning it counterclockwise.

TYPES OF HANDHELD INHALERS

Handheld inhalers use air under pressure to produce a mist containing tiny droplets of medication. Drugs delivered in this form (such as mucolytics and bronchodilators) can travel deep into the lungs.

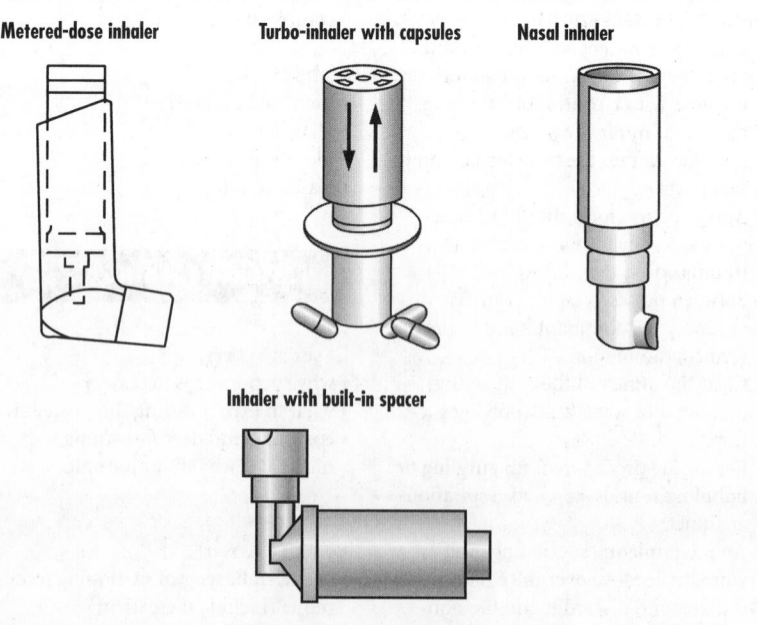

Metered-dose inhaler   Turbo-inhaler with capsules   Nasal inhaler

Inhaler with built-in spacer

- Firmly press the colored portion of the medication capsule into the propeller stem of the mouthpiece.
- Screw the inhaler together again securely.
- Holding the inhaler with the mouthpiece at the bottom, slide the sleeve all the way down and then up again to puncture the capsule and release the medication.
- Have the patient exhale and tilt his head back.
- Tell him to place the mouthpiece in his mouth, close his lips around it, and inhale once—quickly and deeply—through the mouthpiece.
- Tell the patient to hold his breath for several seconds to allow the medication to reach the alveoli.
- Remove the inhaler from the patient's mouth, and tell him to exhale as much air as possible.
- Repeat the procedure until all the medication in the device is inhaled.
- Have the patient gargle with normal saline solution or other appropriate solution, if desired, to remove medication from the mouth and back of the throat.
- Discard the empty medication capsule, put the inhaler in its can, and secure the lid.
- Rinse the inhaler with warm water at least once a week.

USING A NASAL INHALER
- Have the patient blow his nose to clear his nostrils.
- Shake the medication cartridge and insert it in the adapter.
- Remove the protective cap from the adapter tip.
- Hold the inhaler with your index finger on top of the cartridge and your thumb under the nasal adapter with the adapter tip pointing toward the patient.
- Have the patient tilt his head back.
- Next, tell him to place the adapter tip into one nostril while occluding the other nostril with a finger.
- Instruct the patient to inhale gently as he presses the adapter and the cartridge together firmly to release a measured dose of medication.

NURSING ALERT Be sure to follow the manufacturer's instructions; some medications shouldn't be inhaled during administration.
- Tell the patient to remove the inhaler from his nostril and to exhale through his mouth.
- Shake the inhaler, and have the patient repeat the procedure in the other nostril.
- Have the patient gargle with normal saline solution or other appropriate solution to remove medication from his mouth and throat.
- Remove the medication cartridge from the nasal inhaler, and wash the nasal adapter in lukewarm water.
- Let the adapter dry thoroughly before reinserting the cartridge.

✦ SPECIAL CONSIDERATIONS

- When using a turbo-inhaler or a nasal inhaler, make sure the pressurized cartridge isn't punctured or incinerated, and store the medication cartridge below 120° F (48.9° C).
- If you're using a turbo-inhaler, keep the medication capsules wrapped until needed to prevent deterioration.

AGE-RELATED CONCERN Spacer inhalers may provide greater therapeutic benefit for children or the elderly who have difficulty with coordination.

▶ PATIENT TEACHING

Be sure to cover:
- proper use of the inhaler
- how to clean the inhaler
- how to determine how much medication is left in a metered-dose inhaler
- dose and frequency of medication
- adverse drug reactions to report
- (if more than one inhalation is ordered) need to wait at least 2 minutes before repeating the procedure
- need to use the bronchodilator first and wait 5 minutes before using the steroid, if both are prescribed.

●✚ DOCUMENTATION

- Date, time, dose, and name of inhalant administered
- Significant changes in the patient's heart rate and any other adverse reactions
- Patient's ability to perform procedure correctly
- Patient teaching

Selected references

Bower, L.M. "Is Your Patient's Metered Dose Inhaler Technique Up to Snuff?" *Nursing* 35 (8):50-51, August 2005.

Capriotti, T. "Changes in Inhaler Devices for Asthma and COPD," *Medsurg Nursing* 14(3):185-94, June 2005.

Flower, J., and Saewyc, E.M. "Assessing the Capability of School-age Children With Asthma to Safely Self-Carry an Inhaler," *Journal of School Nursing* 21(5):283-92, October 2005.

Joyce, M., et al. "The Use of Nebulized Opioids in the Management of Dyspnea: Evidence Synthesis," *Oncology Nursing Forum* 31(3):551-61, May 2004.

Meadows-Oliver, M., and Banasiak, N.C. "Asthma Medication Delivery Devices," *Journal of Pediatric Health Care* 19(2):121-23, March-April 2005.

Oxygen administration

● OVERVIEW

- Administered in *respiratory emergency,* such as atelectasis and adult respiratory distress syndrome, to reduce ventilatory effort and boost alveolar oxygen levels
- Administered in *cardiac emergency* to meet increased myocardial workload as the heart tries to compensate for hypoxemia, especially when the myocardium is already compromised, such as from myocardial infarction or cardiac arrhythmia
- Administered when *metabolic demand* is high (such as with massive trauma, burns, or high fever), to supply enough oxygen to meet cellular needs
- Indicated when oxygen-carrying capacity of the blood is reduced, such as from carbon monoxide poisoning or sickle cell crisis
- Adequacy determined by arterial blood gas (ABG) analysis, oximetry monitoring, and clinical examination
- Appropriate method determined by patient's disease status, physical condition, and age

Contraindications

- Used cautiously in patients with chronic obstructive pulmonary disease
- Obstructed airway

❖ EQUIPMENT

The equipment needed depends on the type of delivery system ordered. Equipment includes selections from the following: oxygen source (wall unit, cylinder, liquid tank, or concentrator) • flowmeter • adapter, if using a wall unit, or a pressure-reduction gauge, if using a cylinder • sterile humidity bottle and adapters • sterile distilled water • OXYGEN PRECAUTION sign • appropriate oxygen delivery system (a nasal cannula, simple mask, partial rebreather mask, or nonrebreather mask for low-flow and variable oxygen concentrations; a Venturi mask, aerosol mask, T tube, tracheostomy collar, tent, or oxygen hood for high-flow and specific oxygen concentrations) • small-diameter and large-diameter connection tubing • flashlight (for nasal cannula) • water-soluble lubricant • gauze pads and tape (for oxygen masks) • jet adapter for Venturi mask (if adding humidity) • optional: oxygen analyzer

Equipment preparation

- Contact the respiratory therapist to set up the oxygen equipment or, if facility policy indicates, gather the equipment yourself.
- Wash your hands thoroughly.
- Check the oxygen outlet port to verify flow.
- Pinch the tubing near the prongs to ensure that an audible alarm will sound if the oxygen flow stops.

▌▐ ESSENTIAL STEPS

- Confirm the patient's identity using two patient identifiers according to facility policy.
- Explain the procedure to the patient and his family.
- Wash your hands thoroughly
- Assess the patient's condition, and verify the order.
- In an emergency, verify that the patient has an open airway before administering oxygen.
- Check the patient's room to make sure it's safe for oxygen administration.

AGE-RELATED CONCERN When a child is in an oxygen tent, remove all toys that may produce a spark because oxygen supports combustion and the smallest spark can cause a fire.

- Place an OXYGEN PRECAUTION sign over the patient's bed and on the door to his room.
- Place the oxygen delivery device on the patient and make sure it fits properly.
- Check ABG values during initial adjustments of oxygen flow and switch to pulse oximetry when the patient is stabilized.
- Assess frequently for signs of hypoxia, such as decreased level of consciousness, increased heart rate, arrhythmias, restlessness, perspiration, dyspnea, use of accessory muscles, yawning or flared nostrils, cyanosis, and cool, clammy skin.
- Implement measures to prevent skin breakdown on pressure points from the oxygen delivery device.
- Wipe moisture or perspiration from the patient's face and mask as needed.

NURSING ALERT If the patient is to receive oxygen at a concentration greater than 60% for more than 24 hours, watch carefully for signs of oxygen toxicity.

- Remind the patient to cough and deep-breathe frequently to prevent atelectasis.
- To prevent serious lung damage, measure ABG values repeatedly to determine whether high oxygen concentrations are still necessary.

◆ **NURSING ALERT** Never administer oxygen by nasal cannula at more than 2 L/minute to a patient with chronic lung disease, without an order, because high oxygen concentrations can eliminate the stimulus to breath.

- With each change in oxygen flow, monitor the patient closely and check pulse oximetry or measure ABG values in 20 to 30 minutes.
- If the patient is to be discharged with oxygen for the first time, make sure his health insurance covers home oxygen and find out what criteria he must meet to obtain coverage.

Complications

- Oxygen toxicity
- Loss of stimulus to breathe in patients with chronic hypercapnia
- Combustion
- Infection
- Absorption atelectasis
- Bronchopulmonary dysplasia and retrolental fibroplasia in infants

Be sure to cover:
- types of oxygen sources and delivery systems (see *Types of home oxygen therapy*)
- reason the patient is receiving oxygen and the safety issues involved in oxygen administration
- how to properly clean and care for the catheter and insertion site, in the patient receiving transtracheal oxygen therapy
- flow rate and number of hours oxygen is to be used
- how to properly use and clean the equipment and supplies with home use
- signs and symptoms to report
- skin care measures
- follow-up care
- how to perform coughing and deep-breathing exercises, if indicated.

- Date and time of oxygen administration
- Type of delivery device
- Oxygen flow rate
- Vital signs, skin color, respiratory effort, and lung sounds
- Subjective patient response before and after initiation of therapy
- ABG results and pulse oximetry readings
- Patient and family teaching

Selected references

Considine, J. "The Reliability of Clinical Indicators of Oxygenation: A Literature Review," *Contemporary Nurse* 18(3):258-67, April-June 2005.

Demir, F., and Dramali, A. "Requirement for 100% Oxygen Before and After Closed Suction," *Journal of Advanced Nursing* 51(3):245-51, August 2005.

Edwards, M. "Caring for Patients With COPD on Long-Term Oxygen Therapy," *British Journal of Community Nursing* 10(9):404, 406, 408-10, September 2005.

Higgins, D. "Oxygen Therapy," *Nursing Times* 101(4):30-31, January 2005.

Kbar, F.A., and Campbell, L.A. "Oxygen Therapy in Hospitalized Patients: The Impact of Local Guidelines," *Journal of Evaluation in Clinical Practice* 12(1):31-36, February 2006.

Matthews, P.J., et al. "The Latest in Respiratory Care," *Nursing Management* (suppl):18, 20-21, 2005.

TYPES OF HOME OXYGEN THERAPY

Oxygen therapy can be administered at home using an oxygen tank, an oxygen concentrator, or liquid oxygen.

Oxygen tank
Oxygen tanks are commonly used for patients who need oxygen on a standby basis or who need a ventilator at home. An oxygen tank has several disadvantages, including its cumbersome design and the need for frequent refills. Because oxygen is stored under high pressure, the oxygen tank also poses a potential hazard.

Oxygen concentrator
An oxygen concentrator extracts oxygen molecules from room air. It can be used for low oxygen flow (less than 4 L/minute) and doesn't need to be refilled with oxygen. However, because the oxygen concentrator runs on electricity, it won't function during a power failure.

Liquid oxygen
Patients who are oxygen-dependent but still mobile commonly use liquid oxygen. The system includes a large liquid reservoir for home use. When the patient wants to leave the house, he fills a portable unit worn over the shoulder; this supplies oxygen for up to several hours, depending on the flow rate.

Pacemaker (temporary) insertion and care

● OVERVIEW

- Temporary pacemaker consists of external, battery-powered pulse generator connected to a lead or electrode system
- Temporary pacemakers are frequently inserted in emergency situations; commonly used to treat patients with symptomatic bradycardia and conduction defects
- Types of temporary pacemakers include transcutaneous, transvenous, transthoracic (rare), and epicardial
  - In life-threatening situations, *transcutaneous pacing* is used to send an electrical impulse to the heart by two externally applied electrodes attached to the patient's thorax until transvenous pacing can be instituted
  - *Transvenous pacing:* the most common type; involves endocardial stimulation of the right atrium, right ventricle, or both through an electrode introduced into a central vein; best suited for use in urgent situations in which there is adequate time for fluoroscopy
  - *Transthoracic pacing:* used as an elective surgical procedure or as a measure during cardiopulmonary resuscitation
  - *Epicardial pacing:* involves placement of pacing leads directly onto or through the epicardium under direct visualization. Epicardial leads are commonly placed electively in patients undergoing cardiac surgery for postoperative use in the event of bradycardic arrhythmias

Contraindications

- Pulseless electrical activity
- Ventricular fibrillation
- Severe hypothermia

❖ EQUIPMENT

TRANSCUTANEOUS PACING
Transcutaneous pacing generator • transcutaneous pacing electrodes • cardiac monitor

ALL OTHER TYPES OF TEMPORARY PACING
Temporary pacemaker generator with new battery • guide wire or introducer • electrode catheter • sterile gloves • sterile dressings • adhesive tape • povidone-iodine solution • nonconducting tape or rubber surgical glove • emergency cardiac drugs • intubation equipment • defibrillator • cardiac monitor with strip-chart recorder • equipment to start a peripheral I.V. line, if appropriate • I.V. fluids • sedative • optional: elastic bandage or gauze strips, restraints

TRANSVENOUS PACING
All equipment listed for temporary pacing • bridging cable • percutaneous introducer tray or venous cutdown tray • sterile gowns • linen-saver pad • soap • alcohol pads • vial of 1% lidocaine • 5-ml syringe • fluoroscopy equipment, if necessary • fenestrated drape • prepackaged cutdown tray (for antecubital vein placement only) • sutures • receptacle for infectious wastes

TRANSTHORACIC PACING
All equipment listed for temporary pacemaker • transthoracic or cardiac needle

EPICARDIAL PACING
All equipment listed for temporary pacemakers • atrial epicardial wires • ventricular epicardial wires • sterile rubber finger cot • sterile dressing materials

Equipment preparation

- Attach the cardiac monitor to the patient.
- Perform a baseline assessment, including the patient's vital signs, skin color, level of consciousness (LOC), heart rate and rhythm, and emotional state.
- Insert a peripheral I.V. line, if the patient doesn't already have one and begin an infusion at a keep-vein-open rate.
- Insert a new battery into the external pacemaker generator and test it to make sure it has a strong charge.

- Connect the bridging cable to the generator, and align the positive and negative poles.

▌▌▌ ESSENTIAL STEPS

- Confirm the patient's identity using two patient identifiers according to facility policy.
- Explain the procedure to the patient, even if he's unconsciousness.
- Wash your hands thoroughly.
- Maintain asepsis during invasive procedures.
- Wear appropriate personal protective equipment, when necessary, throughout all procedures.
- Make sure the patient has signed a consent form, if appropriate.
- If necessary, clip the hair over the areas of electrode placement.

TRANSCUTANEOUS PACING

- Attach monitoring electrodes to the patient to lead I, II, or III position, even if the patient is already on telemetry monitoring.
- If you select the lead II position, adjust the LL electrode placement to accommodate the anterior pacing electrode and the patient's anatomy.
- Plug the patient's cable into the electrocardiogram (ECG) input connection on the front of the pacing generator.
- Set the selector switch to the MONITOR ON position. You should see the ECG waveform on the monitor.
- Adjust the R-wave beeper volume and press the ALARM ON button.
- Set the alarm for 10 to 20 beats lower and 20 to 30 beats higher than the intrinsic value.
- Press the START/STOP button for a printout of the waveform.
- Make sure the patient's skin is clean and dry.
- Remove the protective strip from the posterior electrode (marked "Back"): apply the electrode on the left side of the back below the scapula and left of the spine.
- The anterior pacing electrode (marked "Front") has two protective strips—one covering the jellied area and one covering the outer rim. Expose the jellied area and apply it to

the skin in the anterior position—to the left side of the precordium in the usual V_2 to V_5 position. (See *Proper electrode placement.*)

- Adjust the electrode to get the best waveform, expose the electrode's outer rim, and firmly press it to the skin.
- After making sure the energy output in milliamperes (mA) is on 0, connect the electrode cable to the monitor output cable.
- Check the waveform, looking for a tall QRS complex in lead II.
- Turn the selector switch to PACER ON.
- Tell the patient that he may feel a thumping or twitching sensation.
- Offer medication if he can't tolerate the discomfort.
- Set the dial to 10 to 20 beats higher than the patient's intrinsic rhythm.
- Look for the pacer artifact or spikes, which will appear as you increase the rate.
- If the patient doesn't have an intrinsic rhythm, set the rate at 60.
- Slowly increase the amount of energy delivered to the heart by adjusting the "Output mA" dial. Do this until capture is achieved—you'll see a pacer spike followed by a widened QRS complex that resembles a premature ventricular contraction. This is the pacing threshold.
- To ensure consistent capture, increase output by 10%.

- With full capture, the patient's heart rate should be approximately the same as the pacemaker rate set on the machine. The usual pacing threshold is betweewn 40 and 80 mA.

TRANSVENOUS PACING

- Check the patient's history for hypersensitivity to local anesthetics.
- Attach the cardiac monitor to the patient, and obtain baselines assessments of vital signs, skin color, level of consciousnses (LOC), heart rate and rhythm, and emotional state.
- Insert a peripheral I.V. catheter if one isn't present.
- Infuse normal saline at a keep-vein-open rate.
- Place the patient in the supine position.
- Open the supply tray while maintaining a sterile field.
- Using sterile technique, clean the insertion site with antimicrobial soap; wipe the area with povidone-iodine solution.
- Cover the insertion site with a fenestrated drape.
- Wear a protective apron if fluoroscopy is used during placement of leadwires.
- Provide the practitioner with the local anesthetic.
- An electrode catheter will be inserted and advanced with a guide wire or an introducer through the brachial, femoral, subclavian, or jugular vein.

- Watch for large P waves and small QRS complexes when the electrode catheter reaches the right atrium.
- Watch for P waves becoming smaller while QRS complexes enlarge as the catheter reaches the right ventricle.
- Watch for elevated ST segments and premature ventricular contractions when the catheter touches the right ventricular endocardium.
- Continuously monitor the patient's cardiac status and treat arrhythmias.
- Assess the patient for jaw pain and earache, which indicate the electrode catheter has moved into the neck instead of the superior vena cava.
- After the electrode catheter is in place, attach the catheter leads to the bridging cable, lining up the positive and negative poles.
- Set the pacemaker as ordered.
- The catheter will be sutured to the insertion site.
- Put on sterile gloves, and apply a sterile dressing to the site.
- Label the dressing with the date and time of application.

TRANSTHORACIC PACING

- Clean the skin to the left of the xiphoid process with povidone-iodine solution. Work quickly because CPR must be interrupted for the procedure.
- A transthoracic needle is inserted through the patient's chest wall to the left of the xiphoid process into the right ventricle.
- The needle is followed with the electrode catheter.
- Connect the electrode catheter to the generator, lining up the positive and negative poles.
- Watch the cardiac monitor for signs of ventricular pacing and capture.
- Apply a sterile $4'' \times 4''$ gauze dressing to the site, and tape it securely.
- Label the dressing with the date and time of application.
- Check the patient's peripheral pulses and vital signs to assess cardiac output. Continue CPR if pulses are absent.
- If the patient has a palpable pulse, assess the patient's vital signs, ECG, and LOC.

PROPER ELECTRODE PLACEMENT

Place the two pacing electrodes for a noninvasive temporary pacemaker at heart level on the patient's chest and back (as shown at right). This placement ensures that the electrical stimulus must travel only a short distance to the heart.

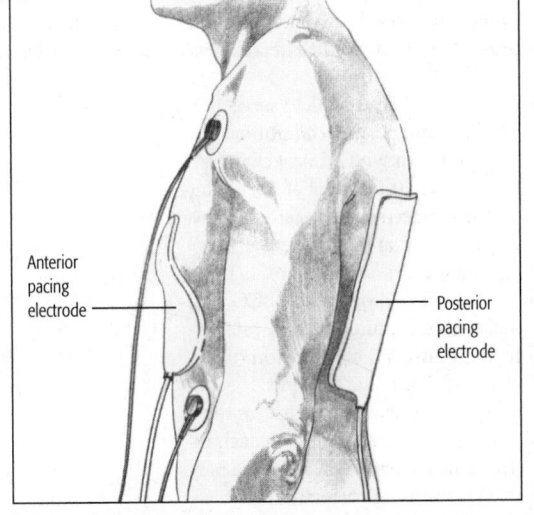

Anterior pacing electrode

Posterior pacing electrode

(continued)

EPICARDIAL PACING

- At the end of cardiac surgery, the surgeon attaches epicardial wires to the epicardium of the atrium, ventricle, or both.
- If indicated, connect the electrode catheter to the generator, lining up the positive and negative poles and set the pacemaker as ordered.
- If the wires won't be connected to an external pulse generator, place them in a sterile rubber finger cot and cover the wires and the insertion site with a sterile, occlusive dressing to protect the patient from microshock and infection.

◆ SPECIAL CONSIDERATIONS

- Prevent microshock by not using any electrical equipment that isn't grounded—such as telephones, electric shavers, televisions, or lamps—around the patient.
- Place a plastic cover supplied by the manufacturer over the pacemaker controls to avoid an accidental setting change.
- Insulate the pacemaker by covering all exposed metal parts, such as electrode connections and pacemaker terminals, with nonconducting tape, or place the pacing unit in a dry, rubber surgical glove.
- Use caution to prevent accidental removal or migration of pacemaker wires.
- During emergency defibrillation, place paddles away from generator and insertion site.
- When using a transcutaneous pacemaker, don't place the electrodes over a bony area because bone conducts current poorly.
- With a female patient, place the anterior transcutaneous electrode under the breast but not over the diaphragm.
- If the physician inserts the electrode through the brachial or femoral vein, immobilize the patient's arm or leg to avoid putting stress on the pacing wires.
- After insertion of any temporary pacemaker, assess the patient's vital signs, skin color, LOC, and peripheral pulses to determine the effectiveness of the paced rhythm.
- Perform a 12-lead ECG to serve as a baseline, and perform additional ECGs daily or with clinical changes.
- Obtain a rhythm strip before, during, and after pacemaker placement as well as any time that pacemaker settings are changed.
- Continuously monitor the ECG reading, noting capture, sensing, rate, intrinsic beats, and competition of paced and intrinsic rhythms.
- Look for the sense indicator on the pulse generator to flash with each intrinsic heart beat, indicating the pacemaker is sensing correctly.

- If the patient has epicardial pacing wires in place, clean the insertion site with povidone-iodine solution (as ordered), inspect for signs of infection, and change the dressing daily.
- Always keep the pulse generator nearby when a patient has epicardial pacing wires in place, in case pacing becomes necessary.

Complications
- Microshock
- Equipment failure
- Competitive or fatal arrhythmias

TRANSCUTANEOUS PACING
- Skin breakdown
- Muscle pain
- Twitching

TRANSVENOUS PACING
- Pneumothorax
- Hemothorax
- Cardiac perforation and tamponade
- Diaphragmatic stimulation
- Pulmonary embolism
- Thrombophlebitis
- Infection
- Venous spasm
- Arrhythmias

TRANSTHORACIC PACING
- Pneumothorax
- Cardiac tamponade
- Embolism
- Sepsis
- Lacerations of myocardium or coronary artery
- Perforation of a cardiac chamber

EPICARDIAL PACING
- Infection
- Cardiac arrest
- Diaphragmatic stimulation
- Major blood vessel injury
- Arrhythmias

Be sure to cover:
- why a pacemaker is needed and how it's inserted
- importance of not changing pacemaker settings or touching the pulse generator or wires
- how to prevent microshock
- monitoring during pacemaker therapy
- possible sensations or discomfort felt with transcutaneous pacing, for which analgesics are available
- signs and symptoms of complications to report to the nurse.

- Date and time of the procedure
- Indications for pacing
- Type of pacemaker inserted
- Pacemaker settings
- Patient's response to the procedure
- Complications and the interventions taken
- Rhythm strips before, during, and after pacemaker placement, and whenever pacemaker settings are changed
- Patient teaching

Selected references

Craig, K. "How to Provide Transcutaneous Pacing," *Nursing* 36(Suppl Cardiac) 22-23, Spring 2006.

Hidaka, N., et al. "Is Intrapartum Temporary Pacing Required for Women with Complete Atrioventricular Block? An Analysis of Seven Cases," *British Journal of Obstetrics and Gynaecology* 113(5):605-607, May 2006.

James, M., et al. "An Unusual Complication of Transvenous Temporary Pacing," *Heart* 89(4):448, April 2003.

Yeh, K. "Two-Dimensional Echocardiography for the Diagnosis of Interventricular Spectrum Perforation by Temporary Pacing Catheter," *American Journal of the Medical Sciences* 331(2):95-96, February 2006.

Passive range-of-motion exercises

● OVERVIEW

- Involve moving the patient's joints through range of motion (ROM) as fully as possible
- Performed to improve or maintain joint mobility and help prevent contractures
- Indicated for patient with temporary or permanent loss of mobility, sensation, or consciousness
- Requires recognition of the patient's limits of motion and support of all joints during movement

Contraindications

- Septic joints
- Acute thrombophlebitis
- Severe arthritic joint inflammation
- Recent trauma with possible hidden fractures or internal injuries

❖ EQUIPMENT

No specific equipment required

▮▮ ESSENTIAL STEPS

- Wash your hands thoroughly.
- Wear gloves if there is wound drainage or open skin lesions.
- Confirm the patient's identity using two patient identifiers according to facility policy.
- Explain the procedure to the patient.
- Provide for privacy.
- Determine which joints need ROM exercises, and consult with the physician or physical therapist about limitations or precautions for specific exercises.
- Perform all exercises slowly, gently, and to the end of the normal ROM or to the point of pain, but no further. (See *Glossary of joint movements*.)
- Before you begin, raise the bed to a comfortable working height.

EXERCISING THE NECK

- Support the patient's head with your hands and extend the neck, flex the chin to the chest, and tilt the head laterally toward each shoulder.
- Rotate the head from right to left.

◈ NURSING ALERT Stop performing passive ROM exercises if there's resistance or muscle spasm or if the patient reports discomfort.

EXERCISING THE SHOULDERS

- Support the patient's arm in an extended, neutral position; then extend the forearm and flex it back.
- Abduct the arm outward from the side of the body, and adduct it back to the side.
- Rotate the shoulder so that the arm crosses the midline, and bend the elbow so that the hand touches the opposite shoulder, then touches the mattress of the bed for complete internal rotation.
- Return the shoulder to a neutral position and, with elbow bent, push the arm backward so that the back of the hand touches the mattress for complete external rotation.

EXERCISING THE ELBOW

- Place the patient's arm at his side with his palm facing up.
- Flex and extend the arm at the elbow.

EXERCISING THE FOREARM

- Stabilize the patient's elbow, and then twist the hand to bring the palm up (supination).
- Twist it back again to bring the palm down (pronation).

EXERCISING THE WRIST

- Stabilize the forearm and flex and extend the wrist.
- Rock the hand sideways for lateral flexion, and rotate the hand in a circular motion.

EXERCISING THE FINGERS AND THUMB

- Extend the patient's fingers, and then flex the hand into a fist; repeat exten-

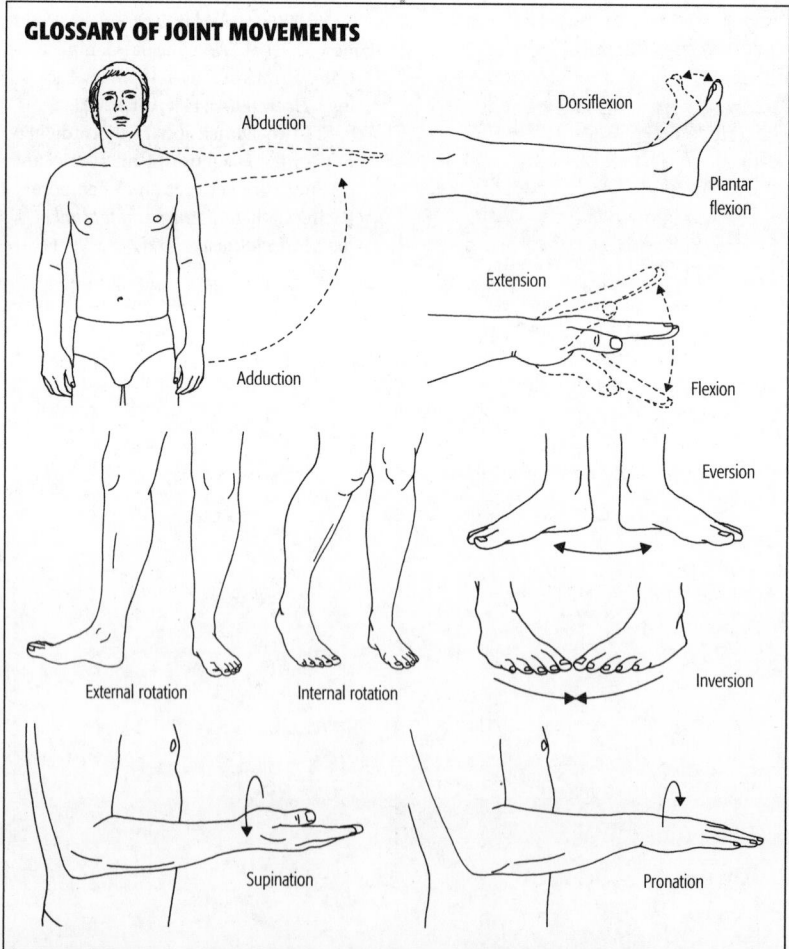

GLOSSARY OF JOINT MOVEMENTS

Abduction
Adduction
External rotation
Internal rotation
Supination
Dorsiflexion
Plantar flexion
Extension
Flexion
Eversion
Inversion
Pronation

sion and flexion of each joint of each finger and thumb separately.

- Spread two adjoining fingers apart (abduction), and then bring them together (adduction).
- Oppose each fingertip to the thumb, and rotate the thumb and each finger in a circle.

EXERCISING THE HIP AND KNEE

- Fully extend the patient's leg, and then bend the hip and knee toward the chest, allowing full joint flexion.
- Move the straight leg sideways, out and away from the other leg (abduction), and then back, over, and across it (adduction).
- Rotate the straight leg internally toward the midline, then externally away from the midline.

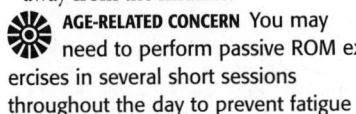 **AGE-RELATED CONCERN** You may need to perform passive ROM exercises in several short sessions throughout the day to prevent fatigue in an elderly patient or one with chronic illness.

EXERCISING THE ANKLE

- Bend the patient's foot so that the toes push upward (dorsiflexion), and then bend the foot so that the toes push downward (plantar flexion).
- Rotate the ankle in a circular motion.
- Invert the ankle so that the sole of the foot faces the midline, and evert the ankle so that the sole faces away from the midline.

EXERCISING THE TOES

- Flex the patient's toes toward the sole, and then extend them back toward the top of the foot.
- Spread two adjoining toes apart (abduction), and bring them together (adduction).

✦ SPECIAL CONSIDERATIONS

- Because joints begin to stiffen within 24 hours of disuse, start passive ROM exercises as soon as possible.
- Perform passive ROM exercises at least once per shift, particularly while bathing or turning the patient.
- Use proper body mechanics, and repeat each exercise at least three times.
- Patients who experience prolonged bed rest or limited activity without profound weakness can also be taught to perform ROM exercises on their own (called active ROM), or they may benefit from isometric exercises.
- If a disabled patient requires long-term rehabilitation after discharge, consult with a physical therapist and teach a family member or caregiver to perform passive ROM exercises.

Complications

- Fatigue
- Joint pain

▶ PATIENT TEACHING

Be sure to cover:

- why the patient needs passive ROM and how it's performed
- signs and symptoms to report
- how to perform isometric exercises, if indicated
- number of repetitions and number of times a day to perform exercises
- incorporation of ROM into a daily routine.

●✛ DOCUMENTATION

- Joints exercised and number of repetitions
- Presence of edema or pressure areas
- Any pain or discomfort resulting from the exercises
- Extent of and limitations of ROM
- Patient's tolerance of the exercises
- Patient teaching

Selected references

Corio, E., et al. "The Effect of Oral and Intrathecal Baclofen Treatment on Passive Range of Motion of the Knee in Children Diagnosed with Cerebral Palsy," *Pediatric Physical Therapy* 17(1):71-72, Spring 2005.

Huang, R.C., et al. "Correlation Between Range of Motion and Outcome After Lumbar Total Disc Replacement: 8.6 Year Follow-up," *Spine* 30(12):1407-11, June 2005.

"Performing Passive Range-of-Motion Exercises," *Nursing* 36(3):50-51, March 2006.

Tully, E. "The Practical Guide to Range of Motion Assessment," *British Journal of Sports Medicine* 39(4):245, April 2005.

Patient-controlled analgesia

● OVERVIEW

- Drug delivery system that provides I.V. analgesia, usually morphine, when the patient presses a call button at the end of a cord (see *Understanding patient-controlled analgesia*)
- Accidental overdosing prevented through a lockout time between doses—usually 6 to 10 minutes; during this interval, patient won't receive any analgesic, even if he pushes button
- Criteria for PCA requiring mental alertness and ability to understand and comply with instructions and procedures

Contraindications

- History of allergy to analgesic
- Limited respiratory reserve
- History of drug abuse or chronic sedative or tranquilizer use, or a psychiatric disorder

❖ EQUIPMENT

PCA system and system-specific tubing • syringe with prescribed medication • alcohol pads • clean gloves • tape

Equipment preparation

- Follow the manufacturer's instructions for setting up the device.
- Obtain the medication and verify the medication order.
- Gather equipment and bring to the patient's bedside.
- Plug the PCA device into an electrical outlet.
- Connect device tubing to the medication syringe and insert syringe into the device.
- Prime the tubing.

||■ ESSENTIAL STEPS

- Wash hands thoroughly.
- Confirm the patient's identity using two patient identifiers according to facility policy.
- Provide for privacy.
- Explain the procedure to the patient and obtain baseline vital signs.

UNDERSTANDING PATIENT-CONTROLLED ANALGESIA

In patient-controlled analgesia (PCA), the patient controls I.V. delivery of an analgesic (usually morphine) by pressing the button on a delivery device so that he receives analgesia at the level he needs and at the time he needs it. The PCA device prevents the patient from accidentally overdosing by imposing a lockout time between doses – usually 6 to 10 minutes. During this interval, the patient won't receive any analgesic, even if he pushes the button.

The device shown here is a reusable, battery-operated peristaltic action pump that delivers a drug dose when the patient presses a call button at the end of a cord.

Indications and advantages

Indicated for patients who need parenteral analgesia, PCA therapy is typically given to trauma patients postoperatively and to terminal cancer patients and others with chronic diseases. To receive PCA therapy, patients must be mentally alert and able to understand and comply with instructions and procedures and have no history of allergy to the analgesic. Patients ineligible for therapy include those with limited respiratory reserve, a history of drug abuse or chronic sedative or tranquilizer use, or a psychiatric disorder. Advantages to PCA therapy include:

- no need for I.M. analgesics
- pain relief tailored to each patient's size and pain tolerance
- sense of control over pain
- ability to sleep at night with minimal daytime drowsiness
- lower opioid use compared with patients not on PCA
- improved postoperative deep breathing, coughing, and ambulation.

PCA setup

To set up a PCA system, the practitioner's order should include:

- medication to be dosed
- appropriate lockout interval
- amount the patient will receive when he activates the device
- maximum amount the patient can receive within a specified time (if an adjustable device is used).

Occasionally the practitioner may order a loading dose and sometimes a base rate will be prescribed.

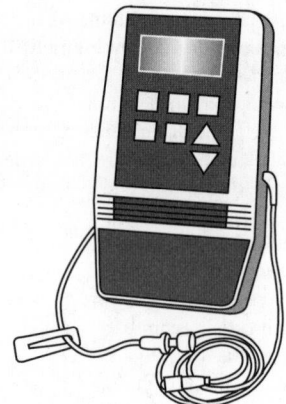

Nursing considerations

Because the primary adverse effect of analgesics is respiratory depression, monitor the patient's respiratory rate routinely. Also, check for infiltration into the subcutaneous tissues and for catheter occlusion, which may cause the drug to back up in the primary I.V. tubing. If the analgesic nauseates the patient, you may need to administer an antiemetic.

Before the patient starts using the PCA device, teach him how it works. Then have the patient practice with a sample device. Explain that he should take enough analgesic to relieve acute pain but not enough to induce drowsiness.

During therapy, monitor and record the amount of analgesic infused, the patient's respiratory rate, and the patient's assessment of pain relief. If the patient reports insufficient pain relief, notify the physician.

- Put on clean gloves.
- If the patient doesn't have an I.V. access site, insert one.
- Connect PCA tubing to the patient's I.V. line or I.V. access device and secure the connection with tape, if necessary.
- Program the device to deliver the prescribed parameters: loading dose, infusion doses, and lockout interval.
- Instruct the patient to push the button each time he has pain and needs relief.
- Monitor vital signs frequently during the initial loading dose and then every 1 to 2 hours throughout therapy.

⬡ **NURSING ALERT** Know the amount the patient will receive when he activates the device and the maximum amount the patient can receive within a specified time (if an adjustable device is used). Have naloxone readily available in case the patient develops respiratory depression.

- Inspect the infusion site for any changes, and check device functioning, including rate, periodically.
- Replace the medication syringe when empty.

✦ SPECIAL CONSIDERATIONS

- Encourage the patient to cough and deep breath to promote ventilation.
- Monitor the I.V. insertion for infiltration into the subcutaneous tissues and for catheter occlusion, which may cause the drug to back up in the primary I.V. tubing.
- If the analgesic nauseates the patient, administer an antiemetic, as ordered.
- Assess the patient's pain using a pain rating scale before therapy and then periodically during therapy. Notify the physician if the patient's pain is not being relieved.

Complications
- Respiratory depression (secondary to drug)
- I.V. infiltration

▶ PATIENT TEACHING

Be sure to cover:
- reason for PCA and expected benefits
- how to use PCA device
- pain assessment methods
- adverse effects of drug therapy
- signs and symptoms of complications and when to report them
- measures to promote ventilation.

●✧ DOCUMENTATION

- Date and time of PCA therapy initiation
- I.V. access device and location
- Baseline vital signs and pain assessment
- Medication doses (loading dose, individual doses, and time interval)
- Ongoing assessments of vital signs, pain, and I.V. site
- Patient's understanding and tolerance of procedure
- Patient teaching

Selected references

Darcy, Y. "Controlling Pain: How to Care for a Surgical Patient with Chronic Pain," *Nursing* 36(3):17, March 2006.

Kennedy, M.S. "PCA Pumps: An Illusion of Safety? Patient-controlled Analgesia Pumps and Errors: There is a Connection," *AJN* 105(2):22, February 2005.

Pasero, C., and McCaffery, M. "Pain Control: Authorized and Unauthorized Use of PCA Pumps: Clarifying the Use of Patient-controlled Analgesia, in Light of Recent Alerts," *AJN* 105(7):30-32, July 2005.

Weir, V.L. "Best-practice Protocols: Preventing Adverse Drug Events," *Nursing Management* 36(9):24-30, September 2005.

Peritoneal dialysis

● OVERVIEW

- Also known as PD
- Indicated for patients with chronic renal failure who cannot tolerate hemodialysis (HD), including those with congestive or ischemic heart disease and extensive vascular disease or those in whom vascular access is problematic, including the majority of young children
- Also indicated for patients who prefer PD or refuse HD; may also be indicated for patients who prefer home dialysis but have no assistant trained for home HD
- Performed by instilling dialysate into the peritoneal cavity by a catheter, to draw waste products, excess fluid, and electrolytes from the blood across the semipermeable peritoneal membrane
- After prescribed period, the dialysate is drained from the peritoneal cavity, removing impurities with it
- Dialysis procedure is then repeated, using a new dialysate each time, until waste removal is complete and fluid, electrolyte, and acid-base balance is restored
- Catheter is inserted in the operating room or at the patient's bedside with a nurse assisting
- With special preparation, nurse may perform dialysis, either manually or using an automatic or semiautomatic cycle machine

❖ EQUIPMENT

All equipment must be sterile. Commercially packaged dialysis kits or trays are available.

CATHETER PLACEMENT AND DIALYSIS
Prescribed dialysate • warmer, heating pad, or water bath • at least three face masks • medication, such as heparin, if ordered • dialysis administration set with drainage bag • two pairs of sterile gloves • I.V. pole • fenestrated sterile drape • vial of 1% or 2% lidocaine • povidone-iodine pads • 3-ml syringe with 25G 1″ • needle scalpel (with #11 blade) • ordered type of multi-eyed, nylon, peritoneal catheter • peritoneal stylet • sutures or hypoallergenic tape • povidone-iodine solution (to prepare abdomen) • precut drain dressings • protective cap for catheter • small, sterile plastic clamp • 4″ × 4″ gauze pads • optional: 10-ml syringe with 22G 1½″ needle, protein or potassium supplement, specimen container, label, laboratory request form

DRESSING CHANGES
One pair of sterile gloves • ten sterile cotton-tipped applicators or sterile • 2″ × 2″ gauze pads • povidone-iodine ointment • two precut drain dressings • adhesive tape • povidone-iodine solution or normal saline solution • two sterile 4″ × 4″ gauze pads

Equipment preparation
- Wash your hands thoroughly before all procedures.
- Bring all equipment to the patient's bedside.
- Make sure the dialysate is at body temperature to reduce discomfort and reduce vasoconstriction of the peritoneal capillaries, which reduces waste clearance into the peritoneal cavity.
- Place the container in a warmer or a water bath, or wrap it in a heating pad set at 98.6° F (37° C) for 30 to 60 minutes to warm the solution.

▌▌▌ ESSENTIAL STEPS

- Confirm the patient's identity using two patient identifiers according to facility policy.
- Explain all procedures to the patient.
- Maintain asepsis throughout all procedures.
- Wear appropriate personal protective equipment, when necessary throughout all procedures.
- Assess and record vital signs, weight, and abdominal girth to establish baseline levels.
- Review recent laboratory values.

CATHETER PLACEMENT AND DIALYSIS
- Have the patient urinate to reduce the risk of bladder perforation during insertion of the peritoneal catheter.
- If the patient can't urinate and you suspect that his bladder isn't empty, obtain an order for straight catheterization.
- Place the patient in the supine position if tolerated and have him put on one of the sterile face masks.
- Inspect the warmed dialysate, which should appear clear and colorless.
- Put on a sterile face mask.
- Add any prescribed medication to the dialysate, using strict sterile technique immediately before the solution is hung and used.
- Prepare the dialysis administration set as shown. (See *Setup for peritoneal dialysis.*)
- Close the clamps on all lines.
- Place the drainage bag below the patient to facilitate gravity drainage and connect the drainage line to it.
- Connect the dialysate infusion lines to the bottles or bags of dialysate.
- Hang the bottles or bags on the I.V. pole at the patient's bedside.
- To prime the tubing, open the infusion lines and allow the solution to flow until all lines are primed, then close all clamps.
- At this point, the physician puts on a mask and a pair of sterile gloves, cleans the patient's abdomen with povidone-iodine solution, and drapes it with a sterile drape.

- Wipe the stopper of the lidocaine vial with povidone-iodine and allow it to dry.
- Invert the vial and hand it to the physician, who withdraws the lidocaine using the 3-ml syringe with the 25G 1″ needle.
- The physician anesthetizes a small area of the patient's abdomen below the umbilicus.
- The physician then makes a small incision with the scalpel, inserts the catheter into the peritoneal cavity—using the stylet to guide the catheter—and sutures or tapes the catheter in place.
- If the catheter is already in place, clean the site with povidone-iodine solution in a circular outward motion, according to your facility's policy, before each dialysis treatment.
- Connect the catheter to the administration set.
- Open the drain dressing and the 4″ × 4″ gauze pad packages.
- Put on the other pair of sterile gloves.
- Apply the precut drain dressings around the catheter, cover them with the gauze pads, and tape them securely.
- Unclamp the lines to the patient and rapidly instill 500 ml of dialysate into the peritoneal cavity to test the catheter's patency.
- Clamp the lines to the patient.
- Immediately unclamp the lines to the drainage bag to allow fluid to drain into the bag.
- Having established the catheter's patency, clamp the lines to the drainage bag and unclamp the lines to the patient to infuse the prescribed volume of solution over a period of 5 to 10 minutes.
- As soon as the dialysate container empties, clamp the lines to the patient immediately to prevent air from entering the tubing.

- Let the solution dwell in the peritoneal cavity for the prescribed time (10 minutes to 4 hours) to allow excess fluid, electrolytes, and accumulated wastes to move from the blood through the peritoneal membrane and into the dialysate.
- Warm the solution for the next infusion.
- At the end of the prescribed dwelling time, unclamp the line to the drainage bag and allow the solution to drain from the peritoneal cavity into the drainage bag (normally 20 to 30 minutes).
- Repeat the infuse-dwell-drain cycle immediately after outflow until the prescribed number of fluid exchanges has been completed.
- If the physician or your facility's policy requires a dialysate specimen, collect one after every 10 infuse-dwell-drain cycles (always during the drain phase), after every 24-hour period, or as ordered.
- To collect a dialysate specimen, attach the 10-ml syringe to the 22G 1½″ needle and insert it into the injection port on the drainage line, using strict sterile technique, and aspirate the drainage sample.
- Transfer the dialysate sample to the specimen container, label it appropriately, and send it to the laboratory with a laboratory request form.
- After completing the prescribed number of exchanges, clamp the catheter, and put on sterile gloves.
- Disconnect the administration set from the peritoneal catheter.
- Place the sterile protective cap over the catheter's distal end.

DRESSING CHANGES
- Remove old dressings carefully, to avoid putting tension on the catheter and accidentally dislodging it and to avoid introducing bacteria into the tract through movement of the catheter.

- Put on the sterile gloves.
- Saturate the sterile applicators or the 2″ × 2″ gauze pads with povidone-iodine, and clean the skin around the catheter, moving in concentric circles from the catheter site outward.
- Remove any crusted material carefully.
- Inspect the catheter site for drainage and the tissue around the site for redness and swelling.
- Apply povidone-iodine ointment to the catheter site with a sterile gauze pad.
- Place two precut drain dressings around the catheter site.
- Tape the 4″ × 4″ gauze pads over them to secure the dressing.

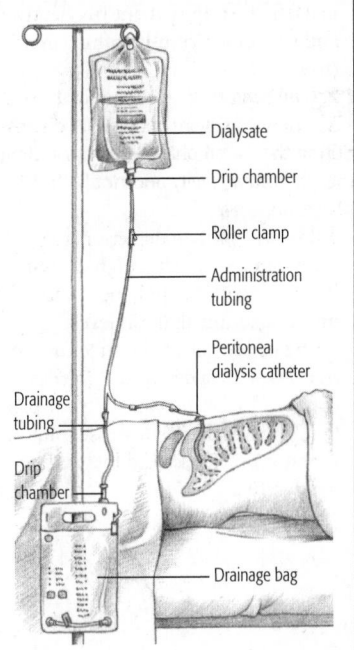

SETUP FOR PERITONEAL DIALYSIS

The proper setup for peritoneal dialysis is illustrated below.

- Dialysate
- Drip chamber
- Roller clamp
- Administration tubing
- Peritoneal dialysis catheter
- Drainage tubing
- Drip chamber
- Drainage bag

(continued)

- During and after dialysis, monitor the patient and his response to treatment.
- Monitor the patient's vital signs every 10 to 15 minutes for the first 1 to 2 hours of exchanges, then every 2 to 4 hours, or more frequently if necessary, and notify the physician of any abrupt changes in the patient's condition.
- Heparin is typically added to the dialysate to prevent an accumulation of fibrin in the catheter.

◈ **NURSING ALERT** To reduce the risk of peritonitis, use strict sterile technique during catheter insertion, dialysis, and dressing changes.

◈ **NURSING ALERT** All personnel in the room should wear masks whenever the dialysis system is opened or entered.

- Change the dressing at least every 24 hours or whenever it becomes wet or soiled to reduce the risk of infection and prevent skin excoriation from any leakage.
- To prevent respiratory distress, position the patient for maximal lung expansion, turn the patient frequently, and encourage deep-breathing exercises.

◈ **NURSING ALERT** If the patient experiences severe respiratory distress during the dwell phase of dialysis, drain the peritoneal cavity and notify the physician.

- To prevent protein depletion, the physician may order a high-protein diet or a protein supplement and monitor serum albumin levels.
- Dialysate is available in three concentrations: 4.25% dextrose, 2.5% dextrose, and 1.5% dextrose. If your patient receives 4.25% dextrose solution, monitor for excess fluid loss and hyperglycemia.

- Patients with low serum potassium levels may require the addition of potassium to the dialysate solution to prevent further losses.
- To help prevent fluid imbalance, monitor fluid volume balance, blood pressure, and pulse and notify the physician if the patient retains 500 ml or more fluid for three consecutive cycles or if he loses at least 1 L of fluid for three consecutive cycles.
- Weigh the patient at the same time each day to help determine how much fluid is being removed during dialysis treatment.
- If inflow and outflow are slow or absent, check the tubing for kinks, raise the I.V. pole, reposition the patient, or apply manual pressure to the lateral aspects of the patient's abdomen. If these maneuvers fail, notify the physician.

◈ **NURSING ALERT** Improper positioning of the catheter or an accumulation of fibrin can obstruct the catheter.

- Normally, outflow fluid (effluent) is clear or pale yellow, but pink-tinged effluent may appear during the first three or four cycles.
- If the effluent is pink-tinged, or if it's grossly bloody, suspect bleeding into the peritoneal cavity and notify the physician.
- If the effluent contains feces, which suggests bowel perforation, or if it's cloudy, which suggests peritonitis, notify the physician and obtain a sample for culture and Gram's stain.
- If the patient experiences pain during the procedure, determine when it occurs, the quality and duration, and whether it radiates to other body parts, and notify the physician.

◈ **NURSING ALERT** Pain during infusion usually results from a dialysate that's too cool or acidic. Pain can also result from rapid inflow; slowing the inflow rate may reduce the pain. Severe, diffuse pain with rebound tenderness and cloudy effluent may indicate peritoneal infection. Pain that radiates to the shoulder often results from air accumulation under the diaphragm. Severe, persistent perineal or rectal pain can result from improper catheter placement.

- To minimize the patient's discomfort, perform daily care during the drain phase of the cycle, when the patient's abdomen is less distended.

Complications
- Abdominal infection and pericatheter infections
- Peritonitis and sclerosing encapsulating peritonitis
- Bladder perforation
- Protein depletion
- Amyloidosis
- Respiratory distress
- Electrolyte imbalances
- Hypotension and shock
- Hyperglycemia
- Bowel perforation
- Tunnel abscess (in continuous ambulatory PD)
- Pulmonary edema
- Catheter occlusion or disconnection

Be sure to cover:
- reason for dialysis and steps involved
- use of sterile technique
- dressing changes and skin care
- signs and symptoms of peritonitis and other complications to report
- daily weight and blood pressure measurements
- accurate intake records
- name and telephone number of a person to call for assistance and questions.
- follow-up home care if PD will continue at home.

- Date and time of dialysis
- Exchange number
- Amount of dialysate infused and drained
- Infusion, dwell, and drain times
- Medications added to the solution
- Color and character of effluent
- Complications and treatment
- Daily weight
- Vital signs before, during, and after dialysis
- Total fluid balance after each exchange
- Pericatheter skin assessment
- Patient's tolerance of procedure
- Reports of unusual pain or discomfort
- Patient teaching

Selected references

Bernardini, J. "Peritoneal Dialysis: Myths, Barriers, and Achieving Optimum Outcomes," *Nephrology Nursing Journal* 31(5):495-98, September-October 2004.

Kelley, K.T. "How Peritoneal Dialysis Works," *Nephrology Nursing Journal* 31(5):481-82, 488-89, September-October 2004.

Redmond, A., and Doherty, E. "Peritoneal Dialysis," *Nursing Standard* 19(4):55-65, June 2005.

Zorzanello, M.M. "Peritoneal Dialysis and Hemodialysis: Similarities and Differences," *Nephrology Nursing Journal* 31(5):588-89, September-October 2004.

Pneumatic compression therapy

● OVERVIEW

- Used to prevent deep vein thrombosis (DVT) in surgical patients
- Massages the legs in a wavelike, milking motion that promotes blood flow and deters thrombosis
- Complements other preventive measures, such as antiembolism stockings and anticoagulant medications
- Used preoperatively and postoperatively because blood clots tend to form during surgery (about 20% of blood clots form in the femoral vein)
- Counteracts blood stasis and coagulation changes, two of the three major factors that promote DVT
- Reduces stasis by increasing peak blood flow velocity, helping to empty the femoral vein's valve cusps of pooled or static blood
- Increases fibrinolytic activity, which stimulates the release of a plasminogen activator

Contraindications

- Acute DVT or DVT diagnosed within the past 6 months
- Severe arteriosclerosis or any other ischemic vascular disease
- Massive edema of the legs resulting from pulmonary edema or heart failure
- Extreme deformity of lower extremity
- Any local condition that the compression sleeves would aggravate such as dermatitis, vein ligation, gangrene, and recent skin grafting

❖ EQUIPMENT

Measuring tape and sizing chart for the brand of sleeves being used • pair of compression sleeves in correct size • connecting tubing • compression controller

Equipment preparation

- Follow the manufacturer's instructions for setting up the device
- Determine the proper sleeve size
  – Measure the circumference of the upper thigh while the patient rests in bed by placing the measuring tape under the thigh at the gluteal furrow (as shown).

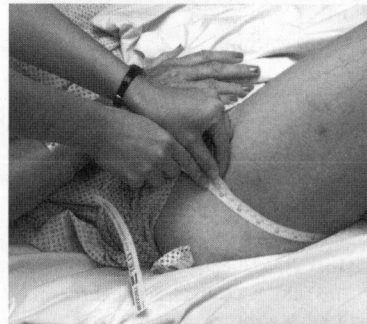

- Hold the tape snugly, but not tightly, around the patient's leg and note the exact circumference.
- Find the patient's thigh measurement on the sizing chart and locate the corresponding size of the compression sleeve.
- Bring equipment to the patient's bedside

▌▌▌ ESSENTIAL STEPS

- Confirm the patient's identity using two patient identifiers according to facility policy.
- Explain the procedure to the patient.
- Wash your hands thoroughly.

APPLYING THE SLEEVES

- Remove the compression sleeves from the package and unfold them.
- Lay the unfolded sleeves on a flat surface with the cotton lining facing up (as shown).

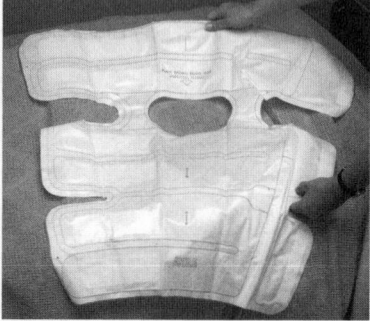

- Position the sleeve at the appropriate ankle or knee landmark.
- Place the patient's leg on the sleeve lining, positioning the back of the knee over the popliteal opening. Make sure the back of the ankle is over the ankle marking.
- Starting at the side opposite the plastic tubing, wrap the sleeve snugly around the patient's leg.
- Fasten the sleeve securely with the Velcro fasteners, starting with the ankle calf sections, and then moving to the thigh.
- Check the fit by inserting two fingers between the sleeve and the patient's leg at the knee opening and loosen or tighten the sleeve to fit snugly, but not tightly, by readjusting the Velcro fastener.

- Using the same procedure, apply the second sleeve (as shown).

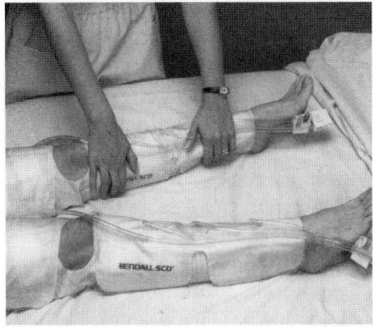

OPERATING THE SYSTEM
- Connect each sleeve to the tubing leading to the controller.
- Line up the blue arrows on the sleeve connector with the arrows on the tubing connectors, and push the ends together firmly, listening for a click signaling a firm connection.
- Make sure the tubing isn't kinked.
- Plug the compression controller into the wall outlet and turn on the power.
- The controller automatically sets the compression sleeve pressure at 45 mm Hg, which is the midpoint of the normal range (35 to 55 mm Hg).

⬙ **NURSING ALERT** Maximum inflation pressure shouldn't exceed the patient's diastolic blood pressure. Recommended range for inflation pressure is 35 to 45 mm Hg. Remove the device if the patient's diastolic pressure falls below 35 mm Hg and notify the physician.

- Observe the patient to see how well he tolerates the therapy and the controller as the system completes its first cycle. (With the instrument shown, each cycle lasts 71 seconds: 11 seconds of compression and 60 seconds of decompression.)
- Check that the green light is lit indicating that the AUDIBLE ALARM is working.
- The compression sleeves should function continuously (24 hours daily) until the patient is fully ambulatory.
- Check the sleeves at least once each shift to ensure proper fit and inflation.

REMOVING SLEEVES
- Remove the sleeves when the patient walks, bathes, or leaves the room for tests or other procedures. Reapply the sleeves immediately after any of these activities.
- Disconnect the sleeves from the tubing by depressing the latches on each side of the connectors and pulling the connectors apart.
- Store the tubing and compression controller according to facility's policy.
- Continue therapy even while patient is sitting in a chair.

◆ SPECIAL CONSIDERATIONS

- The compression controller also has a mechanism to help cool the patient.
- When a malfunction triggers the instrument's alarm, a beeping sound is produced and the system shuts off.
- To respond to the alarm, remove the operator's card from the slot on the top of the compression controller and follow the instructions printed on the card next to the matching code.

⬙ **NURSING ALERT** If signs and symptoms of DVT or pulmonary embolism (PE) develop, discontinue use and notify the physician immediately. If the patient complains of numbness, tingling, discomfort, or tingling in the calf, thigh, or toes, or if distal pulses are absent during maximum inflation, remove the device and notify the physician immediately.

Complications
- Arterial obstruction
- Skin irritation

▶ PATIENT TEACHING

Be sure to cover:
- how therapy helps to prevent DVT
- how device is applied
- signs and symptoms of DVT and PE to report.

◆◆ DOCUMENTATION

- Date and time the device was applied
- Type of sleeve used and knee or thigh length
- Patient's response to and understanding of the procedure
- Maximum inflation pressure and patient's blood pressure
- Reason for removal along with length of time it was removed
- Status of the alarm and cooling settings
- Sleeve cooling mode status
- Proper application of sleeves and connection to air controller
- Skin and circulatory assessment of the lower extremities, including distal pulses
- Whether device was applied to one or both legs, providing rationale if only one leg sleeve was applied
- Patient teaching

Selected references
Bonner, I. "The Prevention and Treatment of Deep Vein Thrombosis," *Nursing Times* 100(29):38-42, July 2004.

Hums, W., and Blostein, P. "A Comparative Approach to Deep Vein Thrombosis Risk Assessment," *Journal of Trauma Nursing* 13(1):28-30, January-March 2006.

Kakkos, S.K., et al. "Comparison of Two Intermittent Pneumatic Compression Systems. A Hemodynamic Study," *International Angiology* 24(4):330-35, December 2005.

Kakkos, S.K., et al. "The Efficacy of a New Portable Sequential Compression Device (SCD Express) in Preventing Venous Stasis," *Journal of Vascular Surgery* 42(2):296-303, August 2005.

Pressure ulcer care

● OVERVIEW

- Pressure ulcers: result when pressure impairs circulation, damaging skin and underlying structures; most develop over bony prominences
- Common sites: the sacrum, coccyx, ischial tuberosities, and greater trochanters; skin over the vertebrae, scapulae, elbows, knees, and heels in bedridden and immobile patients
- Suspected deep tissue injury: purple or maroon localized area of intact skin or blood-filled blister; difficult to detect in dark skin tones
- Stage 1: Nonblanchable erythema of intact skin in individuals with darker skin; discoloration of the skin, warmth edema, induration, or hardness may also be indicators
- Stage 2: Partial-thickness skin loss involving epidermis, dermis, or both; the ulcer is superficial and presents clinically as an abrasion, blister, or shallow crater
- Stage 3: Full-thickness skin loss involving damage to or necrosis of subcutaneous tissue that may extend down to, but not through, underlying fascia; the ulcer presents clinically as a deep crater with or without undermining of adjacent tissue
- Stage 4: Full-thickness skin loss with extensive destruction, tissue necrosis, or damage to muscle, bone, or supporting structures; undermining and sinus tracts
- Unstageable: Full-thickness tissue loss; base of wound covered by slough, eschar, or both
- Pressure ulcer treatment: involves relieving pressure, restoring circulation and resolving or managing related disorders; includes methods to decrease pressure, such as repositioning and use of special equipment to reduce pressure intensity
- Preventive measures: ensuring adequate nourishment and mobility to relieve pressure and promote circulation
- Other therapeutic measures: implementing prescribed wound care procedures.

Contraindications
- None known

❖ EQUIPMENT

Hypoallergenic tape or elastic netting • overbed table • piston-type irrigating system • two pairs of gloves • normal saline solution, as ordered • sterile 4″ × 4″ gauze pads • sterile cotton swabs • selected topical dressing • linen-saver pads • impervious plastic trash bag • disposable wound-measuring device

Equipment preparation
- Wash your hands thoroughly.
- Assemble equipment at the patient's bedside.
- Cut tape into strips.
- Loosen lids on cleaning solutions and medications for easy removal.
- Loosen existing dressing edges and tapes.
- Attach an impervious plastic trash bag to the overbed table to hold used dressings and refuse.

▐▐▐ ESSENTIAL STEPS

- Confirm the patient's identity using two patient identifiers according to facility policy.
- Explain all procedures to the patient and his family.
- Provide for privacy.
- Maintain asepsis and wear personal protective equipment.
- Wash hands thoroughly.

CLEANING A PRESSURE ULCER
- Position the patient for comfort and to allow easy access to the pressure ulcer site.
- Cover the bed linens with a linen-saver pad.
- Open the normal saline solution container and pour normal saline solution into an irrigation container.
- Open the piston syringe and place it into the opening provided in the irrigation container.
- Open the packages of supplies.
- Put on gloves to remove the old dressing and expose the pressure ulcer.
- Discard the soiled dressing in the impervious plastic trash bag.

- Inspect the wound, noting the color, amount, and odor of any drainage and necrotic debris.
- Assess the condition of the skin around the wound.
- Measure the wound perimeter with the disposable wound-measuring device.
- Using the piston syringe, irrigate the pressure ulcer, to remove necrotic debris and reduce bacteria in the wound.
- Remove and discard your soiled gloves and put on a clean pair.
- Insert a sterile cotton swab into the wound to assess wound tunneling or undermining.

> ⬔ **NURSING ALERT** You should see evidence of healing within 2 to 4 weeks in a clean pressure ulcer.

- If adherent necrotic material is in the wound, notify a wound care specialist or physician to ensure appropriate debridement.

> ✳ **AGE-RELATED CONCERN** Expect slower wound healing in elderly patients.

- Apply a topical dressing.
- To apply other dressings or topical agents, follow your facility's protocol or the supplier's instructions.

APPLYING A HYDROCOLLOID DRESSING
- Irrigate the pressure ulcer with normal saline solution.
- Blot the surrounding skin dry.
- Choose a clean, dry, precut dressing, or cut one to overlap the pressure ulcer by about 1″ (2.5 cm).
- Remove the dressing from its package and apply the dressing to the wound.
- To minimize irritation, carefully smooth out wrinkles.
- If the dressing's edges need to be secured with tape, first apply a skin sealant to the intact skin around the ulcer and allow it to dry before taping the dressing in place.
- Remove and discard your gloves in the impervious plastic trash bag.
- Dispose of refuse according to facility policy, and wash your hands.
- Change a hydrocolloid dressing every 2 to 7 days or if it becomes soiled, as needed.
- Discontinue use if signs of infection develop.

APPLYING A TRANSPARENT DRESSING
- Irrigate the pressure ulcer with normal saline solution.
- Blot the surrounding skin dry.
- Select a dressing to overlap the ulcer by 2″ (5 cm).
- Gently lay the dressing over the ulcer.
- To prevent shearing force, don't stretch the dressing.
- Press firmly on the edges of the dressing to promote adherence.
- Although this type of dressing is self-adhesive, you may have to tape the edges to prevent them from curling.
- Change the dressing every 3 to 7 days.

APPLYING AN ALGINATE DRESSING
- Irrigate the pressure ulcer with normal saline solution.
- Blot the surrounding skin dry.
- Apply the alginate dressing to the ulcer surface.
- Cover the area with a second dressing as ordered and secure the dressing with tape or elastic netting.
- If the wound is draining heavily, change the dressing once or twice daily for the first 3 to 5 days decreasing to every 2 to 4 days as drainage decreases.
- When the drainage stops or the wound bed looks dry, stop using alginate dressing.

APPLYING A FOAM DRESSING
- Irrigate the pressure ulcer with normal saline solution.
- Blot the surrounding skin dry.
- Gently lay the foam dressing over the ulcer.
- Use tape, elastic netting, or gauze to hold the dressing in place.
- Change the dressing when the foam no longer absorbs the exudate.

APPLYING A HYDROGEL DRESSING
- Irrigate the pressure ulcer with normal saline solution.
- Blot the surrounding skin dry.
- Apply gel to the wound bed.
- Cover the area with a second dressing.
- Change the dressing daily.
- If the dressing comes in sheet form, cut it to match the wound base.
- Hydrogel dressings also come in a prepackaged, saturated gauze for wounds that require "dead space" to be filled.

PREVENTING PRESSURE ULCERS
- Turn and reposition the patient every 1 to 2 hours unless contraindicated.
- For a patient who can't turn by himself or who is turned on a schedule, use a pressure-reducing device, such as air, gel, or a 4″ (10 cm) foam mattress overlay.
- Low- or high-air-loss therapy may reduce excessive pressure and promote evaporation of excess moisture.
- As appropriate, implement active or passive range-of-motion exercises to relieve pressure and promote circulation.
- When turning the patient, use a turning sheet and get help to lift him rather than slide him because sliding increases friction and shear.
- Use pillows to position the patient.
- Eliminate sheet wrinkles, which increase pressure and cause pain.
- Post a turning schedule at the bedside.
- Avoid placing the patient directly on the trochanters.
- Avoid raising the head of the bed more than 30 degrees, to prevent shearing pressure.
- Direct the patient confined to a chair or wheelchair to shift his weight every 15 minutes to promote blood flow.
- Show a paraplegic patient how to shift his weight by doing push-ups in the wheelchair.

  ⬛ **NURSING ALERT** Don't sit the patient on a rubber or plastic doughnut, which can increase localized pressure at vulnerable points.
- Adjust or pad appliances, casts, or splints as needed, to ensure proper fit and avoid increased pressure.
- Tell the patient to keep his skin from drying out by avoiding harsh soaps and applying lotion after bathing.
- Avoid vigorous massage because it can damage capillaries.
- Recommend a nutritional consultation.
- If diarrhea develops or if the patient is incontinent, clean and dry soiled skin and apply a moisture barrier.
- Make sure the patient, his family, and caregivers learn the importance of prevention and treatment.

◆ SPECIAL CONSIDERATIONS

- Avoid using elbow and heel protectors that fasten with a single narrow strap, which can impair neurovascular function in the involved hand or foot.
- Avoid using artificial sheepskin because it doesn't reduce pressure.
- Repair of stage 3 and 4 ulcers may require surgical intervention, such as direct closure, skin grafting, or flaps.

Complications
- Infection
- Osteomyelitis
- Bacteremia
- Cellulitis

▶ PATIENT TEACHING

Be sure to cover:
- types of treatment and how to perform wound treatments at home
- signs and symptoms of infection
- ways to prevent pressure ulcers.

●◇ DOCUMENTATION

- Date and time of treatment
- Specific treatment
- Color and appearance of wound and surrounding skin
- Amount, odor, and color of drainage
- Condition and temperature of the surrounding skin
- Patient's tolerance of treatment
- Patient teaching

Selected references

Jones, J. "Evaluation of Pressure Ulcer Prevention Devices: A Critical Review of the Literature," *Journal of Wound Care* 14(9):422-25, October 2005.

Niezgoda, J.A., and Mendez-Eastman, S. "The Effective Management of Presure Ulcers," *Advances in Skin & Wound Care* 19(suppl 1):3-15, January-February 2005.

Ohura, N., et al. "Evaluating Dressing Materials for the Prevention of Shear Force in the Treatment of Pressure Ulcers," *Journal of Wound Care* 14(9):401-404, October 2005.

Stevens, J., and Gray, W. "New Guidelines on Preventing and Managing Pressure Ulceres," *Nursing Times* 101(46):40-42, November 2005.

Pulmonary artery pressure and pulmonary artery wedge pressure monitoring

● OVERVIEW

- Provides important information about left ventricular function and preload for monitoring, aiding diagnosis, refining assessment, guiding interventions, and projecting patient outcomes
- Indicated for acutely ill patients, especially those who are hemodynamically unstable, need fluid management or continuous cardiopulmonary assessment, or are receiving multiple or frequently administered cardioactive drugs
- Also indicated for patients with shock, trauma, pulmonary or cardiac disease, or multiorgan disease
- Pulmonary artery pressure (PAP) monitoring catheters have multiple lumens depending on the type, allowing medication and fluid administration; measurement of PAP, pulmonary artery wedge pressure (PAWP), cardiac output, and continuous mixed venous oxygen saturation; and cardiac pacing
- During flow-directed catheter insertion, the catheter follows venous blood flow from right heart chambers into pulmonary artery
- During insertion, the right atrium, right ventricle, pulmonary artery, and wedge position produce characteristic pressures and waveforms that can be observed on the monitor to help track catheter-tip location, especially if image-guidance isn't utilized

Contraindications
- Abnormal bleeding
- Right heart mass
- Tricuspid or pulmonary valve prosthesis
- Endocarditis

❖ EQUIPMENT

Balloon-tipped, flow-directed pulmonary artery catheter • prepared pressure transducer system • I.V. solutions • sterile gloves • alcohol pads • medication-added label • monitor and monitor cable • I.V. pole with transducer mount • emergency resuscitation equipment • electrocardiogram (ECG) monitor • ECG electrodes • armboard • lead aprons • sutures • sterile 4″ × 4″ gauze pads or other dry, occlusive dressing material • prepackaged introducer kit • optional: dextrose 5% in water, shaving materials, small sterile basin, sterile water

IF PREPACKAGED INTRODUCER KIT ISN'T AVAILABLE
An introducer (one size larger than the catheter) • sterile tray containing instruments for procedure • masks • sterile gowns • sterile gloves • sterile drapes • iodine ointment and solution • sutures • two 10-ml syringes • local anesthetic (1% to 2% lidocaine) • one 5-ml syringe • 25G ½″ needle • 1″ and 3″ tape

Equipment preparation
- Make sure the bedside monitor has the correct pressure modules.
- Turn on the monitor before gathering the equipment to give it time to warm up.
- Calibrate the monitor according to the manufacturer's instructions and zero the transducer.
- Wash your hands thoroughly.
- Prepare the pressure monitoring system and position it according to policy.
- Add heparin to the flush, according to your facility's policy.
- To manage any complications from catheter insertion, make sure to have emergency resuscitation equipment on hand, including a chest tube setup.
- Prepare a sterile field, such as on a bedside tray, for insertion of the introducer and catheter.

❙❙❚ ESSENTIAL STEPS

- Confirm the patient's identity using two patient identifiers according to facility policy.
- Explain to the patient and his family the procedure and why it's being done.
- Make sure the patient has signed the appropriate consent form, if indicated.
- Maintain asepsis throughout all procedures.
- Wear appropriate personal protective equipment, as necessary, throughout all procedures.
- Check the patient's chart for heparin sensitivity or history of heparin-induced thrombocytopenia before adding heparin to the flush solution.
- Position the patient at the proper height for catheter placement.
- If the physician will use a superior approach for percutaneous insertion (most commonly using the internal jugular or subclavian vein), remove the pillow and place the patient flat or in a slight Trendelenburg position, with his head turned to the side opposite the insertion site.
- If the physician will use an inferior approach to access a femoral vein, position the patient flat, if tolerated.

PREPARING THE CATHETER
- Clean the insertion site with a povidone-iodine solution and drape it.
- Put on a mask and assist the physician with putting on a sterile mask, gown, and gloves.
- Open the outer packaging of the catheter, revealing the inner sterile wrapping.
- Using sterile technique, the physician opens the inner wrapping and picks up the catheter.
- Take the catheter lumen hubs as he hands them to you.
- Flush the catheter with normal saline solution to remove air and verify patency.
- For multiple pressure lines, ensure the distal PA lumen hub is attached to the pressure line being monitored.
- Inadvertently attaching the distal PA line to the proximal lumen hub will

prevent the proper waveform from appearing during insertion.

- Make sure the scale on the monitor is appropriate for lower pressures. A scale of 0 to 25 mm Hg or 0 to 50 mm Hg (more common) is preferred.
- To verify the integrity of the balloon, the physician inflates it with air (usually 1.5 ml), observing it for symmetrical shape, and, possibly, submerging it in a sterile basin filled with sterile water and observing it for bubbles.

INSERTING THE CATHETER

- Assist the physician as he inserts the introducer to access the vessel by cutdown or (more commonly) percutaneously.

- The physician then inserts the catheter through the introducer. Observe the pressure values and waveforms carefully during insertion, preferably using a scale of 0 to 25 mm Hg or 0 to 50 mm Hg (more common).
- The balloon is inflated when the catheter exits the end of the introducer sheath and reaches the junction of the superior vena cava and right atrium (at the 15- to 20-cm mark on the catheter shaft).
- When the catheter enters the right atrium, the pressure is low (from 2 to 4 mm Hg) and values are read in the mean mode because systolic and diastolic values are similar. (See *Normal pulmonary artery waveforms.*)

- As the physician advances the catheter into the right ventricle (to approximately the 30- to 35-cm mark), the waveform shows sharp systolic upstrokes and lower diastolic dips.
- Record both systolic and diastolic pressures in the right ventricle (systolic pressure normally ranges from 15 to 25 mm Hg; diastolic pressure, from 0 to 8 mm Hg).

◆ **NURSING ALERT** As the catheter passes through the right ventricle, watch the cardiac monitor carefully because irritation can trigger arrhythmias.

- As the catheter floats into the pulmonary artery, note that the upstroke from right ventricular systole is smoother, and systolic pressure is nearly the same as right ventricular systolic pressure.
- With the catheter in the pulmonary artery, record systolic, diastolic, and mean pressures (typically ranging from 8 to 15 mm Hg).

WEDGING THE CATHETER

- To obtain a wedge tracing, the physician lets the inflated balloon float with venous blood flow to a narrow distal branch of the pulmonary artery where it lodges, or wedges (about the 45- to 50-cm mark).
- Note that the tracing resembles the right atrial tracing because the catheter tip is recording left atrial pressure.
- Record PAWP in the mean mode (usually between 6 and 12 mm Hg).

◆ **NURSING ALERT** In a large heart, a longer catheter length — up to 55 cm — typically is required. However, a catheter should generally never be inserted more than 60 cm.

- The physician deflates the balloon, and the catheter drifts out of the wedge position and back into the pulmonary artery.
- To verify balloon deflation, observe the monitor for return of the pulmonary artery tracing.
- Typically, the physician orders a portable chest X-ray to confirm catheter position.
- Apply a sterile occlusive dressing to the insertion site.

(continued)

NORMAL PULMONARY ARTERY WAVEFORMS

During pulmonary artery catheter insertion, the monitor shows various waveforms as the catheter advances through the heart chambers.

Right atrium

When the catheter tip enters the right atrium, a waveform like the one shown below appears on the monitor. Note the two small upright waves. The a waves represent atrial contraction; the v waves, increased pressure or volume in the atrium during ventricular systole.

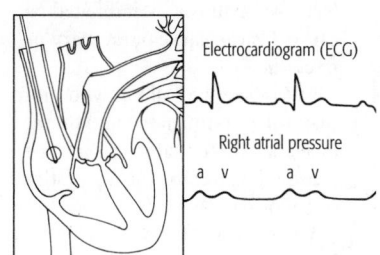

Right ventricle

As the catheter tip reaches the right ventricle, you'll see a waveform with sharp systolic upstrokes and lower diastolic dips.

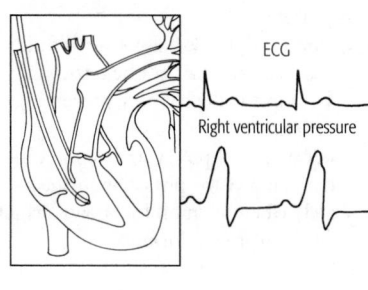

Pulmonary artery

The catheter then floats into the pulmonary artery. The monitor shows a pulmonary artery pressure (PAP) waveform like the one below. Note that the upstroke is smoother than on the right ventricular waveform. The dicrotic notch indicates pulmonic valve closure.

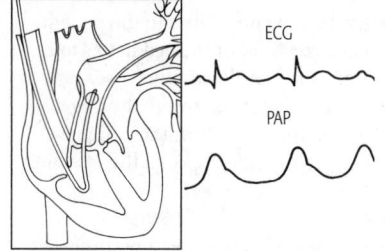

Pulmonary artery, distal branch

Floating into a distal branch of the pulmonary artery, the balloon wedges where the vessel becomes too narrow for it to pass. The monitor now shows a pulmonary artery wedge pressure (PAWP) waveform, with two small uprises from left atrial systole and diastole. The balloon is then deflated and the catheter is left in the pulmonary artery.

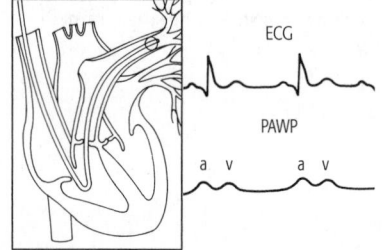

INTERMITTENT PAP MONITORING

- After inserting the catheter and recording initial pressure readings, record subsequent PAP values and monitor waveforms.

NURSING ALERT Be sure to locate and mark the location of the phlebostatic axis on each patient with indelible ink to ensure consistent and accurate pressure measurements.

NURSING ALERT To ensure accurate values, make sure the transducer is properly leveled and zeroed.

- Obtain PAP values at end expiration (when the patient completely exhales).
- If you have trouble identifying end expiration (such as with a rapid respiratory rate), obtain a printout and use the averaged values obtained through the full respiratory cycle.
- To analyze trends accurately, be sure to record values at consistent times during the respiratory cycle.

PAWP MONITORING

- PAWP is recorded by inflating the balloon and letting it float into a distal artery.

NURSING ALERT Some facilities allow only physicians or specially trained nurses to take a PAWP reading because of the risk of pulmonary artery rupture, a rare but life-threatening complication. Know and follow your facility's policy.

- If your facility permits you to perform this procedure, do so with extreme caution and make sure you're thoroughly familiar with intracardiac waveform interpretation.
- Verify that the transducer is properly labeled and zeroed.
- Detach the syringe from the balloon inflation hub and draw 1.5 ml of air into the syringe, and then reattach the syringe to the hub.
- Watching the monitor, inject the air through the hub slowly and smoothly.
- When you see a wedge tracing on the monitor, immediately stop inflating the balloon.

NURSING ALERT When obtaining a PAWP reading, never inflate the balloon beyond the volume needed to obtain a wedge tracing.

- Take the pressure reading at end expiration.
- Note the amount of air needed to change the pulmonary artery tracing to a wedge tracing (normally, 1.25 to 1.5 ml).

NURSING ALERT If the wedge tracing appeared with injection of less than 1.25 ml, suspect that the catheter has migrated into a more distal branch and requires repositioning.

- If the balloon is in a more distal branch, the tracings may move up the oscilloscope, indicating that the catheter tip is recording balloon pressure rather than PAWP and may lead to pulmonary artery rupture.

REMOVING THE CATHETER

- To assist the physician, inspect the chest X-ray for signs of catheter kinking or knotting. (In some states, you may be permitted to remove a pulmonary artery catheter yourself under an advanced collaborative standard of practice.)
- Obtain the patient's baseline vital signs and note the ECG pattern.
- Explain the procedure to the patient.
- Place the head of the bed flat as tolerated, unless ordered otherwise.
- If the catheter was inserted using a superior approach, turn the patient's head to the side opposite the insertion site.
- Gently remove the dressing.
- The physician removes any sutures securing the catheter. (If the introducer is left in place, the physician doesn't remove the sutures.)
- Turn off all stopcocks to the patient.
- The physician puts on sterile gloves.
- After verifying that the balloon is deflated, the physician withdraws the catheter slowly and smoothly; if he feels any resistance, he stops immediately.

- If the patient is conscious, the physician usually tells the patient to hold his breath or to take a deep breath and hold it as the catheter is withdrawn.
- Watch the ECG monitor for arrhythmias.
- If the introducer was removed, apply pressure to the site, and check it frequently for signs of bleeding.
- If the introducer is left in place, observe the diaphragm for blood backflow, which verifies the integrity of the hemostasis valve.
- Dress the site, as necessary.
- Turn off the bedside pressure modules but leave the ECG module on.
- Reassure the patient and his family that he'll be observed closely.
- Tell the patient that the catheter was removed because his condition has improved and he no longer needs it.

✦ SPECIAL CONSIDERATIONS

- Advise the patient to use caution when moving about in bed, to avoid dislodging the catheter.
- Never leave the balloon inflated because this can cause pulmonary infarction.
- Never inflate the balloon with more than the recommended air volume (specified on the catheter shaft) because this can cause loss of elasticity or balloon rupture.

NURSING ALERT If the patient has a suspected intracardial right-to-left shunt, use carbon dioxide to inflate the balloon, as ordered, because it diffuses more quickly than air, thus preventing systemic air embolism if the balloon ruptures.

- Never inflate the balloon with fluids because they may not be retrievable from inside the balloon, preventing deflation.
- Because the tip may irritate the ventricle, notify the physician immediately when the monitor shows a right ventricular waveform.

NURSING ALERT If the wave form appears "wedged," have the patient turn and cough in an attempt to dislodge the wedge.

- To minimize valvular trauma, make sure the balloon is deflated whenever the catheter is withdrawn from the pulmonary artery to the right ventricle or from the right ventricle to the right atrium.
- Change the dressing whenever it's moist or every 24 to 48 hours, according to your facility's policy; change the catheter every 72 hours; change the pressure tubing every 48 hours, and change the flush solution every 24 hours or according to your facility's policy.

Complications
- Pulmonary hemorrhage
- Pulmonary artery perforation
- Pulmonary infarction
- Catheter knotting, entanglement, and fracture
- Local or systemic infection, including endocarditis
- Cardiac arrhythmias
- Balloon rupture with possible air embolism
- Heparin-induced thrombocytopenia
- Thrombosis
- Damage to intracardiac structures, including the pulmonic or tricuspid valvular apparatus

▶ **PATIENT TEACHING**

Be sure to cover:
- why the procedure is being done
- what to expect during catheter insertion (The patient should expect some discomfort at the insertion site, but analgesics are typically ordered.)
- meaning of audible monitor alarms and artifact
- reassurance that the patient will be closely monitored
- why pressure readings are taken periodically
- activity limitations
- symptoms to report immediately to his nurse.

DOCUMENTATION

- Date and time of catheter insertion
- Name of physician who performed the procedure
- Catheter insertion site
- Pressure waveforms and values for the various heart chambers
- Balloon inflation volume required to obtain a wedge tracing
- Type of flush solution and its heparin concentration
- Any arrhythmias occurring during or after the procedure
- Type of dressing applied
- Position of the patient and transducer during pressure measurements
- Calibration of monitor and zeroing of transducer
- Date and time of catheter removal
- Problems encountered during removal
- Patient's tolerance of procedure
- Patient teaching and emotional support

Selected references
Bakker, R. "The Evidence-Based Character of the Pulmonary Artery Catheter (in Cardiac Patients)," *European Journal of Cardiovascular Nursing* 3(2):165-71, July 2004.

Bossert, T., et al. "Swan-Ganz Catheter-Induced Severe Complications in Cardiac Surgery: Right Ventricular Perforation, Knotting, and Rupture of a Pulmonary Artery," *Journal of Cardiac Surgery* 21(3):292-95, May-June 2006.

Harvey S., et al. "Assessment of the Clinical Effectiveness of Pulmonary Artery Catheters in Management of Patients in Intensive Care (PAC-Man): a Randomised Controlled Trial," *Lancet* 366(9484):472-77, August 2005.

Pulse oximetry

- Performed intermittently or continuously for noninvasive monitoring of arterial oxygen saturation
- Photodetector that slipped over the finger that measures transmitted light as it passes through the vascular bed, detects the relative amount of color absorbed by arterial blood, and calculates exact mixed venous oxygen saturation without interference from surrounding venous blood, skin, connective tissue, or bone
- With an ear probe: works by monitoring transmission of light waves through the vascular bed of a patient's earlobe; results inaccurate if the patient's earlobe is poorly perfused, as from low cardiac output (see *How oximetry works*)
- Symbol for arterial oxygen saturation denoted by SpO_2 in oximetry; SaO_2 indicates arterial oxygen saturation measurements collected by an invasive method, such as arterial blood gases (ABGs)

Contraindications
- None known

❖ EQUIPMENT

Oximeter • finger or ear probe • alcohol pads • nail polish remover, if necessary

Equipment preparation
- Review the manufacturer's instructions for assembling the oximeter.

▌▌■ ESSENTIAL STEPS

- Wash your hands thoroughly.
- Confirm the patient's identity using two patient identifiers according to facility policy.
- Explain the procedure to the patient.

PULSE OXIMETRY USING A FINGERTIP SENSOR
- Select a finger for the test without an acrylic fingernail, if possible.
- Remove any nail polish from the test finger, if possible.

⬥ NURSING ALERT Most oximeters can compensate for finger thickness, skin pigmentation, and even most common nail polishes. However, keep in mind that blue or green nail polish can produce erroneous readings, and black or metalic nail polish can block the light completely.

HOW OXIMETRY WORKS

The pulse oximeter allows noninvasive monitoring of the percentage of arterial blood saturated by oxygen, or SpO_2 levels, by measuring the absorption (amplitude) of light waves as they pass through areas of the body that are highly perfused by arterial blood. Oximetry is also used to monitor pulse rate and amplitude.

Light-emitting diodes in a transducer (photodetector) attached to the patient's body (shown here on the index finger) send red and infrared light beams through tissue. The photodetector records the relative amount of each color absorbed by arterial blood and transmits the data to a monitor, which displays the information with each heartbeat. If the SpO_2 level or pulse rate varies from preset limits, the monitor triggers visual and audible alarms.

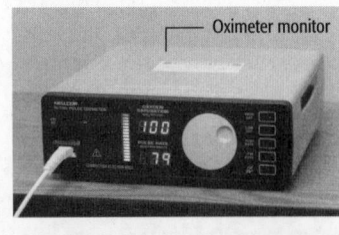
Oximeter monitor

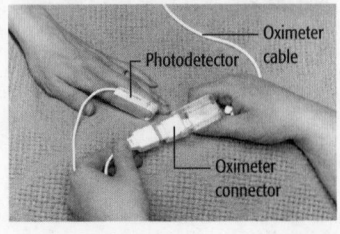
Oximeter cable
Photodetector
Oximeter connector

- Place the photodetector probe over the patient's finger so that light beams and sensors oppose each other. The red and infrared light beams should shine through the nail bed of the finger.
- If the patient has long fingernails, position the probe perpendicular to the finger, if possible, or clip the fingernail.
- Position the patient's hand at heart level to eliminate venous pulsations and to promote accurate readings.

✴ AGE-RELATED CONCERN When testing a neonate or small infant, wrap the probe around the foot so that light beams and detectors oppose each other. For a large infant, use a probe that fits on the great toe and secure it to the foot.
- Turn on the power switch.
- After four to six heartbeats, the SpO_2 and pulse rate displays will supply information with each beat, and the pulse amplitude indicator will begin tracking the pulse.

PULSE OXIMETRY USING EAR CLIP SENSORS
- Using an alcohol pad, massage the patient's earlobe for 10 to 20 seconds until you see mild erythema indicating adequate vascularization.
- Following the manufacturer's instructions, attach the ear probe to the patient's earlobe or pinna.
- Use the ear probe stabilizer for prolonged or exercise testing.
- After the probe has been attached for a few seconds, a saturation reading and pulse waveform will appear on the oximeter's screen.
- Leave the ear probe in place for 3 or more minutes until readings stabilize at the highest point, or take three separate readings and average them.
- After the procedure, remove the probe, turn off and unplug the unit, and clean the probe by gently rubbing it with an alcohol pad.
- Make sure you revascularize the patient's earlobe each time you take a reading.

- An elevated bilirubin level may falsely lower SpO_2 readings, while elevated carboxyhemoglobin or methemoglobin levels (such as occur in heavy smokers and urban dwellers) can cause a falsely elevated SpO_2 reading.
- Certain intravascular substances, such as lipid emulsions and dyes, can also prevent accurate readings.
- Other factors that may interfere with accurate results include excessive light (for example, from phototherapy, surgical lamps, direct sunlight, and excessive ambient lighting), excessive patient movement, excessive ear pigment, hypothermia, hypotension, and vasoconstriction.
- If the patient has compromised circulation in his extremities, you can place a photodetector across the bridge of the nose.
- If SpO_2 is used to guide weaning the patient from forced inspiratory oxygen, obtain ABG analysis occasionally to correlate SpO_2 readings with SaO_2 levels.
- If an automatic blood pressure cuff is used on the same extremity that's used for measuring SpO_2, the cuff will interfere with SpO_2 readings during inflation.
- If light is a problem, cover the probes; if patient movement is a problem, move the probe or select a different probe; and if ear pigment is a problem, reposition the probe, revascularize the site, or use a finger probe. (See *Troubleshooting pulse oximeter problems.*)
- Normal SpO_2 levels for ear and pulse oximetry are 95% to 100% for adults and 93% to 100% by 1 hour after birth for healthy, full-term neonates.

🔲 **NURSING ALERT** If the SpO_2 value drops more than two percentage points—for example, from 97% to 95%—a thorough patient assessment should be performed. If the level drops five or more percentage points, the physician should be notified. If the level drops below 90%, the physician should be notified immediately.

- If your patient has an SpO_2 level below normal that indicates hypoxemia, follow your facility's policy or the physician's orders, which may include increasing oxygen therapy.

Complications
- Skin reactions, burns, and blisters

Be sure to cover:
- purpose of the test and how it's performed (continuously or intermittently)
- reassurance that no pain is involved
- need to keep the test finger still, away from excessive light, and at the level of the heart
- meaning of alarms.

- Indications for SpO_2 monitoring
- Date and time of monitoring, site of measurement, SpO_2 values, and actions taken
- Levels at which high and low alarms are set
- Patient's tolerance of procedure
- Patient teaching

Selected references
Allen, K., "Principles and Limitations of Pulse Oximetry in Patient Monitoring," *Nursing Times* 100(4):34-37, October 2004.

Cooper, R. "Using Finger-Toe Pulse Oximetry to Assess Arterial Blood Flow," *Nursing Times* 101(46):47-49, November 2005.

Giulano, K.K., and Higgins, T.L. "New-Generation Pulse Oximetry in the Case of Critically Ill Patients," *American Journal of Critical Care* 14(1):26-37, January 2005.

Giulano, K.K., and Lieu, L.M. "Knowledge of Pulse Oximetry Among Critical Care Nurses," *Dimensions of Critical Care Nursing* 25(1):44-49, January-February 2006.

McMorrow, R.C., and Mythen, M.G. "Pulse Oximetry," *Current Opinion in Critical Care* 12(3):269-71, June 2006.

TROUBLESHOOTING PULSE OXIMETER PROBLEMS

To maintain a continuous display of arterial oxygen saturation (SpO_2) levels, you need to keep the monitoring site clean and dry. Make sure the skin doesn't become irritated from adhesives used to keep disposable probes in place. You may need to change the site if this happens. Disposable probes that irritate the skin can be replaced by nondisposable models that don't need tape.

A common problem with pulse oximeters is failure of the device to obtain a signal. If this happens, *first check the patient's vital signs*. If they're sufficient to produce a signal, check for the following problems.

Poor connection
Check that the sensors are properly aligned. Make sure that wires are intact and securely fastened and that the pulse oximeter is plugged into a power source.

Inadequate or intermittent blood flow to the site
Check the patient's pulse rate and capillary refill time and take corrective action if blood flow to the site is decreased. This may require you to loosen restraints, remove tight-fitting clothes, take off a blood pressure cuff, or check arterial and I.V. lines. If none of these interventions works, you may need to find an alternate site. Finding a site with proper circulation may be a challenge when the patient is receiving vasoconstrictive drugs.

Equipment malfunction
Remove the pulse oximeter from the patient and attempt to obtain an SpO_2 level on yourself or another healthy person. If you are able to obtain a normal value, the equipment is functioning properly.

Residual limb and prosthesis care

● OVERVIEW

- Performed in immediate postoperative period to monitor drainage from residual limb, position affected limb, assist with exercises prescribed by physical therapist, and wrap and condition the residual limb
- Prosthesis care: includes cleaning, lubricating, and checking for proper fit

Contraindications
- None known

❖ EQUIPMENT

POSTOPERATIVE RESIDUAL LIMB CARE
Pressure dressing • overhead trapeze • 1″ adhesive tape, bandage clips, or safety pins • sandbags or trochanter roll (for a leg) • elastic limb shrinker or 4″ elastic bandage
DAILY RESIDUAL LIMB AND PROSTHESIS CARE
Mild soap • limb socks • two washcloths • two towels • appropriate lubricating oil

Equipment preparation
- Gather all equipment and have readily available at the patient's bedside.

▮▮ ESSENTIAL STEPS

- Explain all procedures to the patient and his family.
- Wash your hands thoroughly.
- Wear appropriate personal protective equipment.
- Perform routine postoperative care.

MONITORING DRAINAGE FROM RESIDUAL LIMB
- Because gravity causes fluid to accumulate at the stump, frequently check the amount of blood and drainage on the dressing and notify the physician if accumulations increase rapidly.
- If excessive bleeding occurs, notify the physician immediately and apply a pressure dressing or compress the appropriate pressure points; keep a tourniquet available, if necessary.

◈ NURSING ALERT Use a tourniquet only as a last resort to control bleeding.
- Monitor the suction drainage equipment, and note the amount and type of drainage.

POSITIONING THE RESIDUAL LIMB
- Elevate the residual limb for the first 24 hours to reduce swelling and promote venous return.
- To prevent contractures, position an arm with the elbow extended and the shoulder abducted.
- To prevent external rotation, position a leg with the foot of the bed slightly elevated and sandbags or a trochanter roll placed against the hip.

◈ NURSING ALERT Don't place a pillow under the thigh to flex the hip because this can cause hip flexion contracture. For the same reason, tell the patient to avoid prolonged sitting.
- After a below-the-knee amputation, maintain knee extension to prevent hamstring muscle contractures.
- Place the patient with a leg amputation on a firm surface in the prone position for at least 2 hours a day, without pillows under his stomach, hips, knees, or the residual limb, unless contraindicated, to prevent hip flexion, contractures, and abduction and stretch the flexor muscles.

ASSISTING WITH PRESCRIBED EXERCISES
- Help the patient with an arm amputation perform isometric and range-of-motion (ROM) exercises for both shoulders, as prescribed by the physical therapist.
- After leg amputation, stand behind the patient and, if necessary, support him with your hands at his waist during balancing exercises.
- Instruct the patient to exercise the affected and unaffected limbs to maintain muscle tone and strength. The patient with a leg amputation may perform push-ups, (in the sitting position, arms at his sides), or pull-ups on the overhead trapeze to strengthen his arms, shoulders, and back.

WRAPPING AND CONDITIONING THE RESIDUAL LIMB
- If the patient doesn't have a rigid cast, apply an elastic limb shrinker to prevent edema and shape the limb in preparation for the prosthesis.

- Wrap the residual limb so that it narrows toward the distal end to help ensure comfort when the patient wears the prosthesis.
- If an elastic shrinker isn't available, wrap the stump in a 4″ elastic bandage by stretching the bandage to about two-thirds its maximum length as you wrap it diagonally around the residual limb, with the greatest pressure distally. (Depending on the size of the leg, you may need to use two 4″ bandages.)
- Secure the elastic bandage with clips, safety pins, or adhesive tape.
- Make sure the bandage covers all portions of the residual limb smoothly because wrinkles or exposed areas encourage skin breakdown. (See *Wrapping a residual limb*.)
- If the patient experiences throbbing after the residual limb is wrapped, remove the bandage immediately and reapply it less tightly because throbbing indicates impaired circulation.
- Check the bandage regularly and rewrap it when it begins to bunch up at the end, or as necessary.
- After removing the bandage to rewrap it, massage the residual limb gently, always pushing toward the suture line rather than away from it to stimulate circulation and prevent scar tissue from adhering to the bone.
- When healing begins, instruct the patient to push the residual limb against a pillow, gradually progressing to pushing against harder surfaces, such as a padded chair, then a hard chair to help the patient adjust to pressure and sensation in the residual limb.

CARING FOR THE HEALED RESIDUAL LIMB
- Bathe the residual limb, but never shave it, to prevent infection.
- Perform bathing at the end of the day, if possible, because warm water may cause swelling, making reapplication of the prosthesis difficult.
- Don't soak the residual limb for long periods of time.
- Don't apply lotion to the residual limb; this may clog follicles, increasing the risk of infection.
- Inspect the residual limb for redness, swelling, irritation, and calluses and report any findings to the physician.

- Tell the patient to avoid putting weight on the residual limb.
- Change the elastic bandages daily to avoid exposing skin to excessive perspiration, which can can cause irritation.
- Wash the elastic bandages in warm water and gentle nondetergent soap; lay them flat on a towel to dry.
- To shape the residual limb, have the patient wear an elastic bandage 24 hours per day except while bathing.

CARING FOR THE PLASTIC PROSTHESIS
- Wipe the plastic socket of the prosthesis with a damp cloth and mild soap to prevent bacterial accumulation.
- Wipe the insert with a dry cloth.
- Dry the prosthesis thoroughly.
- Maintain and lubricate the prosthesis, as instructed by the manufacturer.
- Refer to the prosthetist for malfunctions and adjustments.

APPLYING THE PROSTHESIS
- Apply a residual limb sock, keeping the seams away from bony prominences.
- If the prosthesis has an insert, remove it from the socket, place it over the residual limb, and insert the limb into the prosthesis.

- If the prosthesis has no insert, merely slide the prosthesis over the residual limb.
- Secure the prosthesis according to manufacturer instructions.

◆ SPECIAL CONSIDERATIONS

- As directed by a physical therapist, begin exercising the extremity after surgery.
- If the patient has a rigid dressing, perform normal cast care and make sure it doesn't slip off. If it does, apply an elastic bandage immediately and notify the physician because edema develops rapidly.

Complications
- Hemorrhage
- Contractures
- Swollen or flabby residual limb
- Skin breakdown or infection
- Sebaceous cysts or boils
- Psychological problems
- Phantom limb pain

▶ PATIENT TEACHING

Be sure to cover:
- daily residual limb care
- signs and symptoms to report, such as infection or edema
- importance of massaging stump toward the suture line to mobilize the scar and prevent its adherence to bone
- need to change the elastic bandages or socks daily
- occurance of twitching, spasms, or phantom limb pain as muscles adjust to amputation (patient can reduce these symptoms with heat, massage, or gentle pressure)
- rubbing with a dry washcloth for 4 minutes three times per day if it's sensitive to touch
- performance of prescribed exercises
- positioning to prevent contractures
- caring for the prosthesis properly.

●◆ DOCUMENTATION

- Date and time of residual limb care
- Appearance of the suture line and surrounding tissue
- Amount and type of drainage
- Condition of the dressing and the need for reinforcement
- Signs of skin irritation or infection
- Complications and nursing actions taken
- Patient's tolerance of exercises
- Patient's psychological status
- Patient teaching

Selected references

Gleaves, J.R., and Eldridge, K. "Silicone Sheeting as an Alternative to Elastic Bandages in Dressing Lower Extremity Amputations," *Ostomy and Wound Management* 50(9):8-10, September 2004.

Hayes, D. "How to Wrap an Above-the-Knee Amputation Stump," *Nursing* 03(1):70, January 2003.

Laskowski-Jones, L. "First Aid for Amputation," *Nursing* 36(4):50-52, April 2006.

WRAPPING A RESIDUAL LIMB

Proper care for a residual limb protects the limb, reduces swelling, and prepares the limb for a prosthesis. As you perform the procedure, teach it to the patient.

Start by obtaining two 4" elastic bandages. Center the end of the first 4" bandage at the top of the patient's thigh. Unroll the bandage downward over the residual limb and to the back of the leg (as shown below).

Make three figure-eight turns to adequately cover the ends of the limb. As you wrap, include the roll of flesh in the groin area. Use enough pressure to ensure that the limb narrows toward the end so that it fits comfortably into the prosthesis.

Use the second 4" bandage to anchor the first bandage around the waist. For a below-the-knee amputation, use the knee to anchor the bandage in place. Secure the bandage with clips, safety pins, or adhesive tape. Check the stump bandage regularly, and rewrap it if it bunches at the end.

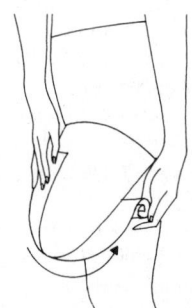
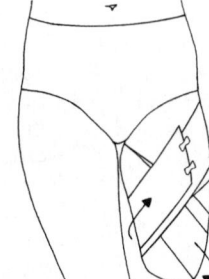
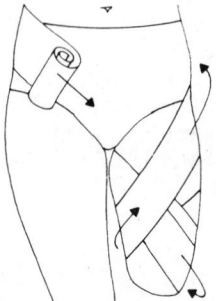

Sitz bath

● OVERVIEW

- Involves immersion of pelvic area in warm or hot water to relieve discomfort, especially after perineal or rectal surgery or childbirth
- Promotes wound healing by cleaning the perineum and anus, increasing circulation, and reducing inflammation
- Also relaxes local muscles

Contraindications
- Symptomatic hypotension

❖ EQUIPMENT

Sitz tub, portable sitz bath, or regular bathtub • bath mat • rubber mat • bath (utility) thermometer • two bath blankets • towels • patient gown • gloves, if the patient has an open lesion or has been incontinent • optional: rubber ring, footstool, overbed table, I.V. pole, wheelchair or cart, dressings

A disposable sitz bath kit is available for single-patient use.

Equipment preparation
- Wash your hands thoroughly.
- Clean and disinfect the sitz tub, portable sitz bath, or regular bathtub or obtain a disposable sitz bath kit.
- Position the bath mat next to the bathtub, sitz tub, or commode.
- If you're using a tub, place the rubber mat on its surface to prevent falls.
- Place the rubber ring on the bottom of the tub to serve as a seat for the patient, and cover the ring with a towel for comfort.

◆ **NURSING ALERT** Keeping the patient elevated improves water flow over the wound site and prevents unnecessary pressure on tender tissues.

- Fill the sitz tub or bathtub one-third to one-half full, so that the water will reach the seated patient's umbilicus.
- Use warm water (94° to 98° F [34.4° to 36.7° C]) for relaxation or wound cleaning and healing and hot water (110° to 115° F [43.3° to 46.1° C]) for heat application, measuring the water temperature using the bath thermometer.
- If you're using a commercial kit, fill the basin to the specified line with water at the prescribed temperature.
- Place the basin under the commode seat, clamp the irrigation tubing to block water flow, and fill the irrigation bag with water of the same temperature as that in the basin.
- To create flow pressure, hang the bag above the patient's head on a hook, towel rack, or I.V. pole.

❚❚■ ESSENTIAL STEPS

- Verify the physician's order and assess the patient's condition.
- Confirm the patient's identity using two patient identifiers according to facility policy.
- Explain the procedure to the patient.
- Provide privacy for the patient.

◆ **NURSING ALERT** Instruct the patient to rise slowly after a sitz bath to prevent dizziness and loss of balance.

- Put on gloves, if necessary.
- Ask the patient to void.
- Assist the patient to the bath area, provide privacy, and make sure the area is warm and free from drafts.
- Help the patient undress, as needed.
- Remove and dispose of any soiled dressings.
- If a dressing adheres to a wound, allow it to soak off in the tub.
- After instructing the patient to use the safety rail for balance, assist him into the tub or onto the commode.
- Explain that the sensation may be unpleasant initially because the wound area is tender and that this discomfort will soon be relieved by the warm water.
- If the patient's feet don't reach the floor (except with a regular bathtub) and the weight of his legs presses against the edge of the equipment, place a small stool under his feet to decrease pressure on local blood vessels.
- Place a folded towel against the patient's lower back to prevent discomfort and promote correct body alignment.
- Drape the patient's shoulders and knees with bath blankets to avoid chills that cause vasoconstriction.
- If you're using the sitz bath kit, open the clamp on the irrigation tubing to allow a stream of water to flow continuously over the wound site.
- Refill the bag with water of the correct temperature, as needed, and encourage the patient to regulate the flow himself.
- If you're using a tub, check the water temperature frequently with the bath thermometer.

- To add warm water to a tub, help the patient stand slowly and instruct him to hold the safety rail for support.
- Run warm water into the tub, check that the water temperature is correct, and help the patient sit down again.
- If necessary, stay with the patient during the bath.
- If the patient can remain alone, show him how to use the call button.
- Check the patient's color and general condition frequently.
- When the prescribed bath time has elapsed—usually 15 to 20 minutes—tell the patient to use the safety rail for balance and help him to a standing position slowly.
- If necessary, help the patient to dry himself.
- Re-dress the wound, as needed.
- Provide a clean gown and assist the patient to bed or back to his room.
- Empty, clean, and disinfect the sitz tub, bathtub, or portable sitz bath.
- Return the commercial kit to the patient's bedside for later use.

◆ SPECIAL CONSIDERATIONS

- Use a regular bathtub only if a special sitz tub, portable sitz bath, or commercial sitz bath kit is unavailable because the application of heat to the extremities causes vasodilation and draws blood away from the perineal area, reducing its effectiveness as a local treatment.
- If the patient will be sitting in a bathtub with his extremities immersed in the hot water, check his pulse before, during, and after the bath to help detect vasodilation that could make him feel faint when he stands up.

  NURSING ALERT If the patient complains of feeling weak, faint, or nauseated or shows signs of cardiovascular distress, discontinue the bath, check the patient's pulse and blood pressure, assist him back to bed using a wheelchair or cart, and notify the physician.

- Tell the patient never to touch an open wound because of the risk of infection.

Complications
- Weakness or faintness
- Irregular or accelerated pulse
- Possible wound contamination and infection

▶ PATIENT TEACHING

Be sure to cover:
- therapeutic effects of a sitz bath
- how the procedure is performed
- proper water temperature
- signs and symptoms to report immediately
- how to use the call button for assistance
- to wait for assistance after the procedure and to rise slowly
- how to perform the procedure at home.

●◆ DOCUMENTATION

- Date and time of the sitz bath
- Type of sitz bath used
- Duration of the procedure
- Temperature of the water
- Wound condition before and after treatment, including color, odor, and amount of drainage; wound care and dressing applied
- Time and name of physician notified of any complications and orders given
- Patient's response to treatment
- Patient teaching

Selected references
Kahraman, A., et al. "Perianal Burn as a Complication of Hemorrhoid Treatment Caused by Hot Water Sitz Bath," *Burns* 30(8):868-70, December 2004.

Leeds, A. "The Art of the Sitz Bath," *Midwifery Today with International Midwife* (65):25-26, Spring 2003.

Tejirian, T., and Abbas, M.A. "Sitz Bath: Where Is the Evidence? Scientific Basis of a Common Practice," *Diseases of the Colon and Rectum* 48(12):2336-40, December 2005.

Skin graft care

● OVERVIEW

- Skin graft: healthy skin taken either from the patient (autograft) or a donor (allograft) and applied to the patient's body to resurface an area damaged by burns, traumatic injury, or surgery
- Care procedures for an autograft or an allograft essentially the same, except autograft requires care for two sites: graft site and donor site
- Types of grafts: split-thickness, full-thickness, or pedicle-flap (see *Types of skin grafts*)
- Successful grafting depends on various factors: clean wound granulation with adequate vascularization, complete contact of the graft with the wound bed, aseptic technique to prevent infection, adequate graft immobilization, and skilled care
- Grafting usually occurs at completion of wound debridement; with enzymatic debridement, grafting may be performed 5 to 7 days after debridement is complete; with surgical debridement, grafting can occur same day as surgery
- Diligent care necessary for donor graft site (see *Caring for a donor graft site*)

Contraindications
- None known

❖ EQUIPMENT

Ordered analgesic • clean and sterile gloves • sterile gown • cap • mask • sterile forceps • sterile scissors • sterile scalpel • sterile 4″ × 4″ gauze pads • Xeroflo gauze • elastic gauze dressing • warm normal saline solution • moisturizing cream • topical medication (such as micronized silver sulfadiazine cream) • optional: sterile, cotton-tipped applicators

Equipment preparation
- Wash your hands thoroughly before all procedures.
- Assemble the equipment on the dressing cart.

◈ **NURSING ALERT** Depending on your facility's policy, a physician or specially trained nurse may change graft dressings.

▮▮ ESSENTIAL STEPS

- Confirm the patient's identity using two patient identifiers according to facility policy.
- Explain the procedure to the patient.
- Provide for privacy.
- Administer an analgesic, as ordered, 20 to 30 minutes before beginning the procedure; alternatively, give an I.V. analgesic immediately before the procedure.
- Put on the sterile gown and the clean mask, cap, and gloves.
- Gently lift off all outer dressings.
- Soak the middle dressings with warm saline solution and remove these carefully and slowly to avoid disturbing the graft site.
- Leave the Xeroflo intact to avoid dislodging the graft.
- Remove and discard the clean gloves, wash your hands, and put on the sterile gloves.
- Maintain asepsis throughout the rest of the procedure.
- Assess the condition of the graft and notify the physician if you see purulent drainage.
- Remove the Xeroflo with sterile forceps, soaking the Xeroflo with warm saline solution to ease removal, if necessary.
- Clean the area gently.
- Inspect an allograft for signs of rejection, such as infection and delayed healing.
- Inspect a sheet graft frequently for blebs and evacuate them carefully with a sterile scalpel, if ordered. (See *Evacuating fluid from a sheet graft.*)
- Apply topical medication if ordered.
- Place fresh Xeroflo over the site to promote wound healing and prevent infection, using sterile scissors to cut the appropriate size.
- Cover the Xeroflo with 4″ × 4″ gauze and elastic gauze dressing.
- Clean completely healed areas and apply a moisturizing cream to them to keep the skin pliable and to retard scarring.

TYPES OF SKIN GRAFTS

A burn patient may receive one or more of the graft types described below.

Split-thickness
A split-thickness graft is the type used most commonly for covering open burns. It includes the epidermis and part of the dermis and may be applied as a sheet (usually on the face or neck to preserve the cosmetic result) or as a mesh. A mesh graft has tiny slits cut in it, which allow the graft to expand up to nine times its original size. Mesh grafts prevent fluids from collecting under the graft and typically are used over extensive full-thickness burns.

Full-thickness
This graft type includes the epidermis and the entire dermis. Consequently, the graft contains hair follicles, sweat glands, and sebaceous glands, which typically aren't included in split-thickness grafts. Full-thickness grafts usually are used for small burns that cause deep wounds.

Pedicle-flap
This full-thickness graft includes not only skin and subcutaneous tissue, but also subcutaneous blood vessels to ensure a continued blood supply to the graft. Pedicle-flap grafts may be used during reconstructive surgery to cover previous defects.

◆ SPECIAL CONSIDERATIONS

- To avoid dislodging the graft, hydrotherapy is usually discontinued, as ordered, for 3 to 4 days after grafting.
- The graft dressings usually stay in place for 3 to 5 days after surgery to avoid disturbing the graft site.
- To protect the graft, avoid using a blood pressure cuff over the graft, don't tug or pull dressings during dressing changes, and keep the patient from lying on the graft.
- If the graft dislodges, apply sterile skin compresses to keep the area moist until the surgeon reapplies the graft.
- If the graft affects an arm or a leg, elevate the affected extremity to reduce postoperative edema and check for bleeding and signs of neurovascular impairment (increasing pain, numbness or tingling, coolness, and pallor).

Complications

- Graft failure from traumatic injury, hematoma or seroma formation, infection, an inadequate graft bed, rejection, or compromised nutritional status.

▶ PATIENT TEACHING

Be sure to cover:
- need for skin graft care and how it's performed
- administration of analgesics before the procedure
- signs and symptoms to report
- caring for the graft at home, including use of sunscreen with a sun protection factor of 20 or higher on all grafted areas.

●◆ DOCUMENTATION

- Time and date of all dressing changes
- Medications administered and patient's response to the medications
- Condition of the graft
- Signs of infection or rejection
- Any additional treatments given
- Patient's reaction to the graft and tolerance of procedure
- Patient teaching

Selected references

Beldon, P. "Comparison of Four Different Dresings on Donor Site Wounds," *British Journal of Nursing* 13(6 Suppl):S38-45, March 2004.

Kairinos, N. "A Short Report on the Prevention of Slippage in Donor Site Dressings," *Journal of Wound Care* 14(1):18, January 2005.

McPhee, H. "Using an Adhesive Retention Tape on Split Skin Graft Donor Areas," *Nursing Times* 101(16):57-58, April 2005.

Shaaban, H. "The Proximal Phalanx: Another Option to Harvest a Skin Graft for Skin Defects on the Fingers," *Plastic & Reconstructive Surgery* 117(6):2104-105, May 2006.

CARING FOR A DONOR GRAFT SITE

Autografts are usually taken from another area of the patient's body with a dermatome, an instrument that cuts uniform, split-thickness skin portions (typically, about 0.013 to 0.05 cm thick). Autografting makes the donor site a partial-thickness wound, which may bleed, drain, and cause pain.

This site needs scrupulous care to prevent infection, which could change the site to a full-thickness wound. Depending on the graft's thickness, tissue may be obtained from the donor site again in as few as 10 days.

Usually, Xeroflo gauze is applied postoperatively. The outer gauze dressing can be taken off on the first postoperative day; the Xeroflo will protect the new epithelial proliferation.

Care for the donor site as you care for the autograft, using dressing changes at the initial stages to prevent infection and promote healing. Follow the guidelines below.

Dressing the wound

- Wash your hands and put on sterile gloves.
- Remove the outer gauze dressings within 24 hours. Inspect the Xeroflo for signs of infection; then leave it open to the air to speed drying and healing.
- Leave small amounts of fluid accumulation alone. Using aseptic technique, aspirate larger amounts through the dressing with a small-gauge needle and syringe.
- Apply a lanolin-based cream daily to completely healed donor sites to keep skin tissue pliable and to remove crusts.

EVACUATING FLUID FROM A SHEET GRAFT

When small pockets of fluid (called blebs) accumulate beneath a sheet graft, evacuate the fluid using a sterile scalpel and sterile cotton-tipped applicators. First, carefully perforate the center of the bleb with the scalpel.

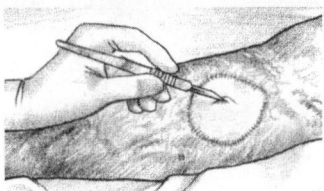

Gently express the fluid with the cotton-tipped applicators.

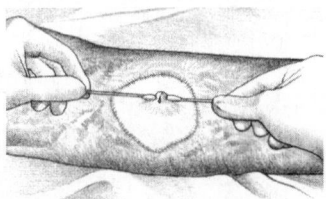

Never express fluid by rolling the bleb to the edge of the graft. This disturbs healing in other areas.

Skin staple, clip, and suture removal

⬤ OVERVIEW

- Skin staples or clips: used instead of sutures to close lacerations or surgical wounds
  - Can secure a wound more quickly than sutures
  - Used where cosmetic results aren't a prime consideration such as the abdomen
  - Distributes tension evenly along the suture line with minimal tissue trauma and compression, facilitating healing and minimizing scarring
- Aims to remove skin sutures from a healed wound without damaging newly formed tissue
- Timing dependent on the shape, size, and location of the sutured incision; absence of inflammation, drainage and infection; and the patient's general condition
- If sufficiently healed, sutures removed 7 to 10 days after insertion
- Techniques for removal dependent on the method of suturing

REMOVING A STAPLE

Position the extractor's lower jaws beneath the span of the first staple, as shown in the first illustration.

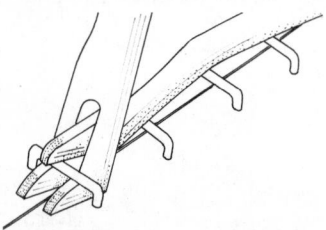

Squeeze the handles until they're completely closed; then lift the staple away from the skin, as shown in the second illustration. The extractor changes the shape of the staple and pulls the prongs out of the intradermal tissue.

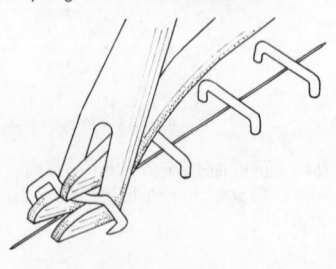

- Usually, physician removes skin staples, clips and sutures; but some facilities permit qualified nurses to remove them

Contraindications
- Insufficient wound healing

❖ EQUIPMENT

Waterproof trash bag • adjustable light • clean gloves, if needed • sterile gloves • sterile gauze pads • sterile staple or clip extractor • sterile forceps or sterile hemostat • sterile curve-tipped suture scissors • antiseptic cleaning agent • normal saline solution • sterile cotton-tipped applicators • optional: butterfly adhesive strips or Steri-Strips, compound benzoin tincture or other skin protectant

Prepackaged, sterile, disposable suture-removal kits are available.

Equipment preparation
- Wash your hands thoroughly.
- Assemble all equipment in the patient's room.
- Check the expiration date on each sterile package and inspect for tears.
- Open the waterproof trash bag, forming a cuff at the top of the bag, and place it near the patient.

▐▐▌ ESSENTIAL STEPS

- Check your policy and procedure manual to determine if your facility allows you to remove skin staples and clips.
- Check the physician's order to confirm the exact timing and details for this procedure.
- Check for patient allergies, especially to adhesive tape and povidone-iodine or other topical solutions or medications.
- Confirm the patient's identity using two patient identifiers according to facility policy.
- Explain the procedure to the patient.
- Provide for privacy and place the patient in a comfortable position that doesn't place undue tension on the incision.

- Adjust the light to shine directly on the incision.
- If the patient's wound has a dressing, put on clean gloves to remove it and discard the dressing and the gloves in the waterproof trash bag.
- Assess the patient's incision and notify the physician of gaping, drainage, inflammation, and other signs of infection.
- Establish a sterile work area with all the equipment and supplies.

STAPLE AND CLIP REMOVAL
- Open the package containing the sterile staple or clip extractor, maintaining asepsis.
- Put on sterile gloves.
- Wipe the incision gently with sterile gauze pads soaked in an antiseptic cleaning agent, or with sterile cotton-tipped applicators, to remove surface encrustations.
- Using the sterile staple or clip extractor, start at one end of the incision and remove the staples or clips. (See *Removing a staple.*)
- Hold the extractor over the trash bag, and release the handle to discard the staple or clip.
- Repeat the procedure for each staple or clip until all are removed.
- Apply a sterile gauze dressing, if needed, to prevent infection and to provide comfort and protection from rubbing.
- Discard your gloves.

SUTURE REMOVAL
- Open the sterile suture removal tray if you're using one.
- Using sterile technique, clean the suture line, which moistens the sutures to ease removal.
- Soften them further, if needed, with normal saline solution.
- Proceed according to the type of suture you're removing.
- The visible part of a suture is contaminated; cut sutures at the skin surface on one side.
- Lift and pull the visible end off the skin.
- If ordered, remove every other suture to maintain support for the incision, and then go back and remove remaining sutures.
- After suture removal, wipe the incision with gauze pads soaked in an anti-

spetic cleaning agent or with a povidone-iodine pad.
- Apply a light sterile gauze dressing, if
needed.
- Discard your gloves.
- According to the practitioner's preference, inform the patient that he may
shower in 1 or 2 days if the incision is
dry and heals well.
- Properly dispose of the solutions and
trash bags: clean or dispose of soiled
equipment and supplies.

◆ SPECIAL CONSIDERATIONS

- Carefully check the physician's order
to determine if you should remove
only alternate staples, clips or sutures
initially and leave the others in place
for an additional day or two to support the incision.
- For interrupted sutures or an incom-
pletely healed suture line, remove only
those sutures specified by the pracit-
tioner.
- Some sutures may be left in place for
1 to 2 days to support the suture line.
- If retention and regular sutures are in
place, check the practitioner's order
for the removal sequence.
- Retention sutures usually remain in
place for 14 to 21 days.
- Retention sutures give added support
to obese or slow-healing patients.
- Carefully clean the suture line before
removing mattress sutures to decrease
the risk of infection when the visible,
contaminated part of the stitch is too
small to cut twice for sterile removal
and must be pulled through the tissue.
- After removing mattress sutures,
monitor the suture line for subsequent infection.
- When removing a staple or clip, place
the extractor's jaws carefully between
the patient's skin and the staple or clip
to avoid patient discomfort.
- Apply butterfly adhesive strips or
Steri-Strips after removing staples or
clips, if appropriate, to give added
support to the incision and prevent
lateral tension from forming a wide
scar, using a small amount of compound benzoin tincture or other skin
protectant to ensure adherence.

- If extraction is difficult, notify the
physician; staples or clips placed too
deeply in the skin or left in place too
long may resist removal.
- If the wound dehisces after staples,
clips, or sutures are removed, apply
butterfly adhesive strips or Steri-Strips
to approximate and support the
edges, and call the physician immediately to repair the wound. (See *Types
of adhesive skin closures.*)

Complications
- Infection
- Dehiscence
- Scarring and keloids

▶ PATIENT TEACHING

Be sure to cover:
- how the procedure is done
- that he may feel a slight pulling or
tickling sensation during removal
- reassurance that the incision is healing
properly and removing the staples,
clips, or sutures won't weaken the incision
- guidelines for showering
- care of the incision at home
- that Steri-Strips or butterfly strips will
fall off in 3 to 5 days, commonly in
the shower, and caution not to pull
them off
- need to call the physician immediately
for signs and symptoms of infection
or dehiscence.

◆ DOCUMENTATION

- Date and time of staple or clip re-
moval
- Number of staples, clips, or sutures
removed or left in place
- Appearance of the incision
- Dressings or butterfly strips applied
- Patient's tolerance of the procedure
- Patient teaching

Selected references

Adams, B., et al. "Frequency of Use of Su-
turing and Repair Techniques Prefereed
by Dermatologic Surgeons," *Dermato-
logic Surgery* 32(5):682-89, May 2006.
Alexander, G., and Al-Rasheed, A.A. "Skin
Staple Removal by Artery Forceps: A
Hazardous Practice?" *Burns* 31(1):116,
February 2005.
Clark, A. "Understanding the Principles of
Suturing Minor Skin Lesions," *Nursing
Times* 100(2):32-34, July 2004.
Holzheimer, R.G. "Adverse Events of Su-
tures: Possible Interactions of Biomate-
rials?" *European Journal of Medical Re-
search* 10(12):521-26, December 2005.
Pullen, R. I. Jr. "Removing Sutures and
Staples," *Nursing* 33(10):18, October
2003.

TYPES OF ADHESIVE SKIN CLOSURES

Steri-Strips are used as a primary means of
keeping a wound closed after suture removal.
They're made of thin strips of sterile, nonwo-
ven, porous fabric tape.

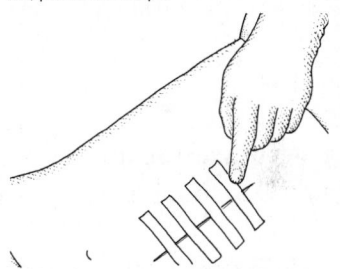

Butterfly closures consist of sterile, waterproof adhesive strips. A narrow, nonadhesive
"bridge" connects the two expanded adhesive
portions. These strips are used to close small
wounds and to assist healing after suture removal.

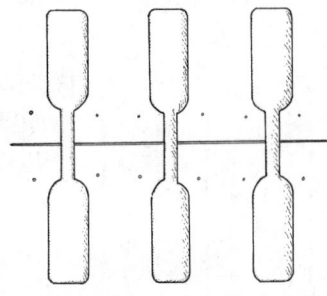

Skull tongs site care

● OVERVIEW

- Skull tongs: immobilize the cervical spine after fracture or dislocation, invasion by tumor or infection, or surgery
- Three types commonly used: Crutchfield, Gardner-Wells, and Vinke (see *Types of skull tongs*)
  - Crutchfield tongs: applied by incising the skin with a scalpel, drilling a hole in the exposed skull, and inserting the pins on the tongs into the hole
  - Gardner-Wells and Vinke tongs: applied less invasively
- Traction created by extending a rope from the center of the tongs over a pulley and attaching weights to establish reduction and maintain alignment

Contraindications
- None known

❖ EQUIPMENT

Three sterile specimen containers • one bottle each of ordered cleaning solution, normal saline solution, and povidone-iodine solution • sterile, cotton-tipped applicators • sandbags or cervical collar (hard or soft) • fine mesh gauze strips • 4″ × 4″ gauze pads • sterile gloves • sterile basin • sterile scissors • hair clippers • optional: turning frame, antibacterial ointment

Equipment preparation
- Wash your hands thoroughly.
- Bring the equipment to the patient's room.
- Place the sterile specimen containers on the bedside table and fill one with a small amount of cleaning solution, one with normal saline solution, and one with povidone-iodine solution.
- Set out the cotton-tipped applicators.
- Keep the sandbags or cervical collar handy for emergency immobilization of the head and neck in case the pins in the tongs slip.

▌▌ ESSENTIAL STEPS

- Confirm the patient's identity using two patient identifiers according to facility policy.
- Explain the procedure to the patient.
- Maintain asepsis throughout all procedures.
- Observe each pin site carefully for loose pins and signs of infection, such as swelling or redness, or purulent drainage.
- Use hair clippers to trim the patient's hair around the pin sites, when necessary, to facilitate assessment.
- Put on gloves, and gently wipe each pin site with a cotton-tipped applicator dipped in cleaning solution to loosen and remove crusty drainage, repeating with a fresh applicator, as needed, for thorough cleaning.
- Use a separate applicator for each site to avoid cross-contamination.
- Next, wipe each site with normal saline solution to remove excess cleaning solution.
- Wipe with povidone-iodine to provide asepsis at the site and prevent infection.
- Check the traction apparatus—rope, weights, and pulleys—at the start of each shift, every 4 hours, and as necessary (for example, after position changes), making sure the rope and weights hang freely.

TYPES OF SKULL TONGS

Skull (or cervical) tongs consist of a stainless steel body with a pin at the end of each arm. Each pin is about ⅛″ (0.3 cm) in diameter with a sharp tip.

On Crutchfield tongs, the pins are placed about 5″ (12.5 cm) apart in line with the long axis of the cervical spine.

On Gardner-Wells tongs, the pins are spring-loaded and inserted farther apart, slightly above the patient's ears.

On Vinke tongs, the pins are placed at the parietal bones, near the widest transverse diameter of the skull, about 1″ (2.5 cm) above the helix.

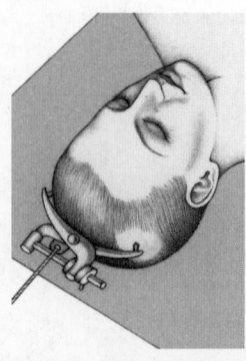 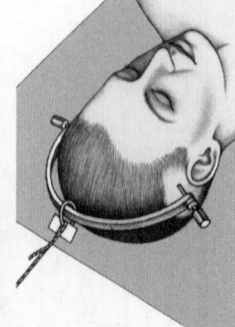 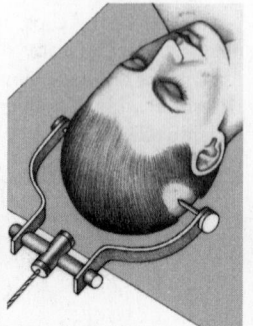

- If an antibacterial ointment is ordered for pin-site care instead of povidone-iodine solution, remove the old ointment, wrap a cotton-tipped applicator with a 4″ × 4″ gauze pad, moisten it with cleaning solution, and gently clean each site.
- If the pin sites are infected, obtain strips of fine mesh gauze, or cut a 4″ × 4″ gauze pad into strips using sterile technique. Soak the strips in a sterile basin of povidone-iodine solution or normal saline solution, as ordered, and squeeze out the excess solution. Wrap one strip securely around each pin site and leave the strip in place to dry. Removing the dried strip aids in debridement and helps clear the infection.
- Keep a box of sterile gauze pads at the patient's bedside.
- Watch for signs and symptoms of loose pins, such as persistent pain or tenderness at pin sites, redness, drainage, or patient reports of feeling or hearing the pins move.
- If you suspect a pin has loosened or slipped, don't turn the patient until the physician examines the skull tongs and fixes them as needed.
- If the pins pull out, immobilize the patient's head and neck with sandbags or apply a cervical collar. Then, carefully remove the traction weights. Apply manual traction to the patient's head by placing your hands on each side of the mandible and pulling very gently, while maintaining proper alignment. Send someone for the physician immediately. When traction is reestablished, take neurologic vital signs.

NURSING ALERT Never add weights to or subtract weights from the traction apparatus without an order from the physician because this can cause a neurologic impairment.

- Take neurologic vital signs at the beginning of each shift, every 4 hours, and after turning or transporting the patient.
- Carefully assess cranial nerve function, which may be impaired by pin placement and note any asymmetry, deviation, or atrophy.

- Review the patient's chart to determine baseline neurologic vital signs on admission to the facility and immediately after the tongs were applied.
- Monitor respirations for signs of respiratory distress, such as unequal chest expansion and an irregular or altered respiratory rate or pattern, and keep suction equipment handy.

NURSING ALERT Monitor the patient's respiratory status closely because injury to the cervical spine can affect respiration.

- If a turning frame is used to facilitate turning without disrupting vertebral alignment, establish a turning schedule to help prevent complications of immobility.
- Never remove a patient from the bed or turning frame when transporting him to another department.

Complications
- Infection
- Cranial nerve damage
- Respiratory distress

Be sure to cover:
- how skull tong site care is done
- that pin sites usually feel tender for several days after the tongs are applied
- signs and symptoms of complications, such as pain at the pin sites or hearing or feeling the pins move, and to notify the physician or nurse if they occur
- how to turn and position himself with skull tongs in place
- reassurance that the patient will be closely monitored.

- Date, time, and type of pin-site care
- Patient's response to the procedure
- Assessment of the site and characteristics of any drainage
- Addition or removal of weights
- Assessment of ropes, weights, and pulleys
- Neurologic vital signs and respiratory status
- Turning schedule
- Patient teaching

Selected references

Awasthy, N., and Chand, K. "Intracranial Bleed Complicating the Use of Crutch-field Tongs," *Journal of Neurosurgical Sciences* 50(1):13-15, March 2006.

Davis, P. "Skeletal Pin Traction: Guidelines on Postoperative Care and Support," *Nursing Times* 99(21):46-48, May-June 2003.

Holmes, S.B., et al. "Skeletal Pin Site Care: National Association of Orthopaedic Nursing," *Orthopaedic Nursing* 2492):99-107, March-April 2005.

Malomo, A.O., et al. "Conservative Management of Third Trimester Cervical Spinal Cord Injury Using Gardner-Wells Tongs Traction," *Nigerian Journal of Clinical Practice* 8(1):46-50, June 2005.

Splint application

● OVERVIEW

- Used to immobilize simple or compound fracture, dislocation, or subluxation (see *Types of splints*)
- Immobilizes injury site, alleviates pain, and allows injury to heal in proper alignment
- Minimizes possible complications, such as excessive bleeding into tissues, restricted blood flow caused by bone pressing against vessels, and possible paralysis from an unstable spinal cord injury
- In case of multiple serious injuries, allows patient to be moved without risking further damage to bones, muscles, nerves, blood vessels, and skin

Contraindications
- For rigid splints, no contraindications
- Traction splints not used for upper extremity injuries and open fractures

❖ EQUIPMENT

Rigid splint, Velcro support splint, spine board, or traction splint • bindings • padding • sandbags or rolled towels or clothing • optional: roller gauze, cloth strips, Velcro straps, sterile compress, ice bag

Several commercial splints are widely available. An inflatable semirigid splint, called an air splint, sometimes can be used to secure an injured extremity.

NURSING ALERT In an emergency, any long, sturdy object, such as a tree limb, mop handle, or broom — even a magazine — can be used to make a rigid splint for an extremity; a door can be used as a spine board. When improvising, avoid using twine or rope, if possible, because these can restrict circulation.

Equipment preparation
- Consult the manufacturer's instructions before applying a splint.

❚❚❚ ESSENTIAL STEPS

- Wash your hands thoroughly.
- Confirm the patient's identity using two patient identifiers according to facility policy.
- Explain all procedures to the patient.
- Maintain asepsis throughout all procedures.
- Wear appropriate personal protective equipment, when necessary, throughout all procedures.
- Obtain a complete history of the injury and perform a head-to-toe assessment, inspecting for obvious deformities, swelling or bleeding.
- Compare the injured extremity with the uninjured extremity.
- Ask the patient if he can move the injured extremity.
- Gently palpate the injured area; inspect for swelling, obvious deformities, bleeding, discoloration, and evidence of fracture or dislocation.
- Remove or cut away clothing from the injury site, if necessary.
- Check neurovascular integrity distal to the site.
- If an obvious bone misalignment causes the patient acute distress or severe neurovascular problems, align the extremity in its normal anatomic position, if possible, but don't continue if this causes further neurovascular deterioration.

NURSING ALERT To avoid damaging displaced vessels and nerves, don't straighten a dislocation.

- Apply sterile compresses to open wounds.

NURSING ALERT Don't reduce a contaminated bone end because this can cause gross contamination of deep tissues and additional laceration of soft tissues, vessels, and nerves.

- Choose a splint that will immobilize the joints above and below the fracture; pad the splint as necessary to protect bony prominences.

APPLYING A RIGID SPLINT
- Support the injured extremity above and below the fracture site while applying firm, gentle traction.
- Have an assistant place the splint under, beside, or on top of the extremity.
- Tell the assistant to apply the bindings to secure the splint without obstructing circulation.
- Assess the neurovascular status of the extremity and reapply the bindings, if necessary.

TYPES OF SPLINTS

Three kinds of splints are commonly used to provide support for injured or weakened limbs or to help correct deformities.

A *rigid splint* is used to immobilize a fracture or dislocation in an extremity, as shown. Ideally, two people should apply a rigid splint to an extremity.

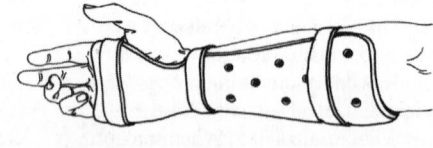

A *traction splint* immobilizes a fracture and exerts a longitudinal pull that reduces muscle spasms, pain, and arterial and neural damage. Used primarily for femoral fractures, a traction splint may also be applied for a fractured hip or tibia. Two trained people should apply a traction splint.

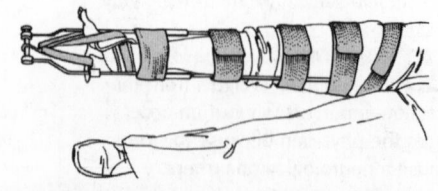

A *spine board,* applied for a suspected spinal fracture, is a rigid splint that supports the injured person's entire body. Three people should apply a spine board.

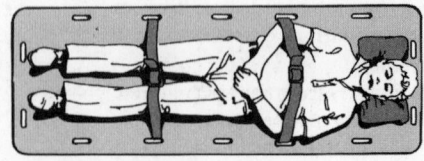

APPLYING A SPINE BOARD

- Pad the spine board (or door) carefully, especially the areas that will support the lumbar region and knees, to prevent uneven pressure and discomfort.
- If the patient is lying on his back, place one hand on each side of his head and apply gentle traction to the head and neck, keeping the head aligned with the body.
- Instruct one assistant to logroll the patient onto his side while another slides the spine board under the patient.
- Then instruct the assistants to roll the patient onto the board while you maintain traction and alignment.
- If the patient is prone, logroll him onto the board so he ends up in a supine position.
- To maintain body alignment, use strips of cloth to secure the patient on the spine board; to keep head and neck aligned, place sandbags or rolled towels or clothing on both sides of his head.

APPLYING A TRACTION SPLINT

- Specialized training is required before applying a traction splint.
- Place the splint beside the injured leg.

NURSING ALERT Never use a traction splint on an arm because the major axillary plexus of nerves and blood vessels can't tolerate countertraction.

- Adjust the splint to the correct length, and then open and adjust the Velcro straps.
- Have an assistant keep the leg motionless while you pad the ankle and foot and fasten the ankle hitch around them. (You may leave the shoe on.)
- Tell the assistant to lift and support the leg at the injury site as you apply firm, gentle traction.
- While you maintain traction, tell the assistant to slide the splint under the leg, pad the groin to avoid excessive pressure on external genitalia, and gently apply the ischial strap.
- Have the assistant connect the loops of the ankle hitch to the end of the splint.
- Adjust the splint to apply enough traction to secure the leg comfortably in the corrected position.

- After applying traction, fasten the Velcro support splints to secure the leg closely to the splint.

NURSING ALERT Don't use a traction splint for a severely angulated femur or knee fracture.

✦ SPECIAL CONSIDERATIONS

- At the scene of an accident, always examine the patient completely for other injuries and avoid unnecessary movement or manipulation, which could cause additional pain or injury.

NURSING ALERT Always consider the possibility of cervical injury in an unconscious patient.

- If possible, apply the splint before repositioning the patient.
- If a rigid splint isn't available, use another body part as a splint. If a leg splint isn't available, for example, pad between the legs and secure the injured leg to the uninjured leg with roller gauze or cloth strips.
- After applying any type of splint, monitor vital signs frequently because bleeding in fractured bones and surrounding tissues can cause shock.
- Monitor the neurovascular status of the fractured limb by assessing skin color, taking the patient's temperature, and checking for pain or numbness in the fingers or toes.

NURSING ALERT Numbness or paralysis distal to the injury may indicate pressure on nerves.

- Immediately transport the patient to a hospital and apply ice to the injury.
- Regardless of the apparent extent of the injury, don't allow the patient to eat or drink anything until the physician evaluates him.
- Apply gentle traction and remove the splint carefully, under a physician's direct supervision, if the patient shows signs of vascular impairment.

Complications
- Fat embolism
- Neurovascular compromise
- Pressure ulcers

▶ PATIENT TEACHING

Be sure to cover:
- an explanation of the procedure
- how to apply and remove the splint
- need to keep the limb elevated and to apply ice for first 24 hours
- signs of neurovascular compromise to report to the physician or nurse
- how to inspect the skin for rubbing and breakdown around splint
- use of analgesics for pain or discomfort
- dates and times of follow-up appointments.

◆ DOCUMENTATION

- Circumstances and cause of the injury
- Patient's complaints, noting whether symptoms are localized
- Neurovascular status before and after applying the splint
- Assessment of splinted area
- Type of wound and the amount and type of drainage, if any
- Level of pain on a scale of 0 to 10
- Use and effectiveness of analgesics
- Date and time of splint application
- Type of splint applied
- Date, time, and name of physician notified and orders given
- Patient teaching

Selected references
Hobman, J.W., and Southern, S.J. "Upper Limb Splints and the Right to Drive—Who Decides?" *British Journal of Plastic Surgery* 57(4):354-57, June 2004.

Miller, N.J., et al. "Improvement in the Emergency Splinting of Fractures after a Simple Educational Exercise," *ANZ Journal of Surgery* 75(9):754-56, September 2005.

Plint, A.C., et al. "A Randomized Controlled Trial of Removable Splinting versus Casting for Wrist Buckle Fractures in Children," *Pediatrics* 117(3):691-97, March 2006.

Vehmeyer-Heeman, M., et al. "Axillary Burns; Extended Grafting and Early Splinting Prevents Contractures," *Journal of Burn Care & Rehabilitation* 26(6):539-42, November-December 2005.

Sputum collection

- Sputum is secreted by mucous membranes lining bronchioles, bronchi, and trachea; helps protect the respiratory tract from infection
- When expelled from respiratory tract, sputum carries saliva, nasal and sinus secretions, dead cells, and normal oral bacteria from the respiratory tract
- Sputum specimens: may be cultured for identification of respiratory pathogens
- Usual method is expectoration; may require ultrasonic nebulization, hydration, or chest percussion and postural drainage
- Less common method, tracheal suctioning and, rarely, bronchoscopy

Contraindications

TRACHEAL SUCTIONING

- Within 1 hour of eating
- Esophageal varices
- Nausea
- Facial or basilar skull fractures
- Laryngospasm
- Bronchospasm

◆ **NURSING ALERT** Tracheal suctioning should be performed cautiously in a patient with heart disease because it can precipitate arrhythmias.

EXPECTORATION
Sterile specimen container with tight-fitting cap • gloves, if necessary • label • laboratory request form • aerosol (10% sodium chloride, propylene glycol, acetylcysteine, or sterile or distilled water), as ordered

TRACHEAL SUCTIONING
#12 to #14 French sterile suction catheter • water-soluble lubricant • laboratory request form • sterile gloves • mask • sterile in-line specimen trap (Lukens trap) • normal saline solution • portable suction machine, if wall suction is unavailable • oxygen therapy equipment
Commercial suction kits have all equipment except the suction machine and an in-line specimen container.

Equipment preparation

- Equipment and preparation depend on the method of collection.
- Wash your hands thoroughly.
- Gather the appropriate equipment for the task.

- Confirm the patient's identity using two patient identifiers according to facility policy.
- Explain the procedure to the patient.
- Wear appropriate personal protective equipment, when necessary.
- Try to collect the specimen early in the morning, before breakfast, to obtain an overnight accumulation of secretions.

COLLECTING SPUTUM BY EXPECTORATION

- Assist the patient to a sitting position; if he can't sit up, place him in a high-Fowler's position.
- Ask the patient to rinse his mouth with water to reduce specimen contamination.

◆ **NURSING ALERT** Don't allow the patient to use mouthwash or toothpaste before obtaining a sputum specimen because these may affect the mobility of organisms in the sputum sample.

- Tell him to cough deeply and expectorate at least 15 ml of sputum directly into the specimen container.
- Put on gloves.
- Cap the container and clean the exterior, if necessary.
- Remove and discard your gloves, and wash your hands thoroughly.
- Label the container with the patient's name and room number, the physician's name, date and time of collection, and initial diagnosis.
- Place the container in a leakproof bag.
- On the laboratory request form, note whether the patient was febrile or taking antibiotics, and whether sputum was induced, because such specimens commonly appear watery and may resemble saliva.
- Send the specimen to the laboratory immediately.

COLLECTING SPUTUM BY TRACHEAL SUCTIONING

- If the patient can't produce an adequate specimen by coughing, prepare to suction him to obtain the specimen.
- Explain the suctioning procedure to him and tell him that he may cough, gag, or feel short of breath during the procedure.

ATTACHING SPECIMEN TRAP TO SUCTION CATHETER

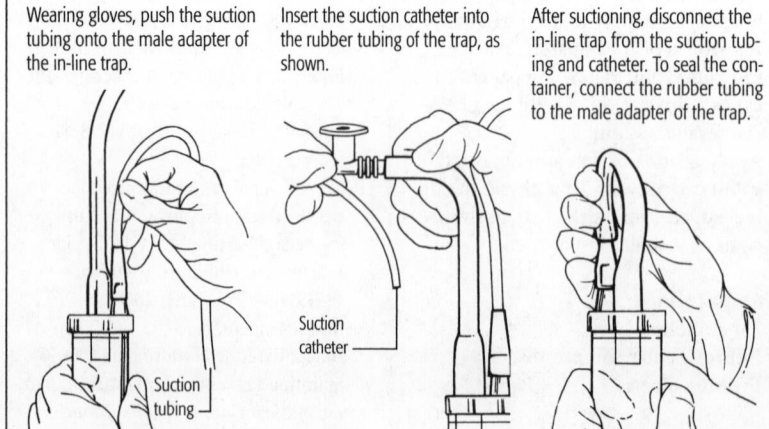

Wearing gloves, push the suction tubing onto the male adapter of the in-line trap.

Insert the suction catheter into the rubber tubing of the trap, as shown.

After suctioning, disconnect the in-line trap from the suction tubing and catheter. To seal the container, connect the rubber tubing to the male adapter of the trap.

Suction tubing

Suction catheter

- Place the patient in high Fowler's or semi-Fowler's position.
- Administer oxygen to the patient before suctioning.
- Wear a mask, gown, and goggles to avoid exposure to pathogens.
- Put on sterile gloves.
- Consider your dominant hand sterile and your nondominant hand clean to prevent cross-contamination.
- Connect the suction tubing to the male adapter of the in-line specimen trap.
- Attach the sterile suction catheter to the rubber tubing of the trap. (See *Attaching specimen trap to suction catheter.*)
- Tell the patient to tilt his head back slightly.
- Lubricate the catheter with normal saline solution, and gently pass it through the patient's nostril without suction.
- When the patient coughs as the catheter reaches the larynx, quickly advance the catheter into the trachea.
- Tell him to take several deep breaths through his mouth to ease insertion.
- To obtain the specimen, apply suction for 5 to 10 seconds.

NURSING ALERT Never suction for longer than 15 seconds because prolonged suction can cause hypoxia.

- If the suctioning must be repeated, let the patient rest for four to six breaths.
- When collection is completed, discontinue the suction, gently remove the catheter, and administer oxygen.
- Detach the catheter from the in-line trap, gather it up in your dominant hand, and pull the glove cuff inside out and down around the used catheter to enclose it for disposal.
- Remove and discard the other glove and your mask, goggles, and gown.
- Detach the trap from the tubing connected to the suction machine.
- Seal the trap tightly by connecting the rubber tubing to the male adapter of the trap.
- Label the trap's container as an expectorated specimen, and send it to the laboratory immediately, in a leakproof bag, with a completed laboratory request form.
- Offer the patient a glass of water or mouthwash.

◆ SPECIAL CONSIDERATIONS

- If you can't obtain a sputum specimen through tracheal suctioning, perform chest percussion to loosen and mobilize secretions, position the patient for optimal drainage, and repeat tracheal suctioning in 20 to 30 minutes.
- Before sending the specimen to the laboratory, examine it to make sure it's actually sputum, not saliva, because saliva will produce inaccurate test results.
- Because expectorated sputum is contaminated by normal mouth flora, tracheal suctioning provides a more reliable specimen for diagnosis.

NURSING ALERT If the patient becomes hypoxic or cyanotic during suctioning, remove the catheter immediately and administer oxygen.

- If the patient has asthma or chronic bronchitis, watch for aggravated bronchospasms with the use of more than a 10% concentration of sodium chloride or acetylcysteine in an aerosol.
- If the patient is suspected of having tuberculosis, don't use more than 20% propylene glycol with water when inducing a sputum specimen because a higher concentration inhibits growth of the pathogen and causes erroneous test results. If propylene glycol isn't available, use 10% to 20% acetylcysteine with water or sodium chloride.

Complications
- Arrhythmias
- Tracheal trauma or bleeding
- Vomiting
- Aspiration
- Hypoxemia

▶ PATIENT TEACHING

Be sure to cover:
- how to cough deeply and expectorate into the specimen container
- need to rinse the mouth before obtaining the specimen
- importance of obtaining the specimen immediately after awakening
- suctioning procedure (if the patient is unable to expectorate a specimen)
- test results and implications.

●✦ DOCUMENTATION

- Date and time of sputum collection
- Collection method
- Color and consistency of the specimen
- Time specimen sent to the laboratory
- Patient's tolerance of the procedure

Selected references
Elkins, M.R., et al. "Effect of Airway Clearance Techniques on the Efficacy of the Sputum Induction Procedure," *European Respiratory Journal* 26(5):904-908, November 2005.
Ko, D.S., et al. "Clinical Implication of Atypical Cells from Sputum in Patients without Lung Cancer," *Respirology* 11(4):362-66, July 2006.
Lumb, R., et al. "An Alternative Method for Sputum Storage and Transport for Mycobacterium Tuberculosis Drug Resistance Surveys," *International Journal of Tuberculosis and Lung Disease* 10(2):172-77, February 2006.

Thoracic drainage

● OVERVIEW

- Uses gravity and, in some cases, suction to restore negative pressure and remove material that collects in the pleural cavity
- Removes accumulated air, fluids (blood, pus, chyle, and serous fluids), or solids (blood clots) from pleural cavity; restores negative pressure in pleural cavity; reexpands partially or totally collapsed lung
- May be performed with disposable drainage system: includes drainage collection, water seal, and suction control in one unit (see *Disposable drainage systems*)
- Underwater seal in drainage system allows air and fluid to escape from the pleural cavity but doesn't allow air to reenter

Contraindications
- None known

❖ EQUIPMENT

Thoracic drainage system such as Pleur-evac, which can function as gravity draining systems or be connected to

---

DISPOSABLE DRAINAGE SYSTEMS

Commercially prepared disposable systems combine drainage collection, water seal, and suction control in one unit, as depicted here. These systems ensure patient safety with positive- and negative-pressure relief valves and have a prominent air-leak indicator. Some systems produce no bubbling sound.

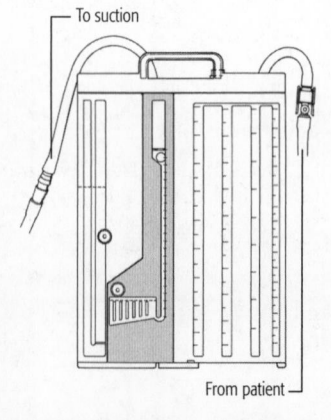

To suction

From patient

---

suction to enhance chest drainage ● sterile distilled water ● adhesive tape ● sterile clear plastic tubing ● bottle or system rack ● two rubber-tipped Kelly clamps ● sterile 50-ml catheter-tip syringe ● suction source, if ordered ● rubber band or safety pin

Equipment preparation
- Check the physician's order to determine the type of drainage system to be used and specific procedures.
- Collect the appropriate equipment, and take it to the patient's bedside.

▌▌ ESSENTIAL STEPS

- Confirm the patient's identity using two patient identifiers according to facility policy.
- Explain the procedure to the patient.
- Wash your hands thoroughly.
- Maintain sterile technique throughout all procedures.
- Wear appropriate personal protective equipment, when necessary, throughout all procedures.

SETTING UP DISPOSABLE SYSTEM
- Open the packaged system and place it on the floor in the rack supplied or hang it from the side of the patient's bed.
- Remove the plastic connector from the short tube attached to the water-seal chamber.
- Using a 50-ml catheter-tip syringe, instill sterile distilled water into the water-seal chamber until it reaches the 2-cm mark or the mark specified by the manufacturer and replace the plastic connector.
- If suction is ordered, remove the cap on the suction-control chamber to open the vent and instill sterile distilled water until it reaches the 20-cm mark or the ordered level, and recap the suction-control chamber.
- Using the long tube, connect the patient's chest tube to the closed drainage collection chamber and secure the connection with tape.
- Connect the short tube on the drainage system to the suction source and turn on the suction.

- Observe for gentle bubbling in the suction chamber, indicating the correct suction level.

MANAGING CLOSED CHEST UNDERWATER SEAL DRAINAGE
- Note the character, consistency, and amount of drainage in the drainage collection chamber.
- Mark the drainage level in the drainage collection chamber every 8 hours (or more often if there's a large amount of drainage).
- Check the water level in the water-seal chamber every 8 hours and add sterile distilled water, if necessary, until the level reaches the 2-cm mark.
- Check for fluctuation of 2″ to 4″ (5 to 10 cm) in the water-seal chamber as the patient breathes, reflecting pressure changes in the pleural space during respiration.
- To check for fluctuation when using a suction system, momentarily disconnect the suction system so the air vent is open, and observe for fluctuation.
- Check for intermittent bubbling in the water-seal chamber that occurs when the system is removing air from the pleural cavity; an absence of bubbling indicates that the pleural space has sealed.

  🔆 **NURSING ALERT** Vigorous bubbling isn't readily apparent in the water-seal chamber during quiet breathing, have the patient take a deep breath or cough.

- Check the water level in the suction-control chamber while the suction source is detached, and add sterile distilled water when the bubbling ceases, if necessary, to bring the level to the 20-cm line or as ordered.
- Check for gentle bubbling in the suction control chamber, indicating that the proper suction level has been reached.

  🔆 **NURSING ALERT** Vigorous bubbling in the suction control chamber increases the rate of water evaporation. Periodically check to make sure the air vent in the system isn't occluded to prevent a buildup of pressure in the system, which could cause a tension pneumothorax.

- Coil the tubing and secure it to the edge of the bed with a rubber band or tape and a safety pin.

- Avoid creating loops, kinks, or pressure on the tubing.
- Avoid lifting the drainage system above the patient's chest because fluid could flow back into the pleural space.
- Keep two rubber-tipped clamps at the bedside to clamp the chest tube if the system cracks or to locate an air leak in the system.
- Encourage the patient to cough frequently and breathe deeply to help drain the pleural space and expand the lungs.
- Instruct the patient to sit upright for optimal lung expansion and to splint the insertion site while coughing to minimize pain.
- Check the rate and quality of respirations and auscultate the patient's lungs periodically to assess air exchange in the affected lung.

◆ **NURSING ALERT** Diminished or absent breath sounds may indicate that the lung hasn't reexpanded.

- Notify the physician immediately if the patient develops cyanosis, rapid or shallow breathing, subcutaneous emphysema, chest pain, or excessive bleeding.
- Check the chest tube dressing at least every 8 hours and change it if necessary, or according to policy.
- Palpate the skin surrounding the chest tube for crepitus or subcutaneous emphysema, indicating that air is leaking into the subcutaneous tissue surrounding the insertion site.
- Encourage active or passive range-of-motion (ROM) exercises for the arm on the affected side if the patient has been splinting the arm to reduce discomfort.
- Give ordered pain medication as needed for comfort and to help with deep breathing, coughing, and ROM exercises.
- To maintain the water seal, remind an ambulatory patient to keep the drainage system below chest level and be careful not to disconnect the tubing.
- With a suction system, remind the patient that he must stay within range of the length of tubing attached to a wall outlet or portable pump.

◆ SPECIAL CONSIDERATIONS

- If there's excessive continuous bubbling in the water-seal chamber, look for a leak in the drainage system by clamping the tube momentarily at various points, starting at the tube's proximal end and working toward the drainage system. The bubbling stops when a clamp is placed between the air leak and the water seal. If you clamp along the tube's entire length and the bubbling doesn't stop, the drainage unit may be cracked and needs replacement.
- If the drainage collection chamber fills, double-clamp the tube close to the insertion site, exchange the system, remove the clamps, and retape the connection.

◆ **NURSING ALERT** Never leave the tubes clamped for more than 1 minute to prevent a tension pneumothorax, which can occur when clamping stops air and fluid from escaping.

- If the system cracks, clamp the chest tube momentarily with the two rubber-tipped clamps placed close to each other, in opposite directions, near the insertion site, and quickly replace the system.

◆ **NURSING ALERT** Make sure that an extra drainage collection system is readily available.

◆ **NURSING ALERT** Never clamp a chest tube except momentarily when changing the chest tube system. Assess for location of air leaks as well as patient's tolerance of chest tube removal.

◆ **NURSING ALERT** If you must clamp a chest tube, even for a brief period, closely observe the patient for altered respirations while the tube is clamped.

- Instead of clamping the tube, you may submerge the distal end of the tube in a container of sterile normal saline solution to create a temporary water seal while you replace the drainage system; check your facility's policy for the proper procedure.

Complications
- Tension pneumothorax
- Infection

▶ PATIENT TEACHING

Be sure to cover:
- what to expect during thoracic drainage care
- why the patient must not lie on, pull on, or disconnect the tubing or touch the equipment
- importance of immediately reporting breathing difficulties
- coughing and deep breathing exercises
- keeping the drainage system below chest level
- how to perform ROM exercises.

●◆ DOCUMENTATION

- Date and time thoracic drainage began
- Type of system used
- Amount of suction applied to the pleural cavity
- Presence or absence of bubbling or fluctuation in the water-seal chamber
- Initial amount, color, consistency, and type of drainage
- Patient's respiratory status
- Site care and dressing changes
- Pulmonary hygiene performed and results
- Patient's level of pain and comfort measures performed
- Complications and nursing actions taken
- Presence and extent of subcutaneous emphysema
- Patient teaching

Selected references
Bruce, F.A., et al. "Chest Drain Removal Pain and Its Management: A Literature Review," *Journal of Clinical Nursing* 15(2):145-54, February 2006.
Carroll, P. "Keeping Up with Mobile Chest Drains," *RN* 68(10):26-31, October 2005.
Roman, M., and Mercado, D. "Review of Chest Tube Use," *Medsurg Nursing* 15(1):41-43, February 2006.

Total parenteral nutrition

OVERVIEW

- Any nutrient solution, including lipids, given through a central venous (CV) line; solution usually contains protein, carbohydrates, electrolytes, vitamins, and trace minerals; lipid emulsion provides necessary fat
- Most total parenteral nutrition (TPN) solutions six times more concentrated than blood and must be delivered through a central venous catheter (CVC) into the superior vena cava
- Peripheral parenteral nutrition (PPN): administered through a peripheral or CV line to supply full caloric needs, or to surpass the patient's caloric requirements; PPN contains 10% or less dextrose to prevent vein sclerosis
- Indicated when a patient can't absorb nutrients (orally or enterally) through GI tract for more than 10 days due to debilitating illness lasting longer than 2 weeks, loss of 10% or more of preillness weight, serum albumin level less than 35 g/dl, renal or hepatic failure, nonfunctioning GI tract for 5 to 7 days in a severely catabolic patient, or excessive nitrogen loss from wound infection, fistulas, or abscesses
- May be indicated in the following conditions: inflammatory bowel disease, radiation enteritis, severe diarrhea, intractable vomiting, moderate to severe pancreatitis, massive small-bowel resection, bone marrow transplantation, high-dose chemotherapy or radiation therapy
- Promotes growth and development in infants with congenital or acquired disorders, such as tracheoesophageal fistula, gastroschisis, duodenal atresia, cystic fibrosis, meconium ileus, diaphragmatic hernia, volvulus, malrotation of the gut, and annular pancreas
- Type of parenteral solution prescribed depends on metabolic needs and the administration route

Contraindications

- Normally functioning GI tract
- Normal function that's expected to resume within 10 days

EQUIPMENT

Bag or bottle of prescribed parenteral nutrition solution • sterile I.V. tubing with attached extension tubing • 0.22-micron filter (or 1.2-micron filter if solution contains lipids or albumin) • infusion pump • reflux valve • alcohol pads • electronic infusion pump • portable glucose monitor • scale • intake and output record • sterile gloves • optional: mask

Equipment preparation

- Wash your hands thoroughly.
- Remove the solution from the refrigerator at least 1 hour before use to avoid pain, hypothermia, venous spasm or constriction.
- Check the solution against the physician's order for correct patient name and formula components.
- Confirm the expiration date.
- Observe the container for cracks and the solution for cloudiness, turbidity, and particles.
- If administering a total nutrient admixture, look for a brown layer on the solution indicating that the lipid emulsion has "cracked," or separated from the solution and return this solution to the pharmacy.
- Confirm the patient's identity using two patient identifiers according to facility policy.
- Explain the procedure to the patient and his family.
- Check the name on the solution container against the name on the patient's wristband.
- Put on gloves and maintain asepsis throughout all procedures.
- Connect the pump tubing, the micron filter with attached extension tubing, and the reflux valve.
- Tape all connections to prevent accidental separation.

> **NURSING ALERT** Accidental separation of tubing connections could result in air embolism, exsanguination, and sepsis.

- Squeeze the I.V. drip chamber and, holding the drip chamber upright, insert the tubing spike into the I.V. bag or bottle, then release the drip chamber.
- Prime the tubing.

- Gently tap the Y-ports to dislodge air bubbles.
- Record the date and time you hung the fluid, and initial the parenteral nutrition solution container.
- Attach the setup to the infusion pump according to the manufacturer's instructions.
- Remove and discard your gloves.
- Flush the catheter according to your facility's policy.

ESSENTIAL STEPS

- To attach the solution to a CV line, clamp the CV line before disconnecting it to prevent air from entering the catheter.

> **NURSING ALERT** To increase intrathoracic pressure and prevent air embolism if a clamp isn't available, ask the patient to perform Valsalva's maneuver just as you change the tubing or, if the patient is being mechanically ventilated, change the I.V. tubing immediately after the machine delivers a breath at peak inspiration.

- Attach the tubing to the designated luer-locking port and remove the clamp.
- Set the infusion pump at the ordered flow rate, and start the infusion.
- Tag the tubing with the date and time of change.

STARTING THE INFUSION

- Because parenteral nutrition often contains a large amount of glucose, start the infusion slowly, if indicated, to allow the patient's pancreatic beta cells time to increase their output of insulin.

> **NURSING ALERT** Administer all TPN with dextrose concentrations greater than 10% through a central line. TPN with concentrations of dextrose between 5% and 10% may be administered through a peripheral I.V. access.

- Initiate therapy at a rate of 40 to 50 ml/hour, as ordered, and increase it by 25 ml/hour every 6 hours (as tolerated) until the desired infusion rate is achieved.
- When the glucose concentration is low, as in most PPN formulas, initiate the rate necessary to infuse the com-

plete 24-hour volume and discontinue the solution without tapering.

CHANGING SOLUTIONS AND TUBING

- Prepare the new solution and I.V. tubing as described earlier. Put on gloves.
- Remove the protective caps from the solution containers; wipe the tops of the containers with alcohol pads; turn off the infusion pump and close the flow clamps.
- Using strict aseptic techniques, remove the spike from the solution container that's hanging and insert it into the new container.
- Hang the new container and tubing alongside the old.
- If attaching the solution to a peripheral line, examine the skin above the insertion site for redness and warmth and assess for pain.

NURSING ALERT If you suspect phlebitis, remove the existing I.V. line and start a line in a different vein. Insert a new line if the I.V. catheter has been in place for 72 hours or more to reduce risk of phlebitis and infiltration.

- Turn off the infusion pump and close the flow clamps.
- Disconnect the tubing from the catheter hub, and connect the new tubing.
- Open the flow clamp on the new container to a moderately slow rate.
- Remove the old tubing from the infusion pump, and insert the new tubing.
- Turn on the infusion pump, set the flow rate, and open the flow clamp completely.
- Remove the old equipment.

◆ SPECIAL CONSIDERATIONS

- Infuse a parenteral nutrition solution at a constant rate without interruption to avoid blood glucose fluctuations.
- Monitor the patient's vital signs every 4 hours or more often if necessary.

NURSING ALERT An increased temperature may be an early sign of catheter-related sepsis.

- Check the patient's blood glucose level every 6 hours to determine the need for supplemental insulin, which the pharmacist may add directly to the solution.
- Record daily intake and output.

- Monitor the results of laboratory tests, such as serum electrolyte, calcium, blood urea nitrogen, creatinine, and blood glucose levels, at least three times weekly; serum magnesium and phosphorus levels, twice weekly; liver function studies, complete blood count and differential, and serum albumin and transferrin levels, weekly; and urine nitrogen balance and creatinine-height index studies, weekly.
- Report abnormal laboratory results to the physician.
- Measure arm circumference and skinfold thickness over the triceps.
- Weigh the patient at the same time each morning and report a weight gain of more than 1 lb (0.5 kg) daily.
- Change the dressing over the catheter according to your facility's policy or whenever the dressing becomes wet, soiled, or nonocclusive using strict sterile technique.
- When performing dressing changes, watch for signs of phlebitis and catheter retraction from the vein and measure the catheter length from insertion site to the hub for verification.
- Change the tubing and filters every 24 hours or according to facility policy.
- Closely monitor the catheter site for swelling, which indicates infiltration.

NURSING ALERT Extravasation of parenteral nutrition solution can lead to tissue necrosis.

- Use caution when using the parenteral nutrition line for other functions.
- Don't use a single-lumen CVC to infuse blood or blood products, give a bolus injection, administer simultaneous I.V. solutions, measure CV pressure, or draw blood.
- Provide regular mouth care and emotional support.

Complications

- Catheter-related sepsis
- Thrombosis
- Phlebitis
- Air embolism
- Tissue necrosis and sloughing
- Hyperglycemia
- Fluid overload

▶ PATIENT TEACHING

Be sure to cover:
- why the patient needs TPN
- how the procedure is performed
- adverse reactions and complications
- managing TPN equipment and site care at home
- mouth care
- need to remain physically active
- how to obtain psychosocial support.

●◆ DOCUMENTATION

- Date and time of all care
- Type and location of the CVC
- Bag number, volume, and rate of the solution infused
- Site care, including description of the insertion site, cleaning of the site, and the type of dressing applied
- Filter, tubing, and solution changes
- Name of physician notified of complication, orders given, and your nursing interventions
- Blood glucose level
- Patient tolerance and teaching and psychosocial support given

Selected references

Driscoll, D.F. "Stability and Compatibility Assessment Techniques for Total Parenteral Nutrition Admixtures: Setting the Bar According to Pharmacopeial Standards," *Current Opinion in Clinical Nutrition & Metabolic Care* 8(3):297-303, May 2005.

Hamilton, H. "Complications Associated with Venous Access Devices: Part One," *Nursing Standard* 20(26):43-50, March 2006.

Muhlebach, S. "Practical Aspects of Multichamber Bags for Total Parenteral Nutrition," *Current Opinion in Clinical Nutrition & Metabolic Care* 8(3):291-95, May 2005.

Tracheal suctioning

● OVERVIEW

- Removes secretions from the trachea or bronchi using a catheter inserted through the mouth or nose, tracheal stoma, a tracheostomy tube, or an endotracheal (ET) tube
- Also performed to stimulate the cough reflex
- Maintains a patent airway to promote exchange of oxygen and carbon dioxide and to prevent pneumonia that results from pooling of secretions
- Performed as often as patient's condition warrants
- Requires strict sterile technique

Contraindications
- Deviated septum
- Nasal obstruction and trauma
- Epistaxis
- Mucosal swelling

❖ EQUIPMENT

Oxygen source (wall or portable unit, and self-inflating ventilation bag with a mask, 15-mm adapter, or a positive end-expiratory pressure [PEEP] valve, if indicated) • wall or portable suction apparatus • collection container • connecting tube • suction catheter kit, or a sterile suction catheter, one sterile glove, one clean glove, and a disposable sterile solution container • 1-L bottle of sterile water or normal saline solution • sterile water-soluble lubricant (for nasal insertion) • syringe for deflating cuff of ET or tracheostomy tube • waterproof trash bag • optional: sterile towel

Equipment preparation
- Wash hands thoroughly.
- Choose a suction catheter with a diameter no larger than one-half the inside diameter of the tracheostomy or ET tube to minimize hypoxia.
- Place the suction apparatus on the patient's overbed table or bedside stand.
- Attach the collection container to the suction unit and the connecting tube to the collection container.
- Set the suction pressure according to facility policy.

- Label and date the normal saline solution or sterile water.
- Open the waterproof trash bag.

▌▌ ESSENTIAL STEPS

- Before suctioning, determine whether your facility requires a physician's order.
- Confirm the patient's identity using two patient identifiers according to facility policy.
- Explain the procedure.
- Continue to reassure the patient throughout the procedure to minimize anxiety, and promote relaxation.
- Maintain asepsis and wear appropriate personal protective equipment, when necessary, throughout all procedures.
- Assess the patient's vital signs, breath sounds, and general appearance to establish a baseline for comparison after suctioning.
- Review the patient's arterial blood gas values and oxygen saturation levels.
- Instruct the patient to cough and deep-breathe to help move secretions up the tracheobronchial tree.
- Place the patient in semi-Fowler's or high Fowler's position to promote lung expansion and productive coughing, unless contraindicated.
- Remove the top from the normal saline solution or water bottle.
- Open the package containing the sterile solution container.
- Open the suction catheter kit, and put on the gloves.
- If using individual supplies, open the suction catheter and the gloves, placing the nonsterile glove on your nondominant hand and the sterile glove on your dominant hand.
- Using your nondominant (nonsterile) hand, pour the normal saline solution or sterile water into the solution container.
- Place a small amount of water-soluble lubricant on the sterile area.
- Place a sterile towel over the patient's chest.
- Using your dominant (sterile) hand, remove the catheter from its wrapper, keeping it coiled so it can't touch a nonsterile object.

- With your other hand, attach the catheter to the connecting tubing.

  ◆ **NURSING ALERT** Suctioning at pressures greater than 80 to 120 mm Hg doesn't enhance secretion removal.
- Occlude the suction port to assess suction pressure.
- Dip the catheter tip in the saline solution and suction a small amount of solution through the catheter, lubricating the inside of the catheter to facilitate passage of secretions and the outside of the catheter to reduce tissue trauma during insertion.
- For nasal insertion, lubricate the tip of the catheter with the sterile, water-soluble lubricant to reduce tissue trauma during insertion.
- Without removing any supplemental oxygen, instruct the patient to take three to six deep breaths to minimize hypoxia during suctioning.
- If the patient is being mechanically ventilated, preoxygenate him with three to six breaths using either a self-inflating ventilation bag (with oxygen set at 15 L/minute) or the sigh mode on the ventilator, adjusting FIO_2 and tidal volume.
- If the patient is being maintained on PEEP, use a self-inflating ventilation bag with a PEEP valve.

NASOTRACHEAL INSERTION FOR NONINTUBATED PATIENT
- Disconnect the oxygen from the patient, if applicable.
- Using your nondominant hand, raise the tip of the patient's nose to straighten the passageway and facilitate insertion of the catheter.
- Insert the catheter into the patient's nostril while gently rolling it between your fingers to help it advance through the turbinates.
- As the patient inhales, quickly advance the catheter as far as possible, without applying suction.
- If the patient coughs as the catheter passes through the larynx, briefly hold the catheter still and then resume advancement when the patient inhales.

NASOTRACHEAL INSERTION FOR INTUBATED PATIENT
- If you're using a closed system, follow the manufacturer's directions.
- Using your nonsterile hand, disconnect the patient from the ventilator.

- Using your sterile hand, insert the suction catheter into the artificial airway.
- Advance the catheter, without applying suction, until you meet resistance.
- If the patient coughs, pause briefly and then resume advancement.

SUCTIONING THE PATIENT

- After inserting the catheter, apply suction intermittently by removing and replacing the thumb of your nondominant hand over the control valve.
- Simultaneously use your dominant hand to withdraw the catheter as you roll it between your thumb and forefinger to prevent the catheter from pulling tissue into the tube as it exits.

◈ **NURSING ALERT** To prevent hypoxia, never suction for more than 10 seconds at a time.

- If the patient is intubated, use your nondominant hand to stabilize the tip of the ET tube as you withdraw the catheter, to prevent mucous membrane irritation or accidental extubation.
- If applicable, reconnect the source of oxygen or ventilation, and hyperoxygenate the patient's lungs before continuing, to prevent or relieve hypoxia.
- Allow the patient to rest for a few minutes before the next suctioning.
- Encourage the patient to cough between suctioning attempts.
- If secretions are thick, clear the catheter by dipping the tip in the saline solution and applying suction.
- Observe the characteristics of the secretions; sputum is watery and sticky.
- If the patient's heart rate and rhythm are being monitored, stop suctioning and ventilate the patient if arrhythmias occur.

AFTER SUCTIONING

- After suctioning, hyperoxygenate the patient on a mechanical ventilator with the self-inflating ventilation bag or the ventilator's sigh mode.
- Readjust the FIO_2 and, for ventilated patients, the tidal volume to the ordered settings.
- After suctioning the lower airway, assess the patient's need for upper airway suctioning.
- If the cuff of the ET or tracheostomy tube is inflated, suction the upper airway before deflating the cuff with a syringe.

- Always change the catheter and sterile glove before resuctioning the lower airway to avoid introducing microorganisms into the lower airway.
- Clear the connecting tubing by aspirating the remaining saline solution or water.
- Discard the gloves and the catheter in the waterproof trash bag.
- Discard and replace suction equipment and supplies according to your facility's policy.
- Wash your hands.
- Auscultate the lungs bilaterally and take vital signs.

◆ SPECIAL CONSIDERATIONS

- Have an assistant raise the patient's nose into the sniffing position to align the larynx and pharynx and facilitate passing the catheter during nasotracheal suctioning.
- If the patient is responsive, ask him to stick out his tongue so he won't swallow the catheter during insertion.
- Because of tracheobronchial anatomy, the suction catheter tends to enter the right mainstem bronchi instead of the left. Using an angled catheter may help you guide the catheter into the left mainstream bronchus.

◈ **NURSING ALERT** Studies have shown that the instillation of normal saline before suctioning has an adverse effect on oxygen saturation and increases the risk of pulmonary infection, especially in intubated patients.

- Observe sputum characteristics; white or translucent color is normal; yellow indicates pus; green indicates retained secretions or *Pseudomonas* infection; brown indicates old blood; red indicates fresh blood; and "red currant jelly" indicates *Klebsiella* infection.
- Don't allow the collection container on the suction machine to become more than three-quarters full.

Complications

- Hypoxemia or hypoxia
- Dyspnea
- Cardiac arrhythmias
- Tracheal or bronchial trauma
- Nasopharyngeal bleeding
- Hypertension or hypotension

- Laryngospasm
- Bronchospasm
- Nosocomial infection
- Increased intracranial pressure (in patients who already have increased ICP)

▶ PATIENT TEACHING

Be sure to cover:
- what to expect during suctioning
- warning that transient coughing or gagging can occur
- deep-breathing exercises
- importance of fluid intake.

●◇ DOCUMENTATION

- Date and time of suctioning
- Technique used
- Reason for suctioning
- Amount, color, consistency, and odor (if any) of the secretions
- Any complications and the nursing action taken
- Patient's tolerance of the procedure
- Patient teaching

Selected references

Bourgault, A.M., et al. "Effects of Endotracheal Tube Suctioning on Arterial Oxygen Tension and Heart Rate Variability," *Biological Research for Nursing* 7(4):268-78, April 2006.

Pruitt, B., and Jacobs, M. "Clearing Away Pulmonary Secretions," *Nursing* 359(7):36-41, July 2005.

Tracheostomy care

- Ensures airway patency by keeping the tracheostomy tube free of mucus buildup, maintains mucous membrane and skin integrity, prevents infection, and provides psychological support
- Performed using sterile technique until stoma has healed to prevent infection; after stoma has healed, clean gloves may be used
- Three types of tracheostomy tube: uncuffed, cuffed, or fenestrated; use depends on patient's condition and physician's preference
  - Uncuffed tube: made of plastic or metal, allows air to flow freely around tracheostomy tube and through the larynx, reducing risk of tracheal damage
  - Cuffed tube: made of plastic, is disposable, and doesn't require periodic deflating to lower pressure because cuff pressure is low and evenly distributed against the tracheal wall, reducing the risk of tracheal damage
  - Plastic fenestrated tube: permits speech through the upper airway when the external opening is capped and the cuff is deflated and allows easy removal of the inner cannula for cleaning

Contraindications
- None known

ASEPTIC STOMA AND OUTER-CANNULA CARE
Waterproof trash bag • two sterile solution containers • normal saline solution • hydrogen peroxide • sterile cotton-tipped applicators • sterile 4″ × 4″ gauze pads • sterile gloves • prepackaged sterile tracheostomy dressing (or 4″ × 4″ gauze pad) • equipment and supplies for suctioning and for mouth care • water-soluble lubricant or topical antibiotic cream • materials as needed for cuff procedures and for changing tracheostomy ties (see below)

ASEPTIC INNER-CANNULA CARE
All of the preceding equipment plus a prepackaged commercial tracheostomy care set, or sterile forceps • sterile nylon brush • sterile 6″ (15-cm) pipe cleaners • clean gloves • a third sterile solution container • disposable temporary inner cannula (for a patient on a ventilator)

CHANGING TRACHEOSTOMY TIES
30″ (76-cm) length of tracheostomy twill tape • bandage scissors • sterile gloves • hemostat

EMERGENCY TRACHEOSTOMY TUBE REPLACEMENT
Sterile tracheal dilator or sterile hemostat • sterile obturator that fits the tracheostomy tube in use • extra sterile tracheostomy tube and obturator in appropriate size • suction equipment and supplies

CUFF PROCEDURES
5- or 10-ml syringe • padded hemostat • stethoscope

Equipment preparation
- Wash your hands thoroughly before all procedures.
- Maintain asepsis throughout all procedures.
- Assemble all equipment and supplies in the patient's room.
- Keep these supplies in full view in the patient's room at all times for easy access in case of emergency.
- Check the expiration date on each sterile package and inspect the package for tears.
- Open the waterproof trash bag, and place it nearby.

NURSING ALERT Tape an emergency sterile tracheostomy tube in a sterile wrapper to the head of the bed for easy access in an emergency.

- Establish a sterile field near the patient's bed, and place equipment and supplies on it.
- Pour normal saline solution, hydrogen peroxide, or a mixture of equal parts of both solutions into one of the sterile solution containers.
- Pour normal saline solution into the second sterile container for rinsing.
- For inner-cannula care, use a third sterile solution container to hold the gauze pads and cotton-tipped applicators saturated with cleaning solution.
- If you'll be replacing the disposable inner cannula, open the package containing the new inner cannula.
- Obtain or prepare new tracheostomy ties, if indicated.

- Confirm the patient's identity using two patient identifiers according to facility policy.
- Explain the procedure, even if the patient is unresponsive, and assess patient's condition.
- Provide for privacy.
- Wear appropriate personal protective equipment, when necessary, throughout all procedures.
- Place the patient in semi-Fowler's position to promote lung expansion.
- Remove any humidification or ventilation device.
- Suction the tracheostomy tube to clear the airway of any secretions that could hinder oxygenation.
- Reconnect the patient to the humidifier or ventilator, if necessary.

CLEANING A STOMA AND OUTER CANNULA

- Put on sterile gloves.
- With your dominant hand, saturate a sterile gauze pad or cotton-tipped applicator with the cleaning solution.
- Squeeze out the excess liquid to prevent aspiration.
- Wipe the patient's neck under the tracheostomy tube flanges and twill tapes.
- Repeat until the skin surrounding the tracheostomy is cleaned.
- Use additional pads or cotton-tipped applicators to clean the stoma site and the tube's flanges.

NURSING ALERT Wipe only once with each pad or applicator, and then discard it to prevent contamination of a clean area with a soiled pad or applicator.

- Rinse away debris and peroxide (if used) with sterile 4" × 4" gauze pads dampened in normal saline solution.
- Dry the area thoroughly with additional sterile gauze pads.
- Apply a new sterile tracheostomy dressing.

CLEANING A NONDISPOSABLE INNER CANNULA

- Put on sterile gloves.
- Using your nondominant hand, remove and discard the patient's tracheostomy dressing.

- With the same hand, disconnect the ventilator or humidification device, and unlock the tracheostomy tube's inner cannula by rotating it counter-clockwise.
- Place the inner cannula in the container of hydrogen peroxide.
- Working quickly, use your dominant hand to scrub the cannula with the sterile nylon brush. If the brush doesn't slide easily into the cannula, use a sterile pipe cleaner.
- Immerse the cannula in the container of normal saline solution, and agitate it for about 10 seconds to rinse it thoroughly.
- Inspect the cannula for cleanliness and repeat the cleaning process if necessary.
- Tap it gently against the inside edge of the sterile container to remove excess liquid and prevent aspiration.
- Don't dry the outer surface because a thin film of moisture acts as a lubricant during insertion.
- Reinsert the inner cannula into the tracheostomy tube, lock it in place, and gently pull on it to make sure it's secure.
- Reconnect the mechanical ventilator.
- Apply a new sterile tracheostomy dressing.
- If the patient can't tolerate being disconnected from the ventilator for the time it takes to clean the inner cannula, replace the inner cannula with a clean one and reattach the mechanical ventilator.
- Then clean the cannula just removed from the patient, and store it in a sterile container for the next time.

CARING FOR A DISPOSABLE INNER CANNULA

- Put on clean gloves.
- Using your dominant hand, remove the patient's inner cannula.
- After evaluating the secretions in the cannula, discard it properly.
- Pick up the new inner cannula, touching only the outer locking portion.
- Insert the cannula into the tracheostomy and lock it securely.

CHANGING TRACHEOSTOMY TIES

- Obtain assistance from another nurse or a respiratory therapist to prevent accidental tube expulsion.

NURSING ALERT Obtain assistance when changing tracheostomy ties because patient movement or coughing can dislodge the tube.

- Put on sterile gloves.
- If commercial ties aren't available, prepare new ties from a 30" (76-cm) length of twill tape by folding one end back 1" (2.5 cm) on itself. Then with the bandage scissors, cut a ½" (1.3 cm) slit down the center of the tape from the folded edge.
- Prepare the other end of the tape the same way.
- Hold both ends together and, using scissors, cut the resulting circle of tape so that one piece is approximately 10" (25 cm) long and the other is about 20" (51 cm) long.
- Assist the patient into semi-Fowler's position.
- Instruct your gloved-assistant to hold the tracheostomy tube in place to prevent its expulsion during replacement of the ties.
- If you must perform the procedure without assistance, fasten the clean ties in place before removing the old ties to prevent tube expulsion.
- Remove and discard the old ties; if you use scissors, be careful not to cut the tube of the pilot balloon.
- Thread the slit end of one new tie a short distance through the eye of one tracheostomy tube flange from the underside.
- Thread the other end of the tie completely through the slit end, and pull it taut so it loops firmly through the flange to avoid knots that can cause throat discomfort, tissue irritation, pressure, and necrosis at the patient's throat.
- Fasten the second tie to the opposite flange in the same manner.
- Instruct the patient to flex his neck while you bring the ties to the side, and tie them together with a square knot because flexion produces the same neck circumference as coughing and helps prevent an overly tight tie.
- Instruct your assistant to place one finger under the tapes as you tie them to ensure that they're tight enough to avoid slippage but loose enough to prevent choking or jugular vein constriction.

(continued)

- Placing the closure on the side allows easy access and prevents pressure necrosis at the back of the neck when the patient is recumbent.
- After securing the ties, cut off the excess tape with the scissors and instruct your assistant to release the tracheostomy tube.

◆ **NURSING ALERT** Check tension on the tracheostomy-tie frequently on patients with traumatic injury, radical neck dissection, restlessness, or heart failure.

✹ **AGE-RELATED CONCERN** Check a neonate frequently because ties can loosen and cause tube dislodgment.

DEFLATING AND INFLATING A TRACHEOSTOMY CUFF

- Read the cuff manufacturer's instructions because cuff types and procedures vary widely.
- Help the patient into semi-Fowler's position or place him in a supine position so secretions above the cuff site will be pushed up into his mouth if he's receiving positive-pressure ventilation.
- Suction the oropharyngeal cavity to prevent any pooled secretions from descending into the trachea after cuff deflation.
- Release the padded hemostat clamping the cuff inflation tubing, if a hemostat is present.
- Insert a 5- or 10-ml syringe into the cuff pilot balloon, and very slowly withdraw all air from the cuff because slow deflation allows positive lung pressure to push secretions upward from the bronchi.
- Leave the syringe attached to the tubing for reinflation of the cuff.

◆ **NURSING ALERT** Cuff deflation may stimulate the patient's cough reflex, producing additional secretions.

- Remove any ventilation device.
- Suction the lower airway to remove all secretions.
- Reconnect the patient to the ventilation device.
- Maintain cuff deflation for the prescribed time.

- Observe the patient for adequate ventilation, and suction as necessary.
- If the patient has difficulty breathing, reinflate the cuff immediately by depressing the syringe plunger very slowly.
- Use a stethoscope to listen over the trachea for the air leak, and then inject the least amount of air necessary to achieve an adequate tracheal seal.
- When inflating the cuff, you may use the minimal-leak technique or the minimal occlusive volume technique to help gauge the proper inflation point.
- If you're inflating the cuff using cuff pressure measurement, the recommended cuff pressure is about 18 mm Hg, but don't to exceed 25 mm Hg.

◆ **NURSING ALERT** If cuff pressure exceeds 25 mm Hg, notify the physician because you may need to change to a larger size tube, use higher inflation pressures, or permit a larger air leak.

- After you've inflated the cuff, if the tubing doesn't have a one-way valve at the end, clamp the inflation line with a padded hemostat, and remove the syringe.
- Check for a minimal-leak cuff seal; you shouldn't feel air coming from the patient's mouth, nose, or tracheostomy site, and a conscious patient shouldn't be able to speak.

◆ **NURSING ALERT** Suspect an air leak from the cuff if injection of air fails to inflate the cuff or increase cuff pressure, if you're unable to inject the amount of air you withdrew, if the patient can speak, if ventilation fails to maintain adequate respiratory movement with pressures or volumes previously considered adequate, or if air escapes during the ventilator's inspiratory cycle.

- Note the exact amount of air used to inflate the cuff to detect tracheal malacia if more air is consistently needed.

CONCLUDING TRACHEOSTOMY CARE

- Replace any humidification device.
- Provide oral care because the oral cavity can become dry and malodorous or develop sores from encrusted secretions.

- Observe soiled dressings and any suctioned secretions for amount, color, consistency, and odor.
- Properly clean or dispose of all equipment, supplies, solutions, and trash, according to policy.
- Remove and discard your gloves.
- Make sure the patient is comfortable and can easily reach the call button.
- Make sure all necessary supplies are readily available at the bedside.
- Change the dressing as often as necessary because a wet dressing with exudate or secretions predisposes the patient to skin excoriation, breakdown, and infection.

✦ SPECIAL CONSIDERATIONS

- Keep appropriate equipment at the patient's bedside for immediate use in an emergency.

  ⬖ NURSING ALERT Follow facility policy if a tracheostomy is expelled or the outer cannula becomes blocked. If breathing is obstructed, call the appropriate code and provide manual resuscitation with a handheld resuscitation bag or reconnect the patient to the ventilator. Don't remove the tracheostomy tube because the airway may close completely. Use caution when reinserting to avoid tracheal trauma, perforation, compression, and asphyxiation.

- Don't change the tracheostomy ties unnecessarily during the immediate postoperative period before the stoma track is well formed (usually 4 days) to avoid accidental dislodgment and explusion of the tube. Unless secretions of drainage are a problem, ties can be changed once per day.

- Refrain from changing a single-cannula tracheostomy tube or the outer cannula of a double-cannula tube, this is usually performed by the physician.

- If the patient's neck or stoma is excoriated or infected, apply a water-soluble lubricant or topical antibiotic cream as ordered.

- Don't use a powder or an oil-based substance on or around a stoma because aspiration of such substances can lead to infection and abscess.

Complications
- Hemorrhage
- Tracheal edema
- Aspiration
- Pneumothorax
- Hypoxia, acidosis
- Subcutaneous emphysema
- Skin excoriation and infection
- Airway obstruction
- Tracheal erosion and necrosis

▶ PATIENT TEACHING

Be sure to cover:
- what to expect during tracheostomy care
- need to remain still and avoid vigorous coughing when ties are being changed
- signs and symptoms of complications to report
- care of the tracheostomy at home.

●◆ DOCUMENTATION

- Date and time of the tracheostomy care
- Type of care performed
- Amount, consistency, color, and odor of secretions
- Stoma and skin condition
- Respiratory status
- Change of the tracheostomy tube by the physician
- Duration of any cuff deflation, amount of any cuff inflation; and cuff pressure readings and specific body position
- Complications and the nursing action taken
- Patient's tolerance of the treatment
- Patient or family teaching and their comprehension

Selected references

Edgtton-Winn, M., and Wright, K. "Tracheostomy: A Guide to Nursing Care," *Australian Nursing Journal* 13(5):17-20, November 2005.

Lewis, T., and Oliver, G. "Improving Tracheostomy Care for Ward Patients," *Nursing Standard* 19(19):33-37, January 2005.

Roman, M. "Tracheostomy Tubes," *Medsurg Nursing* 14(2):143-45, April 2005.

Russell, C. "Providing the Nurse with a Guide to Trachestomy Care and Management," *British Journal of Nursing* 4(8):328-33, April 2005.

St. John, R.E., and Malen, J.F. "Contemporary Issues in Adult Tracheostomy Management," *Critical Care Nursing Clinics of North America* 16(3):413-30, ix-x, September 2004.

Wilson, M. "Tracheostomy Management," *Paediatric Nursing* 17(3):38-43, April 2005.

Transabdominal tube feeding and care

● OVERVIEW

- Tube placed surgically or percutaneously through the patient's abdominal wall to access the stomach, duodenum, or jejunum
- Gastrostomy or jejunostomy tube: usually inserted during abdominal surgery to provide feeding during immediate postoperative period or for long-term enteral access
- Percutaneous endoscopic gastrostomy (PEG) or jejunostomy (PEJ) tube: inserted endoscopically in the endoscopy suite or at patient's bedside
- PEG or PEJ tube may be used for nutrition, drainage, and decompression
- With either type of tube placement, feedings may begin after 24 hours or when peristalsis resumes
- When tube needs replacement, indwelling urinary catheter, mushroom catheter, or gastrostomy button may be inserted

Contraindications

- Obstruction (such as an esophageal stricture or duodenal blockage)
- Previous gastric surgery
- Morbid obesity
- Ascites

❖ EQUIPMENT

FEEDING
Feeding formula • large-bulb or catheter-tip syringe • 120 ml of water • 4″ × 4″ gauze pads • soap • skin protectant • hypoallergenic tape • gravity-drip administration bags • mouthwash, toothpaste, or mild salt solution • stethoscope • gloves • optional: enteral infusion pump

DECOMPRESSION
Suction apparatus with tubing and straight drainage collection set

Equipment preparation
- Wash your hands thoroughly.
- Check the expiration date on commercially prepared feeding formulas.
- If the formula was prepared by the dietitian or pharmacist, check the preparation time and date.

NURSING ALERT Discard any opened formula that's more than 1 day old.
- Place the desired amount of formula into the gavage container and purge air from the tubing.
- To avoid contamination, hang only a 4- to 6-hour supply of formula at a time.

▌▌▌ ESSENTIAL STEPS

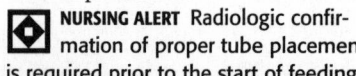

- Confirm the patient's identity using two patient identifiers according to facility policy.
- Explain the procedure to the patient.
- Wear appropriate personal protective equipment, when necessary, throughout all procedures.

NURSING ALERT Radiologic confirmation of proper tube placement is required prior to the start of feedings.
- Provide for privacy.
- Assess bowel sounds before feeding and check for abdominal distention.
- Assist the patient into a sitting or semi-Fowler's position to prevent esophageal reflux and pulmonary aspiration of the formula.
- For an intermittent feeding, keep the patient upright for 30 minutes to 1 hour after the feeding.
- Attach the syringe to the feeding tube and aspirate to measure residual gastric contents.
- If the residual contents measure more than twice the amount infused, hold the feeding and recheck in 1 hour; if residual contents remain too high, notify the physician.

NURSING ALERT Residual contents are minimal with PEJ tube feedings.
- Allow 30 ml of water to flow into the feeding tube to establish patency.
- Administer formula at room temperature because a cold formula may cause cramping.

INTERMITTENT FEEDINGS
- Allow gravity to help the formula flow over 30 to 45 minutes.

NURSING ALERT Infusing the feeding too quickly can cause bloating, cramps, or diarrhea.
- Begin intermittent feeding with a low volume (200 ml) daily.

- Increase the volume per feeding, as tolerated, to reach the desired calorie intake.
- When the feeding finishes, flush the feeding tube with 30 to 60 ml of water to maintain patency and provide hydration.
- Cap the tube to prevent leakage.
- Rinse the feeding administration set thoroughly with hot water to avoid contaminating subsequent feedings and allow it to dry between feedings.

CONTINUOUS FEEDINGS
- Measure residual gastric contents every 4 hours.
- To administer the feeding with a pump, set up the equipment according to the manufacturer's guidelines, and fill the feeding bag.
- To administer the feeding by gravity, fill the container with formula and purge air from the tubing.
- Monitor the gravity drip rate or pump infusion rate frequently to ensure accurate delivery of formula.
- Flush the feeding tube with 30 to 60 ml of water every 4 hours to maintain patency and to provide hydration.
- Monitor intake and output to detect fluid imbalances.

DECOMPRESSION
- To decompress the stomach, connect the PEG port to the suction device with tubing or straight gravity drainage tubing.
- Jejunostomy feeding may be given simultaneously via the PEJ port of the dual-lumen tube.

TUBE EXIT SITE CARE
- Provide daily skin care.
- Gently remove the dressing; never use scissors because you risk cutting the tube or the sutures.
- Clean the skin around the tube using a 4″ × 4″ gauze pad soaked in the prescribed cleaning solution.
- When healed, wash the skin around the exit site daily with soap, rinse with water, and pat dry.
- Apply skin protectant, if necessary.
- Anchor a gastrostomy or jejunostomy tube to the skin with hypoallergenic tape to prevent peristaltic migration of the tube and tension on the sutures.
- Coil the tube, if necessary, and tape it to the abdomen. (PEG and PEJ tubes have toggle-bolt-like internal and ex-

ternal bumpers that make tape anchors unnecessary). (See *Caring for a PEG or PEJ site*.)

✦ SPECIAL CONSIDERATIONS

- If the patient vomits or complains of nausea, feeling too full, or regurgitation, stop the feeding and restart it in 1 hour (measure residual gastric contents first), possibly at a reduced volume or rate.

◈ **NURSING ALERT** Monitor for signs and symptoms of aspiration during feeding, including shortness of breath and changes in breath sounds. Have suction equipment readily available.

- If the patient develops dumping syndrome, which includes nausea, vomiting, cramps, pallor, and diarrhea, reduce the rate of feedings.
- Control diarrhea resulting from dumping syndrome by using continuous pump or gravity-drip infusions, diluting the feeding formula, or adding antidiarrheal medications.
- Provide oral hygiene frequently.
- Administer most tablets and pills through the tube by crushing them and diluting as necessary.

◈ **NURSING ALERT** Don't crush enteric-coated or sustained-released drugs for administration through a feeding tube.

Complications

- Cramping, nausea, vomiting, bloating, and diarrhea or constipation
- Pulmonary aspiration
- Infection at the tube exit site
- Tube dislodgment or obstruction
- Vitamin and mineral deficiencies
- Fluid and electrolyte imbalances

▶ PATIENT TEACHING

Be sure to cover:
- all aspects of enteral feedings, including tube maintenance and site care
- signs and symptoms to report to the physician
- administering medications through a feeding tube
- adverse effects and actions to take
- that tube may eventually be replaced with a gastrostomy button or a latex, indwelling, or mushroom catheter
- performing syringe feedings.

●◇ DOCUMENTATION

- Verification of proper tube placement
- Date, time, and amount of each feeding and the water volume instilled
- Type of formula, the infusion method and rate, and delivery method
- Patient's tolerance of the procedure and formula
- Amount of residual gastric contents
- Complications and actions taken
- Date and time physician notified of complications and orders given
- Abdominal assessment findings, including bowel sounds
- Breath sounds
- Condition of exit site and site care
- Laboratory test results
- Patient teaching

Selected references

Carey, T.S., et al. "Expectations and Outcomes of Gastric Feeding Tubes," *American Journal of Medicine* 119(6):527, e11-16, June 2006.

Todd, V., et al. "Percutaneous Endoscopic Gastrostomy (PEG): The Role and Perspective of Nurses," *Journal of Clinical Nursing* 14(2):187-94, February 2005.

Williams, T.A., and Leslie, G.D. "A Review of the Nursing Care of Enteral Feeding Tubes in Critically Ill Adults: Part I," *Intensive & Critical Nursing* 20(6):330-43, December 2004.

CARING FOR A PEG OR PEJ SITE

The exit site of a percutaneous endoscopic gastrostomy (PEG) or percutaneous endoscopic jejunostomy (PEJ) tube requires routine observation and care. Follow these care guidelines:

- Change the dressing daily while the tube is in place
- After removing the dressing, carefully slide the tube's outer bumper away from the skin (as shown below) about ½" (1.5 cm).

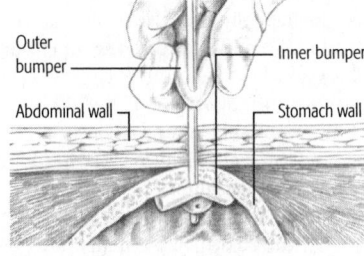

Outer bumper — Inner bumper
Abdominal wall — Stomach wall

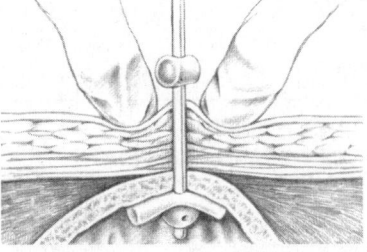

- Examine the skin around the tube. Look for redness and other signs of infection or erosion.
- Gently depress the skin surrounding the tube and inspect for drainage (as shown above right). Expect minimal wound drainage initially after implantation. This should subside in about 1 week.
- Inspect the tube for wear and tear. (A tube that wears out will need replacement.)
- Clean the site with the prescribed cleaning solution.

- Apply povidone-iodine ointment over the exit site, according to facility guidelines.
- Rotate the outer bumper 90 degrees (*to avoid repeating the same tension on the same skin area*), and slide the outer bumper back over the exit site.
- If leakage appears at the PEG site, or if the patient risks dislodging the tube, apply a sterile gauze dressing over the site. Don't put sterile gauze underneath the outer bumper. Loosening the anchor this way allows the feeding tube free play, which could lead to wound abscess.
- Write the date and time of the dressing change on the tape.

Transcranial Doppler monitoring

● OVERVIEW

- Noninvasive method of monitoring blood flow in the intracranial vessels, specifically the circle of Willis
- Used in intensive care to monitor patients with cerebrovascular disorders, such as stroke, head trauma, or subarachnoid hemorrhage
- Detects intracranial stenosis, vasospasm, and arteriovenous malformations as well as assesses collateral pathways
- Allows monitoring of continuous waveform, for use in intraoperative monitoring of cerebral circulation (see *Understanding transcranial Doppler monitoring*)
- Performed to monitor the effect of intracranial pressure changes on the cerebral circulation; to monitor patient response to various medications; to evaluate carbon dioxide reactivity; which may be impaired or lost from arterial obstruction or trauma; and to confirm brain death
- Benefits include instantaneous, real-time information about cerebral blood flow and that it's noninvasive, painless, portable, and easy to use
- Major disadvantage is that it relies on the ability of ultrasound waves to penetrate thin areas of the cranium
- Requires specialized training to ensure accurate vessel identification and correct interpretation of the signals

Contraindications
- None known

❖ EQUIPMENT

Transcranial Doppler unit • transducer with an attachment system • terry cloth headband • ultrasonic coupling gel • marker

Equipment preparation
- Turn on the Doppler unit and observe as it performs a self-test; the screen should show six parameters: PEAK (CM/S), MEAN (CM/S), DEPTH (M/M), DELTA (%), EMBOLI (AGR), and PI+.
- Enter the patient's name and identification number in the appropriate place on the Doppler unit. You may also need to enter additional information, such as the patient's diagnosis or the physician's name.
- Indicate the vessel that you wish to monitor (usually the right or left middle cerebral artery [MCA]).
- Set the approximate depth of the vessel within the skull (50 mm for the MCA).
- Use the keypad to increase the power level to 100% to initially locate the signal, decreasing it later, as needed, depending on the thickness of the patient's skull.

UNDERSTANDING TRANSCRANIAL DOPPLER MONITORING

The transcranial Doppler unit transmits pulses of high-frequency ultrasound, which are then reflected back to the transducer by the red blood cells moving in the vessel being monitored. This information is then processed by the instrument into an audible signal and a velocity waveform, which is displayed on the monitor.

The displayed waveform is actually a moving graph of blood flow velocities with TIME displayed along the horizontal axis, VELOCITY displayed along the vertical axis, and AMPLITUDE represented by various colors or intensities within the waveform. The heart's contractions speed up the movement of blood cells during systole and slow it down during diastole, resulting in a waveform that varies in velocity over the cardiac cycle.

❚❚❙ ESSENTIAL STEPS

- Confirm the patient's identity using two patient identifiers according to facility policy.
- Explain the procedure to the patient.
- Wash your hands thoroughly.
- Place the patient in the proper position, usually the supine position.

AGE-RELATED CONCERN Transcranial Doppler monitoring may be less reliable in an elderly patient, due to thickening of the temporal bone.

- Examine the temporal region of the patient's head, and mentally identify the three windows of the transtemporal access route: posterior, middle, and anterior.
- Apply a generous amount of ultrasonic gel at the level of the temporal bone between the tragus of the ear and the end of the eyebrow, over the area of the three windows.
- Place the transducer on the posterior window and angle the transducer slightly in an anterior direction, and slowly move it in a narrow circle (commonly called the flashlighting technique).
- As you hold the transducer at an angle and perform flashlighting, begin to very slowly move the transducer forward across the temporal area, listening for the audible signal with the highest pitch. This sound corresponds to the highest velocity signal, which corresponds to the signal of the vessel you're assessing.
- Use headphones to better evaluate the audible signal and provide patient privacy.
- After you've located the highest-pitched signal, use a marker to draw a circle around the transducer head on the patient's temple.
- Note the angle of the transducer so that you can duplicate it after the transducer attachment system is in place.
- Place the plate of the transducer attachment system over the patient's temporal area; matching the circular opening in the plate exactly with the circle drawn on the patient's head.
- Holding the plate in place, encircle the patient's head with the straps attached to the system.

- Tighten the straps so that the transducer attachment system stays in place on the patient's head.
- Fill the circular opening in the plate with the ultrasonic gel.
- Place the transducer in the gel-filled opening in the attachment system plate.
- Using the plastic screws provided, loosely secure the two plates together, holding the transducer in place but allowing it to rotate for the best angle.
- Adjust the position and angle of the transducer until you again hear the highest-pitched audible signal.
- Look at the monitor screen for a clear waveform with a bright white line (called an envelope) at the upper edge of the waveform; the envelope exactly follows the contours of the waveform itself.
- If the envelope doesn't follow the waveform's contours, adjust the GAIN setting.
- If the signal is wrapping around the screen, use the SCALE key to increase the scale and the BASELINE key to drop the baseline.
- When you have the strongest, highest-pitched signal and the best waveform, lock the transducer in place at the angle you've chosen by tightening the plastic screws.
- Disconnect the transducer handle.
- Place a wide terry cloth headband over the transducer attachment system, and secure it around the patient's head to provide additional stability for the transducer.
- Make sure you can see a waveform and read the numeric values of the peak, mean velocities, and pulsatility index (PI+) above the displayed waveform on the monitor screen; the shape of the waveform reveals more information.

✦ SPECIAL CONSIDERATIONS

- Velocity changes in the transcranial Doppler signal correlate with changes in cerebral blood flow and are reflected in the mean velocity.
- Establish a baseline for the mean velocity. As the patient's velocity increases or decreases, the value (%) will change negatively or positively from the baseline.
- Emboli appear as high-intensity transients occurring randomly during the cardiac cycle, making a distinctive "clicking," "chirping," or "plunking" sound.
- Set up an emboli counter, as indicated, to count either the total number of emboli aggregates or the rate of embolic events per minute.
- Various screens can be stored on the system's hard drive and can be recalled or printed.
- Before using the transcranial Doppler system, remove turban head dressings or thick dressings over the test site.
- The transcranial Doppler unit should always be used with its power set at the lowest level needed to provide an adequate waveform.

Complications
- None known

▶ PATIENT TEACHING

Be sure to cover:
- why the procedure is being performed
- equipment used
- sounds that may be heard
- that the procedure is painless and noninvasive.

●◆ DOCUMENTATION

- Date and time monitoring began
- Artery being monitored and the results
- Patient's tolerance of the procedure
- Patient teaching

Selected references

Demchuk, A.M., et al. "Transcranial Doppler in Acute Stroke," *Neuroimaging Clinics of North America* 15(3):473-80, August 2005.

Evans, D.H. "Embolus Differentiation Using Multifrequency Transcranial Doppler," *Stroke* 37(7):1641, July 2006.

Kirkness, C.J. "Cerebral Blood Flow Monitoring in Clinical Practice," *AACN Clinical Issues* 15(4):476-87, October-December 2005.

White, H., and Venkatesh, B. "Application of Transcranial Doppler in the ICU: A Review," *Intensive Care Medicine* 32(7):981-94, July 2006.

Transcutaneous electrical nerve stimulation

● OVERVIEW

- Based on the gate control theory of pain, which proposes that painful impulses pass through a "gate" in the brain
- Performed with a portable, battery-powered device that transmits painless electrical current to peripheral nerves or directly to a painful area over relatively large nerve fibers
- Alters the patient's perception of pain by blocking painful stimuli traveling over smaller fibers
- Reduces the need for analgesic drugs and allows the patient to resume normal activities in postoperative patients and those with chronic pain
- Typically, treatments last 3 to 5 days
- Also known as *TENS*
- Some conditions, such as phantom limb pain, may require continuous stimulation; other conditions, such as a painful arthritic joint, require shorter periods (3 to 4 hours) (see *Uses for transcutaneous electrical nerve stimulation*)

Contraindications
- Cardiac pacemakers
- Pregnant patients
- Dementia

NURSING ALERT TENS electrodes shouldn't be placed on the head or neck of a patient with a vascular or seizure disorder.

❖ EQUIPMENT

TENS device • alcohol pads • electrodes • electrode gel • warm water and soap • leadwires • charged battery pack • battery recharger • adhesive patch or hypoallergenic tape
Commercial TENS kits are available.

Equipment preparation
- Test the battery pack to make sure it's fully charged.

USES FOR TRANSCUTANEOUS ELECTRICAL NERVE STIMULATION

Transcutaneous electrical nerve stimulation (TENS) must be prescribed by a physician and is most successful if it's administered and taught to the patient by a therapist skilled in its use. TENS has been used for temporary relief of acute pain, such as postoperative pain, and for ongoing relief of chronic pain such as sciatica.

Types of pain that respond to TENS include:
- arthritis
- bone fracture pain
- bursitis
- cancer-related pain
- lower back pain
- musculoskeletal pain
- myofascial pain
- neuralgias and neuropathies
- phantom limb pain
- postoperative incision pain
- sciatica
- whiplash.

▌▌█ ESSENTIAL STEPS

- Wash your hands thoroughly before all procedures.
- Provide for privacy.
- Confirm the patient's identity using two patient identifiers according to facility policy.
- Explain the procedure to the patient.
- Make sure the patient has signed the appropriate consent form.

BEFORE TENS TREATMENT
- With an alcohol pad, clean the skin where the electrode will be applied and dry the site. Clip hair at the site, if necessary.
- Apply electrode gel to the bottom of each electrode.
- Place the ordered number of electrodes on the proper skin area, leaving at least 2″ (5 cm) between them. (See *Positioning TENS electrodes.*)
- Secure the electrodes with the adhesive patch or hypoallergenic tape.
- Tape all sides evenly so that the electrodes are firmly attached to the skin.
- Plug the pin connectors into the electrode sockets, holding the connectors—not the cords themselves—during insertion.
- Turn the channel controls to the OFF position or as recommended in the operator's manual.
- Plug the leadwires into the jacks in the control box.
- Turn the amplitude and rate dials slowly as the manual directs. (The patient should feel a tingling sensation.)
- Adjust the controls to the prescribed settings or to settings that are most comfortable, most commonly frequencies of 60 to 100 Hz.
- Attach the TENS control box to part of the patient's clothing, such as a belt, pocket, or bra.
- Monitor the patient for signs of excessive stimulation, such as muscle twitches, and for signs of inadequate stimulation, signaled by the patient's inability to feel any mild tingling sensation.

NURSING ALERT Controls set too high can lead to pain; if controls are set too low, pain won't be relieved.

AFTER TENS TREATMENT
- Turn off the controls, and unplug the electrode lead wires from the control box.
- If another treatment will be given soon, leave the electrodes in place; if not, remove them.
- Clean the electrodes with soap and water, and clean the patient's skin with alcohol pads. (Don't soak the electrodes in alcohol because it will damage the rubber.)
- Remove the battery pack from the unit, and replace it with a charged battery pack.
- Recharge the used battery pack so it's ready for use.

◆ SPECIAL CONSIDERATIONS

- If you must move the electrodes during the procedure, turn off the controls first.
- Follow the physician's orders regarding electrode placement and control settings.

  ◈ NURSING ALERT Incorrect placement of the electrodes results in inappropriate pain control.
- If TENS is used continuously for postoperative pain, remove the electrodes at least daily to check for skin irritation, and provide skin care.
- If appropriate, let the patient study the operator's manual.

  ◈ NURSING ALERT Never place the electrodes near the patient's eyes or over the nerves that innervate the carotid sinus or laryngeal or pharyngeal muscles, to avoid interference with critical nerve function.

Complications
- Skin irritation
- Pain
- Inadequate pain relief

▶ PATIENT TEACHING

Be sure to cover:
- how TENS relieves pain
- how the electrodes are applied
- how the TENS unit is used
- adverse effects and how to correct them.

●◆ DOCUMENTATION

- Date and time of TENS treatment
- Electrode sites and the control settings
- Patient's tolerance to treatment
- Assessment of pain control before and after treatment

Selected references
Kapur. S., et al. "Assessment of the Efficacy of Electronic Nerve Modulation (ENM) in Comparison to TENS in Patients with Chronic Low Back Pain," *Neuromodulation* 9(2);161-62, April 2006.

Khadilkar. A., et al. "Transcutaneous Electrical Nerve Stimulation for the Treatment of Chronic Low Back Pain: A Systematic Review," *Spine* 30(23):2657-66, December 2005.

Limoges, M.F., and Rickabaugh, B. "Evaluation of TENS During Screening Flexible Sigmoidoscopy," *Gastroenterology Nursing* 27(2):61-68, March-April 2004.

Siddle, L. "The Challenge and Management of Phantom Limb Pain after Amputation," *British Journal of Nursing* 13(11):664-67, June 2004.

POSITIONING TENS ELECTRODES

In transcutaneous electrical nerve stimulation (TENS), electrodes placed around peripheral nerves (or an incisional site) transmit mild electrical pulses to the brain. The current is thought to block pain impulses. The patient can influence the level and frequency of his pain relief by adjusting the controls on the device.

Typically, electrode placement varies even though patients may have similar complaints. Electrodes can be placed in several ways:
- To cover the painful area or surround it, as with muscle tenderness or spasm or painful joints
- To "capture" the painful area between electrodes, as with incisional pain.

In peripheral nerve injury, electrodes should be placed proximal to the injury (between the brain and the injury site) to avoid increasing pain. Placing electrodes in a hypersensitive area also increases pain. In an area lacking sensation, electrodes should be placed on adjacent dermatomes.

The illustrations show combinations of electrode placement (black squares) and areas of nerve stimulation (shaded gray) for lower back and leg pain.

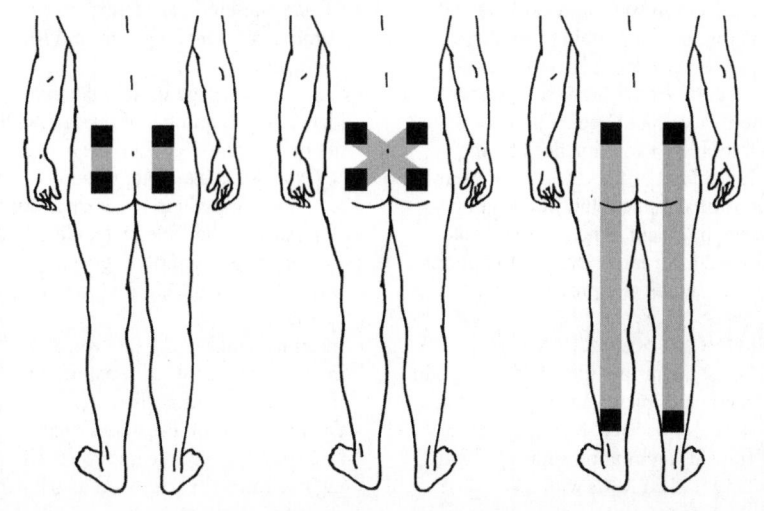

Transfusion of whole blood and packed cells

● OVERVIEW

- Whole blood transfusion: replenishes volume and oxygen-carrying capacity of circulatory system
- Transfusion of packed red blood cells (RBCs): restores only oxygen-carrying capacity
- Both types of transfusions: increase hemoglobin levels and hematocrit; each unit of whole blood or RBCs contains enough hemoglobin to raise hemoglobin concentration in average-sized adult by 1 g/dL (about 3%)
- Whole blood usually used when decreased levels result from hemorrhage; packed RBCs used when depressed levels accompany normal blood volume, avoiding possible fluid and circulatory overload
- Both whole blood and packed RBCs: contain cellular debris, requiring in-line filtration during administration
- Washed packed RBCs: commonly used for patients previously sensitized to transfusions; rinsed with special solution that removes white blood cells and platelets, decreasing chance of transfusion reaction

Contraindications

- Religious practices that may prohibit transfer of blood or blood products

❖ EQUIPMENT

Blood administration set (170 to 260 micron filter and tubing with drip chamber for blood, or combined set; straight line and Y-type sets most commonly used) • I.V. pole • gloves • gown • face shield • multiple-lead tubing • whole blood or packed RBCs • 250 ml of normal saline solution • venipuncture equipment, if necessary (should include 20G or larger catheter) • optional: ice bag, warm compresses

Equipment preparation

- Select the proper filter. Filters come in mesh and microaggregate types; the latter is preferred, especially when transfusing multiple units of blood.
- Give packed RBCs with a Y-type set.
- Piggybacking increases the chance of harmful microorganisms entering the tubing because the blood line is connected to the established line.
- Prepare the equipment when you're ready to start the infusion.

❚❚▌ ESSENTIAL STEPS

- Wash your hands thoroughly.
- Confirm the patient's identity using two patient identifiers according to facility policy.
- Explain the procedure to the patient.
- Make sure the patient has signed the appropriate consent form.

◈ NURSING ALERT If the patient is a Jehovah's Witness, a transfusion requires special written permission.

- Maintain asepsis throughout all procedures.
- Wear appropriate personal protective equipment throughout all procedures.
- Record the patient's baseline vital signs.
- Obtain whole blood or packed RBCs within 30 minutes of starting the transfusion.
- Check the expiration date on the blood bag, and observe for abnormal color, RBC clumping, gas bubbles, and extraneous material.
- Return outdated or abnormal blood to the blood bank.
- Compare the name and number on the patient's wristband with those on the blood bag label.
- Check the blood bag identification number, ABO blood group, and Rh compatibility.
- Compare the patient's blood bank identification number, if present, with the number on the blood bag.

◈ NURSING ALERT Identification of blood and blood products is done at the patient's bedside by two licensed professionals, according to policy.

- Using a Y-type set, close all the clamps on the set.
- Insert the spike of the line you're using for the normal saline solution into the bag of saline solution.
- Open the port on the blood bag, and insert the spike of the line you're using to administer the blood or cellular component into the port.
- Hang the bag of normal saline solution and blood or cellular component on the I.V. pole, open the clamp on the line of saline solution, and squeeze the drip chamber until it's half full.
- Remove the adapter cover at the tip of the blood administration set, open the main flow clamp, and prime the tubing with saline solution.
- If you're administering packed RBCs with a Y-type set, you can add saline solution to the bag to dilute the cells by closing the clamp between the patient and the drip chamber and opening the clamp from the blood.
- Lower the blood bag below the saline container and let 30 to 50 ml of saline solution flow into the packed cells.
- Close the clamp to the blood bag, re-hang the bag, rotate it gently to mix the cells and saline solution, and close the clamp to the saline container.
- If the patient doesn't have an I.V. line in place, perform a venipuncture, using a 20G or larger-diameter catheter.
- Avoid using an existing line for transfusion if the needle or catheter lumen is smaller than 20G.
- Consider the patient's central venous access device for transfusion therapy.
- If you're administering whole blood, gently invert the bag several times to mix the cells.
- Attach the prepared blood administration set to the venipuncture device, and flush it with normal saline solution.
- Close the clamp to the saline solution, and open the clamp between the blood bag and the patient.
- Adjust the flow rate to no greater than 5 ml/minute for the first 15 minutes of the transfusion.
- Remain with the patient and watch for signs and symptoms of a transfusion reaction.

◈ NURSING ALERT If the patient develops an adverse reaction to the blood transfusion, he may exhibit a variety of signs and symptoms, including fever, chills, nausea, vomiting, and dyspnea. If a transfusion reaction is suspected, stop the transfusion immediately, start a saline infusion using a new I.V. administration set to maintain vascular access, notify the physician, and follow your facility's policy for transfusion reaction management.

- If no signs of a reaction appear within 15 minutes, adjust the flow, clamp to the ordered infusion rate, which should be as rapid as his circulatory system can tolerate.
- After completing the transfusion, put on gloves and remove and discard the used infusion equipment.
- Reconnect the original I.V. fluid, if necessary, or discontinue the I.V. infusion.
- Return the empty blood bag to the blood bank, if facility policy dictates, and discard the tubing and filter.
- Record the patient's vital signs.

◆ SPECIAL CONSIDERATIONS

- Although some microaggregate filters can be used for up to 10 units of blood, always replace the filter and tubing if more than 1 hour elapses between transfusions.
- Use of highly effective leukocyte removal filters can postpone sensitization to transfusion therapy when transfusing blood and packed RBCs.

■ **NURSING ALERT** Potential transplant candidates who require blood transfusions need special restrictions related to the blood product in order to decrease antibody development. These may include the use of leukocyte-depleted and cytomegalovirus (CMV)–safe blood products.

- When administering multiple units of blood under pressure, use a blood warmer to avoid hypothermia, warming the blood to no more than 107.6° F (42° C).
- For rapid blood replacement, you may need to use a pressure bag.

■ **NURSING ALERT** Excessive pressure may develop when using a pressure bag, leading to broken blood vessels and extravasation, with hematoma and hemolysis of the infusing RBCs.

- If the infusion rate must be so slow that the entire unit can't be infused within 4 hours, consider discussing with your facility's blood bank the possibility of dividing the unit and keeping one portion refrigerated until it can be safely administered.
- If the transfusion becomes sluggish or stops:

– check that the I.V. container is at least 3′ (1 m) above the I.V. site
– make sure that the flow clamp is open and that blood completely covers the filter; if it doesn't, squeeze the drip chamber until it does
– gently rock the bag back and forth to agitate blood cells that may have settled
– untape the dressing over the I.V. site to check needle placement; reposition the needle, if necessary
– flush the line with normal saline solution and restart the transfusion. Using a Y-type set, close the flow clamp to the patient and lower the blood bag; next, open the saline clamp and allow some normal saline solution to flow into the blood bag; rehang the blood bag, open the flow clamp to the patient, and reset the flow rate.

- If a hematoma develops at the I.V. site, immediately stop the infusion, remove the I.V. cannula, notify the physician, and expect to place ice on the site intermittently for 8 hours. A new I.V. line will need to be started to allow completion of the transfusion.
- If the blood bag empties before the next one arrives, administer normal saline solution slowly. If you're using a Y-type set, close the blood-line clamp, open the saline clamp, and let the normal saline solution run slowly until the new blood arrives. Decrease the flow rate or clamp the line before attaching the new unit of blood.

Complications
- Transfusion reaction
- Infectious disease transmission
- Circulatory overload
- Hemolytic, allergic, febrile, and pyrogenic reactions
- Coagulation disturbances
- Citrate intoxication
- Hyperkalemia
- Acid-base imbalance
- Loss of 2,3-diphosphoglycerate
- Ammonia intoxication
- Hypothermia

▶ PATIENT TEACHING

Be sure to cover:
- reason for transfusion
- how a transfusion is performed
- typing and crossmatching of blood
- associated risks and interventions performed to reduce those risks
- monitoring that will occur before, during, and after transfusion
- signs and symptoms to report during and after transfusion.

●◆ DOCUMENTATION

Before administering the transfusion, document that you matched the label on the blood bag to:
- patient's name and medical record number
- patient's blood group or type
- patient's and donor's Rh factor
- crossmatch data
- blood bank identification number
- expiration date of the product.

Document that the blood and blood component were identified by two health professionals, both of whom sign the slip that comes with the blood and verify that the information is correct.

On the transfusion record, document:
- date and time transfusion was started and completed
- name of the health care professional who verified the information
- type and gauge of the catheter
- total amount of the transfusion
- vital signs before, during, and after the transfusion
- infusion device used and its flow rate
- blood-warming unit used.

Selected references

Davis, K., et al. "Transfusing Safely: A 2006 Guide for Nurses," *Australian Nursing Journal* 13(6):17-20, December 2005-January 2006.

Hughes, M. "Using Guidelines to Minimise the Hazards of Blood Transfusion," *Nursing Times* 101(4):36, January 2005.

Sandler, S.G., et al. "Bar Code Technology Improves Positive Patient Identification and Transfusion Safety," *Development in Biologicals* 120:19-24, 2005.

Transfusion reaction management

● **OVERVIEW**

- Transfusion reaction: typically, a result of a major antigen-antibody reaction; can result from single or massive transfusion of blood or blood products
- Many reactions occur during transfusion or within 96 hours afterward
- Requires immediate recognition and prompt nursing action to prevent further complications and, possibly, death (see *Guide to transfusion reactions*)

Contraindications
- None known

❖ **EQUIPMENT**

Normal saline solution • I.V. administration set • sterile urine specimen container • needle, syringe, and tubes for blood samples • transfusion reaction report form • optional: oxygen, epinephrine, hypothermia blanket, leukocyte removal filter

Equipment preparation
- Have all equipment readily available at the bedside.

▐▌▐ **ESSENTIAL STEPS**

- As soon as you suspect an adverse reaction, stop the transfusion and start the saline infusion, using a new I.V. administration set at a keep-vein-open rate to maintain venous access.
- Notify the physician immediately.
- Monitor vital signs every 15 minutes or as indicated by the severity and type of reaction.
- Compare the labels on all blood containers with corresponding patient identification forms to verify that the transfusion was the correct blood or blood product.
- Notify the blood bank of a possible transfusion reaction and collect blood samples, as ordered.
- Immediately send the samples, all transfusion containers (even if empty), and the administration set to the blood bank for testing to further evaluate the reaction.
- Collect the first posttransfusion urine specimen, mark the collection slip "Possible transfusion reaction," and send it to the laboratory immediately to determine the presence of hemoglobin, indicating a hemolytic reaction.
- Monitor intake and output closely because hemoglobin deposition in the renal tubules can cause renal damage.
- If prescribed, administer oxygen, epinephrine, or other drugs and apply a hypothermia blanket to reduce fever.
- Make the patient as comfortable as possible and provide reassurance as necessary. Provide emotional support.

(Text continues on page 855.)

GUIDE TO TRANSFUSION REACTIONS

Any patient receiving a transfusion of processed blood products risks certain complications – hemosiderosis and hypothermia, for example. The chart below describes *endogenous reactions,* those caused by an antigen-antibody reaction in the recipient, and *exogenous reactions,* those caused by external factors in administered blood.

Reaction and causes	Signs and symptoms	Nursing interventions
ENDOGENOUS		
ALLERGIC • Allergen in donor blood • Donor blood hypersensitive to certain drugs	• Anaphylaxis (chills, facial swelling, laryngeal edema, pruritus, urticaria, wheezing), fever, nausea and vomiting	• Administer antihistamines, as prescribed. • Monitor patient for anaphylactic reaction, and administer epinephrine and corticosteroids as ordered. • As prescribed, premedicate patient with diphenhydramine before subsequent transfusion.
FEBRILE • Bacterial lipopolysaccharides • Antileukocyte recipient antibodies directed against donor white blood cells	• Fever up to 104° F (40° C), chills, headache, facial flushing, palpitations, cough, chest tightness, increased pulse rate, flank pain	• Relieve symptoms with an antipyretic, an antihistamine, or meperidine, as ordered. • If the patient requires further transfusions, use frozen red blood cells (RBCs), add a special leukocyte removal filter to the blood line, or premedicate him with acetaminophen, as ordered, before starting another transfusion.
HEMOLYTIC • ABO or Rh incompatibility • Intradonor incompatibility • Improper cross-matching • Improperly stored blood	• Chest pain, dyspnea, facial flushing, fever, chills, shaking, hypotension, flank pain, hemoglobinuria, oliguria, bloody oozing at the infusion site or surgical incision site, burning sensation along vein receiving blood, shock, renal failure	• Monitor blood pressure. • Manage shock with I.V. fluids, oxygen, epinephrine, a diuretic, and a vasopressor, as ordered. • Obtain posttransfusion-reaction blood samples and urine specimens for analysis. • Observe for signs of hemorrhage resulting from disseminated intravascular coagulation.
PLASMA PROTEIN INCOMPATIBILITY • Immunoglobulin-A incompatibility	• Abdominal pain, diarrhea, dyspnea, chills, fever, flushing, hypotension	• Administer oxygen, fluids, epinephrine, or a corticosteroid, as ordered.
EXOGENOUS		
BACTERIAL CONTAMINATION • Organisms that can survive cold, such as *Pseudomonas* or *Staphylococcus*	• Chills, fever, vomiting, abdominal cramping, diarrhea, shock, signs of renal failure	• Provide broad-spectrum antibiotics, corticosteroids, or epinephrine, as prescribed. • Maintain strict blood-storage control. • Change blood administration set and filter every 4 hours or after every 2 units. • Infuse each unit of blood over 2 to 4 hours; stop the infusion if the time span exceeds 4 hours. • Maintain sterile technique when administering blood products.
BLEEDING TENDENCIES • Low platelet count in stored blood, causing thrombocytopenia	• Abnormal bleeding and oozing from a cut, a break in the skin surface, or the gums; abnormal bruising and petechiae	• Administer platelets, fresh frozen plasma, or cryoprecipitate, as ordered. • Monitor platelet count.
CIRCULATORY OVERLOAD • May result from infusing whole blood too rapidly	• Increased plasma volume, back pain, chest tightness, chills, fever, dyspnea, flushed feeling, headache, hypertension, increased central venous pressure and jugular vein pressure	• Monitor blood pressure. • Use packed RBCs instead of whole blood. • Administer diuretics, as ordered.
ELEVATED BLOOD AMMONIA LEVEL • Increased ammonia level in stored donor blood	• Confusion, forgetfulness, lethargy	• Monitor ammonia level in blood. • Decrease the amount of protein in the patient's diet. • If indicated, give neomycin.

(continued)

GUIDE TO TRANSFUSION REACTIONS *(continued)*

Reaction and causes	Signs and symptoms	Nursing interventions
EXOGENOUS *(continued)*		
HEMOSIDEROSIS • Increased level of hemosiderin (iron-containing pigment) from RBC destruction, especially after many transfusions	• Iron plasma level exceeding 200 mg/dl	• Perform a phlebotomy to remove excess iron.
HYPOCALCEMIA • Citrate toxicity occurs when citrate-treated blood is infused rapidly. Citrate binds with calcium, causing a calcium deficiency, or normal citrate metabolism becomes impeded by hepatic disease	• Arrhythmias, hypotension, muscle cramps, nausea and vomiting, seizures, tingling in fingers	• Slow or stop the transfusion, depending on the patient's reaction. Expect a more severe reaction in hypothermic patients or patients with elevated potassium levels. • Slowly administer calcium gluconate I.V., if ordered.
HYPOTHERMIA • Rapid infusion of large amounts of cold blood, which decreases body temperature	• Chills; shaking; hypotension; arrhythmias, especially bradycardia; cardiac arrest, if core temperature falls below 86° F (30° C)	• Stop the transfusion. • Warm the patient with blankets. • Place the patient in a warm environment if necessary. • Obtain an electrocardiogram (ECG). • Warm blood if the transfusion is resumed.
INCREASED OXYGEN AFFINITY FOR HEMOGLOBIN • Decreased level of 2,3-diphosphoglycerate in stored blood, causing an increase in the oxygen's hemoglobin affinity. When this occurs, oxygen stays in the patient's bloodstream and isn't released into body tissues	• Depressed respiratory rate, especially in patients with chronic lung disease	• Monitor arterial blood gas levels, and provide respiratory support, as needed.
POTASSIUM INTOXICATION • An abnormally high level of potassium in stored plasma caused by hemolysis of RBCs	• Diarrhea, intestinal colic, flaccidity, muscle twitching, oliguria, renal failure, bradycardia progressing to cardiac arrest, ECG changes with tall, peaked T waves	• Obtain an ECG. • Administer sodium polystyrene sulfonate (Kayexalate) orally or by enema. • Administer glucose 50% and insulin, bicarbonate, or calcium, as ordered, to force vitamin K into cells.

- Treat all transfusion reactions as serious until proved otherwise.
- If a transfusion reaction is anticipated, such as one that may occur in a leukemia patient, administer prophylactic treatment with antihistamines or antipyretics before blood administration, as ordered.
- To avoid a possible febrile reaction, the physician may order the blood washed to remove as many leukocytes as possible, or a leukocyte removal filter may be used during the transfusion.

Complications
- Anaphylaxis
- Sepsis
- Fever
- Shock
- Disseminated intravascular coagulation
- Heart failure
- Death

Be sure to cover:
- how a transfusion reaction occurs
- care being performed to prevent further complications
- signs and symptoms to report immediately.

- Time and date of the transfusion reaction
- Type and amount of infused blood or blood products
- Time transfusion was started and stopped
- Clinical signs of the transfusion reaction, in order of occurrence
- Vital signs
- Urine and blood samples sent to the laboratory
- Time and name of physician notified and orders given
- Treatment given and the patient's response to treatment
- Blood transfusion equipment sent to the blood bank
- Completion of a transfusion reaction form (if required by facility policy)
- Follow-up care
- Patient teaching

Selected references
"Documenting a Transfusion Reaction," *Nursing* 35(3):25, March 2005.

Narvios, A.B., et al. "Underreporting of Minor Transfusion Reactions in Cancer Patients," *Medscape General Medicine* 6(2):17, May 2004.

Sandler, S.G. "How I Manage Patients Suspected of Having had an IgA Anaphylactic Transfusion Reaction," *Transfusion* 46(1):10-13, January 2006.

Szymanski, I., and Seder, R. "Acute Pancreatitis Associated with Massive Hemolysis Due to a Delayed Hemolytic Transfusion Reactions," *Transfusion* 45 (10):1691-92, October 2005.

Weinstein, S.M. *Plumer's Principles and Practice of Intravenous Therapy,* 8th ed. Philadelphia: Lippincott Williams & Wilkins, 2006.

Tube feedings

OVERVIEW

- Involves delivery of a liquid feeding formula directly to the stomach (known as gavage feedings), duodenum, or jejunum
- Indicated for patient with dysphagia, oral or esophageal obstruction or injury; also for unconscious or intubated patient or patient recovering from GI tract surgery
- Duodenal or jejunal feedings: decrease risk of aspiration because the formula bypasses the pylorus
- Jejunal feedings: result in reduced pancreatic stimulation
- Patients usually receive gastric feedings on intermittent schedule; for duodenal or jejunal feedings, most patients tolerate continuous slow drip
- Liquid nutrient solutions: come in various formulas for administration through nasogastric tube, small-bore feeding tube, gastrostomy or jejunostomy tube, percutaneous endoscopic gastrostomy or jejunostomy tube, or gastrostomy feeding button
- Bulb syringe or large catheter-tip syringe: may be substituted for a gavage bag if the patient tolerates a gravity drip infusion
- Infusion pump possibly ordered to ensure accurate delivery of the prescribed formula

Contraindications
- Absent bowel sounds
- Intestinal obstruction (suspected)

EQUIPMENT

GASTRIC FEEDINGS
Feeding formula • graduated container • 120 ml of water • gavage bag with tubing and flow regulator clamp • pH test strip • towel or linen-saver pad • 60-ml syringe • optional: infusion controller and tubing set, adapter to connect gavage tubing to feeding tube
DUODENAL OR JEJUNAL FEEDINGS
Feeding formula • enteral administration set containing a gavage container, drip chamber, roller clamp or flow regulator, and tube connector • I.V. pole • 60-ml syringe with adapter tip • water • optional: pump administration set, Y-connector

Equipment preparation
- Refrigerate formulas prepared in the dietary department or pharmacy.
- Refrigerate commercial formulas only after opening them.
- Check the date on each formula container and discard expired formulas.
- Use powdered formula within 24 hours of mixing and always shake the container well to mix the solution.
- Allow the formula to warm to room temperature before administration.

⬥ NURSING ALERT Administering a cold formula increases the risk of diarrhea. Never warm the formula over direct heat or in a microwave. Heat may curdle the formula or change its chemical composition.

- Pour 60 ml of water into the graduated container.
- After closing the flow clamp on the administration set, pour the formula into the gavage bag.
- Hang no more than a 4- to 6-hour supply at one time to prevent bacterial growth.
- Open the flow clamp on the administration set to remove air from the lines.

ESSENTIAL STEPS

- Wash your hands thoroughly.
- Wear appropriate personal protective equipment, as necessary.
- Provide for privacy.
- Confirm the patient's identity using two patient identifiers according to facility policy.
- Explain the procedure to the patient.
- If the patient has a nasal or oral tube, cover his chest with a towel.
- Assess the patient's abdomen for bowel sounds and distention.
- Elevate the head of the bed and place the patient in low Fowler's position.

DELIVERING GASTRIC FEEDING
- Check tube patency and position. Remove the cap or plug and attach the syringe.

⬥ NURSING ALERT Never give a tube feeding until you're sure the tube is properly positioned in the patient's stomach. Administering a feeding through a misplaced tube can cause formula to enter the patient's lungs.

- Aspirate stomach contents. Examine aspirate and place a small amount on pH test strip. Aspirate of gastric fluid commonly appears grassy-green, clear, colorless with mucus shreds, or brown and has a pH of 5 or less.
- To assess gastric emptying, aspirate residual gastric contents and hold the feeding if residual volume is greater than the amount specified in the physician's order. Reinstill any aspirate obtained.
- Connect the gavage bag tubing to the feeding tube.
- When using a bulb or catheter-tip syringe, remove the bulb or plunger and attach the syringe to the pinched-off feeding tube to prevent excess air from entering the patient's stomach.
- When using an infusion controller, thread the tube from the formula container through the controller, purge the tubing of air, and attach it to the feeding tube.
- Open the regulator clamp on the gavage bag tubing and adjust the flow rate appropriately.
- When using a bulb syringe, fill the syringe with formula and release the feeding tube to allow formula to flow through it.
- Regulate the flow rate by adjusting the height at which you hold the syringe.
- To prevent air from entering the tube and the patient's stomach, never allow the syringe to empty completely.
- When using an infusion controller, set the flow rate according to the manufacturer's directions.
- Always administer a tube feeding slowly depending on the patient's tolerance and the physician's order to prevent sudden stomach distention, which can cause nausea, vomiting, cramps, or diarrhea.
- After administering the formula, flush the tubing to maintain patency by adding about 60 ml of water to the gavage bag or bulb syringe, or manually flush it using a barrel syringe.
- When administering a continuous feeding, flush the feeding tube every

4 hours to help prevent tube occlusion.

- Monitor gastric emptying during a continuous feeding every 4 hours.
- To discontinue gastric feeding, close the regulator clamp on the gavage bag tubing and turn off the infusion controller or disconnect the syringe from the feeding tube.
- Plug the end of the feeding tube.
- Leave the patient in semi-Fowler's or high Fowler's position for at least 30 minutes.
- Rinse all reusable equipment with warm water.
- Dry the equipment and store it in a convenient place for the next feeding.
- Change equipment every 24 hours or according to the facility's policy.

DELIVERING DUODENAL OR JEJUNAL FEEDING

- Open the enteral administration set and hang the gavage container on the I.V. pole.
- If you're using a nasoduodenal tube, measure its length to check tube placement.

NURSING ALERT Residual solution may be absent when you aspirate through a nasoduodenal tube.

- Open the flow clamp and regulate the flow to the desired rate.
- To regulate the rate using a volumetric infusion pump, follow the manufacturer's directions.
- Flush the tube every 4 hours with water.
- A needle catheter jejunostomy tube may require flushing every 2 hours to prevent formula buildup inside the tube. A Y-connector may be useful for frequent flushing.
- Change equipment according to facility policy.

◆ SPECIAL CONSIDERATIONS

- If the feeding solution doesn't initially flow through a bulb syringe, attach the bulb and squeeze it gently to start the flow, and then remove the bulb.
- During continuous feedings, assess the patient for abdominal distention.
- If the patient becomes nauseated or vomits, stop the feeding immediately.

- If the patient develops diarrhea, give small, frequent, less concentrated feedings, or give bolus feedings over a longer time. Antidiarrheals or a change in formula may be ordered.
- If the patient is constipated, the pracitioner may increase fruit, vegetable, or sugar content of the formula.
- Assess the patient's hydration status; increase fluid intake as necessary. If the condition persists, give an appropriate drug or enema, as ordered.
- After consulting with a pharmacist, administer drugs through the feeding tube by crushing tablets or opening and diluting capsules in water before administering them; finish by flushing the tube to ensure full instillation of medication.

NURSING ALERT There have been many documented formula-medication interactions. Be especially cautious when administering phenytoin, warfarin, and ciprofloxacin.

NURSING ALERT Never crush enteric-coated drugs or time-released medications to administer by feeding tube.

- Keep in mind that some drugs may change the osmolarity of the feeding formula and cause diarrhea.
- Because a small-bore feeding tube can kink, change the patient's position or withdraw the tube a few inches and restart. Never use a guide wire to reposition the tube.
- Monitor blood glucose levels to assess glucose tolerance and serum electrolytes, blood urea nitrogen, and serum osmolality.
- Check the flow rate hourly.
- For duodenal or jejunal feeding, most patients tolerate a continuous drip better than bolus feedings.
- Until the patient acquires a tolerance, you may need to dilute formula to one-half or three-quarter strength.

Complications

- Erosion of esophageal, tracheal, nasal, or oropharyngeal mucosa
- Bloating and retention
- Dehydration, diarrhea, vomiting, and constipation; dumping syndrome
- Hyperglycemia
- Hyperosmolar dehydration
- Pneumonia
- Tube occlusion or displacement

▶ PATIENT TEACHING

Be sure to cover:
- using an infusion control device
- use of the syringe or bag and tubing
- care of the tube and insertion site
- formula preparation and storage
- signs and symptoms that require notifying the physician.

●◆ DOCUMENTATION

- Date and time of all care
- Abdominal assessment
- Amount of residual gastric contents
- Verification of tube placement
- Amount, type, and time of feeding
- Tube patency
- Patient's tolerance to the feeding
- Hydration status
- Drugs given through the tube
- Administration set changes
- Oral and nasal hygiene
- Laboratory results
- Name of physician notified of complications, orders given, and your actions
- Patient teaching

Selected references

Ellet, M.L., "Important Facts about Intestinal Feeding Tube Placement," *Gastroenterology Nursing* 29(2):112-24, March-April 2006.

Evans-Smith, P. *Taylor's Clinical Nursing Skills.* Philadelphia: Lippincott Williams & Wilkins, 2005.

Ista, F., and Joosten, K. "Nuritional Assessment and Enteral Support of Critically Ill Children," *Critical Care Nursing Clinics of North America* 17(4):385-93, December 2005.

Metheny, N.A., et al. "Indicators of Tubesite During Feedings," *Journal of Neuroscience Nursing* 37(6):320-35, December 2005.

Urinary diversion stoma care

● OVERVIEW

- Provides an alternative route for urine flow when a disorder, such as an invasive bladder tumor, impedes normal drainage
- Usually requires the patient to wear a urine-collection appliance and to care for a stoma created during surgery
- Permanent urinary diversion is indicated in any condition that requires total cystectomy
- Urinary diversions may also be indicated for patients with neurogenic bladder, congenital anomaly, traumatic injury to the lower urinary tract, or severe chronic urinary tract infection
- Two types of permanent urinary diversions with stomas: Ileal conduit and continent urinary diversion (see *Types of permanent urinary diversion*)

Contraindications
- None known

❖ EQUIPMENT

Soap and warm water • waterproof trash bag • linen-saver pad • hypoallergenic paper tape • povidone-iodine solution • urine-collection container • rubber catheter (usually #14 or #16 French) • ruler • scissors • urine-collection appliance (with or without antireflux valve) • graduated cylinder • cottonless gauze pads (some rolled, some flat) • washcloth • skin barrier in liquid, paste, wafer, or sheet form • appliance belt • stoma covering (nonadherent gauze pad or panty liner) • two pairs of gloves • optional: adhesive solvent, irrigating syringe, tampon, hair dryer, electric razor, regular gauze pads, vinegar, and deodorant tablets

Commercially packaged stoma care kits are available. In place of soap and water, you can use adhesive remover pads, if available, or cotton gauze saturated with adhesive solvent.

Equipment preparation
- Wash your hands thoroughly.
- Assemble all the equipment on the patient's overbed table.
- Open the waterproof trash bag and place it near the patient's bed.
- Provide for privacy.
- Measure the diameter of the stoma.
- Cut the opening of the appliance with the scissors to no more than ⅛″ to ⅙″ (0.3 to 0.4 cm) larger than the diameter of the stoma.

- Moisten the faceplate of the appliance with a small amount of solvent or water to prepare it for adhesion.

III ESSENTIAL STEPS

- Wash hands again.
- Confirm the patient's identity using two patient identifiers according to facility policy.
- Explain the procedure to the patient.
- Wear appropriate personal protective equipment.
- Place the bed in low Fowler's position so the patient's abdomen is flat, eliminating skin folds that could cause the appliance to slip or irritate the skin.
- Put on gloves and place the linen-saver pad under the patient's side, near the stoma.
- Open the drain valve of the appliance being replaced to empty the urine into the graduated cylinder.
- To remove the appliance, use a washcloth to apply soap and water or adhesive solvent as you gently push the skin back from the pouch.
- If the appliance is disposable, discard it in the waterproof trash bag; if it's reusable, clean it with soap and lukewarm water and let it air-dry.
- If adhesive remains on the skin, gently rub it off with a dry gauze pad.

◆ **NURSING ALERT** To avoid irritating the patient's stoma, don't touch it with the adhesive solvent.

- To keep the skin dry while you're changing the appliance, wick the urine with an absorbent, lint-free material. (See *Wicking urine from a stoma.*)
- Use water to wash off any crystal deposits that formed around the stoma.
- If urine has stagnated and has a strong odor, use soap to wash it off.
- Rinse thoroughly to remove any oily residue that could cause the appliance to slip.
- Dry the peristomal area thoroughly with a gauze pad because moisture will keep the appliance from sticking.
- Remove any hair from the area with scissors or an electric razor to prevent hair follicles from becoming irritated when the pouch is removed, which can cause folliculitis.

TYPES OF PERMANENT URINARY DIVERSION

The steps involved in creating an ileal conduit or a continent urinary diversion are described here.

Ileal conduit
A short segment of the ileum is excised, and the intestine is reanastomosed. One end of the excised section is closed, and the ureters are dissected from the bladder and anastomosed to the ileal segment. The open end of the ileal segment is brought out to the abdominal wall as a stoma. Urine will now pass through this conduit and out the opening in the abdomen.

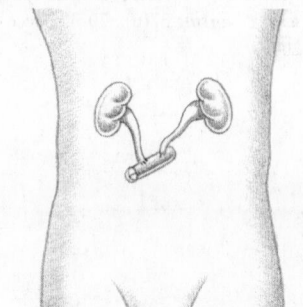

Continent urinary diversion
A tube is formed from part of the ascending colon and ileum. One end of the tube is brought to the skin to form the stoma. At the internal end of this tube, a nipple valve is constructed so urine won't drain out unless a catheter is inserted through the stoma into the newly formed bladder pouch. The urethral neck is sutured closed.

Another type of continent urinary diversion (not pictured here) is "hooked" back to the urethra, obviating the need for a stoma.

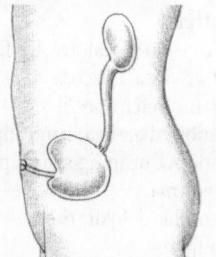

- Note the size, color, and shape of the stoma.
- Check the color and the appearance of the suture line and examine any moisture or effluent.
- Inspect the peristomal skin for redness, irritation, and intactness.
- When applying a skin barrier, cut it to fit over the stoma, remove any protective backing and set the barrier aside with the adhesive side up.
- When applying a liquid barrier (such as Skin-Prep), saturate a gauze pad and coat the peristomal skin, moving in concentric circles outward from the stoma until you've covered an area 2″ (5.1 cm) larger than the wafer. Let the skin dry for several minutes; it should feel tacky.
- Gently press the wafer around the stoma, sticky side down, smoothing from the stoma outward.
- If you're using a barrier paste, squeeze a ribbon of paste directly onto the peristomal skin making several concentric circles starting about ½″ (1.5 cm) from the stoma. Dip your fingers into lukewarm water and smooth the paste until the skin is completely covered from the edge of the stoma to 3″ to 4″ (7.5 to 10 cm) outward. The paste should be ¼″ to ½″ (0.5 to 1.5 cm) thick. Discard the gloves, wash your hands, and put on new gloves.
- Remove the material used for wicking urine and place it in the trash bag.
- Place the appliance over the stoma, leaving only a small amount (⅜″ to ¾″ [1 to 2 cm]) of skin exposed.
- Secure the faceplate of the appliance to the skin with paper tape, if recommended.
- Apply the appliance belt, if one is being used, loose enough to insert two fingers under it and making sure that it's on a level with the stoma so it doesn't break the bag's seal or rub against the stoma.
- Dispose of the used materials appropriately.

◆ SPECIAL CONSIDERATIONS

- Provide emotional support as the patient adjusts to the stoma.
- When positioned correctly, most appliances remain in place for at least 3 days without leakage but should be changed after 5 days.
- Empty the appliance when it's one-third to one-half full because the weight of the urine can loosen the seal around the stoma and separate the appliance from the skin.
- Some devices don't require a belt; instead, the pouch has a ridge that fits over the rim of barrier adhesive and snaps securely into place.
- Wash a reusable appliance with soap and lukewarm water; rinse and allow to air dry. Soaking a reusable appliance in vinegar and water or placing deodorant tablets in it can dissipate stubborn odors.
- Encourage an acid-ash diet that includes ascorbic acid and cranberry juice to increase urine acidity and reduce bacterial action and fermentation, the underlying causes of odor.
- Encourage fluid intake to reduce odor and the risk of infection.
- Be aware that mucus may be present in the urine.
- Monitor the patient with a continent urinary diversion for reduced urinary output, which may indicate obstruction.

Complications
- Mucosal bleeding
- Peristomal skin excoriation and irritation
- Infection

▶ PATIENT TEACHING

Be sure to cover:
- care for stoma and appliance at home
- types of and how to use equipment
- how to recognize problems and correct them
- importance of increasing fluid intake and consuming an acid-ash diet
- emotional adjustment to a stoma
- support services provided by ostomy clubs and American Cancer Society
- follow-up with a visiting nurse or an enterostomal therapist.

●◆ DOCUMENTATION

- Date, time, and location of stoma care
- Condition of the stoma, noting any redness, irritation, breakdown, bleeding, or other unusual conditions
- Whether the stoma is inverted, flush with the skin, or protruding (noting how much it protrudes)
- Appearance and condition of the peristomal skin
- Stoma care provided
- Appearance of urine
- Type of appliance used, appliance size, type of adhesive and skin protectant
- Whether the appliance was changed
- Patient teaching and ability to provide self-care
- Emotional support given

Selected references

Burch, J. "The Pre- and Postoperative Nursing Care for Patients with a Stoma," *British Journal of Nursing* 14(6):310-18, March-April 2005.

Gray, E.H., et al. "Stoma Care in the School Setting," *Journal of School Nursing* 22(2):74-80, April 2006.

Gray, N., et al. "Counseling Patients Undergoing Urinary Diversion: Does the Type of Diversion Influence Quality of Life," *Journal of Wound, Ostomy, and Continence Nursing* 21(1):7-15, January-February 2005.

WICKING URINE FROM A STOMA

Use a piece of rolled, cotton-free gauze or a tampon to wick urine from a stoma. Working by capillary action, wicking absorbs urine while you prepare the patient's skin to hold a urine-collection appliance.

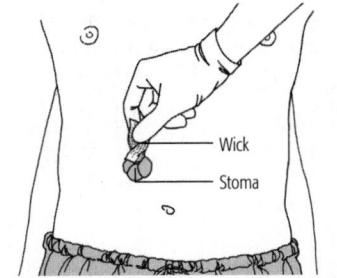

Venipuncture

● OVERVIEW

- Performed to obtain a venous blood sample
- Involves piercing a vein with a needle and collecting blood in a syringe or evacuated tube, most commonly from the antecubital fossa
- May involve other sites, such as veins in the dorsal forearm, the dorsum of the hand or foot, or another accessible location

Contraindications

- Extremity with arteriovenous (AV) fistula
- Ipsilateral extremity of mastectomy
- Infected site
- Sites with edema
- Sites of previous hematomas or vascular injury

❖ EQUIPMENT

Tourniquet • gloves • syringe or evacuated tubes and needle holder • alcohol or povidone-iodine pads • 20G or 21G needle for the forearm or 25G needle for the hand, and ankle, and for children • color-coded collection tubes containing appropriate additives • labels • laboratory request form • 2″ × 2″ gauze pads • adhesive bandage

Equipment preparation

- When using evacuated tubes, open the needle packet, attach the needle to its holder, and select the appropriate tubes.
- When using a syringe, choose one large enough to hold all the blood required for the test, and attach the appropriate needle.
- Label all collection tubes with the patient's name and room number, physician's name, and date and time of collection.

▌▌▌ ESSENTIAL STEPS

- Wash hands thoroughly and put on gloves.
- Confirm the patient's identity using two patient identifiers according to facility policy.
- Explain the procedure to the patient.
- Wear appropriate personal protective equipment throughout the procedure.
- Assess patient for complaints of faintness, dizziness, diaphoresis or nausea with previous blood draws.
- If the patient is on bed rest, ask him to lie supine, with his head slightly elevated and his arms at his sides.
- Ask the ambulatory patient to sit in a chair and support his arm securely on an armrest or table.
- Assess the patient's veins to determine the best puncture site. (See *Common venipuncture sites.*)
- Observe the skin for the vein's blue color, or palpate the vein for a firm rebound sensation.
- Tie a tourniquet 2″ (5 cm) proximal to the area chosen to produce venous dilation.
- If the tourniquet fails to dilate the vein, have the patient open and close his fist repeatedly. Next, ask him to close his fist as you insert the needle and to open it again when the needle is in place.
- Clean the venipuncture site with an alcohol or povidone-iodine pad.

◈ **NURSING ALERT** Don't wipe off the povidone-iodine with alcohol because alcohol cancels the effect of povidone-iodine.

- Wipe in a circular motion, spiraling outward from the site to avoid introducing potentially infectious skin flora into the vessel during the procedure.
- If you use alcohol, apply it with friction for 30 seconds, or until the final pad comes away clean.
- Allow the skin to dry before performing venipuncture.

✴ **AGE-RELATED CONCERN** When performing venipuncture on a child, apply a topical anesthetic, such as lidocaine-prilocaine emulsion (EMLA cream), to the site 1 hour before the procedure to reduce pain. Check for sensitivity or allergy to local anesthetics,

such as lidocaine, before using EMLA cream.

- Immobilize the vein by pressing just below the venipuncture site with your thumb and drawing the skin taut.
- Position the needle holder or syringe with the needle bevel up and the shaft parallel to the path of the vein and at a 30-degree angle to the arm.
- Insert the needle into the vein.
- When using a syringe, venous blood appears in the hub; withdraw the blood slowly, pulling the plunger of the syringe gently until you obtain the required sample.

◈ **NURSING ALERT** When using a needle and syringe to draw blood, pulling the plunger too forcibly can collapse the vein.

- When using a needle holder and an evacuated tube, grasp the holder securely to stabilize it in the vein, and push down on the collection tube until the needle punctures the rubber stopper, and blood will flow into the tube automatically.
- Remove the tourniquet as soon as blood flows adequately to prevent stasis and hemoconcentration, which can impair test results.

◈ **NURSING ALERT** If the flow is sluggish, leave the tourniquet in place longer, but always remove it before withdrawing the needle. Don't leave the tourniquet on for longer than 3 minutes.

- Continue to fill the required tubes, removing one and inserting another.
- Gently rotate each tube as you remove it to help mix the additive with the sample.
- After you've drawn the sample, place a gauze pad over the puncture site, and slowly and gently remove the needle from the vein.
- When using an evacuated tube, remove it from the needle holder to release the vacuum before withdrawing the needle from the vein.
- Apply gentle pressure to the puncture site for 2 or 3 minutes or until bleeding stops.
- After bleeding stops, apply an adhesive bandage.
- To transfer the sample to a collection tube, if you've used a syringe, detach the needle from the syringe, open the collection tube, and gently empty the

sample into the tube to avoid foaming, which can cause hemolysis.
- Discard syringes, needles, and used gloves in the appropriate containers.

◆ SPECIAL CONSIDERATIONS

- Never draw a venous sample from an arm or leg that's already being used for I.V. therapy or blood administration because this may affect test results.
- Don't collect a venous sample from an infection site because this may introduce pathogens into the vascular system.
- Avoid drawing blood from edematous areas, AV shunts, or sites of previous hematoma or vascular injury.
- If the patient has large, distended, and highly visible veins, perform venipuncture without a tourniquet to minimize the risk of hematoma formation.
- If the patient has a clotting disorder or is receiving anticoagulant therapy, maintain firm pressure on the venipuncture site for at least 5 minutes after withdrawing the needle to prevent hematoma formation.

AGE-RELATED CONCERN Use pediatric tubes for collecting specimens on infants and children; the volumes are less than volumes collected on adults. Pediatric tubes may also be used in elderly patients or others with low blood volume, as indicated. Check facility policy.

- Avoid using veins in the patient's legs for venipuncture, if possible, because this increases the risk of thrombophlebitis.

Complications
- Hematoma
- Infection

▶ PATIENT TEACHING

Be sure to cover:
- how the test will be performed and what sensations the patient can expect
- laboratory tests being performed
- need to report bleeding, hematoma formation, or signs and symptoms of infection at the site
- when the dressing can be removed.

●◆ DOCUMENTATION

- Date and time of venipuncture
- Site of venipuncture
- Name of the test
- Time the sample was sent to the laboratory
- Amount of blood collected
- Patient's temperature
- Adverse reactions to the procedure
- Patient's tolerance of the procedure
- Patient teaching

Selected references
Higgins, D. "Venepuncture," *Nursing Times* 100(39):30-31, September-October 2004.

Melhuisj, S., and Payne, H. "Nurses' Attitudes to Pain Management During Routine Venepuncture in Young Children," *Paediatric Nursing* 18(2):20-23, March 2006.

Rosenthal, K. "Tips for Venipuncture in Children," *Nursing* 35(12):31, December 2005.

Thurgate, C., and Heppell, S. "Needle Phobia—Changing Venepuncture Practice in Ambulatory Care," *Paediatric Nursing* 17(9)15-8, November 2005.

COMMON VENIPUNCTURE SITES

The illustrations below show the anatomic locations of veins commonly used for venipuncture. The most commonly used sites are on the forearm, followed by those on the hand.

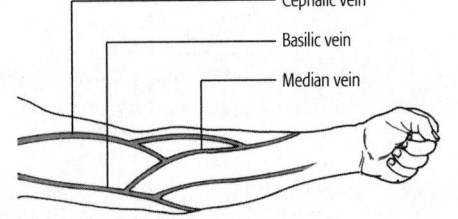

Cephalic vein
Basilic vein
Median vein

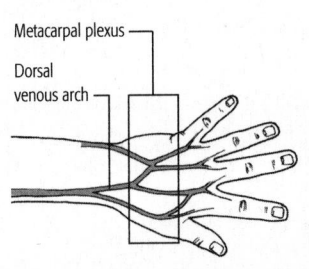

Metacarpal plexus
Dorsal venous arch

Wound care, dehiscence and evisceration

● OVERVIEW

- Surgical wounds: usually heal well; however, edges of a wound may fail to join or may separate even after they seem to be healing normally, which may lead to more serious complications of evisceration, in which a portion of the viscera (usually a bowel loop) protrudes through the incision
- Evisceration: may lead to peritonitis and septic shock
- Dehiscence and evisceration: most likely to occur 6 or 7 days after surgery, when sutures may have been removed and the patient can cough easily and breathe deeply, which strain the incision (see *Recognizing dehiscence and evisceration*)
- Caused by:
  - poor nutrition (from inadequate intake or condition such as diabetes mellitus)
  - chronic pulmonary or cardiac disease and metastatic cancer, because the injured tissue doesn't get needed nutrients and oxygen
  - localized wound infection that may limit closure, delay healing, and weaken the incision
  - stress on the incision from coughing or vomiting that may cause abdominal distention or severe stretching

Contraindications
- None known

❖ EQUIPMENT

Two sterile towels • 1 L of sterile normal saline solution • sterile irrigation set, including basin, solution container, and 50-ml catheter-tip syringe • several large abdominal dressings • sterile, waterproof drape • linen-saver pads • sterile gloves

RETURN TO THE OPERATING ROOM
All previous equipment • I.V. administration set and I.V. fluids • equipment for nasogastric (NG) intubation • sedative, as ordered • suction apparatus

Equipment preparation
- Gather all equipment quickly and ensure that it's readily available at the bedside.
- Wash hands thoroughly.

▌▌ ESSENTIAL STEPS

- Confirm patient's identity using two patient identifiers according to facility policy.
- Provide reassurance and support to ease the patient's anxiety.
- Tell the patient to stay in bed. If possible, stay with him while someone else notifies the practitioner and collects the necessary equipment.
- Place a linen-saver pad under the patient to keep sheets dry when you moisten the exposed viscera.
- Using sterile technique, unfold a sterile towel to create a sterile field.
- Open the package containing the irrigation set, and place the basin, solution container, and 50-ml syringe on the sterile field.
- Open the bottle of normal saline solution and pour about 400 ml into the solution container. Also pour about 200 ml into the sterile basin.
- Open several large abdominal dressings and place them on the sterile field.
- Put on the sterile gloves and place one or two of the large abdominal dressings into the basin to saturate them with normal saline solution.
- Place the moistened dressings over the exposed viscera; place a sterile, waterproof drape over the dressings to prevent the sheets from getting wet.

RECOGNIZING DEHISCENCE AND EVISCERATION

In wound dehiscence, the layers of the surgical wound separate. With evisceration, the viscera (in this case, a bowel loop) protrude through the surgical incision.

Wound dehiscence

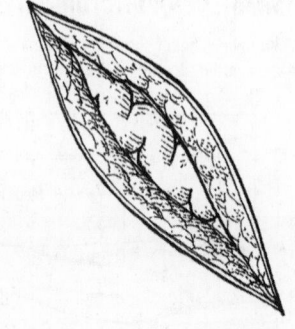

Evisceration of bowel loop

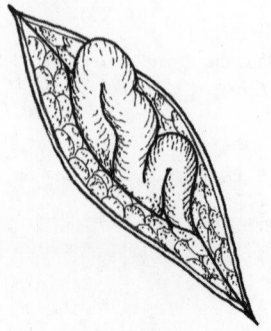

- Moisten the dressings every hour by drawing normal saline solution into a syringe and squirting solution on the dressings.
- When you moisten the dressings, inspect the color of the viscera.

⬥ NURSING ALERT If the viscera appears dusky or black, notify the practitioner immediately. With its blood supply interrupted, a protruding organ may become ischemic and necrotic.

- Keep the patient on absolute bed rest in low Fowler's position (no more than 20 degrees' elevation) with his knees flexed to prevent injury and reduce stress on an abdominal incision.

⬥ NURSING ALERT Don't allow the patient to have anything by mouth to decrease risk of aspiration during surgery.

- Monitor the patient's pulse, respirations, blood pressure, and temperature every 15 minutes to detect shock.
- If necessary, prepare him to return to the operating room. After gathering the appropriate equipment, start an I.V. infusion, as ordered.
- Insert an NG tube and connect it to continuous or intermittent low suction, as ordered. NG intubation may make the patient gag or vomit, causing further evisceration; therefore, the practitioner may choose to have the NG tube inserted in the operating room with the patient under anesthesia.
- Give preoperative drugs to the patient, as ordered.
- Continue to reassure the patient while you prepare him for surgery.
- Make sure the patient has signed a consent form and the operating room staff has been informed about the procedure.

✦ SPECIAL CONSIDERATIONS

- If you're caring for a postoperative patient who's at risk for poor healing, make sure he gets an adequate supply of protein, vitamins, and calories. Monitor his dietary deficiencies; discuss problems with the practitioner and dietitian.
- When changing wound dressings, always use sterile technique.
- Inspect the incision with each dressing change; if you recognize early signs of infection, start treatment before dehiscence or evisceration can occur.
- If local infection develops, clean the wound, as necessary, to eliminate a buildup of purulent drainage.
- Make sure bandages aren't so tight that they limit blood supply to the wound.

Complications
- Infection
- Peritonitis
- Septic shock
- Necrosis

▶ PATIENT TEACHING

Be sure to cover:
- what has happened
- procedures being performed.

◆ DOCUMENTATION

- Time of event
- Patient's activity preceding the problem
- Patient's condition and the time the practitioner was notified
- Appearance of the wound or eviscerated organ; the amount, color, consistency, and odor of drainage; and nursing actions taken
- Vital signs, the patient's response to the incident, and the practitioner's actions
- Changes to the care plan that reflect nursing actions taken to promote proper healing

Selected references
Banwell, P.E., et al. "Treatment of Dehisced and Infected Wounds," *Journal of Wound Care* 14(3):110, March 2005.
Moz, T. "Wound Dehiscence and Evisceration," *Nursing* 34(5):88, May 2004.
Penn, E., and Rayment, S. "Management of a Dehisced Abdominal Wound with VAC Therapy," *British Journal of Nursing* 13(4):194-201, February-March 2004.

Wound care, traumatic

- Types of traumatic wounds:
  - abrasion: scraped skin, with partial loss of skin surface
  - laceration: torn skin with jagged, irregular edges; severity dependent on size, depth, and location
  - puncture wound: occurs when a pointed object penetrates the skin
  - amputation: involves removal of part of the body (limb or part of a limb)
- Assessment of patient's ABCs: (airway, breathing, and circulation) top priority
- When ABCs are stabilized, bleeding controlled with firm, direct pressure and elevation of the extremity
- If bleeding continues, application of pressure to pressure point
- Management and cleaning technique usually dependent on specific type of wound and degree of contamination

Contraindicatons
- None known

Sterile basin • normal saline solution • sterile 4″ × 4″ gauze pads • sterile gloves • clean gloves • dry sterile dressing • nonadherent pad, or petroleum gauze • linen-saver pad • scissors • towel • goggles, mask, gown • 50-ml catheter-tip syringe • surgical scrub brush • antibacterial ointment • porous tape • sterile forceps • sutures and suture set • optional: hydrogen peroxide

Equipment preparation
- Place a linen-saver pad under the area to be cleaned and remove clothing covering the wound.
- If necessary, clip hair around the wound with scissors.
- Assemble needed equipment at the patient's bedside.
- Fill a sterile basin with normal saline solution.
- Make sure the treatment area has enough light to allow close observation of the wound.
- Depending on the nature and location of the wound, wear sterile or clean gloves to avoid spreading infection.

- Confirm the patient's identity using two patient identifiers according to facility policy.
- Check the patient's medical history for previous tetanus immunization and, if needed and ordered, arrange for immunization.
- Administer medication for pain, if ordered.
- Wash your hands thoroughly.
- Use appropriate protective equipment, such as a gown, gloves, mask, and goggles, if spraying or splashing of body fluids is possible.

ABRASION
- Flush the scraped skin with normal saline solution.
- Remove dirt or gravel with a sterile 4″ × 4″ gauze pad moistened with normal saline solution. Rub in the opposite direction from which the dirt or gravel became embedded.
- If the wound is extremely dirty, use a surgical brush to clean it.
- Allow a small wound to dry and form a scab. A larger wound may need to be covered with a nonadherent pad or petroleum gauze and a light dressing.
- Apply antibacterial ointment, if ordered.

LACERATION
- Moisten a sterile 4″ × 4″ gauze pad with normal saline solution and clean the wound, working outward from its center to about 2″ (5 cm) beyond its edges.
- Discard the soiled gauze pad and use a fresh one, as necessary, until the wound is clean.
- If the wound is dirty, irrigate with a 50-ml catheter-tip syringe and normal saline solution.
- Help the practitioner suture the wound edges using the suture kit, or apply sterile strips of porous tape.
- Apply prescribed antibacterial ointment to help prevent infection.
- Apply a dry sterile dressing over the wound to absorb drainage and help prevent bacterial contamination.

PUNCTURE WOUND

- If the wound is minor, allow it to bleed for a few minutes before cleaning it; for a larger puncture wound, irrigate it before applying a dry dressing.
- Stabilize an embedded foreign object until the practitioner can remove it.
- Clean the wound as you would clean a laceration.

AMPUTATION

- Apply a gauze pad moistened with normal saline solution to the amputation site. Elevate the affected part, and immobilize it for surgery.
- Recover the amputated part, and prepare it for transport to a facility where microvascular surgery is performed.

◆ SPECIAL CONSIDERATIONS

- When irrigating a traumatic wound, avoid using more than 8 psi of pressure. High-pressure irrigation can seriously interfere with healing, kill cells, and allow bacteria to infiltrate the tissue.
- Use normal saline solution or hydrogen peroxide—its foaming action facilitates debris removal. However, peroxide should never be instilled into a deep wound because of risk of embolism from evolving gases.
- Solutions such as hydrogen peroxide or sodium hypochloraite may damage tissue and delay healing.
- Rinse your hands thoroughly after using hydrogen peroxide.

  NURSING ALERT Avoid cleaning a traumatic wound with alcohol because it causes pain and tissue dehydration. Avoid using antiseptics for wound cleaning because they can impede healing. Never use a cotton ball or cotton-filled gauze pad to clean a wound because cotton fibers left in the wound can cause contamination.

- After a wound has been cleaned, the practitioner may want to debride it to remove dead tissue and reduce risk of infection and scarring. If this is to be done, pack the wound with gauze pads soaked in normal saline solution until debridement.
- Observe for signs and symptoms of infection, such as warm red skin at the site or purulent discharge. Infection of a traumatic wound can delay healing, increase scar formation, and trigger systemic infection such as septicemia.
- Observe dressings. If edema is present, adjust the dressing to avoid impairing circulation to the area.

Complications

- Temporary increase in the patient's pain during cleaning and care of traumatic wounds
- Further disruption of tissue integrity during excessive, vigorous cleaning

▶ PATIENT TEACHING

Be sure to cover:
- reason for the procedure.
- follow-up wound care, if appropriate.

●○ DOCUMENTATION

- Date and time of the procedure
- Wound size and condition, drug administration, and specific wound care measures
- Patient's response to the procedure
- Patient teaching.

Selected references

Chavez, B. "Making the Case for Using a Silicone Dressing in Burn Wound Management," *Ostomy/Wound Management* 51(11A Suppl):17-18, November 2005.

Clontz, A.S., et al. "Trauma Nursing: Amputation," *RN* 67(7):38-43, July 2004.

Eckert, K.L. "Penetrating and Blunt Abdominal Trauma," *Critical Care Nursing Quarterly* 28(1):41-59, January-March 2005.

Hoban, V. "Wound Care: What Every Nurse Should Know," *Nursing Times* 101(12):20-22, March 2005.

Worley, C.A. "Assessment and Terminology: Critical Issues in Wound Care," *Dermatology Nursing* 16(5):451-52, 457, October 2004.

Wound irrigation

● OVERVIEW

- Cleans tissues and flushes cell debris and drainage from an open wound
- Promotes wound healing from inner tissue layers outward to the skin surface and prevents premature surface healing over abscess pocket or infected tract
- Requires strict sterile technique
- Usually followed by packing of open wound to absorb additional drainage

Contraindications

- None known

IRRIGATING A DEEP WOUND

When irrigating a wound, attach a 19G needle or catheter to a 35-ml piston syringe. This set-up delivers an irrigation pressure of 8 psi, which is effective in cleaning the wound and reducing the risk of trauma and wound infection. To prevent tissue damage or, in an abdominal wound, intestinal perforation, avoid forcing the needle or catheter into the wound.

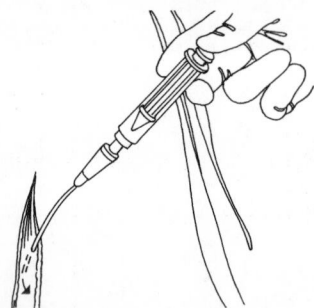

Irrigate the wound with gentle pressure until the solution returns clean. Then position the emesis basin under the wound to collect any remaining drainage.

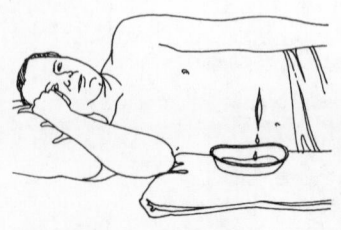

❖ EQUIPMENT

Waterproof trash bag • linen-saver pad • emesis basin • clean gloves • sterile gloves • facemask • gown, if indicated • prescribed irrigant such as sterile normal saline solution • sterile water or normal saline solution • soft rubber or plastic catheter • sterile container • materials as needed for wound care • sterile irrigation and dressing set • commercial wound cleanser • 35-ml piston syringe with 19G needle or catheter • skin-protectant wipe

Equipment preparation

- Wash your hands thoroughly.
- Assemble all equipment in the patient's room.
- Check the expiration date on each sterile package and inspect for tears.
- Check the sterilization date and the date that each bottle of irrigating solution was opened.

  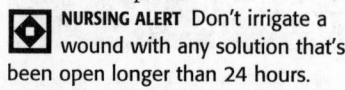 **NURSING ALERT** Don't irrigate a wound with any solution that's been open longer than 24 hours.
- Using aseptic technique, dilute the prescribed irrigant to the correct proportions with sterile water or normal saline solution, if necessary.
- Let the solution stand until it reaches room temperature, or warm it to 90° to 95° F (32.2° to 35° C).
- Open the waterproof trash bag, and place it near the patient's bed.

❚❚❚ ESSENTIAL STEPS

- Confirm the patient's identity using two patient identifiers according to facility policy.
- Explain the procedure to the patient and family members.
- Wear appropriate personal protective equipment.

  NURSING ALERT Always follow the standard precautions guidelines of the Centers for Disease Control and Prevention (CDC).
- Maintain asepsis throughout the procedure.
- Check the physician's order, and assess the patient's condition.
- Identify the patient's allergies, especially to povidone-iodine or other topical solutions or medications.
- Provide privacy, and position the patient correctly for the procedure so that the solution flows from the clean to the dirty area of the wound to prevent contamination of clean tissue by exudate.
- Place the linen-saver pad under the patient.
- Place the emesis basin below the wound to catch the irrigating solution.
- Wash hands thoroughly and put on clean gloves and gown.
- Remove the soiled dressing, and discard the dressing and gloves in the trash bag.
- Establish a sterile field with all the equipment and supplies you need for irrigation and wound care.
- Pour the prescribed amount of irrigating solution into a sterile container.
- Put on sterile gloves, gown, and face mask, if indicated.
- Fill the syringe with the irrigating solution, and connect the catheter to the syringe.
- Gently instill a slow, steady stream of irrigating solution into the wound until the syringe empties. (See *Irrigating a deep wound.*)
- Make sure the solution reaches all areas of the wound and flows from the clean to dirty area of the wound.
- Refill the syringe, reconnect it to the catheter, and repeat the irrigation.
- Continue to irrigate the wound until you've administered the prescribed

amount of solution or until the solution returns clear.

- Note the amount of solution administered and returned.
- Remove and discard the catheter and syringe in the waterproof trash bag.
- Keep the patient positioned to allow further wound drainage into the basin.
- Clean the area around the wound with normal saline solution.
- Wipe intact skin with a skin protectant wipe and allow it to dry well to help prevent skin breakdown and infection.
- Pack the wound, if ordered, and apply a sterile dressing.
- Remove and discard your gloves and gown.
- Make sure the patient is comfortable.
- Properly dispose of drainage, solutions, and trash bag, and clean or dispose of soiled equipment and supplies according to your facility's policy and CDC guidelines.

◆ SPECIAL CONSIDERATIONS

- Use only the irrigant specified by the physician because others may be erosive or otherwise harmful.
- Follow your facility's policy and CDC guidelines concerning wound and skin precautions.

⬦ **NURSING ALERT** When irrigating wounds, use minimal mechanical force, typically with pressures between 4 and 15 pounds per square inch. Remember, the greater the size of the syringe, the lower the pressure; the greater the size of the needle, the greater the flow and the greater the pressure.

- If the wound is small or not especially deep, you may want to use just the syringe for irrigation.

Complications

- Infection
- Excoriation
- Increased pain
- Wound trauma

▶ PATIENT TEACHING

Be sure to cover:
- why irrigation is necessary for wound healing
- how irrigation is performed
- how to perform irrigation at home using strict sterile technique, if appropriate
- signs and symptoms of wound infection or failure to heal to report to the physician or nurse
- follow up with visiting nurse and physician.

● DOCUMENTATION

- Date and time of irrigation
- Amount and type of irrigant
- Appearance of the wound
- Any sloughing tissue or exudate
- Amount of solution returned
- Skin care performed around the wound
- Dressings applied
- Patient's tolerance of the treatment
- Patient teaching

Selected references

Al-Ramashi, M., et al. "Saline Irrigation and Wound Infection in Abdominal Gyncologic Surgery," *International Journal of Gynecology and Obstetrics* 94(1):33-36, July 2006.

Draeger, R.W., and Dahners, L.E., "Traumatic Wound Debridement: A Comparison of Irrigation Methods," *Journal of Orthopaedic Trauma* 20(2):83-88, February 2006.

Todkar, M. "Comparison of Soap and Antibiotic Solutions for Irrigation of Lower-Limb Open Fracture Wounds," *Journal of Bone and Joint Surgery* 88(2):452, February 2006.

Wound management, surgical

● OVERVIEW

- Helps to prevent infection by stopping pathogens from entering the wound
- Promote patient comfort and protect the skin surface from maceration and excoriation caused by contact with irritating drainage
- Also allow for measurement of wound drainage to monitor healing and fluid and electrolyte balance
- Two primary methods of wound management: dressing and pouching
- Dressing preferred unless caustic or excessive drainage is compromising skin integrity
  – Lightly seeping wounds with drains and wounds with minimal purulent drainage managed with packing and gauze dressings
  – Some wounds, such as those that become chronic, possibly requiring an occlusive dressing
- Wound with copious, excoriating drainage requiring pouching to protect surrounding skin

Contraindications
- None known

❖ EQUIPMENT

Waterproof trash bag • clean gloves • sterile gloves • gown and face shield or goggles, if indicated • sterile 4″ × 4″ gauze pads • large absorbent dressings, if indicated • sterile cotton-tipped applicators • sterile dressing set • povidone-iodine swabs • topical drug, if ordered • adhesive or other tape • soap and water • skin protectant; nonadherent pads; collodion spray or acetone-free adhesive remover; sterile normal saline solution; graduated container; Montgomery straps; fishnet tube elasticized dressing support; or T-binder (optional)

DRESSING A DRAIN
Sterile scissors • sterile 4″ × 4″ gauze pads without cotton lining • sump drain • ostomy pouch or another collection bag • sterile pre-cut tracheostomy pads or drain dressings • adhesive tape (paper or silk tape if patient is hypersensitive) • surgical mask

POUCHING A WOUND
Collection pouch with drainage port • sterile gloves • skin protectant • sterile gauze pads

Equipment preparation
- Assess the patient's condition and identify his allergies, especially to adhesive tape, povidone-iodine or other topical solutions, or drugs.
- Assemble the equipment in his room.
- Check the expiration date on each sterile package, and inspect for tears.
- Put the waterproof trash bag near the patient to avoid reaching across the sterile field or the wound when disposing of soiled items.
- Turn down the top of the trash bag to provide a wide opening and prevent contamination of instruments or gloves by only touching the bag's edge.

TAILORING WOUND CARE TO WOUND COLOR

If your patient has an open wound, you can assess how well it's healing by inspecting its color, which will guide management of the wound.

Red wounds
Red indicates normal healing. When a wound begins to heal, a layer of pale pink granulation tissue covers the wound bed. As it thickens, it becomes beefy red.

Cover a red wound, keep it moist and clean, and protect it from trauma. Use a transparent dressing (such as Tegaderm or Op-site), a hydrocolloidal dressing (such as DuoDerm), or a gauze dressing moistened with sterile normal saline solution or impregnated with petroleum jelly or an antibiotic.

Yellow wounds
Yellow is the color of exudate produced by microorganisms in an open wound. Exudate usually appears whitish yellow, creamy yellow, yellowish green, or beige. Water content influences shade: Dry exudate appears darker.

If the wound is yellow, clean it and remove exudate, using high-pressure irrigation; then cover it with a moist dressing. Use absorptive products (for example, Debrisan beads and paste) or a moist gauze dressing with or without an antibiotic. You may also use hydrotherapy with whirlpool or high-pressure irrigation.

Black wounds
Black, the least healthy color, signals necrosis. Dead, avascular tissue slows healing and provides a site for microorganisms to proliferate.

You should debride a black wound. After removing dead tissue, apply a dressing to keep the wound moist and guard against external contamination. As ordered, use enzyme products, surgical debridement, hydrotherapy with whirlpool or high-pressure irrigation, or a moist gauze dressing.

Multicolored wounds
You may note two or even all three colors in a wound. In this case, classify the wound according to the least healthy color present. For example, if his wound is red and yellow, classify it as a yellow wound.

▐▌ ESSENTIAL STEPS

- Check the practitioner's order for specific wound care and drug instructions. Note the location of surgical drains to avoid dislodging them during the procedure.
- Confirm the patient's identity using two patient identifiers according to facility policy.
- Explain the procedure to the patient to lessen his fear and gain his cooperation.
- Provide for privacy, position him as necessary, and expose the wound site.
- Use the color of the wound to help determine which type of dressing to apply. (See *Tailoring wound care to wound color.*)
- Wash your hands and put on a gown, clean gloves, and a face shield, if necessary.
- Loosen the soiled dressing by holding the patient's skin and pulling the tape or dressing toward the wound. This protects the newly formed tissue and prevents stress on the incision.
- Moisten the tape with acetone-free adhesive remover, if necessary, to make tape removal less painful (particularly if the skin is hairy).

◈ **NURSING ALERT** Don't apply solvents to the incision because they can contaminate the wound.

- Slowly remove the soiled dressing.
- If the gauze adheres to the wound, loosen the gauze by moistening it with sterile normal saline solution.
- Observe the dressing for amount, type, color, and odor of drainage.
- Discard the dressing and gloves in the waterproof trash bag.

CARING FOR THE WOUND

- Wash your hands.
- Establish a sterile field with the equipment and supplies you'll need for suture-line care and dressing change, including a sterile dressing set and povidone-iodine swabs.
- If the practitioner has ordered ointment, squeeze the needed amount onto the sterile field.

- If using an antiseptic from an unsterile bottle, pour the antiseptic cleaning agent into a sterile container so you won't contaminate your gloves.
- Put on sterile gloves.
- Saturate the sterile gauze pads with the prescribed cleaning agent.

◈ **NURSING ALERT** Avoid using cotton balls because they may shed fibers in the wound, causing irritation, infection, or adhesion.

- If ordered, obtain a wound culture; then proceed to clean the wound.
- Pick up the moistened gauze pad or swab and squeeze out excess solution.
- Working from the top of the incision, wipe once to the bottom, and then discard. Wipe a second moistened pad from top to bottom in a vertical path next to the incision. Continue to work outward from the incision in lines running parallel to it. Always wipe from the clean area toward the less clean area (usually from top to bottom).
- Use each gauze pad or swab for only one stroke.
- Use sterile cotton-tipped applicators for efficient cleaning of tight-fitting wire sutures, deep and narrow wounds, or wounds with pockets. Wipe only once with each applicator.

◈ **NURSING ALERT** If the patient has a surgical drain, clean the drain's surface last. Moist drainage promotes bacterial growth; the drain is considered the most contaminated area. Clean skin around the drain by wiping in half or full circles from the drain site outward.

- Clean all areas of the wound to wash away debris, pus, blood, and necrotic material. Try not to disturb sutures or irritate the incision.
- Clean to at least 1″ (2.5 cm) beyond the end of the new dressing. If you aren't applying a new dressing, clean to at least 2″ (5 cm) beyond the incision.
- Check to make sure the edges of the incision are lined up properly, and check for signs of infection, dehiscence, or evisceration.

◈ **NURSING ALERT** If you see signs of infection or the patient reports pain at the wound, notify the practitioner.

- Irrigate the wound, as ordered.
- Wash skin surrounding the wound with soap and water, and pat dry using a sterile 4″ × 4″ gauze pad. Avoid oil-based soap; it may interfere with pouch adherence. Apply prescribed topical drug.
- Apply a skin protectant, if needed.
- If ordered, pack the wound with gauze pads or strips folded to fit, using sterile forceps.

◈ **NURSING ALERT** Avoid using cotton-lined gauze pads. Cotton fibers can adhere to the wound surface and cause complications.

- Pack the wound using the wet-to-damp method. Soaking the packing material in solution and wringing it out so it's slightly moist provides a moist wound environment that absorbs debris and drainage. Pack the wound loosely to prevent damaging the wound. Removing the packing won't disrupt new tissue.

APPLYING A FRESH GAUZE DRESSING

- Place sterile 4″ × 4″ gauze pads at the center of the wound, and move progressively outward to the edges of the wound site.
- Extend the gauze at least 1″ beyond the incision in each direction, and cover the wound evenly with enough sterile dressings (usually two or three layers) to absorb drainage until the next dressing change.
- Use large absorbent dressings to form outer layers, if needed, to provide greater absorbency.
- Secure the dressing's edges to the patient's skin with strips of tape to maintain sterility of the wound site, or secure the dressing with a T-binder or Montgomery straps to prevent skin excoriation, which may occur with repeated tape removal necessitated by frequent dressing changes.
- If the wound is on a limb, secure the dressing with a fishnet tube elasticized dressing support.

(continued)

- Make sure the patient is comfortable.
- Properly dispose of the solutions and trash bag. Clean or discard soiled equipment and supplies according to facility policy.

◈ **NURSING ALERT** If the patient's wound has purulent drainage, don't return unopened sterile supplies to the sterile supply cabinet; this could crosscontaminate other equipment.

DRESSING A WOUND WITH A DRAIN

- Prepare a drain dressing by using sterile scissors to cut a slit in a sterile 4″ × 4″ gauze pad.
- Fold the pad in half; then cut inward from the center of the folded edge.
- Don't use a cotton-lined gauze pad. Cutting the gauze opens the lining and releases cotton fibers into the wound.
- Prepare a second pad the same way, or use commercially pre-cut gauze.
- Press one folded pad close to the skin around the drain so that the tubing fits into the slit. Press the second folded pad around the drain from the opposite direction so that the two pads encircle the tubing.
- Layer as many uncut sterile 4″ × 4″ gauze pads or large absorbent dressings around the tubing, as needed, to absorb expected drainage. Tape the dressing in place, or use a T-binder or Montgomery straps.

POUCHING A WOUND

- If the patient's wound is draining heavily, or if drainage may damage surrounding skin, apply a pouch.
- Measure the wound. Cut an opening ⅜″ (0.3 cm) larger than the wound in the facing of the collection pouch.
- Apply a skin protectant, as needed.
- Plan to position the pouch's drainage port so that gravity facilitates drainage.
- Make sure the drainage port at the bottom of the pouch is closed firmly to prevent leaks.

- Gently press the contoured pouch opening around the wound, starting at its lower edge, to catch drainage.
- To empty the pouch, put on gloves and a face shield or mask and goggles to avoid splashing.
- Insert the pouch's bottom one-half into a graduated biohazard container, and open the drainage port. Note the color, consistency, odor, and amount of fluid.
- If ordered, obtain a culture specimen and send it to the laboratory immediately.
- Remember to follow Centers for Disease Control and Prevention standard precautions when handling infectious drainage.
- Wipe the bottom of the pouch and drainage port with a gauze pad and reseal the port.
- Change the pouch only if it leaks or fails to adhere.

◆ **SPECIAL CONSIDERATIONS**

- If the patient has two wounds in the same area, cover each wound separately with layers of sterile 4″ × 4″ gauze pads. Cover each site with a large absorbent dressing secured to the patient's skin with tape.
- Don't use a single large absorbent dressing to cover both sites because drainage quickly saturates a pad, promoting cross-contamination.
- Avoid overlapping damp packing onto surrounding skin because it macerates the intact tissue.
- To save time when dressing a wound with a drain, use precut tracheostomy pads or drain dressings to fit around the drain.
- If the patient is sensitive to adhesive tape, use paper or silk tape.
- Use a surgical mask to cradle a chin or jawline dressing.
- If ordered, use a collodion spray or similar topical protectant instead of a gauze dressing.
- If a sump drain isn't adequately collecting wound secretions, reinforce it with an ostomy pouch or another collection bag.
- Use waterproof tape to strengthen a spot on the front of the pouch near the adhesive opening; then cut a small "X" in the tape. Feed the drain catheter into the pouch through the "X" cut.
- Seal the cut around the tubing with more waterproof tape; then connect the tubing to the suction pump.
- If you use more than one collection pouch for a wound or wounds, record drainage volume separately for each pouch.
- Avoid using waterproof material over the dressing.
- Many practitioners prefer to change the first postoperative dressing themselves to check the incision; don't change the first dressing unless you have specific instructions.
- If you have no such order and drainage comes through the dressings, reinforce the dressing with fresh sterile gauze. Request an order to change the dressing, or ask the practitioner to change it as soon as possible. A reinforced dressing shouldn't remain in

place longer than 24 hours because it's a medium for bacterial growth.
- For the recent postoperative patient or a patient with complications, check the dressing every 15 to 30 minutes, or as ordered. For the patient with a properly healing wound, check the dressing at least once every 8 hours.
- If the dressing becomes wet from the outside, replace it as soon as possible to prevent wound contamination.

Complications
- Allergic reaction
- Skin redness, rash, or excoriation
- Infection
- Skin tears

▶ PATIENT TEACHING

Be sure to cover:
- reason for wound care and procedure being done
- importance of using aseptic technique
- signs and symptoms of infection and other complications
- wound care methods for use after discharge.

●◆ DOCUMENTATION

- Appearance of dressing before change
- Date, time, and type of wound management procedure
- Amount of soiled dressing and packing removed
- Wound appearance (including size, condition of margins, and presence of necrotic tissue) and odor (if present)
- Type, color, consistency, and amount of drainage (for each wound); presence and location of drains
- Additional procedures, such as irrigation, packing, or application of a topical drug
- Type and amount of new dressing or pouch applied
- Patient's tolerance of the procedure
- Special or detailed wound care instructions and pain management steps

Selected references
Harvey, C. "Wound Healing," *Orthopaedic Nursing* 24(2):143-57, March-April 2005.

Hoban, V. "Wound Care: What Every Nurse Should Know," *Nursing Times* 101(12):20-22, March 2005.

Worley, C.A. "Assessment and Terminology: Critical Issues in Wound Care," *Dermatology Nursing* 16(5):451-52, 457, October 2004.

Part IV ▶ DIAGNOSTIC STUDIES

Amniocentesis

- Sterile needle aspiration of fluid from the amniotic sac for analysis
- Performed during any trimester of pregnany, but most commonly in the second trimester between weeks 16 to 18

Purpose

- To detect fetal abnormalities, particularly chromosomal and neural tube defects
- To detect hemolytic disease of the fetus
- To diagnose metabolic disorders, amino acid disorders, and mucopolysaccharidosis
- To assess fetal age and lung maturity during the third trimester
- To detect the presence of meconium or blood
- To measure amniotic levels of estriol and fetal thyroid hormone
- To identify gender of fetus

Patient preparation

- Make sure that the patient has signed an appropriate consent form.
- Confirm the patient's identity using two patient identifiers according to facility policy.
- Note and report allergies.
- Check Rh status.
- Tell the patient that dietary restrictions aren't necessary.
- Check the patient's history for hypersensitivity to local anesthetics.
- Tell the patient that an ultrasound will be done first.
- Have the patient empty her bladder just before the procedure.

TEACHING POINTS

Be sure to cover:
- purpose of the study and how it's done
- who will perform the test and where
- that the fetus will be monitored closely during the study.

- The patient is placed supine on the examining table and draped so that only the abdomen is exposed.
- During the test, fetal heart rate and rhythm and maternal vital signs are monitored.
- A baseline recording of fetal heart rate is obtained.
- A pocket of amniotic fluid is identified via ultrasound.
- The skin is prepared with antiseptic and alcohol and a local anesthetic is given.
- A 20G spinal needle with a stylet is inserted into the pocket and fluid is withdrawn and placed in a test tube that's protected from exposure to light.
- The needle is removed and pressure is applied to the site.
- A sterile dressing is applied and specimens are sent to the laboratory immediately.

Postprocedure care

- Position the patient so that she's as comfortable as possible.

AMNIOTIC FLUID ANALYSIS FINDINGS

Amniotic fluid analysis can provide information about the condition of the mother, fetus, and placenta. This table shows normal findings and abnormal results and their implications.

Test component	Normal findings	Abnormal results
Color	Clear, with white flecks of vernix caseosa in a mature fetus	Blood of maternal origin is usually harmless. "Port wine" fluid may indicate abruptio placentae. Fetal blood may indicate damage to the fetal, placental, or umbilical cord vessels.
Bilirubin	Absent at term	High levels indicate hemolytic disease of the neonate.
Meconium	Absent	Presence indicates fetal hypotension or distress.
Creatinine	More than 2 mg/dl (SI, 177 μmol/L in a mature fetus)	Decrease may indicate fetus less than 37 weeks.
Lecithin-sphingomyelin ratio	More than 2	Less than 2 indicates pulmonary immaturity.
Phosphatidyl glycerol	Present	Absence indicates pulmonary immaturity.
Glucose	Less than 45 mg/dl (SI, 2.3 mmol/L)	Excessive increases at term or near term indicate hypertrophied fetal pancreas.
Alpha-fetoprotein	Variable, depending on gestational age and laboratory technique	Inappropriate increases indicate neural tube defects, such as spina bifida or anencephaly, impending fetal death, congenital nephrosis, or contamination of fetal blood.
Bacteria	Absent	Presence indicates chorioamnionitis.
Chromosome	Normal karyotype	Abnormal karyotype indicates fetal chromosome disorders.
Acetylecholinesterase	Absent	Presence may indicate neural tube defects, exomphalos, or other serious malformations.

- Administer RhoD immune globulin (RhoGAM) I.M. if the woman is Rh negative.
- Instruct the patient to rest after returning home and engage in only light activity for 24 hours after the procedure.
- Encourage the patient to report any abdominal pain or cramping, uterine contractions, chills, fever, vaginal bleeding or leakage of serous vaginal fluid, or fetal hyperactivity or unusual fetal lethargy.
- Tell the patient that the physician will call her with the results, which may take up to 3 weeks.

MONITORING
- Maternal vital signs
- Fetal heart rate
- Insertion site
- Leakage of amniotic fluid

Precautions
- A full bladder increases the risk of inadvertent bladder puncture.
- Because the patient may be anxious about the possible results, offer support.
- Because of the potential severity of possible complications, amniocentesis is contraindicated as a general screening test.

Complications
- Spontaneous abortion
- Fetal or placental trauma
- Bleeding
- Preterm labor
- Infection
- Rh sensitization

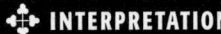 **INTERPRETATION**

Normal findings
- Clear fluid, possibly with white flecks of vernix, is evident when fetus is near term.

Abnormal results
See *Amniotic fluid analysis findings.*

Antegrade pyelography

- Radiographic procedure that allows examination of the upper collecting system when ureteral obstruction rules out retrograde ureteropyelography, or when cystoscopy is contraindicated
- Also indicated when excretory urography or renal ultrasonography demonstrates hydronephrosis and the need for therapeutic nephrostomy

Purpose
- To evaluate obstruction of the upper collecting system
- To evaluate hydronephrosis
- To evaluate function of the upper collecting system after ureteral surgery or urinary diversion
- To assess renal functional reserve before surgery
- To allow placement of a percutaneous nephrostomy tube

Patient preparation
- Make sure that the patient has signed an appropriate consent form.
- Note and report all allergies, especially to contrast media, iodine, or shellfish.
- Explain that fasting may be required for 6 to 8 hours before the test.
- Explain that antimicrobials may be given before and after the procedure.
- Warn the patient that mild discomfort may be felt during injection of the local anesthetic and contrast medium, which can also cause transient burning and flushing.
- Tell the patient that the radiograph machine makes loud clacking sounds as films are taken.

TEACHING POINTS
Be sure to cover:
- purpose of the study and how it's done
- who will perform the test and where
- that the test takes 1 to 2 hours
- that a tube may be left in the kidney for drainage.

- A sedative may be administered.
- The patient is placed in a prone position on the radiograph table, the skin over the kidney is cleaned with antiseptic solution, and a local anesthetic is injected.
- Previous urographic films or ultrasound recordings are studied for anatomic landmarks in order to determine angle of needle entry.
- Under the guidance of fluoroscopy or ultrasound, the needle is inserted below the 12th rib at the level of the transverse process of the second lumbar vertebra with a stylet.
- Aspiration of urine confirms that the needle has reached the dilated collecting system.
- Flexible tubing is connected to the needle to prevent displacement during the procedure.
- If intrarenal pressure is to be measured, a manometer is connected to the tubing.
- Urine may be collected for cultures and cytologic studies.
- An amount of urine equal to the amount of contrast medium to be injected is withdrawn to prevent overdistention of the collecting system.
- The contrast medium is injected directly into the renal pelvis or calyces.
- Radiographs are taken at various angles.
- Ureteral peristalsis is observed to evaluate obstruction.
- A percutaneous nephrostomy tube is inserted, if needed, or the catheter is withdrawn and a sterile dressing is applied.

Postprocedure care
- For bleeding, apply direct pressure.
- For a hematoma, apply warm soaks.
- Report urine leakage to the physician immediately.
- Report hematuria if it persists after the third voiding.
- Notify the physician if the patient doesn't void within 8 hours.
- Irrigate nephrostomy tube, if present, with 5 to 7 ml of sterile saline, as ordered.
- Administer antibiotics and analgesics, as ordered.

MONITORING
- Vital signs
- Intake and output
- Signs and symptoms of hypersensitivity to contrast medium
- Puncture site for bleeding, hematoma, or urine leakage
- Hematuria
- Nephrostomy tube patency and drainage
- Results of recent surgery or urinary diversion

Precautions
Inform the physician of:
- patient's history of bleeding disorders
- potential for pregnancy
- any history of hypersensitivity reactions to contrast media, iodine, or shellfish.

◈ **NURSING ALERT** Watch for and report signs and symptoms of sepsis such as chills, fever, rapid pulse or respiratory rate, shortness of breath, and hypotension.

Complications
- Puncture of adjacent organs
- Pneumothorax
- Bleeding at puncture site
- Hematoma

Normal findings
- The upper collecting system should fill uniformly and appear normal in size and course.
- Normal structures should be clearly outlined.

Abnormal results
- Enlargements of the upper collecting system and parts of the ureteropelvic junction suggest obstruction from calculi, scarring, or tumor.
- Marked distention of the ureteropelvic junction suggests hydronephrosis.
- Intrarenal pressures that exceed 20 cm H_2O suggest obstruction.
- Urine culture or cytology may suggest antegrade pyelonephrosis or malignant tumor.

Arterial blood gas analysis

● OVERVIEW

- Used to evaluate gas exchange in the lungs
- Measures oxygen content (O_2CT), arterial oxygen saturation (SaO_2), and bicarbonate (HCO_3^-) values
- pH: hydrogen ion (H^+) concentration, indicating acidity or alkalinity of the blood
- $PaCO_2$: concentration of arterial carbon dioxide in the blood; reflects the adequacy of alveolar ventilation and respiratory response to acid-base balance
- PaO_2: amount of oxygen crossing the alveolar capillary membrane and the concentration of arterial oxygen in the blood
- HCO_3^-: measure of the metabolic component of acid-base balance
- SaO_2: ratio of the amount of oxygen in the blood combined with hemoglobin to the total amount of oxygen that the hemoglobin can carry

Purpose
- To evaluate efficiency of pulmonary gas exchange
- To assess integrity of the ventilatory control system
- To determine acid-base balance
- To monitor response to respiratory therapy
- To monitor pathophysiologic changes influencing ventilatory effort or gas exchange

Patient preparation
- Make sure that the patient has signed an appropriate consent form.
- Restriction of food or fluids isn't necessary.
- Explain that the study requires an arterial blood sample and that brief cramping or throbbing pain may be felt at the puncture site.
- Before the puncture, evaluate the arterial blood supply to the hand by performing the Allen test.
- Note and report all allergies.

TEACHING POINTS
Be sure to cover:
- the purpose of the test and how it's done
- who will perform the test and where

- that the procedure takes less than 10 minutes.

▶ PROCEDURE

- The blood sample is obtained from either a percutaneous arterial puncture or from an arterial line.
- A heparinized blood gas syringe is used to draw the sample.
- All air is eliminated from the sample; it's placed on ice immediately and is transported for analysis.
- The following information is included on the laboratory request:
  - room air or amount of oxygen and method of delivery
  - ventilator settings if on mechanical ventilation
  - patient's temperature.

Postprocedure care
- Apply direct manual pressure to the puncture site for 3 to 5 minutes or until hemostasis is obtained.
- Apply a sterile dressing.

MONITORING
- Vital signs
- Peripheral vascular status
- Bleeding or hematoma formation at the puncture site

🔲 **NURSING ALERT** Observe for signs of circulatory impairment, such as swelling, discoloration, pain, numbness, or tingling in the extremity used for the puncture.

Precautions
- Maintain standard precautions.
- Exposing the sample to air affects PaO_2 and $PaCO_2$, interfering with accurate results.
- Failure to comply with correct specimen handling procedures will adversely affect the test results.
- Venous blood in the sample will render lower PaO_2 and elevate $PaCO_2$.
- Drugs including bicarbonates, ethacrynic acid, hydrocortisone, metolazone, prednisone, and thiazides may elevate $PaCO_2$.
- Drugs including acetazolamide, methicillin, nitrofurantoin, and tetracycline may decrease $PaCO_2$.

- Wait at least 20 minutes before drawing arterial blood gas in the following situations:
  - after initiating, changing, or discontinuing oxygen therapy
  - after initiating or changing settings of mechanical ventilation
  - after extubation.

Complications
- Hematoma
- Bleeding
- Infection
- Thrombosis
- Nerve damage

✜ INTERPRETATION

Normal findings
- pH: 7.35 to 7.45 (SI, 7.35 to 7.45)
- $PaCO_2$: 35 to 45 mm Hg (SI, 4.7 to 5.3 kPa)
- PaO_2: 75 to 100 mm Hg (SI, 10.6 to 13.3 kPa)
- HCO_3^-: 22 to 26 mEq/L (SI, 22 to 25 mmol/L)
- SaO_2: 94% to 100% (SI, 0.94 to 1)
- O_2CT: 15% to 23% (SI, 0.15 to 0.23)

Abnormal results
- Low PaO_2, O_2CT, and SaO_2 levels in combination with a high $PaCO_2$ suggest conditions that impair respiratory function, such as respiratory muscle weakness or paralysis, respiratory center inhibition, and airway obstruction.
- Low PaO_2 and SaO_2, with a normal $PaCO_2$ suggest impaired diffusion between alveoli and blood, or an arteriovenous shunt that permits blood to bypass the lungs.
- Decreased levels may result from bronchiole obstruction caused by asthma or emphysema; from an abnormal ventilation-perfusion ratio caused by partially blocked alveoli or pulmonary capillaries; or from alveoli that are damaged or filled with fluid because of disease, hemorrhage, or near drowning.

Arthrocentesis

● OVERVIEW

- Synovial fluid aspiration
- Fluid specimen obtained by insertion of sterile needle into a joint space, most commonly the knee, under sterile conditions
- Indicated in undiagnosed articular disease and symptomatic joint effusion

Purpose
- To analyze synovial fluid
- To aid differential diagnosis of arthritis, especially septic or crystal-induced arthritis
- To identify cause or nature of joint effusion
- To relieve pain and distention from joint effusion
- To allow administration of local drug therapy, such as corticosteroids

Patient preparation
- Make sure that the patient has signed an appropriate consent form.
- Note and report all allergies.
- If glucose testing of synovial fluid is ordered, advise fasting for 6 to 12 hours before the test; otherwise, there's no need to restrict food and fluids before the test.
- Warn the patient that transient pain may be felt when the needle penetrates the joint capsule.
- Administer sedation as ordered.

TEACHING POINTS
Be sure to cover:
- purpose of the study and how it's done
- who will perform the test and where
- that the test takes less than 15 minutes.

▶ PROCEDURE

- The patient is properly positioned and instructed to maintain this position throughout the procedure.
- The skin over the puncture site is cleaned and prepared.
- After a local anesthetic is administered, an aspirating needle is quickly inserted through the skin, subcutaneous tissue, and synovial membrane into the joint space.
- As much fluid as possible is aspirated into the syringe, preferably at least 15 ml.
- The joint (except for the area around the puncture site) may be wrapped with an elastic bandage to compress the free fluid into this portion of the sac, ensuring maximal collection of fluid.
- If a corticosteroid is being injected, the syringe is detached, leaving the needle in the joint, the syringe con-

SYNOVIAL FLUID FINDINGS IN VARIOUS DISORDERS

Disease	Color	Clarity	Viscosity	Mucin clot
GROUP 1 NONINFLAMMATORY				
Traumatic arthritis	Straw to bloody to yellow	Transparent to cloudy	Variable	Good to fair
Osteoarthritis	Yellow	Transparent	Variable	Good to fair
GROUP II INFLAMMATORY				
Systemic lupus erythematosus	Straw	Clear to slightly cloudy	Variable	Good to fair
Rheumatic fever	Yellow	Slightly cloudy	Variable	Good to fair
Pseudogout	Yellow	Slightly cloudy (if acute)	Low (if acute)	Fair to poor
Gout	Yellow to milky	Cloudy	Low	Fair to poor
Rheumatoid arthritis	Yellow to green	Cloudy	Low	Fair to poor
GROUP III SEPTIC				
Tuberculous arthritis	Yellow	Cloudy	Low	Poor
Septic arthritis	Gray or bloody	Turbid, purulent	Low	Poor

taining the steroid is attached to the needle, and the steroid is injected.
- The needle is withdrawn and pressure is applied to the puncture site until hemostasis is obtained.
- The puncture site is cleaned and a sterile dressing is applied.
- If synovial fluid glucose is being measured, venipuncture is performed to obtain a specimen for blood glucose analysis.

Postprocedure care
- Apply ice or cold packs to the affected joint for 24 to 36 hours after aspiration to decrease pain and swelling.
- Use pillows to support the joint.
- If a large quantity of fluid was aspirated, apply an elastic bandage as ordered to prevent fluid from accumulating again.
- If the patient's condition permits, resume the patient's normal activities and diet immediately after the procedure.

- Warn the patient to avoid excessive use of the joint for a few days after the test, even if pain and swelling have subsided. Excessive use can cause transient pain, swelling, and stiffness.

MONITORING
- Vital signs
- Pain
- Fever
- Puncture site

Precautions
- Failure to adhere to dietary restrictions can affect glucose levels.
- Failure to mix specimen and anticoagulant adequately or to send the specimen to the laboratory immediately may cause inaccurate test results.
- Don't perform the test in areas of skin or wound infections.
- Use strict sterile technique throughout aspiration to prevent contamination of the joint space or the synovial fluid specimen.
- Send the properly labeled specimens to the laboratory immediately. If a

white blood cell (WBC) count is ordered, clearly label the specimen "Synovial fluid" and "Caution: Don't use acid diluents" because these can alter the count.

Complications
- Joint infection
- Hemorrhage
- Hemarthrosis

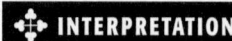 **INTERPRETATION**

Normal findings
- With gross examination:
  - Color: colorless to pale yellow
  - Clarity: clear
  - Quantity (in knee): 0.3 to 3.5 ml
  - pH: 7.2 to 7.4
  - Mucin clot: good

Abnormal results
See *Synovial fluid findings in various disorders.*

WBC count; % neutrophils	Cartilage debris	Crystals	Rheumatoid arthritis cells	Bacteria
1,000; 25%	None	None	None	None
700; 15%	Usually present	None	None	None
2,000; 30%	None	None	Lupus erythematosus (LE) cells	None
14,000; 50%	None	None	Possibly LE cells	None
15,000; 70%	Usually present	Calcium pyrophosphate	None	None
20,000; 70%	None	Urate	None	None
20,000; 70%	None	Occasionally, cholesterol	Usually present	None
20,000; 60%	None	None	None	Usually present
90,000; 90%	None	None	None	Usually present

Arthrography

● OVERVIEW

- Radiographic examination of a joint after injection of a radiopaque dye, air, or both (double-contrast arthrography)

Purpose
- To outline joint contour and soft-tissue structures
- To evaluate persistent unexplained joint discomfort or pain
- To identify acute or chronic abnormalities of the joint capsule or supporting ligaments of the knee, shoulder, ankle, hip, or wrist
- To detect internal joint derangements
- To locate synovial cysts
- To evaluate damage from recurrent dislocations

Patient preparation
- Make sure that the patient has signed an appropriate consent form.
- Note and report all allergies.
- Restriction of food or fluids isn't necessary.
- Warn the patient that a tingling sensation, burning, or pressure in the joint may be felt with contrast injection.

TEACHING POINTS
Be sure to cover:
- purpose of the study and how it's done
- who will perform the study and where
- that the study takes about 45 minutes
- that some swelling, discomfort, or crepitant noises may occur in the joint after the study; that these usually disappear after 1 to 2 days; and to contact the physician if symptoms persist.

▶ PROCEDURE

- The skin around the puncture site is cleaned with an antiseptic solution and injected with a local anesthetic.
- A needle is inserted into the joint space.
- Fluid may be aspirated and sent to the laboratory for analysis.
- When fluoroscopic examination demonstrates correct needle placement, contrast medium is injected into the joint space.
- The needle is removed and the puncture site is covered with a sterile dressing.
- The joint is put through its range of motion to distribute the contrast medium in the joint space.
- A series of radiographs is rapidly taken before the joint tissue can absorb the contrast medium.

Postprocedure care
- Rest the joint for 6 to 12 hours.
- Wrap the knee in an elastic bandage as ordered for several days if knee arthrography was performed.
- Apply ice to the joint for swelling.
- Administer analgesics as ordered.
- Report signs and symptoms of infection.

MONITORING
- Vital signs
- Pain
- Puncture site
- Infection
- Swelling of joint

Precautions
- Incomplete aspiration of joint effusion dilutes the contrast medium and diminishes film quality.
- Check the patient's history for hypersensitivity to:
  - local anesthetics
  - iodine
  - contrast media.
- Contraindications include:
  - pregnancy
  - active arthritis
  - joint infection
  - previous hypersensitivity to iodinated contrast media.

Complications
- Hypersensitivity reactions to contrast medium
- Persistent joint swelling, pain, or crepitus
- Infection

✛ INTERPRETATION

Normal findings
- A knee arthrogram shows a characteristic wedge-shaped shadow pointed toward the interior of the joint, indicating a normal medial meniscus.
- A shoulder arthrogram shows the bicipital tendon sheath, redundant inferior joint capsule, and intact subscapular bursa.

Abnormal results
- Structural abnormalities of the knee commonly suggest tears and lacerations of the meniscus.
- Extrameniscal lesions may suggest osteochondral fractures, cartilaginous abnormalities, synovial abnormalities, cruciate ligament tears, and joint capsule and collateral ligament disruptions.
- Shoulder abnormalities may suggest adhesive capsulitis, bicipital tenosynovitis or rupture, and rotator cuff tears.

Arthroscopy

● OVERVIEW

- Visual examination of the interior of a joint using a fiber-optic endoscope
- Most commonly used to examine the knee joint
- Permits concurrent surgery or biopsy using triangulation, in which instruments are passed through a separate cannula
- Usually an outpatient procedure

Purpose

- To evaluate suspected or confirmed joint disease
- To provide a safe, convenient alternative to open surgery (arthrotomy) and separate biopsy
- To detect and diagnose meniscal, patellar, condylar, extrasynovial, and synovial diseases

Patient preparation

- Make sure that the patient has signed an appropriate consent form.
- Note and report all allergies.
- Instruct the patient that fasting is required after midnight before the procedure.
- Warn the patient that transient discomfort may be felt from injection of the local anesthetic and pressure of the tourniquet on the leg.
- Explain that a thumping sensation may be felt as the cannula is inserted into the joint capsule.

TEACHING POINTS

Be sure to cover:
- purpose of the study and how it's done
- who will perform the study and where
- that the study takes about 1 hour
- the need to avoid tub baths until after the postoperative visit. (Showers are permitted 48 hours after the study.)

▶ PROCEDURE

- Arthroscopic techniques vary depending on the surgeon and the type of arthroscope used.

- An area 5″ (12.7 cm) above and below the joint is prepared and draped.
- A sedative may be administered.
- Local or regional anesthesia is administered; general anesthesia is used for more extensive surgery.
- As much blood as possible is usually drained from the leg by wrapping it in an elastic bandage and elevating it.
- A mixture of lidocaine, epinephrine, and sterile normal saline solution may be injected to distend the knee, reduce bleeding, and provide a better view.
- A cannula is passed through a small incision and positioned in the joint cavity.
- The arthroscope is inserted through the cannula.
- The knee structures are visually examined.
- Photographs are taken for further study, if indicated.
- A synovial biopsy or appropriate surgery is performed, if indicated.
- The arthroscope is removed and the joint is irrigated.
- An adhesive strip and compression bandage are applied to the site.

Postprocedure care

- Administer analgesics as ordered.
- Elevate the leg and apply ice for the first 24 hours.
- Report any fever, bleeding, drainage, or increased swelling or pain in the joint.
- Limit weight bearing by using a walker, cane, or crutches for 48 hours.
- Apply an immobilizer if ordered.
- Resume the patient's usual diet.

MONITORING

- Fever
- Swelling
- Increased pain
- Localized inflammation
- Neurovascular status of the extremity

Precautions

- Check the patient's history for hypersensitivity to the anesthetic or sedation.
- Contraindications include:
  - fibrous ankylosis with flexion of less than 50 degrees
  - local skin or wound infections.

Complications

- Infection
- Hematoma
- Thrombophlebitis
- Joint injury

✛ INTERPRETATION

Normal findings

- The knee is a diarthrodial joint surrounded by muscles, ligaments, cartilage, and tendons and lined with synovial membrane.

  AGE-RELATED CONCERN In a child, the menisci are smooth and opaque, with their thick outer edges attached to the joint capsule and their inner edges lying snugly against the condylar surfaces, unattached.

- Articular cartilage appears smooth and white.
- Ligaments and tendons appear cable-like and silvery.
- The synovium is smooth and marked by a fine vascular network.
- Degenerative changes begin during adolescence.

Abnormal results

- Meniscal abnormalities may suggest torn medial or lateral meniscus.
- Patellar abnormalities may suggest chondromalacia, dislocation, subluxation, fracture, or parapatellar synovitis.
- Condylar abnormalities may suggest degenerative articular cartilage, osteochondritis dissecans, or loose bodies.
- Extrasynovial abnormalities may suggest torn anterior cruciate or tibial collateral ligaments, Baker's cyst, and ganglion cyst.
- Synovial abnormalities may suggest synovitis and rheumatoid and degenerative arthritis
- Foreign bodies may suggest gout, pseudogout, and osteochondromatosis.

Barium enema

● OVERVIEW

- Radiographic examination of the large intestine after rectal instillation of barium sulfate (single-contrast technique), or barium sulfate and air (double-contrast technique)
- Single-contrast technique: provides a profile view of the large intestine
- Double-contrast technique: provides profile and frontal views

Purpose

- Aids in diagnosing colorectal cancer and inflammatory bowel disease
- To detect polyps, diverticula, and changes in the large intestine

Patient preparation

- Make sure that the patient has signed an appropriate consent form.
- Note all allergies.
- Administer a bowel preparation as ordered.
- Dairy products are restricted (liquid diet 24 hours before the test).
- Instruct the patient to drink five 8-oz (240-ml) glasses of clear liquids in the 12 to 24 hours before the test to ensure adequate hydration.
- Withhold breakfast before the procedure; clear liquids allowed if the test is scheduled for late afternoon.
- Warn the patient that cramps or the urge to defecate may be experienced as the barium or air is introduced into the intestine.
- Explain that the anal sphincter should be tightly contracted against the rectal tube to hold the tube in position and prevent the barium from leaking.

◈ **NURSING ALERT** Various diets, laxatives, and cleansing enemas may be used, but some conditions, such as ulcerative colitis and active GI bleeding, may preclude the use of laxatives and enemas.

TEACHING POINTS

Be sure to cover:
- the purpose of the study
- who will perform the test and where
- that the study takes 30 to 45 minutes
- accurate test results depend on following the prescribed bowel preparation
- that stools will be light-colored for 24 to 72 hours after the test.

▶ PROCEDURE

- The patient is placed in a supine position on a tilting radiograph table and spot films of the abdomen are taken.
- A well-lubricated rectal tube is inserted through the anus after patient is placed in the Sims' position.
- Barium is then administered slowly and the filling process is monitored fluoroscopically.
- The table may be tilted or the patient assisted to supine, prone, and lateral decubitus positions to aid the filling process.
- Overhead films of the abdomen are taken when the intestine is filled with barium.
- The rectal tube is withdrawn and the patient is escorted to the toilet or provided with a bedpan and instructed to expel as much barium as possible.
- After evacuation, an additional overhead film is taken to record the mucosal pattern of the intestine and to evaluate the efficiency of colonic emptying.
- In patients with a colostomy or ileostomy, barium (or barium and air) is instilled through the stoma.
- A double-contrast barium enema may directly follow this examination or may be performed separately.

Postprocedure care

- Encourage extra oral fluid intake to prevent dehydration and help eliminate the barium.
- Administer a mild cathartic or an enema because barium retention can cause intestinal obstruction or fecal impaction.

MONITORING

- Vital signs
- Intake and output
- Stools
- Abdominal distension
- Bowel sounds

Precautions

- Flexible sigmoidoscopy provides the best view of the rectosigmoid region, where most colon cancers occur.
- Barium enema should precede barium swallow and the upper GI and small-bowel series because retained barium in the GI tract may interfere with subsequent radiographic studies.
- Contraindications include fulminant ulcerative colitis associated with systemic toxicity and megacolon, suspected bowel perforation, and pregnancy.
- Barium enema is performed cautiously with bowel obstruction, acute inflammatory conditions, acute vascular insufficiency of the bowel, acute fulminant bloody diarrhea, and suspected pneumatosis cystoids intestinalis.

Complications

- Perforation of the colon
- Water intoxication
- Barium granulomas
- Intraperitoneal and extraperitoneal extravasation of barium

✛ INTERPRETATION

Normal findings

SINGLE-CONTRAST TEST

- Intestine is uniformly filled with barium and colonic haustral markings are clearly apparent.
- Intestinal walls collapse as the barium is expelled.
- Mucosa has a regular, feathery appearance on the post-evacuation film.

DOUBLE-CONTRAST TEST

- Intestine is uniformly distended with air, with a thin layer of barium providing detail of the mucosal pattern.

Abnormal results

- Localized filling defects, with transition between normal and necrotic mucosa, suggests carcinoma.
- Diffuse inflammatory lesions originating in the anal region and ascending through the intestine suggest ulcerative colitis.
- Diffuse inflammatory lesions originating in the cecum and terminal ileum and then descending through the intestine suggest granulomatous colitis.
- Structural abnormalities suggest many possible disorders, such as saccular adenomatous polyps, broad-based villous polyps, intussusception, sigmoid volvulus, and sigmoid torsion.

Basal gastric secretion

- Used to measures basal gastric secretion under fasting conditions by aspirating stomach contents through a nasogastric (NG) tube
- Indicated for patients with epigastric pain, anorexia, and weight loss

Purpose
- To determine gastric output in the fasting state

Patient preparation
- Make sure that the patient has signed an appropriate consent form.
- Note all allergies.
- Withhold antacids, anticholinergics, cholinergics, histamine-2 (H_2) receptor antagonists, proton pump inhibitors, reserpine, adrenergic blockers, and adrenocorticosteroids for 24 hours before the test as ordered. If these medications must be continued, note this on the laboratory request.
- Explain the need for food restrictions for 12 hours before the test, and oral fluid and smoking restrictions for 8 hours before the test.
- Warn the patient that some initial discomfort and coughing or gagging may be experienced as tube is passed.

TEACHING POINTS
Be sure to cover:
- test's purpose and how it's done
- who will perform the test and where
- that the test takes 1½ hours.

▶ PROCEDURE

- An NG tube is inserted and a 20-ml syringe is attached.

◆ NURSING ALERT During insertion, make sure the NG tube enters the esophagus, not the trachea; remove it immediately if the patient develops respiratory distress or paroxysmal coughing.

- To ensure complete emptying, stomach contents are aspirated while the patient assumes three positions (supine and right and left lateral decubitus).
- Stomach contents are placed in a specimen container labeled "Residual contents."
- The NG tube is then connected to a suction machine.
- Gastric contents are aspirated by continuous low suction for 1 to 1½ hours.
- A specimen is collected every 15 minutes.
- The first two specimens are discarded to eliminate any influence by the stress of the intubation.
- The color and odor of each specimen are recorded, and the presence of food, mucus, bile, or blood is noted.
- These specimens are labeled "Basal contents," and numbered 1 to 4.
- If the NG tube is to be left in place, it's clamped or attached to low intermittent suction as ordered.

Postprocedure care
- Provide soothing lozenges for a sore throat.
- Resume the patient's usual diet and medications, unless the gastric acid stimulation test will also be conducted.

MONITORING
- Vital signs
- Abdominal distention

Precautions
- Basal gastric secretion is contraindicated in patients with conditions that prohibit NG intubation.
- Failure to adhere to pretest restrictions and psychological stress increases basal secretion.
- Instruct the patient to expectorate excess saliva to prevent contamination of gastric specimens with saliva.
- Send the specimens to the laboratory as soon as the collection is completed.
- Cholinergics, reserpine, alcohol, adrenergic blockers, and adrenocorticosteroids increase basal secretion.
- Antacids, anticholinergics, H_2-receptor antagonists, and proton pump inhibitors depress basal secretion.
- An insulin gastric analysis (the Hollander test) can be used to evaluate the effectiveness of the surgery in a patient who had a vagotomy to reduce gastric acid secretion. (See *The Hollander test*.)

Complications
- Nausea and vomiting
- Abdominal distention or pain

⬥ INTERPRETATION

Normal findings
- Basal gastric secretion ranges from 1 to 5 mEq/hour in males, and from 0.2 to 3.8 mEq/hour in females.

Abnormal results
- Abnormal findings are nonspecific and must be correlated with results of the gastric acid stimulation test.
- Increased secretion may suggest duodenal or jejunal ulcer (after partial gastrectomy).
- Markedly increased secretion may suggest Zollinger-Ellison syndrome.
- Decreased secretion may indicate gastric carcinoma or benign gastric ulcer.
- Absence of secretion may indicate pernicious anemia.

THE HOLLANDER TEST

I.V. injection of insulin in a patient with normal blood glucose levels causes hypoglycemia by promoting cellular absorption of glucose. Hypoglycemia, in turn, affects the vagus nerve, which stimulates acid secretion by the parietal and chief cells. A vagotomy eliminates this neural stimulus for gastric acid secretion.

The Hollander test is used to evaluate the effectiveness of vagotomy and is most effective when performed 3 to 6 months after surgery. In this test, gastric contents are aspirated under fasting conditions through a nasogastric (NG) tube before and after a dose of insulin and are then compared; at the same time, blood glucose levels are determined before and after the insulin injection.

If the acid output after the insulin injection exceeds the preinjection acid output, the vagotomy is likely to be incomplete; if acid output fails to increase after the insulin injection, the vagotomy is considered complete. Failure to increase acid output is significant only if achlorhydria persists after blood glucose falls below 50 mg/dl.

The test is contraindicated in coronary artery or cerebrovascular disease, hypoglycemia, or conditions that prohibit NG intubation. It isn't useful in patients with achlorhydria, as demonstrated by the gastric acid stimulation test, because such patients fail to respond to insulin injection.

Blood culture

OVERVIEW

- Performed by inoculating a culture medium with a blood sample and incubating it for isolation and identification of the causative pathogens in bacteremia and septicemia
- Used to identify about 67% of pathogens within 24 hours, and up to 90% within 72 hours
- Timing of specimen collection: varies, usually depending on type of suspected bacteremia and whether drug therapy needs to be started regardless of test results

Purpose
- To confirm bacteremia
- To identify the causative organism in bacteremia and septicemia
- To determine the cause of a fever of unknown origin

Patient preparation
- Note and report all allergies.
- Restriction of food and fluids isn't necessary.
- Explain that transient discomfort may be felt from the needle punctures and pressure of the tourniquet.
- Confirm patient's identity using two patient identifiers according to facility policy.

TEACHING POINTS
Be sure to cover:
- the purpose of the study and how it's done
- who will perform the test and where
- that the test usually takes less than 5 minutes
- the number of samples the test requires.

PROCEDURE

- Wash your hands thoroughly.
- Maintain asepsis throughout the test.
- Wear protective equipment throughout the test.
- Clean the venipuncture site first with an alcohol swab, and then with a povidone-iodine swab, starting at the site and working outward in a circular motion.
- Wait at least 1 minute for the skin to dry.
- Apply the tourniquet.
- Perform a venipuncture.
- Draw 10 to 20 ml of blood for an adult, or 2 to 6 ml for a child.
- Clean the diaphragm tops of the culture bottles with alcohol or iodine and change the needle on the syringe.
- If broth is used, add blood to each bottle until a 1:5 or 1:10 dilution is achieved. For example, add 10 ml of blood to a 100-ml bottle. Note that the size of the bottle may vary depending on hospital protocol.
- If a special resin is used, add blood to the resin in the bottles, according to facility protocol, and invert gently to mix.
- Draw the blood directly into a special collection-processing tube if the lysis-centrifugation technique (Isolator) is used.
- Document the tentative diagnosis and any current or recent antimicrobial therapy on the laboratory request.
- To detect most causative agents, blood cultures are ideally performed on 2 consecutive days.

Postprocedure care
- Use alcohol to remove the iodine from the venipuncture site.
- Apply warm soaks if a hematoma develops at the venipuncture site.

MONITORING
- Bleeding
- Hematoma
- Signs and symptoms of infection

Precautions
- Maintain standard precautions when performing the procedure and handling specimens.
- Send each sample to the laboratory immediately after collection.

- Collect blood cultures prior to administration of antimicrobial agents whenever possible because previous or current antimicrobial therapy may give false-negative results.
- Improper collection techniques may contaminate the sample.
- Removal of culture bottle caps may prevent anaerobic growth.
- Use of an incorrect bottle and media may prevent aerobic growth and may also result in rejection of the specimen by the laboratory.

Complications
- Bleeding
- Hematoma
- Infection

INTERPRETATION

Normal findings
- Blood cultures are normally sterile.
- For negative specimens, reports should be made at 24 hours, 48 hours, and 1 week of incubation.

Abnormal results
- Positive blood cultures don't necessarily confirm pathologic septicemia. Mild, transient bacteremia may occur during the course of many infectious diseases or may complicate other disorders.
- Persistent, continuous, or recurrent bacteremia reliably confirms the presence of serious infection.
- Although 2% to 3% of cultured blood samples are contaminated by skin bacteria, such as *Staphylococcus epidermidis,* diphtheroids, and propionibacterium, these organisms may be clinically significant when isolated from multiple cultures or from immunocompromised patients.
- Debilitated or immunocompromised patients may have isolates of *Candida albicans.*

Bone biopsy

- Removal of a piece or a core of bone for histologic examination
- Performed using a special drill needle under local anesthesia, or by surgical excision under general anesthesia
- Indicated in patients with bone pain and tenderness after a bone scan, a computed tomography scan, radiographs, or arteriography reveals a mass or deformity
- Excision provides larger specimen than drill biopsy and permits immediate surgical treatment if rapid histologic analysis of the specimen reveals malignant tumor

Purpose
- To distinguish between benign and malignant bone tumors

Patient preparation
- Make sure that the patient has signed an appropriate consent form.
- Note and report all allergies.
- Fasting overnight before the test is necessary with open biopsy. Food and fluids restriction isn't generally necessary with drill biopsy.
- A local anesthetic is administered before drill biopsy.
- Warn the patient that some discomfort and pressure will be experienced when the biopsy needle enters the bone in drill biopsy.

TEACHING POINTS
Be sure to cover:
- the purpose of the study and how it's done
- who will perform the biopsy and where
- that it should take no longer than 30 minutes.

DRILL BIOPSY
- The biopsy site is prepared and draped.
- A small incision (usually about 3 mm) is made following administration of a local anesthetic.
- The biopsy needle is pushed into the bone using firm, even pressure.
- The needle is engaged in the bone and rotated about 180 degrees while maintaining steady pressure.
- When the bone core is obtained, the trocar is withdrawn by reversing the drilling motion.
- The specimen is placed in a properly labeled container with 10% formalin solution or Zenker's acetic acid solution.
- Pressure is applied to the site with a sterile gauze pad until hemostasis is obtained.
- A sterile dressing is applied.

OPEN BIOPSY
- After the patient is anesthetized, the biopsy site is prepared and draped.
- An incision is made and a piece of bone is removed and sent to the laboratory for immediate histologic analysis.
- The incision is closed and a sterile dressing is applied.

Postprocedure care
- Notify the physician of excessive drainage or bleeding at the biopsy site.
- Administer analgesics as ordered.
- Resume the patient's usual diet after full recovery from anesthesia.

MONITORING
- Vital signs
- Biopsy site
- Signs and symptoms of infection

◈ **NURSING ALERT** For several days after the biopsy, watch for indications of bone infection, including fever, headache, pain on movement, and tissue redness or abscess at or near the biopsy site. Notify the physician if these symptoms develop.

Precautions
- Check the patient's history for hypersensitivity to the anesthetic.

- Bone biopsy is performed cautiously in patients with uncorrected coagulopathy.
- Send the specimen to the laboratory immediately.
- Failure to obtain a representative bone specimen or to use the proper fixative may alter test results.

Complications
- Bone fracture
- Damage to surrounding tissue
- Infection (osteomyelitis)

Normal findings
- Bone tissue is classified as one of two histologic types: compact or cancellous.
- Compact bone has dense, concentric layers of mineral deposits, or lamellae.
- Cancellous bone has widely spaced lamellae with osteocytes and red and yellow marrow between them.

Abnormal results
- Well-circumscribed and nonmetastasizing lesions suggest benign tumors, such as osteoid osteoma, osteoblastoma, osteochondroma, unicameral bone cyst, benign giant cell tumor, and fibroma.
- Irregularly and rapidly spreading lesions suggest malignant tumors, such as multiple myeloma and osteosarcoma.

Bone densitometry

● OVERVIEW

- A noninvasive means to measure bone mass
- Uses a radiography tube and computer-analyzed images to measure bone mineral density (BMD)
- Performed in the radiology department, a physician's office, or a clinic
- Exposes the patient to minimal radiation
- Also known as *dual energy X-ray absorptiometry* or *DEXA*

Purpose
- To determine bone mineral density
- To identify people at risk for osteoporosis
- To evaluate clinical response to therapy aimed at reducing the rate of bone loss

Patient preparation
- Remove all metal objects from the area to be scanned.

TEACHING POINTS
Be sure to cover:
- who will perform the test and where
- the purpose of the test and how it's done
- that the test is painless and exposure to radiation is minimal
- that the test takes from 10 minutes to 1 hour, depending on the areas scanned.

▶ PROCEDURE

- The patient is positioned on a table located under the scanning device, with the radiation source below him and the detector above.
- The lumbar spine and the proximal femur, two sites at high risk for fracture, may be scanned.
- The distal forearm may be scanned because research shows a high correlation between bone mineral density of this area and the bone mineral density of the spine and femur.
- Bone size, thickness, and volumetric density are calculated to determine potential resistance to mechanical stress.
- The bone's absorption of the radiation is measured by the detector and a digital readout is registered.

Postprocedure care
- No specific postprocedure care is required.

Precautions
- Bone densitometry is contraindicated during pregnancy.
- The accuracy of test results may be influenced by:
  - osteoarthritis
  - fractures
  - size of the region to be scanned
  - fat tissue distribution.

Complications
- None known

⊕ INTERPRETATION

Normal findings
- T-score is above −1.

Abnormal results
- A T-score between −1 and −2.5 may suggest osteopenia.
- A T-score at or below −2.5 may suggest osteoporosis.

Bone marrow aspiration and biopsy

⬤ OVERVIEW

- Involves collection of a specimen of the soft tissue in the medullary canals of long bone and interstices of cancellous bone for histologic and hematologic examination
- Performed by aspiration or needle biopsy under local anesthesia
- Aspiration biopsy: involves removal of a fluid specimen from the bone marrow
- Needle biopsy: involves removal of a core of marrow cells, not fluid
- Both methods commonly used concurrently to obtain the best possible marrow specimens

Purpose

- To diagnose thrombocytopenia, leukemias, granulomas, and anemias
- To diagnose primary and metastatic tumors
- To determine causes of infection
- To aid in disease staging, such as with Hodgkin's disease
- To evaluate chemotherapy
- To monitor myelosuppression

Patient preparation

- Make sure that the patient has signed an appropriate consent form.
- Note all allergies.
- Explain that a blood sample will be collected before the biopsy for laboratory testing.
- Explain that pressure on insertion of the biopsy needle and a brief, pulling pain on removal of the marrow will be felt.
- Administer a mild sedative 1 hour before the test as ordered.

TEACHING POINTS

Be sure to cover:

- the purpose of the study and how it's done
- that it usually takes only 5 to 10 minutes
- which bone site (sternum, anterior or posterior iliac crest, vertebral spinous process, rib, or tibia) will be used.

▷ PROCEDURE

- The patient is positioned and instructed to remain as still as possible.
- The biopsy site is prepared and draped.

ASPIRATION BIOPSY

- A local anesthetic is injected.
- The marrow aspiration needle is inserted through the skin, subcutaneous tissue, and bone cortex, using a twisting motion.
- The stylet is removed from the needle, and a 10- to 20-ml syringe is attached.
- 0.2 to 0.5 ml of marrow is aspirated and the needle is withdrawn.
- If the specimen is inadequate, the needle may be repositioned within the marrow cavity or removed and reinserted in another anesthetized site.
- If the second attempt fails, a needle biopsy may be necessary.

NEEDLE BIOPSY

- The skin at the site is marked with an indelible pencil or marking pen.
- A local anesthetic is injected intradermally, subcutaneously, and at the surface of the bone.
- The biopsy needle is inserted into the periosteum and the needle guard is set as indicated.
- Alternately rotating the inner needle clockwise and counterclockwise directs the needle into the marrow cavity.
- A tissue plug is removed and the needle assembly is withdrawn.
- The marrow is expelled into a labeled bottle containing a special fixative.

Postprocedure care

- While marrow slides are being prepared, apply pressure to site until hemostasis is obtained.
- Clean biopsy site and apply sterile dressing.

MONITORING

- Vital signs
- Biopsy site for bleeding
- Signs and symptoms of hemorrhage
- Signs and symptoms of infection

Precautions

- Bone marrow biopsy is contraindicated in patients with bleeding disorders.

- Check the patient's history for hypersensitivity to the local anesthetic.
- Failure to obtain a representative specimen, to use a fixative for histologic analysis, or to immediately send the specimen to the laboratory may alter test results.

Complications

- Infection
- Hemorrhage
- Puncture of the mediastinum (sternum)

⟐ INTERPRETATION

Normal findings

- Yellow marrow contains fat cells and connective tissue.
- Red marrow contains hematopoietic cells, fat cells, and connective tissue.
- The iron stain, which measures hemosiderin (storage iron), has a +2 level.
- The Sudan black B (SBB) stain, which shows granulocytes, is negative.
- The periodic acid-Schiff (PAS) stain, which detects glycogen reactions, is negative.

Abnormal results

- Decreased hemosiderin levels in an iron stain may indicate a true iron deficiency.
- Increased hemosiderin levels may suggest other types of anemias or blood disorders.
- A positive SBB stain can differentiate acute myelogenous leukemia from acute lymphoblastic leukemia (negative SBB) and may also suggest granulation in myeloblasts.
- A positive PAS stain may suggest acute or chronic lymphocytic leukemia, amyloidosis, thalassemia, lymphoma, infectious mononucleosis, iron-deficiency anemia, or sideroblastic anemia.

Bone scan

● OVERVIEW

- Permits imaging of the skeleton by a scanning camera after I.V. injection of a radioactive tracer compound
- Tracer of choice is radioactive technetium diphosphonate
- Increased concentrations of tracer collect in bone tissue at sites of abnormal metabolism; when scanned, these sites appear as hot spots (commonly detectable months before radiography reveals lesion)
- May be performed with gallium scan to promote early detection of lesions
- Primary indications:
  – Symptoms of metastatic bone disease
  – Bone trauma
  – Known degenerative disorders that require monitoring for signs of progression

Purpose

- To detect malignant bone lesions when radiographic findings are normal but cancer is confirmed or suspected
- To rule out suspected bone lesions
- To detect occult bone trauma associated with pathologic fractures
- To monitor degenerative bone disorders
- To detect infection
- To evaluate unexplained bone pain
- To assist in staging cancer

Patient preparation

- Make sure that the patient has signed an appropriate consent form, if required.
- Note all allergies.
- There are no dietary restrictions.
- Instruct the patient to drink fluids to maintain hydration and to reduce the radiation dose to the bladder after tracer injection and before scanning.
- Explain the importance of holding still during scanning.

TEACHING POINTS
Be sure to cover:
- the purpose of the study and how it's done
- who will perform the test and where
- that the scan is painless and takes about 1 hour

- that the radioactive isotope emits less radiation than a standard radiograph machine
- that analgesics will be given as ordered for positional discomfort.

▶ PROCEDURE

- The I.V. tracer and imaging agent are administered 3 hours before the scan.
- Increased fluid intake is encouraged for the next 1 to 3 hours to facilitate renal clearance of circulating free tracer, not picked up by bone.
- The patient is instructed to urinate immediately before the procedure or a urinary catheter may be inserted to empty the bladder.
- The patient is positioned on the scanner table.
- The scanner moves over the patient's body, detects low-level radiation emitted by the skeleton, and translates this into a two-dimensional picture.
- The scanner takes as many views as needed to cover the specified area.
- The patient may have to be repositioned several times during the test to obtain adequate views.

✳ **AGE-RELATED CONCERN** Children unable to hold still for the scan may need to be sedated.

Postprocedure care

- Instruct the patient to drink additional fluids and to empty his bladder frequently for the next 24 to 48 hours.

MONITORING
- Signs and symptoms of infection at injection site
- Intake and output

Precautions

- A bone scan is contraindicated during pregnancy or lactation.
- Allergic reactions to the radionuclide are rare.
- A bone scan doesn't distinguish between normal and abnormal bone formation.
- Antihypertensives may affect test results.
- A distended bladder may obscure pelvic detail.

- Improper injection technique allows the tracer to seep into muscle tissue, producing erroneous hot spots.
- Avoid scheduling additional radionuclide tests for the next 24 to 48 hours.

Complications

- Infection at the injection site
- Allergic reactions to radionuclide (rare)

✛ INTERPRETATION

Normal findings

- Uptake of the tracer is symmetrical and uniform.
- The tracer concentrates at sites of new bone formation or increased metabolism.
- The epiphyses of growing bone are normal sites of high concentration or hot spots.

Abnormal results

- Increased uptake of tracer where bone formation is occurring faster than in surrounding bone may suggest:
  – all types of bone cancer
  – infection
  – fracture
  – additional disorders when used in conjunction with the patient's medical and surgical history, radiographic findings, and laboratory test results.

Breast biopsy

OVERVIEW

- Allows histologic examination of breast tissue to confirm or rule out cancer
- Needle biopsy or fine-needle biopsy: used to obtain a core of tissue or a fluid aspirate
- Both needle biopsy and fine-needle biopsy limit diagnostic values because of small and unrepresentative specimens possibly obtained
- Open biopsy provides complete tissue specimen; allows specimen to be sectioned, allowing more accurate evaluation
- Breast tissue analysis usually includes estrogen and progesterone receptor assay to aid in selecting therapy if mass is malignant
- Indications:
  - Palpable masses
  - Suspicious areas on mammography
  - Bloody discharge from the nipples
  - Persistently encrusted, inflamed, or eczematoid breast lesions

Purpose
- To differentiate between benign and malignant breast tumors

Patient preparation
- Make sure that the patient has signed an appropriate consent form.
- Note and report all allergies.
- A nothing-by-mouth after midnight order is necessary with general anesthesia. No dietary restrictions are necessary with local anesthesia.
- Obtain and report abnormal results of pre-biopsy studies, such as blood tests, urine tests, and radiographs of the chest.

TEACHING POINTS
Be sure to cover:
- the purpose of the study and how it's done
- that the test takes 15 to 30 minutes
- that breast masses don't always indicate cancer
- the need to wear a support bra at all times after the study until healing is complete.

PROCEDURE

- The biopsy site is prepared and draped.

NEEDLE BIOPSY
- A local anesthetic is administered.
- The syringe is introduced into the lesion.
- Aspirated fluid is placed into a labeled, heparinized tube.
- The aspiration procedure is both diagnostic and therapeutic if cyst fluid is clear yellow and the mass disappears; the aspirate is discarded.
- If cyst aspiration yields no fluid or if the lesion recurs two or three times, an open biopsy is appropriate.
- Tissue is placed in a labeled specimen bottle containing normal saline solution or formalin.
- With fine-needle aspiration, a slide is made for cytology and viewed immediately under a microscope.
- Pressure is applied to the biopsy site until hemostasis is obtained.
- A sterile dressing is applied.

OPEN BIOPSY
- A local or general anesthetic is administered.
- An incision is made in the breast to expose the mass.
- A portion of tissue or the entire mass is excised.
- Benign-appearing masses smaller than ¾″ (2 cm) in diameter are usually excised.
- A specimen is usually incised before larger or malignant-appearing masses are excised.
- Incisional biopsy generally provides an adequate specimen for histologic analysis.
- Specimens are placed in properly labeled specimen bottles containing 10% formalin solution.
- Malignant-appearing tissue is sent for frozen section and receptor assays.
- The biopsy site is sutured and a sterile dressing is applied.

Postprocedure care
- Administer analgesics as ordered.
- Apply an ice bag for discomfort at the site.
- Provide emotional support.

MONITORING
- Vital signs
- Bleeding
- Signs and symptoms of infection at the biopsy site

Precautions
- Check the patient's history for hypersensitivity to anesthetics.
- Open breast biopsy is contraindicated in patients with conditions that preclude surgery.
- All specimens should be sent to the laboratory immediately.
- Needle biopsy should be restricted to fluid-filled cysts and advanced malignant lesions.

Complications
- Bleeding
- Infection

INTERPRETATION

Normal findings
- Breast tissue consists of cellular and noncellular connective tissue, fat lobules, and various lactiferous ducts.
- Breast tissue is pink, more fatty than fibrous, and shows no abnormal development of cells or tissue elements.

Abnormal results
- Benign tumors may suggest:
  - fibrocystic disease
  - adenofibroma
  - intraductal papilloma
  - mammary fat necrosis
  - plasma cell mastitis.
- Malignant tumors may suggest:
  - adenocarcinoma
  - cystosarcoma
  - intraductal or infiltrating carcinoma
  - inflammatory carcinoma
  - medullary or circumscribed carcinoma
  - colloid carcinoma
  - lobular carcinoma
  - sarcoma
  - Paget's disease.

Bronchoscopy

OVERVIEW

- Direct visualization of the larynx, trachea, and bronchi using a rigid or fiber-optic bronchoscope
- Flexible fiber-optic bronchoscope: allows a better view of the segmental and subsegmental bronchi with less risk of trauma
- Large, rigid bronchoscope: used to remove foreign objects, excise endobronchial lesions, and control massive hemoptysis; requires general anesthesia
- Brush, biopsy forceps, or catheter passed through bronchoscope to obtain specimen for cytology or microbiologic examination

Purpose
- To allow visual examination of tumors, obstructions, secretions, or foreign bodies in the tracheobronchial tree
- To diagnose bronchogenic carcinoma, tuberculosis, interstitial pulmonary disease, and fungal or parasitic pulmonary infections
- To obtain specimens for microbiological and cytologic examination
- To locate bleeding sites in the tracheobronchial tree
- To remove foreign bodies, malignant or benign tumors, mucous plugs, and excessive secretions from the tracheobronchial tree

Patient preparation
- Make sure that the patient has signed an appropriate consent form.
- Note all allergies.
- Instruct the patient to fast for 6 to 12 hours before the test.
- Obtain results of preprocedure studies; report any abnormal results.
- Obtain baseline vital signs.
- An I.V. sedative may be given.
- Remove the patient's dentures.

TEACHING POINTS
Be sure to cover:
- test's purpose and how it's done
- who will perform the test and where
- that the test takes 45 to 60 minutes
- that the airway isn't blocked
- that hoarseness, loss of voice, hemoptysis, and sore throat may occur.

PROCEDURE

- The patient is properly positioned.
- Supplemental oxygen by nasal cannula is given if ordered.
- Pulse oximetry, vital signs, and cardiac rhythm are monitored.
- Local anesthetic is sprayed into the patient's mouth and throat to suppress the gag reflex.
- The bronchoscope is inserted through the patient's mouth or nose; a bite block is placed in the mouth if the oral approach is used.
- When the bronchoscope is just above the vocal cords, about 3 to 4 ml of 2% to 4% lidocaine is flushed through the inner channel of the scope to the vocal cords to anesthetize deeper areas.
- A fiber-optic camera is used to take photographs for documentation.
- Tissue specimens are obtained from suspect areas.
- Suction apparatus may remove foreign bodies or mucous plugs.
- Bronchoalveolar lavage may remove thickened secretions or be used to diagnose infectious causes of infiltrates.
- Specimens are properly prepared and immediately sent to the laboratory.

Postprocedure care
- Position a conscious patient in semi-Fowler's position.
- Position an unconscious patient on one side, with the head of the bed slightly elevated to prevent aspiration.
- Instruct the patient to spit out saliva rather than swallow it.
- Observe for bleeding.
- Resume the patient's usual diet, beginning with sips of clear liquid or ice chips, when the gag reflex returns.
- Provide lozenges or a soothing liquid gargle to ease discomfort when the gag reflex returns.
- Check follow-up chest X-ray to rule out pneumothorax.

MONITORING
- Vital signs
- Characteristics of sputum
- Respiratory status

NURSING ALERT Immediately report subcutaneous crepitus around the patient's face, neck, or chest because these may indicate tracheal or bronchial perforation or pneumothorax.

NURSING ALERT Watch for and immediately report symptoms of respiratory difficulty associated with laryngeal edema or laryngospasm, such as laryngeal stridor and dyspnea.

Precautions
- Check the patient's history for hypersensitivity to the anesthetic.
- Failure to observe pretest dietary restrictions may result in aspiration.
- Bronchoscopy findings must be correlated with clinical signs and symptoms and radiographic and cytologic findings.

Complications
- Tracheal or bronchial perforation
- Hypoxemia
- Cardiac arrhythmias
- Bleeding
- Infection
- Bronchospasm
- Laryngeal edema

INTERPRETATION

Normal findings
- The bronchi appear structurally similar to the trachea.
- The right bronchus is slightly larger and more vertical than the left.
- Smaller segmental bronchi branch off from the main bronchi.

Abnormal results
- Structural abnormalities of the bronchial wall suggest inflammation, ulceration, tumors, and enlargement of submucosal lymph nodes.
- Structural abnormalities of endotracheal origin suggest stenosis, compression, ectasia, and diverticulum.
- Structural abnormalities of the trachea or bronchi suggest calculi, foreign bodies, masses, and paralyzed vocal cords.
- Abnormal results of tissue and cell studies suggest interstitial pulmonary disease, infection, carcinoma, and tuberculosis.

Camera endoscopy

- Records video images of stomach and small intestine, using a tiny video camera with light source and transmitter inside a capsule propelled through digestive tract by peristalsis
- Modality that's able to travel and record where other diagnostic techniques may not reach or make visible (see *Detecting disorders in the stomach and small intestine*)

Purpose
- To detect polyps or cancer
- To detect the causes of bleeding and anemia

Patient preparation
- Usually no bowel preparation is involved, but some patients may benefit from it.
- Inform the patient that he may need to fast for 12 hours before the test but may have fluids for up to 2 hours before the test.
- Explain to the patient that he'll need to swallow the camera "pill" and that it will send information to a receiver he'll wear on his belt.

TEACHING POINTS
Be sure to cover:
- purpose of the study and how it's done
- who will perform the test and where
- that the test is painless and that after swallowing the pill he can go home or go to work
- that walking helps facilitate movement of the pill
- need to return to the facility in 24 hours (or as directed) so the recorder can be removed from his belt
- that he will excrete the pill normally in his feces within 8 to 72 hours.

- The patient ingests the camera pill, and a receiver is attached to his belt.
- The pill records images for up to 6 hours along its path through the stomach, small intestine, and mouth of the large intestine, transmitting the information to a data recorder in a belt worn around the patient's waist.
- The patient returns to the facility, as instructed, so the images can be transmitted to the computer, where they're displayed on the screen.

Postprocedure care
- After the images are obtained, tell the patient to resume his usual diet.

MONITORING
- None necessary

Precautions
- The procedure is contraindicated in patients with a suspected obstruction, fistula, or stricture and in infants, young children, and others who can't swallow capsules.
- Because the battery is short lived, images of the large intestine can't be obtained.
- The capsule can't stop bleeding, take tissue samples, remove growths, or repair other detected problems (other invasive studies may be needed).

Complications
- None known

Normal findings
- Anatomy of the stomach and small intestine is normal.

Abnormal results
- Bleeding sites or abnormalities of the stomach and small bowel, such as erosions, Crohn's disease, celiac disease, benign and malignant tumors of the small intestine, vascular disorders, medication-related small bowel injuries, and pediatric small bowel disorders may be seen.

DETECTING DISORDERS IN THE STOMACH AND SMALL INTESTINE

With camera endoscopy, the patient swallows the camera capsule, which then travels through the body by the natural movement of the digestive tract. A receiver worn outside the body records the images. The strength of the signal indicates the capsule's location.

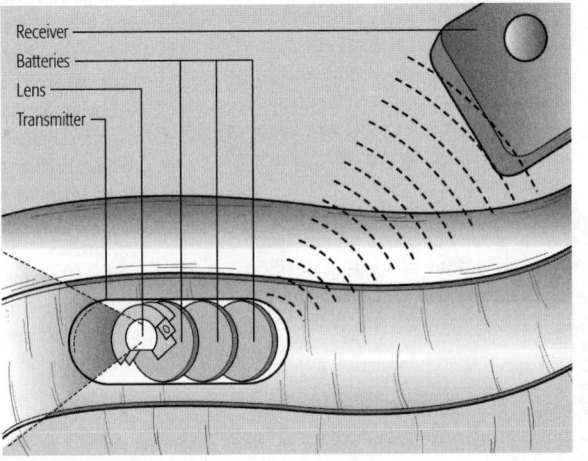

Receiver
Batteries
Lens
Transmitter

Cardiac blood pool imaging

● OVERVIEW

- A noninvasive evaluation of regional and global ventricular performance after I.V. injection of human serum albumin, or red blood cells (RBCs), tagged with the isotope technetium Tc 99m pertechnetate
- First-pass imaging: scintillation camera records the radioactivity emitted by the isotope in its initial pass through the left ventricle, allowing calculation of the ejection fraction
- Gated cardiac blood pool imaging: performed after first-pass imaging or as a separate test; commonly uses signals from an electrocardiogram (ECG) to trigger the scintillation camera
- Two-frame gated imaging: the camera records left ventricular end-systole and end-diastole for 500 to 1,000 cardiac cycles, allowing assessment of left ventricular contractility
- Multiple-gated acquisition (MUGA) scanning: the camera records 14 to 64 points of a single cardiac cycle; used to evaluate regional wall motion and determine indices of cardiac function
- Stress MUGA test: MUGA scanning done at rest and after exercise to detect changes in ejection fraction and cardiac output
- Nitro MUGA test: the camera records points in the cardiac cycle after sublingual administration of nitroglycerin; used to assess the drug's effect on ventricular function
- Blood pool imaging: involves less risk than left ventriculography in assessing cardiac function

Purpose
- To evaluate left ventricular function
- To detect and evaluate myocardial wall-motion abnormalities (areas of akinesia or dyskinesia)
- To detect and evaluate intracardiac shunting

Patient preparation
- Make sure that the patient has signed an appropriate consent form.
- Note all allergies.
- Restriction of food and fluids isn't necessary.
- Warn the patient that the needle puncture may cause transient discomfort, but that the imaging procedure is painless.

TEACHING POINTS
Be sure to cover:
- the purpose of the study and how it's done
- who will perform the test and where
- that the study takes about 1½ hours
- that the tracer used for the study poses no radiation hazard, and rarely produces adverse effects
- that the patient will need to remain silent and motionless, unless instructed otherwise.

▶ PROCEDURE

- The patient is placed in a supine position beneath the detector of a scintillation camera.
- The radioisotope is injected.
- The scintillation camera records the first pass of the isotope through the heart to locate the aortic and mitral valves.
- Using the ECG, the camera is gated for selected 60-msec intervals, representing end-systole and end-diastole, and 500 to 1,000 cardiac cycles are recorded on radiograph or film.
- The patient may be assisted to a modified left anterior oblique position to observe septal and posterior wall motion.
- The patient may be assisted to a right anterior oblique position and given 0.4 mg of nitroglycerin sublingually.
- The scintillation camera records additional gated images to evaluate abnormal contraction in the left ventricle.
- The patient may be instructed to exercise as the scintillation camera records gated images.

✹ **AGE-RELATED CONCERN** If the patient is elderly or physically compromised, assist him to a sitting position and make sure he isn't dizzy. Then assist him in getting off the examination table.

Postprocedure care
- No specific postprocedure care is required.

Precautions
- Cardiac blood pool imaging is contraindicated during pregnancy.

Complications
- Adverse reaction to tracer (rare)

✥ INTERPRETATION

Normal findings
- The left ventricle contracts symmetrically.
- The isotope appears evenly distributed.
- The ejection fraction is 55% to 65%.

Abnormal results
- Globally reduced ejection fractions suggest possible cardiomyopathy.
- Prolongation of the radioisotope's activity may indicate a left-to-right shunt.
- Early arrival of radioisotope activity in the left ventricle or aorta may signify a right-to-left shunt.
- Segmental abnormalities of ventricular wall motion suggest possible coronary artery disease or myocarditis.
- Ejection fraction less than 35% to 40% suggests left ventricular systolic dysfunction.

Cardiac catheterization

● OVERVIEW

- Involves passage of a catheter into the right, left, or both sides of the heart
- Used to measure pressures in chambers of the heart; records films of the ventricles (contrast ventriculography) and arteries (coronary arteriography)
- Left-sided heart catheterization: used to assess patency of the coronary arteries and function of left ventricle
- Right-sided heart catheterization: used to assess pulmonary artery pressures

Purpose

- To evaluate valvular insufficiency or stenosis, septal defects, congenital anomalies, myocardial function, myocardial blood supply, and cardiac wall motion
- To aid in diagnosing left ventricular enlargement, aortic root enlargement, ventricular aneurysms, and intracardiac shunts

Patient preparation

- Make sure that the patient has signed an appropriate consent form.
- Note and report all allergies.
- Discontinue anticoagulant therapy to reduce complications of bleeding.
- Restrict food and fluids for at least 6 hours before the test.
- Explain that if a mild sedative is given the patient remains conscious.
- Warn the patient that a transient hot, flushing sensation or nausea may occur.
- Stress the need to cough or breathe deeply.

TEACHING POINTS

Be sure to cover:
- test's purpose and how it's done
- that the test will take 1 to 2 hours.

▷ PROCEDURE

- The patient is placed in a supine position on a padded table and his heart rate and rhythm, respiratory status, and blood pressure are monitored throughout the procedure.
- An I.V. line is started if not already in place and a local anesthetic is injected at the insertion site.

- A small incision is made into the artery or vein, depending on if left-side or right-side studies are performed.
- The catheter is passed through the sheath into the vessel and guided using fluoroscopy.
- In right-sided heart catheterization, the catheter is inserted into the antecubital or femoral vein and advanced through the vena cava into the right side of the heart and into the pulmonary artery.
- In left-sided heart catheterization, the catheter is inserted into the brachial or femoral artery and advanced retrograde through the aorta into the coronary artery ostium and left ventricle.
- When the catheter is in place, the contrast medium is injected to visualize the cardiac vessels and structures.
- Nitroglycerin is given to eliminate catheter-induced spasm or observe its effect on the coronary arteries.
- Direct pressure is applied to the incision site after the catheter is removed, until hemostasis is achieved and a sterile dressing is applied.

Postprocedure care

- Reinforce the dressing as needed.
- Enforce bed rest for 8 hours.
- If the femoral route was used for catheter insertion, keep the leg straight at the hip for 6 to 8 hours.
- If the antecubital fossa route was used, keep the arm straight at the elbow for at least 3 hours.
- Resume medications and administer analgesics as ordered.
- Encourage fluid intake.

MONITORING

- Vital signs
- Intake and output
- Cardiac rhythm
- Neurologic and respiratory status
- Peripheral vascular status distal to the puncture site
- Catheter insertion site and dressings
- Signs and symptoms of infection

Precautions

- Notify the physician of hypersensitivity to shellfish, iodine, or contrast media.
- Contraindications to right- and left-heart catheterization include uncor-

rected coagulopathy, poor renal function, and debilitation.
- Contraindications to right-heart catheterization include left bundle-branch block, unless a temporary pacemaker is inserted to counteract possible ventricular asystole.
- The brachial artery causes a higher incidence of complications.
- Prophylactic antibiotics prevent infective endocarditis in a patient with valvular heart disease.

Complications

- With left-or right-sided catheterization: myocardial infarction, arrhythmias, cardiac tamponade, infection, hypovolemia, pulmonary edema, hematoma, blood loss, adverse reaction to contrast media, and vasovagal response
- With left-sided catheterization: arterial thrombus or embolism, and stroke
- With right-sided catheterization: thrombophlebitis and pulmonary embolism

✛ INTERPRETATION

Normal findings

- There are no abnormalities of heart valves, chamber size, pressures, configuration, wall motion or thickness, and blood flow.
- Coronary arteries have a smooth and regular outline.

Abnormal results

- Coronary artery narrowing greater than 70% suggests significant coronary artery disease.
- Narrowing of the left main coronary artery and occlusion or narrowing high in the left anterior descending artery suggests the need for revascularization surgery.
- Impaired wall motion suggests myocardial incompetence.
- A pressure gradient, or difference in pressures above and below a heart valve indicates valvular heart disease.
- Retrograde flow of the contrast medium across a valve during systole indicates valvular incompetence.

Cardiac magnetic resonance imaging

● OVERVIEW

- Magnetic resonance imaging (MRI): noninvasive procedure that enables visualization of cross-sectional images of bone and delineation of fluid-filled soft tissue in great detail; produces images of organs and vessels in motion
- Most commonly relies on the magnetic properties of hydrogen, the most abundant and magnetically sensitive of the body's atoms
- Cardiac MRI: involves placing the patient in a magnetic field, obtaining cross-sectional images of the heart and related structures in multiple planes, and recording them for permanent record
- Magnetic fields and radiofrequency (RF) energy used for MRI are imperceptible to the patient; no harmful effects have been documented
- Optimal magnetic fields and RF waves for each type of tissue under investigation

Purpose

- To identify anatomic sequelae related to myocardial infarction, such as formation of ventricular aneurysm and mural thrombus
- To detect and evaluate cardiomyopathy
- To detect and evaluate pericardial disease
- To identify paracardiac or intracardiac masses
- To detect and evaluate congenital heart disease, such as atrial or ventricular septal defects and malposition of the great vessels
- To identify vascular disease such as thoracic aortic aneurysm and dissection
- To assess the structure of the pulmonary vasculature

Patient preparation

- Make sure that the patient has signed an appropriate consent form.
- Note and report all allergies.
- Restriction of food and fluids isn't necessary.
- Have the patient remove all metal objects.
- Make sure the patient doesn't have a pacemaker or surgically implanted

joints, pins, clips, valves, or pumps containing metal that could be attracted to the strong MRI magnet.
- Ask if the patient has ever worked with metals or has any metal in his eyes.
- Explain that MRI is painless, but discomfort may be associated with remaining still inside a small space throughout the test.
- The patient may be given earplugs because the scanner makes clicking, whirring, and thumping noises as it moves.
- Provide reassurance that the patient will be able to communicate with the technician at all times, and the procedure will be stopped if he feels claustrophobic.
- Administer a sedative if ordered, especially for a claustrophobic patient.

TEACHING POINTS

Be sure to cover:
- the purpose of the study and how it's done
- who will perform the test and where
- that the test takes up to 90 minutes
- importance of remaining still.

▶ PROCEDURE

- The patient is checked for metal objects.
- He's placed in a supine position on a narrow, padded, nonmetallic bed that slides to the desired position inside the scanner.
- During the procedure the patient is asked to remain still.
- The response of the patient to the enclosed environment is assessed and reassurance is provided if necessary.
- RF energy is directed at the patient's chest.
- Resulting images are displayed on a monitor and recorded for permanent storage.

Postprocedure care

- No specific postprocedure care is usually required unless the patient required sedation.

MONITORING

◆ NURSING ALERT Monitor the sedated patient's hemodynamic, cardiac, respiratory, and mental status

until the effects of the sedative have worn off.

Precautions

- If claustrophobia is an issue, the patient may need sedation, or may not be able to tolerate the procedure.
- Monitor cardiac patients for signs of ischemia secondary to anxiety.
- No metal can enter the testing area because the MRI works through a powerful magnetic field.
- MRI can't be performed on patients with pacemakers, intracranial aneurysm clips, or other ferrous metal implants.
- Ventilators, I.V. infusion pumps, and other metallic or computer-based equipment cannot be used in the MRI area.
- Unstable patients need an I.V. access without metal components, and all equipment must be MRI-compatible.
- Excessive patient movement can blur images.
- If necessary, monitor the patient's oxygen saturation, cardiac rhythm, and respiratory status during the test.
- A member of the anesthesia department may be needed to monitor a heavily sedated patient.
- A nurse or radiology technician should maintain verbal contact with a conscious patient.

Complications

- Panic attacks related to claustrophobia
- Adverse reactions to sedation

✛ INTERPRETATION

Normal findings

- No cardiovascular anatomic and structural abnormalities are present.

Abnormal results

- Cardiovascular anatomic or structural abnormalities may suggest:
  - cardiomyopathy and pericardial disease
  - atrial or ventricular septal defects
  - congenital defects
  - paracardiac or intracardiac masses
  - pericardiac or vascular disease.

Cardiac positron emission tomography

- Combines elements of both computed tomography scanning and conventional radionuclide imaging
- Works by measuring emissions of particles of injected radioisotopes, called positrons, and converting them to tomographic images
- Unlike conventional radionuclide imaging, uses radioisotopes of biologically important elements, oxygen, nitrogen, carbon, and fluorine
- Positron emitters: can be chemically tagged to biologically active molecules, such as carbon monoxide, neurotransmitters, hormones, and metabolites (particularly glucose), allowing study of their uptake and distribution in tissue
- Radiation is 25% of that received by computed tomography scan
- Costly because of short half-lives of the radioisotopes, which must be produced at an on-site cyclotron and attached quickly to the desired tracer molecules
- Also known as *PET scanning*

Purpose
- To detect coronary artery disease
- To evaluate myocardial metabolism
- To distinguish viable from infarcted cardiac tissue, especially during early stages of myocardial infarction

Patient preparation
- Make sure that the patient has signed an appropriate consent form.
- Note and report all allergies.
- Provide reassurance that the test is painless, other than possible minor discomfort if an I.V. access is inserted.
- Fasting after midnight the night before the test may be required.
- Abstinence from caffeinated beverages, alcohol, and tobacco products may be required for 24 hours before the test.
- Stress the importance of remaining still during the study.

TEACHING POINTS
Be sure to cover:
- the purpose of the study and how it's done
- who will perform the test and where
- that the test takes 1 to 1½ hours.

- The patient is placed in a supine position with his arms above his head.
- An attenuation scan, lasting about 30 minutes, is performed.
- The appropriate positron emitter is administered and scanning is completed.
- An additional different positron emitter may be given if comparative studies are needed.

Postprocedure care
- Instruct the patient to move slowly immediately after the procedure to avoid postural hypotension.
- Encourage increased oral fluid intake to help flush the radioisotope from the bladder.

MONITORING
- Vital signs
- Cardiac status

Precautions
- Carefully screen female patients of childbearing age because the radioisotope may be harmful to a fetus.
- Failure of the patient to maintain proper positioning can prevent accurate imaging.

Complications
- Postural hypotension

Normal findings
- No areas of ischemic tissue are present.
- If the patient receives two tracers, the flow and distribution should match, indicating normal tissue.

Abnormal results
- Reduced blood flow, with increased glucose use, indicates ischemia.
- Reduced blood flow, with decreased glucose use, indicates necrotic, scarred tissue.

Celiac and mesenteric arteriography

● OVERVIEW

- Radiographic examination of abdominal vasculature after intra-arterial injection of a contrast medium through a catheter
- Catheter passed through the femoral artery into the abdominal aorta and positioned in the celiac, superior mesenteric, or inferior mesenteric artery using fluoroscopic guidance

Purpose

- To locate the source of and control GI bleeding when other measures fail
- To distinguish between benign and malignant neoplasms
- To evaluate cirrhosis and portal hypertension
- To evaluate vascular damage after abdominal trauma
- To detect vascular abnormalities

Patient preparation

- Make sure that the patient has signed an appropriate consent form.
- Note and report all allergies.
- Obtain results of preprocedure tests and report abnormal results.
- Fasting is required for 8 hours before the test.
- I.V. moderate sedation and a local anesthetic will be given. Warn the patient that he may feel a brief, stinging sensation when it's injected.
- Warn that transient burning may be felt as the contrast is injected.
- Administer a sedative if ordered.

TEACHING POINTS

Be sure to cover:

- the purpose of the test
- how the test will be performed
- who will perform the test and where
- that the test can take from 30 minutes to 3 hours, depending on the number of vessels studied.

▶ PROCEDURE

- The patient is placed in a supine position on the radiograph table and an I.V. infusion is started.
- Vital signs and cardiac rhythm are monitored and peripheral pulses are palpated and marked.

- The puncture site, usually the right groin, is cleaned and prepared.
- Local anesthetic is injected.
- The needle is inserted into the femoral artery.
- A series of films is taken as contrast is injected through the catheter.
- After filming, the catheter is withdrawn and firm pressure applied.
- The site is observed for hematoma formation and peripheral pulses are reassessed.
- The site is cleaned and a sterile dressing applied.

Postprocedure care

- Maintain bed rest and keep the affected leg straight for 4 to 6 hours.
- Raise the head of the bed 30 degrees.
- Assist the patient in rolling side to side.
- The unaffected leg may be used to help in repositioning.
- Resume usual diet as ordered.
- Encourage fluid intake.

MONITORING

- Vital signs
- Intake and output

◈ **NURSING ALERT** Monitor peripheral pulses, color, temperature, and sensation of the leg that was used for the test. Immediately notify the physician of any changes.

◈ **NURSING ALERT** Check the puncture site for bleeding or expanding hematoma. If either develops, apply direct manual pressure to the site and notify the physician immediately.

Precautions

- Check the patient's history for hypersensitivity to iodine, shellfish, or contrast medium.

◈ **NURSING ALERT** Celiac and mesenteric arteriography should be performed cautiously in patients with uncorrected coagulopathy and those who are taking anticoagulant drugs.

◈ **NURSING ALERT** Reactions to the contrast medium occur within 30 minutes. Watch for cardiovascular shock or arrest, flushing, laryngeal stridor, and urticaria.

- Celiac and mesenteric arteriography is contraindicated in pregnancy.
- Gas, stool, or barium present from a previous procedure can affect the accuracy of test results.

- Atherosclerotic lesions in the vessel to be cannulated may prevent entry and passage of the catheter.

Complications

- Hemorrhage, thrombosis, and emboli
- Cardiac arrhythmias and infection

✛ INTERPRETATION

Normal findings

- Arteries taper in size.
- Contrast spreads evenly within the sinusoids (it empties from the intestine into the superior mesenteric vein and into the portal vein).

Abnormal results

- Extravasation of contrast from damaged vessels suggests GI hemorrhage.
- Angiographic findings suggesting abdominal neoplasm include: invasion, encasement, distortion, or displacement of blood vessels; areas of necrosis appearing as puddles of contrast; a tumor blush or stain produced by contrast remaining longer in the neoplasm; and arteriovenous (AV) shunting, depending on tumor size and location.
- Angiographic findings suggesting cirrhosis include: diminished portal venous flow, dilated and tortuous collateral veins, and reversed portal venous flow.
- Angiographic findings suggesting splenic injury include: displaced intrasplenic arterial branches, contrast leakage from splenic arteries into splenic pulp, displaced splenic arteries and veins by enlarged spleen, and stretched intrasplenic arteries and compressed splenic pulp by an avascular mass indicating a subcapsular hematoma.
- Angiographic findings suggesting hepatic injury include: vascular distortion, displaced and stretched intrahepatic arteries by intrahepatic and subcapsular hematomas, and AV fistulas between the hepatic artery and portal vein.
- Narrowed or occluded arterial lumens suggest atherosclerotic plaque, vessel spasm, or emboli.

Cerebral angiography

● OVERVIEW

- Radiographic examination of the cerebral vasculature after injection of intra-arterial contrast medium
- Most common approach: the femoral artery; other approaches include a direct carotid or vertebral artery puncture, or the brachial, axillary, or subclavian artery
- Indicated for suspected abnormalities of the cerebral vasculature, commonly supported by other imaging study results

Purpose
- To detect cerebrovascular abnormalities, such as aneurysm or arteriovenous malformation, thrombosis, narrowing, or occlusion
- To evaluate vascular displacement caused by tumor, hematoma, edema, herniation, vasospasm, increased intracranial pressure, or hydrocephalus
- To locate clips applied to blood vessels during surgery and to evaluate the postoperative status of such vessels
- To evaluate the presence and degree of carotid artery disease

Patient preparation
- Make sure that the patient has signed an appropriate consent form.
- Note and report all allergies.
- Have the patient fast for 8 to 10 hours before the test.
- Tell the patient his head will be immobilized and he'll need to lie still.
- A local anesthetic will be administered.
- Warn the patient that nausea, warmth, or burning may occur with contrast injection.
- Initiate an I.V. access and administer I.V. fluids as ordered.
- Administer a sedative as ordered.
- Have the patient void.
- Document baseline vital signs and neurologic assessment data.

TEACHING POINTS
Be sure to cover:
- the purpose of the study and how it's done
- who will perform the test and where
- that it takes 2 to 4 hours.

▶ PROCEDURE

- The patient is placed in a supine position on a radiographic table.
- The access site is prepared and draped and a local anesthetic is injected.
- The artery is punctured with the appropriate needle and catheterized under fluoroscopic guidance.
- Catheter placement is verified by fluoroscopy and a contrast medium is injected.
- A series of radiographs is taken and reviewed.
- Arterial catheter patency is maintained by continuous or periodic flushing.
- Vital signs and neurological status are continuously monitored.
- The catheter is removed, firm pressure is applied to the access site until hemostasis is achieved, and a pressure dressing is applied.

Postprocedure care
- Enforce bed rest and apply an ice bag as ordered.
- If active bleeding or expanding hematoma occurs, apply firm pressure to the puncture site and inform the physician immediately.
- Ensure adequate hydration to assist in clearing the contrast material through the kidneys.
- Provide analgesia as ordered.
- Resume usual diet as ordered.

MONITORING
- Vital signs
- Intake and output
- Neurovascular status of extremity distal to the access site
- Neurologic and respiratory status
- Puncture site for active bleeding or expanding hematoma

◈ **NURSING ALERT** If the femoral approach was used, keep the involved leg straight at the hip and check pulses distal to the site (dorsalis pedis, posterior tibial, and popliteal) as ordered. Check the temperature, color, and sensation of the affected leg because thrombosis, embolism, or hematoma can occlude distal blood flow.

◈ **NURSING ALERT** If the carotid artery was used as the access site, watch for dysphagia or respiratory distress, which can result from hematoma

or edema. Also watch for disorientation, weakness, or numbness in the extremities (signs of neurovascular compromise) and for arterial spasms, which produce symptoms of transient ischemic attacks (TIAs). Notify the physician immediately if abnormal signs develop.

◈ **NURSING ALERT** If the brachial artery was used, keep the arm straight at the elbow and assess distal pulses (radial and ulnar) as ordered. Avoid venipuncture and blood pressures in the affected arm. Observe the extremity for changes in color, temperature, or sensation. If it becomes pale, cool, or numb, notify the physician immediately.

Precautions
- Check for allergy to iodine or other contrast media and notify the physician.
- Cerebral angiography is contraindicated in patients with severe renal or thyroid disease, recent anticoagulation therapy, and recent thrombotic or embolic events.
- Head movement affects the clarity of the angiographic images.

Complications
- Adverse reaction to contrast media
- Embolism
- Bleeding
- Infection
- Hematoma at the puncture site
- Vasospasm
- Thrombosis
- TIA or stroke

✛ INTERPRETATION

Normal findings
- Cerebral vasculature is normal.
- During the arterial phase of perfusion, the contrast medium fills and opacifies superficial and deep arteries and arterioles.
- During the venous phase, the contrast medium opacifies superficial and deep veins.

Abnormal results
- Changes in the caliber of vessel lumina suggest vascular disease.
- Vessel displacement suggests a possible tumor.

Cerebrospinal fluid analysis

- Commonly obtained by lumbar puncture; rarely, by cisternal or ventricular puncture (for qualitative analysis)
- May also be obtained during other neurologic tests such as myelography

Purpose

- To measure cerebrospinal fluid (CSF) pressure as an aid in detecting an obstruction of CSF circulation
- To help diagnose viral or bacterial meningitis, subarachnoid or intracranial hemorrhage, tumors, and brain abscesses
- To help diagnose neurosyphilis and chronic central nervous system infections
- To check for Alzheimer's disease

Patient preparation

- No dietary restrictions are needed.
- Make sure that the patient or a responsible family member has signed an informed consent form.
- Confirm the patient's identity using two patient identifiers according to facility policy.
- Explain to the patient that this test analyzes the fluid around the spinal cord.
- Advise the patient that a headache is the most common adverse effect of a lumbar puncture, but reassure him that his cooperation during the test helps minimize this effect.
- Tell the patient that when the spinal needle is inserted, he may feel slight local pain as the needle transverses the dura mater.
- If the patient is unusually anxious, assess and report his vital signs.
- Instruct the patient to report pain or sensations that differ from or continue after this expected discomfort because such sensations may indicate irritation or puncture of a nerve root, thus requiring needle repositioning.

TEACHING POINTS
Be sure to cover:
- purpose of the study and how it's done
- who will perform the test and where
- importance of remaining still and breathing normally because movement and hyperventilation can alter pressure readings or cause injury
- that the test should take less than 3 minutes.

FINDINGS IN CEREBROSPINAL FLUID ANALYSIS

Test	Normal	Abnormality	Implications
Pressure	50 to 180 mm H_2O	Increase	Increased intracranial pressure
		Decrease	Spinal subarachnoid obstruction above puncture site
Appearance	Clear, colorless	Cloudy	Infection
		Xanthochromic or bloody	Subarachnoid, intracerebral, or intraventricular hemorrhage; spinal cord obstruction; traumatic tap (usually noted only in initial specimen)
		Brown, orange, or yellow	Elevated protein levels, red blood cell (RBC) breakdown (blood present for at least 3 days)
Protein	15 to 50 mg/dl (SI, 0.15 to 0.5 g/L)	Marked increase	Tumors, trauma, hemorrhage, diabetes mellitus, polyneuritis, blood in cerebrospinal fluid (CSF)
		Marked decrease	Rapid CSF production
Gamma globulin	3% to 12% of total protein	Increase	Demyelinating disease, neurosyphilis, Guillain-Barré syndrome
Glucose	50 to 80 mg/dl (SI, 2.8 to 4.4 mmol/L)	Increase	Systemic hyperglycemia
		Decrease	Systemic hypoglycemia, bacterial or fungal infection, meningitis, mumps, postsubarachnoid hemorrhage
Cell count	0 to 5 white blood cells	Increase	Active disease: meningitis, acute infection, onset of chronic illness, tumor, abscess, infarction, demyelinating disease
	No RBCs	RBCs	Hemorrhage or traumatic lumbar puncture
Venereal Disease Research Laboratories, test for syphilis, and other serologic tests	Nonreactive	Positive	Neurosyphilis
Chloride	118 to 130 mEq/L (SI, 118 to 130 mmol/L)	Decrease	Infected meninges
Gram stain	No organisms	Gram-positive or gram-negative organisms	Bacterial meningitis

- During the procedure, observe closely for adverse reactions, such as elevated pulse rate, pallor, or clammy skin, and report any significant changes immediately.
- Position the patient on his side at the edge of the bed with his knees drawn up to his abdomen and his chin on his chest.
- Provide pillows to support the spine on a horizontal plane. This position allows full flexion of the spine and easy access to the lumbar subarachnoid space. Help him maintain this position by placing one arm around his knees and the other arm around his neck.
- If the sitting position is preferable, have the patient sit up and bend his chest and head toward his knees. Help him maintain this position throughout the procedure.
- The skin is prepared for injection and the area is draped.
- The anesthetic is injected, and the spinal needle is inserted in the midline, between the spinous processes of the vertebrae (usually between the third and fourth lumbar vertebra). At this point, initial (or opening) CSF pressure is measured and a specimen is obtained.
- After the specimen is collected, label the containers in the order in which they were filled.
- Record the collection time on the test request form. Send the labeled specimens to the laboratory immediately after collection.
- A final pressure reading is taken, and the needle is removed.
- The puncture site is cleaned with a local antiseptic, such as povidone-iodine solution, and a small adhesive bandage is applied.

Postprocedure care

- Check whether the patient must lie flat or if the head of his bed may be slightly elevated.
- In most cases, instruct the patient to keep lying flat for 8 hours after the lumbar puncture. Sometimes, a 30-degree elevation at the head of the bed is allowed. Remind the patient that although he must not raise his head, he can turn from side to side.
- Encourage the patient to drink fluids.
- Provide a flexible straw.

MONITORING
- Puncture site
- Neurologic status

Precautions

⬥ **NURSING ALERT** Monitor the patient for complications of lumbar puncture, such as reaction to the anesthetic, meningitis, bleeding into the spinal canal, cerebellar tonsillar herniation, and medullary compression.

- Infection at the puncture site contraindicates removal of CSF; in patients with increased intracranial pressure, CSF should be removed with extreme caution because the rapid reduction in pressure can cause cerebellar tonsillar herniation and medullary compression.

Complications

- Reaction to the anesthetic
- Meningitis
- Bleeding into the spinal canal
- Cerebellar tonsillar herniation
- Medullary compression

⬥ **INTERPRETATION**

Normal findings

- See *Findings in cerebrospinal fluid analysis.*

Abnormal results

- See *Findings in cerebrospinal fluid analysis.*

Cervical punch biopsy

● OVERVIEW

- Excision by sharp forceps of a tissue specimen from the cervix for histologic examination
- Multiple biopsies usually obtained from all areas with abnormal tissue
- Performed when the cervix is least vascular (usually 1 week after menses)
- Biopsy sites selected by direct visualization of the cervix with a colposcope (the most accurate method); also selected by Schiller's test (normal squamous epithelium stains dark mahogany while abnormal tissue fails to change color)

Purpose
- To evaluate suspicious cervical lesions
- To diagnose cervical cancer

Patient preparation
- Make sure that the patient has signed an appropriate consent form.
- Note and report all allergies.
- Just before the biopsy, ask the patient to void.

TEACHING POINTS
Be sure to cover:
- the purpose of the study and how it's done
- who will perform the biopsy and where
- that it takes about 15 minutes
- that mild discomfort during and after the biopsy may be experienced
- that an outpatient should have someone accompany her home after the biopsy.

▶ PROCEDURE

- The patient is placed in the lithotomy position.
- A nonlubricated speculum is inserted.

DIRECT VISUALIZATION
- The colposcope is inserted through the speculum.
- The biopsy site is located.
- The cervix is cleaned with a swab soaked in 3% acetic acid solution.
- Biopsy forceps are inserted through the speculum or the colposcope.
- Tissue is removed from lesion or selected sites, starting from the posterior lip to avoid obscuring other sites with blood.
- Each specimen is immediately put in 10% formalin solution in a labeled bottle.
- The cervix is swabbed with 5% silver nitrate solution (cautery or sutures may be used instead) to control bleeding.
- The examiner may insert a tampon if bleeding persists.

SCHILLER'S TEST
- An applicator stick saturated with iodine solution is inserted through the speculum. This stains the cervix to identify lesions for biopsy.

Postprocedure care
- Instruct the patient to avoid strenuous exercise for 8 to 24 hours.
- Encourage the outpatient to rest briefly before leaving the office.
- Tell the patient to leave the tampon (if used) in place for 8 to 24 hours as ordered.
- Inform the patient that some bleeding may occur, but to report heavy bleeding (heavier than menstrual) to the physician.
- Warn the patient to avoid using additional tampons, which can irritate the cervix and provoke bleeding, according to her physician's directions.
- Tell the patient to avoid douching.
- Tell the patient to refrain from sexual intercourse for up to 2 weeks, or as directed, if cryotherapy or laser treatment was also done.
- Inform the patient that a foul-smelling, gray-green vaginal discharge

is normal for several days after the biopsy and may persist for 3 weeks.

MONITORING
- Vaginal bleeding
- Pain and discomfort

Precautions
- Send the specimens to the laboratory immediately.

Complications
- Bleeding
- Infection

✦ INTERPRETATION

Normal findings
- No dysplasia and abnormal cell growth are present.
- Normal cervical tissue is composed of:
  - columnar and squamous epithelial cells
  - loose connective tissue
  - smooth-muscle fibers.

Abnormal results
- Dysplasia or abnormal cell growth on histologic examination of a cervical tissue specimen may suggest:
  - intraepithelial neoplasia
  - invasive cancer.

Chest radiography

● OVERVIEW

- A noninvasive and relatively inexpensive study
- X-ray beams penetrate the chest and react on specially sensitized film; air is radiolucent, so thoracic structures appear as different densities on the film
- Commonly known as *chest X-ray*

Purpose

- To establish a baseline for future comparison
- To detect pulmonary disorders such as pneumonia
- To detect mediastinal abnormalities such as tumors
- To verify correct placement of pulmonary artery catheters, endotracheal (ET) tubes, and chest tubes
- To determine location of swallowed or aspirated radiopaque foreign bodies
- To determine location and size of lesions
- To evaluate response to interventions such as diuretic therapy

Patient preparation

- Make sure that the patient has signed an appropriate consent form.
- Restriction of food and fluids isn't necessary.
- Move cardiac monitoring cables, oxygen tubing, I.V. tubing, pulmonary artery catheter lines, and other equipment out of the radiographic field.
- Explain that the patient will be asked to take a deep breath and hold it momentarily while the film is being taken.

TEACHING POINTS

Be sure to cover:
- the purpose of the study
- who will perform the test
- that the test takes less than 5 minutes

▶ PROCEDURE

- The patient stands or sits in front of a stationary radiography machine.
- Posteroanterior and left lateral views are obtained.
- A portable radiography machine is used at patient's bedside if he can't travel to radiology.

- Because an upright chest radiograph is preferable, move the patient to the head of the bed if this position can be tolerated.
- Elevate the head of the bed for maximum upright positioning.

Postprocedure care

- Check that no tubes have been dislodged during positioning.

MONITORING

- None necessary

Precautions

- Chest radiography is usually contraindicated during the first trimester of pregnancy.
- Whenever possible, place a lead apron over the patient's abdomen to protect the gonads.
- To avoid radiation exposure, leave the area or wear lead shielding while the films are being taken.
- Portable films may be less reliable than stationary radiographs.
- Inability to take a full inspiration will decrease the quality of radiographs.

Complications

- Potential for dislodging tubes or wires, such as the ET tube or pacemaker wires during positioning

✥ INTERPRETATION

Normal findings

TRACHEA

- There's a visible midline in the anterior mediastinal cavity.
- It has a translucent, tubelike appearance.

HEART

- It's visible in the anterior left mediastinal cavity.
- It appears solid because of its blood content.

AORTIC KNOB

- It's visible as water density.
- It's formed by the aortic arch.

MEDIASTINUM (MEDIASTINAL SHADOW)

- It's visible as the space between the lungs.
- It has a shadowy appearance, widening at the hilum.

RIBS

- They're visible as thoracic cavity encasement.

SPINE

- It has a visible midline in the posterior chest that's best seen on a lateral view.

CLAVICLES

- They're visible in the upper thorax.
- They're intact and equidistant in properly centered films.

HILA (LUNG ROOTS)

- They're visible above the heart.
- They're found where pulmonary vessels, bronchi, and lymph nodes join the lungs.
- They appear as small, white, bilateral branching densities.

MAINSTEM BRONCHUS

- It's visible as part of the hila.
- It has a translucent, tubelike appearance.

BRONCHI

- They aren't usually visible.

LUNG FIELDS

- They aren't usually visible, except for blood vessels.

HEMIDIAPHRAGM

- It's rounded and visible.
- The right side is 1 to 2 cm higher than the left side.

Abnormal results

Deviations from normal findings should be correlated with additional tests and physical findings and include the following:
- Deviation of trachea from midline suggests possible tension pneumothorax or pleural effusion.
- Right heart hypertrophy suggests possible cor pulmonale or heart failure.
- A tortuous aortic knob suggests atherosclerosis.
- Gross widening of the mediastinum suggests neoplasm or aortic aneurysm.
- A break or misalignment of bones suggests fracture.
- Visible bronchi suggest bronchial pneumonia.
- Flattening of the diaphragm suggests emphysema or asthma.
- Irregular, patchy infiltrates in the lung fields suggest pneumonia.

Cholangiography, postoperative

● OVERVIEW

- Radiographic and fluoroscopic examination of the biliary ducts after injection of contrast medium
- Performed through a T-shaped rubber tube inserted into the common bile duct, immediately after cholecystectomy or common bile duct exploration, to facilitate drainage
- Also known as T-tube cholangiography

Purpose

- To assess size and patency of the biliary ducts
- To detect obstructions overlooked during surgery
- To detect calculi, strictures, neoplasms, and fistulae in the biliary ducts

Patient preparation

- Make sure that the patient has signed an appropriate consent form.
- Check the patient's history for hypersensitivity to iodine, seafood, or contrast media.
- Note and report all allergies.
- Clamp the T-tube the day before the procedure if ordered.
- Withhold the meal just before the test.
- Administer an enema about 1 hour before the procedure if ordered.
- Warn the patient that a bloating sensation in the right upper quadrant may be experienced as the contrast is injected.

TEACHING POINTS
Be sure to cover:
- the purpose of the study and how it's done
- who will perform the test and where
- that the test takes approximately 15 minutes.

▶ PROCEDURE

- The patient is placed in a supine position on the radiograph table.
- The injection area of the T tube is cleaned.
- A needle attached to a long transparent catheter is inserted into the end of the T tube.
- Injecting air into the biliary tree is avoided because air bubbles may affect the clarity of the radiograph films.
- A contrast medium is injected under fluoroscopic guidance.
- A series of radiographs is taken.
- The T tube is clamped and additional films are taken in the erect position (to distinguish air bubbles from calculi).
- Final films are taken to record emptying of contrast-laden bile into the duodenum.

Postprocedure care

- Reattach T-tube to the drainage system as ordered.
- Resume a normal diet.

MONITORING
- Vital signs
- Intake and output
- T-tube drainage

Precautions

- Cholangiography is contraindicated in patients who are hypersensitive to iodine, seafood, or contrast media.
- Marked gas overlying the biliary ducts may interfere with the test.

Complications

- Adverse reaction to contrast media
- Infection

✛ INTERPRETATION

Normal findings

- Filling of the bile ducts with contrast medium is homogeneous.
- The diameter of the biliary ducts is normal.
- The flow of contrast into the duodenum is unimpeded.

Abnormal results

- Biliary duct filling defects, associated with dilation, suggest calculi or neoplasms.
- Abnormal channels of contrast medium from biliary ducts suggest possible fistulae.

Cholecystography, oral

- Radiographic examination of the gallbladder after administration of contrast medium
- Indicated for patients with symptoms of biliary tract disease
- Commonly performed to confirm gallbladder disease

Purpose

- To detect gallstones
- To aid diagnosis of inflammatory disease and tumors of gallbladder

Patient preparation

- Make sure that the patient has signed an appropriate consent form.
- Note and report all allergies.
- Instruct the patient to eat a meal containing fat at noon the day before the test as ordered to stimulate release of bile from the gallbladder.
- Instruct the patient to eat a fat-free meal in the evening as ordered to inhibit gallbladder contraction and to promote bile accumulation.
- The patient may have nothing to eat or drink, except water, after the evening meal.
- Give the patient an oral contrast agent (usually tablets) as ordered 2 to 3 hours after the evening meal.

◆ **NURSING ALERT** Examine any vomitus or diarrhea for undigested tablets. If noted, notify the physician and the radiography department.

- Administer an enema the morning of the test if ordered.

TEACHING POINTS
Be sure to cover:
- the purpose of the study and how it's done
- who will perform the test and where
- that it usually takes 30 to 45 minutes.

- Fluoroscopic examination is performed to evaluate gallbladder opacification.
- Various positions are used to detect filling defects.
- A fat stimulus, such as a high-fat meal or a synthetic fat-containing agent may be given.
- The emptying of the gallbladder is observed in response to the fat stimulus and spot films are taken to visualize the common bile duct.
- If the gallbladder empties slowly or not at all, delayed films are taken.

Postprocedure care

- If the test results are normal, the patient may resume his usual diet as ordered.
- If gallstones are discovered, the physician orders an appropriate diet, usually fat-restricted, to help prevent acute attacks.
- If oral cholecystography must be repeated, the low-fat diet must be continued until a definitive diagnosis can be made.

MONITORING
- Diet
- Signs and symptoms of gall bladder disease

Precautions

- Oral cholecystography should precede barium studies to prevent retained barium from interfering with subsequent radiograph films.
- Oral cholecystography is contraindicated in patients with severe renal or hepatic damage, and in those with a hypersensitivity to iodine, seafood, or other contrast media.
- Oral cholecystography is contraindicated in pregnant patients because of possible teratogenic effects of radiation.

Complications

- Adverse reaction to contrast medium

Normal findings

- Opacification of the gallbladder is normal.
- The gallbladder appears pear-shaped with smooth, thin walls.

Abnormal results

- Filling defects may indicate gallstones.
- Fixed defects may indicate polyps or a benign tumor.
- Failed or faint opacification may indicate inflammatory disease, such as cholecystitis, with or without gallstones.
- Failure of the gallbladder to contract following stimulation by a fatty meal may indicate cholecystitis or common bile duct obstruction.

Colonoscopy

- Visual examination of the lining of the large intestine with a flexible fiber-optic endoscope
- Indicated for patients with a history of constipation or diarrhea, persistent rectal bleeding, or lower abdominal pain; for colorectal cancer screening

Purpose

- To detect and evaluate inflammatory and ulcerative bowel disease
- To locate the origin of lower GI bleeding
- To aid diagnosis of colonic strictures and benign or malignant lesions

Patient preparation

- Make sure that the patient has signed an appropriate consent form.
- Note and report all allergies.
- A clear liquid diet is required for 24 to 48 hours before the test.
- Nothing by mouth after midnight.
- Administer bowel preparation as ordered the day before the test.
- The large intestine must be thoroughly cleaned to be clearly visible.
- Warn the patient that an urge to defecate may be experienced when the scope is inserted and advanced.
- Explain that air is introduced through the colonoscope to distend the intestinal wall and facilitate the test.
- Explain that I.V. sedation will be administered.

TEACHING POINTS

Be sure to cover:
- the purpose of the test and how it's done
- who will perform the test and where
- that the test takes 30 to 60 minutes.

PROCEDURE

- I.V. sedation is administered before insertion of colonoscope.
- The patient is positioned on his left side with knees flexed, or in Sim's position and the colonoscope is inserted anally and advanced through the large intestine under direct vision.

- A small amount of air is insufflated to locate the bowel lumen, and the scope is advanced through the rectum.
- Fluoroscopy and abdominal palpation may facilitate passage of the endoscope through the bends in the large intestine.
- Incremental administration of sedatives reduces the incidence of respiratory depression and cardiac adverse effects.

NURSING ALERT Monitor vital signs throughout the procedure. If the patient has cardiovascular disease, continuous monitor cardiac rhythm should be instituted. Continuous pulse oximetry is advisable, particularly in high-risk patients with possible respiratory depression secondary to sedation.

- The patient is placed in various positions as needed until the colonoscope reaches the ascending colon and cecum.
- Suction may be used to remove blood or excessive secretions.
- Specimens for histologic and cytologic examination may be obtained.
- An electrocautery snare may be used to remove polyps.

Postprocedure care

- Provide a safe environment until the patient has recovered from sedation.
- Resume a usual diet as ordered.
- Inform the patient that he may pass large amounts of flatus after air insufflation.

NURSING ALERT If a polyp has been removed, inform the patient that there may be some blood in his stool and that he should report excessive bleeding immediately.

MONITORING

- Vital sign
- Respiratory status
- Level of consciousness
- Abdominal distension
- Bowel sounds
- Bleeding
- Stools

NURSING ALERT Observe the patient closely for signs of bowel perforation: malaise, rectal bleeding, abdominal pain and distention, fever, and mucopurulent drainage. Notify the physician immediately if such signs develop.

NURSING ALERT Watch closely for adverse effects of the sedative,

such as respiratory depression, hypotension, bradycardia, and confusion. Have emergency resuscitation equipment immediately available as well as a narcotic antagonist such as naloxone.

Precautions

- Colonoscopy is contraindicated in pregnancy and in patients who have recently had an acute myocardial infarction or abdominal surgery.
- Colonoscopy is contraindicated in patients who have ischemic bowel disease, acute diverticulitis, peritonitis, fulminant granulomatous colitis, fulminant ulcerative colitis, or a perforated viscus.
- Patients shouldn't drive, operate any machinery, or ingest alcohol for 24 hours after sedation.
- Poor bowel preparation greatly impairs visual examination.
- Retained barium from previous diagnostic studies impairs accurate visual examination.
- Fixation of the sigmoid colon from inflammatory bowel disease, surgery, or radiation therapy may inhibit passage of the colonoscope.

Complications

- Perforation of the large intestine
- Excessive bleeding from a biopsy or polypectomy site
- Retroperitoneal emphysema

INTERPRETATION

Normal findings

- Large intestine mucosa beyond the sigmoid colon appears light pink with semilunar folds and deep tubular pits.
- Blood vessels are visible beneath the intestinal mucosa, which glistens from mucus secretion.

Abnormal results

- Structural abnormalities detected by colonoscopy alone suggest diverticular disease or lower GI bleeding.
- Structural abnormalities detected by colonoscopy, in conjunction with histologic and cytologic test results, may indicate: proctitis, granulomatous and ulcerative colitis, Crohn's disease, or malignant and benign lesions.

Colposcopy

⬤ OVERVIEW

- Visual examination of the cervix and vagina by means of a colposcope, an instrument with a magnifying lens and light source

Purpose
- To confirm cervical intraepithelial neoplasia or invasive carcinoma after an abnormal Papanicolaou (Pap) test
- To evaluate vaginal or cervical lesions
- To monitor conservatively treated cervical intraepithelial neoplasia
- To monitor patients whose mothers received diethylstilbestrol during pregnancy

Patient preparation
- Make sure that the patient has signed an appropriate consent form.
- Note and report all allergies.
- Restriction of food and fluids is unnecessary.
- Instruct the patient not to douche, use tampons or vaginal medication, or have sexual intercourse for 2 days before the study.

TEACHING POINTS
Be sure to cover:
- the purpose of the study and how it's done
- who will perform the test and where
- that the test is safe and painless and takes 10 to 15 minutes
- that the procedure is similar to a routine pelvic examination, except the practitioner looks through the colposcope
- that minimal bleeding and mild cramping may be experienced with biopsy and endocervical curettage, if performed.

▶ PROCEDURE

- The patient is placed in the lithotomy position.
- A speculum is inserted into the vagina.
- A Pap test is performed, if indicated.
- A small amount of dilute vinegar solution is applied to the cervix to aid in differentiating the cell types; it makes abnormal areas more readily visible.
- The cervix and vagina are visually examined.
- A biopsy is performed on areas that appear abnormal.
- Endocervical curettage is done to sample the cells just inside the cervical canal.
- Bleeding is controlled by applying pressure or hemostatic solutions or by cautery.

Postprocedure care
- After biopsy, instruct the patient to:
  – abstain from sexual intercourse until the biopsy site heals
  – avoid inserting anything into the vagina (such as tampons) until the biopsy site heals (approximately 10 days)
  – expect a watery vaginal discharge, which is normal during healing.

MONITORING
- Vaginal drainage

Precautions
- Failure to clean the cervix of foreign materials, such as creams and medications, may impair visualization.
- Oral contraceptives may affect test results.

Complications
- Bleeding (especially during pregnancy)
- Infection

✛ INTERPRETATION

Normal findings
- Surface contour of the cervical vessels should be smooth and pink.
- Columnar epithelium should appear grapelike.
- Different tissue types should be sharply demarcated.

Abnormal results
- White epithelium or punctuation and mosaic patterns may indicate underlying cervical intraepithelial neoplasia.
- Keratinization in the transformation zone may indicate cervical intraepithelial neoplasia or invasive carcinoma.
- Atypical vessels may indicate invasive carcinoma.
- Inflammatory changes suggest possible infection.
- Condyloma suggests human papillomavirus.

Computed tomography

● OVERVIEW

- Combines radiologic and computer technology to produce cross-sectional images of various layers of tissue
- Reconstructs cross-sectional, horizontal, sagittal, and coronal plane images
- I.V. or oral contrast medium accentuates differences in tissue density
- Also known as CT scan

Purpose

- To produce tissue images not readily seen on standard radiographs

Patient preparation

- Make sure that the patient has signed an appropriate consent form.
- Note and report all allergies.
- The specific type of CT scan dictates the need for oral or I.V. contrast medium.
- Warn about transient discomfort from the needle puncture and a warm or flushed feeling if an I.V. contrast medium is used.
- Instruct the patient to remain still during the test because movement can limit the accuracy of results.
- Tell the patient he may experience minimal discomfort because of lying still.

NURSING ALERT Tell the patient to immediately report feelings of nausea, vomiting, dizziness, headache, itching, or hives. Check the patient's history for hypersensitivity to iodine or contrast media used in other diagnostic tests.

TEACHING POINTS

Be sure to cover:

- the purpose of the study and how it's done
- who will perform the test and where
- that the study takes from 5 minutes to 1 hour depending on the type of CT scan ordered and the patient's ability to remain still.

▶ PROCEDURE

- The patient is positioned on an adjustable table inside a scanning gantry.
- A series of transverse radiographs is taken and recorded.
- The information is reconstructed by a computer and selected images are photographed.
- After the images are reviewed, an I.V. contrast enhancement may be ordered.
- Additional images are obtained after I.V. contrast injection.
- The patient is carefully observed for adverse reactions to the contrast medium.

Postprocedure care

- Normal diet and activities may be resumed, unless otherwise ordered.

MONITORING

- None necessary

Precautions

- CT scan isn't usually recommended during pregnancy because of potential risk to the fetus.
- Check the patient's history for hypersensitivity to shellfish, iodine, or iodinated contrast media, and document such reactions on the patient's chart.
- Inform the physician of any sensitivities because prophylactic medications may be ordered or contrast enhancement may not be used.
- Oral or I.V. contrast media use in previous diagnostic tests may obscure the images.

Complications

- Adverse reaction to contrast media

✛ INTERPRETATION

Normal findings

- The specific type of CT scan performed dictates normal findings.
- Structures are evaluated according to their density, size, shape, and position.
- Tissue densities appear as black, white, or shades of gray on the CT scan image. Bone, the densest tissue, appears white. Cerebrospinal fluid, the least dense, appears black.

Abnormal results

- The specific type of CT scan performed dictates abnormal findings.

Computed tomography, abdomen and pelvis

that the test takes about 35 to 40 minutes.

● OVERVIEW

- Combines radiologic and computer technology to produce cross-sectional images of various layers of tissue
- Computed tomography (CT) of abdomen: includes the area between the dome of the diaphragm and iliac crests
- Pelvic CT: includes the area between the iliac crests and the perineum
- In males, pelvic viscera include the bladder and prostate
- In females, pelvic viscera include the bladder and adnexa
- CT of abdomen performed with or without CT of pelvis
- Spiral CT scans of the abdomen and pelvis also possible (see *Spiral CT*)

Purpose
- To evaluate soft tissue and organs of the abdomen, pelvis, and retroperitoneal space
- To evaluate inflammatory disease
- To aid staging of neoplasms
- To evaluate trauma
- To detect tumors, cysts, hemorrhage, or edema
- To evaluate response to chemotherapy

Patient preparation
- Make sure that the patient has signed an appropriate consent form.
- Note and report all allergies.
- Restriction of food and fluids for 4 hours before the test is usually required if contrast medium is used; no restrictions are necessary for noncontrast study.
- Stress the need to remain still during testing because movement can limit the test's accuracy. The patient may experience minimal discomfort because of lying still.
- Warn about transient discomfort from the needle puncture and a warm or flushed feeling or metallic taste if an I.V. contrast medium is used.
- Inform the patient that clacking sounds are heard as the table is moved into the scanner.

TEACHING POINTS
Be sure to cover:
- the purpose of the study and how it's done
- who will perform the test and where

▶ PROCEDURE

- Oral contrast material is usually required to outline the intestines.
- The patient is placed in a supine position with his arms above his head.
- An I.V. contrast agent may be injected into a vein to help define certain tissues.
- The table will advance slightly between each scan.
- Cross-sectional images are obtained and reviewed by the radiologist.

Postprocedure care
- Normal diet and activities may be resumed unless otherwise ordered.

MONITORING
- None necessary

Precautions
- CT of the abdomen and pelvis isn't usually recommended during pregnancy because of potential risk to the fetus.
- Check the patient's history for hypersensitivity to shellfish, iodine, or iodinated contrast media, and document such reactions on the patient's chart.
- Inform the physician of any sensitivity so that prophylactic medications may be ordered; the physician may choose not to use contrast enhancement.

Complications
- Adverse reaction to contrast medium

✛ INTERPRETATION

Normal findings
- Organs are normal in size and position.
- There are no masses or other abnormalities.

Abnormal results
- Well-circumscribed or poorly defined areas of slightly lower density than normal parenchyma suggest possible primary and metastatic neoplasms.
- Relatively low-density, homogeneous areas, usually with well-defined borders suggest possible abscesses.
- Sharply defined round or oval structures, with densities less than that of abscesses and neoplasms, suggest cysts.
- Dilatation of the biliary ducts suggests obstructive disease from tumor or calculi.

SPIRAL CT

The recent development of noncontrast spiral, or helical, computed tomography (CT) has many advantages. It has replaced excretory pyelography as first-line imaging for suspected acute renal colic. It enables accurate diagnosis of flank pain in less than 1 minute and efficient calculation of stone size. Contrast agents are avoided, so this eliminates any complications they may cause. Imaging results aren't affected by operator experience, which is another advantage over excretory pyelography. Preliminary studies show a 94% to 100% overall diagnostic accuracy rate.

Spiral CT aids in the differential diagnosis of abdominal aortic aneurysms, masses in the adnexal uteri, appendicitis, diverticulitis, gallstones, and hernias.

Computed tomography, intracranial

● OVERVIEW

- Provides a series of tomograms, translated by a computer and displayed on an oscilloscope screen; contrast enhancement commonly used
- Provides layers of cross-sectional images of the brain
- Reconstructs cross-sectional, horizontal, sagittal, and coronal-plane images
- Also known as *CT of the brain* or *head*

Purpose
- To diagnose intracranial lesions and abnormalities
- To monitor effects of surgery, radiotherapy, or chemotherapy in treatment of intracranial tumors
- To guide cranial surgery
- To assess focal neurologic abnormalities
- To evaluate suspected head injury such as subdural hematoma

Patient preparation
- Make sure that the patient has signed an appropriate consent form.
- Note and report all allergies.
- Explain restriction of food and fluids with contrast enhancement as ordered.
- Stress remaining still during the test because movement can limit accuracy of the test.
- Warn the patient that minimal discomfort may be experienced because of lying still and immobilizing the head.
- Warn about transient discomfort from the needle puncture and a warm or flushed feeling if an I.V. contrast medium is used.
- Caution that clacking sounds are heard as the head of the table is moved into the scanner, which rotates around the patient's head.

TEACHING POINTS
Be sure to cover:
- the purpose of the study and how it's done
- who will perform the test and where
- that the test takes 15 to 30 minutes.

▶ PROCEDURE

- The patient is helped into the supine position on the X-ray table.
- The patient's head is immobilized by straps and he's instructed to lie still.
- The head of the table is moved into the scanner, which rotates around the patient's head, taking radiographs.
- When the initial series of scans is complete, the I.V. contrast enhancement is performed if ordered.
- Usually, 50 to 100 ml of contrast medium is injected by I.V. bolus or infusion.
- The patient is observed for hypersensitivity reactions.
- Another series of scans is taken.
- Selected views are taken for further study.

Postprocedure care
- No specific postprocedure care is necessary if the test was performed without contrast enhancement.
- If a contrast agent was used, watch for delayed adverse reactions.
- Resume the usual diet and medications unless otherwise ordered.

MONITORING
- None necessary

Precautions
- Intracranial CT isn't usually recommended during pregnancy because of potential risk to the fetus.
- Check the patient's history for hypersensitivity to shellfish, iodine, or iodinated contrast media, and document such reactions on the patient's chart.
- Inform the physician of any sensitivities because prophylactic medications may be ordered or because contrast enhancement may not be used.

Complications
- Adverse reaction to contrast media

✛ INTERPRETATION

Normal findings
- Brain matter appears in shades of gray.
- Ventricular and subarachnoid cerebrospinal fluid appears black.

Abnormal results
- Enlarged ventricles with large sulci suggest cerebral atrophy.

☀ AGE-RELATED CONCERN In children, enlargement of the fourth ventricle usually indicates hydrocephalus.
- Areas of marked generalized lucency suggest cerebral edema.
- Cerebral vessels appearing with slightly increased density suggest possible arteriovenous malformation.
- Areas of altered density or displaced vasculature or other structures may indicate:
  - intracranial tumors
  - intracranial hematoma
  - cerebral atrophy, infarction, edema
  - congenital anomalies such as hydrocephalus.

◆ NURSING ALERT If test results are abnormal, provide psychological support to the patient. If the etiology of the abnormality indicates an emergency, the patient will likely need preparation for a surgical procedure.

Computed tomography, liver and biliary tree

● OVERVIEW

- Combines radiologic and computer technology to produce cross-sectional images of various layers of tissue
- Penetrates the upper abdomen with multiple X-rays, while a detector records the differences in tissue thickness, displayed as an image on a screen
- Distinguishes the biliary tree and the liver, if the ducts are large
- Indicated for obese patients and in those with livers positioned high under the rib cage because excessive fat and bone can hinder ultrasound transmission

Purpose

- To distinguish between obstructive and nonobstructive jaundice
- To detect intrahepatic tumors and abscesses, subphrenic and subhepatic abscesses, cysts, and hematomas

Patient preparation

- Check the patient's history for hypersensitivity to iodine, seafood, or contrast media used in other diagnostic tests.
- Make sure that the patient has signed an appropriate consent form.
- Give the patient the oral contrast medium supplied by the radiology department. The patient should drink the contrast medium and fast until after the examination.
- If the test involves an I.V. contrast medium, tell the patient that he may experience transient discomfort from the needle puncture and a localized feeling of warmth upon injection as well as a salty or metallic taste.
- Inform the patient that he'll lie on an adjustable table inside a scanning gantry.
- Stress the importance of remaining still during the test because movement can cause artifacts, thereby prolonging the test and limiting its accuracy.
- Describe possible adverse reactions to the medium, such as nausea, vomiting, dizziness, headache, and hives, and tell him to report these symptoms.

TEACHING POINTS

Be sure to cover:
- purpose of the study and how it's done
- who will perform the test and where
- need to remain still during the test and periodically hold his breath
- that the test takes about 30 minutes.

▶ PROCEDURE

- The patient is helped into the supine position on the X-ray table, and the table is positioned within the opening in the scanning gantry.
- A series of transverse X-rays is taken and recorded on magnetic tape.
- This information is reconstructed by a computer and appears as a series of images on a monitor.
- When the first series of X-rays is completed, the images are then reviewed.
- If contrast enhancement is ordered, the contrast medium is injected. A second series of X-rays is taken. The patient is observed carefully for an allergic reaction.

Postprocedure care

- No specific postprocedure care is required.

Precautions

◆ NURSING ALERT Tell the patient to immediately report feelings of nausea, vomiting, dizziness, headache, itching, or hives.
- The test is contraindicated during pregnancy due to potential risk to the fetus.

Complications

- Adverse reactions to contrast medium

✦ INTERPRETATION

Normal findings

- The liver has a uniform density that's slightly greater than that of the pancreas, kidneys, and spleen.
- Linear and circular areas of slightly lower density, representing hepatic vascular structures, may interrupt this uniform appearance.
- The portal vein is usually visible, but not the hepatic artery.
- I.V. contrast medium enhances the isodensity of vascular structures and liver parenchyma.
- Intrahepatic biliary radicles aren't visible, but the common hepatic and bile ducts may be visible as low-density structures. Because bile has the same density as water, use of an I.V. contrast medium improves demarcation of the biliary tract by enhancing the surrounding parenchyma and vascular structures.
- Like the biliary ducts, the gallbladder is visible as a round or elliptic low-density structure.

Abnormal results

- Most focal hepatic defects appear less dense than the normal parenchyma, and CT scans can detect small lesions.
- Primary and metastatic neoplasms may appear as well-circumscribed or poorly defined areas of slightly lower density than the normal parenchyma.
- Especially large neoplasms may distort the liver's contour.
- Hepatic abscesses appear as relatively low-density, homogeneous areas, usually with well-defined borders.
- Hepatic cysts appear as sharply defined round or oval structures and have a density lower than abscesses and neoplasms.
- Subcapsular hematomas are usually crescent-shaped and compress the liver away from the capsule.
- Absence of dilation indicates nonobstructive jaundice.
- Biliary duct dilation indicates obstructive jaundice.
- Dilated intrahepatic bile ducts appear as low-density linear and circular branching structures.
- Dilation of the common hepatic duct, common bile duct, and gallbladder may also be apparent, depending on the site and severity of obstruction.

Computed tomography, pancreas

● OVERVIEW

- Combines radiologic and computer technology to produce cross-sectional images of various layers of tissue of the pancreas
- Penetrates the upper abdomen with multiple X-rays, while a detector records the differences in tissue thickness, displayed as an image on a screen
- Accurately distinguishes the pancreas and surrounding organs and vessels if enough fat is present between the structures
- More accurate than ultrasonography; shows general swelling that accompanies acute inflammation of the gland (in retroperitoneal disorders, specifically when pancreatitis is suspected)
- Easily detects calcium deposits commonly missed by simple radiography, particularly in obese patients (in chronic cases)

Purpose

- To detect pancreatic carcinoma or pseudocysts
- To detect or evaluate pancreatitis
- To distinguish between pancreatic disorders and disorders of the retroperitoneum

Patient preparation

- Check the patient's history for recent barium studies and for hypersensitivity to iodine, seafood, or contrast media used in previous tests.
- Make sure that the patient has signed an appropriate consent form.
- The test may require an I.V. or oral contrast medium, or both, to enhance visualization of the pancreas.
- Give the oral contrast medium, if ordered.
- Instruct the patient to fast after receiving oral contrast medium; if the patient is to receive I.V. contrast, tell him to fast for 4 hours before the test.
- Describe possible adverse reactions to the medium, such as nausea, flushing, dizziness, and sweating, and tell him to report these symptoms.

TEACHING POINTS

Be sure to cover:
- purpose of the study and how it's done
- who will perform the test and where
- that the procedure is painles.
- that he'll need to remain still during the test and periodically hold his breath
- that the test takes about 20 minutes.

▶ PROCEDURE

- The patient is helped into the supine position on the X-ray table, and the table is positioned within the opening in the scanning gantry.
- A series of transverse X-rays is taken and recorded on magnetic tape. The images are studied, and selected ones are photographed.
- After the first series of X-rays is complete, the images are reviewed. Contrast enhancement may be ordered.
- After the contrast medium is given, another series of X-rays is taken. The patient is observed for an allergic reaction, such as itching, hypotension, hypertension, diaphoresis, or dyspnea.

Postprocedure care

- Instruct the patient to resume his usual diet, as ordered.

MONITORING
- None necessary

Precautions

◆ **NURSING ALERT** Tell the patient to immediately report feelings of nausea, vomiting, dizziness, headache, itching, or hives.
- The test is contraindicated during pregnancy due to potential risk to the fetus.

Complications

- Delayed allergic reaction to the contrast dye, such as urticaria, headache, and vomiting

✛ INTERPRETATION

Normal findings

- The pancreatic parenchyma displays a uniform density, especially when an I.V.. contrast medium is used.
- The gland thickens from tail to head and has a smooth surface.

Abnormal results

- Because the tissue density of pancreatic carcinoma resembles that of the normal parenchyma, changes in pancreatic size and shape help demonstrate carcinoma and pseudocysts.
- Usually, a carcinoma first appears as a localized swelling of the head, body, or tail of the pancreas and may spread to obliterate the fat plane, dilate the main pancreatic duct and common bile duct by obstructing them, and produce low-density focal lesions in the liver from metastasis.
- Use of an I.V. contrast medium helps detect metastases by opacifying the pancreatic and hepatic parenchyma.
- Cystadenoma and cystadenocarcinoma, usually multilocular, occur most frequently in the body and tail of the pancreas and can appear as low-density focal lesions marked by internal septa.
- Acute pancreatitis, either edematous (interstitial) or necrotizing (hemorrhagic), produces diffuse enlargement of the pancreas.
- In acute edematous pancreatitis, parenchyma density is uniformly decreased; in acute necrotizing pancreatitis, the density is nonuniform because of the presence of necrosis and hemorrhage. The areas of tissue necrosis have diminished density.
- Abscesses, within or outside the pancreas, appear as low-density areas and are most readily detected when they contain gas.
- Pseudocysts, which may be unifocal or multifocal, appear as sharply circumscribed, low-density areas that may contain debris.
- In chronic pancreatitis, the pancreas may appear normal, enlarged, or atrophic, depending on disease severity.

Computed tomography, renal

● OVERVIEW

- Combines radiologic and computer technology to produce cross-sectional images of layers of tissue
- Reveals masses and other lesions by measuring the amount of radiation the kidney tissue absorbs
- Highly accurate test to investigate diseases initially found by other tests, such as excretory urography

Purpose

- To detect and evaluate renal abnormalities, such as tumor, obstruction, calculi, polycystic disease, congenital anomalies, and abnormal fluid accumulation
- To evaluate the retroperitoneum

Patient preparation

- Make sure that the patient has signed an appropriate consent form.
- Check the patient's history for hypersensitivity to shellfish, iodine, or contrast media.
- Have the patient put on a gown and remove any metallic objects that could interfere with the scan.
- Tell the patient that flushing, metallic taste, and headache may occur after the contrast medium is injected.
- Advise the patient that the scanner may make loud clacking sounds as it rotates around his body.
- If the patient will receive a contrast medium, instruct him to fast for 4 hours before the test.
- Give the patient any prescribed sedatives.

TEACHING POINTS

Be sure to cover:
- purpose of the study and how it's done
- who will perform the test and where
- that the test takes about 30 minutes.

▶ PROCEDURE

- The patient is helped into the supine position on the X-ray table and secured with straps.
- The scanner rotates around the patient, taking multiple images at different angles within each cross-sectional slice.
- When one series of scans is complete, the I.V. contrast enhancement may be performed. Another series of scans is then taken.
- After the I.V. contrast medium is given, the patient is monitored for signs and symptoms of an allergic reaction, such as respiratory difficulty, urticaria, or skin eruptions.

Postprocedure care

- If calculi are present, strain the urine, hydrate the patient, and discuss nutritional adaptations.
- Support the patient and his family if surgery is indicated for a neoplasm.
- After the test, instruct the patient to resume his usual diet, as ordered.

MONITORING

- Renal function
- Vital signs
- Hypersensitivity reaction

Precautions

⬙ NURSING ALERT Tell the patient to immediately report feelings of nausea, vomiting, dizziness, headache, itching, or hives.
- The test is contraindicated during pregnancy due to potential risk to the fetus.

Complications

- Adverse reaction to contrast medium

⬥ INTERPRETATION

Normal findings

- Renal parenchyma appears more dense than hepatic parenchyna, but less dense than bone, which appears white on a computed tomography scan.
- The density of the collecting system is generally low (black), unless a contrast medium enhances it to a higher density (more white).
- Evaluating kidney position depends on the surrounding structures; counting cuts between the superior and inferior poles and following the contour of the kidneys' outline gives size and shape.

Abnormal results

- Renal masses appear as areas of different density than normal parenchyma, possibly altering the shape of the kidneys or projecting beyond their margins.
- Renal cysts appear as smooth, sharply defined masses with thin walls and a lower density than normal parenchyma.
- Tumors, such as renal cell carcinoma, usually aren't well delineated; they have thick walls and nonuniform density.
- With contrast enhancement, solid tumors appear more dense than renal cysts but less dense than normal parenchyma.
- Tumors with hemorrhage, calcification, or necrosis appear more dense; vascular tumors are more clearly defined with contrast enhancement.
- Obstructions, calculi, polycystic kidney disease, congenital anomalies, and abnormal accumulations of fluid around the kidneys, such as hematomas, lymphoceles, and abscesses can also be identified.
- After nephrectomy, scanning can detect abnormal masses, such as recurrent tumors in a renal fossa that should be empty.

Computed tomography, spine

● OVERVIEW

- Provides detailed high-resolution images in the cross-sectional, longitudinal, sagittal, and lateral planes
- Multiple X-ray beams from computerized body scanner directed at spine from different angles, which pass through body and strike radiation detectors, producing electrical impulses that computer converts into three-dimensional image on monitor
- Allows electronic recreation and manipulation of the image, creating a permanent record that enables reexamination without repeating the procedure
- Helps define lesions causing spinal cord compression and diagnose conditions, such as metastatic disease and discogenic disease with osteophyte formation and calcification

Purpose
- To diagnose spinal lesions and abnormalities
- To monitor the effects of spinal surgery or therapy

Patient preparation
- Make sure that the patient has signed an appropriate consent form.
- Have the patient wear a radiologic examining gown and remove all metal objects and jewelry.
- Check the patient's history for hypersensitivity reactions to iodine, shellfish, or contrast media. Note them in the chart; also notify the physician, who may order prophylactic medications or choose not to use contrast enhancement.
- If the patient will receive a contrast medium, instruct him to fast for 4 hours before the test; otherwise, dietary restrictions aren't necessary.
- If the patient will receive a contrast medium, tell him that he may feel flushed and warm and may experience a transient headache, a salty taste, and nausea or vomiting after the injection. Reassure him that these reactions are normal.
- If the patient appears restless or apprehensive about the procedure, a mild sedative may be prescribed.

- For the patient with significant back pain, give prescribed analgesics before the scan.

TEACHING POINTS
Be sure to cover:
- purpose of the test and how it's done
- who will perform the test and where
- that the test takes about 30 minutes.

▶ PROCEDURE

- The patient is helped into the supine position on an X-ray table and asked to lie as still as possible.
- If the patient becomes claustrophobic or anxious inside the computed tomography (CT) body scanner, give him a mild sedative to help relieve these symptoms.
- The table slides into the circular opening of the CT scanner and the scanner revolves around the patient, taking radiographs at preselected intervals.
- After the first set of scans is taken, the patient is removed from the scanner. Contrast medium may be given.
- Observe the patient for signs and symptoms of a hypersensitivity reaction, including pruritus, rash, and respiratory difficulty, for 30 minutes after injection of the contrast medium.
- After the contrast medium is injected, the patient is moved back into the scanner, and another series of scans is taken.

Postprocedure care
- Instruct the patient to resume his usual diet, as ordered.

MONITORING
- Residual effects, such as headache, nausea, and vomiting

Precautions
⬙ **NURSING ALERT** Tell the patient to immediately report feelings of nausea, vomiting, dizziness, headache, itching, or hives.
- The test is contraindicated during pregnancy due to potential risk to the fetus.

Complications
- Claustrophobia or anxiety (when inside the CT body scanner)
- Adverse reaction to contrast medium

⬥ INTERPRETATION

Normal findings
- The spinal tissue appears white, black, or gray, depending on its density.
- Vertebrae, the densest of tissues, appear white; cerebrospinal fluid appears black; and soft tissues appear in shades of gray.

Abnormal results
- Spinal lesions and other abnormalities are visualized on the scan.
- Tumors appear as masses varying in density. Measuring this density and noting the configuration and location relative to the spinal cord can usually identify the type of tumor. For example, a neurinoma (schwannoma) appears as a spherical mass dorsal to the cord. A darker, wider mass lying more lateral or ventral to the cord may be a meningioma.
- Degenerative processes and structural changes appear in detail.
- A herniated nucleus pulposus shows as an obvious herniation of disk material with unilateral or bilateral nerve root compression; if the herniation is midline, spinal cord compression will be evident.
- Cervical spondylosis shows as cervical cord compression; lumbar stenosis, as hypertrophy of the lumbar vertebrae.
- Facet disorders show as soft-tissue changes, bony overgrowth, and spurring of the vertebrae.
- Fluid-filled arachnoidal and other paraspinal cysts show as dark masses displacing the spinal cord.
- Vascular malformations, evident after contrast, show as masses or clusters, usually on the dorsal aspect of the spinal cord.
- Congenital spinal malformations show as abnormally large, dark gaps between the white vertebrae.

Cystometry

- Measures pressure and volume of fluid in the bladder during filling, storing, and voiding
- Used to assess neuromuscular function of bladder
- Results supported by results of other urologic tests, such as cystourethrography and excretory urography
- Also called *CMG*

Purpose

- To evaluate detrusor muscle function and tonicity
- To determine cause of bladder dysfunction
- To measure bladder reaction to thermal stimulation
- To detect the cause of involuntary bladder contractions and incontinence

Patient preparation

- Make sure that the patient has signed an appropriate consent form.
- Note and report all allergies.
- Check the medication history for drugs that may affect test results such as antihistamines.
- Restriction of food and fluids isn't necessary.
- Ask the patient to urinate before test.
- Assess for signs and symptoms of urinary tract infection.
- Tell the patient he may feel a strong urge to urinate during the test.
- Warn the patient that the procedure may cause embarrassment and be uncomfortable.

TEACHING POINTS
Be sure to cover:
- the purpose of the study and how it's done
- who will perform the test and where
- that the test takes about 40 minutes.

PROCEDURE

- The patient is placed in a supine position on an examining table.
- A catheter is passed into the bladder to measure residual urine.
- To test the response to thermal sensation, 30 ml of room-temperature physiologic saline solution or sterile water is instilled into the bladder.
- An equal volume of warm fluid (110° to 115° F [43.3° to 46.1° C]) is then instilled.
- The patient is asked to report symptoms, such as the need to urinate, nausea, or a flushed feeling.
- The fluid is drained from the bladder and the catheter is connected to the cystometer.
- Normal saline solution, sterile water, or gas (usually carbon dioxide) is slowly introduced into the bladder.
- The patient is asked to indicate when an urge to void is felt.
- Related pressures and volumes are automatically plotted on a graph.
- When the bladder reaches its full capacity, the patient is asked to urinate.
- The maximal intravesical voiding pressure is then recorded.
- The bladder is drained.
- If abnormal bladder function is caused by muscle incompetence or disrupted innervation, an anticholinergic or cholinergic medication may be injected and the study repeated in 20 to 30 minutes.

Postprocedure care

- Administer a sitz bath or warm tub bath for discomfort.
- Encourage oral fluid intake (unless contraindicated) to relieve dysuria.
- Notify the physician if hematuria persists after the third voiding.
- Administer antibiotics as ordered.

MONITORING
- Vital signs
- Intake and output
- Hematuria
- Signs and symptoms of infection

Precautions

- CMG is contraindicated in acute urinary tract infections.
- Straining with urination could cause ambiguous cystometric readings.
- Drugs, such as antihistamines, may interfere with bladder function and alter test results.
- Inability to urinate in a supine position will interfere with test results.
- Inconclusive results are likely if performed within 6 to 8 weeks after surgery for spinal cord injury.

Complications
- Infection
- Bleeding

INTERPRETATION

Normal findings
- Ability to start and stop micturition
- No residual urine
- Positive vesical sensation
- First urge to void at 150 to 200 ml
- Bladder capacity: 400 to 500 ml
- No bladder contractions
- Low intravesical pressure
- Positive bulbocavernosus reflex
- Positive saddle sensation test
- Positive ice water test result
- Positive anal reflex
- Positive heat sensation and pain

Abnormal results
- Inability to stop micturition, early first urge to void, decreased bladder capacity, bladder contractions, increased intravesical pressure, and positive bethanechol sensitivity test suggest inhibited neurogenic bladder.
- Inability to start and stop micturition, residual urine, absent vesical sensation, absent first urge to void, decreased bladder capacity, bladder contractions, increased intravesical pressure, increased bulbocavernosus reflex, negative saddle sensation test, and absent heat sensation and pain suggest reflex neurogenic bladder.
- Inability to start and stop micturition, residual urine, absent vesical sensation, increased bladder capacity, decreased intravesical pressure, absent bulbocavernosus reflex, negative saddle sensation test, negative ice water test, absent anal reflex, and absent heat sensation and pain suggests autonomous neurogenic bladder.
- Residual urine, absent vesical sensation, delayed first urge to void, increased bladder capacity, decreased intravesical pressure, negative ice water test, variable anal reflex, and absent heat sensation and pain suggests sensory paralytic bladder.
- Inability to start and stop micturition, residual urine, negative ice water test, and variable anal reflex suggest motor paralytic bladder.

Cystourethroscopy

● OVERVIEW

- Allows visual examination of the bladder, urethra, ureter orifice, ureters, and prostate in males
- Combines two endoscopic techniques, cystoscopy and urethroscopy
- Cystoscope is used to examine the bladder
- Urethroscope, or panendoscope, is used to examine bladder neck and urethra
- The cystoscope and urethroscope pass through a common sheath inserted into the urethra to obtain the desired view
- Usually preceded by kidney-ureter-bladder radiography, excretory urography, and the bladder tumor antigen (BTA) urine test

Purpose
- To diagnose and evaluate urinary tract disorders by direct visualization of urinary structures
- To facilitate biopsy, lesion resection, removal of calculi, dilatation of a constricted urethra, and catheterization of the renal pelvis for pyelography

Patient preparation
- Make sure that the patient has signed an appropriate consent form.
- Note and report all allergies.
- Administer a sedative if ordered.
- Instruct the patient to urinate.
- Restriction of food and fluids is unnecessary unless general anesthesia ordered.
- If only local anesthesia is used, the patient may complain of:
  - a burning sensation when the instrument is passed through the urethra
  - an urgent need to urinate as the bladder fills with irrigating solution.
- Some discomfort after the procedure may be experienced, including a slight burning when the patient urinates.

TEACHING POINTS
Be sure to cover:
- the purpose of the study and how it's done
- who will perform the test and where
- that the test takes about 20 to 30 minutes.

▶ PROCEDURE

- General or regional anesthesia may be administered.
- The patient is placed in lithotomy position on a cystoscopic table.
- Genitalia are cleaned with an antiseptic solution and the patient is draped.
- The urethra is visually examined with a urethroscope.
- The urethroscope is removed and a cystoscope is inserted into the bladder.
- The bladder is filled with irrigating solution and the entire bladder surface wall and ureteral orifices are examined.
- The cystoscope is removed and the urethroscope reinserted.
- The bladder neck and various portions of the urethra, including the internal and external sphincters are examined as the urethroscope is withdrawn.
- A urine specimen is taken from the bladder for culture and sensitivity testing.
- Residual urine volume is measured.
- Urine for cytologic examination is taken if a tumor is suspected.
- If a tumor is found, biopsy may be performed.
- If a urethral stricture is present, urethral dilatation may be necessary before cystourethroscopy.

Postprocedure care
- Provide postoperative general anesthesia care as indicated.
- Encourage oral fluid intake and administer I.V. fluids as ordered.
- Administer analgesia as ordered.
- Administer antibiotics as ordered.
- ◉ **NURSING ALERT** Report flank or abdominal pain, chills, fever, an elevated white blood cell count, or low urine output to the physician immediately.
- Notify the physician if the patient doesn't void within 8 hours after the test or if bright red blood persists after three voidings.
- Instruct the patient to abstain from alcohol for 48 hours.
- Apply heat to the lower abdomen to relieve pain and muscle spasm (if ordered).

- Administer a warm sitz bath as ordered.

MONITORING
- Vital signs
- Intake and output
- Bleeding
- Hematuria
- Signs and symptoms of infection
- Bladder distention

Precautions
- Cystourethroscopy is contraindicated in acute forms of urethritis, prostatitis, or cystitis.
- Cystourethroscopy is contraindicated in bleeding disorders.

Complications
- Sepsis
- Infection
- Bleeding

✛ INTERPRETATION

Normal findings
- Urethra, bladder, and ureteral orifices appear normal in size, shape, and position.
- Mucosal lining of the lower urinary tract appears smooth and shiny.
- There's no evidence of erythema, cysts, or other abnormalities.
- There are no obstructions, tumors, or calculi in the bladder.

Abnormal results
- Structural abnormalities suggest various disorders, including enlarged prostate gland in older men, urethral strictures, calculi, tumors, diverticula, ulcers, and polyps.

Digital subtraction angiography, cerebral

⬤ OVERVIEW

- Sophisticated radiographic technique that uses video equipment and computer-assisted image enhancement to provide high-contrast view of blood vessels without interfering images or shadows of bone and soft tissue
- Also referred to as DSA
- Has several advantages over conventional angiography, including superior image quality and intravenous administration of contrast media, instead of intra-arterial administration
- Used to study peripheral and renal vascular disease, but is most useful for evaluating cerebrovascular disorders

Purpose
- To visualize extracranial and intracranial cerebral blood flow
- To detect and evaluate cerebrovascular abnormalities
- To aid postoperative evaluation of cerebrovascular surgery

Patient preparation
- Make sure that the patient has signed an appropriate consent form.
- Note and report all allergies.
- Provide instructions for fasting 4 hours before the test as ordered.
- Stress the importance of lying still during the procedure; even swallowing can interfere with imaging. The patient is required to hold his breath for 10-second intervals at various times during the study.
- Warn the patient that a feeling of warmth, headache, metallic taste, nausea, or vomiting may be experienced after injection of contrast medium.

TEACHING POINTS
Be sure to cover:
- the purpose of the study and how it's done
- who will perform the test and where
- that the test may take 1 to 2 hours.

▷ PROCEDURE

- The patient is placed in a supine position on a radiography table with his arms at his sides.
- An initial series of fluoroscopic pictures (mask images) is taken.
- The access site is prepared and draped (a vein or artery may be used).
- A local anesthetic is administered.
- I.V. sedation may be administered as ordered.
- The vessel is cannulated and a catheter is inserted and advanced to the area to be studied.
- Contrast medium is injected and films are taken in various views.

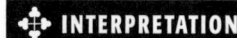 **NURSING ALERT** The patient's vital signs and neurologic status are monitored, and he's observed for signs of a hypersensitivity reaction, such as urticaria, pruritus, and respiratory distress.

Postprocedure care
- The patient should drink at least 1 L of fluid on the day of the procedure because contrast medium acts as a diuretic. Extra fluid intake also aids excretion of the contrast medium.
- If bleeding occurs, apply firm pressure to the puncture site and tell the physician immediately.
- Resume a normal diet as ordered.

MONITORING
- Vital signs
- Intake and output
- Neurologic status
- Puncture site
- Signs and symptoms of infection
- Bleeding
- Delayed hypersensitivity reaction to the contrast medium
- Thrombotic events

Precautions
- Check the patient's history for hypersensitivity to iodine, iodine-containing substances such as shellfish, and contrast media.
- Note previous hypersensitivity on the patient's medical record and tell the physician.
- The procedure may be contraindicated in a patient with:
  - hypersensitivity to iodine or contrast media

  - poor cardiac function
  - renal, hepatic, or thyroid disease
  - severe diabetes
  - multiple myeloma.

Complications
- Bleeding
- Infection
- Thrombotic and embolic events

✛ INTERPRETATION

Normal findings
- Contrast medium should fill and opacify all superficial and deep arteries, arterioles, and veins.

Abnormal results
- Vascular filling defects may indicate arteriovenous occlusion or stenosis.
- Outpouchings in vessel lumina may reflect aneurysms.
- Vessel displacement or vascular masses may indicate tumor.

Echocardiography

● OVERVIEW

- Noninvasive test to examine the size, shape, and motion of cardiac structures
- Transducer directs ultra-high-frequency sound waves toward cardiac structures, which reflect these waves; the transducer picks up the echoes, converts them to electrical impulses, and relays them to an echocardiography machine for display
- In M-mode (motion mode): a single, pencil-like ultrasound beam strikes the heart and produces a vertical view; useful for recording the motion and dimensions of intracardiac structures
- In two-dimensional echocardiography: a cross-sectional view of cardiac structures is used for recording lateral motion and spatial relationship between structures

Purpose
- To diagnose and evaluate valvular abnormalities
- To measure and evaluate the size of the heart's chambers and valves
- To aid the diagnosis of cardiomyopathies and atrial tumors
- To evaluate cardiac function or wall motion after myocardial infarction
- To detect pericardial effusion or mural thrombi

Patient preparation
- Restriction of food and fluids isn't necessary.
- Explain that the patient may be asked to breathe in and out slowly, to hold his breath, or to inhale a gas with a slightly sweet odor (amyl nitrite) while changes in heart function are recorded.
- Warn about possible adverse effects of amyl nitrite (dizziness, flushing, and tachycardia), but provide reassurance that such effects quickly subside.
- Stress the need to remain still during the test because movement may distort results.

TEACHING POINTS
Be sure to cover:
- the purpose of the study and how it's done
- who will perform the test and where
- that the test takes 15 to 30 minutes.

▶ PROCEDURE

- The patient is placed in a supine position and conductive gel is applied to the third or fourth intercostal space to the left of the sternum, and the transducer is placed directly over it.
- The transducer is systematically angled to direct ultrasonic waves at specific parts of the patient's heart.
- During the test, the oscilloscope screen is observed; significant findings are recorded on a strip chart recorder or on a videotape recorder.
- For a left lateral view, the patient may be positioned on his left side.
- Doppler echocardiography may also be used in which color flow simulates red blood cell flow through the heart valves; sound of the blood flow may also be used to assess heart sounds and murmurs as they relate to cardiac hemodynamics.

Postprocedure care
- Remove the conductive gel from the patient's skin.
MONITORING
- None necessary

Precautions
- None known

Complications
- None known

✛ INTERPRETATION

Normal findings
MITRAL VALVE
- Anterior and posterior mitral valve leaflets separate in early diastole and attain maximum excursion rapidly, then move toward each other during ventricular diastole; after atrial contraction, they come together and remain so during ventricular systole.
AORTIC VALVE
- Aortic valve cusps move anteriorly during systole and posteriorly during diastole.
TRICUSPID VALVE
- Motion of the tricuspid valve resembles that of the mitral valve.

PULMONIC VALVE
- The pulmonic valve moves posteriorly during atrial systole and during ventricular systole. During right ventricular ejection, the cusp moves anteriorly, attaining its most anterior position during diastole.
VENTRICULAR CAVITIES
- The left ventricular cavity normally appears as an echo-free space between the interventricular septum and the posterior left ventricular wall.
- The right ventricular cavity normally appears as an echo-free space between the anterior chest wall and the interventricular septum.

Abnormal results
- In mitral stenosis, the valve narrows abnormally because of the leaflets' thickening and disordered motion; during diastole both mitral valve leaflets move anteriorly instead of posteriorly.
- In mitral valve prolapse, one or both leaflets balloon into the left atrium during systole.
- In aortic insufficiency, leaflet fluttering of the aortic valve during diastole occurs.
- In stenosis, the aortic valve thickens and thus generates more echoes.
- In bacterial endocarditis, valve motion is disrupted and fuzzy echoes usually appear on or near the valve.
- A large chamber size may indicate cardiomyopathy, valvular disorders, or heart failure.
- A small chamber may indicate restrictive pericarditis.
- Hypertrophic cardiomyopathy can be identified by systolic anterior motion of the mitral valve and asymmetrical septal hypertrophy.
- Myocardial ischemia or infarction may cause absent or paradoxical motion in ventricular walls.
- Pericardial effusion is suggested when fluid accumulates in the pericardial space, causing an abnormal echo-free space to appear. In large effusions, pressure exerted by excess fluid can restrict pericardial motion.

Echocardiography, exercise

● OVERVIEW

- Involves the use of two-dimensional echocardiography and exercise to detect changes in cardiac wall motion
- Allows imaging both before and immediately after exercise stress testing
- Specificity and sensitivity is an adjunct to results obtained in exercise electrocardiography
- Also known as *stress echocardiography*

Purpose

- To identify causes of chest pain
- To determine chamber size and functional capacity of the heart
- To screen for asymptomatic cardiac disease
- To set limits for an exercise program
- To diagnose and evaluate valvular and wall motion abnormalities
- To detect atrial tumors, mural thrombi, vegetative growth on valve leaflets, pericardial effusions
- To evaluate myocardial perfusion, coronary artery disease (CAD) and obstructions, extent of myocardial damage following myocardial infarction (MI)

Patient preparation

- Make sure that the patient has signed an appropriate consent form.
- Note and report all allergies.
- Instruct the patient to refrain from eating, smoking, or drinking alcoholic or caffeine-containing beverages at least 3 to 4 hours before the test or as directed by the physician.
- Withhold current medications before testing as directed.
- Warn the patient that he might feel tired, diaphoretic, and slightly short of breath. Provide reassurance that if symptoms become severe or if chest pain develops, the test will be terminated.

TEACHING POINTS
Be sure to cover:
- the purpose of the study and how it's done.
- who will perform the test and where
- that the test takes approximately 60 minutes.

▶ PROCEDURE

- The patient is placed in a supine position on a litter and a baseline echocardiogram is obtained.
- An initial baseline ECG is obtained with an initial blood pressure reading.
- The patient is placed on the treadmill at slow speed until he becomes acclimated to it.
- The work rate is increased every 3 minutes as tolerated (increasing the speed of the machine slightly and increasing the degree of incline by 3% each time).
- The cardiac monitor is observed continuously for changes and blood pressure is monitored at predetermined intervals.
- The rhythm strip is checked at preset intervals for arrhythmias, premature ventricular contractions, ST-segment changes, and T-wave changes.
- The test level and the amount of time it took to reach that level are marked on each strip.
- Common responses to maximal exercise include dizziness, light-headedness, leg fatigue, dyspnea, diaphoresis, and a slightly ataxic gait. If symptoms become severe, the test is stopped.
- After the patient has reached the maximum predicted heart rate, the treadmill is slowed.
- While the patient's heart rate is still elevated, he's assisted off the treadmill and placed on a litter for a second echocardiogram.

Postprocedure care

- Remove electrodes and conductive gel.

MONITORING
- Vital signs
- ECG
- Heart sounds

Precautions

■ **NURSING ALERT** Testing should be stopped for significant ECG changes, arrhythmias, or symptoms including hypertension, hypotension, or angina.

- Wolff-Parkinson-White syndrome, electrolyte imbalance, or the use of digoxin preparations may cause false-positive results.

- Conditions that cause left ventricular hypertrophy may interfere with testing for ischemia.
- The procedure may be contraindicated in ventricular or dissecting aortic aneurysms, uncontrolled arrhythmias, pericarditis, myocarditis, severe anemia, uncontrolled hypertension, unstable angina, and heart failure.

■ **NURSING ALERT** The procedure shouldn't be performed without a physician and emergency resuscitation equipment readily available.

Complications

- Angina
- Cardiac arrhythmias
- Myocardial ischemia or MI
- Cardiac arrest
- Death

✢ INTERPRETATION

Normal findings

- Contractility of the ventricular walls increases and results in hyperkinesis associated with sympathetic and catecholamine stimulation.
- Heart rate increases in direct proportion to the workload and metabolic oxygen demand. Systolic blood pressure also increases as workload increases.
- The endurance level appropriate for the patient's age and exercise is attained.

Abnormal results

- Exercise-induced myocardial ischemia suggests disease in the coronary artery supplying the involved area of myocardium. Hypokinesis or akinesis of the myocardium suggests significant CAD.
- Exercise-induced hypotension, ST-segment depression of 2 mm or more, or downsloping ST segments appearing within the first 3 minutes of exercise and lasting 8 minutes into the posttest recovery period may indicate multivessel or left coronary artery disease.
- ST-segment elevation may indicate critical myocardial ischemia or injury.

Echocardiography, non-exercise stress

● OVERVIEW

- Detects changes in regional cardiac wall motion
- Increases myocardial contractility and stroke volume, permitting study of heart under stress conditions without need for the patient to exercise
- Imaging done during infusion of increasing amounts of dobutamine until maximum predicted heart rate reached

Purpose
- To identify causes of anginal symptoms
- To measure chambers of the heart and determine functional capacity
- To help set limits for an exercise program
- To diagnose and evaluate valvular and wall motion abnormalities
- To detect atrial tumors, mural thrombi, vegetative growth on valve leaflets, and pericardial effusions
- To evaluate myocardial perfusion, coronary artery disease and obstruction, and the extent of myocardial damage following myocardial infarction (MI)

Patient preparation
- Make sure that the patient has signed an appropriate consent form.
- Note and report all allergies.
- Explain the need to refrain from eating, smoking, or drinking alcoholic or caffeine-containing beverages at least 4 hours before the test or as directed by the physician.
- Withhold current medications before testing as directed.
- Warn the patient that when the dobutamine infusion is started, the patient may feel palpitations, some mild shortness of breath, and some fatigue.
- Instruct the patient to report all symptoms experienced during the study.

TEACHING POINTS
Be sure to cover:
- test's purpose and how it's done
- who will perform the test and where
- that the entire test should take 60 to 90 minutes.

▶ PROCEDURE

- The patient is placed in a supine position on a litter and an echocardiogram obtained.
- An initial electrocardiogram (ECG) is obtained.
- Continuous ECG monitoring is performed during the procedure.
- Initial and serial blood pressure readings are recorded.
- After I.V. access is obtained, dobutamine infusion is administered in increasing amounts, usually up to a maximum of 30 mcg/kg/minute.
- The infusion continues until the patient reaches his maximum predicted heart rate or becomes symptomatic.
- If the maximum predicted heart rate is not reached with maximum dobutamine, I.V. atropine may be administered.
- As the maximum predicted heart rate is achieved, a second (stress) echocardiogram is obtained.
- After the dobutamine infusion is completed, a third (recovery) echocardiogram is completed.

Postprocedure care
- If heart rate doesn't return to baseline or the patient becomes symptomatic, an I.V. beta-adrenergic blocker may be administered.
- Remove electrodes and conductive gel from the patient's chest.

MONITORING
- Vital signs
- ECG
- Heart sounds
- Anginal symptoms
- Respiratory status

Precautions
- Contraindications for dobutamine stress testing include:
  - MI within 10 days of testing
  - acute myocarditis or pericarditis
  - ventricular or atrial arrhythmias
  - severe aortic or mitral stenosis
  - hyperthyroidism or severe anemia
  - ventricular or dissecting aortic aneurysms
  - clinical heart failure
  - acute severe infections.

NURSING ALERT Testing should be stopped for significant ECG changes, hypertension, hypotension, angina, dyspnea, syncope, or other critical symptoms.

NURSING ALERT Dobutamine stress echocardiography should never be performed without a physician and emergency resuscitation equipment immediately available.

Complications
- Angina
- Hypertension
- Hypotension
- Cardiac arrhythmias
- Myocardial ischemia

✛ INTERPRETATION

Normal findings
- Ventricular wall contractility increases.

Abnormal results
- Abnormal regional wall motion may indicate cardiac ischemia or infarction.

Electrocardiography

● OVERVIEW

- Graphically records the electrical current generated by the heart and measured by electrodes connected to an amplifier and strip chart recorder
- Standard resting electrocardiogram (ECG): measures the electrical potential from 12 different leads: the standard limb leads (I, II, III), the augmented limb leads (aV_F, aV_L, and aV_R), and the precordial, or chest, leads (V_1 through V_6)
- Also known as *ECG*

Purpose

- To identify conduction abnormalities, cardiac arrhythmias, myocardial ischemia or infarction (MI)
- To monitor recovery from MI
- To document pacemaker performance

Patient preparation

- Explain the need to lie still, relax, and breathe normally during the procedure.
- Note current cardiac drug therapy on the test request form as well as any other pertinent clinical information, such as chest pain or pacemaker

TEACHING POINTS

Be sure to cover:
- the purpose of the study and how it's done
- who will perform the test and where
- that the test is painless and takes 5 to 10 minutes.

▶ PROCEDURE

- Place the patient in a supine position or semi-Fowler's position.
- Expose the chest, ankles, and wrists.
- Place electrodes on the inner aspect of wrists, medial aspect of lower legs, and on the chest.
- Connect the leadwires after all electrodes are in place.
- Press the START button and input any required information.
- Make sure that all leads are represented in the tracing. If not, determine which electrode has come loose, reattach it, and restart the tracing.

Postprocedure care

- Disconnect the equipment, remove the electrodes, and remove the gel with a moist cloth towel.
- Electrode patches are left in place if the patient is having recurrent chest pain or if serial ECGs are ordered.

MONITORING
- None necessary

Precautions

- All recording and other nearby electrical equipment should be properly grounded.
- Ensure that electrodes are firmly attached.

Complications

- Skin sensitivity to electrodes

✛ INTERPRETATION

Normal findings

Common, basic findings include:
- ECG tracings normally consist of P wave, QRS complex, and T wave. (See *ECG waveform components.*)
- The normal cardiac rate is 60 to 100 beats/minute.
- The cardiac rhythm should be normal sinus rhythm (NSR).
- The P wave precedes each QRS complex.
- The PR interval has a duration of 0.12 to 0.20 second.
- The QRS complex has a duration of 0.06 to 0.10 second.
- The ST segment is usually not more than 0.1 mV.
- The T wave is usually rounded and smooth and is usually positive in leads I, II, V_3, V_4, V_5, and V_6.
- The duration of the QT interval varies but usually lasts 0.36 to 0.44 second.

Abnormal results

Common, basic findings include:
- A heart rate below 60 beats/minute is bradycardia.
- A heart rate greater than 100 beats/minute is tachycardia.
- Abnormalities in cardiac rhythm suggest arrhythmias.
- Missing P waves may indicate atrioventricular (AV) block, atrial arrhythmia, or junctional rhythm.
- A short PR interval may indicate a junctional arrhythmia; a prolonged PR interval may indicate AV block.
- A prolonged QRS complex may indicate intraventricular conduction defects; missing QRS complexes may indicate AV block or ventricular asystole.
- ST-segment elevation of 0.2 mV or more above baseline may indicate myocardial injury; ST-segment depression may indicate myocardial ischemia or injury.
- T-wave inversion in leads I, II, V_3 to V_6 may indicate myocardial ischemia; peaked T waves may indicate hyperkalemia or myocardial ischemia; variations in T wave amplitude may indicate electrolyte imbalances.
- A prolonged QT interval may suggest life-threatening ventricular arrhythmias.

ECG WAVEFORM COMPONENTS

The electrocardiogram (ECG) renders the heart's electrical activity. The illustration represents the electrical activity during one normal cardiac cycle, with the locations of the various waveform components.

Major components

Three basic waveforms make up all ECG tracings: the P wave, the QRS complex, and the T wave. These units of electrical activity can be further broken down into the following segments and intervals: the PR interval, the ST segment, and the QT interval.

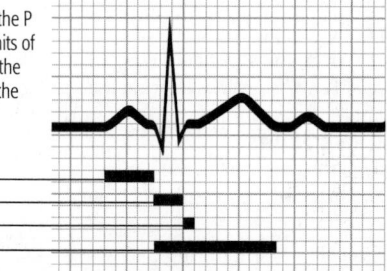

PR interval
QRS complex
ST segment
QT interval

Electrocardiography, exercise

● OVERVIEW

- Monitors patient's electrocardiogram (ECG) and blood pressure while the patient walks on a treadmill or pedals a stationary bicycle; response to a constant or increasing workload is observed
- Used to evaluate the heart during physical stress
- Also known as *exercise stress test*

Purpose

- To diagnose the cause of chest pain
- To determine functional capacity of the heart
- To screen for asymptomatic coronary artery disease
- To help set limitations for an exercise program
- To identify cardiac arrhythmias that develop during physical exercise
- To evaluate effectiveness of antiarrhythmic or antianginal therapy
- To evaluate myocardial perfusion

Patient preparation

- Make sure that the patient has signed an appropriate consent form.
- Note and report all allergies.
- Check the patient's history for a recent physical examination (within 1 week) and for baseline 12-lead ECG results.
- Instruct the patient not to eat, smoke, or drink alcoholic or caffeine-containing beverages before the test as ordered.
- Continue medications unless the physician directs otherwise.
- Warn the patient that he might feel fatigued, slightly breathless, and sweaty during the test.
- Provide reassurance that the test may be stopped if the patient experiences significant symptoms such as chest pain.
- Instruct the patient to wear comfortable socks and shoes and loose, lightweight shorts or slacks during the procedure.

TEACHING POINTS

Be sure to cover:
- the purpose of the study and how it's done
- who will perform the test and where
- that the test takes about 30 minutes.

▶ PROCEDURE

- Baseline ECG and blood pressure readings are taken.
- ECG and blood pressure readings are taken while the patient walks on a treadmill or pedals a stationary bicycle.
- Unless complications develop, the test continues until the patient reaches the target heart rate, determined by an established protocol (usually 85% of maximum predicted heart rate for the patient's age and gender).
- The cardiac monitor is observed continuously for changes in the heart's electrical activity.
- The rhythm strip is checked at preset intervals for arrhythmias, premature ventricular contractions (PVCs), ST-segment changes, and T-wave changes.
- Blood pressure is monitored at predetermined intervals (usually at the end of each test level).
- The test is stopped when the patient reaches the target heart rate or if symptoms become severe.

Postprocedure care

- Assist the patient to a chair and continue monitoring heart rate and blood pressure for 10 to 15 minutes or until the ECG returns to baseline.
- Remove the electrodes and clean the application sites.
- Resume a normal diet and activities as ordered.

MONITORING

- Vital signs
- ECG
- Heart sounds
- Anginal symptoms

Precautions

- The procedure may be contraindicated in a patient with:
  - ventricular or dissecting aortic aneurysm
  - uncontrolled arrhythmias
  - pericarditis
  - myocarditis
  - severe anemia
  - uncontrolled hypertension
  - unstable angina
  - heart failure.

◆ **NURSING ALERT** Stop the test immediately if the ECG shows significant arrhythmias or increase in ectopy, if systolic blood pressure falls below resting level, if the heart rate falls 10 beats/minute or more below resting level, or if the patient becomes exhausted or experiences severe symptoms such as chest pain.

- Conditions that cause left ventricular hypertrophy may interfere with testing for ischemia.
- The test may be stopped for new bundle-branch block, ST-segment depression exceeding 1.5 mm, or frequent or multifocal PVCs; if blood pressure fails to rise above resting level; if systolic pressure exceeds 220 mm Hg; or if the patient experiences angina.
- The test may also be stopped if the examiner suspects that persistent ST-segment elevation may indicate myocardial injury.

Complications

- Angina
- Cardiac arrhythmias
- Myocardial ischemia or infarction

✛ INTERPRETATION

Normal findings

- The heart rate increases in direct proportion to the workload and metabolic oxygen demand.
- Systolic blood pressure increases as workload increases.
- The patient attains the endurance levels appropriate for his age and the exercise protocol.

Abnormal results

- T-wave inversion or ST-segment depression may signify ischemia.
- Significant coronary artery disease may be indicated by:
  - exercise-induced hypotension
  - ST-segment depression of 2 mm or more
  - downsloping ST segments
- ST-segment elevation may indicate myocardial injury.

Electroencephalography

● OVERVIEW

- Involves recording a portion of the brain's electrical activity through electrodes attached to the scalp
- Electrical impulses are transmitted to electroencephalograph, magnified, and recorded as brain waves
- Intracranial electrodes are sometimes surgically implanted to record EEG changes for localization of seizure focus
- Also known as *EEG*

Purpose
- To determine the presence and type of epilepsy
- To aid diagnosis of intracranial lesions
- To evaluate brain activity in metabolic disease, head injury, meningitis, encephalitis, and psychological disorders
- To help confirm brain death

Patient preparation
- Make sure that the patient has signed an appropriate consent form.
- Note and report all allergies.
- Wash and dry the patient's hair to remove hair sprays, creams, or oils.
- Withhold tranquilizers, barbiturates, and other sedatives for 24 to 48 hours before the test as ordered.
- Minimize sleep (4 to 5 hours) the night before the study if ordered.
- If a sleep EEG is ordered, administer a sedative to promote sleep during the test as ordered.
- There's no need to restrict food and fluids before the test, but stimulants such as caffeine-containing beverages, chocolate, and smoking are not permitted for 8 hours before the study.
- Provide reassurance that the electrodes won't shock the patient.
- If needle electrodes are used, warn the patient that he might feel pricking sensations during insertion.

◈ **AGE-RELATED CONCERN** Infants and very young children may require sedation to prevent crying and restlessness; however, these drugs may alter test results.

TEACHING POINTS
Be sure to cover:
- test's purpose and how it's done
- who will perform the test and where
- that the test takes about 1 hour.

▶ PROCEDURE

- The patient is positioned and electrodes are attached to the scalp.
- During recording, the patient is carefully observed; blinking, swallowing, talking, or other movements that can cause artifacts are noted.
- The patient may be tested in various stress situations including hyperventilation and photic stimulation to elicit abnormal patterns not obvious in the resting stage.

Postprocedure care
- Resume medications as ordered.
- Provide a safe environment.
- Maintain seizure precautions
- Help the patient remove electrode paste from his hair.
- If brain death is confirmed, provide emotional support for the family.

MONITORING
- Seizure activity
- Adverse effects of sedation if used

Precautions
- Skipping the meal before the test can cause hypoglycemia and alter brain wave patterns.
- Anticonvulsants, tranquilizers, barbiturates, and other sedatives can interfere with the accuracy of test results.

Complications
- Adverse effects of sedation
- Possible seizure activity

✣ INTERPRETATION

Normal findings
- Alpha waves:
  - occur at frequencies of 8 to 13 cycles/second in a regular rhythm
  - are present only in the waking state when the patient's eyes are closed but he's mentally alert
  - usually disappear with visual activity or mental concentration
  - are decreased by apprehension or anxiety
  - are most prominent in the occipital leads.
- Beta waves (13 to 30 cycles/second):
  - indicate normal activity when the patient is alert with eyes open
  - are seen most readily in the frontal and central regions of the brain.
- Theta waves (4 to 7 cycles/second):
  - are most common in children and young adults
  - appear primarily in the parietal and temporal regions
  - indicate drowsiness or emotional stress in adults.
- Delta waves (less than 4 cycles/second):
  - are seen in deep sleep stages and in serious brain dysfunction.

Abnormal results
- Spikes and waves at a frequency of 3 cycles/second suggest absence seizures.
- Multiple, high-voltage, spiked waves in both hemispheres suggest generalized tonic-clonic seizures.
- Spiked waves in the affected temporal region suggest temporal lobe epilepsy.
- Localized, spiked discharges suggest focal seizures.
- Slow waves (usually delta waves, but possibly unilateral beta waves) suggest intracranial lesions.
- Focal abnormalities in the injured area suggest vascular lesions.
- Generalized, diffuse, and slow brain waves suggest metabolic or inflammatory disorders or increased intracranial pressure.
- Absent EEG pattern or a "flat" tracing (except for artifacts) may indicate brain death.

Electromyography

● OVERVIEW

- Records the electrical activity of selected skeletal muscle groups at rest and during voluntary contraction
- Nerve conduction time often measured simultaneously (see *Nerve conduction studies*)
- Also known as *EMG*

Purpose
- To differentiate between primary muscle disorders such as muscular dystrophies and certain metabolic disorders
- To identify diseases characterized by central neuronal degeneration such as amyotrophic lateral sclerosis (ALS)
- To aid in diagnosis of neuromuscular disorders such as myasthenia gravis
- To aid in diagnosis of radiculomyopathies

Patient preparation
- Make sure that the patient has signed an appropriate consent form.
- Note and report all allergies.
- Check for and note medications that may interfere with test results (cholinergics, anticholinergics, anticoagulants, and skeletal muscle relaxants).
- Foods and fluids aren't withheld before this test. Cigarettes, coffee, tea, and cola may be restricted for 2 to 3 hours before the test as ordered.
- Warn the patient that he might experience some discomfort as a needle is inserted into selected muscles.

TEACHING POINTS
Be sure to cover:
- the purpose of the study and how it's done
- who will perform the test and where
- that the test takes at least 1 hour.

▶ PROCEDURE

- The patient is positioned so the muscle to be tested is at rest.
- Needle electrodes are quickly inserted into the selected muscle.
- A metal plate is placed under the patient to serve as a reference electrode.
- The resulting electrical signal is recorded during rest and contraction, amplified 1 million times, and displayed on an oscilloscope or computer screen.
- Leadwires are usually attached to an audio-amplifier so that voltage fluctuations within the muscle can be heard.

Postprocedure care
- Apply warm compresses and administer analgesics as ordered for discomfort.
- Resume medications or substances that were withheld before the test as ordered.

MONITORING
- Infection
- Pain and response to analgesics

Precautions
- Electromyography may be contraindicated in patients with bleeding disorders.

Complications
- Infection

✛ INTERPRETATION

Normal findings
- At rest, a normal muscle exhibits minimal electrical activity.
- During voluntary contraction, electrical activity increases markedly.
- A sustained contraction, or one of increasing strength, produces a rapid "train" of motor unit potentials.

Abnormal results
- Short (low amplitude) motor unit potentials, with frequent, irregular discharges suggest possible primary muscle disease such as muscular dystrophies.
- Isolated and irregular motor unit potentials with increased amplitude and duration suggest possible disorders, such as ALS and peripheral nerve disorders.
- Initially normal motor unit potentials, which progressively diminish in amplitude with continuing contractions suggest possible myasthenia gravis.

NERVE CONDUCTION STUDIES

Nerve conduction studies aid diagnosis of peripheral nerve injuries and diseases affecting the peripheral nervous system such as peripheral neuropathies. To measure nerve conduction time, a nerve is stimulated electrically through the skin and underlying tissues. The patient experiences a mild electric shock with each stimulation. At a known distance from the point of stimulation, a recording electrode detects the response from the stimulated nerve.

The time between stimulation of the nerve and the detected response is measured on an oscilloscope. The speed of conduction along the nerve is then calculated by dividing the distance between the point of stimulation and the recording electrode by the time between stimulus and response. In peripheral nerve injuries and diseases such as peripheral neuropathies, nerve conduction time is abnormal.

Electromyography, external sphincter

● OVERVIEW

- Measures electrical activity of the external urinary sphincter
- Activity measured in three ways: by skin electrodes (most commonly used), by needle electrodes inserted in perineal or periurethral tissues, or by electrodes in an anal plug
- Often used with cystometry and voiding urethrography as part of full urodynamic study

Purpose
- To evaluate incontinence
- To assess neuromuscular function of the external urinary sphincter
- To assess functional balance between bladder and sphincter muscle activity

Patient preparation
- Make sure that the patient has signed an appropriate consent form.
- Note and report all allergies.
- If the patient is taking cholinergic or anticholinergic drugs, notify the physician and discontinue medications as ordered.
- If needle electrodes are used, warn the patient that discomfort may be felt during insertion.
- Provide reassurance that there's no danger of electric shock.
- If an anal plug is used, provide reassurance that only the tip of the plug will be inserted into the rectum; the patient may feel fullness but no discomfort.

TEACHING POINTS
Be sure to cover:
- the purpose of the study and how it's done
- who will perform the test and where
- that the test takes 30 to 60 minutes
- that a female patient may notice slight bleeding with the first voiding after the procedure.

▶ PROCEDURE

- The patient is placed in the lithotomy position for electrode placement, then may lie in a supine position.
- Electrode paste is applied to the ground plate, which is taped to the thigh and grounded and electrodes are applied and connected to electrode adapters.
- For a female patient, skin electrodes are placed in the periurethral area; for a male, in the perineal area beneath the scrotum.
- For a female patient, needle electrodes are inserted periurethrally; for a male, through the perineal skin toward the apex of the prostate.
- The electrodes are connected to adapters inserted into the preamplifier and recording begins.
- The patient is asked to alternately relax and tighten the sphincter.
- The patient is asked to bear down and exhale while the anal plug and needle electrodes are removed.
- Cystometrography is sometimes done with electromyography (EMG) for a thorough evaluation of detrusor and sphincter coordination.

Postprocedure care
- Clean and dry the area.
- Report hematuria after the first voiding in a female patient tested with needle electrodes.
- Report signs and symptoms of mild urethral irritation, including dysuria, hematuria, and urinary frequency.
- Advise the use of warm sitz baths and increased oral fluids (2 to 3 qt [2 to 3 L]/day), unless contraindicated.

MONITORING
- Urinary complaints
- Intake and output
- Pain

Precautions
- Cholinergic or anticholinergic drugs may interfere with test results.

Complications
- Bleeding
- Infection

✛ INTERPRETATION

Normal findings
- Muscle activity is increased when the external urinary sphincter is tightened.
- Muscle activity is decreased when the external urinary sphincter is relaxed.
- If EMG and cystometrography are done together, a comparison of results shows:
  - muscle activity of the sphincter that increases as the bladder fills, during voiding, and with bladder contraction
  - muscle activity that decreases as the sphincter relaxes.

Abnormal results
- Failure of the sphincter to relax or increased muscle activity during voiding indicates detrusor-sphincter dyssynergia.

Electrophysiology studies

- Permits measurement of discrete conduction intervals
- Records electrical conduction during the slow withdrawal of an electrode catheter from the right ventricle through the bundle of His to the sinoatrial node
- Also known as *EPS* or *bundle of His electrography*

Purpose

- To diagnose arrhythmias and conduction anomalies
- To determine the need for an implanted pacemaker, internal cardioverter-defibrillator, and cardioactive drugs
- To locate the site of a bundle-branch block, especially in asymptomatic patients with conduction disturbances
- To determine the presence and location of accessory conducting pathways

Patient preparation

- Make sure that the patient has signed an appropriate consent form.
- Note and report all allergies.
- Instruct the patient to restrict food and fluids for at least 6 hours before the test.
- Provide reassurance that the patient remains conscious during the test. Instruct him to report any discomfort or pain.

TEACHING POINTS

Be sure to cover:

- the purpose of the study and how it's done
- who will perform the test and where
- that the test takes 1 to 3 hours.

▶ PROCEDURE

- The patient is placed in a supine position on a special table.
- Electrogardiogram (ECG) monitoring is initiated.
- The insertion site is prepared and draped (usually the groin or antecubital fossa).
- Local anesthetic is injected, and a catheter is inserted intravenously, using fluoroscopic guidance.

- The catheter is advanced into the right ventricle, then slowly withdrawn.
- Recordings of conduction intervals are taken from each pole of the catheter, either simultaneously or sequentially.
- After recordings and measurements are complete, the catheter is removed.
- The insertion site is cleaned and a sterile dressing is applied.

Postprocedure care

- Enforce bed rest, as ordered.
- If bleeding occurs, apply pressure and inform the physician immediately.
- Resume a usual diet, as ordered.
- Obtain a 12-lead resting ECG.

MONITORING

- Vital signs
- Insertion site
- Bleeding
- Signs and symptoms of infection
- Cardiac arrhythmias
- Anginal symptoms
- Signs and symptoms of embolism
- ECG changes

Precautions

- The procedure is contraindicated in a patient with:
  - severe uncorrected coagulopathy
  - recent thrombophlebitis
  - acute pulmonary embolism.

◆ **NURSING ALERT** Emergency resuscitation equipment should be immediately available in case of arrhythmias during the test.

Complications

- Arrhythmias
- Pulmonary emboli
- Thromboemboli
- Hemorrhage
- Infection

✛ INTERPRETATION

Normal findings

- The HV interval (conduction time from the bundle of His to the Purkinje fibers) is 35 to 55 msec.
- The AH interval (conduction time from the atrioventricular node to the bundle of His) is 45 to 150 msec.

- The PA (intra-atrial) interval is 20 to 40 msec. (See *Normal bundle of His electrogram.*)

Abnormal results

- A prolonged HV interval suggests possible acute or chronic disease.
- AH interval delays suggest atrial pacing, chronic conduction system disease, carotid sinus pressure, recent myocardial infarction, and use of certain drugs.
- PA interval delays suggest possible acquired, surgically induced, or congenital atrial disease and atrial pacing.

NORMAL BUNDLE OF HIS ELECTROGRAM

In a normal bundle of His electrogram (shown here), atrial activation appears as a sharp diphasic or triphasic wave (A) during the P wave, followed by bundle of His deflection (H) and ventricular activation (V). By measuring the interval between the beginning of the P wave and bundle of His activation (PH interval), or the interval between the beginning of the atrial wave and bundle of His activation (AH interval), abnormally prolonged AV nodal conduction can be detected.

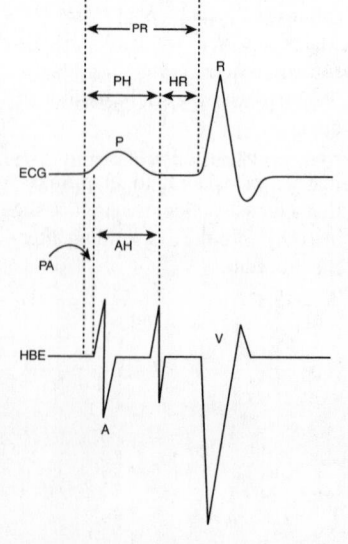

Endoscopic retrograde cholangiopancreatography

● OVERVIEW

- Radiographic examination of the pancreatic ducts and hepatobiliary tree after injection of contrast medium into the duodenal papilla
- Also known as *ERCP*

Purpose
- To evaluate obstructive jaundice
- To diagnose cancer of the duodenal papilla, pancreas, and biliary ducts
- To locate calculi and stenosis in pancreatic ducts and hepatobiliary tree

Patient preparation
- Make sure that the patient has signed an appropriate consent form.
- Note and report all allergies.
- Administer a sedative as ordered.
- Instruct the patient to fast before the study as ordered.
- Explain the use of a local anesthetic spray to suppress the gag reflex and the use of a mouth guard to protect the teeth.
- Provide reassurance that oral insertion of the endoscope doesn't obstruct breathing and that the patient remains conscious during the procedure.

TEACHING POINTS
Be sure to cover:
- the purpose of the study and how it's done
- who will perform the study and where
- that the study takes 1 to 1½ hours; longer if a procedure such as stent placement is performed
- that the patient may have a sore throat for 3 to 4 days after the examination
- that belching and passing flatus occur after the test
- that avoidance of alcohol and driving is necessary for 24 hours after the study.

▶ PROCEDURE

- An I.V. infusion is started.
- A local anesthetic and I.V. sedation are administered.
- Vital signs, cardiac rhythm, and pulse oximetry are continuously monitored.
- The patient is placed in a left lateral position.
- The endoscope is inserted into the mouth and advanced using fluoroscopic guidance, into the stomach and duodenum.
- The patient is assisted to the prone position.
- An I.V. anticholinergic or glucagon may be administered to decrease GI motility.
- A cannula is passed through the biopsy channel of the endoscope, into the duodenal papilla, and into the ampulla of Vater.
- Contrast medium is injected.
- The pancreatic duct and hepatobiliary tree are visualized.
- Rapid-sequence radiographs are taken after each contrast injection.
- Tissue specimen or fluid may be aspirated for histologic and cytologic examination.
- Therapeutic measures (sphincterectomy, stent placement, stone removal, or balloon dilatation) may be performed before endoscope withdrawal, as indicated.
- After the films have been reviewed the cannula is removed.

Postprocedure care
- Withhold food and fluids until the gag reflex returns; resume diet as ordered.
- Provide soothing lozenges and warm saline gargles for sore throat.

MONITORING
- Vital signs
- Cardiac rhythm
- Pulse oximetry
- Level of consciousness
- Abdominal distention and bowel sounds
- Adverse drug reactions
- Signs and symptoms of:
  - Perforation
  - Respiratory depression
  - Urinary retention

- Ascending cholangitis
- Pancreatitis

Precautions
- Inform the physician about hypersensitivity to iodine, seafood, or iodinated contrast media.
- The procedure is contraindicated in:
  - pregnancy
  - stricture or obstruction of the esophagus or duodenum
  - acute pancreatitis or cholangitis
  - severe cardiorespiratory disease.

◈ **NURSING ALERT** Emergency resuscitation equipment and a benzodiazepine and narcotic antagonist should be immediately available during the test.

Complications
- Ascending cholangitis
- Pancreatitis
- Adverse drug reactions
- Cardiac arrhythmias
- Perforation of the bowel
- Respiratory depression

✥ INTERPRETATION

Normal findings
- Duodenal papilla appears as a small red or pale erosion protruding into the lumen.
- Pancreatic and hepatobiliary ducts usually join and empty through the duodenal papilla; separate orifices are sometimes present.
- Contrast agent uniformly fills the pancreatic duct, hepatobiliary tree, and gallbladder.

Abnormal results
- Hepatobiliary tree filling defects, strictures, or irregular deviations suggest possible biliary cirrhosis, primary sclerosing cholangitis, calculi, or cancer of the bile ducts.
- Filling defects, strictures, and irregular deviations of pancreatic duct suggest possible pancreatic cysts and pseudocysts, pancreatic tumors, chronic pancreatitis, pancreatic fibrosis, calculi, or papillary stenosis.

Endoscopic ultrasound

● OVERVIEW

- Combines ultrasonography and endoscopy to visualize the GI wall and adjacent structures
- Allows ultrasound imaging with high resolution
- Also known as an *EUS*

Purpose

- To evaluate or stage lesions of the esophagus, stomach, duodenum, pancreas, ampulla, biliary ducts, and rectum
- To evaluate submucosal tumors

Patient preparation

- Make sure that the patient has signed an appropriate consent form.
- Note and report all allergies.
- Fasting is necessary for 6 to 8 hours before the test.
- For a sigmoid EUS, warn the patient that the scope is inserted through the anus. He may have to take a laxative the evening before and may feel an urge to defecate during the study.
- An I.V. sedative may be administered to help the patient relax before the endoscope is inserted.

TEACHING POINTS

Be sure to cover:
- the purpose of the study and how it's done
- who will perform the test and where
- that the test takes 30 to 90 minutes.

▶ PROCEDURE

- Vital signs are monitored throughout the procedure.
- Oxygen saturations and cardiac rhythm are monitored if I.V. sedation is used.
- Follow the procedures for esophagogastroduodenoscopy (EGD) or sigmoidoscopy, depending on which type of EUS is to be performed.

Postprocedure care

- Follow the procedures for EGD or sigmoidoscopy, depending on which type of EUS is to be performed.
- Resume activity and diet as ordered.

MONITORING
- Vital signs
- Level of consciousness
- Cardiac rhythm
- Bleeding
- Signs and symptoms of perforation

Precautions

- The patient should avoid alcohol and driving for 24 hours after the test if I.V. sedation was used.
- Esophageal stricture hinders passage of the endoscope.

Complications

- Perforation
- Bleeding

✛ INTERPRETATION

Normal findings

- Normal anatomy is found, with no evidence of tumor.

Abnormal results

- Results may show evidence of acute or chronic ulcers, benign or malignant tumors, or inflammatory disease.

Endoscopy

● OVERVIEW

- Direct visualization of the lining of a hollow viscus using an endoscope
- Cablelike cluster of glass fibers in endoscope transmits light into the viscus; image is then returned to the scope's optical head or video monitor

Purpose
- To diagnose inflammatory, ulcerative, and infectious diseases
- To diagnose benign and malignant tumors and other lesions of the mucosa

Patient preparation
- Make sure that the patient has signed an appropriate consent form.
- Note and report all allergies.
- An I.V. sedative may be given to help the patient relax before the endoscope is inserted.

TEACHING POINTS
Be sure to cover:
- the purpose of the study and how it's done
- who will perform it and where
- that the study takes about 1 hour.

▶ PROCEDURE

- I.V. access is initiated if indicated.
- Vital signs, pulse oximetry, and cardiac rhythm are monitored throughout the procedure.
- Follow the procedure for the specific endoscopy to be performed (arthroscopy, bronchoscopy, colonoscopy, colposcopy, cystourethroscopy, endoscopic retrograde cholangiopancreatography, esophagogastroduoentoscopy, sigmoidoscopy, hysteroscopy, laparoscopy, laryngoscopy, mediastinoscopy, protosigmoidoscopy, thoracoscopy).

Postprocedure care
- Provide a safe environment.
- Withhold food and fluids until the gag reflex returns.
- Resume the patient's diet as ordered.

MONITORING
- Vital signs
- Respiratory status
- Neurologic status
- Cardiac rhythm
- Complications

Precautions
- For a patient on anticoagulation therapy, adjustments to medications may be necessary.
- For high-risk procedures, warfarin should be discontinued 3 to 5 days before the procedure and appropriate medication ordered such as low molecular weight heparin.
- Discontinue aspirin or nonsteroidal anti-inflammatory drugs 3 to 7 days before the study as ordered.

Complications
- Adverse reaction to sedation
- Cardiac arrhythmias
- Respiratory suppression
- Bleeding

✛ INTERPRETATION

Normal findings
See the specific endoscopy procedure.

Abnormal results
See the specific endoscopy procedure.

Esophageal acidity test

- A sensitive indicator of gastric reflux
- Indicated for patients who complain of persistent heartburn with or without regurgitation
- Esophageal sphincter pressure also measured
- Newer method developed for monitoring pH (see *Monitoring pH with the Bravo system*)

Purpose

- To evaluate the competence of the lower esophageal sphincter
- To measure intra-esophageal pH

Patient preparation

- Make sure that the patient has signed an appropriate consent form.
- Note and report all allergies.
- Withhold antacids, anticholinergics, cholinergics, beta-adrenergic blockers, alcohol, corticosteroids, histamine-2 receptor antagonists, proton pump inhibitors, and reserpine for 24 hours before the test, as ordered.
- Instruct the patient to fast and avoid smoking after midnight before the test.
- Warn the patient that he might experience slight discomfort and may cough or gag during passage of a tube through his mouth and into the stomach.

TEACHING POINTS

Be sure to cover:
- the purpose of the study and how it's done
- who will perform the test and where
- that the test takes about 45 minutes.

- The patient is placed in high Fowler's position.
- A catheter, with pH electrode, is inserted into the mouth and advanced to the lower esophageal sphincter.
- The patient performs a Valsalva's maneuver or lifts his legs to stimulate reflux.
- The intraesophageal pH is determined.

Postprocedure care

- Resume medications and diet as ordered.
- Provide soothing lozenges for a sore throat.

MONITORING

- Vital signs
- Pain

Precautions

NURSING ALERT During insertion, the catheter may inadvertently enter the trachea; if respiratory distress or paroxysmal coughing occurs, remove the catheter immediately.
- Clamp the catheter before removal to prevent aspiration.

Complications

- Respiratory distress
- Aspiration of gastric contents

Normal findings

- pH of the esophagus is greater than 5.0.

Abnormal results

- Intraesophageal pH of 1.5 to 2.0 indicates gastric acid reflux due to incompetence of the lower esophageal sphincter.

MONITORING pH WITH THE BRAVO SYSTEM

Traditional testing for esophageal acid levels typically uses an esophageal catheter that's inserted for a 24-hour period. Recently, however, a new technique called the *Bravo pH monitoring system* was developed to measure acid levels in the esophagus via a capsule (about the size of a gel cap). The capsule is temporarily attached to the patient's esophageal wall using an endoscope and collects pH data, which are then transmitted to a pager-sized receiver that the patient wears. Data are collected for 48 hours, downloaded from the receiver, and analyzed with special software.

The Bravo method is more accurate than catheter methods because the patient can eat normally and maintain regular activities during testing. The additional 24 hours also provides more information for diagnosing certain esophageal disorders.

In 7 to 10 days, the capsule spontaneously detaches from the esophageal wall and is passed through the patient's digestive system.

Esophagogastroduodenoscopy

● OVERVIEW

- Visual examination of the lining of the esophagus, stomach, and upper duodenum, using a flexible fiber-optic endoscope
- Also known as *EGD* or *ESD* (*esophagus, stomach, duodenum*)

Purpose

- To detect small or surface lesions missed by radiography
- To diagnose and treat upper GI bleeding
- To diagnose and treat inflammatory disease, tumors, ulcers, and structural abnormalities
- To evaluate the stomach and duodenum postoperatively
- To obtain specimens for laboratory evaluation
- To allow removal of foreign bodies by suction, snare, or forceps

Patient preparation

- Make sure that the patient has signed an appropriate consent form.
- Note and report all allergies.
- Remove the patient's dentures.
- Instruct the patient to fast for 6 to 12 hours before the test.
- Inform the patient that the procedure involves passing a flexible tube through the mouth.
- Explain that a bitter-tasting local anesthetic will be sprayed into the mouth and throat to suppress the gag reflex.
- Tell the patient that an I.V. line will be started to allow administration of a sedative or I.V. fluids.
- A mouth guard is inserted to protect the patient's teeth from the endoscope.
- Explain to the patient that he'll remain conscious during the procedure.

TEACHING POINTS
Be sure to cover:
- the purpose of the study and how it's done
- who will perform the test and where
- that the test takes about 30 minutes
- that belching of insufflated air after the test is normal
- sore throat (3 to 4 days after the test)

▶ PROCEDURE

- Vital signs, cardiac rhythm, and pulse oximetry are monitored throughout the procedure.
- When emergent EGD is performed, stomach contents are aspirated through a nasogastric tube.
- The patient is placed in a left lateral position.
- The endoscope is inserted into the mouth and advanced under direct vision to examine the esophagus and the cardiac sphincter, then advanced into the stomach.
- After examination of the stomach, the endoscope is advanced into the duodenum for examination.
- Air may be instilled to open the bowel lumen and flatten tissue folds during the test.
- The endoscope is slowly withdrawn and suspicious areas reexamined.
- Tissue specimens obtained are sent to the laboratory for analysis.

Postprocedure care

- Provide a safe environment until the patient has recovered from sedation.
- Withhold food and fluids until the gag reflex returns (within 1 hour).
- Provide throat lozenges and warm saline gargles for sore throat.
- Instruct the patient to avoid alcohol, operating any machinery, and driving for 24 hours after I.V. sedation.
- Instruct the patient to report persistent difficulty swallowing, pain, fever, black stools, or bloody vomitus.

◆ **NURSING ALERT** Observe for and report evidence of aspiration of gastric contents, which could precipitate aspiration pneumonia.

MONITORING
- Vital signs
- Cardiac rhythm
- Signs and symptoms of perforation
- Intake and output

◆ **NURSING ALERT** Observe for and immediately report signs and symptoms of perforation. Perforation in the cervical area of the esophagus produces pain on swallowing and neck movement; thoracic perforation causes substernal or epigastric pain that increases with breathing or with movement of the trunk; diaphragmatic perfo-

ration produces shoulder pain and dyspnea; gastric perforation causes abdominal or back pain, fever, or pleural effusion.

Precautions

- EGD is contraindicated in patients with a large aortic aneurysm, a recent ulcer perforation, known or suspected viscus perforation, unstable cardiac or pulmonary condition.
- EGD shouldn't be performed within 2 days after an upper GI series because barium can obscure visual examination.
- Observe closely for medication adverse effects and have emergency resuscitation equipment immediately available.

Complications

- Perforation of the esophagus, stomach, or duodenum
- Adverse reaction to sedation
- Aspiration of gastric contents
- Aspiration pneumonia

✥ INTERPRETATION

Normal findings

- The esophageal mucosa is smooth and yellow-pink with fine vascular markings.
- The gastric mucosa is orange-red beginning at the Z line, an irregular transition line slightly above the esophagogastric junction.
- Rugae are present in the stomach.
- The duodenal bulb mucosa is reddish and marked by a few shallow longitudinal folds.
- The distal duodenum has prominent circular folds, lined with villi.

Abnormal results

- Anatomic abnormalities of the esophagus suggest tumors, varices, Mallory-Weiss syndrome, esophageal stenoses, and esophageal hiatal hernia.
- Anatomic abnormalities of the stomach and duodenum suggest acute or chronic ulcers, benign or malignant tumors, or diverticula.
- Inflammatory changes suggest esophagitis, gastritis, and duodenitis.

Evoked potential studies

- Measurement of the brain's electrical response to stimulation of the sensory organs or peripheral nerves
- Allows evaluation of visual, somatosensory, and auditory nerve pathways
- Electrodes attached the scalp and skin over various peripheral sensory nerves detect and record electronic impulses
- Computer extracts low-amplitude impulses from background brain wave activity and averages the signals from repeated stimuli
- Can be used during therapeutic coma and in trauma brain-injured patients

Purpose

- To aid diagnosis of nervous system lesions and abnormalities
- To monitor spinal cord function during spinal surgery
- To assess neurologic function
- To evaluate neurologic function in infants
- To monitor comatose or anesthetized patients.

Patient preparation

- Make sure that the patient has signed an appropriate consent form.
- Note and report all allergies.
- Provide reassurance that the electrodes won't hurt him, but he may feel a small shock when somatosensory evoked responses are done.
- Encourage the patient to relax because tension can affect the test results.

TEACHING POINTS

Be sure to cover:
- the purpose of the study and how it's done
- who will perform the test and where
- that the test takes 45 to 60 minutes.

- The patient is positioned in a reclining or straight-backed chair or on a bed.
- The patient is instructed to relax and remain still.
- Electrodes are attached, depending on the specific type of evoked potentials performed.
- Visual evoked potentials, produced by exposing the eye to a rapidly reversing checkerboard pattern, help evaluate demyelinating disease (such as multiple sclerosis), traumatic injury, and puzzling visual complaints. One eye may be covered at a time with procedure then repeated on the other eye.
- Somatosensory evoked potentials, produced by electrically stimulating a peripheral sensory nerve, help diagnose peripheral nerve disease and locate brain and spinal cord lesions.
- Auditory brain stem evoked potentials, produced by delivering clicks to the ear, are used in locating auditory lesions and evaluating brain stem integrity and in assessing brainstem integrity when cranial nerve testing is inconclusive or cannot be performed.
- A computer amplifies and averages the brain's response to each stimulus and results are plotted as a waveform.

Postprocedure care

- No specific posttest care is necessary.

Precautions

- Extremely poor visual acuity can hinder accurate determination of visual evoked potentials.

Complications

- None known

Normal findings

VISUAL EVOKED POTENTIALS

- On the waveform, the most significant wave is P100, a positive wave appearing about 100 msec after the pattern-shift stimulus is applied.
- Normal results vary greatly among laboratories and patients.

SOMATOSENSORY EVOKED POTENTIALS

- The waveforms vary, depending on locations of the stimulating and recording electrodes.

Abnormal results

VISUAL EVOKED POTENTIALS

- Abnormal (extended) P100 latencies confined to one eye suggest a visual pathway lesion anterior to the optic chiasm.
- Bilateral abnormal P100 latencies suggest possible disorders, such as multiple sclerosis, optic neuritis, retinopathies, and amblyopia.

SOMATOSENSORY AND AUDITORY EVOKED POTENTIALS

- Changes in the electrical waveforms may indicate damaged or degenerated nerve pathways to the brain from the eyes, ears, or limbs.
- Absence of activity in a pathway may mean complete loss of nerve function in that pathway.
- Other changes may provide evidence of the type and location of nerve damage.
- Abnormal upper-limb interwave latencies suggest possible cervical spondylosis, intracerebral lesions, or sensorimotor neuropathies.
- Abnormalities in the lower limb suggest peripheral nerve and root lesions, such as those in Guillain-Barré syndrome, compressive myelopathies, multiple sclerosis, and traumatic spinal cord injury.

Excretory urography

● OVERVIEW

- Allows visualization of the renal parenchyma, calyces, and pelvis as well as the ureters, bladder and, in some cases, the urethra after I.V. administration of a contrast medium
- Also known as *intravenous pyelography* or *IVP*

Purpose

- To evaluate the structure and excretory function of the kidneys, ureters, and bladder
- To support a differential diagnosis of renovascular hypertension

Patient preparation

- Make sure that the patient has signed an appropriate consent form.
- Note and report all allergies.
- Check the patient's history for hypersensitivity to iodine, iodine-containing foods, or iodinated contrast media.
- Instruct the patient to fast for 8 hours before the test.
- Administer a laxative, if ordered, the night before the test.
- Obtain and report any abnormal results of renal function test, such as blood urea nitrogen and creatinine.
- Warn the patient that he might experience a transient burning sensation and metallic taste when the contrast agent is injected.

TEACHING POINTS

Be sure to cover:
- the purpose of the study and how it's done
- who will perform the test and where
- that the test takes about 30 to 45 minutes.

▶ PROCEDURE

- The patient is placed in a supine position.
- A kidney-ureter-bladder radiograph is performed.
- I.V. contrast medium is injected.
- Radiographs are obtained at regular intervals.
- Ureteral compression is performed after the 5-minute film to facilitate retention of the contrast medium by the upper urinary tract.
- After the 10-minute film, ureteral compression is released.
- Another film is taken of the lower halves of both ureters and bladder.
- The patient voids and final films are taken immediately to visualize residual bladder contents or mucosal abnormalities of the bladder or urethra.

Postprocedure care

- Observe for delayed reactions to the contrast medium.
- Continue I.V. fluids or provide oral fluids to promote hydration.

MONITORING

- Intake and output
- Allergic reactions

Precautions

- Excretory urography is contraindicated in a patient with abnormal renal function.
- Antibiotics may be ordered if pyelonephritis is identified.
- Fecal matter, gas, or retained barium in the colon from a previous diagnostic study may interfere with results.

※ **AGE-RELATED CONCERN** Excretory urography is contraindicated in children and elderly patients with actual or potential dehydration.

Complications

- Adverse reaction to contrast media
- Dehydration
- Impaired renal function

✥ INTERPRETATION

Normal findings

- Kidneys, ureters, and bladder show no gross evidence of soft- or hard-tissue lesions.
- Visualization of the contrast medium in the kidneys occurs promptly.
- Bilateral renal parenchyma and pelvi-calyceal systems have normal conformity.
- There's no post-voiding mucosal abnormality and little residual urine.

Abnormal results

- Anatomic abnormalities may suggest:
  - renal and ureteral calculi
  - supernumerary or absent kidney
  - polycystic kidney disease
  - redundant pelvis or ureter
  - space-occupying lesions or tumors
  - renal, bladder, or ureteral hematoma, laceration, or trauma
  - hydronephrosis.

Exophthalmometry

- Used to determine the relative forward protrusion of the eye from its orbit, or the anteroposterior position of the globe in the orbit
- Exophthalmometer: consists of horizontal calibrated bar with movable carriers holding mirrors inclined at a 45 degree angle; used to measure the distance from the apex of the cornea to the lateral orbital margin

Purpose

- To measure the amount of forward protrusion of the eye
- To evaluate progression or regression of exophthalmos
- To provide information in any condition that displaces the eye in the orbit, such as thyroid disease, tumors of the eye, cavernous sinus thrombosis, and orbital filtration from leukemia

Patient preparation

- Make sure that the patient has signed an appropriate consent form.
- Note and report all allergies.

TEACHING POINTS

Be sure to cover:
- the purpose of the study and how it's done
- who will perform the study and where
- that the study takes 5 to 10 minutes.

- The patient sits upright facing the examiner with his eyes on the same level.
- The horizontal bar of the exophthalmometer is held in front of the patient's eyes, parallel to the floor.
- The device's two small concave mirrors are moved against the lateral orbital margins at its deepest angle.
- The calibrated bar reading is recorded for a baseline reading.
- The patient fixates his right eye on the examiner's left eye.
- Using the inclined mirrors, the apex of the right cornea is superimposed on the millimeter scale.
- Left eye, right eye, and biocular readings are obtained, representing the eye's relative forward displacement from its orbit.
- The patient fixates his left eye on the examiner's right eye and the procedure is repeated.

Postprocedure care

- Refer the patient to an appropriate specialist as needed.

◈ **NURSING ALERT** Exophthalmos may result from a systemic disorder, such as thyroid disease, xanthomatosis, or a blood dyscrasia, in which case a complete medical examination is indicated.

MONITORING
- None necessary

Precautions

- For follow-up examinations, the calibrated bar is set at the baseline reading.
- Avoid excessive or prolonged pressure on the lateral orbital rim.

Complications

- None known

Normal findings

- Average readings are 15 to 17 mm for adults, with a range of 12 to 22 mm.
- Measurements for each eye are similar, usually differing by 1.5 mm or less and rarely by more than 3 mm.
- Repeated readings shouldn't vary more than 1 mm.

Abnormal results

- A difference between the eyes of more than 2 mm suggests exophthalmos or enophthalmos.
- A single reading that exceeds 20 mm may indicate exophthalmos.
- Readings less than 12 mm may indicate enophthalmos.
- Bilateral exophthalmos suggests a possible systemic disorder such as thyroid disease as well as xanthomatosis or a blood dyscrasia.

Fluorescein angiography

● OVERVIEW

- Rapid-sequence blue-colored flash photographs of the fundus taken with a special camera after I.V. injection of a vegetable-based dye, sodium fluorescein
- Fluorescein dye and sophisticated photographic equipment enhance the visibility of microvascular structures of the retina and choroids
- Allows evaluation of the entire retinal vascular bed, including retinal circulation
- May be used in conjunction with a photographic technique called indocyanine green—or ICG—angiography in certain diseases to obtain further information

Purpose

- To document retinal circulation and the layers beneath the retina
- To aid in evaluating intraocular abnormalities, such as retinopathy, tumors, or inflammatory disorders

Patient preparation

- Make sure that the patient has signed an appropriate consent form.
- Note and report all allergies.
- Check the patient's history for glaucoma.
- Don't administer miotic eyedrops on the day of the test.
- Warn the patient that he may experience a strobe-light effect during the test.

TEACHING POINTS

Be sure to cover:
- the purpose of the study and how it's done
- who will perform the test and where
- that the test takes about 30 minutes.
- that the study is fairly painless and adverse effects are uncommon but may include nausea and mild urticaria
- that skin and urine may appear yellow for 24 to 48 hours.

▶ PROCEDURE

- Mydriatic eyedrops are administered.
- The patient is positioned in an examination chair facing the camera with his chin on the chin rest and his forehead against the bar.
- He opens his eyes as widely as possible and stares straight ahead.
- Contrast medium is injected rapidly into the antecubital vein.
- 25 to 30 photographs are taken in rapid sequence (1 second apart).
- Photographs may be taken up to 1 hour after the injection.

Postprocedure care

- Encourage oral fluid intake to help excrete the dye.
- Caution the patient that near vision will be blurred for up to 12 hours.
- Instruct the patient to avoid direct sunlight and driving during blurred vision.
- Instruct the patient that his skin and urine will be slightly discolored for 24 to 48 hours after the test.

MONITORING

- Vision
- Allergic response

Precautions

- Serious adverse effects (laryngeal edema, bronchospasm, and respiratory arrest) are possible. Have emergency resuscitation equipment at hand.
- Extravasation of the dye is painful and toxic to the tissues.

Complications

- Extravasation of contrast agent
- Laryngeal edema
- Bronchospasm
- Respiratory arrest

✛ INTERPRETATION

Normal findings

- After rapid injection, sodium fluorescein reaches the retina in 12 to 15 seconds (filling phase).
- The retinal background appears evenly mottled (choroidal flush) during choroidal vessel and choriocapillary filling.
- The contrast fills the arteries (arterial phase).
- No leakage of contrast from retinal vessels is visible.

Abnormal results

- Abnormalities in the early filling phase suggest possible microaneurysms, arteriovenous shunts, and neovascularization.
- Delayed or absent flow of the dye through the arteries may indicate arterial stenosis or occlusion.
- Dilation of the vessels and fluorescein leakage may suggest venous occlusion.
- Recanalization and collateral circulation suggests chronic obstruction.
- Increased vascular tortuosity suggests hypertensive retinopathy.
- Leaking of fluorescence, surrounded by hard, yellow exudate, suggest possible aneurysms and capillary hemangiomas.
- Vascular leakage in the disk area suggests papilledema.

Fluoroscopy, thoracic

● OVERVIEW

- Provides visualization of physiologic or pathologic structural motion of thoracic contents
- Dynamic shadows of the heart, lungs, and diaphragm on a fluorescent screen created by a continuous stream of X-rays passing through the patient

Purpose

- To assess lung expansion and contraction
- To assess movement of the diaphragm and chest wall
- To assist with placement of tubes or catheters such as a pulmonary artery catheter

Patient preparation

- Make sure that the patient has signed an appropriate consent form.
- Note and report all allergies.
- Advise the patient that he will be asked to breathe deeply and cough during imaging.
- Explain the need to remove all metallic objects (including jewelry) in the X-ray field.
- Explain the need to wear a lead apron to protect gonads.

TEACHING POINTS

Be sure to cover:
- the purpose of the study and how it's done
- who will perform the test and where
- that the test usually takes 5 minutes.

▶ PROCEDURE

- The patient is placed in a supine position on the fluoroscopy table or upright to best visualize diaphragmatic motion.
- Equipment may be used to intensify the images or a videotape recording may be made for later study.

Postprocedure care

- No specific posttest care is necessary.

Precautions

- Thoracic fluoroscopy is contraindicated during pregnancy.
- Check that no tubes have been dislodged during positioning.
- If you must stay in the area, wear a lead-lined apron.

Complications

- Inadvertent dislodgement of patient lines or tubes

✛ INTERPRETATION

Normal findings

- Diaphragmatic movement is synchronous and symmetrical.
- Diaphragmatic excursion ranges from 5 to 6 cm.

Abnormal results

- Diminished diaphragmatic movement may indicate pulmonary disease or phrenic nerve injury.
- Increased lung translucency may indicate loss of elasticity or bronchiolar obstruction.
- Diminished or paradoxical diaphragmatic movement may indicate phrenic paralysis.

Gallium scanning

- Total body scan that's usually performed 24 to 72 hours after I.V. injection of radioactive gallium GA 67 citrate
- With acute inflammatory conditions, scan possibly performed within 4 to 6 hours of injection

Purpose

- To detect primary or metastatic neoplasms
- To detect inflammatory lesions, abscesses, or infections
- To evaluate malignant lymphoma
- To identify recurrent tumors
- To clarify focal defects in the liver when scanning and ultrasonography are inconclusive
- To evaluate bronchogenic carcinoma
- To screen for cause of "fever of unknown origin"

Patient preparation

- Make sure that the patient has signed an appropriate consent form.
- Note and report all allergies.
- The patient need not restrict food or fluids.
- Administer a laxative or cleansing enema (or both) as ordered.

TEACHING POINTS

Be sure to cover:

- the purpose of the study and how it's done
- who will perform the test and where
- that the test takes 30 to 60 minutes
- that radiation exposure is minimal.

- Various patient positions may be used depending on the condition.
- Scans or scintigraphs are taken from various views 24, 48, and 72 hours after injection of gallium.
- If bowel disease is suggested and additional scans are necessary, a cleansing enema may be administered.

Postprocedure care

- Resume previous activity as ordered.

MONITORING

- None necessary

Precautions

- Gallium scanning is contraindicated in children and in pregnant or breast-feeding women unless benefit outweighs the risks.
- Hepatic and splenic uptake may obscure the detection of abnormal para-aortic nodes in Hodgkin's disease, causing false-negative scans.
- Barium studies within 1 week before this scan can interfere with visualization of gallium activity in the bowel.
- Other isotope studies may be postponed for up to 7 days after gallium scan due to slow elimination of gallium.
- Previous treatment with antibiotics or high doses of steroids may decrease the inflammatory response and result in false negative gallium imaging.

Complications

- Infection at injection site

Normal findings

- Gallium activity is normally demonstrated in the liver, spleen, bones, and large bowel.

Abnormal results

- Abnormally high activity suggests inflammatory bowel disease and colon cancer.
- Abnormal activity in one or more lymph nodes or in extranodal locations suggest possible Hodgkin's disease and non-Hodgkin's lymphoma.
- Localization of gallium suggests possible hepatoma, abscess, or tumor.

Gastric acid stimulation

● OVERVIEW

- Used to measure secretion of gastric acid for 1 hour after subcutaneous injection of pentagastrin or a similar drug that stimulates gastric acid output
- Usually performed immediately after a basal secretion test suggests abnormal gastric secretion

Purpose

- To aid diagnosis of duodenal ulcer, Zollinger-Ellison syndrome, pernicious anemia, and gastric carcinoma

Patient preparation

- Make sure that the patient has signed an appropriate consent form.
- Note and report all allergies.
- Check the patient's history for hypersensitivity to pentagastrin.
- Withhold antacids, anticholinergics, beta-adrenergic blockers, histamine-2 receptor antagonists, corticosteroids, proton pump inhibitors, and reserpine before the test as ordered.
- Instruct the patient to refrain from eating, drinking, and smoking after midnight before the test.
- Tell the patient to report adverse effects (abdominal pain, nausea, vomiting, flushing, transitory dizziness, faintness, and numbness of the extremities) immediately.

TEACHING POINTS

Be sure to cover:
- the purpose of the study and how it's done
- who will perform the test and where
- that the test takes 1 hour.

▶ PROCEDURE

- A nasogastric (NG) tube is inserted.
- Basal gastric secretions are collected using the NG tube.
- Pentagastrin is injected subcutaneously.
- After 15 minutes a specimen is collected every 15 minutes for 1 hour.
- The color, odor, and presence of food, mucus, bile, or blood in specimens is noted and recorded.
- All specimens are labeled "Stimulated contents," and numbered 1 through 4.
- Specimens are sent to the laboratory immediately.

Postprocedure care

- If the NG tube is to be left in place, clamp it or attach it to low intermittent suction, as ordered.
- Watch for and report nausea, vomiting, abdominal distention or pain after removal of the NG tube.
- For a sore throat, provide soothing lozenges.
- Diet and medications may be resumed as ordered.

MONITORING

- Abdominal distention
- NG patency and function, if appropriate
- Pain

Precautions

- Gastric acid stimulation is contraindicated in hypersensitivity to pentagastrin.
- Gastric acid stimulation is contraindicated in conditions that prohibit NG intubation.
- Observe for adverse effects of pentagastrin.
- Prevent contamination of specimens with saliva.

Complications

- Adverse effects of pentagastrin

✛ INTERPRETATION

Normal findings

- Gastric secretion following stimulation ranges from 18 to 28 mEq/hour for males and from 11 to 21 mEq/hour for females.

Abnormal results

- Elevated gastric secretion may indicate duodenal ulcer.
- Markedly elevated secretion suggests Zollinger-Ellison syndrome.
- Depressed secretion may indicate gastric carcinoma.
- Achlorhydria may indicate pernicious anemia.

Holter monitoring

- Continuous recording of heart activity as the patient follows his normal routine, usually for 24 hours
- Patient-activated monitor: worn for 5 to 7 days, allows patient to manually initiate recording of heart activity when symptoms are experienced
- Also known as *ambulatory electrocardiogram (ECG)* or *dynamic monitoring*

Purpose
- To detect cardiac arrhythmias
- To evaluate chest pain
- To evaluate effectiveness of antiarrhythmic drug therapy
- To monitor pacemaker function
- To correlate symptoms and palpitations with actual cardiac events and patient activities
- To detect sporadic arrhythmias missed by an exercise or resting ECG

Patient preparation
- Make sure that the patient has signed an appropriate consent form.
- Note and report all allergies.
- Provide bathing instructions because some equipment must not get wet.
- Instruct the patient to avoid magnets, metal detectors, high-voltage areas, and electric blankets.

TEACHING POINTS
Be sure to cover:
- the purpose of the study and how it's done
- routine activities during the monitoring period
- the importance of logging activities as well as emotional upsets, physical symptoms, and ingestion of medication, in a diary
- how to mark the tape at the onset of symptoms if applicable
- how to check the recorder to make sure it's working properly.

- Electrodes are applied to the chest wall and attached securely to the lead-wires and monitor.
- A new or fully charged battery is inserted in the recorder.
- A tape is inserted and the recorder turned on.
- The electrode attachment circuit is tested by connecting the recorder to a standard ECG machine, noting artifact during normal patient movement.

Postprocedure care
- Remove all chest electrodes.
- Clean the electrode sites.

MONITORING
- None necessary

Precautions
- Avoid placing electrodes over large muscles masses, such as the pectorals, to limit artifact.

Complications
- Skin sensitivity to the electrodes

Normal findings
- The ECG shows no significant arrhythmias or ST-segment changes.
- Changes in heart rate occur during various activities.

Abnormal results
- Abnormalities in cardiac rate or rhythm suggest possible serious arrhythmias, which may be symptomatic or asymptomatic.
- ST-T wave changes may coincide with patient symptoms or increased patient activity, and suggest possible myocardial ischemia.

Hypersensitivity skin tests, delayed

● OVERVIEW

- Evaluates the cell-mediated immune response
- Assesses status of a patient's immune system in severe infection, cancer, pre-transplantation, and malnutrition
- Previous exposure to antigen and intact immune system required for accurate response
- Most commonly used recall antigen: *Mycobacterium tuberculosis* (purified protein derivative Mantoux test)
- Other antigens: *Candida, Trichophyton*, and mumps (antigens previously used for delayed-type hypersensitivity testing, such as fungi and streptococci, no longer available or recommended)
- Involves applying antigenic material to the skin; helps confirm allergic contact sensitization and isolates the causative agent

✺ AGE-RELATED CONCERN Hypersensitivity skin testing has only limited value in infants because their immune systems are immature and inadequately sensitized.

Purpose
- To evaluate primary and secondary immune responses
- To diagnose fungal, bacterial, and viral diseases
- To monitor the course of certain diseases (Hodgkin's disease)

Patient preparation
- Make sure that the patient has signed an appropriate consent form.
- Note and report all allergies.
- Check history for hypersensitivity to any of the test antigens.
- Check for history of tuberculosis or previous bacille Calmette-Guérin vaccination.
- Restriction of food or fluids before the test isn't necessary.

TEACHING POINTS
Be sure to cover:
- the purpose of the study and how it's done
- who will perform the test and where
- that the test takes about 10 minutes for each antigen to be administered and reactions appear in 48 to 72 hours

- that some antigens are administered again after 2 weeks and, if negative, a stronger dose of antigen may be given.

▶ PROCEDURE

- Wash your hands thoroughly.
- Maintain asepsis throughout the procedure.
- Wear personal protective equipment.
- Inject each antigen being tested intradermally, using a separate tuberculin syringe, on the patient's forearm.
- Inject control allergy diluent on the other forearm.
- Circle each injection site with a skin marker and label each according to the antigen given.
- Instruct to avoid washing off the circles until the test is completed.
- Inspect sites for reactivity after 48 and 72 hours.

Postprocedure care
- Record induration and erythema in millimeters.
- Administer corticosteroids as ordered.

◈ NURSING ALERT Watch closely for severe local reactions that may occur at the test site, such as pain, blistering, swelling, induration, itching, and ulceration. Scarring or hyperpigmentation may also result.

- A negative test at the first concentration of antigen should be confirmed using a higher concentration.
- Tell the patient experiencing hypersensitivity that corticosteroids will control the reaction but that skin lesions may persist for 10 to 14 days.
- Tell the patient to avoid scratching.

MONITORING
- Vital signs
- Induration and erythema
- Severe local reactions

◈ NURSING ALERT Watch for swelling and tenderness in lymph nodes at elbow or axillary region. Check for tachycardia and fever, although these rarely occur. Symptoms typically appear in 15 to 30 minutes.

Precautions
- Store antigens in lyophilized (freeze-dried) form at 39.2° F (4° C), protected from light.

- Reconstitute antigens shortly before use; check expiration dates.
- If the patient is suspected of being hypersensitive to the antigens, apply them first in low concentrations.
- If the forearms aren't free from disease use other sites such as the back.

Complications
- Severe local and systemic reactions

◈ NURSING ALERT Anaphylactic shock may occur with respiratory distress and hypotension. Administer epinephrine and notify the physician immediately.

✧ INTERPRETATION

Normal findings
- A positive response (5 mm or more of induration) appears 48 hours after injection.

Abnormal results
- In the recall antigen test, diminished delayed hypersensitivity may be indicated by a positive response to less than two of the six test antigens, persistent unresponsiveness to intradermal injection of higher-strength antigens, or a generalized diminished reaction (causing less than 10 mm combined induration).

Hysterosalpingography

● OVERVIEW

- Radiologic examination that visualizes the uterine cavity, fallopian tubes, and peritubal area
- Fluoroscopic radiographs: obtained as contrast medium flows through the uterus and the fallopian tubes
- Performed as part of an infertility study

Purpose
- To confirm tubal abnormalities such as adhesions
- To confirm uterine abnormalities such as congenital malformations
- To confirm the presence of fistulas or peritubal adhesions
- To evaluate the cause of repeated miscarriage or infertility

Patient preparation
- Make sure that the patient has signed an appropriate consent form.
- Note and report all allergies, including iodinated contrast media.
- Check the patient's history for recent pelvic infection and ensure patient is not pregnant.
- A test for pelvic infections may be ordered before the study.
- Antibiotics may be prescribed before the test.
- The procedure should take place 2 to 5 days after menstruation ends.
- Warn the patient that he might experience moderate cramping.
- Tell patient she may be asked to restrict oral intake for 4 to 6 hours before the test.
- Explain that she may receive a mild sedative or a nonprescription prostaglandin inhibitor, if ordered, 30 minutes before the procedure.

TEACHING POINTS
Be sure to cover:
- the purpose of the study and how it's done
- who will perform the test and where
- that the test takes about 15 minutes
- that a small amount of vaginal bleeding and pelvic cramping is normal for a few days after the study.

▶ PROCEDURE

- The patient is placed in the lithotomy position and a scout film is taken.
- A bimanual examination is done to determine uterine size and position.
- A speculum is inserted in the vagina and the vagina and cervix are cleaned.
- A cannula is inserted into the cervix and anchored to a tenaculum.
- Contrast medium is injected through the cannula.
- Uterus and the fallopian tubes are viewed fluoroscopically and radiographs are taken.
- The table may be tilted or the patient asked to change position, for oblique views.
- Films may be taken later to evaluate spillage of contrast medium into the peritoneal cavity.

Postprocedure care
- Instruct the patient to return to pretest activities gradually.
- Tell the patient that additional tests and studies may be required to establish a precise diagnosis.

MONITORING
- Vital signs
- Signs and symptoms of infection and uterine perforation
- Bleeding
- Adverse reaction to the contrast medium

Precautions
- Hysterosalpingography contraindicated in:
  - menstruation
  - undiagnosed vaginal bleeding
  - pelvic inflammatory disease
  - pregnancy

Complications
- Uterine perforation
- Infection
- Bleeding
- Adverse reaction to contrast media

✛ INTERPRETATION

Normal findings
- The uterine cavity is symmetrical.
- The fallopian tubes are a normal caliber.
- Contrast spills freely into the peritoneal cavity.
- Contrast doesn't leak from the uterus.

Abnormal results
- Asymmetrical uterus suggests intrauterine adhesions or masses.
- Impaired contrast flow through the fallopian tubes suggests partial or complete blockage.
- Leakage of contrast medium through the uterine wall suggests fistulas.

Hysteroscopy

- Involves use of small-diameter endoscope to visualize interior of the uterus
- Usually performed as an office procedure using a local anesthetic or mild sedation during the first week after the end of the patient's menstrual cycle

Purpose
- To investigate abnormal uterine bleeding
- To remove polyps
- To evaluate infertile patients
- To direct removal of intrauterine devices
- To aid in diagnosis and treatment of intrauterine adhesions
- To diagnose uterine fibroids

Patient preparation
- Make sure that the patient has signed an appropriate consent form.
- Note and report all allergies.
- Check the patient's history for hypersensitivity to the anesthetic.
- Obtain the results of the last Papanicolaou test.
- Food and fluids may be restricted before the test.
- The physician will perform a complete pelvic examination.
- Cultures of the vagina and cervix may be taken.
- Instruct the patient to empty her bladder before the test.
- Warn the patient that the physician may inflate her uterus with carbon dioxide (CO_2), which will be absorbed and may cause upper abdominal or shoulder pain lasting 24 to 36 hours after the test.

TEACHING POINTS
Be sure to cover:
- that some vaginal bleeding and mild abdominal cramping occur after the test
- a recommendation that a friend or relative drive her home.

- The patient is placed in a modified dorsal lithotomy position with her legs in stirrups.
- A local anesthetic is administered.
- The vagina is cleaned and the hysteroscope is inserted.
- Visualization begins at the level of the internal os.
- In contact hysteroscopy, the uterus isn't distended; only the area in direct contact with the hysteroscope can be viewed.
- In panoramic hysteroscopy, an external illumination source and media (such as CO_2) for distention are used; allows visualization of the tissue from a distance.
- Cultures of vagina and cervix may be done.

Postprocedure care
- Provide a sanitary pad if needed.
- Provide analgesics as needed.

MONITORING
- Vital signs
- Bleeding
- Adverse reaction to medications
- Signs and symptoms of infection

Precautions
- Severe cramps, dyspnea, upper abdominal and right shoulder pain can develop if CO_2 passes into the peritoneal cavity.
- Heavy bleeding or a distended bladder may interfere with visualization.

Complications
- Bleeding
- Adverse reaction to medications
- Infection
- Perforation of uterus

Normal findings
- The interior of the uterus is normal in size and shape and free from adhesions and lesions.

Abnormal results
- Uterine anatomical abnormalities suggest possible polyps, uterine wall tumors, and adhesions.

Impedance plethysmography

● OVERVIEW

- Reliable noninvasive test for measuring venous flow in the limbs
- Also known as *occlusive impedance phlebography*
- Records changes in electrical resistance (impedance) caused by blood volume variations (the result of normal respiration or venous occlusion)

Purpose
- To detect deep vein thrombosis in the proximal deep veins of the leg
- To screen patients at high risk for thrombophlebitis
- To evaluate patients with suspected pulmonary embolism

Patient preparation
- Make sure that the patient has signed an appropriate consent form.
- Note and report all allergies.
- Inform the patient that both legs will be tested.
- The patient need not restrict food, fluids, or medications before the test.
- A mild analgesic may be ordered.
- Instruct patient to void just before the test.
- Emphasize that accurate testing requires leg muscles to be relaxed and breathing to be normal.

TEACHING POINTS
Be sure to cover:
- the purpose of the study and how it's done
- who will perform the test and where
- that the test takes 30 to 45 minutes
- that test is painless and safe.

▶ PROCEDURE

- The patient is placed in a supine position with the tested leg elevated 30 to 35 degrees with calf above heart level.
- Electrodes from a plethysmograph are applied to the patient's leg.
- A pressure cuff is wrapped snugly around the thigh about 2″ (5 cm) above the knee.
- The pressure cuff is inflated with 45 to 60 cm of water and maintained for 45 seconds until tracing stabilizes.
- The cuff pressure is rapidly deflated.
- The test is repeated for the other leg.
- Three to five tracings for each leg may be obtained.

Postprocedure care
- Remove the conductive jelly from the patient's skin.

MONITORING
- None necessary

Precautions
- Decreased peripheral arterial blood flow may interfere with test results.
- Extrinsic venous compression may alter test results.
- Cold extremities can alter test results.

Complications
- None known

✛ INTERPRETATION

Normal findings
- Temporary venous occlusion normally produces a sharp rise in venous volume.
- Release of the occlusion produces rapid venous outflow.

Abnormal results
- When clots in a major deep vein obstruct venous outflow, calf vein pressure rises; these veins become distended and can't expand futher when more pressure is applied with an occlusive thigh cuff.
- Blockage of major deep veins also decreases the rate at which blood flows from the leg.
- If significant thrombi are present in major deep vein of the lower leg (such as the popliteal, femoral or iliac vein), calf vein filling and venous outflow rates are reduced. The physician will evaluate the need for further treatment, such as anticoagulant therapy, taking the patient's overall condition into consideration.

Kidney-ureter-bladder radiography

● OVERVIEW

- Used to survey the abdomen without requiring intact renal function
- Also known as a *flat plate of the abdomen* or *KUB radiography*

Purpose

- To evaluate the size, structure, and position of the kidneys and bladder
- To screen for abnormalities, such as calcifications, in the region of the kidneys, ureters, and bladder

Patient preparation

- Make sure that the patient has signed an appropriate consent form.
- Note and report all allergies.
- Restriction of food or fluids isn't necessary.

TEACHING POINTS

Be sure to cover:
- the purpose of the study and how it's done
- who will perform the test and where
- that the test only takes a few minutes.

▶ PROCEDURE

- The patient is placed in a supine position on an X-ray table. (See *Positioning the patient for KUB radiography.*)
- Symmetrical positioning of the iliac crests is noted.
- A single radiograph is taken.

Postprocedure care

- No specific posttest care is necessary.

Precautions

- The procedure shouldn't follow recent instillation of barium, which obscures the urinary system.
- A male patient should have gonadal shielding.
- A female patient's ovaries can't be shielded because they're too close to the kidneys, ureters, and bladder.

Complications

- None known

✛ INTERPRETATION

Normal findings

- Kidney shadows appear bilaterally, the right slightly lower than the left.
- Both kidneys should be approximately the same size, with the superior poles tilted slightly toward the vertebral column, paralleling the shadows of the psoas muscles.
- The bladder's shadow isn't as clearly visible as the kidneys' shadows.

Abnormal results

- Bilateral renal enlargement suggests possible polycystic kidney disease, multiple myeloma, lymphoma, amyloidosis, hydronephrosis, or compensatory renal hypertrophy.
- Unilateral renal enlargement suggests possible a tumor, cyst, or hydronephrosis.
- Abnormally small kidneys suggests possible end-stage glomerulonephritis or bilateral atrophic pyelonephritis.
- An apparent decrease in the size of one kidney suggests possible congenital hypoplasia, atrophic pyelonephritis, or ischemia.
- Renal displacement may be caused by a retroperitoneal tumor.
- Obliteration or bulging of a portion of the psoas muscle stripe suggest possible tumor, abscess, or hematoma.
- Abnormal location or absence of a kidney suggest possible congenital anomalies.
- A lobulated edge or border suggest possible polycystic kidney disease or patchy atrophic pyelonephritis.
- Opaque bodies suggest possible calculi, vascular calcification, cystic tumors, fecaliths, foreign bodies, soft tissue mass, or abnormal fluid or gas collection.

POSITIONING THE PATIENT FOR KUB RADIOGRAPHY

For kidney-ureter-bladder (KUB) radiography, the patient is instructed to lie in a supine position with his arms extended over his head. To prevent motion and ensure films of good quality, he is asked to lie still for the few seconds it takes to make the exposure. An obese patient may be asked to exhale and then hold his breath during the brief procedure. As an added precaution, the gonads of male patients should be shielded.

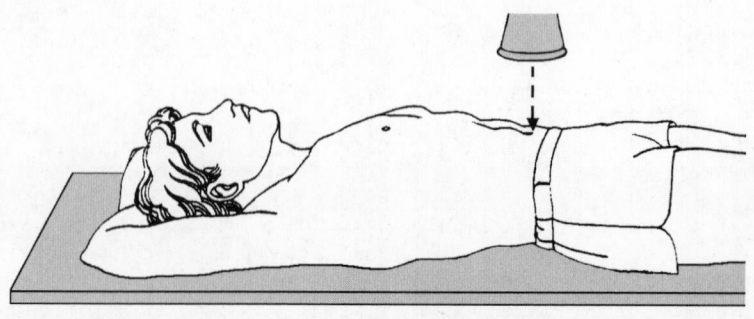

Laparoscopy, peritoneal cavity

● OVERVIEW

- Permits visualization of the peritoneal cavity through a small fiber-optic telescope (laparoscope) inserted through the anterior abdominal wall
- Requires only a small incision; results in less cost and faster recovery
- Allows many concurrent types of abdominal surgery, such as tubal ligation and cholecystectomy

Purpose

- To identify the cause of pelvic pain
- To detect endometriosis, ectopic pregnancy, or pelvic inflammatory disease (PID)
- To remove ectopic pregnancy, uterine fibroids, or adhesions
- To fulgurate endometrial implants
- To evaluate pelvic masses
- To evaluate infertility
- To stage carcinoma

Patient preparation

- Make sure that the patient has signed an appropriate consent form.
- Note and report all allergies.
- Check the patient's history for hypersensitivity to the anesthetic.
- Inform the physician if the patient takes aspirin, nonsteroidal anti-inflammatory drugs, or other drugs which affect clotting.
- Fasting is required after midnight before the test or for at least 8 hours before surgery.
- Explain the use of a local or general anesthetic.
- Warn the patient that she may experience pain at the puncture site and in the shoulder.
- Instruct the patient to empty her bladder just before the test.

TEACHING POINTS
Be sure to cover:
- the purpose of the study and how it's done
- who will perform the procedure and where
- that the test takes 15 to 30 minutes.

▶ PROCEDURE

- The patient is anesthetized and placed in lithotomy position.
- The bladder may be catheterized.
- A bimanual examination of the pelvic area may be performed to detect abnormalities.
- An incision is made at the inferior rim of the umbilicus.
- The peritoneal cavity is insufflated with carbon dioxide or nitrous oxide.
- A laparoscope is inserted to examine the pelvis and abdomen.
- A second incision may be made just above the pubic hair line for some procedures.
- After the examination, minor surgical procedures, such as ovarian biopsy, may be performed.

Postprocedure care

- Resume usual diet as ordered.
- Instruct the patient to restrict activity for 2 to 7 days as ordered.
- Explain that abdominal and shoulder pain should disappear within 24 to 36 hours.
- Provide analgesics as ordered.

MONITORING
- Vital signs
- Adverse reactions to medications
- Intake and output
- Bleeding
- Infection

Precautions

- Laparoscopy of peritoneal cavity is contraindicated with:
  - advanced abdominal wall cancer
  - advanced respiratory or cardiovascular disease
  - intestinal obstruction
  - palpable abdominal mass
  - large abdominal hernia
  - history of peritonitis
  - chronic tuberculosis.

Complications

- Punctured visceral organ
- Peritonitis

✛ INTERPRETATION

Normal findings

- The uterus and fallopian tubes are a normal size and shape, free from adhesions, and mobile.
- The ovaries are a normal size and shape.
- There are no cysts or endometriosis.

Abnormal results

- A bubble on the surface of the ovary suggests possible ovarian cyst.
- Sheets or strands of tissue suggests possible adhesions.
- Small, blue powder burns on the peritoneum or serosa suggests endometriosis.
- Growths on the uterus suggests fibroids.
- An enlarged fallopian tube suggests possible hydrosalpinx.
- Enlarged or ruptured fallopian tube suggests possible ectopic pregnancy.
- Infection or abscess suggests possible PID.

Laryngoscopy, direct

● OVERVIEW

- Visualization of the larynx using a fiber-optic endoscope, or laryngoscope, passed through the mouth or nose and pharynx to the larynx
- Usually follows indirect laryngoscopy, a more common procedure

Purpose
- To detect lesions, strictures, or foreign bodies in the larynx
- To aid diagnosis of laryngeal cancer or vocal cord impairment
- To remove benign lesions or foreign bodies from the larynx
- To examine the larynx when the view provided by indirect laryngoscopy is inadequate
- To evaluate symptoms of pharyngeal or laryngeal disease (stridor or hemoptysis)

Patient preparation
- Make sure that the patient has signed an appropriate consent form.
- Note and report all allergies.
- Check the patient's history for hypersensitivity to the anesthetic.
- Fasting is required for 6 to 8 hours before the test.
- Sedation is administered to help the patient relax. Dentures and contact lenses need to be removed before sedation is given.
- Medication is administered to reduce secretions.
- A general or local anesthetic is administered to numb the gag reflex.

TEACHING POINTS
Be sure to cover:
- the purpose of the study and how it's done
- who will perform test and where
- that the study takes about 30 minutes; longer if minor surgery is performed at the same time.

▶ PROCEDURE

- The patient is placed in a supine position.
- A general anesthetic is administered, or the mouth or nose and throat are sprayed with local anesthetic
- The laryngoscope is inserted through the mouth.
- The larynx is examined for abnormalities.
- Specimens may be collected for further study.
- Minor surgery (polyp removal) may be performed at this time.

Postprocedure care
- Place the patient on his side with his head slightly elevated to prevent aspiration.
- Restrict food and fluids until the gag reflex returns (usually 2 hours).
- Reassure the patient that voice loss, hoarseness, and sore throat are most likely temporary.
- Provide throat lozenges or a soothing liquid gargle after gag reflex returns.
- Immediately report any adverse reaction to the anesthetic or sedative.
- Apply an ice collar to prevent or minimize laryngeal edema.
- Observe sputum for blood and notify the physician immediately if excessive bleeding or respiratory compromise occurs.
- After biopsy, instruct the patient to refrain from clearing the throat and coughing, and to avoid smoking as ordered.

NURSING ALERT Immediately report subcutaneous crepitus around the patient's face and neck—a sign of tracheal perforation.

NURSING ALERT Observe the patient with epiglottitis for signs of airway obstruction. Immediately report signs of respiratory difficulty, such as laryngeal stridor or dyspnea. Keep emergency resuscitation equipment and a tracheotomy tray readily available for 24 hours.

MONITORING
- Vital signs
- Respiratory status
- Voice quality
- Adverse reaction to medications

- Edema
- Sputum
- Subcutaneous emphysema
- Bleeding

Precautions
- Direct laryngoscopy is contraindicated in patients with epiglottiditis unless performed in the operating room with resuscitative equipment immediately available.

Complications
- Tracheal perforation
- Adverse reaction to medications
- Airway obstruction
- Bleeding

✛ INTERPRETATION

Normal findings
- There's no evidence of inflammation, lesions, strictures, or foreign bodies.

Abnormal results
- Combined with results of biopsy, abnormal lesions suggests possible laryngeal cancer or benign lesions.
- Narrowing suggests stricture.
- Inflammation suggests possible laryngeal edema secondary to radiation or tumor.
- Asynchronous vocal cords suggests possible vocal cord dysfunction.

Liver biopsy, percutaneous

● OVERVIEW

- Needle aspiration of a core of liver tissue for histologic analysis
- Generally performed under local anesthesia with image-guidance

Purpose

- To diagnose hepatic parenchymal disease
- To diagnose malignant tumors and granulomatous infections

Patient preparation

- Make sure that the patient has signed an appropriate consent form.
- Note and report all allergies.
- Check the patient's history for hypersensitivity to the local anesthetic.
- Report any abnormal coagulation study results to the physician.
- Ensure that all aspirin products, nonsteroidal anti-inflammatory drugs, antiplatelets such as clopidogrel (Plavix), and anticoagulants were discontinued at least 5 days before the study.
- Food and fluids are restricted for 4 to 8 hours before the test.
- Warn the patient that right shoulder pain may be experienced.

TEACHING POINTS

Be sure to cover:

- the purpose of the study and how it's done
- who will perform the biopsy and where
- that the test takes about 10 to 15 minutes.

▶ PROCEDURE

- The patient is placed in a supine position with his right hand under his head.
- The biopsy site is selected and local anesthetic is injected.
- The patient takes a deep breath, exhales, then holds his breath at the end of expiration.
- The biopsy needle is quickly inserted into the liver and withdrawn in 1 second during breath holding. (See *Using a Menghini needle.*)
- After the needle is withdrawn, the patient resumes normal respirations.
- The tissue specimen is then placed in a properly labeled specimen cup.

Postprocedure care

- Apply direct pressure to the biopsy site to stop bleeding.
- Maintain bed rest as ordered.
- Administer analgesia as ordered.
- Resume normal diet as ordered.

MONITORING

- Vital signs
- Bleeding
- Respiratory distress

NURSING ALERT Watch for and immediately report bleeding or signs and symptoms of bile peritonitis (tenderness and rigidity around the biopsy site).

NURSING ALERT Watch for symptoms of pneumothorax (tachypnea, decreased breath sounds, dyspnea, persistent shoulder pain, pleuritic chest pain).

Precautions

- Extrahepatic obstruction should be ruled out before biopsy.
- Abdominal pain or dyspnea after the biopsy may indicate perforation of an abdominal organ or pneumothorax.
- Percutaneous liver biopsy is contraindicated in uncorrected coagulopathies, severe anemia, vascular tumor, hepatic angioma, hydatid cyst, tense ascites, and empyema of the lungs, pleurae, peritoneum, biliary tract, or liver.

Complications

- Perforation of an abdominal organ
- Pneumothorax
- Peritonitis
- Bleeding
- Infection

⬥ INTERPRETATION

Normal findings

- A reticulin framework supports sheets of hepatocytes.

Abnormal results

- Diffuse hepatic disease suggests possible cirrhosis or hepatitis.
- Granulomatous infections suggests possible tuberculosis.
- Primary malignant tumors suggests possible hepatocellular carcinoma, cholangiocellular carcinoma, and angiosarcoma.

USING A MENGHINI NEEDLE

In percutaneous liver biopsy, a Menghini needle attached to a 5-ml syringe containing normal saline solution is introduced through the chest wall and intercostal space. First, negative pressure is created in the syringe. Then the needle is pushed rapidly into the liver and, finally, pulled out of the body entirely to obtain a tissue specimen.

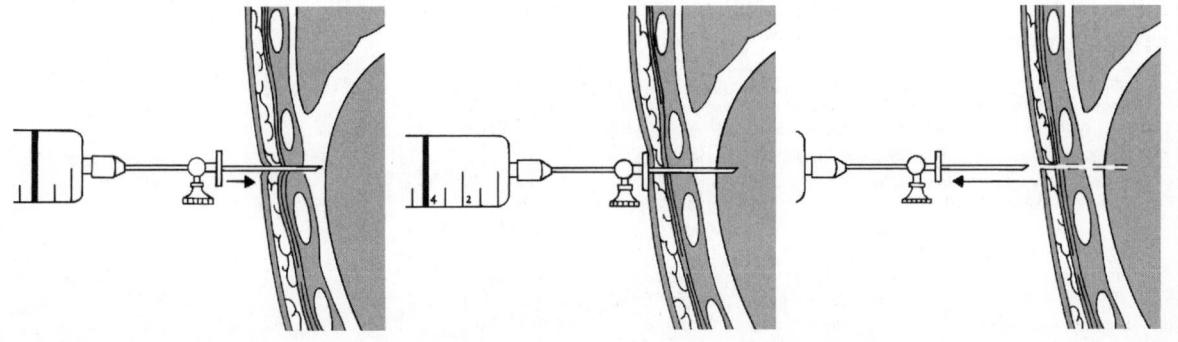

Liver-spleen scan

● OVERVIEW

- Distribution of radioactivity within the liver and spleen, recorded by a gamma camera after I.V. injection of a radioactive colloid, technetium-99m (^{99m}Tc)
- Demonstrates focal disease nonspecifically as a cold spot (a defect that fails to take up the colloid)
- In conjunction with flow studies, may help to distinguish between metastases, tumors, cysts, and abscesses (see *Flow studies*)

Purpose

- To screen for hepatic metastases and hepatocellular disease
- To detect focal disease (tumors, cysts, abscesses)
- To demonstrate hepatomegaly, splenomegaly, and splenic infarcts
- To assess condition of liver and spleen after abdominal trauma

Patient preparation

- Make sure that the patient has signed an appropriate consent form.
- Note and report all allergies.
- There's no need to restrict food or fluids before the test.
- Stress the importance of lying still during the study.

TEACHING POINTS

Be sure to cover:
- the purpose of the study and how it's done
- who will perform the test and where
- that the test takes about 1 hour
- that the procedure involves only trace amounts of radioactivity, and adverse reactions are rare.

▶ PROCEDURE

- ^{99m}Tc is injected I.V.
- After 10 to 15 minutes the abdomen is scanned using various views.
- Scintigraphs are reviewed for clarity.
- Additional views are obtained as needed.

Postprocedure care

◆ **NURSING ALERT** Watch for anaphylactoid or pyrogenic reactions that may result from a stabilizer, such as dextran or gelatin, added to ^{99m}Tc.
- Encourage oral fluid intake (unless contraindicated) to assist elimination of the radioactive material.
- Instruct the patient to flush the toilet immediately after urinating.

MONITORING
- Vital signs
- Intake and output
- Respiratory status

Precautions

✺ **AGE-RELATED CONCERN** The procedure is contraindicated in children and pregnant or breast-feeding women.
- Scanning may fail to reveal focal lesions smaller than 2 cm in diameter.
- Scanning may fail to disclose early hepatocellular disease.
- More than one radionuclide scan shouldn't be scheduled for the same day.

Complications

- Anaphylactoid reactions
- Pyrogenic reactions

✛ INTERPRETATION

Normal findings

- The liver and spleen appear equally bright on images.
- The distribution of radioactive colloid is generally more homogeneous in the spleen than in the liver.

Abnormal results

- A uniformly decreased or patchy appearance suggests hepatocellular disease.
- Uniformly decreased distribution of the colloid suggests possible hepatitis.
- Failure to take up the radioactive colloid and the appearance of solitary or multiple focal defects suggests cysts, abscesses, and tumors.
- Lentiform defects on the periphery of the liver suggests possible subcapsular hematoma.
- Linear defects suggests possible hepatic laceration.
- Focal defects in or next to the spleen, which may transect it, suggests possible splenic hematoma.

FLOW STUDIES

In contrast to liver-spleen scanning, which provides static nuclear images, flow studies (dynamic scintigraphy) record in rapid sequence the stages of perfusion after I.V. injection of a radionuclide such as technetium sulfide-99m. Because flow studies demonstrate the vascularity of a nonspecific focal defect, they sometimes help distinguish among metastases, tumors, cysts, and abscesses.

In flow studies, a hot defect will show early increased uptake of the radionuclide when compared with the surrounding parenchyma, then will appear as a filling defect, or cold spot, on later routine images. Cysts and abscesses, which are avascular, fail to take up the radionuclide; hemangiomas appear characteristically hot because of their enlarged vessels.

Tumors and metastases are generally more difficult to evaluate because their vascularity is more variable. Although vascular metastases may appear hot, most metastases demonstrate poor uptake of the radionuclide. Hepatomas can also appear hot or can show perfusion similar to normal parenchyma.

Lumbar puncture

● OVERVIEW

- Permits sampling of cerebral spinal fluid (CSF) for qualitative analysis
- More common than cisternal or ventricular puncture
- Also known as a spinal tap

Purpose
- To measure CSF pressure
- To aid diagnosis of viral or bacterial meningitis
- To aid diagnosis of subarachnoid or intracranial hemorrhage
- To aid diagnosis of tumors and brain abscesses
- To aid diagnosis of neurosyphilis and chronic CNS infections

Patient preparation
- Make sure that the patient has signed an appropriate consent form.
- Note and report all allergies.
- Restriction of food and fluids isn't necessary.

TEACHING POINTS
Be sure to cover:
- the purpose of the study and how it's done
- who will perform the test and where
- that the test takes at least 15 minutes.
- that headache is the most common adverse effect.

▶ PROCEDURE

- Position the patient on his side at the edge of the bed with his knees drawn up to his abdomen and his chin tucked against his chest (the fetal position); or position the patient sitting while leaning over a bedside table.
- If the patient is in a supine position, provide pillows to support the spine on a horizontal plane.
- The skin site is prepared and draped.
- The local anesthetic is injected.
- The spinal needle is inserted in the midline between the spinous processes of the vertebrae (usually between the third and fourth lumbar vertebrae or between the fourth and fifth vertebrae).

- The stylet is removed from the needle; CSF will drip out of the needle if properly positioned.
- A stopcock and manometer are attached to the needle to measure the initial (opening) CSF pressure.
- Specimens are collected and placed in the appropriate containers.
- The needle is removed and a small sterile dressing applied.

◆ **NURSING ALERT** During the procedure, observe closely for signs of an adverse reaction (elevated pulse rate, pallor, or clammy skin).

Postprocedure care
- Keep the patient lying flat for 4 to 6 hours as ordered.
- Inform him that he can turn from side to side.
- Encourage and assist the patient to drink fluids.
- Administer analgesics as ordered.

MONITORING
- Vital signs
- Intake and output
- Neurologic status
- Puncture site for redness, swelling, and drainage
- Bleeding
- Infections
- Complaints of headache

Precautions
- Lumbar puncture is contraindicated in skin infections at the puncture site.

◆ **NURSING ALERT** In a patient with increased intracranial pressure (ICP), CSF should be removed with extreme caution because cerebellar herniation and medullary compression can result.

Complications
- Adverse reaction to the anesthetic
- Infection
- Meningitis
- Bleeding into the spinal canal
- Leakage of CSF
- Cerebellar herniation
- Medullary compression
- Spinal headache

✛ INTERPRETATION

Normal findings
- Pressure: 50 to 180 mm H_2O
- Appearance: clear, colorless
- Protein: 15 to 45 mg/dl (SI, 150 to 450 mg/L)
- Gamma globulin: 3% to 12% of total protein
- Glucose: 40 to 70 mg/dl (SI, 2.2 to 3.9 mmol/L)
- Cell count: 0 to 5 white blood cells (WBCs); no red blood cells (RBCs)
- Venereal Disease Research Laboratories (VDRL): nonreactive
- Chloride: 118 to 130 mEq/L (SI, 118 to 130 mmol/L)
- Gram stain: no organisms

Abnormal results
PRESSURE
- Increased ICP: tumor, hemorrhage, or edema caused by trauma
- Decreased ICP: spinal subarachnoid obstruction

APPEARANCE
- Cloudy: infection
- Xanthochromic or bloody: intracranial hemorrhage or spinal cord obstruction
- Brown, orange: increased protein levels or RBC breakdown

PROTEIN
- Increased: tumor, trauma, diabetes mellitus, or blood in CSF
- Decreased: rapid CSF production

GAMMA GLOBULIN
- Increased: demyelinating disease or Guillian-Barré syndrome

GLUCOSE
- Increased: hyperglycemia
- Decreased: hypoglycemia, infection, or meningitis

CELL COUNT
- Increased: meningitis, tumor, abscess, demyelinating disease
- RBCs: hemorrhage, traumatic tap

VDRL
- Positive: neurosyphilis

CHLORIDE
- Decreased: infected meninges

GRAM STAIN
- Gram-positive or gram-negative organisms: bacterial meningitis

Lung biopsy

● OVERVIEW

- Used to obtain a pulmonary tissue specimen for histologic examination
- Needle biopsy: performed when the lesion is readily accessible, originates in the lung parenchyma, or is affixed to the chest wall
- Transbronchial biopsy: removal of multiple tissue specimens through a fiber-optic bronchoscope; performed in diffuse infiltrative pulmonary disease, tumors, or when severe debilitation contraindicates open biopsy
- Open biopsy: appropriate for the study of a well-circumscribed lesion that may require resection

Purpose
- To confirm diagnosis of diffuse parenchymal pulmonary disease
- To confirm diagnosis of pulmonary lesions

Patient preparation
- Make sure that the patient has signed an appropriate consent form.
- Note and report all allergies.
- Obtain results of pre-study tests; report abnormal results to the physician.
- Check the patient's history for hypersensitivity to local anesthetic.
- Fasting is required after midnight before the procedure.
- Chest X-ray and blood studies will be performed before the biopsy.
- Administer a mild sedative as ordered 30 minutes before the biopsy.

TEACHING POINTS
Be sure to cover:
- the purpose of the study and how it's done
- who will perform the biopsy and where
- that the test takes 30 to 60 minutes.

▶ PROCEDURE

- The procedure depends on the type of approach: percutaneous, transbronchial, or open biopsy.
- Tissue specimens are obtained for histologic examination.
- Specimens are placed in appropriate and properly labeled containers.

Postprocedure care
- Repeat chest X-ray immediately after the biopsy is completed.
- Resume a normal diet as ordered.

MONITORING
- Vital signs
- Intake and output
- Respiratory status
- Pulse oximetry
- Breath sounds
- Infection
- Bleeding

Precautions
- Lung biopsy is contraindicated in patients with:
  – severe uncorrected coagulopathy
  – severe pulmonary or cardiac disease.
- Coughing or movement during the biopsy can cause pneumothorax.
- Failure to obtain a representative tissue specimen may affect test results.

Complications
- Bleeding
- Infection
- Pneumothorax

✛ INTERPRETATION

Normal findings
- Pulmonary tissue exhibits uniform texture of the alveolar ducts, alveolar walls, bronchioles, and small vessels.

Abnormal results
- Histologic examination of a pulmonary tissue specimen reveals possible squamous cell or oat cell carcinoma and adenocarcinoma.

Lung perfusion scan

- Produces a visual image of pulmonary blood flow after I.V. injection of a radiopharmaceutical
- Human serum albumin microspheres (particles) or macroaggregated albumin, bonded to technetium, possibly used

Purpose

- To assess arterial perfusion of the lungs
- To detect pulmonary emboli
- To evaluate pulmonary function

Patient preparation

- Make sure that the patient has signed an appropriate consent form.
- Note and report all allergies.
- No restriction of food and fluids is necessary before the test.
- Stress the importance of lying still during imaging.

TEACHING POINTS

Be sure to cover:

- the purpose of the study and how it's performed
- who will perform the test and where
- that the test takes about 30 minutes
- that the amount of radioactivity is minimal.

- The patient is placed in a supine position on a nuclear medicine table.
- The radiopharmaceutical is injected I.V. over 5 to 10 seconds.
- A gamma camera takes a series of images in various view.
- Images projected on an oscilloscope screen show the distribution of radioactive particles.

Postprocedure care

- Apply warm soaks if a hematoma develops at the injection site.

MONITORING

- Vital signs
- Injection site
- Respiratory status

Precautions

- Lung perfusion scan is contraindicated in hypersensitivity to the radiopharmaceutical.

Complications

- Sensitivity to the radiopharmaceutical

Normal findings

- Hot spots (areas of high uptake) indicate normal blood perfusion.
- The uptake pattern is uniform.

Abnormal results

- Cold spots (areas of low uptake) indicate poor perfusion, suggesting an embolism.
- Decreased regional blood flow, without vessel obstruction, suggests possible pneumonitis.

Lung ventilation scan

● OVERVIEW

- A nuclear scan performed after inhalation of air mixed with radioactive gas
- Differentiates areas of ventilated lung from areas of underventilated lungs

Purpose

- To diagnose pulmonary emboli when used in combination with lung perfusion scan
- To identify areas of the lung that are capable of ventilation
- To evaluate regional respiratory function
- To locate regional hypoventilation

Patient preparation

- Make sure that the patient has signed an appropriate consent form.
- Note and report all allergies.
- Restriction of food or fluids isn't necessary.
- Stress the importance of lying still during imaging.
- Explain that the patient wears a tight-fitting mask during the study.

TEACHING POINTS

Be sure to cover:
- the purpose of the study and how it's done
- who will perform the test and where
- that the test takes 15 to 30 minutes.

▷ PROCEDURE

- The patient is properly placed in a supine position on a nuclear medicine table.
- A mask is applied, covering the patient's nose and mouth.
- The patient inhales air mixed with a small amount of radioactive gas through the tightly fitted mask.
- Distribution of the gas in the lungs is monitored on a nuclear scanner.
- The patient's chest is scanned as the gas is exhaled.

Postprocedure care

- Reinstate any oxygen therapy previously ordered.

MONITORING

- Vital signs
- Respiratory status

Precautions

- Leaks in the closed system of radioactive gas can contaminate the surrounding atmosphere.

Complications

- Panic attacks from wearing the mask

✛ INTERPRETATION

Normal findings

- Gas should be equally distributed in both lungs.

Abnormal results

- Unequal gas distribution in both lungs suggests poor ventilation or airway obstruction in areas with low radioactivity.
- When performed with a lung perfusion scan, vascular obstruction with normal ventilation suggests decreased perfusion such as in pulmonary embolism.
- Both ventilation and perfusion abnormalities suggest possible parenchymal disease.

Lymph node biopsy

● OVERVIEW

- Surgical excision of an active lymph node or the needle aspiration of a nodal specimen for histologic examination

Purpose
- To determine cause of lymph node enlargement
- To distinguish between benign and malignant lymph node tumors
- To stage metastatic cancer

Patient preparation
- Make sure that the patient has signed an appropriate consent form.
- Note and report all allergies.
- Check the patient's history for hypersensitivity to anesthetic.
- For excisional biopsy, instruct the patient to restrict food from midnight, and to drink only clear liquids.
- If a general anesthetic will be used, fluids are restricted.
- For a needle biopsy, no restriction of food or fluids is necessary.

TEACHING POINTS
Be sure to cover:
- the purpose of the study and how it's done
- who will perform the biopsy and where
- that the test takes 15 to 30 minutes.

▶ PROCEDURE

EXCISIONAL BIOPSY
- The skin over the biopsy site is prepared and draped.
- The anesthetic is administered.
- An incision is made and an entire node removed.
- The specimen is placed in an appropriate, properly labeled container.
- The wound is sutured, and a sterile dressing applied.

NEEDLE BIOPSY
- The biopsy site is prepared and draped.
- A local anesthetic is administered.
- The biopsy needle is directed into the node and a small core specimen obtained.
- The specimen is placed in a properly labeled container.
- Pressure is applied to the biopsy site to control bleeding.
- A dressing is applied after hemostasis is obtained.

Postprocedure care
- Resume diet and activity as ordered.

MONITORING
- Vital signs
- Bleeding
- Infection
- Biopsy site

Precautions
- Place the tissue specimen in normal saline instead of in 10% formalin solution.

Complications
- Bleeding
- Infection

✛ INTERPRETATION

Normal findings
- The lymph node is encapsulated by collagenous connective tissue.
- The lymph node is divided into smaller lobes by tissue strands called trabeculae.
- The outer cortex is composed of lymphoid cells and nodules or follicles containing lymphocytes.
- The inner medulla is composed of reticular phagocytic cells.

Abnormal results
- Histologic examination may be used to distinguish between malignant and nonmalignant causes of lymph node enlargement. (See *Staging non-Hodgkin's lymphoma*.)
- A lymphoma affecting the entire lymph system suggests possible Hodgkin's disease.
- Lymph node malignancy suggests possible metastatic cancer.

STAGING NON-HODGKIN'S LYMPHOMA

Stage I: Involvement of a single lymph node region or of a single extralymphatic organ or site

Stage II: Involvement of two or more lymph node regions on the same side of the diaphragm, or localized involvement of an extralymphatic organ or the site of one or more lymph node regions on the same side of the diaphragm

Stage III: Involvement of lymph node regions on both sides of the diaphragm, which may also be accompanied by localized involvement of an extralymphatic organ or site or of the spleen (or both)

Stage IV: Diffuse or disseminated involvement of one or more extralymphatic organs or tissue with or without associated lymph node enlargement

Lymphoscintigraphy

- Uses a radiopharmaceutical agent to visualize the lymphatic system via a gamma camera and computer
- Creates images of lymph flow and calculates speed of uptake
- Considered the safest and most accepted method for evaluating the lymphatic system

Purpose

- To diagnose lymphedema
- To evaluate lymph flow in an extremity
- To identify the sentinel node preoperatively in breast cancer and malignant melanoma

Patient preparation

- Make sure that the patient has signed an appropriate consent form.
- Have the patient remove all clothing and jewelry from the waist up.
- No dietary restrictions are necessary unless surgery will follow immediately after study.
- Encourage the patient to remain still during the test.

TEACHING POINTS

Be sure to cover:

- purpose of the study and how it's done
- who will perform the test and where
- that the length of the test depends on how many images are needed.

PROCEDURE

- The patient is positioned supine on the scanning table.
- The radiopharmaceutical agent is injected.
  - For lymphedema, injection is given into the skin between the first and second fingers or toes of each hand or foot.
  - For breast cancer, injections are given through the skin near the tumor or around the areola.
  - For melanoma, three to five injections are given into the skin surrounding the site of the melanoma.
- Images are obtained after the injection and repeated at 5-minute intervals for 45 to 60 minutes for lymphedema and 2 to 4 hours for breast cancer and melanoma.
- For lymphedema, the patient may be asked to exercise lightly (such as walking for leg evaluation or handgrip exercises for arm evaluation) for about 10 minutes; additional images may be taken after exercise and at 1- to 2-hour intervals for up to 6 hours.
- For breast cancer, images are obtained of the axillary, breast, and chest regions; for melanoma, images are obtained of the axillary region, head, neck, and both groins. Marks are made on the skin to identify where the lymph nodes are located.
- Movement of the radiopharmaceutical is followed on a computer screen.
- Lymph node biopsy may be performed immediately after the test for patients with breast cancer or melanoma.

Postprocedure care

- Resume regular activities after the procedure.
- Offer emotional support as the patient may be anxious about the results.

MONITORING

- Injection site
- Allergic reaction

Precautions

- Extravasation of the radiopharmaceutical may occur, causing hot spots in the area of the axillary lymph nodes.
- Allergic reactions to the radiopharmaceutical are rare.

Complications

- Pain and redness at injection site

INTERPRETATION

Normal findings

- No abnormal lymph nodes are present.

Abnormal results

- Leakage into adjacent tissue, bluish discoloration around affected node, and unusual collateral lymph flow paths indicate abnormal nodes.
- Impaired flow or obstruction to radiopharmaceutical suggests lymphedema.

Magnetic resonance imaging

● OVERVIEW

- Uses a powerful magnetic field and radiofrequency waves to produce computerized images of internal organs and tissues
- Eliminates the risks associated with exposure to X-ray beams and causes no harm to cells
- Also known as *MRI*

Purpose
- To obtain images of internal organs and tissues not readily seen on standard X-rays

Patient preparation
- Make sure that the patient has signed an appropriate consent form.
- Note and report all allergies.
- No special diet or fluid restrictions are necessary.
- Instruct the patient to remove any metal objects he's carrying or wearing.
- Warn the patient that the machine makes loud clacking sounds.
- Advise the patient that he'll be asked to remain still during the procedure.

TEACHING POINTS
Be sure to cover:
- the purpose of the study and how it's done
- who will perform the test and where
- that the test takes about 30 to 90 minutes.

▶ PROCEDURE

- If a contrast medium is used, an I.V. line is started and the medium is administered before the procedure.
- The patient is checked for metal objects at the scanner room door.
- The patient is placed in a supine position on a padded scanning table.
- The table is positioned in the opening of the scanning gantry.
- A call bell or intercom is used to maintain verbal contact.
- The patient may wear earplugs if desired.
- Varying radiofrequency waves are directed at the area being scanned.
- A computer reconstructs information as images on a television screen.

Postprocedure care
- A normal diet and activities may be resumed unless otherwise indicated.

MONITORING
- Vital signs
- Postural hypotension

Precautions
- Claustrophobic patients may require sedation or open MRI. (See *Open MRI.*)
- MRI is contraindicated in:
  - pregnancy
  - patients with metal implants, rods, screws, prosthetic devices, or pacemakers
  - extremely obese patients.
- All metal objects, such as jewelry, hairpins, and dentures, must be removed before the test.
- Patients requiring life support equipment, including ventilators, require special preparation; contact MRI staff ahead of time.

Complications
- Postural hypotension
- Claustrophobia
- Anxiety

✣ INTERPRETATION

Normal findings
- See "Normal findings" for the specific type of MRI.

Abnormal results
- See "Abnormal results" for the specific type of MRI.

OPEN MRI

With an open magnetic resonance imaging (MRI) unit, the patient isn't completely enclosed in a tunnel. This is ideal for patients with claustrophobia. Open MRI units are low-field units (0.2 to 0.5 Tesla) as opposed to closed MRI units, which are typically high-field units (1.0 to 1.5 or greater Tesla). The image quality is almost always better in a high-field unit, not only because of the field strength, but also because of the gradient speed/strength, surface coils, and software.

Accurate diagnosis may be difficult unless the interpreting radiologist has experience reading low-field units. If results with an open MRI are equivocal, a repeat closed MRI should be done. For small body parts (such as the hand, wrist, foot, ankle, or elbow), a high-resolution closed MRI is recommended. Some clinicians prefer a high-resolution MRI for the cervical spine as well because small extradural defects in the neural foramina are difficult to see even when using a high-field unit.

Magnetic resonance imaging, bone and soft tissue

● OVERVIEW

- Noninvasive technique producing clear and sensitive tomographic images of bone and soft tissue
- Provides superior contrast of body tissues and allows imaging of multiple planes, including direct sagittal and coronal views
- Eliminates the risks associated with exposure to radiation from X-rays and causes no known harm to cells

Purpose

- To evaluate bony and soft-tissue tumors
- To identify changes in the bone marrow cavity
- To identify spinal disorders

Patient preparation

- Make sure the patient has signed an appropriate consent form.
- Note and report all allergies.
- Make sure the scanner can accommodate the patient's weight and abdominal girth.
- Screen for surgically implanted joints, pins, clips, valves, pumps, or pacemakers containing metal.
- Discontinue I.V. infusion pumps, feeding tubes with metal tips, pulmonary artery catheters, and similar devices before the test as ordered.
- Explain that the patient will hear the scanner clicking, whirring, and thumping, so he may use earplugs.
- Provide reassurance to the patient that he'll be able to communicate with the technician at all times.
- An I.V. may be started for injection of a contrast agent for certain types of magnetic resonance imaging (MRI).
- If the patient is claustrophobic, sedation or an open scanner may be used.
- Stress the importance of removing all metallic objects, such as jewelry, hairpins, and a watch.

TEACHING POINTS

Be sure to cover:
- the purpose of the study and how it's done
- who will perform the test and where
- that no dietary restrictions are necessary
- that the test takes 30 to 90 minutes

- that MRI is painless and involves no exposure to radiation.

▶ PROCEDURE

- The patient is checked for metal objects at the scanner room door.
- The patient is placed on a narrow, padded, nonmetallic table that moves into the scanner tunnel.
- A call bell or intercom is used to maintain verbal contact.
- The patient is instructed to remain still during the procedure.
- The area to be studied is stimulated with radiofrequency waves.
- A computer measures resulting energy changes at these body sections and uses them to generate images.

Postprocedure care

- Provide comfort measures as needed.
- Resume normal activities as ordered.

MONITORING

- Vital signs
- Postural hypotension

Precautions

- Monitor for claustrophobia and anxiety.
- MRI involves using a powerful magnetic field, so don't allow any metal objects, such as I.V. pumps, ventilators, and other metallic equipment, or computer-based equipment to enter the MRI area.

  ◆ **NURSING ALERT** If the patient is unstable, make sure an I.V. line without metal components is in place and that all equipment is compatible with MRI imaging; monitor oxygen saturation, cardiac rhythm, and respiratory status during the test. An anesthesiologist may be needed to monitor a heavily sedated patient.

Complications

- Claustrophobia
- Anxiety
- Postural hypotension

✛ INTERPRETATION

Normal findings

- There's no evidence of pathology in bone, muscles, and joints.

Abnormal results

- Structural abnormalities suggest possible primary and metastatic tumors and various disorders of the bone, muscles, and joints.

Magnetic resonance imaging, neurologic system

● OVERVIEW

- Produces cross-sectional images of the brain and spine in multiple planes
- Enables ability to "see through" bone and to delineate fluid-filled soft tissue
- May use angiography with MRI (called magnetic resonance angiography [MRA]) to image neurologic system (see *MRI techniques*)

Purpose

- To aid diagnosis of intracranial and spinal lesions
- To aid diagnosis of soft-tissue abnormalities
- To detect small tumors and hemorrhages and cerebral infarction earlier than computed tomography scanning

Patient preparation

- Make sure the patient has signed an appropriate consent form.
- Note and report all allergies.
- Screen for any surgically implanted joints, pins, clips, valves, pumps, or pacemakers containing metal.
- Remove all metallic objects from the patient.
- Explain the need to remain still for the entire procedure.
- Warn the patient that clicking, whirring, and thumping sounds will be heard during the procedure.
- Advise the patient that he might receive earplugs.
- Provide reassurance that the patient will be able to communicate at all times during the procedure.

TEACHING POINTS

Be sure to cover:
- the purpose of the study and how it's done
- who will perform the test and where
- that no dietary restrictions are needed
- that the test takes up to 90 minutes
- that magnetic resonance imaging (MRI) is painless and involves no exposure to radiation.

▶ PROCEDURE

- The patient is placed in a supine position on a narrow table.
- The table is moved to the desired position inside the scanner.
- Radio-frequency energy is directed at the head or spine.
- Resulting images are displayed on a monitor.
- Images are recorded on film or magnetic tape.

Postprocedure care

- Provide comfort measures, as needed.
- Resume normal activity, as ordered.

MONITORING

- Vital signs
- Postural hypotension

Precautions

- Because of powerful magnetic fields, MRI is contraindicated in patients with pacemakers, intracranial clips, ferrous metal implants, or gunshot wounds to the head.
- Metallic or computer-based equipment (for example, ventilators and I.V. pumps) must not enter the MRI area.
- If the patient is claustrophobic, sedation or an open scanner may be used.

Complications

- Claustrophobia
- Postural hypotension
- Anxiety

✛ INTERPRETATION

Normal findings

- Brain and spinal cord structures appear distinct and sharply defined.

Abnormal results

- Structural changes that increase tissue water content suggest possible cerebral edema, demyelinating disease, and pontine and cerebellar tumors.
- Areas of demyelination (curdlike gray or gray-white areas) around the edges of ventricles suggest multiple sclerosis lesions.
- Changes in normal anatomy suggest possible tumors.

MRI TECHNIQUES

Magnetic resonance imaging (MRI) is used to provide clear images of parts of the brain, such as the brain stem and cerebellum that are difficult to image by other methods. Four MRI techniques are available to examine other aspects of the brain.

Magnetic resonance angiography

Magnetic resonance angiography allows the visualization of blood flowing through the cerebral vessels. Images of blood vessels done with magnetic resonance angiography aren't as clear as those obtained by angiography, but this technique is less invasive.

Magnetic resonance spectroscopy

Magnetic resonance spectroscopy creates images over time that show the metabolism of certain chemical markers in a specific area of the brain. Some researchers have dubbed this test a "metabolic biopsy" because it reveals pathologic neurochemistry over time.

Diffusion-perfusion imaging

Diffusion-perfusion imaging uses a stronger-than-normal magnetic gradient to reveal areas of focal cerebral ischemia within minutes. Currently used in stroke research, this MRI technique may be used by diagnosticians to distinguish permanent from reversible ischemia.

Neurography

Neurograms provide a three-dimensional image of nerves. They may be used to find the exact location of nerves that are damaged, crimped, or in disarray.

Magnetic resonance imaging, urinary tract

⬤ OVERVIEW

- Uses radiofrequency waves and magnetic fields to show specific structures (kidney or prostate), which are then converted to computer-generated images
- May reveal blood vessel size and anatomy when imaging soft-tissue structures of kidneys; not useful for detecting calculi or calcified tumors

Purpose
- To diagnose urinary tract disorders
- To evaluate genitourinary tumors and abdominal or pelvic masses
- To detect prostate calculi and cysts
- To detect cancer invasion into seminal vesicles and pelvic lymph nodes

Patient preparation
- Make sure that the patient or family member has signed an appropriate consent form.
- If the patient will receive a contrast medium, obtain a history of allergies or hypersensitivity to these drugs. Mark sensitivities on the chart and notify the practitioner.
- Ask the patient if he has any implanted metal devices or prostheses, such as vascular clips, shrapnel, pacemakers, joint implants, filters, and intrauterine devices. If so, the patient may not be able to have the test.
- Instruct the patient to avoid alcohol, caffeine-containing beverages, and tobacco for at least 2 hours, and food for at least 1 hour, before the test.
- Tell the patient to continue taking medications, except for iron, which interferes with the imaging.
- Before the test, tell the patient that he'll need to remove all clothing, jewelry, and metallic objects and wear a special hospital gown without snaps or closures.
- Inform the patient that he won't feel pain but may feel claustrophobic while lying supine in the tubular magnetic resonance imaging (MRI) chamber.
- Tell him the practitioner may order an anxiolytic.
- Tell the patient that he'll hear loud noises from the machine during the test but may receive earplugs or a music headset to decrease this noise.
- Inform the patient that, although his face remains uncovered to allow him to see out, to keep his eyes closed to promote relaxation and prevent a closed-in feeling.
- If the patient feels nauseated because of claustrophobia, encourage him to take deep breaths.
- Just before the procedure, have the patient void.

TEACHING POINTS
Be sure to cover:
- purpose of the study and how it's done
- who will perform the test and where
- that the test takes between 30 and 90 minutes.

▶ PROCEDURE

- The patient is placed in the supine position on a narrow, flat table.
- If the patient will receive a contrast medium, an I.V. line is started so that the medium is infused before the procedure.
- The table is moved to the enclosed cylindrical scanner.
- The patient is encouraged to lie still in the scanner while the images are being produced.
- Varying radiofrequency waves are directed at the area being scanned.

Postprocedure care
- If the patient received a sedative, maintain safety precautions until the patient is awake and responsive.
- Allow patient to resume his usual diet, fluids, and medications, once awake and responsive.

MONITORING
- Vital signs
- Adverse reactions to the contrast medium (such as flushing, nausea, urticaria, and sneezing)

Precautions
- Because of powerful magnetic fields, MRI is contraindicated in patients with pacemakers, intracranial clips, ferrous metal implants, or gunshot wounds to the head.
- Metallic or computer-based equipment (such as ventilators and I.V. pumps) must not enter the MRI area.

Complications
- Anxiety
- Adverse reactions to contrast medium

✛ INTERPRETATION

Normal findings
- The soft tissue structures of the kidneys are visible.
- Blood vessels can be seen.

Abnormal results
- Visual images suggest tumors, strictures, stenosis, thrombosis, malformations, abscess, inflammation, edema, fluid collection, bleeding, hemorrhage, or organ atrophy.

Mammography

● OVERVIEW

- Radiographic technique used to detect breast cysts or tumors, especially those not palpable on physical examination
- Xeromammography: electrostatically charged plate records the radiographic images and transfers them to special paper
- Questionable finding on mammography possible indication for ultrasound (see *Using ultrasound to detect breast cancer*)
- Guidelines for using mammography established by American Cancer Society
- Digital imaging: approved by U.S. Food and Drug Administration; used similarly to mammography (see *Digital mammography*)

Purpose

- To screen for malignant breast tumors
- To investigate breast masses, breast pain, or nipple discharge
- To differentiate between benign breast disease and malignant tumors
- To monitor patients with breast cancer treated with breast-conserving surgery and radiation

Patient preparation

- Make sure the patient has signed an appropriate consent form.
- Note and report all allergies.
- Instruct the patient to avoid using underarm deodorant or powder the day of the exam.
- When scheduling the test, inform the staff of breast implants.

TEACHING POINTS

Be sure to cover:

- the purpose of the study and how it's done

- who will perform the test and where
- that the test takes about 15 minutes
- that no dietary restrictions are necessary
- that the patient may be asked to wait while the films are checked.

▶ PROCEDURE

- The patient rests one breast on a table above radiograph cassette.
- The compressor is placed on the breast.
- The patient holds her breath.
- A radiograph is taken of the craniocaudal view.
- The machine is rotated and the breast is compressed again.
- A radiograph is taken in the lateral view.
- The procedure is repeated for the other breast.
- The films are developed and checked for quality.

Postprocedure care

- No specific posttest care is necessary.

Precautions

- Mammography is never a substitute for biopsy; it may not reveal clinical cancer.
- Many false-positive results are found.

Complications

- Possible vasovagal reaction during compression

✛ INTERPRETATION

Normal findings

- Normal ducts, glandular tissue, and fat architecture are found.
- No abnormal masses or calcifications are found.

Abnormal results

- Irregular, poorly outlined, opaque areas suggest malignant tumor, especially if solitary and unilateral.
- Well-outlined, regular, clear spots may be benign, especially if bilateral.

DIGITAL MAMMOGRAPHY

Digital mammography produces pictures of the breast using X-rays. Instead of film, this process uses detectors that change the X-rays into electrical signals, which are then converted to an image. Digital mammography is used for screening and diagnosis. For the patient, the procedure is the same as with ordinary mammography.

Digital mammography may offer advantages over conventional mammography:

- The images can be stored and retrieved electronically, which makes long-distance consultations with other mammography specialists easier.
- Because the images can be adjusted by the radiologist, subtle differences between tissues may be noted.
- The number of follow-up procedures required may be reduced.
- The need for fewer exposures with digital mammography can reduce the already low levels of radiation.

The U.S. Food and Drug Administration has recently approved the Lorad Digital Breast Imager to be used with the Lorad M-IV Mammography X-ray System for this digital procedure.

Digital mammography has been shown to be effective in the detection of breast cancer and other abnormalities.

USING ULTRASOUND TO DETECT BREAST CANCER

Ultrasonography is especially useful for diagnosing tumors less than ¼" (0.635 cm) diameter. It's also helpful in distinguishing cysts from solid tumors in dense breast tissue. As in other ultrasound techniques, a transducer is used to focus a beam of high-frequency sound waves through the patient's skin and into the breast. The sound waves then bounce back to the transducer as an echo that varies in strength with the density of the underlying tissues. A computer processes these echoes and displays the resulting image on a screen for interpretation.

Ultrasound can show all areas of a breast, including the area close to the chest wall, which is difficult to study with X-rays. When used as an adjunct to mammography, ultrasound increases diagnostic accuracy; when used alone, it's more accurate than mammography in examining the denser breast tissue of young patients.

Mediastinoscopy

● OVERVIEW

- Operative procedure that directly visualizes mediastinal structures through a mediastinoscope with a built-in light source
- Used when sputum cytology, lung scans, radiography, and bronchoscopic biopsy fail to confirm a diagnosis

Purpose
- To detect bronchogenic carcinoma, lymphoma, and sarcoidosis
- To stage lung cancer
- To permit biopsy of paratracheal and carinal lymph nodes

Patient preparation
- Make sure the patient has signed an appropriate consent form.
- Note and report all allergies.
- Check the patient's history for hypersensitivity to the anesthetic.
- Fasting is required after midnight before the test.
- Explain that the patient will be given a general anesthetic.
- Warn the patient that he may have temporary chest pain, tenderness at the incision site, and sore throat (from intubation).
- Explain that he'll have an incision above the suprasternal notch.

TEACHING POINTS
Be sure to cover:
- the purpose of the study and how it's done
- who will perform the procedure and where
- that the test takes about 1 hour.

▶ PROCEDURE

- The patient is intubated and anesthetized.
- A small transverse suprasternal incision is made.
- A channel is formed using finger dissection and lymph nodes are palpated.
- The mediastinoscope is inserted.
- Tissue specimens are collected and sent to the laboratory for frozen section examination.
- If analysis confirms malignancy of a resectable tumor, thoracotomy and pneumonectomy may follow immediately.

Postprocedure care
- Administer the prescribed analgesic, as ordered.
- Resume diet and activity, as ordered.

MONITORING
- Vital signs
- Intake and output
- Bleeding
- Infection
- Incision and dressings
- Respiratory status
- Neurologic status

NURSING ALERT Observe for signs and symptoms of complications: fever (mediastinitis); crepitus (subcutaneous emphysema); dyspnea, cyanosis, and diminished breath sounds (pneumothorax); or tachycardia and hypotension (hemorrhage or cardiac tamponade).

Precautions
- Study is contraindicated during pregnancy unless benefit outweighs risk.
- Check for a history of adverse reaction to anesthetics.
- Antineoplastics may affect test results.

Complications
- Pneumothorax
- Perforated esophagus
- Mediastinitis
- Infection
- Hemorrhage
- Left recurrent laryngeal nerve damage
- Cardiac tamponade

✛ INTERPRETATION

Normal findings
- Lymph nodes appear as small, smooth, flat oval bodies of lymphoid tissue.

Abnormal results
- Anatomical abnormalities suggest possible various disorders including lung or esophageal cancer, and lymphomas such as Hodgkin's disease.

Myelography

● OVERVIEW

- Combines fluoroscopy and radiography to evaluate the spinal subarachnoid space after injection of a contrast medium
- Fluoroscopy: used to visualize flow of the contrast medium and outline of subarachnoid space

Purpose

- To demonstrate lesions partially or totally blocking cerebrospinal fluid flow in the subarachnoid space (tumors and herniated intervertebral disks)
- To detect arachnoiditis, spinal nerve root injury, or tumors in the posterior fossa of the skull
- To evaluate cause of neurologic signs and symptoms

Patient preparation

- Make sure the patient has signed an appropriate consent form.
- Note and report all allergies.
- Check the patient's history for hypersensitivity to iodine and iodine-containing substances (such as shellfish) and contrast media.
- Notify the radiologist if there's a history of epilepsy or antidepressant or phenothiazine use.

  NURSING ALERT Phenothiazines in combination with metrizamide given during myelography increases the risk of toxicity.
- An enema may be ordered for a patient undergoing lumbar puncture.
- Administer a sedative and anticholinergic as ordered.
- Explain the need to restrict food and fluids before the test as ordered.
- Warn the patient that transient burning may be felt as the contrast medium is injected and that he may experience flushing and warmth, a headache, a salty taste, or nausea and vomiting.

TEACHING POINTS

Be sure to cover:
- the purpose of the study and how it's done
- who will perform the test and where
- that the test takes at least 1 hour.

▶ PROCEDURE

- The patient is positioned on his side at the edge of the table with his knees drawn up to his abdomen and his chin on his chest.
- A cisternal puncture may be done if lumbar deformity or infection at puncture site present.
- A lumbar puncture is performed.
- Fluoroscopy verifies proper needle position in the subarachnoid space.
- Some CSF may be removed for routine laboratory analysis.
- The patient is turned to the prone position.
- The contrast medium is injected.
- If a subarachnoid space obstruction blocks the upward flow of the contrast medium, a cisternal puncture may be performed.
- The flow of the contrast medium is studied with fluoroscopy.
- X-rays are taken.
- The contrast medium is withdrawn, if oil-based, and the needle is removed.
- The puncture site is cleansed and a small dressing applied.
- If a spinal tumor is confirmed, the patient may go directly to the operating room

Postprocedure care

- Determine the type of contrast medium used for the test.
- If an oil-based contrast agent was used, keep the patient flat in bed for 8 to 12 hours.
- If a water-based contrast agent was used, elevate the head of the bed for 6 to 8 hours.
- Maintain bed rest as ordered.
- Encourage oral fluid intake to assist the kidneys in eliminating the contrast media.
- Notify the doctor if the patient fails to void within 8 hours.
- Resume a usual diet and activities the day after the test as ordered.

  NURSING ALERT If a water-based contrast is used, care must be taken that the large dye load doesn't reach the surface of the brain; to prevent this, the patient's head is kept elevated for 30 to 45 degrees after the procedure.

MONITORING

- Vital signs
- Intake and output
- Neurologic status
- Puncture site
- Bleeding
- Infection
- Seizure activity

  NURSING ALERT If radicular pain, fever, back pain, or signs and symptoms of meningeal irritation (headache, irritability, or neck stiffness) develops, inform the doctor immediately. Keep the room quiet and dark, and provide an analgesic or an antipyretic as ordered.

Precautions

- Myelography is contraindicated in:
  – increased intracranial pressure
  – hypersensitivity to contrast media
  – infection at the puncture site.
- Improper positioning after the test may affect recovery.

Complications

- Bleeding
- Infection
- Meningeal irritation
- Seizures
- Dehydration

✛ INTERPRETATION

Normal findings

- Contrast medium flows freely through the subarachnoid space.
- No obstruction or structural abnormality is found.

Abnormal results

- Extradural lesions suggest possible herniated intervertebral disks, or metastatic tumors.
- Lesions within the subarachnoid space suggest possible neurofibromas or meningiomas.
- Lesions within the spinal cord suggest possible ependymomas or astrocytomas.
- Fluid-filled cavities in the spinal cord and widening of the cord itself suggest possible syringomyelia.

Myocardial perfusion imaging, radiopharmaceutical

● OVERVIEW

- Alternative method of assessing coronary arteries for patients who can't tolerate exercise stress tests
- A drug (adenosine, dobutamine, or dipyridamole) is used to chemically stress the patient; this simulates the effects of exercise by increasing blood flow in the coronary arteries or by increasing heart rate and contractility
- Radiopharmaceutical is injected and resting and stress images are obtained and compared to evaluate coronary perfusion
- Also known as chemical stress test imaging

Purpose

- To assess the presence and degree of coronary artery disease
- To evaluate myocardial perfusion
- To evaluate patient's response after therapeutic procedures (such as bypass surgery and coronary angioplasty)

Patient preparation

- Make sure the patient has signed an appropriate consent form.
- Note and report all allergies.
- Confirm that the patient isn't pregnant.
- Weigh the patient to determine the appropriate drug dosage.
- Withhold nitrates 6 hours before testing as ordered.
- Fasting for 3 to 4 hours is required before the test; the patient may have water.
- A cardiologist, nurse, electrocardiogram (ECG) technician, and nuclear medicine technologist are usually present during test.
- Warn the patient that he may experience flushing, shortness of breath, dizziness, headache, chest pain, increased heart rate or palpitations during the infusion, depending on the drug used.
- Provide reassurance that emergency equipment will be available if needed.

ADENOSINE OR DIPYRIDAMOLE ADMINISTRATION

- Withhold all theophylline medications for 24 to 36 hours before the examination as ordered.

- Instruct the patient to avoid all caffeine-containing products for 12 hours before testing.

DOBUTAMINE ADMINISTRATION

- Withhold beta-adrenergic blockers for 48 hours before the test as ordered.
- Administer medications, such as antihypertensives, as ordered.

TEACHING POINTS

Be sure to cover:
- the purpose of the study and how it's done
- who will perform the test and where
- that the study takes 1 to 2 hours, and the time can be longer depending on the type of nuclear medicine equipment
- that signs and symptoms generally stop as soon as the infusion ends.

▶ PROCEDURE

- The patient is placed in a supine position on an examination table.
- I.V. access is obtained.
- Baseline ECG and vital signs are obtained.
- The chemical stress medication is infused as ordered.
- During the infusion, vital signs and cardiac rhythm are monitored continuously.
- At the appropriate time, the radiopharmaceutical is injected.
- Rest imaging may be done before stress imaging or 3 to 4 hours afterwards, depending on the radiopharmaceutical used.
- After the images are completed, the I.V. access is removed.

Postprocedure care

- Regular diet and activity are resumed as ordered.

MONITORING

- Vital signs
- ECG
- Cardiac rhythm
- Respiratory status
- Anginal symptoms
- Heart sounds
- Breath sounds

Precautions

- Keep resuscitation equipment readily available.

- Screen for bronchospastic lung disease or asthma (adenosine and dipyridamole are contraindicated).
- Screen for the presence of a pacemaker; dobutamine may be contraindicated.
- Reversal agents that should be readily available include:
  - I.V. aminophylline for adenosine and dipyridamole
  - I.V. beta-adrenergic blocker for dobutamine.
- Contraindications include:
  - myocardial infarction within 10 days of testing
  - acute myocarditis and pericarditis
  - unstable angina
  - arrhythmias
  - hypertension or hypotension
  - severe aortic or mitral stenosis
  - hyperthyroidism.

Complications

- Serious arrhythmias
- Myocardial ischemia or infarction

✛ INTERPRETATION

Normal findings

- No perfusion defects are found on imaging.
- No ischemic changes are found on ECG.

Abnormal results

- Cold spots, indicating areas of decreased uptake, may suggest:
  - coronary artery disease (most common)
  - myocardial fibrosis
  - attenuation caused by soft tissue (breast and diaphragm)
  - coronary spasm.

Nephrotomography

● OVERVIEW

- Tomographic technique that presents images as "slices" or linear layers of the kidneys; structures in front of and behind the selected planes appear blurry
- Used to produce film images of renal arterial network and parenchyma before and after opacification with contrast medium
- A separate procedure or adjunct to excretory urography (I.V. pyelography, or IVP)

Purpose

- To differentiate between a simple renal cyst and solid neoplasm
- To assess renal lacerations
- To assess posttraumatic nonperfused areas of the kidneys
- To localize adrenal tumors
- To visualize space-occupying lesions

Patient preparation

- Make sure the patient has signed an appropriate consent form.
- Note and report all allergies.
- Check the patient's history for hypersensitivity to iodine or iodine-containing foods (such as shellfish) or to iodinated contrast media.
- Check the serum creatinine level and inform the doctor if it's greater than 1.5 mg/dl. (I.V. fluids may be ordered.)
- Fasting is required for 8 hours before the test.
- Advise that the patient may hear loud, clacking sounds as the films are exposed.
- Warn the patient that he may experience transient adverse effects from the injection of the contrast medium (burning, stinging at the injection site, flushing, and a metallic taste).

TEACHING POINTS

Be sure to cover:
- the purpose of the study and how it's done
- who will perform the test and where
- that the test takes less than 1 hour.

▶ PROCEDURE

- A plain film of the kidneys is obtained.
- Preliminary tomograms are obtained and reviewed.
- Contrast medium is administered I.V. using either a bolus or infusion method.
- Serial tomograms are obtained.

Postprocedure care

- Ensure adequate hydration.
- Resume normal diet and activity as ordered.

MONITORING

- Vital signs
- Intake and output
- Serum creatinine levels

◆ **NURSING ALERT** Observe for signs and symptoms of a posttest allergic reaction to contrast medium (flushing, nausea, urticaria, and sneezing) or an anaphylactic reaction.

Precautions

- Nephrotomography is performed with extreme caution in patients with:
  - hypersensitivity to iodine-based compounds
  - cardiovascular disease
  - multiple myeloma
  - impaired renal function (serum creatinine levels greater than 1.5 mg/dl), especially in elderly and dehydrated patients.
- If the patient has a history of I.V. contrast hypersensitivity, inform the doctor so prophylaxis (such as diphenhydramine) or a low osmolar contrast agent can be used.

- Residual barium from a recently performed barium study may obscure the kidneys.

Complications

- Adverse reaction to contrast media
- Impaired renal function

✛ INTERPRETATION

Normal findings

- Normal size, shape, and position of the kidneys are found.
- No space-occupying lesions or other abnormalities are found.

Abnormal results

- Various structural abnormalities are demonstrated by nephrotomography, such as simple cysts and solid tumors, renal sinus-related lesions, ectopic renal lobes, adrenal tumors, areas of nonperfusion, and trauma-related renal lacerations. (See *Distinguishing between simple cysts and solid tumors.*)

DISTINGUISHING BETWEEN SIMPLE CYSTS AND SOLID TUMORS

Feature	Cysts	Tumors
Consistency	Homogeneous	Irregular
Contact with healthy renal tissue	Sharply distinct	Poorly resolved
Density	Radiolucent	Variable radiolucent patches (or same as normal renal parenchyma)
Shape	Spherical	Variable
Wall of lesion	Thin and well defined	Thick and irregular

Nuclear medicine scans

● OVERVIEW

- Imaging of specific body organs or systems by a scintillating scanning camera after I.V. injection, inhalation, or oral ingestion of a radioactive tracer compound.

Purpose
- To produce tissue analysis and images not readily seen on standard X-rays
- To detect or rule out malignant lesions when X-ray findings are normal or questionable

Patient preparation
- Make sure the patient has signed an appropriate consent form.
- Note and report all allergies.
- Note any prior nuclear medicine procedures.
- Make sure the patient isn't scheduled for more than one radionuclide scan on the same day.
- Advise that the patient will be asked to take various positions on a scanner table.
- Stress the need to remain still during the procedure.

TEACHING POINTS
Be sure to cover:
- the purpose of the study and how it's done
- who will perform the test and where
- that dietary restrictions may be necessary depending on the specific scan
- that the study takes approximately 1½ hours, but the time varies depending on the specific nuclear medicine scan

▶ PROCEDURE

- If an intravenous tracer isotope is used, an I.V. line is started.
- The detector of a scintillation camera is directed at the area being scanned and displayed on a monitor.
- Scintigraphs are obtained and reviewed for clarity .
- If necessary, additional views are obtained.

Postprocedure care
- Resume normal diet and activities as ordered.

MONITORING
- Vital signs
- Injection site
- Infection
- Postural hypotension.

Precautions
- Nuclear medicine scans are contraindicated during pregnancy.

Complications
- Postural hypotension
- Infection

⊹ INTERPRETATION

Normal findings
- See "Normal findings" for the specific nuclear medicine scan.

Abnormal results
- See "Abnormal results" for the specific nuclear medicine scan.

Ophthalmoscopy, handheld

⬤ OVERVIEW

- Magnified examination of living vascular and nerve tissue of the fundus, including the optic disk, retinal vessels, macula, and retina
- Ophthalmoscope: used directly or indirectly; direct model is easier to use than indirect model

Purpose

- To detect and evaluate eye disorders
- To detect and evaluate ocular manifestations of systemic disease, such as diabetes mellitus and hypertension
- To identify opacities of the cornea, lens, and vitreous, as well as lesions of the retina and optic nerve

Patient preparation

- Confirm the patient's identity using two patient identifiers according to facility policy.
- Note and report all allergies.
- Check the patient's history for previous use of dilating eyedrops.
- Check the patient's history for angle-closure glaucoma.
- Advise the patient that eyedrops may be instilled to dilate the pupils.

TEACHING POINTS

Be sure to cover:
- the purpose of the study and how it's done
- who will perform the test and where
- that the test takes less than 5 minutes; headband binocular indirect ophthalmoscopy usually takes 20 to 30 minutes following drug instillation.

▶ PROCEDURE

- The patient sits upright in the examination chair.
- The room is darkened.
- The right eye is examined with the ophthalmoscope.
- The patient looks straight ahead at a specific object 20′ (6 m) away, and is instructed not to move his eyes.
- The light beam of the ophthalmoscope is directed into the pupil.
- The examiner slowly approaches the patient at an angle of about 15 degrees temporal to the patient's line of vision.
- The red reflex is observed.
- The optic disk is examined.
- The physiologic cup is located.
- The retinal vessels emerging from the optic disk are examined.
- The macula and fovea are examined.
- The patient looks up, down, and to each side to examine the extreme periphery.
- The superior, inferior, temporal, and nasal portions of the retina are examined.
- The patient's left eye is examined in the same manner.

Postprocedure care

- If the eyes are dilated, protect the eyes from bright lights and explain the need to avoid driving or operating machinery until vision returns to normal.

MONITORING

- Vision

Precautions

🔲 **NURSING ALERT** Don't administer dilating eyedrops to a patient who has angle-closure glaucoma or a history of hypersensitivity reactions to the drops. Don't dilate the patient's pupils if head trauma or acute disease of the central nervous system is suspected.

Complications

- Adverse reaction to mydriatics, if used, including photophobia and increased intraocular pressure

✛ INTERPRETATION

Normal findings

- A visible red reflex is found.
- A slightly oval optic disk, measuring 5 mm vertically lies to the nasal side of the fundus center. It's usually pink with darker edges at its nasal border.
- The physiologic cup varies in size and tends to be larger in myopia and smaller in hyperopia; appears as a central depression in the surface of the disc.
- A semitransparent retina surrounds the optic disk.
- Retinal vessels branch out from the disk, including venules and the slightly smaller arterioles.
- Vessel diameter progressively decreases with distance from the optic disk.
- Retinal arterioles are medium red in color; venules appear dark red or blue.
- The macula, a small avascular area, appears darker than the surrounding retina, is located approximately two and a half disk diameters temporal from the optic disk; may appear slightly yellow due to the xanthophyll pigment in the retina.
- In the macula's center lies a small, even darker spot, the fovea.
- A tiny light reflex can be seen at the center of the fovea.

Abnormal results

- Absent or diminished red reflex suggests possible gross corneal lesions, dense opacities of the aqueous or vitreous humor, cataracts, or detached retina.
- Cloudy vitreous humor suggests possible inflammatory disease of the optic disk, retina, or uvea.
- An elevated, increased vascular optic disk suggests possible optic neuritis.
- A white-appearing disk suggests possible optic nerve atrophy.
- Abnormal elevation of the disk, blurring of disk margins, engorged vessels, and hemorrhages suggest papilledema.
- An enlarged physiologic cup appearing gray, with white edges suggests glaucoma.
- A milky-white retina suggests the acute phase of central retinal artery occlusion.
- Widespread retinal hemorrhage, patches of white exudate, and disk elevation suggest central retinal vein occlusion.
- Gray, elevated areas suggest retinal detachment.
- A dark lesion suggests possible a choroidal tumor.
- Vasospasm, sclerosis, and eventual occlusion of retinal arterioles, leading to retinal edema and hemorrhage, and papilledema suggest hypertension.
- Retinal fibroses, patches of white exudate, and microaneurysms suggest complications of diabetes mellitus.

Orbital radiography

● OVERVIEW

- X-rays of the orbital structures, eyebrow, bridge of the nose, and the cheekbone
- Tomograms may be taken with standard X-rays

Purpose
- To identify orbital fractures and pathology
- To locate intraorbital or intraocular foreign bodies and changes to the structure of the eye, which may indicate various diseases
- To detect problems resulting from injury and trauma to the eye

Patient preparation
- Make sure the patient has signed an appropriate consent form.
- Note and report all allergies.
- Have the patient remove any jewelry or metal objects that may interfere with a clear image.
- Advise the patient that positioning may cause some discomfort.

TEACHING POINTS
Be sure to cover:
- the purpose of the study and how it's done
- who will perform the test and where

- that no dietary restrictions are necessary
- that the test takes about 15 minutes.

▶ PROCEDURE

- The patient is placed in a supine position on the radiographic table or seated in a chair.
- A series of orbital X-rays is taken, including projections of the optical canal.
- Films are developed and checked for quality.
- Images of the unaffected eye may also be taken to compare its shapes and structures to those of the affected eye.
- If the patient is in severe pain due to injury or trauma, a pain medication may be given during positioning.

Postprocedure care
- No specific posttest care is necessary.

MONITORING
- Response to test
- Vision

Precautions
- Female patients are screened for pregnancy.

Complications
- None known

✛ INTERPRETATION

Normal findings
- Each orbit is composed of a roof, floor, and medial and lateral walls.
- The medial walls of both orbits parallel each other.
- The lateral walls of both orbits project toward each other.
- The superior orbital fissure lies in the back of the orbit, between the lateral wall and the roof. (See *Radiographic view of orbital structures.*)

Abnormal results
- Enlargement of an orbit suggests the presence of a lesion.
- Superior orbital fissure enlargement suggests possible orbital meningioma, intracranial conditions (such as pituitary tumors) or vascular anomalies.
- Optic canal enlargement suggests possible extraocular extension of a retinoblastoma, or indicates irritation from an injury or foreign body.
- Destruction of the orbital walls suggests possible malignant neoplasm or infection.

✹ **AGE-RELATED CONCERN** A child's orbit is more likely to be enlarged by a fast-growing lesion because the orbital bones aren't fully developed.
- Clear-cut local indentations of the orbital wall suggest a benign tumor or cyst.
- Increased bone density suggests possible conditions, such as osteoblastic metastasis, sphenoid ridge meningioma, or Paget's disease.

RADIOGRAPHIC VIEW OF ORBITAL STRUCTURES

Illustrated below are the structures demonstrated by orbital radiography.

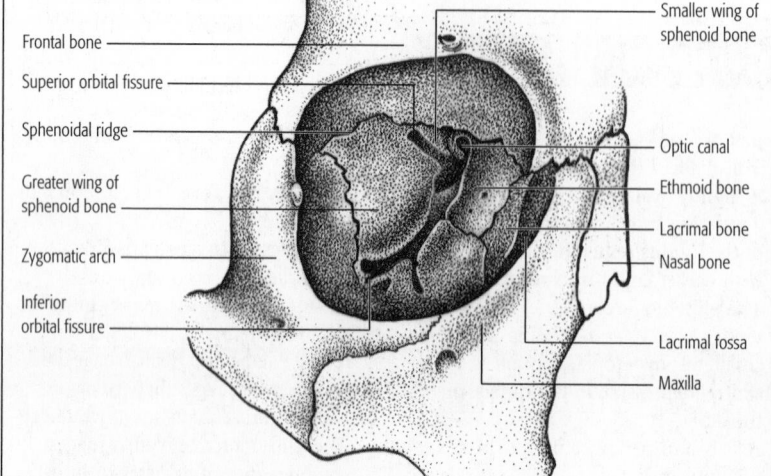

Frontal bone

Superior orbital fissure

Sphenoidal ridge

Greater wing of sphenoid bone

Zygomatic arch

Inferior orbital fissure

Smaller wing of sphenoid bone

Optic canal

Ethmoid bone

Lacrimal bone

Nasal bone

Lacrimal fossa

Maxilla

Otoscopy

● OVERVIEW

- Direct visualization of the external auditory canal and tympanic membrane (TM) through use of an otoscope
- Indirectly provides information about the eustachian tube and middle ear cavity

Purpose

- To detect foreign bodies, cerumen, or stenosis in the external canal
- To detect external or middle ear pathology (infection or perforation)
- To evaluate integrity and appearance of the TM

Patient preparation

- Confirm the patient's identity using two patient identifiers according to facility policy.
- Warn the patient that with pneumatic otoscopy, he may experience dizziness with nystagmus.

TEACHING POINTS

Be sure to cover:
- the purpose of the study and how it's done
- who will perform the test and where
- that the test takes less than 5 minutes to perform.

▶ PROCEDURE

- The patient is positioned with his head tilted slightly away from the examiner so that the ear to be examined is pointed upward.
- The auricle is pulled upward, backward, and slightly away from the head to straighten the ear canal.

  ◈ **NURSING ALERT** To straighten a child's ear canal, the auricle is pulled downward to allow the best view.

- The largest speculum that will comfortably fit the patient is selected.

  ◈ **NURSING ALERT** If the patient has ear pain, the unaffected ear is assessed first; the affected ear is then carefully assessed.

- The otoscope is gently inserted into the ear canal with a downward and forward motion.
- The TM is located and examined.

- The malleus is located, which should be partially visible through the translucent TM.
- The TM and surrounding fibrous rim (annulus) is examined.

Postprocedure care

- No specific postprocedure care is necessary.

Precautions

- The otoscope should be held securely in the dominant hand.
- The otoscope should be advanced slowly and gently.
- Obstruction of the ear canal by cerumen or foreign matter obscures the TM.

  ◈ **NURSING ALERT** Continuing to insert an otoscope against resistance can cause a perforation or other injury.

Complications

- Perforation of TM

✥ INTERPRETATION

Normal findings

- The TM is thin, translucent, shiny, and slightly concave. It appears pearl gray or pale pink, and reflects light in its inferior portion (cone of light) with clearly defined landmarks.
- The short process of the malleus, manubrium, and umbo are visible but not prominent.
- Blood vessels should be visible only in the periphery.

Abnormal results

- Scarring, discoloration, retraction or bulging of the TM as well as the presence of drainage and scaly surface areas suggests pathology.
- Movement of the TM in tandem with respiration suggests abnormal patency of the eustachian tube. (See *Common abnormalities of the tympanic membrane.*)
- A dry, flaky auditory canal lining may suggest eczema.
- An inflamed, swollen, and narrowed auditory canal, possibly with discharge, suggests otitis externa.

COMMON ABNORMALITIES OF THE TYMPANIC MEMBRANE

Visual examination of the tympanic membrane may reveal abnormal findings. This table lists some of the more common findings and their typical causes.

ABNORMAL FINDINGS	USUAL CAUSE
Bright red	Inflammation (otitis media)
Yellowish	Pus or serum behind the tympanic membrane (acute or chronic otitis media)
Bubble behind tympanic membrane	Serous fluid in middle ear (serous otitis media)
Absent light reflection	Bulging tympanic membrane (acute otitis media)
Absent or diminishing landmarks	Thickened tympanic membrane (chronic otitis media, otitis externa, or tympanosclerosis)
Oval dark areas	Perforated or scarred tympanic membrane (otitis media or trauma)
Prominent malleus	Retracted tympanic membrane (nonfunctional eustachian tube)
Reduced mobility	Stiffened middle ear system (serous otitis media or, more rarely, middle ear adhesions), negative pressure, middle ear fluid

Papanicolaou test

● OVERVIEW

- Widely used for early detection of cervical cancer
- Permits cytologic evaluation of the vaginal pool, prostatic secretions, urine, gastric secretions, cavity fluids, bronchial aspirates, sputum, and solid tumor cells obtained by fine-needle aspiration
- Also known as a *Pap test* or *ThinPrep Pap test*

Purpose
- To detect malignant cells
- To detect inflammatory changes in tissue
- To assess response to chemotherapy and radiation therapy
- To detect viral, fungal and, occasionally, parasitic invasion

Patient preparation
- Make sure the patient has signed an appropriate consent form.
- Note and report all allergies.
- Schedule the study for midcycle of the menstrual cycle.
- Advise the patient that she might experience slight discomfort from the speculum.
- Explain the need to avoid activities that can wash away cellular deposits and change vaginal pH, including:
  - sexual intercourse for 24 hours
  - douching for 48 hours
  - using vaginal creams or medications for 1 week.

TEACHING POINTS
Be sure to cover:
- the purpose of the study and how it's done
- who will perform the test and when
- that the test takes 5 to 10 minutes.

▶ PROCEDURE

- The patient is placed in the lithotomy position with her feet in stirrups.
- An unlubricated speculum is inserted into the vagina.
- The cervix is located.
- Secretions from the cervix and material from the endocervical canal are collected with an endocervical brush and a wooden spatula.
- Specimens are spread on slides and immediately immersed in a fixative or sprayed with a fixative.
- Specimens are appropriately labeled; date of last menstrual period, collection site, and method are included.

Postprocedure care
- If bleeding occurs, supply the patient with a sanitary napkin.
- Schedule a return appointment for her next Pap test.

Precautions
- If vaginal or vulval lesions are present, scrapings taken directly from the lesion are preferred.
- Preserve the slides immediately with fixative.

Complications
- Bleeding

✛ INTERPRETATION

Normal findings
- No malignant cells or abnormalities are present.

Abnormal results
- Cells with relatively large nuclei, only small amounts of cytoplasm, abnormal nuclear chromatin patterns, and marked variation in size, shape, and staining properties, with prominent nucleoli suggests malignancy.
- Atypical but non-malignant cells suggest a benign abnormality.
- Atypical cells may suggest dysplasia.
- Human papillomavirus (HPV) has been identified as a major risk factor for cervical cancer. A test is available that detects the types of HPV via their deoxyribonucleic acid. (See *Testing for cervical cancer.*)

TESTING FOR CERVICAL CANCER

ThinPrep test
Cervical cells for ThinPrep test analysis may be collected in the same manner as those of a Papanicolaou (Pap) test, using a cytobrush and plastic spatula. The specimens are deposited in a bottle provided with a fixative and sent to the laboratory. A filter is then inserted into the bottle, and excess mucus, blood, and inflammatory cells are filtered out by centrifuge. Remaining cells are then placed on a slide in a uniform, thin layer and read as a Pap test. This procedure causes fewer slides to be classified as unreadable, significantly reducing the incidence of false negatives and the need for repeat tests.

HPV DNA test
When using the ThinPrep test, screening can also be easily done for the human papillomavirus (HPV), of which certain strains have been identified as the primary cause of cervical cancer. The Digene hc2 HPV deoxyribonucleic acid (DNA) test has been approved by the U.S. Food and Drug Administration to determine if those identified at high risk for developing cervical cancer have been exposed to HPV. The specimen is collected as a Pap smear, but is dispersed with ThinPrep solution. Separate aliquots are used for each test, from brushings of the endocervix. The brush is then inserted into the specialized tube, snapped off at the shaft, and capped securely. The target solution in the tube disrupts the virus and releases target DNA, which combines with specific ribonucleic acid (RNA) probes creating RNA:DNA hybrids. The hybrids are captured, bound, and magnified and measured using a luminometer.

If the patient is found to be positive for HPV, she has been infected with the virus. Depending on the type of HPV found through DNA testing, the patient harboring high-risk HPV strains has a higher risk of developing cervical cancer. It's recommended that the patient undergo colposcopy, in which the cervix is viewed under a microscope and a biopsy is taken from the tissue sample.

Paracentesis

● OVERVIEW

- A method of obtaining samples of ascitic fluid for diagnostic and therapeutic purposes by insertion of a trocar and cannula through the abdominal wall
- May be performed using image-guidance
- Four-quadrant tap: aspiration of fluid from each quadrant of the abdomen to verify abdominal trauma and need for surgery
- Peritoneal fluid analysis: examination of gross appearance, red blood cell (RBC) and white blood cell (WBC) counts, cytologic studies, microbiological studies for bacteria and fungi, and determinations of protein, glucose, amylase, ammonia, and alkaline phosphatase levels

Purpose
- To determine cause of ascites
- To detect abdominal trauma
- To remove accumulated ascitic fluid

Patient preparation
- Make sure the patient has signed an appropriate consent form.
- Note and report all allergies.
- Restriction of food and fluids before the test isn't necessary.
- Inform the patient that a local anesthetic will be used.
- If the patient has severe ascites, inform him that the procedure will relieve his discomfort and allow him to breathe easier.
- Advise the patient that a blood sample may be taken for laboratory analysis.

TEACHING POINTS
Be sure to cover:
- purpose of study and how it's done
- who will perform the test and where
- that the test takes 45 to 60 minutes.

▶ PROCEDURE

- Obtain baseline vital signs, weight, and abdominal girth measurements.
- The patient is positioned in a chair or in bed in high Fowler's position.
- The puncture site is prepared and draped.

- A local anesthetic is injected.
- The needle or trocar and cannula are inserted, usually 1″ to 2″ (2.5 to 5 cm) below the umbilicus, or in each quadrant of the abdomen.
- Fluid samples are aspirated.
- Specimens are placed in appropriately labeled containers.
- The trocar or needle is removed and a dressing applied.

Postprocedure care
- Resume previous activity as ordered.
- Administer I.V. infusions and albumin as ordered.

MONITORING
- Vital signs
- Intake and output
- Puncture site and drainage
- Daily weight
- Daily abdominal girth measurement
- Bleeding
- Infection
- Hematuria, which may indicate bladder trauma
- Serum electrolyte (especially sodium) and protein levels

🔲 **NURSING ALERT** If a large amount of fluid was removed, watch for signs of vascular collapse (tachycardia, tachypnea, hypotension, dizziness, and mental status changes).

🔲 **NURSING ALERT** Watch for signs and symptoms of hemorrhage and shock and for increasing pain and abdominal tenderness. These may indicate a perforated intestine or, depending on the site of the tap, puncture of the inferior epigastric artery, hematoma of the anterior cecal wall, or puncture of the iliac vein or bladder.

🔲 **NURSING ALERT** Observe the patient with severe hepatic disease for signs of hepatic coma, which may result from loss of sodium and potassium accompanying hypovolemia. Watch for mental status changes, drowsiness, and stupor. Such a patient is also prone to uremia, infection, hemorrhage, and protein depletion.

Precautions
- Paracentesis is contraindicated in pregnancy and in bleeding tendencies.

Complications
- Bleeding, hemorrhage
- Infection

- Bladder trauma
- Shock
- Perforated intestine
- Inferior epigastric artery puncture
- Anterior cecal wall hematoma
- Iliac vein puncture

✛ INTERPRETATION

Normal findings
- Peritoneal fluid is odorless and clear to pale yellow.

Abnormal results
- Milk-colored fluid may indicate chylous ascites.
- Bloody fluid may indicate:
  - benign or malignant tumor
  - hemorrhagic pancreatitis
  - perforated intestine or duodenal ulcer
  - traumatic injury.
- Cloudy or turbid fluid may indicate peritonitis or an infectious process.
- RBC count greater than 100/µl (SI, > 100/L) suggests possible neoplasm or tuberculosis.
- RBC count greater than 100,000/µl (SI, > 100,000/L) suggests intra-abdominal trauma.
- WBC count greater than 300/µl, with more than 25% neutrophils, suggests possible spontaneous bacterial peritonitis or cirrhosis.
- A high percentage of lymphocytes suggests tuberculous peritonitis or chylous ascites.
- A protein ascitic fluid/serum ratio of > 0.5 or a lactate dehydrogenase ascitic fluid/serum ratio > 0.6 suggests malignant, tuberculous, or pancreatic ascites.
- Protein levels rise above 3 g/dl (SI, > 3 g/L) in malignancy and above 4 g/dl (SI, > 4 g/L) in tuberculosis.
- An albumin gradient between ascitic fluid and serum greater than 1 g/dl (SI, > 1 g/L) indicates chronic hepatic disease.
- Gram-positive cocci commonly indicate primary peritonitis; gram-negative organisms indicate secondary peritonitis.
- Fungi may indicate histoplasmosis, candidiasis, or coccidioidomycosis.

Percutaneous transhepatic cholangiography

● OVERVIEW

- Fluoroscopic examination of the biliary ducts after injection of an iodinated contrast medium directly into a biliary radicle
- Used in patients with previous gastrointestinal surgery and endoscopically inaccessible bilio-enteric anastomosis to perform a contrast study of the biliary ducts
- May be performed for unsuccessful endoscopic cholangiopancreatography
- Also called PTHC

Purpose
- To evaluate upper abdominal pain after cholecystectomy
- To evaluate patients with severe jaundice
- To distinguish between obstructive and nonobstructive jaundice
- To determine location, extent and, in many cases, cause of mechanical obstruction

Patient preparation
- Make sure the patient has signed an appropriate consent form.
- Note and report all allergies.
- Check the patient's history for abnormal coagulation study results
- Check the patient's history for hypersensitivity to iodine, seafood, the local anesthetic, and iodinated contrast media.
- Fasting is required for 8 hours before the test.
- Explain the possible need for a laxative the night before and a cleansing enema the morning of the test.
- Explain the need to use a local anesthetic and I.V. sedation.
- Possible transient pain as the liver capsule is entered.
- Warn the patient that injection of the contrast medium may cause a sensation of pressure and epigastric fullness.

◆ **NURSING ALERT** In patients with severely disturbed coagulation, transjugular needle cholangiography should be considered.

TEACHING POINTS
Be sure to cover:
- the purpose of the study and how it's done

- who will perform the test and where
- that the test takes about 1 to 2 hours.

▶ PROCEDURE

- Preprocedure antibiotics are administered if ordered.
- Sedation and analgesia are administered if ordered.
- The patient is positioned supine on the table.
- Right upper quadrant of the abdomen is prepared and draped.
- The skin, subcutaneous tissue, and liver capsule are infiltrated with local anesthetic.
- A flexible needle is inserted, under fluoroscopic guidance, through the 10th or 11th intercostal space at the right midclavicular line.
- A contrast medium is injected.
- Spot films of significant findings are taken in various views.
- A drainage tube may be inserted to allow percutaneous drainage of bile, if dilated ducts are due to obstruction.
- An internal stent may be inserted to allow bile drainage into the bowel, when the dilation and inflammation have diminished.

Postprocedure care
- Apply sterile dressing to puncture site.
- Enforce bed rest, as ordered, for at least 6 hours with patient lying on right side.
- Resume usual diet, as ordered.

MONITORING
- Vital signs
- Intake and output
- Insertion site
- Bleeding
- Infection
- Drainage

◆ **NURSING ALERT** Check the puncture site for bleeding, swelling, and tenderness. Watch for signs and symptoms of peritonitis: chills, temperature of 102° to 103° F (38.9° to 39.4° C), and abdominal pain, tenderness, and distention. Notify the doctor immediately if such complications develop.

Precautions
- Contraindications include: cholangitis, massive ascites, uncorrected coag-

ulopathy, or hypersensitivity to iodine; pregnancy because of the possible teratogenic effects of radiation.
- The possible adverse effects of contrast agents may also accompany intraductal injection.

Complications
- Adverse effects of iodinated contrast media
- Adverse effects of sedation
- Pneumothorax
- Vasovagal reactions
- Peritonitis
- Bleeding
- Infection or sepsis
- Bile leakage

✥ INTERPRETATION

Normal findings
- Biliary ducts are of normal diameter and appear as regular channels homogeneously filled with contrast medium.

Abnormal results
- Dilated biliary ducts may suggest:
  - cholelithiasis
  - biliary tract cancer
  - cancer of the pancreas
  - cancer of the ampulla of Vater.
- Persistent filling defects may suggest calculi.
- A short and irregular stricture, commonly producing a rat-tail appearance with gross dilation of the proximal ducts, may suggest pancreatic or biliary carcinoma.
- Diffuse intrahepatic and extrahepatic stricture may suggest advanced sclerosing cholangitis or infiltrating cholangiocarcinoma.
- Ducts filled with debris, with possible abscesses of various size in communication with the ducts, may suggest acute suppurative cholangitis.

pH test, 24-hour

● OVERVIEW

- Also known as a 24-hour ambulatory pH monitoring study
- Most sensitive indicator of gastric reflux
- Currently considered the gold standard to diagnose or confirm a diagnosis of gastroesophageal reflux disease
- New method of measuring esophageal pH using a small capsule (see *Monitoring pH with the Bravo System*)

Purpose
- To measure esophageal pH for a total of 24 hours, while a probe is in place
- To determine presence of gastroesophageal reflux
- To evaluate control of gastroesophageal reflux while on proton pump inhibition
- To determine if reflux episodes can be correlated to symptoms such as chest pain

Patient preparation
- Make sure the patient has signed an appropriate consent form.
- Note and report all allergies.
- Explain the need for fasting and the avoidance of cigarette smoking after midnight the night before test.
- Advise that the patient may experience slight discomfort and possible gagging or coughing during probe insertion.
- Explain the need for possible withholding of certain GI medications.
- If performed to document reflux, explain the need for withholding of certain medications including all proton pump inhibitors generally for 7 days before the procedure. Other medications that may be withheld include histamine-2 receptor antagonists, calcium channel blockers, beta-blockers, metoclopramide, erythromycin, nitroglycerin, belladonna alkaloids/phenobarbital, hyoscyamine sulfate, and bethanechol. These medications are generally discontinued for at least 48 hours before the procedure.
- If being done to document adequacy of control with proton pump inhibition (PPI), explain the need for fasting after midnight and resumption of routine medications including PPI after probe placement.

TEACHING POINTS
Be sure to cover:
- the purpose of the study and how it's done
- who will perform the test and where
- that the test takes up to 15 minutes
- the need for keeping a diary while the probe is in place.

▷ PROCEDURE

- The patient is placed in high Fowler's position.
- A probe, with a pH electrode, is inserted gently into one of his nostrils.
- The probe is advanced to the lower esophageal sphincter.
- After it's appropriately placed, the probe is taped to his cheek and placed behind his ear with the unit attached to the recorder.
- The patient is instructed when to return to have the probe removed.

Postprocedure care
- Resume usual diet and medications as ordered.
- Schedule a return visit in 24 hours for probe removal.

MONITORING
- Comfort level
- Respiratory status

Precautions
- Failure to withhold certain medications may alter test results.
- Use caution in a patient with uncorrected coagulopathies or nasal anatomical abnormalities.

◆ **NURSING ALERT** During probe insertion, the catheter may inadvertently enter the trachea; if respiratory distress or paroxysmal coughing occurs, remove the catheter immediately.

Complications
- Inadvertent positioning of the probe into the trachea
- Epitaxis (rare)

✛ INTERPRETATION

Normal findings
- A pH less than 4.0 occurs less than 4% of the total 24 hours.

Abnormal results
- A pH of less than 4.0 occurring more than 4% of the total 24 hours suggests gastroesophageal reflux disease.

MONITORING pH WITH THE BRAVO SYSTEM

Traditional testing for esophageal acid levels typically uses an esophageal catheter that's inserted for a 24-hour period. Recently, a new technique called the Bravo pH monitoring system was developed to measure acid levels in the esophagus via a capsule (about the size of a gel cap). The capsule is temporarily attached to the patient's esophageal wall using an endoscope and collects pH data, which are transmitted to a pager-sized receiver that the patient wears. Data are collected for 48 hours, downloaded from the receiver, and analyzed with special software.

The Bravo method is more accurate than catheter methods because the patient can eat normally and maintain regular activities during testing. The additional 24 hours also provides more information for diagnosing certain esophageal disorders.

In 7 to 10 days, the capsule spontaneously detaches from the esophageal wall and is passed through the patient's digestive system.

Pleural biopsy

● OVERVIEW

- Removal of a sample of pleural tissue by needle biopsy or open biopsy for histologic examination
- Percutaneous needle pleural biopsy: performed under local anesthesia; frequently done using image-guidance
- Open pleural biopsy: performed in the operating room; permits direct visualization of the pleura and the underlying lung

Purpose
- To differentiate between nonmalignant and malignant disease
- To diagnose viral, fungal, or parasitic disease
- To diagnose collagen vascular disease of the pleura

Patient preparation
- Make sure the patient has signed an appropriate consent form.
- Note and report all allergies.
- Explain the need for fasting before the biopsy.
- Advise the patient that chest X-rays will be taken before and after the biopsy.
- Explain the administration of an anesthetic.
- Provide reassurance that the patient should experience minimal pain.

TEACHING POINTS
Be sure to cover:
- the purpose of the study and how it's done
- who will perform the biopsy and where
- that the test takes 30 to 45 minutes.

▶ PROCEDURE

PERCUTANEOUS PLEURAL BIOPSY
- Patient is positioned based on biopsy location.
- The skin site is cleaned and prepared.
- A local anesthetic is administered.
- The needle or trocar is inserted through the appropriate intercostal space into the biopsy site. (See *Using Cope's needle*.)
- The specimen is withdrawn and immediately put in 10% neutral buffered

formalin solution in a labeled specimen bottle.
- The skin around the biopsy site is cleaned and dressed.

Postprocedure care
- Obtain a chest X-ray immediately after the biopsy.
- Resume previous diet and activity as ordered.

MONITORING
- Vital signs
- Intake and output
- Pulse oximetry
- Respiratory status
- Breath sounds
- Subcutaneous emphysema

◆ **NURSING ALERT** Watch for signs and symptoms of pneumothorax, such as dyspnea, pleuritic chest pain, apprehension, agitation, decreased breath sounds, tracheal deviation, subcutaneous emphysema, or signs of decreased cardiac output.

Precautions
- Contraindications include:
  – uncorrected severe bleeding disorders
  – patients requiring mechanical ventilation.

Complications
- Pneumothorax
- Hemorrhage
- Vasovagal reaction
- Infection

✛ INTERPRETATION

Normal findings
- Pleura consists primarily of mesothelial cells, flattened in a uniform layer.
- Layers of areolar connective tissue contain blood vessels, nerves, and lymphatics.

Abnormal results
- Lesions that are fibrous and epithelial suggest primary neoplasms.
- Specific histologic results from tissue analysis suggest possible disorders including:
  – malignant disease
  – tuberculosis
  – viral, fungal, parasitic disease
  – collagen vascular disease.

USING COPE'S NEEDLE

Cope's needle, which is used to obtain a pleural biopsy specimen, consists of three parts: a sharp obturator (A) and a cannula (B), which when fitted together are called a trocar, and a blunt-ended, hooked stylet (C). The trocar is used to gain access to the pleural cavity. Then the obturator is removed, leaving the cannula in place. The stylet is passed through the cannula to excise a tissue specimen, as shown below.

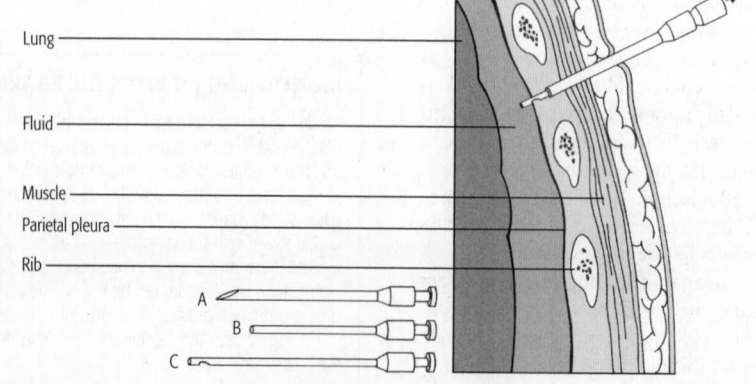

Positron emission tomography

● OVERVIEW

- Nuclear medicine scan that measures the metabolic process of the organ being observed
- Radioactive chemicals administered to patient; positrons emitted from the chemicals in organs are detected by sensors placed around patient during the scan
- Positron counts, with computed tomography, helping record the image of the organ in a two- or three-dimensional image
- Yields information about anatomy and physiology of an organ by demonstrating glucose metabolism, blood flow, tissue perfusion, and oxygenation of a specific area
- Used mostly in cardiology, neurology, and oncology
- Also known as *PET*

Purpose

- To detect strokes or aneurysms by decreased blood flow and oxygen consumption
- To diagnose Parkinson's disease and Huntington's disease based on decreased cerebral metabolism
- To evaluate cranial tumor preoperatively and postoperatively to help determine treatment
- To assess the size of myocardial infarcts
- To assess the presence of coronary artery disease as seen by decreased metabolism during ischemia and after angina
- To evaluate the presence or recurrence of cancer or tumors
- To evaluate the presence of metastases of a cancerous tumor
- To monitor the effectiveness of therapy

Patient preparation

- Make sure the patient has signed an appropriate consent form.
- Instruct him to void before beginning the test.
- If the patient has diabetes, have him take his insulin at the usual time and eat a meal 4 hours before the test.
- Have all other patients fast for 4 hours before the test and avoid alcohol, caffeine, and tobacco for 24 hours before the test.
- Warn him not to take a sedative or tranquilizer before the test.

TEACHING POINTS

Be sure to cover:
- the purpose of the study and how it's done
- who will perform the test and where
- need for two I.V. access sites
- that exposure to radioactive material will be minimal.
- that the test takes 45 to 90 minutes.

▶ PROCEDURE

- Position the patient, as appropriate, for the organs to be scanned.
- Radioactive material is injected through an I.V. line.
- The gamma rays that are able to penetrate the tissue are recorded outside the body by a series of detectors and are displayed on a computer screen.
- If the patient is having a brain scan done, he may be asked to perform a series of cognitive activities.
- The imaging is done at periodic intervals for up to 1 hour.

Postprocedure care

- Remove the I.V. access, as ordered.
- Have the patient increase his fluid intake for 24 to 48 hours to help flush the radionuclide from the body, unless otherwise ordered.

MONITORING

- I.V. access site for swelling, hematoma, or redness
- Adverse reactions to radioactive agent

Precautions

- Gloves must be worn when handling the radionuclide.
- Have emergency resuscitation equipment available during the procedures in case the patient experiences a reaction to the radioactive agent.

Complications

- I.V. infiltration
- Reaction to the radioactive agents

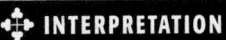 INTERPRETATION

Normal findings

- Normal organ anatomy and physiology, including tissue metabolism, oxygenation, and blood flow, are noted.

Abnormal results

- Abnormalities vary depending on the organ being scanned.
- A brain scan will show abnormalities including strokes, metastasis, dementia, head trauma, migraines, seizure disorders, and tumors.
- Cardiac scan abnormalities indicate necrotic tissue, hypertrophic left ventricle, myocardial ischemia, pulmonary edema, and chronic obstructive pulmonary disease.
- Increased radionuclide uptake is seen in abnormal lymph nodes, tumors, and metastasis.

Proctosigmoidoscopy

⬤ OVERVIEW

- Endoscopic examination of the lining of the distal sigmoid colon, the rectum, and the anal canal
- Involves three separate steps: digital examination, sigmoidoscopy, and proctoscopy
- Specimens obtained from suspicious areas of the mucosa by biopsy, lavage or cytology brush, or culture swab

Purpose

- To aid diagnosis of inflammatory, infectious, and ulcerative bowel disease
- To diagnose hemorrhoids, hypertrophic anal papilla, polyps, fissures, fistulas, and abscesses within the rectum and anal canal
- To evaluate recent changes in bowel habits, lower abdominal and perineal pain, prolapse on defecation, pruritus ani, or passage of mucus, blood, or pus in the stool

Patient preparation

- Make sure the patient has signed an appropriate consent form.
- Note and report all allergies.
- Check the patient's history for barium tests within the past week.
- Warn about a possible urge to defecate during insertion of the scope.
- Instruct the patient to maintain a clear liquid diet for 24 to 48 hours before the test as ordered.
- Explain the need for fasting the morning of the procedure if ordered.
- Explain the need for administration of an enema 3 to 4 hours before the procedure as ordered.
- Advise the patient that air may be introduced through the endoscope to distend the walls of the intestine. Flatus may escape around the endoscope and he shouldn't attempt to control it.
- Warn about possible blood in the stool if a biopsy or polypectomy is performed.
- Explain the need for sedation administration to help the patient relax.

TEACHING POINTS

Be sure to cover:
- the purpose of the study and how it's done
- who will perform the test and where
- that the test takes 15 to 30 minutes.

▶ PROCEDURE

- The patient is placed in a knee-to-chest or left lateral position with his knees flexed.
- The patient is asked to breathe deeply and slowly through his mouth.
- A well-lubricated, gloved index finger is inserted into the anus.
- The anal canal is palpated for induration and tenderness.
- The rectal mucosa is palpated.
- The sigmoidoscope is inserted into the anus and passed through the anal sphincters, anal canal and into the rectum.
- At the rectosigmoid junction, a small amount of air may be insufflated to open the bowel lumen.
- The scope is advanced to its full length into the distal sigmoid colon.
- As the sigmoidoscope is slowly withdrawn, air is carefully insufflated and the intestinal mucosa is thoroughly examined.
- Specimens may be obtained from a suspicious area of the intestinal mucosa.
- Polyps may be removed for histologic examination by insertion of an electrocautery snare through the sigmoidoscope.
- After the sigmoidoscope is withdrawn, the proctoscope is inserted through the anus and gently advanced to its full length.
- After examination, the proctoscope is withdrawn.

Postprocedure care

- Resume previous diet and activity when fully awake as ordered.

MONITORING

- Vital signs
- Intake and output
- Abdominal distention
- Bowel sounds
- Stools
- Bleeding

◉ **NURSING ALERT** Observe the patient closely for signs of bowel perforation (abdominal distention and pain, nausea, vomiting, and fever) and for vasovagal reaction (hypotension, pallor, diaphoresis, and bradycardia). Notify the doctor immediately if such signs or symptoms develop.

Precautions

- In general, anticoagulant therapy isn't a contraindication for this procedure (with or without a biopsy) because the procedure is considered low-risk for those who need to maintain an International Normalized Ratio between 1.5 and 2.5.
- Aspirin and most nonsteroidal anti-inflammatory drugs in standard doses don't generally increase the risk of significant bleeding.
- The presence of barium in the colon from previous barium studies makes accurate examination impossible.

Complications

- Rectal bleeding
- Bowel perforation

✤ INTERPRETATION

Normal findings

- The mucosa of the sigmoid colon appears light pink-orange and is marked by semilunar folds and deep tubular pits.
- The rectal mucosa appears redder because of its rich vascular network, deepens to a purple hue at the pectinate line (the anatomic division between the rectum and anus), and has three distinct valves.
- The lower two-thirds of the anus (anoderm) is lined with smooth gray-tan skin and joins with the hair-fringed perianal skin.

Abnormal results

- Biopsy results may suggest the presence of malignant tumors.
- Inflammatory changes suggest possible ulcerative and ischemic colitis.
- Visual examination and palpation are used to disclose possible abnormalities of the anal canal and rectum, including:
  - internal and external hemorrhoids
  - hypertrophic anal papillae
  - anal fissures and fistulas
  - anorectal abscesses.

Prostate gland biopsy

● OVERVIEW

- Needle excision of a prostate tissue specimen for histologic examination
- Three possible approaches: perineal, transrectal, or transurethral; transrectal approach usually for high prostatic lesions

Purpose
- To confirm prostate cancer
- To determine cause of prostatic hypertrophy

Patient preparation
- Make sure the patient has signed an appropriate consent form.
- Note and report all allergies.
- For a transrectal approach, administer enemas until the return is clear as ordered.
- Administer antibiotics as ordered.
- Administer a sedative before study as ordered.
- Explain the need to use a local anesthetic.
- Depending on the approach used, the patient may need to fast for 6 to 8 hours before the test.

TEACHING POINTS
Be sure to cover:
- the purpose of the study and how it's done
- who will perform the biopsy and where
- that the test takes less than 30 minutes.

▶ PROCEDURE

PERINEAL APPROACH
- The patient is placed in the left lateral, knee-chest, or lithotomy position.
- The perineal skin is cleansed and prepared.
- A 2-mm incision is made into the perineum.
- The biopsy needle is introduced into a prostate lobe.
- Specimens are obtained from several different areas of the prostate.
- Specimens are placed immediately in a labeled specimen bottle containing 10% formalin solution.
- Hemostasis is obtained, and a dressing applied.

TRANSRECTAL APPROACH
- The patient is placed in a left lateral position.
- A curved needle guide (or a spring powered device for cone biopsy) is attached to the finger palpating the rectum.
- The biopsy needle is pushed along the guide, into the prostate.
- The needle is rotated to cut the tissue and withdrawn.

TRANSURETHRAL APPROACH
- An endoscopic instrument with a cutting loop is passed through the urethra.
- The endoscope permits direct viewing of the prostate and passage of a cutting loop.
- Specimens are obtained and placed immediately in a labeled specimen bottle containing 10% formalin solution.

Postprocedure care
- Administer analgesics as ordered.
- Gradually resume normal diet and activity as tolerated.

MONITORING
- Vital signs
- Intake and output
- Urinary retention
- Bleeding
- Infection
- Biopsy site
- Hematuria

◆ **NURSING ALERT** Observe the biopsy site for and immediately report hematoma and signs of infection, such as redness, swelling, and pain.

Precautions
- Failure to obtain an adequate tissue specimen may affect accuracy of results.
- Check the patient's history for reaction to anesthetics.

◆ **NURSING ALERT** Watch for and immediately report urinary retention, frequency, or hematuria.

Complications
- Bleeding into the prostatic urethra and bladder
- Infection
- Urinary retention

✛ INTERPRETATION

Normal findings
- The prostate gland normally consists of a thin, fibrous capsule surrounding the stroma, which is made up of elastic and connective tissues and smooth-muscle fibers.
- The epithelial glands, found in these tissues and muscle fibers, drain into the chief excreting ducts.
- No cancer cells are present.

Abnormal results
- Increased acid phosphatase levels suggest possible metastatic prostate cancer.
- Low acid phosphatase levels suggest possible cancer that is confined to the prostatic capsule.
- Histologic examination of the tissue reveals various possible disorders, including:
  – prostate, rectal, and bladder cancer
  – benign prostatic hyperplasia
  – prostatitis
  – tuberculosis
  – lymphomas.

Pulmonary angiography

● OVERVIEW

- Radiographic examination of the pulmonary circulation after injection of a radiopaque contrast agent into the pulmonary artery or one of its branches
- May be used to diagnose pulmonary embolism when lung ventilation perfusion scans are indeterminate
- May be performed to administer local thrombolytic therapy in patients with pulmonary embolism (PE)
- Also known as *pulmonary arteriography*

Purpose

- To detect pulmonary embolism in a symptomatic patient with an equivocal lung scan
- To evaluate pulmonary circulation abnormalities
- To provide accurate preoperative evaluation of patients with shunt physiology caused by congenital heart disease
- To treat identified PE with thrombolysis

Patient preparation

- Make sure the patient has signed an appropriate consent form.
- Note and report all allergies.
- Check the patient's history for hypersensitivity to iodine, seafood, or iodinated contrast agents.
- Check for and report history of anticoagulation.
- Check for and report history of renal insufficiency.
- Note and inform the doctor of any abnormal laboratory results.
- Discontinue heparin infusion 3 to 4 hours before the test as ordered.
- Fasting is required for 8 hours before the test or as ordered.
- Explain the need to use a local anesthetic.
- Warn about a possible urge to cough, flushed feeling, or salty taste for 3 to 5 minutes after the injection.

TEACHING POINTS

Be sure to cover:
- the purpose of the study and how it's done
- who will perform the test and where
- that the test takes about 1½ to 2 hours

- that the patient will be monitored during the study.

▶ PROCEDURE

- The patient is placed in a supine position.
- The access site, usually the right groin, is cleaned and prepared.
- A local anesthetic is injected.
- The vein is accessed and a catheter is introduced under image-guidance.
- The catheter is advanced through the right atrium, the right ventricle, and into the pulmonary artery.
- Pulmonary artery pressures are measured and blood samples may be drawn from various regions of the pulmonary circulation.
- The contrast agent is injected and images are obtained.
- Thrombolysis is initiated if indicated.
- After the catheter is removed, hemostasis is obtained.
- The access site is cleaned and dressed.

Postprocedure care

- Maintain bed rest for 6 hours, as ordered.
- Resume usual diet, as ordered.
- Restart anticoagulation, as ordered.
- Encourage oral fluid intake, or administer I.V. fluids, as ordered, to help eliminate the contrast agent.

MONITORING

- Vital signs
- Intake and output
- Catheter insertion site
- Bleeding
- Infection
- Hematoma formation
- Renal function studies
- Adverse reaction to contrast agent

◈ **NURSING ALERT** Observe the site for bleeding and swelling. If these occur, maintain pressure at the insertion site for at least 10 minutes and notify the radiologist.

Precautions

- Pulmonary angiography is contraindicated during pregnancy.
- Ventricular arrhythmias may be caused by passage of the catheter through the heart chambers.

Complications

- Myocardial perforation or rupture
- Ventricular arrhythmias and conduction defects
- Acute renal failure
- Bleeding and hematoma formation
- Infection
- Adverse reaction to contrast agent
- Cardiac valve damage
- Right-sided heart failure

✛ INTERPRETATION

Normal findings

- The contrast agent should flow symmetrically and without interruption through the pulmonary circulation.

Abnormal results

- Interruption of blood flow and filling defects suggests possible acute pulmonary embolism.
- Arterial webs, stenoses, irregular occlusions, wall-scalloping, and "pouching" defects (a concave edge of thrombus facing the opacified lumen) suggest chronic pulmonary embolism.

Pulmonary artery catheterization

● OVERVIEW

- Uses a balloon-tipped, flow-directed catheter to provide intermittent occlusion of the pulmonary artery
- Permits measurement of pulmonary artery pressure (PAP) and pulmonary artery wedge pressure (PAWP)
- PAWP: generally accurately reflects left atrial pressure and left ventricular end-diastolic pressure
- Also known as *Swan-Ganz catheterization*

Purpose

- To assess right- and left-sided heart failure
- To monitor therapy for complications of acute myocardial infarction
- To monitor fluid status in patients with serious burns, renal disease, noncardiogenic pulmonary edema, or adult respiratory distress syndrome
- To establish baseline pressures preoperatively in patients with existing cardiac disease
- To differentiate between noncardiac and cardiac pulmonary edema
- To monitor the effects of cardiovascular drugs

Patient preparation

- Make sure the patient has signed an appropriate consent form.
- Note and report all allergies.
- Explain the use of a local anesthetic.
- Explain that the catheter will remain in place, causing little or no discomfort, for 48 to 72 hours.

TEACHING POINTS

Be sure to cover:
- the purpose of the study and how it's done
- who will perform the test and where
- that the test takes about 30 minutes.

▶ PROCEDURE

- The patient is placed in a supine position with his head and shoulders slightly lower than his trunk.
- The catheter is introduced into the vein percutaneously.
- The catheter is directed into the right atrium.

- The catheter balloon is partially inflated.
- Venous flow carries the catheter tip through the right atrium and tricuspid valve into the right ventricle and into the pulmonary artery.
- The monitor is observed for characteristic pressure waveform changes as the catheter enters each heart chamber.

◉ NURSING ALERT As the catheter is passed into the chambers on the right side of the heart, the monitor screen is observed for frequent premature ventricular contractions, ventricular tachycardia, and other arrhythmias. If arrhythmias occur, the catheter may be partially withdrawn or medication administered to suppress the arrhythmias.

RECORDING PAWP

- The catheter balloon is carefully inflated with the specified amount of air (no more than 1.5 cc), until a PAWP waveform is obtained.
- After PAWP is recorded, the air from the balloon is allowed to return to the syringe.
- The monitor screen is observed for a PA waveform.
- The catheter may be sutured to the skin and a dressing applied.

◉ NURSING ALERT The balloon catheter shouldn't be overinflated, which could distend the pulmonary artery, causing vessel rupture. If the balloon can't be fully deflated after recording the PAWP, it shouldn't be reinflated unless the physician is present; balloon rupture can cause a life-threatening air embolism.

Postprocedure care

- Obtain a chest X-ray to verify proper catheter placement and to assess for complications such as pneumothorax.
- After each PAWP reading, make sure the balloon is completely deflated.
- Notify the doctor if difficulty in flushing the system is encountered.
- Maintain 300 mm Hg pressure in the pressure bag to permit 3 to 6 ml/hour fluid flow to flush the system continuously.

◉ NURSING ALERT If a damped waveform occurs, the catheter may need to be withdrawn slightly. Pulmonary infarct can occur if the catheter is allowed to remain in a wedged position

MONITORING

- Vital signs
- Cardiac arrhythmias
- PAP and PAWP pressures and waveforms
- Right atrial and right ventricular pressures and waveforms
- Cardiac output
- Infection of insertion site
- Bleeding

◉ NURSING ALERT Watch for signs and symptoms of pulmonary emboli, pulmonary artery perforation, and arrhythmias.

Precautions

- Pulmonary artery catheterization is performed cautiously in a patient with left bundle-branch block or an implanted pacemaker.

✛ INTERPRETATION

Normal findings

- Right atrial (RA) pressure is 1 to 6 mm Hg.
- Right ventricular (RV) systolic pressure is 20 to 30 mm Hg.
- RV diastolic pressure is less than 5 mm Hg.
- Systolic PAP is 20 to 30 mm Hg.
- Diastolic PAP is 10 to 15 mm Hg.
- Mean PAP is less than 20 mm Hg.
- PAWP is 6 to 12 mm Hg.
- Left atrial pressure is 10 mm Hg.

Abnormal results

- Elevated RA pressures may suggest pulmonary disease, right-sided heart failure, fluid overload, or cardiac tamponade.
- Elevated RV pressures may suggest pulmonary hypertension, pulmonary valvular stenosis, right-sided heart failure, pericardial effusion, or ventricular septal defects.
- Elevated PAP may suggest atrial or ventricular septal defects, pulmonary hypertension, mitral stenosis, chronic obstructive pulmonary disease, pulmonary edema or embolus, or left-sided heart failure.
- Elevated PAWP may suggest left-sided heart failure or cardiac tamponade.
- Decreased PAWP may suggest hypovolemia.

Pulmonary function tests

● OVERVIEW

- Evaluation of pulmonary function through a series of spirometric measurements
- Also known as *PFTs*

Purpose
- To assess effectiveness of a specific therapeutic regimen
- To differentiate between obstructive and restrictive pulmonary disease
- To evaluate pulmonary status before surgery
- To stage a disease process
- To determine disability
- To assess diffusion capacity
- To evaluate baseline function as part of screening for certain occupations

Patient preparation
- Make sure the patient has signed an appropriate consent form.
- Note and report all allergies.
- Withhold bronchodilators for 8 hours.
- Stress the need to avoid a heavy meal before the tests.
- Stress the need to avoid smoking for 12 hours before the tests.
- Tell the patient to wear loose clothing.
- Provide reassurance that the procedure is painless and the patient can rest between tests.

TEACHING POINTS
Be sure to cover:
- the purpose of the study and how it's done
- who will perform the test and where
- that the study takes 1 to 2 hours.

▶ PROCEDURE

TIDAL VOLUME
- The patient breathes normally into the mouthpiece 10 times.

EXPIRATORY RESERVE VOLUME
- The patient breathes normally for several breaths and then exhales as completely as possible.

VITAL CAPACITY
- The patient inhales as deeply as possible and exhales into the mouthpiece as completely as possible. Repeat three times; result showing the largest volume is used.

INSPIRATORY CAPACITY
- The patient breathes normally for several breaths and inhales as deeply as possible.

FUNCTIONAL RESIDUAL CAPACITY
- The patient breathes normally into a spirometer. After a few breaths, the concentrations of gas in the spirometer and the lungs reach equilibrium. The functional residual capacity (FRC) is calculated by subtracting the spirometer volume from the original volume.

FORCED VITAL CAPACITY AND FORCED EXPIRATORY VOLUME
- The patient inhales as slowly and deeply as possible and then exhales into the mouthpiece as quickly and completely as possible. Repeated three times; largest volume is recorded. The volume of air expired at 1 second (FEV_1), at 2 seconds (FEV_2), and at 3 seconds (FEV_3) during all three repetitions is recorded.

MAXIMAL VOLUNTARY VENTILATION
- The patient breathes into the mouthpiece as quickly and deeply as possible for 15 seconds.

DIFFUSING CAPACITY FOR CARBON MONOXIDE
- The patient inhales a gas mixture with a low concentration of carbon monoxide and holds his breath for 10 to 15 seconds before exhaling.

Postprocedure care
- Resume medications, diet, and activities as ordered.

MONITORING
- Respiratory status

Precautions
- Accuracy of the study may be diminished with chest pain, abdominal pain, or cough.

  ◆ **NURSING ALERT** Pulmonary function tests may be contraindicated in patients with acute coronary insufficiency, angina, or recent myocardial infarction. Watch for respiratory distress, changes in pulse rate; blood pressure, coughing, and bronchospasm.

Complications
- Respiratory distress
- Bronchospasm
- Physical exhaustion

✛ INTERPRETATION

Normal findings
- Normal values are predicted for each patient based on age, height, weight, and sex and are expressed as a percentage:
  - Tidal volume (V_T) is 5 to 7 mg/kg of body weight.
  - Expiratory reserve volume (ERV) is 25% of vital capacity (VC).
  - Inspiratory capacity (IC) is 75% of VC.
  - FEV_1 is 83% of VC after 1 second.
  - FEV_2 is 94% of VC after 2 seconds.
  - FEV_3 is 97% of VC after 3 seconds.

Abnormal results
- FEV_1 less than 80% suggests obstructed pulmonary disease.
- FEV_1/FVC ratio greater than 80% suggests restrictive pulmonary disease.
- Decreased V_T suggests possible restrictive disease.
- Decreased minute volume (MV) suggests possible disorders such as pulmonary edema.
- Increased MV suggests possible acidosis, exercise, or low compliance states.
- Reduced CO_2 response suggests possible emphysema, myxedema, obesity, hypoventilation syndrome, or sleep apnea.
- Residual volume greater than 35% of total lung capacity after maximal expiratory effort suggests obstructive disease.
- Decreased IC suggests restrictive disease.
- Increased FRC suggests possible obstructive pulmonary disease.
- Low total lung capacity (TLC) suggests restrictive disease.
- High TLC suggests obstructive disease.
- Decreased forced vital capacity suggests flow resistance from obstructive disease or from restrictive disease.
- Low forced expiratory flow suggests obstructive disease of the small and medium-sized airways.
- Decreased peak expiratory flow rate suggests upper airway obstruction.
- Decreased diffusing capacity for carbon monoxide suggests possible interstitial pulmonary disease.

Pure tone audiometry

OVERVIEW

- Provides a record of the lowest intensity levels at which a patient can hear a set of test tones about 50% of the time
- Test tones: introduced through earphones or a bone conduction vibrator
- Pure tones: have energy concentrated at discrete frequencies and are compared to established norms of various frequencies
- Octave frequencies used to obtain air conduction thresholds
- Comparison of air and bone conduction thresholds: suggests possible conductive, sensorineural, or mixed hearing loss but not the cause of the loss
- Pure tone average: suggests possible need for referral for evaluation of communication difficulties (see *Implications of pure tone average*)

Purpose
- To document patient's auditory acuity
- To determine the presence, type, and degree of hearing loss
- To assess communication abilities and rehabilitation needs
- To accurately determine pure tone and speech reception threshold

Patient preparation
- Make sure the patient has signed an appropriate consent form.
- Note and report all allergies.
- Obtain and document a complete aural history, including possible hearing loss, noise exposure, and use of hearing protection.
- Explain the importance of responding to even faint tones.
- Instruct the patient to remove all potential obstructions (such as earrings) to permit proper earphone placement.

TEACHING POINTS
Be sure to cover:
- the purpose of the study and how it's done
- who will perform the test and where
- that the test takes about 20 minutes.

PROCEDURE

- The ear canal is checked for impacted cerumen.
- Earphones are positioned and the headband is tightened.
- The examiner familiarizes the patient with the test tone by presenting it to his better ear a level 15 to 25 dB above the expected threshold to avoid cross-hearing.
- If the patient responds to the tone, air conduction testing is begun.
- After testing the better ear, the poorer ear is tested.
- In each ear, test or retest differences may be ±5 dB.
- For bone conduction testing, the earphones are removed, a small plastic vibrator is placed on the mastoid process.
- Ascending and descending tones are used as in air conduction testing, using 250 Hz, 500 Hz, 1,000 Hz, 2,000 Hz, and 4,000 Hz and 8,000 Hz.

Postprocedure care
- No specific posttest care is necessary.

Precautions
- False responses include failure to indicate when a tone has been heard or responding when no tone has been heard, which can be misleading and can influence interpretation of test results.
- If patient has been exposed to noises within the past 16 hours that are loud enough to cause tinnitus or make face-to-face communication difficult, postpone the test.
- Normal test results don't rule out pathology.
- Alcohol and other drugs can interfere with testing.
- The patient may feign results to receive compensation.

Complications
- None known

INTERPRETATION

Normal findings
- An audiogram displays frequency on the x-axis (horizontal) and dB of hearing loss on the y-axis (vertical).
- An adult's normal range of hearing sensitivity is −10 to +15 dB.

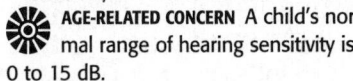 **AGE-RELATED CONCERN** A child's normal range of hearing sensitivity is 0 to 15 dB.

Abnormal results
- Depressed threshold responses for air and bone conduction tones suggest sensorineural loss.
- Depressed threshold responses for air and unchanged bone thresholds suggest conductive loss.
- Abnormal threshold responses for air and bone conduction tones, with air conduction more depressed than bone conduction, suggests mixed hearing loss.

IMPLICATIONS OF PURE TONE AVERAGE

The patient's pure tone average helps determine his degree of hearing loss as well as the audibility of speech in a quiet environment.

PURE TONE AVERAGE	DEGREE OF HEARING LOSS	SPEECH AUDIBILITY
0 to 25 dB	Normal limits	No significant difficulty
26 to 40 dB	Mild	Difficulty with faint or distant speech
41 to 55 dB	Moderate	Difficulty with conversational speech
56 to 70 dB	Moderately severe	Speech must be loud; difficulty with group conversation
71 to 90 dB	Severe	Difficulty with loud speech; understands only shouted or amplified speech
91+ dB	Profound	May not understand amplified speech

Purified protein derivative (PPD) testing

● OVERVIEW

- Screen for previous infection by the tubercle bacillus
- Performed when radiographic findings suggest tuberculosis (TB)
- Purified protein derivative (PPD) test: intradermal injection of tuberculin antigen that causes a delayed hypersensitivity reaction in patients with active or dormant TB
- Mantoux test: uses a single-needle intradermal injection of PPD, permitting precise dose measurement
- Multipuncture tests (such as the tine test, Mono-Vacc tests, and Aplitest): used for screening; intradermal injections with tines impregnated with PPD; require less skill and are more rapidly given; positive result confirmed by follow-up Mantoux test

Purpose
- To distinguish TB from blastomycosis, coccidioidomycosis, and histoplasmosis
- To identify people who need diagnostic investigation for TB because of possible exposure

Patient preparation
- Check the patient's history for active TB, the results of previous skin tests, and hypersensitivities.
- **◆ NURSING ALERT** If the patient has had TB, don't perform a skin test. Don't administer the skin test to patients who received the baciile Calmette-Guérin vaccine (commonly administered in other countries).
- If the patient has had a positive reaction to previous skin tests, consult the practitioner or follow facility policy.
- Tell the patient that the test requires an intradermal injection, which may cause him discomfort.
- Inform the patient that a positive reaction to a skin test appears as a red, hard, raised area at the injection site. Although the area may itch, instruct him not to scratch it.

TEACHING POINTS
Be sure to cover:
- purpose of the test and how it's done
- who will perform the test and where
- when to return to have the results read, as necessary

that a positive reaction doesn't always indicate active TB.

▶ PROCEDURE

- Confirm the patient's identity using two patient identifiers according to facility policy.
- Ask the patient to sit and support his extended arm on a flat surface.
- Clean the volar surface of the upper forearm with alcohol and allow the area to dry completely.

MANTOUX TEST
- Perform an intradermal injection.

MULTIPUNCTURE TEST
- Remove the protective cap on the injection device to expose the four tines.
- Hold the patient's forearm in one hand, stretching the skin of the forearm tightly.
- With your other hand, firmly depress the device into the patient's skin without twisting it.
- Hold the device in place for at least 1 second before removing it.
- If you've applied sufficient pressure, you'll see four puncture sites and a circular depression made by the device on the patient's skin.

Postprocedure care
- Record where the test was given, the date and time, and when the results are to be read.
- Expect to read tuberculin skin tests generally 48 to 72 hours after injection; the Mono-Vacc tests can be read 48 to 96 hours after the test.
- If an ulceration or necrosis develops at the injection site, apply cold soaks or a topical steroid.

MONITORING
- Injection site

Precautions
- Have epinephrine available to treat a possible anaphylactic or acute hypersensitivity reaction.
- Don't perform a skin test in areas with excessive hair, acne, or insufficient subcutaneous tissue, such as over a tendon or bone.
- Corticosteroids, other immunosuppressants, and live vaccine viruses (such as measles, mumps, rubella, and

polio within 4 to 6 weeks before the test) may suppress skin reaction.

Complications
- Ulceration or necrosis at the injection site
- Anaphylactic or acute hypersensitivity reaction

✛ INTERPRETATION

Normal findings
- In tuberculin skin tests, negative or minimal reactions are noted.
- In the Mantoux test, there's no induration or induration is less than 5 mm in diameter.
- In the tine test and Aplitest, there's no vesiculation or induration or induration is less than 2 mm in diameter.
- In the Mono-Vacc tests, there's no induration.

Abnormal results
- A positive tuberculin reaction indicates previous infection by tubercle bacilli. It doesn't distinguish between an active and a dormant infection or provide a definitive diagnosis.
- If a positive reaction occurs, sputum smear and culture and chest radiography are needed.
- In the Mantoux test, induration of 5 to 9 mm in diameter indicates a borderline reaction; larger induration, a positive reaction.
- Because patients infected with atypical mycobacteria, other than tubercle bacilli, may have borderline reactions, repeat testing is needed.
- In the tine test or Aplitest, vesiculation indicates a positive reaction; induration of 2 mm in diameter without vesiculation requires confirmation by the Mantoux test. Any induration in the Mono-Vacc tests indicates a positive reaction; this reaction should be confirmed by the Mantoux test.

Radioactive iodine uptake

● OVERVIEW

- Used to evaluate thyroid function by measuring the amount of orally ingested radioactive isotopes of iodine, ^{123}I or ^{131}I, that accumulate in the thyroid gland after 2, 6, and 24 hours
- Used to accurately diagnose hyperthyroidism (about 90%), but less accurate for hypothyroidism; also used to distinguish between permanent causes of hyperthyroidism (Grave's disease) and temporary causes such as thyroiditis
- Also known as *RAIU test*
- Perchlorate suppression test possibly used in addition to RAIU in patient with suspected Hashimoto's disease (see *Perchlorate suppression test*)

Purpose
- To evaluate thyroid function
- To aid diagnosis of hyperthyroidism or hypothyroidism
- To distinguish between primary and secondary thyroid disorders
- To differentiate Graves' disease from hyperfunctioning toxic adenoma, when performed concurrently with radionuclide thyroid imaging and the triiodothyronine resin uptake test

Patient preparation
- Make sure the patient has signed an appropriate consent form.
- Note and report all allergies.
- Check the patient history for past or present iodine exposure, including use of iodine preparations or thyroid medication, which may interfere with test results.
- Check for previous radiologic tests using contrast media or nuclear medicine procedures.
- Instruct the patient to fast from midnight before the test
- Provide reassurance that the study is painless.

TEACHING POINTS
Be sure to cover:
- the purpose of the study and how it's done
- that the patient needs to stop thyroid medications 5 to 7 days before the test
- who will perform the test and where
- that test takes 1 to 1½ hours

- that radiation exposure is minimal and harmless.

▶ PROCEDURE

- An oral dose of radioactive iodine is administered.
- The thyroid gland is scanned 2, 6, and 24 hours after the radioactive iodine dose.
- The amount of radioactivity detected is compared to the amount in the original dose.
- The percentage of radioactive iodine retained by the thyroid is determined.

Postprocedure care
- Resume a light diet 2 hours after taking the oral dose of ^{123}I or ^{131}I as ordered.
- Have patient resume usual diet when study is completed.
- Have the patient wash hands and flush toilet twice after urinating for at least the first 24 hours.

Precautions
- An iodine-deficient diet or ingestion of phenothiazines can increase iodine uptake, affecting the accuracy of test results.
- Contraindications include:
  - pregnancy
  - iodine or shellfish allergy.

Complications
- None known

✛ INTERPRETATION

Normal findings
- After 2 hours, 4% to 12% of the radioactive iodine should accumulate in the thyroid; after 6 hours, 5% to 20%; after 24 hours, 8% to 29%.
- Local variations in the normal range of iodine uptake may stem from regional differences in dietary iodine intake or procedural differences among individual laboratories.

Abnormal results
- Below-normal percentages of iodine uptake may suggest:
  - hypothyroidism
  - subacute thyroiditis
  - iodine overload.
- Above-normal percentages may suggest:
  - hyperthyroidism
  - early Hashimoto's disease
  - hypoalbuminemia
  - ingestion of lithium
  - iodine-deficient goiter.
- In hyperthyroidism, the rate of turnover may be so rapid that a falsely normal measurement occurs at 24 hours.

PERCHLORATE SUPPRESSION TEST

The perchlorate suppression test is used to evaluate patients with suspected Hashimoto's disease or to demonstrate an enzyme deficiency within the thyroid gland. Because potassium perchlorate competes with and displaces the iodide ions that aren't organified, this study can identify defects in the iodide organification process within the thyroid.

In this procedure, a small dose of radioactive iodine is administered orally. A radioactive iodine uptake test is performed 2 to 4 hours afterward. After uptake test, the patient receives 10 mg/kg of potassium perchlorate orally. Uptake tests are performed every 30 to 60 minutes. The total test time is 2 to 4 hours.

The results of the uptake tests performed after administration of potassium perchlorate are compared with those of the uptake test before perchlorate was administered. In a normal person, the uptake of radioactive iodine won't change significantly after administration of perchlorate. Patients with either Hashimoto's disease or an enzyme deficiency will experience a decrease in uptake. Those with an enzyme deficiency will experience a drop in their uptake of more than 15% after administration of perchlorate.

Renal angiography

● OVERVIEW

- Radiographic examination of renal vasculature and parenchyma after arterial injection of contrast medium
- Follows standard aortography, which shows individual variations in the number, size, and condition of the main renal arteries and relationship of the renal arteries to the aorta

Purpose

- To demonstrate renal vasculature configuration before surgical procedures
- To determine cause of renovascular hypertension
- To evaluate chronic renal disease or renal failure
- To investigate renal masses and renal trauma
- To identify complications after a kidney transplant
- To differentiate highly vascular tumors from avascular cysts

Patient preparation

- Make sure the patient has signed an appropriate consent form.
- Note and report all allergies.
- Evaluate peripheral pulse sites and mark them for postprocedure assessment.
- Verify adequate renal function and adequate clotting ability.
- Instruct the patient to fast for 8 hours before the test.
- Advise the patient to drink extra fluids the day before the test and after the test to maintain adequate hydration.
- Instruct the patient to use a laxative or an enema the night before the test.
- Warn the patient that transient flushing, burning, and nausea may be experienced during injection of the contrast medium.

TEACHING POINTS

Be sure to cover:
- the purpose of the study and how it's done
- who will perform the test and where
- that the test takes about 1 hour.

▶ PROCEDURE

- The patient is placed in the supine position, and a peripheral I.V. infusion is started. The skin over the arterial puncture site is cleaned with antiseptic solution and a local anesthetic is injected.
- Using Seldinger technique, the femoral artery is cannulated and with fluroscopic guidance, a catheter is advanced to the aorta.
- The guide wire is removed, and the catheter is flushed. The constrast medium is injected, and screening aortograms are obtained.
- When the aortographic study is completed, a renal catheter is exchanged for the vascular catheter.
- To determne the position of the renal arteries, a test bolus (3 to 5 ml) of contrast medium is injected.
- If the patient has no adverse reaction to the contrast medium, 20 to 25 ml of the substance is injected just below the origin of the renal arteries.
- A series of rapid-sequence X-ray films of the filling of the renal vascular tree is exposed.
- If the films are satisfactory, the catheter is removed.
- Patient's blood pressure is monitored when the arterial line is removed.
- Hemostasis is obtained and a sterile dressing applied to the puncture site.

Postprocedure care

- Maintain bed rest for 6 hours with the affected leg straight at the hip, as ordered.
- If active bleeding or expanding hematoma occurs, apply direct manual pressure and notify the doctor promptly.
- Apply cold compresses to the puncture site to lessen edema and pain as ordered.
- Encourage oral fluid intake to prevent nephrotoxicity from the contrast medium.

MONITORING

- Vital signs
- Intake and output
- Puncture site
- Bleeding, hematoma formation
- Infection

- Peripheral pulses, neurovascular status of extremities
- Renal function
- Adverse reaction to contrast media

Precautions

- Renal angiography is contraindicated in:
  - pregnancy
  - hypersensitivity to contrast media
  - uncorrected dehydration
  - uncorrected coagulopathies.

Complications

- Adverse reaction to contrast media
- Bleeding, hematoma
- Infection
- Arterial dissection

✛ INTERPRETATION

Normal findings

- Normal renal vascular tree and normal architecture of renal parenchyma are found.

Abnormal results

- Hypervascular areas suggest possible renal tumors.
- Clearly delineated, radiolucent masses suggest possible renal cysts.
- Constriction in the blood vessel suggests possible vasospasm or renal artery stenosis.
- Characteristic "beads-on-a-string appearance" suggests possible presence of alternating aneurysms and stenotic regions in renal artery dysplasia.
- The appearance of absent or cut off blood vessels suggests possible renal infarction.
- Abnormal widening of the artery suggests possible renal artery aneurysm.
- Direct connection between the renal artery and renal vein suggests a renal arteriovenous fistula.
- An increase in capsular vessels with abnormal intrarenal circulation suggests possible renal abscesses or inflammatory masses.
- Intrarenal hematoma, parenchymal laceration, shattered kidney, and areas of infarction suggests possible renal trauma.

Renal biopsy, percutaneous

● OVERVIEW

- Needle aspiration of a core kidney tissue specimen for histologic examination
- Provides valuable information about glomerular and tubular function
- Ultrasound commonly used to direct biopsy toward the lower pole of the kidney, avoiding major vessels

Purpose
- To aid diagnosis of diffuse renal parenchymal disease
- To monitor progression of renal disease and assess effectiveness of treatment
- To diagnose renal transplant rejection

Patient preparation
- Make sure the patient has signed an appropriate consent form.
- Note and report all allergies.
- Check the patient history for bleeding tendencies.
- Restriction of food and fluids is required for 8 hours before the test.
- A 24-hour hospital stay is usually required.
- Preprocedure laboratory work may be ordered.
- Explain the use of a local anesthetic.
- Warn of a pinching pain when the needle is inserted through the back into the kidney.

TEACHING POINTS
Be sure to cover:
- the purpose of the study and how it's done
- who will perform the biopsy and where
- that the test takes 15 to 30 minutes.

▶ PROCEDURE

- The patient is placed in a prone position.
- The biopsy site is prepared and draped.
- A local anesthetic is injected.
- A small incision is made in the anesthetized skin.
- A biopsy needle is inserted through the incision, down the tract of the infiltrating needle.
- The patient may be asked to hold his breath for approximately 30 seconds during needle insertion.
- Specimens are obtained while the patient is instructed to hold his breath.
- Specimens are placed in the appropriate properly labeled container.
- If an adequate tissue specimen hasn't been obtained, the procedure is repeated.
- Pressure is applied to the biopsy site until hemostasis is obtained.
- The site is cleaned and a sterile dressing is applied.

Postprocedure care
- Maintain bed rest as ordered.
- Notify the doctor of gross hematuria.
- Encourage oral fluid intake as ordered.
- Resume normal diet as ordered.
- Discourage strenuous activities for several days after the procedure to prevent possible bleeding.

MONITORING
- Vital signs
- Intake and output
- Biopsy site
- Bleeding
- Infection
- Hematuria

Precautions
- Percutaneous renal biopsy is contraindicated in:
  - hypersensitivity to contrast media
  - severe uncorrected bleeding disorder.

Complications
- Bleeding
- Hematoma
- Infection
- Arteriovenous fistula

⬥ INTERPRETATION

Normal findings
- Kidney tissue shows Bowman's capsule, the glomerular tuft, and the capillary lumen.
- The proximal tubule is one layer of epithelial cells with microvilli that form a brush border.
- The descending loop of Henle has flat, squamous epithelial cells.
- The ascending, distal convoluted, and collecting tubules are lined with squamous epithelial cells.

Abnormal results
- Histologic examination of renal tissue suggests possible malignancy such as renal cell carcinoma.
- Characteristic histologic changes suggest possible renal disease, such as:
  - disseminated lupus erythematosus
  - amyloid infiltration
  - acute and chronic glomerulonephritis
  - renal vein thrombosis
  - pyelonephritis.

Renal imaging, radionuclide

● OVERVIEW

- I.V. injection of a radionuclide followed by scintiphotography to evaluate the kidneys
- Used to assess renal blood flow, nephron and collecting system function, and renal structure
- Often includes double-isotope technique to obtain a sequence of perfusion and function studies, followed by static images
- May also be substituted for excretory urography in patients with a hypersensitivity to iodinated contrast agents

Purpose
- To detect and assess functional and structural renal abnormalities
- To assess renal transplantation status
- To assess renal injury caused by trauma
- To evaluate urinary tract obstruction

Patient preparation
- Make sure the patient has signed an appropriate consent form.
- Note and report all allergies.
- Withhold antihypertensives before the test as ordered.
- Encourage the patient to drink extra fluids before the test, if ordered.

TEACHING POINTS
Be sure to cover:
- the purpose of the study and how it's done
- who will perform the test and where
- that the test takes about 2 hours
- that radiation exposure is minimal and the radionuclide is usually excreted by the body within 24 hours.

▶ PROCEDURE

- The patient is positioned appropriately and instructed to hold still.
- A perfusion study is performed to evaluate renal blood flow.
- Technetium is administered I.V. and rapid-sequence images are taken for 1 minute.
- A function study is performed to measure the transit time of the radionuclide through the kidneys' functional units.
- Static images are obtained 4 or more hours later, after the radionuclide has drained through the pelvicaliceal system.

Postprocedure care
- Instruct the patient to flush the toilet for 24 hours immediately after urinating, as a radiation precaution.
- Resume medications and activities as ordered.

MONITORING
- Intake and output
- Renal function studies
- Fluid and electrolytes

Precautions
- Radionuclide renal imaging is contraindicated in pregnancy.

Complications
- None known

✛ INTERPRETATION

Normal findings
- Immediately evident renal perfusion after uptake of technetium in the abdominal aorta is found.
- A normal renal circulation pattern appears within 1 to 2 minutes.
- The radionuclide delineates the kidneys simultaneously, symmetrically, and with equal intensity.
- Normal size, shape, and position of kidneys are found.
- Effective renal plasma flow is 420 ml/minute or greater.
- The percentage of the dose excreted in urine at 30 to 35 minutes is greater than 66%.

Abnormal results
- Perfusion defects reflect impeded renal circulation and suggest possible renal artery stenosis or infarction.
- Increased areas of vascularity suggest possible renal tumors.
- Reduced radionuclide activity in the collecting system suggests possible markedly decreased tubular function.
- Decreased radionuclide activity in the tubules, with increased activity in the collecting system suggests possible outflow obstruction and level of ureteral obstruction.
- Space-occupying lesions within or surrounding the kidney suggests possible tumor, infarct, or abscess.
- Areas of infarction, rupture, or hemorrhage suggest possible traumatic injury.
- A lower-than-normal total concentration of the radionuclide suggests a diffuse renal disorder such as acute tubular necrosis.
- Decreased radionuclide uptake in a kidney transplant patient suggests organ rejection.
- Failure of visualization may indicate congenital ectopia or aplasia.

Renal venography

● OVERVIEW

- Radiographic examination of the main renal veins and their tributaries after injection of contrast media
- Renin assays of blood samples may be used in the differential diagnosis of hypertension

Purpose

- To detect renal vein thrombosis
- To evaluate renal vein compression caused by extrinsic tumors or retroperitoneal fibrosis
- To assess renal tumors and detects invasion of the renal vein or inferior vena cava
- To detect venous anomalies and defects
- To differentiate renal agenesis from a small kidney
- To allow collection of renal vein blood samples for evaluation of renovascular hypertension

Patient preparation

- Make sure the patient has signed an appropriate consent form.
- Note and report all allergies.
- Restrict dietary sodium intake.
- Fasting is required for 4 hours before the test if ordered.
- Discontinue antihypertensive drugs, diuretics, estrogen, and oral contraceptives as ordered.
- Obtain and report any abnormal kidney function study results.
- Explain the use of sedation and local anesthesia.
- Warn about transient burning and flushing with injection of the contrast medium.

TEACHING POINTS

Be sure to cover:
- the purpose of the study and how it's done
- who will perform the test and where
- that the test takes about 1 hour.

▶ PROCEDURE

- The patient is placed in a supine position.
- Typically, the right groin is prepared and draped.
- A local anesthetic is administered.
- The femoral vein is cannulated.
- Under fluoroscopic guidance, a catheter is advanced into the inferior vena cava.
- A test bolus of contrast medium is injected to ensure that the vena cava is patent.
- The catheter is advanced into the right renal vein and contrast medium is injected.
- When studies of the right renal vasculature are completed, the catheter is withdrawn into the vena cava.
- The catheter is guided into the left renal vein.
- Contrast is injected and images obtained.
- Blood specimens from the renal veins may be obtained for renin assays.
- The catheter is removed and hemostasis obtained.
- The site is cleaned and dressed.

Postprocedure care

- Encourage oral fluid intake (unless contraindicated) to help excrete contrast media.
- Resume normal diet and medications as ordered.
- Maintain bed rest for 2 hours as ordered.
- If bleeding occurs, apply direct manual pressure and notify the doctor.

MONITORING

- Vital signs
- Intake and output
- Puncture site
- Bleeding
- Infection
- Adverse reaction to contrast agent

Precautions

- Renal venography is contraindicated in:
  - severe uncorrected bleeding disorders
  - hypersensitivity to the contrast medium.

Complications

- Vein perforation
- Embolism
- Adverse reaction to contrast agent
- Adverse reaction to sedation
- Bleeding
- Infection

✛ INTERPRETATION

Normal findings

- Opacification of the renal vein and tributaries occurs as soon as the contrast agent is injected.
- Renin content of venous blood in an adult in a supine position is 1.5 to 1.6 ng/ml/hour.

Abnormal results

- Occlusion of the renal vein near the inferior vena cava or kidney suggests renal vein thrombosis.
- Filling defects suggests possible stenosis or thrombosis of the vessel or obstruction or compression by an extrinsic tumor or retroperitoneal fibrosis.
- Prolonged transit time of the contrast media through the renal veins suggests vessel occlusion.
- A filling defect with a sharply defined border suggests possible renal tumor that invades the renal vein or inferior vena cava.
- Opacification of abnormally positioned or clustered vessels suggests possible venous anomalies.
- Absence of a renal vein suggests possible renal agenesis.
- Elevated renin content in renal venous blood suggests possible essential renovascular hypertension when assay results correspond for both kidneys.
- Elevated renin levels in one kidney suggests a possible unilateral renal artery stenosis.

Retrograde cystography

● OVERVIEW

- Instillation of contrast medium into the bladder, followed by radiographic examination
- Performed if excretory urography hasn't adequately visualized the bladder
- Voiding cystourethrography: commonly performed concomitantly

✳ AGE-RELATED CONCERN Retrograde cystography is performed when cystoscopic examination is impractical such as in male infants.

Purpose
- To evaluate the structure and integrity of the bladder
- To determine the location and extent of bladder rupture
- To aid diagnosis of neurogenic bladder, recurrent urinary tract infections, suspected vesicoureteral reflux, vesical fistulas, diverticula, and tumors

Patient preparation
- Make sure the patient has signed an appropriate consent form.
- Note and report all allergies.
- Restriction of food or fluids isn't necessary.
- Warn the patient that some discomfort may be experienced during catheter insertion.

TEACHING POINTS
Be sure to cover:
- the purpose of the study and how it's done
- who will perform the test and where
- that the test takes about 1 hour.

▶ PROCEDURE

- The patient is placed in a supine position on the examining table.
- A preliminary kidney-ureter-bladder radiograph is taken and reviewed.
- The bladder is catheterized, and 200 to 300 ml of contrast medium instilled.

✳ AGE-RELATED CONCERN In an infant, 50 to 100 ml of contrast medium is instilled after catheterization of the bladder.

- The catheter is clamped.
- With the patient in a supine position, an anteroposterior film is taken. The patient is then tilted to one side, then the other, and two posterior oblique (and sometimes lateral) views are taken.
- If the patient's condition permits, he's assisted into the jackknife position. A posteroanterior film is taken. A space-occupying vesical lesion may require additional exposures. Rarely, to enhance visualization, 100 to 300 ml of air may be insufflated into the bladder by syringe after removal of the contrast medium (double-contrast technique)
- The catheter is then unclamped, the bladder fluid is allowed to drain, and an X-ray is obtained to detect urethral diverticula, reflux into the ureters, fistulous tracts into the vagina, or intraperitoneal or extraperitoneal extravasation of the contrast medium.

Postprocedure care.
- Resume previous activity as ordered.
- Record time of voidings.
- Notify the doctor if hematuria persists after the third voiding.
- Prepare the patient for surgery and urinary diversion, if indicated.
- Strain urine if calculi are detected.
- Administer medications as ordered (baclofen for spasms; bethanechol chloride for hypotonic bladder).
- Teach self-catheterization if indicated for neurogenic bladder.

MONITORING
- Vital signs
- Intake and output
- Urine characteristics, especially hematuria
- Infection

- Calculi
- Urinary retention, especially with neurogenic bladder

◈ NURSING ALERT Watch for and report signs and symptoms of urinary sepsis from urinary tract infection (chills, fever, elevated pulse and respiration rates, and hypotension).

Precautions
- Retrograde cystography contraindications include the following:
  - obstruction preventing passage of a urinary catheter
  - patients with hypersensitivity to contrast media.

Complications
- Urinary sepsis
- Urethral evulsion or transection

✛ INTERPRETATION

Normal findings
- The bladder has normal contours, capacity, integrity, and urethrovesical angle.
- No evidence of tumor, diverticula, or rupture is found.
- Vesicoureteral reflux is absent.
- There's no bladder displacement or external compression.
- The bladder wall is smooth and not thickened.

Abnormal results
- Anatomical abnormalities may suggest:
  - vesical trabeculae or diverticula
  - space-occupying lesions (tumors)
  - calculi or gravel
  - blood clots.
- Functional abnormalities may suggest:
  - vesicoureteral reflux
  - hypotonic or hypertonic bladder.

Retrograde ureteropyelography

● OVERVIEW

- Radiographic examination of the renal collecting system after injection of a contrast medium through a ureteral catheter during cystoscopy
- Preferred for patients with hypersensitivity to iodine
- Used when visualization of the renal collecting system by excretory urography is inadequate

Purpose

- To assess the structure and integrity of the renal collecting system (calyces, renal pelvis, and ureter)

Patient preparation

- Make sure the patient has signed an appropriate consent form.
- Note and report all allergies.
- Administer premedication if ordered.
- Fasting is required for 8 hours before the test if a general anesthetic is ordered.
- If awake for the procedure, warn the patient that he may feel pressure as the instrument is passed and an urge to void.

TEACHING POINTS

Be sure to cover:
- the purpose of the study and how it's done
- who will perform the test and where
- that the test takes about 1 hour.

▶ PROCEDURE

- The patient is placed in the lithotomy position.
- After the patient is anesthetized, a cystoscopic examination is performed.
- After visual inspection of the bladder, one or both ureters are catheterized with opaque catheters.
- The renal pelvis is emptied by gravity drainage or aspiration.
- Contrast medium is slowly injected through the catheter.
- Films are taken and immediately developed.
- The ureters are visualized with additional contrast, as the catheter is slowly withdrawn.

- Delayed films are taken to check for retention of the contrast medium.
- If ureteral obstruction is present, the ureteral catheter may be left in place for drainage.

Postprocedure care

- Report gross hematuria or hematuria after the third voiding.
- Notify the physician if the patient doesn't void in 8 hours or if the bladder is distended.
- Protect ureteral catheters (if present) from dislodgment.
- Note output amounts for each catheter (indwelling urinary, ureteral) separately.

◆ **NURSING ALERT** If irrigation of ureteral catheters is ordered, use 5 to 10 ml of sterile saline solution.

MONITORING

- Vital signs
- Intake and output
- Infection
- Hematuria
- Bladder distension
- Ureteral catheter patency and output (if present)

◆ **NURSING ALERT** Watch for and report severe pain in the area of the kidneys as well as any signs or symptoms of sepsis (such as chills, fever, and hypotension).

Precautions

- Retrograde ureteropyelography is contraindicated in pregnancy.

Complications

- Bleeding
- Infection
- Ureteral catheter obstruction

✛ INTERPRETATION

Normal findings

- Opacification of the renal pelvis and calyces is found.
- Structures are clearly outlined and symmetrical.
- Ureters fill uniformly and appear normal in size and course.

Abnormal results

- Incomplete or delayed drainage suggests obstruction, usually at the ureteropelvic junction.
- Enlargement of the components of the collecting system or delayed emptying of the contrast medium suggests possible obstruction caused by tumor, blood clot, stricture, or calculi.
- Fixation of the kidney on the same side suggests possible perinephric inflammation or suppuration.
- Upward, downward, or lateral renal displacement suggests possible renal abscess, tumor, or perinephric abscess.
- Displacement of either pole or of the entire kidney suggests possible neoplasms. (See *What ureteropyelography reveals.*)

WHAT URETEROPYELOGRAPHY REVEALS

Ureteropyelography may be used to detect obstruction of urine flow in the calyces, pelvis, or ureter of the renal collecting system. Such obstruction may result from stricture, neoplasm, blood clot, or calculi, as depicted below. Small calculi may remain in the calyces and pelvis, or pass down the ureter. A staghorn calculus (a cast of the calyceal and pelvic collecting system) may form from a stone that stays in the kidney.

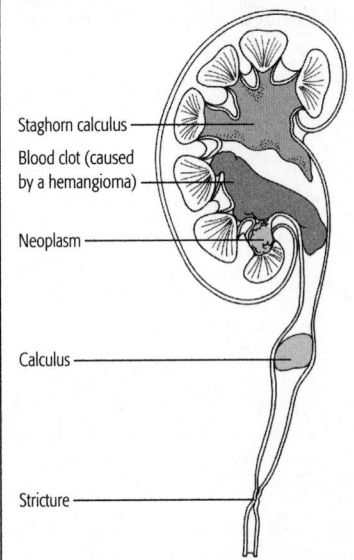

Staghorn calculus

Blood clot (caused by a hemangioma)

Neoplasm

Calculus

Stricture

Retrograde urethrography

- Instillation or injection of a contrast medium into the urethra to permit visualization of its membranous, bulbar, and penile portions
- May be used in females with suspected urethral diverticula

Purpose

- To diagnose urethral strictures, lacerations, diverticula, and congenital anomalies
- To allow follow-up after surgical repair of the urethra
- To assess urethral lacerations or other trauma

Patient preparation

- Make sure the patient has signed an appropriate consent form.
- Note and report all allergies.
- Restriction of food or fluids isn't necessary.
- Warn the patient that he might experience some discomfort when the catheter is inserted.
- Give sedative, as ordered, before procedure
- Have patient void before leaving for procedure.

TEACHING POINTS

Be sure to cover:

- the purpose of the study and how it's done
- who will perform the test and where
- that the test takes about 30 minutes.

- The patient is placed in a recumbent position on the examining table.
- Anteroposterior radiographs of the bladder and urethra are taken and reviewed.
- In males, the glans and meatus are cleaned with an antiseptic solution.
- The catheter is filled with contrast medium before insertion to eliminate air bubbles.
- In females, a double-balloon catheter is inserted, which occludes the bladder neck from above and the external meatus from below.
- The catheter is inserted until the balloon portion is inside the meatus.
- The balloon is inflated with 1 to 2 ml of water, which prevents the catheter from slipping out of position.
- The patient assumes the right posterior oblique position with his right thigh drawn up to a 90-degree angle and the penis placed along its axis. The left thigh is extended.
- The contrast medium is injected through the catheter. After three-fourths of the contrast medium have been injected, the first X-ray film is exposed while the remainder of the contrast medium is being injected. Left lateral oblique views may also be taken.
- Flouroscopic control may be helpful, especially for evaluating urethral injury.

Postprocedure care

- Observe the patient for adverse effects to the contrast media.
- Instruct the patient to return to pretest activities gradually.

MONITORING

- Vital signs
- Intake and output
- Sepsis
- Urinary tract infection

Precautions

- Check for hypersensitivity to iodine-based contrast media or iodine-containing foods such as shellfish.

Complications

- Sepsis
- Urinary tract infection

Normal findings

- Membranous, bulbar, and penile portions of the urethra appear normal in size, shape, and course.

Abnormal results

- Structural abnormalities may suggest:
  - urethral diverticula, fistulas, and strictures
  - false passages and calculi
  - lacerations
  - congenital anomalies such as urethral valves
  - tumors.

Sentinel lymph node biopsy

- Sentinel lymph node: the first node in the lymphatic basin into which a primary tumor site drains; histology of sentinel node reflects histology of the other nodes in that basin
- Usually performed by combining two techniques (lymphoscintigraphy and blue dye injection) to increase the chance of identifying the sentinel node

Purpose

- To identify the sentinel lymph node and evaluate it for the presence or absence of tumor cells indicating nodal metastasis

Patient preparation

- Make sure the patient has signed an appropriate consent form.
- Note and report all allergies.
- Explain that a radioactive substance will be injected under the skin. Provide reassurance that the patient won't be radioactive; radiation exposure is less than that of a routine chest radiograph.
- Inform the patient that surgery may follow soon after the biopsy.

TEACHING POINTS
Be sure to cover:
- the purpose of the study and how it's done
- who will perform the test and where
- that the test is usually done in conjunction with surgery.

- The patient is positioned on the table in the nuclear medicine suite.
- A standard dose of technetium-99m (^{99m}Tc) pyrophosphate is injected circumferentially around the margins of a palpable mass, using a 25G needle.
- For a nonpalpable mass, injections are guided with ultrasound or mammographic techniques.
- Images of the axilla are taken with a gamma camera. The location of the sentinel node is marked on the skin in indelible ink and noted on a data sheet.
- The patient is transported to the operating room and placed under appropriate anesthesia.
- Blue dye is injected circumferentially in the tissue immediately surrounding the biopsy site using a 25G needle.
- A small incision is made in the axilla over the suspected location of the sentinel lymph node.
- The node having the highest radioactivity is deemed the sentinel node and removed.
- The axilla is then checked for remaining radioactivity; if none is noted, the surgical procedure concludes.
- Because of the radioactivity, the sentinel lymph node is maintained in formalin for 24 to 48 hours before it is processed.

Postprocedure care

- Other than routine postoperative care, no special posttest care is required for this procedure.

Precautions

- Because ^{99m}Tc is a radioactive substance, all radiation precautions must be implemented. Staff members need to be monitored for radiation exposure. Radiation levels need to be determined in both the nuclear medicine suite and the operating room postsurgically.

◆ **NURSING ALERT** Rare cases of allergy to ^{99m}Tc or blue dye have been noted; patients should be observed for signs of allergic reaction (skin changes and respiratory difficulties).

Complications

- Adverse reaction to ^{99m}Tc or blue dye (rare)

Normal findings

- Normal findings are the same as for a normal lymph node biopsy.

Abnormal results

- Abnormal pathology indicates the presence of melanoma or breast cancer cells.
- The presence of cancer cells suggests lymph node metastasis.

Sigmoidoscopy, flexible

● OVERVIEW

- Endoscopic examination of the lining of the descending colon, sigmoid colon, rectum, and anal canal, using a flexible sigmoidoscope
- Allows several methods for obtaining specimens from suspicious areas of the mucosa: biopsy, cytology brush, or aspirate
- Used in colorectal screening (starting at age 50 for normal risk individuals without family history of colorectal cancer or adenomatous colon polyps)

Purpose
- To aid in diagnosis of acute or chronic diarrhea and rectal bleeding
- To evaluate changes in bowel habits or stool characteristics
- To aid in the assessment of known ulcerative colitis

Patient preparation
- Make sure the patient has signed an appropriate consent form.
- Note and report all allergies.
- Check the patient's history for barium tests within the last week because barium in the colon makes accurate examination impossible.
- Warn about a possible urge to defecate during the procedure.
- Advise the patient that air may be introduced through the endoscope to distend the walls of the colon, which causes flatus.
- Fasting before the procedure may be required.
- A laxative or enema before the examination may be required.
- Discuss the possible use of sedation to help the patient relax.

TEACHING POINTS
Be sure to cover:
- the purpose of the study and how it's done
- that the test may be performed in an endoscopy laboratory or the physician's office
- that the test takes 10 to 30 minutes.

▷ PROCEDURE

- The patient is placed in Sims' position on the examination table.
- Before the procedure, the endoscopist visually inspects the anus and perineum.
- Digital rectal examination is performed.
- The flexible sigmoidoscope is slowly advanced to the splenic flexure, if possible, or as far as the patient can tolerate with only mild discomfort.
- Specimens may be obtained from any suspicious area of the intestinal mucosa.
- Polyps may be biopsied for histologic diagnosis or removed by the insertion of an electrocautery snare through the endoscope and submitted for histological examination.
- Stool aspirate may be obtained when indicated for laboratory analysis.
- Before withdrawal of the scope, retroflexion is performed, allowing examination of the internal anal verge and the adjacent rectal mucosa.
- The scope is withdrawn, the lining of the colon is thoroughly examined, and air is removed.

Postprocedure care
- Resume the previous diet as ordered.
- If the patient has received sedation, don't resume diet and activity until the patient is fully awake.
- Encourage the patient to expel flatus.
- If a biopsy or polypectomy was performed, tell the patient he may notice a minute amount of blood in his stool.

MONITORING
- Vital signs
- Stools
- Abdominal distention
- Bleeding
- Bowel sounds

◉ **NURSING ALERT** Observe the patient closely for any signs of bowel perforation (abdominal distention and pain, nausea, vomiting, and fever) and for vasovagal reaction (hypotension, pallor, diaphoresis, and bradycardia). Notify the endoscopist immediately for any of these signs.

Precautions
- Flexible sigmoidoscopy is contraindicated when there's evidence of a perforated viscus and acute diverticulitis.
- Usual dosages of aspirin and most nonsteroidal anti-inflammatory medications don't significantly increase the risk of bleeding from a biopsy or polypectomy site.
- Anticoagulant therapy isn't contraindicated for the procedure because it's considered low-risk for those who need to maintain an International Normalized Ratio between 1.5 and 2.5.

Complications
- Rectal bleeding
- Bowel perforation
- Vasovagal reaction
- Adverse reaction to sedation

✥ INTERPRETATION

Normal findings
- Mucosa of the anal canal is pearly white or pigmented, depending on the patient's race.
- Mucosa of the rectum is pink and may appear velvety due to the prevalence of lymphoid tissue.
- The rich vascular network becomes less prominent at the rectosigmoid junction.
- Three semilunar valves (Houston's valves) are present in the proximal half of the rectum.
- Mucosa of the sigmoid and descending colon is light pink-orange.

Abnormal results
- Biopsy results suggest possible benign, precancerous, or malignant polyps or tumors and various forms of colitis.
- Visual inspection of the anus and perineum may disclose abnormalities, such as external hemorrhoids, anal fissure, anorectal cellulitis or abscess, and perirectal skin tag.
- Digital rectal examination may disclose rectal mass, internal hemorrhoids, or anorectal abscess.
- Inflammatory change suggests possible diverticulitis.
- Melanosis coli (a brownish discoloration of the colon) suggests possible chronic laxative use.

Single photon emission computed tomography

- Nuclear medicine scan that measures the blood flow through the organ being observed
- Radionuclide administered to patient picked up by the tissues as radionuclide circulates in the blood; photons, the radionuclide particles, detected by the gamma camera
- Information transferred to a computer converting data into images in three-dimensional view
- Used mostly in cardiology, neurology, and oncology
- Also known as *SPECT*

Purpose
- To detect neurologic conditions such as strokes, seizures, or brain injury
- To help in differentiating between types of dementia
- To evaluate blood flow to the organ such as the brain or heart
- To diagnose ischemic heart disease
- To identify presence or recurrence of cancers or tumors
- To evaluate for presence of metastasis
- To monitor the effectiveness of therapy

Patient preparation
- Make sure the patient has signed an informed consent form.
- Note and report any allergies
- Instruct him to void before beginning the test.
- Tell the patient about any possible dietary restrictions (depending on the organ being studied)
- Inform the patient that the test requires an injection of a small amount of radioactive tracer I.V. but that the radiation exposure is minimal
- Stress the need for remaining still during the testing because movement can interfere with accuracy.

TEACHING POINTS
Be sure to cover:
- purpose of the study and how it is done
- who will perform the test and where
- that an I.V. will be started to administer the radioactive tracer and that he may feel slight discomfort from the puncture

that the test can last from 1 to 2 hours.

▶ PROCEDURE

- The patient is positioned, as appropriate, for the organs to be scanned.
- An I.V. line is started and radioactive contrast medium is injected.
- The scanner camera rotates around the patient picking up the radioactive material, transferring data to a computer screen where images are converted to a three-dimensional view.

Postprocedure care
- Remove the I.V. access, as ordered.
- Have patient increase his fluid intake for 24 to 48 hours to help flush the radionuclide from the body, unless otherwise ordered.
- Allow patient to resume normal activities and diet, unless ordered otherwise.

MONITORING
- I.V. site
- Adverse reactions to radionuclide

Precautions
- Pregnant or breast-feeding women shouldn't undergo SPECT scanning.

Complications
- I.V. infiltration
- Reaction to the radioactive agents

✛ INTERPRETATION

Normal findings
- Normal blood flow through the organ is evident.
- No evidence of masses or other abnormalities is noted.

Abnormal results
- Deviation in normal rate of absorption suggests abnormal metabolic activity or function of the organ being studied.
- Increased radionuclide uptake is associated with tumors and metastasis.

Site-of-lesion tests

- Performed to identify the location of a lesion suggested by patient history or pure tone audiometry
- Indications include history of difficulty understanding speech, disproportionate to the degree of pure tone loss; dizziness, tinnitus, or sudden or fluctuating hearing loss\ or other neural symptoms; primary indication from pure tone audiometry is a difference between ears in the sensorineural components
- Used to distinguish cochlear from retrocochlear lesions and to localize lesions in the retrocochlear system at the eighth nerve, in the extra-axial (peripheral) or intra-axial brain stem, and in the cortex

Purpose
- To distinguish cochlear from retrocochlear hearing loss
- To localize lesions in the retrocochlear component of the auditory system

Patient preparation
- Make sure the patient has signed an appropriate consent form.
- Note and report all allergies.

TEACHING POINTS
Be sure to cover:
- the purpose of the study and how it's done
- that no dietary restrictions are required
- that the study is performed by an audiologist and takes about 90 minutes.

▶ PROCEDURE

- Earphones are used for each test.
- For *alternate binaural loudness:* A tone is presented to one ear and then the other. The tone in one ear is held at a constant intensity of 90 dB hearing level (HL); the other tone is varied. The patient indicates when the tones sound equally loud to both ears.
- For *simultaneous binaural midplane localization:* A 90-dB HL tone is presented to one ear and tones of varying intensity are simultaneously presented to the other ear. The patient indicates when he perceives a single tone in the center of his head.
- For *Rosenburg tone decay:* A tone is presented at or near threshold and the patient indicates how long he can hear it. If the tone becomes inaudible or changes to a buzzing or hissing sound, the tone is raised 5 dB, which produces a tone that the patient should again be able to hear. The process is repeated until the patient hears the tone continuously for 60 seconds.
- For *Suprathreshold Adaptation Test:* The tone is presented at 110 dB HL, rounded to 100 dB HL at 500 and 2,000 Hz and to 105 dB HL at 1,000 Hz.
- For *Békésy audiometry:* The patient controls the tone intensity by depressing a response button whenever he hears a tone. When the tone softens and disappears, he releases the button; the tone then becomes louder. The patient repeats this procedure for several minutes and the resulting audiometric tracing shows excursions above and below the actual threshold. Tracings are obtained for pulsed and continuous tones. The relationship between these two categories can be grouped into diagnostic patterns.
- For *masking level differences:* A 500-Hz tone and a narrow-band masking noise are presented to both ears at the same time. The noise is held at a constant intensity and the patient's threshold for the tonal stimulus in that noise is determined. Then the phase of the tone to one ear is changed by 180 degrees.
- For *difficult speech discrimination tasks:* An example of this type of test is speech discrimination in white noise. A speech stimulus is presented to one ear and the result is scored; then white noise and speech stimulus are simultaneously presented to the same ear and the result is scored. The two scores are compared; then the task is repeated for the other ear and its scores are compared. Finally, each ear's score is compared with the other's and with normal range.
- For *auditory brain stem electrical response measures:* Electrodes are placed at the vertex of the patient's scalp (active), the mastoid process or earlobe of the stimulated ear (reference), and the mastoid process or earlobe of the opposite ear (ground).Clicks or rapid rise time (1 millisecond) tone pips are presented at 10/second until 2,000 time-locked responses are collected and averaged. This tests mainly the 1,000 to 4,000 Hz frequency.
- For *competing message tasks:* A different message is presented to each ear and the patient is asked to discriminate between the messages. In a gross measure test, such as the Northwestern University test #20, speech discrimination words are presented to one ear and the patient is asked to repeat them. Then speech discrimination words are presented to the same ear and short sentences are simultaneously presented to the other ears, the patient is asked to repeat the words and ignore the sentences. The patient's scores on each task are then compared.
- In a *precise message test* such as the dichotic nonsense syllables test: carefully aligned nonsense syllables are presented to both ears at once and the patient is asked to repeat or write both syllables. The number of syllables correctly identified in one ear is compared with the number of syllables correctly identified in the other ear as well as with a normal range.

Postprocedure care
- No specific posttest care is necessary.

Complications
- None known

✛ INTERPRETATION

Normal findings
- Sensory and neural deficits are absent.

Abnormal results
- Sensory deficits suggest lesions of the auditory portions of the inner ear (cochlea).
- Neural deficits suggest lesions beyond the inner ear (retrocochlea).
- Abnormal adaptation to a continuous tone in tone decay tests suggests the presence of retro-cochlear lesions.

Skin biopsy

- Removal of a small piece of tissue, under local anesthesia, from a lesion suspected of being malignant
- Specimen for histologic examination may be obtained by shave, punch, or excision biopsy
- Fully developed lesions: selected for biopsy whenever possible because they provide more diagnostic information than resolving lesions or those in early developing stages

Purpose

- To allow differential diagnosis of basal cell carcinoma, squamous cell carcinoma, malignant melanoma, and benign growths
- To diagnose chronic bacterial or fungal skin infections

Patient preparation

- Make sure the patient has signed an appropriate consent form.
- Note and report all allergies.
- Restriction of food and fluids isn't necessary.
- Inform the patient that a local anesthetic will be used to minimize pain during the procedure.

TEACHING POINTS

Be sure to cover:

- the purpose of the study and how it's done
- who will perform the test and where
- that the test takes about 15 minutes.

- The patient is positioned comfortably and the biopsy site is cleaned.
- A local anesthetic is administered.
- For *shave biopsy:* The protruding growth is cut off at the skin line with a #15 scalpel, and the tissue is placed immediately in a properly labeled specimen bottle containing 10% formalin solution. Pressure is applied to the area to stop the bleeding.
- For *punch biopsy:* The skin surrounding the lesion is pulled taut, and the punch is firmly introduced into the lesion and rotated to obtain a tissue specimen. The plug is lifted with forceps or a needle and is severed as deeply into the fat layer as possible. The specimen is placed in a properly labeled specimen bottle containing 10% formalin solution or, if indicated, in a sterile container. The method used to close the wound depends on the size of the punch.
- For *excision biopsy:* A #15 scalpel is used to excise the lesion completely; the incision is made as wide and as deep as necessary. The examiner removes the tissue specimen and places it immediately in a properly labeled specimen bottle containing 10% formalin solution. Pressure is applied to the site to stop the bleeding. The wound is closed and if the incision is large, skin graft may be required.

Postprocedure care

- If the patient experiences pain at the biopsy site, administer analgesia as ordered.
- Advise the patient with sutures to keep the area clean and as dry as possible. Facial sutures will be removed in 3 to 5 days; trunk sutures, in 7 to 14 days.
- Instruct the patient with adhesive strips to leave them in place for 14 to 21 days or until they fall off.

MONITORING

- Pain
- Vital signs
- Biopsy site

Complications

- Bleeding
- Infection

Normal findings

- Normal skin consists of squamous epithelium (epidermis) and fibrous connective tissue (dermis).

Abnormal results

- Histologic examination of the tissue specimen suggests possible benign lesions such as dermatofibromas, or malignant lesions such as malignant melanoma.
- Cultures can be used to determine chronic bacterial and fungal infections.

Slit-lamp examination

● OVERVIEW

- Slit-lamp: an instrument equipped with a special lighting system and a binocular microscope (see *Understanding biomicroscopic examination*)
- Allows ophthalmologist to visualize in detail the anterior segment of the eye, including eyelids, eyelashes, conjunctiva, sclera, cornea, tear film, anterior chamber, iris, crystalline lens, and vitreous face
- Used to evaluate normally transparent or nearly transparent ocular fluids and tissues

Purpose

- To detect and evaluate abnormalities of the anterior segment tissues and structures

Patient preparation

- Make sure the patient has signed an appropriate consent form.
- Note and report all allergies.
- Instruct the patient to remove contact lenses before the test, unless the test is being done to evaluate the fit of the contact lens.
- Explain the need to remain still during the test.
- Mydriatics aren't used for a routine eye examination because the slit lamp's bright light would hurt the dilated eyes.
- Some diseases, such as iritis, require pupillary dilation to alleviate pain and allow the ophthalmologist to examine the eyes with adequate illumination.

TEACHING POINTS
Be sure to cover:
- the purpose of the study and how it's done
- that the test takes 5 to 10 minutes
- that the examination is painless.

  ◈ **NURSING ALERT** Don't instill mydriatic drops into the eyes of a patient with angle-closure glaucoma or a patient who has had a hypersensitivity reaction to the drops.

▷ PROCEDURE

- The patient is seated in the examining chair with both feet on the floor

- The patient is assessed before the examination for the presence of obvious signs, such as different corneal diameters or heterochromia.
- His chin is placed on the rest and his forehead against the bar.
- The room lights are dimmed.
- The ophthalmologist examines the patient's eyes — starting with the lids and lashes and progressing to the vitreous face — altering light and magnification as necessary.
- A special camera may be attached to the slit lamp to photograph portions of the eye.
- If a corneal abrasion or ulcer is detected, a fluorescein stain allows better viewing of the area.
- If a tearing deficiency is suspected, the ophthalmologist may examine the eye after applying a fluorescein or rose bengal stain; he may also perform the Schirmer tearing test.

Postprocedure care

- If dilating drops were instilled, tell the patient that his near vision will be blurred for 40 minutes to 2 hours.

MONITORING
- Vision

Complications

- Increased intraocular pressure with mydriatic drops are used in angle-closure glaucoma
- Hypersensitivity reaction to eyedrops

⬥ INTERPRETATION

Normal findings

- No abnormalities of anterior segment tissues and structures are found.

Abnormal results

- Irregular corneal shape suggests possible keratoconus.
- A parchmentlike consistency of the lid skin, with redness, minor swelling, and moderate itching, suggests a possible hypersensitivity reaction.
- Early-stage lens opacities suggest the possible development of cataracts.
- Fluorescein stain suggests possible corneal abrasion or ulcer.
- A Schirmer tearing test suggests a possible tearing deficiency.

UNDERSTANDING BIOMICROSCOPIC EXAMINATION

The patient shown at right is undergoing a slit-lamp biomicroscopic examination. The slit lamp directs an intense, narrow beam of light on optic tissue, allowing the ophthalmologist to see the patient's cornea and lens as layers of different optical densities, not transparent structures. This method permits accurate detection of pathologic conditions in the eye's anterior segment.

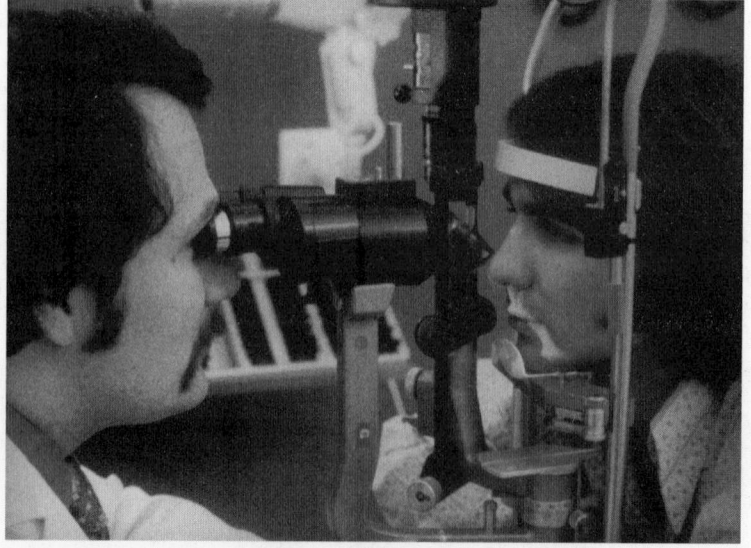

Small-bowel biopsy

● OVERVIEW

- Use of a capsule to obtain larger tissue samples for histologic analysis than in endoscopic biopsy
- Allows removal of tissue from areas beyond an endoscope's reach
- Although an invasive procedure, it causes little pain and complications are rare

Purpose

- To evaluate diseases of the intestinal mucosa, which may cause malabsorption or diarrhea
- To confirm the diagnosis of some diseases, such as Whipple's disease and tropical sprue

Patient preparation

- Make sure the patient has signed an appropriate consent form.
- Note and report all allergies.
- Ensure that coagulation tests have been performed and abnormal results were reported to the doctor.
- Withhold aspirin and anticoagulants as ordered.
- Restriction of food and fluids is required for at least 8 hours before the test.

TEACHING POINTS

Be sure to cover:
- the purpose of the study and how it's done
- who will perform the biopsy and where
- that the biopsy takes 45 to 60 minutes but causes little discomfort.

▶ PROCEDURE

- The tubing and the capsule are lightly lubricated with a water-soluble lubricant and the mercury bag moistened with water.
- The back of the patient's throat is sprayed with a local anesthetic to decrease gagging during passage of the tube.
- With the patient seated upright, the capsule is placed in his pharynx and he is asked to flex his neck and swallow as the doctor advances the tube about 20″ (50 cm). (If a local anes-

thetic is used to control the gag reflex, the patient must not receive any fluids to help him swallow the capsule.)
- The patient is positioned on his right side; the tube is advanced another 20″.
- The tube's position is checked by fluoroscopy or by instilling air through the tube and listening with a stethoscope for air to enter the stomach.
- Next, the tube is advanced 2″ to 4″ (5 to 10 cm) at a time to pass the capsule through the pylorus.
- Food is discussed with the patient to stimulate the pylorus and help the capsule pass.
- When fluoroscopy confirms that the capsule has passed the pylorus, the patient is maintained on his right side to allow the capsule to move into the second and third portions of the small bowel.
- The patient is instructed that he may hold the tube loosely to one side of his mouth if it makes him more comfortable.
- Capsule position is checked again by fluoroscopy and the biopsy site is determined.
- The patient is placed in a supine position so the capsule's position can be verified fluoroscopically.
- A glass syringe is placed on the end of the tube and steady suction is applied to close the capsule and cut off a tissue specimen.
- Suction is maintained on the syringe as the tube and capsule are removed; then the suction is released.
- The specimen is gently removed with forceps, placed mucosal side up on a piece of mesh and placed in a biopsy bottle with required fixative.
- The specimen is immediately sent to the laboratory.

Postprocedure care

- Resume diet after return of the gag reflex as ordered.
- Instruct the patient to report abdominal pain or bleeding.

MONITORING

- Vital signs
- Bleeding
- Infection
- Aspiration
- Abdominal distention
- Bowel sounds

NURSING ALERT Watch for and immediately report signs and symptoms of hemorrhage, bacteremia, and bowel perforation.

Precautions

- Keep suction equipment nearby to prevent aspiration.
- Biopsy is contraindicated in uncooperative patients, those taking aspirin or anticoagulants, and those with uncorrected coagulation disorders.

Complications

- Hemorrhage
- Bacteremia
- Bowel perforation

✛ INTERPRETATION

Normal findings

- A normal small-bowel biopsy specimen consists of fingerlike villi, crypts, columnar epithelial cells, and round cells.

Abnormal results

- Histologic changes in cell structure suggest possible Whipple's disease, abetalipoproteinemia, lymphoma, lymphangiectasia, eosinophilic enteritis, and parasitic infections, such as giardiasis and coccidiosis.
- Histologic abnormalities may also suggest celiac disease, tropical sprue, infectious gastroenteritis, intraluminal bacterial overgrowth, folate and B_{12} deficiency, radiation enteritis, and malnutrition, requiring further investigation.

Sputum culture

● OVERVIEW

- Bacteriologic examination of sputum
- Usual method of specimen collection: expectoration
- Other methods of specimen collection: tracheal suctioning
- Examination of acid-fast sputum smear: may disclose evidence of mycobacterial infection such as tuberculosis (TB)

Purpose

- To isolate and identify causes of pulmonary infections
- To aid diagnosis of respiratory diseases, such as bronchitis, TB, lung abscess, and pneumonia

Patient preparation

- The test requires a sputum specimen.
- Explain that specimens may be collected on at least 3 consecutive mornings if the suspected organism is *Mycobacterium tuberculosis.*

TEACHING POINTS
Be sure to cover:
- the purpose of the study and how it's done
- who will perform the test and where
- results available in 48 to 72 hours
- results for TB cultures take up to 2 months.

▶ PROCEDURE

- Confirm the patient's identity using two patient identifiers according to facility policy.
- Wash your hands thoroughly.
- Maintain asepsis.
- Wear personal protective equipment.

EXPECTORATION
- Instruct the patient to cough deeply and expectorate into the container.
- If the cough is nonproductive, use chest physiotherapy or nebulization to induce sputum as ordered.
- Close the container securely.
- Dispose of equipment properly; seal the container in a leakproof bag before sending it to the laboratory.

TRACHEAL SUCTIONING
- Administer oxygen to the patient before and after the procedure as necessary.
- Attach the sputum trap to the suction catheter.
- Lubricate the catheter with normal saline solution and pass the catheter through the patient's nostril without suction.
- Advance the catheter into the trachea.
- Apply suction while withdrawing the catheter, not during catheter insertion.
- Suction for only 5 to 10 seconds at a time to obtain the specimen.

NURSING ALERT If the patient becomes hypoxic or cyanotic during suctioning, remove the catheter immediately and administer oxygen while monitoring pulse oximetry.
- Stop suction and remove the catheter.
- Discard the catheter in the proper receptacle.
- Detach the in-line sputum trap from the suction apparatus and cap the opening.

Postprocedure care
- Label the container with the patient's name, the nature and origin of the specimen, the date and time of collection, the initial diagnosis, and any current antimicrobial therapy.
- Send the specimen to the laboratory immediately after collection.
- Provide mouth care.

MONITORING
- Vital signs
- Respiratory status
- Oxygen saturations with pulse oximetry

Precautions
- Tracheal suctioning is contraindicated in patients with esophageal varices or cardiac disease.
- During passage through the throat and oropharynx, sputum specimens are commonly contaminated with indigenous bacterial flora.
- Don't use more than 20% propylene glycol with water as an inducer for a specimen scheduled for TB culturing, since higher concentrations inhibit the growth of *M. tuberculosis.* (If propylene glycol isn't available, use 10% to 20% acetylcysteine with water or sodium chloride.)
- A Gram stain of expectorated sputum must be examined to ensure that it's a representative specimen of secretions from the lower respiratory tract (many white blood cells [WBCs], few epithelial cells) rather than one contaminated by oral flora (few WBCs, many epithelial cells).

Complications
- Hypoxemia
- Cardiac arrhythmias
- Laryngospasm
- Bronchospasm
- Pneumothorax
- Perforation of the trachea or bronchus
- Trauma to respiratory structures
- Bleeding

✛ INTERPRETATION

Normal findings
- Flora commonly found in the respiratory tract include alpha-hemolytic streptococci, *Neisseria* species, and diphtheroid; however, the presence of normal flora doesn't rule out infection.

Abnormal results
- Because sputum is invariably contaminated with normal oropharyngeal flora, a culture isolate must be interpreted in light of the patient's overall clinical condition.
- Isolation of *M. tuberculosis* suggests TB.
- Isolation of pathogenic organisms most often includes *Streptococcus pneumoniae, M. tuberculosis, Klebsiella pneumoniae* (and other Enterobacteriaceae), *Haemophilus influenzae, Staphylococcus aureus,* and *Pseudomonas aeruginosa.*

Stool culture

● OVERVIEW

- Bacteriologic examination of the feces
- Identification of organisms: prevention of possibly fatal complications (especially in a debilitated patient), and confinement of infectious diseases
- Used to detect viruses, such as enterovirus, which can cause aseptic meningitis
- Sensitivity testing may follow isolation of pathogen

Purpose

- To identify pathogenic organisms causing GI disease, such as typhus and dysentery
- To identify carrier states

Patient preparation

- Obtain patient history for dietary patterns, recent antimicrobial therapy, and recent travel that might suggest an endemic infection or infestation.
- Collect specimens before starting antimicrobial therapy.
- No restriction of food and fluids.
- Advise the patient that testing may require the collection of a stool specimen on 3 consecutive days.

TEACHING POINTS

Be sure to cover:
- the purpose of the study and how it's done.

▶ PROCEDURE

- Confirm the patient's identity using two patient identifiers according to facility policy.
- Wear personal protective equipment.
- Collect stool specimen directly in the container.
- If the patient isn't ambulatory, collect it in a clean, dry bedpan; use a tongue blade to transfer the specimen.
- If you must collect the specimen by rectal swab, insert the swab beyond the anal sphincter, rotate it gently, and withdraw it. Place the swab in the appropriate container.
- Check with the laboratory for the proper collection procedure before obtaining a specimen for a virus test.

- Label the specimen with the patient's name, doctor's name, hospital number, and date and time of collection.

Postprocedure care

- Ensure perirectal skin integrity.

Precautions

- Send the specimen to the laboratory immediately; be sure to include mucoid and bloody portions. The specimen must always represent the first, middle, and last portion of the feces passed.
- If specimens can't be transported within 1 hour, refrigerate or place it in transport media.
- If the patient uses a bedpan or a diaper, avoid contaminating the stool specimen with urine.
- Put the specimen in a leakproof bag before sending it to the laboratory.
- Indicate the suspected cause of the patient's GI disorder and current antimicrobial therapy on the request.

Complications

- None known

✥ INTERPRETATION

Normal findings

- More than 95% of normal fecal flora consists of anaerobes, including non–spore-forming bacilli, clostridia, and anaerobic streptococci. The remainder consists of aerobes, including gram-negative bacilli (predominantly

Escherichia coli and other Enterobacteriaceae, plus small amounts of Pseudomonas), gram-positive cocci (mostly enterococci), and a few yeasts.

Abnormal results

- Isolation of some pathogens (such as *Salmonella, Shigella, Campylobacter, Yersinia,* and *Vibrio*) suggests bacterial infection in patients with acute diarrhea. (See *Pathogens of the GI tract.*)
- Because normal fecal flora may include *Clostridium difficile, Escheria coli,* and other organisms, isolation of these may require further tests to demonstrate invasiveness or toxin production.
- Isolation of pathogens such as *C. botulinum* suggests food poisoning, although the pathogens must also be isolated from the contaminated food.
- In patients undergoing long-term antimicrobial therapy as well as those with acquired immunodeficiency syndrome or who are taking immunosuppressant drugs, isolation of large numbers of *Staphylococcus aureus* or such yeasts as Candida suggests possible infection.
- Isolation of enteroviruses suggests possible aseptic meningitis.
- A highly increased polymorphonuclear leukocyte count in fecal material suggests a possible invasive pathogen.

PATHOGENS OF THE GI TRACT

The presence of the following pathogens in a stool culture may indicate certain disorders:

- *Aeromonas hydrophila:* gastroenteritis, which causes diarrhea, especially in children
- *Bacillus cereus:* food poisoning, acute gastroenteritis (rare)
- *Campylobacter jejuni:* gastroenteritis
- *Clostridium botulinum:* food poisoning and infant botulism (a possible cause of sudden infant death syndrome)
- Toxin-producing *Clostridium difficile:* pseudomembranous enterocolitis
- *Clostridium perfringens:* food poisoning
- Enterotoxigenic *Escherichia coli:* gastroenteritis (resembles cholera or shigellosis)
- *Salmonella:* gastroenteritis, typhoid fever, nontyphoidal salmonellosis, paratyphoid fever, enteric fever
- *Shigella:* shigellosis, bacillary dysentery
- *Staphylococcus aureus:* food poisoning, suppression of normal bowel flora from antimicrobial therapy
- *Vibrio cholerae:* cholera
- *Vibrio parahaemolyticus:* food poisoning, especially seafood
- *Yersinia enterocolitica:* gastroenteritis, enterocolitis (resembles appendicitis), mesenteric lymphadenitis, ileitis

Sweat test

● OVERVIEW

- Quantitative measurement of electrolyte concentrations (primarily sodium and chloride) in sweat, usually through pilocarpine iontophoresis (pilocarpine is a sweat inducer)
- Used mainly in children to confirm cystic fibrosis, a congenital condition that increases sodium and chloride electrolyte levels in sweat
- Genetic testing for cystic fibrosis (CF) available (see *Tag-It Cystic Fibrosis Kit*)

Purpose
- To confirm CF
- To exclude the diagnosis in siblings of those with CF

Patient preparation
- Make sure the patient, or parent if the patient is a minor, has signed an appropriate consent form.
- Note and report all allergies.
- No restrictions of diet, medications, or activity are necessary before the test.
- Warn the patient that a slight tickling sensation may be experienced during the procedure.

TEACHING POINTS
Be sure to cover:
- the purpose of the study and how it's done
- who will perform the test and where
- that the test takes 20 to 45 minutes and is painless.

▶ PROCEDURE

- The area to be tested (flexor surface of the right forearm or, if the arm is too small to secure electrodes, as with an infant, the right thigh) is cleaned using distilled water, and dried thoroughly.
- A gauze pad saturated with premeasured pilocarpine solution is placed on the positive electrode.
- A gauze pad saturated with normal saline solution is placed on the negative electrode.
- Both electrodes are applied to the area to be tested and secured with straps.

- Leadwires to the analyzer are given a current of 4 mA in 15 to 20 seconds. This process (iontophoresis) is continued at 15- to 20-second intervals for 5 minutes.
- After iontophoresis, both electrodes are removed.
- The pads are discarded, the patient's skin cleaned with distilled water and dried.
- Using forceps, a dry gauze pad or filter paper (previously weighed on a gram scale) is placed on the area where the pilocarpine was used.
- The pad or filter paper is covered with a slightly larger piece of plastic and the edges of the plastic are sealed with waterproof adhesive tape.
- The gauze pad or filter paper is left in place for about 45 minutes. (The appearance of droplets on the plastic usually indicates induction of an adequate amount of sweat.)
- The pad or filter paper is removed with the forceps and placed immediately in the weighing bottle.
- Carefully seal the gauze pad or filter paper in the weighing bottle and send the bottle to the laboratory at once.
- The difference between the first and second weights indicates the weight of the sweat specimen collected.

Postprocedure care
- Wash the tested area with soap and water, and dry it thoroughly.
- If the area looks red, reassure the patient that this is normal and that the redness will disappear within a few hours.
- Tell the patient that he may resume his usual activities.

Precautions
⬦ **NURSING ALERT** Never perform iontophoresis on the chest, especially in a child, because the current can induce cardiac arrest.
- To prevent electric shock, use battery-powered equipment if possible.
- Make sure at least 100 mg of sweat is collected in 45 minutes.

⬦ **NURSING ALERT** Stop the test immediately if the patient complains of a burning sensation, which usually indicates that the positive electrode is exposed or positioned improperly. Adjust the electrode and continue the test.

Complications
- Possible electric shock if improperly performed

✛ INTERPRETATION

Normal findings
- Sodium values in sweat range from 10 to 30 mEq/L (SI, 10 to 30 mmol/L).
- Chloride values in sweat range from 10 to 35 mEq/L (SI, 10 o 35 mmol/L).
- In females, sweat electrolyte levels fluctuate cyclically: Chloride concentrations usually peak 5 to 10 days before onset of menses and most women retain fluid before menses.

Abnormal results
- Sodium and chloride concentrations of 50 to 60 mEq/L (SI, 50 to 60 mmol/L) strongly suggest CF.
- Levels greater than 60 mEq/L (SI, > 60 mmol/L) with topical signs and symptoms confirm the diagnosis.
- Elevated sweat electrolyte levels may also suggest untreated adrenal insufficiency as well as type I glycogen storage disease, vasopressin-resistant diabetes insipidus, meconium ileus, and renal failure.

TAG-IT CYSTIC FIBROSIS KIT

The U.S. Food and Drug Administration approved the use of a deoxyribonucleic acid (DNA) test for diagnosing cystic fibrosis (CF). The test, called the *Tag-It Cystic Fibrosis Kit,* is a blood test that screens for genetic mutations and variations in the cystic fibrosis transmembrane conductance regulator (CFTR) gene. This test identifies 23 genetic mutations and 4 variations in the CFTR gene. It also screens for 16 additional mutations in the gene that are involved in many cases of CF.

The test is recommended for use in detecting and identifying these mutations and variations in the gene as a means for determining carrier status in adults, screening neonates, and for confirming diagnostic testing in neonates and children. There are over 1,300 genetic variations in the CFTR gene responsible for causing CF. Therefore, the test isn't recommended as the only means for diagnosing CF. Test results need to be viewed with the patient's condition, ethnic background, and family history. Additionally, genetic counseling is suggested to help patients understand the results and their implications.

Synovial membrane biopsy

● OVERVIEW

- Needle excision of a tissue specimen of the thin epithelial layer lining the diarthrodial joint capsules for histologic examination
- Performed when analysis of synovial fluid (a viscous, lubricating fluid contained within the synovial membrane) is nondiagnostic or when the fluid is absent
- Preliminary arthroscopy: used to aid selection of biopsy site in a large joint such as the knee

Purpose

- To diagnose gout, pseudogout, bacterial infections and lesions, and granulomatous infections
- To aid diagnosis of rheumatoid arthritis, systemic lupus erythematosus, or Reiter's syndrome
- To monitor joint pathology

Patient preparation

- Make sure the patient has signed an appropriate consent form.
- Note and report all allergies.
- Administer a sedative if ordered.
- Restriction of food or fluids isn't necessary.
- Provide reassurance that a local anesthetic will be used to minimize discomfort.
- Warn about transient pain when the needle enters the joint.

TEACHING POINTS

Be sure to cover:
- the purpose of the study and how it's done
- who will perform the test and where
- that the test takes about 30 minutes
- which site was selected for biopsy (usually, the most symptomatic joint): knee (most common), elbow, wrist, ankle, or shoulder
- that test results are usually available in 1 or 2 days
- that complications are rare but may include infection and bleeding into the joint.

▶ PROCEDURE

- The patient is properly positioned.
- The biopsy site is prepared and draped.
- Local anesthetic is injected into the joint space.
- The trocar is forcefully thrust into the joint space, away from the site of anesthetic infiltration.
- The biopsy needle is inserted through the trocar.
- While the trocar is held stationary, the biopsy needle is twisted to cut off a tissue segment.
- Then the needle is withdrawn and the specimen is placed in a properly labeled sterile container or a specimen bottle containing heparin or absolute ethyl alcohol.
- Several specimens can be obtained without reinserting the trocar.
- The trocar is then removed, the biopsy site is cleaned, and a dressing is applied.

Postprocedure care

- Administer analgesics as ordered.
- Instruct the patient to rest the joint from which the tissue specimen was removed for 1 day before resuming normal activities.

MONITORING

- Vital signs
- Bleeding into the joint
- Biopsy site
- Infection

Precautions

- Synovial membrane biopsy shouldn't be performed in areas of skin or wound infection.

Complications

- Bleeding into the joint
- Infection

✛ INTERPRETATION

Normal findings

- Synovial membrane contains cells identical to those found in other connective tissue.
- Membrane surface is relatively smooth, except for villi, folds, and fat pads that project into the joint cavity.
- Membrane tissue produces synovial fluid and contains a capillary network, lymphatic vessels, and a few nerve fibers.

Abnormal results

- Results of histologic examination of synovial tissue can suggest coccidioidomycosis, gout, pseudogout, hemochromatosis, tuberculosis, sarcoidosis, amyloidosis, pigmented villonodular synovitis or synovial tumors.

Tangent screen examination

- Evaluation of a patient's central visual field through systematic movement of a test object across a tangent screen, usually a piece of black felt with concentric circles and lines radiating from a central fixation point, much like a spider web
- Monocular visual field examinations: important in detecting and following the progression of ocular diseases, such as glaucoma and optic neuritis; also used to detect and evaluate neurologic disorders, such as brain tumors and strokes; localization of specific visual field defect often points to underlying pathology

Purpose
- To detect central visual field loss and evaluate its progression or regression

Patient preparation
- Make sure the patient has signed an appropriate consent form.
- Note and report all allergies.
- Inform the patient that the test involves no pain but requires his full cooperation.
- Instruct the patient to wear normal corrective lenses during the test.

TEACHING POINTS
Be sure to cover:
- the purpose of the study and how it's done
- who will perform the test and where
- that the test takes about 30 minutes.

▶ PROCEDURE

- The patient is seated comfortably about 3′ (1 m) from the tangent screen so the eye being tested is directly in line with the central fixation target on the screen.
- The patient's left eye is covered and he's instructed that while he fixates on the central target, a test object will be moved into his visual field.
- He's instructed not to look for the test object, but to wait for it to appear and then signal when he sees it.
- The examiner stands to the side of the eye being tested.

- The test object is moved inward from the periphery of the screen at 25- to 30-degree intervals, as represented by the radiating lines on the screen.
- Using black-tipped straight pins the points on the screen at which the patient can see the object (areas of equal visual acuity) are plotted.
- To guarantee the adequacy of fixation the blind spot (projection of optic nerve into the visual field) is clearly identified.
- How well the patient can see within his visual field is tested by turning the test object to the black side.
- The object is turned over within each 25- to 30-degree interval and the patient is asked to signal when he sees the test object.
- Areas in which the patient has failed to identify the test object are plotted for size, shape, and density.
- The patient's visual field is recorded, and marked in degrees, noting any abnormal areas within the field.
- Because isopters (boundary of a visual field for a specific target size and distance) vary with the patient's age, visual acuity, and pupil size; the size and color of the test object; and the distance between the patient and the screen, careful recording of all measurements is required.
- The patient's right eye is covered and the test is repeated.

Postprocedure care
- No specific posttest care is necessary.

Precautions
- Remind the patient that he must maintain fixation on the central target on the tangent screen.
- The test measures only the central 30 degrees of visual field.

Complications
- None known

Normal findings
- The central visual field normally forms a circle, extending 25 degrees superiorly, nasally, inferiorly, and temporally.
- The physiologic blind spot lies 12 to 15 degrees temporal to the central fixation point, approximately 1.5 degrees below the horizontal meridian. It extends approximately 7.5 degrees in height and 5.5 degrees in width.
- The test object should be visible throughout the patient's entire central visual field except within the physiologic blind spot.

Abnormal results
- Inability to see the test object within the temporal half of the central visual field suggests possible bitemporal hemianopsia.
- Bitemporal hemianopsia suggests possible lesions of the optic chiasm (commonly caused by pituitary tumor), craniopharyngiomas in the young, and meningiomas or aneurysm of the circle of Willis.
- Bilateral homonymous hemianopsia suggests possible multiple thrombosis in the posterior cerebral circulation.
- An enlarged blind spot, a central scotoma, or a centrocecal scotoma suggests possible diseases involving the optic nerve such as glaucoma.
- A ring scotoma (a scotoma 10 or more degrees away from the fixation point) suggests retinitis pigmentosa, a slowly progressive disease that leads to night blindness.

Technetium-99m pyrophosphate scanning

● OVERVIEW

- Used to detect and determine extent of recent myocardial infarction (MI)
- I.V. tracer isotope (^{99m}Tc pyrophosphate) accumulates in damaged myocardial tissue (possibly by combining with calcium in the damaged myocardial cells), where it forms a hot spot on a scan made with a scintillation camera
- Useful when serum cardiac enzyme tests are unreliable or when patients have equivocal electrocardiograms (ECGs) such as in left bundle-branch block
- Also known as hot spot myocardial imaging and infarct avid imaging

Purpose
- To confirm recent MI
- To define size and location of recent MI
- To assess prognosis after acute MI

Patient preparation
- Make sure the patient has signed an appropriate consent form.
- Note and report all allergies.
- Restriction of food and fluids isn't necessary.
- Provide reassurance that only transient discomfort will be felt during isotope injection; the scan itself is painless.
- Stress the need to remain quiet and motionless during scanning.

TEACHING POINTS
Be sure to cover:
- the purpose of the study and how it's done
- who will perform the 30- to 60-minute test and where
- that radiation exposure is minimal.

▶ PROCEDURE

- ^{99m}Tc pyrophosphate is injected into the antecubital vein.
- After 2 to 3 hours the patient is placed in a supine position.
- ECG electrodes are attached for continuous monitoring during the test.
- Scans are usually taken with the patient in several positions, including anterior, left anterior oblique, right anterior oblique, and left lateral.
- Each scan takes about 10 minutes.

Postprocedure care
- No specific posttest care is necessary.

Precautions
- Remind the patient he must remain motionless during the scanning.

Complications
- None known

✛ INTERPRETATION

Normal findings
- No isotope is found in the myocardium.

Abnormal results
- Isotope is taken up by the sternum and ribs, and their activity is compared with the heart's; 2+, 3+, and 4+ activity (equal to or greater than bone) suggests a positive myocardial scan.
- Areas of isotope accumulation, or hot spots, suggest damaged myocardium.

Tensilon test

- Involves I.V. administration of Tensilon (edrophonium chloride), a rapid, short-acting anticholinesterase that improves muscle strength by increasing muscle response to nerve impulses

Purpose

- To aid diagnosis of myasthenia gravis
- To differentiate between myasthenic and cholinergic crises
- To monitor oral anticholinesterase therapy

Patient preparation

- Make sure the patient has signed an appropriate consent form.
- Note and report all allergies.
- Check the patient's history for use of medications that affect muscle function.
- If the patient is receiving anticholinesterase therapy, note this on the requisition form along with the last dose he received and the time it was administered.
- Withhold medications as ordered.
- Start an I.V. infusion of dextrose 5% in water or normal saline solution.
- Restriction of food and fluids isn't necessary.
- Warn about possible transient unpleasant adverse effects from the Tensilon, including nausea, dizziness, and blurred vision.
- Provide reassurance that someone will stay with the patient at all times.
- Inform the patient that the test may need to be repeated several times.

TEACHING POINTS
Be sure to cover:
- the purpose of the study and how it's done
- who will perform the test and where
- that the study takes 15 to 30 minutes.

PROCEDURE

TO DIAGNOSE MYASTHENIA GRAVIS

- 2 mg of Tensilon is administered initially. Infants and children require a dosage adjustment.

- Before the rest of the dose is administered, the doctor may want to tire the muscles by asking the patient to perform various exercises, such as looking up until ptosis develops, or holding his arms above his shoulders until they drop.
- When the muscles are fatigued, the remaining 8 mg of Tensilon is administered over 30 seconds.
- If a placebo is used (to evaluate the patient's muscle response more accurately) the placebo is administered and the patient is observed.
- After administration of Tensilon, the patient is asked to perform repetitive muscular movements, such as opening and closing his eyes and crossing and uncrossing his legs.
- The patient is closely observed for improved muscle strength.
- If muscle strength doesn't improve within 3 to 5 minutes, the test may be repeated.

TO DIFFERENTIATE BETWEEN MYASTHENIC CRISIS AND CHOLINERGIC CRISIS

- 1 to 2 mg of Tensilon is infused.
- After infusion, the patient's vital signs are continuously monitored.
- The patient is watched closely for respiratory distress.
- If muscle strength doesn't improve, more Tensilon is infused cautiously— 1 mg at a time up to a maximum of 5 mg—and the patient is observed for distress.
- Neostigmine is administered immediately if the test demonstrates myasthenic crisis; atropine is administered for cholinergic crisis.

TO EVALUATE ORAL ANTICHOLINESTERASE THERAPY

- 2 mg of Tensilon is infused 1 hour after the patient's last dose of the anticholinesterase.
- The patient is observed carefully for adverse reactions and muscle response.
- After administration of Tensilon, the I.V. line is kept open at a rate of 20 ml/hour until all the patient's responses have been evaluated.

Postprocedure care

- When the test is complete, discontinue the I.V. infusion as ordered.
- Resume medications discontinued before the test as ordered.

MONITORING
- Vital signs
- Muscle strength
- Respiratory status
- Adverse effects of Tensilon

Precautions

- Because of the systemic adverse reactions Tensilon may produce, this test may be contraindicated in patients with hypotension, bradycardia, apnea, or mechanical obstruction of the intestine or urinary tract.

  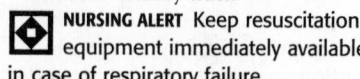 **NURSING ALERT** Keep resuscitation equipment immediately available in case of respiratory failure.

- Patients with respiratory disorders, such as asthma, should receive atropine, as ordered, during the test to minimize Tensilon's adverse effects.
- The test provides inconsistent results when myasthenia gravis affects only ocular muscles, as in mild or early forms of the disorder.

Complications

- Seizures
- Bradycardia, heart block, cardiac arrest
- Paralysis of respiratory muscles
- Bronchospasm, laryngospasm
- Respiratory depression
- Respiratory arrest

INTERPRETATION

Normal findings

- Development of fasciculations in response to Tensilon is found.

Abnormal results

- Improvement in muscle strength (a positive response) with Tensilon administration suggests myasthenia gravis.
- A positive response may also suggest motor neuron disease, some neuropathies, and myopathies.
- Patients in myasthenic crisis show a brief improvement in muscle strength after Tensilon administration.
- In patients in cholinergic crisis, Tensilon promptly exaggerates muscle weakness.

Thoracentesis

● OVERVIEW

- Performed diagnostically to obtain specimens of pleural fluid for analysis, or therapeutically to relieve respiratory symptoms caused by the accumulation of excess pleural fluid
- Specimens are examined for color, consistency, pH, glucose and protein content, cellular composition, and the enzymes lactate dehydrogenase (LD) and amylase; also examined cytologically for malignant cells and cultured for pathogens
- Also known as pleural fluid aspiration

Purpose
- To provide pleural fluid specimens to determine the cause and nature of pleural effusion
- To provide symptomatic relief with large pleural effusion

Patient preparation
- Make sure the patient has signed an appropriate consent form.
- Note and report all allergies.
- Record baseline vital signs.
- Food and fluids may be restricted if sedation will be used.
- Explain to the patient that pleural fluid may be located by chest X-ray or ultrasound study.
- Explain that a local anesthetic will be used. Warn about a stinging sensation felt on injection of the anesthetic and some pressure during withdrawal of the fluid.
- Instruct the patient to avoid coughing, deep breathing, or moving during the test to minimize the risk of injury to the lung.

TEACHING POINTS
Be sure to cover:
- the purpose of the study and how it's done
- who will perform the test and where
- that the study takes about 1 hour

▶ PROCEDURE

- The patient is properly positioned to widen the intercostal spaces and allow easier access to the pleural cavity.

- If the patient can't sit up, he's positioned on his unaffected side with the arm on the affected side elevated.
- After the patient is properly positioned the site is prepared and draped.
- A local anesthetic is injected into the subcutaneous tissue and the thoracentesis needle is inserted.
- When the needle reaches the pocket of fluid, it's attached to a 50-ml syringe or a vacuum bottle and the fluid is removed.
- During aspiration, the patient is monitored for signs of respiratory distress and hypotension.
- Pleural fluid characteristics and total volume are noted.
- After the needle is withdrawn, pressure is applied until hemostasis is obtained and a small dressing is applied.
- Specimens are placed in the proper containers, appropriately labeled, and immediately sent to the laboratory.

Postprocedure care
- Elevate the head of the bed to facilitate breathing.
- Obtain a chest X-ray as ordered.

NURSING ALERT Tell the patient to immediately report difficulty breathing. Immediately report signs and symptoms of pneumothorax, tension pneumothorax, and pleural fluid reaccumulation.

NURSING ALERT Monitor the patient for reexpansion pulmonary edema (RPE), a rare but serious complication of thoracentesis. Thoracentesis should be halted if the patient has sudden chest tightness or excessive coughing.

MONITORING
- Vital signs
- Pulse oximetry
- Breath sounds
- Puncture site and dressings
- Subcutaneous emphysema
- Pleural pressure

Precautions
- Supplemental oxygen is administered and pulse oximetry is monitored closely during thoracentesis.

NURSING ALERT Thoracentesis is contraindicated in patients with uncorrected bleeding disorders or anticoagulant therapy. The benefits of the procedure should outweigh the risks for

a patient taking an anticoagulant with an International Normalized Ratio of 1.5 to 2.5.
- Note the patient's temperature and use of antimicrobial therapy.

NURSING ALERT Pleural fluid for pH determination must be collected anaerobically, heparinized, kept on ice, and analyzed promptly.

Complications
- Laceration of intercostal vessels
- Pneumothorax
- Mediastinal shift
- Reexpansion pulmonary edema
- Bleeding and infection

✛ INTERPRETATION

Normal findings
- The pleural cavity should maintain negative pressure and contain less than 50 ml of serous fluid.

Abnormal results
- Bloody fluid suggests possible hemothorax, malignancy, or traumatic tap.
- Milky fluid suggests chylothorax.
- Fluid with pus suggests empyema.
- Transudative effusion suggests heart failure, hepatic cirrhosis, or renal disease.
- Exudative effusion suggests lymphatic drainage abstraction, infections, pulmonary infarctions, and neoplasms.
- Positive cultures suggest infection.
- Predominating lymphocytes suggest tuberculosis or fungal or viral effusions.
- Elevated LD levels in a nonpurulent, nonhemolyzed, nonbloody effusion suggest possible malignant tumor.
- Pleural fluid glucose levels that are 30 to 40 mg/dl lower than blood glucose levels may indicate cancer, bacterial infection, or metastasis.
- Increased amylase suggests pleural effusions associated with pancreatitis.

Thoracoscopy

● OVERVIEW

- Insertion of an endoscope directly into the chest wall allowing visualization of the pleural space
- Used for both diagnostic and therapeutic purposes; can sometimes replace traditional thoracotomy
- Reduces morbidity (by avoiding open chest surgery) and postoperative pain, decreases surgical and anesthesia time, and allows faster recovery

Purpose

- To diagnose pleural disease
- To obtain biopsy specimens from the mediastinum, lung, or pericardium
- To facilitate treatment of pleural conditions, such as cysts, blebs, and effusions
- To allow resection such as wedge biopsy

Patient preparation

- Make sure the patient has signed an appropriate consent form.
- Note and report all allergies.
- Make sure appropriate preoperative tests (such as pulmonary function and coagulation tests, electrocardiogram, and chest X-ray) have been performed; report abnormal results to the doctor.
- Explain that general anesthesia is frequently used.
- Restriction of food and fluids is required for 10 to 12 hours before the procedure.
- Explain the placement of a chest tube and use of a chest tube drainage system.

TEACHING POINTS

Be sure to cover:
- purpose of the study and how it's done
- how the study will be performed
- that analgesics will be available postoperatively.

▶ PROCEDURE

- The patient is anesthetized and a double-lumen endobronchial tube is inserted.
- The lung on the operative side is collapsed and a small intercostal incision is made, through which a trocar is inserted.
- A lens is inserted to view the area and assess thoracoscopy access.
- Two or three more small incisions are made and trocars are placed for insertion of suctioning and dissection instruments.
- The camera lens and instruments are moved from site to site as needed.
- After thoracoscopy, the lung is reexpanded and a chest tube is placed through one incision site.
- The other incisions are closed with adhesive strips and dressed.
- A water-seal drainage system is attached to the chest tube.

Postprocedure care

- Administer analgesics as ordered.
- Resume diet and activity as ordered.
- Send specimens to the laboratory immediately.

MONITORING

- Vital signs
- Intake and output
- Respiratory status
- Patency of the chest tube and drainage system
- Bleeding
- Infection

Precautions

- Thoracoscopy is contraindicated in patients with:
  - uncorrected coagulopathies
  - lesions near major blood vessels
  - history of previous thoracic surgery
  - inability to be adequately oxygenated with one lung.
- Excessive bleeding during the procedure may necessitate open thoracotomy.
- Extensive or inaccessible pathology may prevent thoracoscopy.

Complications

- Hemorrhage
- Nerve injury
- Perforation of the diaphragm
- Air emboli
- Tension pneumothorax

✛ INTERPRETATION

Normal findings

- The pleural cavity should contain a small amount of lubricating fluid that facilitates movement of the lung and chest wall.
- The parietal and visceral layers should be lesion-free and able to separate from each other.

Abnormal results

- Lesions adjacent to or involving the pleura or mediastinum suggest possible malignancy; will be biopsied for diagnosis and determination of treatment.
- Blebs suggest possible presence of chronic lung disease; can be removed by wedge resection to reduce the risk of spontaneous pneumothorax.
- The presence of increased pleural fluid indicates pleural effusion; specimens can be obtained for analysis and diagnosis of cause of pleural effusion.

Throat culture

- Requires swabbing the throat, streaking a culture plate, and allowing organisms to grow for isolation and identification of pathogens
- Preliminary identification possibly obtained through Gram-stained smear; used to guide clinical management and determine the need for further tests
- Rapid nonculture antigen testing methods: used to detect group A streptococcal antigen in as little as 5 minutes; all negative specimens should be cultured

Purpose

- To isolate and identify pathogens, especially group A beta-hemolytic streptococci
- To screen asymptomatic carriers of pathogens, especially *Neisseria meningitidis*

Patient preparation

- Make sure the patient has signed an appropriate consent form.
- Confirm the patient's identity using two patient identifiers according to facility policy.
- Note and report all allergies.
- Wash your hands thoroughly.
- Maintain asepsis throughout all procedures.
- Wear personal protective equipment throughout the procedure.
- Check the patient's history for recent antimicrobial therapy.
- Determine immunization history if pertinent to the preliminary diagnosis.
- Obtain a specimen before beginning antimicrobial therapy.
- Restriction of food and fluids before the test isn't necessary.
- Warn the patient that gagging may be experienced during the swabbing.

TEACHING POINTS

Be sure to cover:
- purpose of the test and how it's done
- who will perform the test and where
- that the test takes less than 30 seconds
- that results should be available in 2 or 3 days.

- Tell the patient to tilt his head back and close his eyes.
- With the throat well illuminated, check for inflamed areas, using a tongue blade.
- Swab the tonsillar areas from side to side; include any inflamed or purulent sites. Don't touch the tongue, cheeks, or teeth with the swab.
- Immediately place the swab in the culture tube. If a commercial sterile collection and transport system is used, crush the ampule and force the swab into the medium to keep it moist.
- Note recent antimicrobial therapy on the laboratory request. Label the specimen with the patient's name, doctor's name, date and time of collection, and origin of the specimen. Also indicate the suspected organism, especially *Corynebacterium diphtheriae* (requires two swabs and a special growth medium), and *N. meningitidis* (requires enriched selective media).

Postprocedure care

- No specific posttest care is necessary.

Precautions

- Use standard precautions.
- Send the specimen to the laboratory immediately.
- Unless a commercial sterile collection and transport system is used, keep the container upright during transport.

Complications

- None known

Normal findings

- Throat flora include nonhemolytic and alpha-hemolytic streptococci, Neisseria species, staphylococci, diphtheroids, some Haemophilus species, pneumococci, yeasts, enteric gram-negative organisms, spirochetes, Veillonella species, and Micrococcus species.

Abnormal results

- Group A beta-hemolytic streptococci *(Streptococcus pyogenes),* suggests possible scarlet fever or pharyngitis.
- *Candida albicans* suggests possible thrush.
- *C. diphtheriae* suggests possible diphtheria.
- *Bordetella pertussis* suggests possible whooping cough.
- *Legionella* species and *Mycoplasma pneumoniae* suggests bacterial pneumonia.
- *Histoplasma capsulatum, Coccidioides immitis,* and *Blastomyces dermatitidis* suggest fungal infections.
- Adenovirus, enterovirus, herpesvirus, rhinovirus, influenza virus, and parainfluenza virus suggest viral infections.

Thyroid biopsy

- The excision of a thyroid tissue specimen for histologic examination
- May be indicated for patients with thyroid enlargement or nodules; breathing and swallowing difficulties; vocal cord paralysis, weight loss, hemoptysis, or a sensation of fullness in the neck
- Commonly performed when noninvasive tests, such as thyroid ultrasonography and scans, are abnormal or inconclusive
- Specimens obtained with hollow needle under local anesthesia or during open (surgical) biopsy under general anesthesia

Purpose
- To differentiate between benign and malignant thyroid disease
- To diagnose Hashimoto's disease, hyperthyroidism, and nontoxic nodular goiter

Patient preparation
- Make sure the patient has signed an appropriate consent form.
- Note and report all allergies.
- Obtain results of coagulation studies and report abnormal results to the doctor.
- Restriction of food and fluids isn't necessary unless a general anesthetic will be used.
- Explain the use of a local anesthetic.
- Warn the patient that he might experience some pressure when the tissue specimen is obtained.
- Administer sedation, as ordered.

TEACHING POINTS
Be sure to cover:
- the purpose of the study and how it's done
- who will perform the biopsy and where
- that the test takes 15 to 30 minutes
- that results should be available in 48 to 72 hours
- that sore throat is possible the day after the test.

- The patient is placed in a supine position with a pillow under his shoulder blades. This position pushes the trachea and thyroid forward and allows the neck veins to fall backward.
- The biopsy site is prepared and draped.
- Local anesthetic is administered.
- The carotid artery is palpated, and the biopsy needle is inserted parallel to and about 1″ (2.5 cm) from the thyroid cartilage to prevent damage to the deep structures and the larynx.
- After the specimen is obtained, the needle is removed and the specimen is immediately placed in formalin.
- Pressure is applied to the biopsy site until hemostasis is obtained.
- The biopsy site is cleaned and dressed.

Postprocedure care
- Place the patient in semi-Fowler's position.
- Teach the patient to avoid undue strain on the biopsy site by putting both hands behind his neck when he sits up.
- Keep the biopsy site clean and dry.

MONITORING
- Vital signs
- Respiratory status
- Neck circumference
- Swallowing ability
- Bleeding
- Infection
- Voice quality

⬙ **NURSING ALERT** Observe for difficulty breathing associated with edema or hematoma, with resultant tracheal compression. Also check the back of the patient's neck and his pillow for bleeding every hour for 8 hours. Report bleeding immediately.

Precautions
- Thyroid biopsy is used cautiously in patients with uncorrected coagulation defects.
- Because cell breakdown in the tissue specimen begins immediately after excision, the specimen must be placed in formalin solution immediately.
- Bleeding may persist in a patient with abnormal prothrombin time or abnormal activated partial thromboplastin time or in a patient with a large, vascular thyroid and distended veins.

Complications
- Bleeding
- Infection
- Respiratory compromise

Normal findings
- Fibrous networks divide the gland into pseudolobules that consist of follicles and capillaries.
- Cuboidal epithelium lines the follicle walls and contains the protein thyroglobulin, which stores triiodothyronine and thyroxine.

Abnormal results
- Well-encapsulated, solitary nodules of uniform but abnormal structure suggest possible malignant tumors.
- Hypertrophy, hyperplasia, and hypervascularity suggest possible benign conditions such as nontoxic nodular goiter.
- Characteristic histologic patterns suggest possible subacute granulomatous thyroiditis, Hashimoto's disease, and hyperthyroidism.

Thyroid imaging, radionuclide

● OVERVIEW

- Allows visualization of the thyroid gland by a gamma camera after administration of a radioisotope (usually ^{123}I, ^{131}I, or technetium-99m [^{99m}Tc] pertechnetate); ^{123}I and ^{131}I: used most often because of their short half-lives (which limit exposure to radiation) and to enable measurement of thyroid function
- Usually recommended after discovery of a palpable mass, enlarged gland, or asymmetrical goiter
- Usually performed concurrently with measurement of serum triiodothyronine (T_3) and serum thyroxine levels and thyroid uptake tests

Purpose
- To assess size, structure, and position of the thyroid gland
- To evaluate thyroid function in conjunction with other thyroid tests

Patient preparation
- Make sure the patient has signed an appropriate consent form.
- Note and report all allergies.
- Determine if the patient has undergone tests that used radiographic contrast media within the past 60 days; note such tests or the use of drugs that may interfere with iodine uptake on the radiograph request.
- Two to three weeks before the test, discontinue administration of thyroid hormones, thyroid hormone antagonists, and iodine preparations (Lugol's solution, some multivitamins, and cough syrups), phenothiazines, corticosteroids, salicylates, anticoagulants, and antihistamines as ordered.
- Instruct the patient to avoid iodized salt, iodinated salt substitutes, and seafood for 14 to 21 days as ordered.
- Discontinue liothyronine, propylthiouracil, and methimazole 3 days before the test as ordered.
- Discontinue thyroxine 10 days before the test as ordered.
- Tell the patient to fast after midnight the night before the test (if scheduled to receive an oral dose of ^{123}I or ^{131}I); fasting is necessary for another 2 hours after it's administered.

- There's no need to fast if the patient will receive an I.V. injection of ^{99m}Tc pertechnetate.

TEACHING POINTS
Be sure to cover:
- the purpose of the study and how it's done
- who will perform the test and where
- that the test takes only 30 minutes and that radiation exposure is minimal.

▶ PROCEDURE

- The test is performed 24 hours after oral administration of ^{123}I or ^{131}I, or 20 to 30 minutes after I.V. injection of ^{99m}Tc pertechnetate.
- Just before the test, tell the patient to remove his dentures and any jewelry that could interfere with visualization of the thyroid.
- The patient is placed in a supine position with his neck extended.
- The patient's thyroid gland is palpated.
- The gamma camera is placed over the anterior portion of the neck; the radioactive substance within the thyroid gland projects an image of the gland on an oscilloscope screen and X-ray film.
- Three views of the thyroid are obtained: one straight-on anterior view and two bilateral oblique views.

Postprocedure care
- Resume medications as ordered.
- Resume a normal diet as ordered.

MONITORING
- Vital signs

Precautions
- Contraindications include:
  - pregnancy
  - lactation
  - previous allergy to iodine, shellfish, or radioactive tracers.

Complications
- Adverse reaction to the radioactive tracer (rare)

✛ INTERPRETATION

Normal findings
- Thyroid gland should be about 2″ (5 cm) long and 1″ (2.5 cm) wide, with uniform uptake of the radioisotope and without tumors.
- The gland should be butterfly-shaped, with the isthmus located at the midline.
- Occasionally, a third lobe called the pyramidal lobe may be present; this is a normal variant.

Abnormal results
- Areas of excessive iodine uptake, appearing as black regions called hot spots, suggest hyperfunctioning nodules.
- White or light gray regions, appearing as areas of little or no iodine uptake called cold spots, suggest hypofunctioning nodules.

Transcranial Doppler studies

● OVERVIEW

- Provide information about the presence, quality, and changing nature of circulation to an area of the brain by measuring the velocity of blood flow through cerebral arteries
- Commonly not definitive but advantageous because it provides diagnostic information in a noninvasive manner
- After transcranial Doppler study and before surgery: the patient may undergo cerebral angiography to further define cerebral blood flow patterns and to locate the exact vascular abnormality

Purpose
- To measure velocity of blood flow through certain cerebral vessels
- To detect and monitor progression of cerebral vasospasm
- To determine presence of collateral blood flow before surgical ligation or radiologic occlusion of diseased blood vessels

Patient preparation
- Make sure the patient has signed an appropriate consent form.
- Note and report all allergies.
- Fasting before the test isn't necessary.

TEACHING POINTS
Be sure to cover:
- the purpose of the study and how it's done
- who will perform the test and where
- that the test usually takes less than 1 hour, depending on the number of vessels to be examined and any interfering factors.

▶ PROCEDURE

- The patient reclines in a chair or on a stretcher or bed.
- A small amount of gel is applied to the transcranial "window" (temporal, transorbital, and through the foramen magnum) where bone is thin enough to allow the Doppler signal to enter and be detected.
- The technologist directs the signal toward the artery being studied and then records the velocities detected and the direction of the blood flow.
- In a complete study, the middle cerebral arteries, anterior cerebral arteries, ophthalmic arteries, carotid siphon, vertebral arteries, and basilar artery are studied.
- The Doppler signal can be transmitted to varying depths. Waveforms may be printed for later analysis.

Postprocedure care
- Remove any remaining gel from the patient's skin.

Precautions
- Dressings over the test site may prevent insonation.

Complications
- None known

⊹ INTERPRETATION

Normal findings
- Normal waveforms and velocities are found.

Abnormal results
- High velocities suggest that the vessel is stenotic or in vasospasm. Highly turbulent blood flow may suggest the presence of arteriovenous malfunction. (See *Comparing velocity waveforms*.)

COMPARING VELOCITY WAVEFORMS

A normal transcranial Doppler signal is usually characterized by mean velocities that fall within the normal reported values. Additional information can be gathered by evaluating the shape of the velocity waveform.

Effect of significant proximal vessel obstruction
A delayed systolic upstroke can be seen in a waveform when significant proximal vessel obstruction is present.

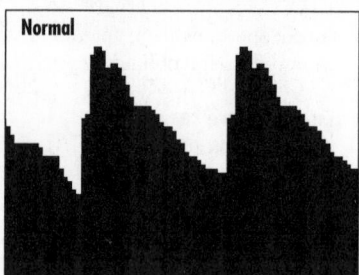

Normal

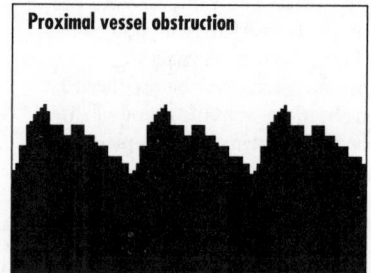

Proximal vessel obstruction

Effect of increased cerebrovascular resistance
Changes in cerebrovascular resistance, as occur with increased intracranial pressure, cause a decrease in diastolic flow.

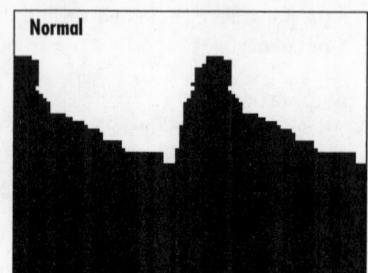

Normal

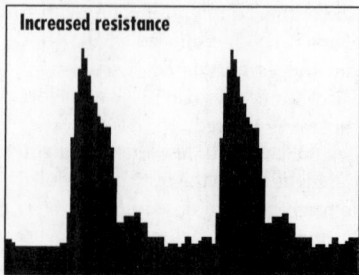

Increased resistance

Transesophageal echocardiography

- Combines ultrasonography with endoscopy to provide a better view of the heart's structures
- Involves small transducer attached to the end of a gastroscope and inserted into the esophagus, allowing images to be taken from the posterior aspect of the heart
- Causes less tissue penetration and interference from chest wall structures and produces high-quality images of the thoracic aorta, except for the superior ascending aorta, which is shadowed by the trachea

Purpose

- To visualize and evaluate many disorders:
  - Thoracic and aortic disorders, such as dissection and aneurysm
  - Valvular disease (especially of the mitral valve)
  - Endocarditis
  - Congenital heart disease
  - Intracardiac thrombi
  - Cardiac tumors
  - Cardiac tamponade
  - Ventricular dysfunction

Patient preparation

- Make sure the patient has signed an appropriate consent form.
- Note and report all allergies.
- Review the patient's medical history and report possible contraindications to the test, such as esophageal obstruction or varices, GI bleeding, previous mediastinal radiation therapy, or severe cervical arthritis.
- Note and report loose teeth.
- Fasting is required for 6 hours before the procedure.
- Instruct the patient to remove dentures or oral prostheses.
- Explain the use of a topical anesthetic throat spray.
- Warn about possible gagging when the tube is inserted.
- Explain the need for I.V. sedation and continuous monitoring during the study.

TEACHING POINTS
Be sure to cover:
- the purpose of the study and how it's done

- who will perform the test and when
- that the study takes about 2 hours including preparation and recovery.

▶ PROCEDURE

- The patient is connected to monitors for continual blood pressure, heart rate, and pulse oximetry assessment.
- The patient is positioned supine on his left side and the ordered sedative is administered.
- The back of his throat is sprayed with a topical anesthetic.
- A bite block is placed in the patient's mouth and he's instructed to close his lips around it.
- The endoscope is inserted and advanced 12″ to 14″ (30 to 35 cm) to the level of the right atrium.
- To visualize the left ventricle, the scope is advanced 16″ to 18″ (40 to 45 cm).
- Ultrasound images are obtained and reviewed.

Postprocedure care

- Ensure patient safety and patent airway until the sedative wears off.
- Withhold food and water until his gag reflex returns.
- Keep resuscitation equipment immediately available.
- Keep suction equipment immediately available to avoid aspiration if vomiting occurs.
- Observe closely for a vasovagal response, which may occur with gagging.
- Use pulse oximetry to detect hypoxia.
- If the procedure is done on an outpatient basis, advise the patient to have someone drive him home.

MONITORING
- Level of consciousness
- Vital signs
- Respiratory status
- Cardiac arrhythmias
- Bleeding
- Gag reflex

Precautions

- If bleeding occurs, stop the procedure immediately.
- Laryngospasm, arrhythmias, or bleeding increases the risk of complica-

tions. If any of these occurs, postpone the test.
- Possible contraindications include esophageal obstruction or varices, GI bleeding, previous mediastinal radiation therapy, or severe cervical arthritis.

Complications
- Laryngospasm
- Cardiac arrhythmias
- Bleeding
- Adverse reaction to sedation

✣ INTERPRETATION

Normal findings
- The heart is without structural abnormalities.
- No vegetations or thrombus is visible.
- No tumors are visible.

Abnormal results
- Structural thoracic and aortic abnormalities suggest possible endocarditis, congenital heart disease, intracardiac thrombi, or tumors.
- Congenital defects suggest possible patent ductus arteriosus.

Ultrasonography

● OVERVIEW

- Involves use of a transducer to send sound waves through targeted tissue
- After passing through tissue, sound waves reflect back to the transducer, where they're converted into electrical impulses, which are amplified and displayed on a screen
- Sound waves travel at varying speeds, depending on density of tissue they're passing through; images on the display screen reflect this difference

Purpose
- To measure organ size and evaluate structure
- To detect foreign bodies and differentiate between a cyst and solid tumor
- To monitor tissue response to radiation or chemotherapy

Patient preparation
- Make sure the patient has signed an appropriate consent form.
- Note and report all allergies.
- Stress the importance of remaining still during scanning to prevent a distorted image.

TEACHING POINTS
Be sure to cover:
- the purpose of the study and how it's done
- who will perform the test and where
- how long the test will take
- that the procedure is painless and safe; no radiation exposure is involved.

▶ PROCEDURE

- The patient is placed in a supine position; pillows may be used to support the area to be examined.
- The target area is coated with a gel. The transducer is used to scan the area, projecting the images on the oscilloscope screen. The image on the screen is recorded for subsequent examination.
- The patient may be placed in right or left lateral positions for subsequent views, if indicated.

Postprocedure care
- Remove the gel from the patient's skin.

Complications
- None known

✛ INTERPRETATION

Normal findings
- See "Normal findings" for specific ultrasonography procedure.

Abnormal results
- See "Abnormal results" for specific ultrasonography procedure.

Ultrasonography, abdominal aorta

- Used to confirm a suspected aortic aneurysm and method of choice for determining its diameter; performed to detect expansion of a known aneurysm because the risk of rupture is high when aneurysmal diameter is 5.0 to 5.5 cm or greater
- Used every 6 months to monitor changes in patient's status
- Transducer directs high-frequency sound waves into the abdomen over a wide area from the xiphoid process to the umbilical region; sound waves echoing to transducer from tissue of different densities are transmitted as electrical impulses and displayed on a monitor to reveal internal organs, the vertebral column and, most important, the size and course of the abdominal aorta and other major vessels

Purpose
- To detect and measure a suspected abdominal aortic aneurysm
- To monitor expansion of a known abdominal aortic aneurysm

Patient preparation
- Make sure the patient has signed an appropriate consent form.
- Note and report all allergies.
- Administer simethicone to reduce bowel gas if ordered.
- Fasting is required for 8 hours before the test to minimize bowel gas and motility.
- Inform the patient that he will feel slight pressure during the study
- Instruct the patient to remain still during scanning and to hold his breath when requested.

TEACHING POINTS
Be sure to cover:
- the purpose of the study and how it's done
- who will perform the test and where
- that the test takes 30 to 45 minutes.

- The patient is placed in a supine position.
- Gel is applied to the abdomen.
- Longitudinal scans are then made at 0.5- to 1-cm intervals to the left and right of midline until the entire abdominal aorta is outlined.
- Transverse scans are made at 1- to 2-cm intervals from the xiphoid process to the bifurcation at the common iliac arteries.
- The patient may be placed in right and left lateral positions.
- Appropriate views are recorded.

Postprocedure care
- Remove gel from the skin.
- Resume the patient's usual diet and medications as ordered.
- ◆ **NURSING ALERT** Remember that sudden onset of constant abdominal or back pain accompanies rapid expansion of the aneurysm; sudden, excruciating pain with weakness, sweating, tachycardia, and hypotension signals rupture.

Complications
- None known

Normal findings
- In adults, the abdominal aorta tapers about ½″ to 1″ (1 to 2.5 cm) in diameter along its length from the diaphragm to the bifurcation.
- The abdominal aorta descends through the retroperitoneal space, anterior to the vertebral column and slightly left of the midline.
- Four of the abdominal aorta's major branches are usually well visualized: the celiac trunk, the renal arteries, the superior mesenteric artery, and the common iliac arteries.

Abnormal results
- Luminal diameter of the abdominal aorta greater than 1″ (3 cm) indicates an aneurysm.
- Luminal diameter of the abdominal aorta greater than 2″ (5 cm) indicates an aneurysm with a high risk of rupture.

Ultrasonography, Doppler

● OVERVIEW

- Noninvasive imaging and nonimaging test to evaluate blood flow in major veins and arteries of arms, legs, and extracranial cerebrovascular system and abdomen
- High-frequency sound waves directed by handheld transducer to artery or vein; sound waves reflect from blood flow moving through vessels
- Measures speed, direction, and pattern of blood flow and vein abnormalities to help detect peripheral arterial occlusive disease

Purpose

- To help diagnose venous insufficiency, superficial and deep vein thromboses, and peripheral arterial occlusive disease and aneurysm
- To monitor arterial reconstruction and bypass graft patients
- To detect abnormalities of carotid artery blood flow
- To evaluate arterial trauma

Patient preparations

- Make sure the patient has signed an appropriate consent form.
- Note and report any allergies.

TEACHING POINTS

Be sure to cover:

- purpose of the test and how it's done
- who will perform the test and where
- that the test takes 30 to 60 minutes.

▶ PROCEDURE

- Doppler ultrasonography is usually performed bilaterally.
- The patient is assisted into the supine position on the examination table with his arms at his sides.
- Water-soluble gel is applied.

PERIPHERAL ARTERIAL EVALUATION

- For peripheral arterial evaluation in the leg, the usual test sites are the common and superficial femoral, popliteal, posterior tibial, and dorsalis pedis arteries.
- For peripheral arterial evaluation in the arm, the usual test sites are the subclavian, axillary, brachial, radial, and ulnar arteries.

- Brachial blood pressure is measured, and the transducer is placed at various points along the test arteries.
- The Doppler signals are obtained and waveforms recorded.
- The blood flow velocity is monitored and recorded from the test artery.
- Segmental limb blood pressures may be obtained to localize arterial occlusive disease.
- For extracranial cerebrovascular imaging, the usual test sites are the common, external, and internal carotid arteries; the vertebral arteries; subclavian artery, and jugular veins.

PERIPHERAL VENOUS EVALUATION

- For peripheral venous evaluation in the leg, the usual test sites are the popliteal, femoral and common femoral, and posterior tibial veins.
- The transducer is placed over the appropriate vessel, waveforms are recorded, and respiratory modulations are noted.
- Limb compression maneuvers are performed to detect thrombus
- Augmentation after release of compression is noted to evaluate venous valve competency
- For tests involving the legs, patient is asked to perform Valsalva's maneuver and venous blood flow is recorded.

Postprocedure care

- Remove the gel from the patient's skin.

Precautions

- Don't place the Doppler probe or transducer over an open or draining lesion.

Complications

- Bradyarrhythmia (if probe placed near carotid sinus)

✛ INTERPRETATION

Normal findings

- Arterial dethysmographic waveforms of the arms and legs are multiphasic, with a prominent systolic component and one or more diastolic sounds.
- Proximal thigh pressure is 20 to 30 mm Hg greater than arm pressure.
- Venous blood flow velocity is phasic with respiration, with a lower pitch than arterial flow.
- Venous blood flow velocity increases with distal compression or release of proximal limb compression.
- Valsalva's maneuver interrupts venous return.
- In arterial testing, a triphasic velocity signal is present.
- In the common carotid artery, blood flow velocity increases in diastole.
- Ankle-brachial index (ABI) is 0.9.

Abnormal results

- Reduced blood flow velocity signal implies proximal arterial stenosis or occlusion.
- Absent velocity signal suggests complete occlusion.
- ABI of 0.5 to 0.9 indicates claudication; ABI<0.5, resting ischemic pain; and ABI< 0.2, gangrenous foot or leg.
- High-velocity, turbulent arerial spectral waveforms indicate critical stenosis.
- Incompressible veins without spontaneous, phasic Doppler signals indicate venous thrombosis.
- Reversed flow velocity signal suggests chronic venous insufficiency.

Ultrasonography, gallbladder and biliary system

● OVERVIEW

- Focused beam of high-frequency sound waves passes into the right upper quadrant of the abdomen, creating echoes that vary with changes in tissue density
- Images reveal the size, shape, structure, and position of gallbladder and biliary system
- Ultrasound of gallbladder is procedure of choice for evaluating jaundice and for emergency diagnosis of patients with signs of acute cholecystitis such as right upper quadrant pain with or without local tenderness
- When ultrasonography fails to clearly define the site of biliary obstruction: necessitates percutaneous transhepatic cholangiography or endoscopic retrograde cholangiopancreatography

Purpose
- To confirm diagnosis of cholelithiasis
- To diagnose acute cholecystitis
- To distinguish between obstructive and nonobstructive jaundice

Patient preparation
- Make sure the patient has signed an appropriate consent form.
- Note and report all allergies.
- Provide a fat-free meal in the evening before the study.
- Fasting is required for 8 to 12 hours before the procedure, if possible; this promotes accumulation of bile in the gallbladder and enhances ultrasonic visualization.
- Instruct the patient to remain as still as possible during the procedure and to hold his breath when requested; this ensures that the gallbladder is in the same position for each scan.

TEACHING POINTS
Be sure to cover:
- purpose of the test
- a darkened room aids visualization
- that the test takes 15 to 30 minutes.

▶ PROCEDURE

- The patient is placed in a supine position.
- A water-soluble gel is applied to the face of the transducer, and transverse scans of the gallbladder are taken at 1-cm intervals, starting at the level of the xiphoid and moving laterally to the right subcostal area.
- Longitudinal oblique scans are taken at 5-mm intervals parallel to the long axis of the gallbladder marked on the patient's skin, beginning medial to the gallbladder and continuing through to its lateral border.
- During each scan the patient is asked to exhale deeply and hold his breath.
- If the gallbladder is positioned deeply under the right costal margin, a scan may be taken through the intercostal spaces, while the patient inhales deeply and holds his breath.
- The patient is placed in a left lateral decubitus position and scanned beneath the right costal margin. This allows for displacing stones lodged in the cystic duct region, which escape detection in the supine position.
- Scanning with the patient erect helps demonstrate mobility or fixation of suspicious echogenic areas.
- Oscilloscopic views are obtained and photographed for later study.

Postprocedure care
- Remove the gel from the patient's skin.
- Resume the patient's normal diet.

Precautions
- Fasting before the study prevents the excretion of bile in the gallbladder.

Complications
- None known

✛ INTERPRETATION

Normal findings
- The normal gallbladder is sonolucent; it appears circular on transverse scans and pear-shaped on longitudinal scans.

- Although the gallbladder's size varies, its outer walls normally appear sharp and smooth.
- Intrahepatic radicles seldom appear because the flow of sonolucent bile is very fine.
- The cystic duct may be indistinct because of folds known as Heister's valves that line the cystic duct lumen.
- When visualized, the cystic duct has a serpentine appearance.
- The common bile duct has a linear appearance but is sometimes obscured by overlying bowel gas.

Abnormal results
- Mobile, echogenic areas, usually associated with an acoustic shadow, suggests gallstones within the gallbladder lumen or the biliary system.
- When the gallbladder is shrunken or fully impacted with gallstones, inadequate bile may make gallstone detection difficult and the gallbladder itself may fail to be visualized. In this case, the presence of an acoustic shadow in the gallbladder fossa suggests cholelithiasis.
- An acoustic shadow in the cystic and common bile ducts suggests possible choledocholithiasis.
- Fixed echogenic areas within the gallbladder lumen suggests possible polyps or tumors; polyps usually appear as sharply defined, echogenic areas; carcinoma appears as a poorly defined mass commonly associated with a thickened gallbladder wall.
- A fine layer of echoes that slowly gravitates to the dependent portion of the gallbladder as the patient changes position, suggests biliary sludge within the gallbladder lumen.
- An enlarged gallbladder with thickened, double-rimmed walls, usually accompanied by gallstones within the lumen, suggests acute cholecystitis.
- A contracted gallbladder with thickened walls suggests chronic cholecystitis.
- A dilated biliary system and, usually, a dilated gallbladder suggests obstructive jaundice.

Ultrasonography, kidney and perirenal structures

● OVERVIEW

- High-frequency sound waves (usually 1 to 5 million cycles/second) are transmitted from transducer and through the kidneys and perirenal structures; resulting echoes are amplified and converted into electrical impulses and displayed on aa monitor as anatomic images
- Usually performed with other urologic tests to detect abnormalities or provide more information about abnormalities detected by other tests
- A safe, painless procedure, it's especially valuable when excretory urography is ruled out—for example, because of hypersensitivity to the contrast medium or the need for serial examinations
- Doesn't require adequate renal function (unlike excretory urography) and therefore useful in patients with renal failure
- Evaluation of urologic disorders may also include ultrasonography of ureter, bladder, and gonads

Purpose

- To determine the size, shape, and position of the kidneys, their internal structures, and perirenal tissues
- To evaluate and localize urinary obstruction and abnormal accumulation of fluid
- To assess and diagnose complications after kidney transplantation
- To detect renal or perirenal masses
- To differentiate between renal cysts and solid masses
- To verify placement of a nephrostomy tube

Patient preparation

- Explain that the test is used to detect abnormalities in the kidneys.
- Food and fluids need not be restricted before the test.

TEACHING POINTS
Be sure to cover:
- the purpose of the study and how it's done
- who will perform the test and where
- that the test takes about 30 minutes
- that the test is safe and painless.

▶ PROCEDURE

- The patient is placed in the prone position and the area to be scanned is exposed.
- Gel is applied to the area before the scanning begins.
- The longitudinal axis of the kidneys is located using measurements from excretory urography or by performing transverse scans through the upper and lower renal poles.
- These points are marked on the skin and connected with straight lines.
- Sectional images (1 to 2 cm apart) can then be obtained by moving the transducer longitudinally and transversely or at any other angle required.
- During the test the patient may be asked to breathe deeply to visualize upper portions of the kidney.

Postprocedure care

- After the procedure, remove the gel from the patient's skin.
- If bladder abnormalities are found, prepare the patient for further testing.

MONITORING
- If rejection of a transplanted kidney is suspected or diagnosed, monitor intake and output, blood pressure, blood urea nitrogen and creatinine levels, and vital signs
- If an adrenal tumor is detected, check for adrenal dysfunction (hypotension, decreased urine output, and electrolyte imbalances)
- If a nephrostomy tube has been placed, monitor the amount and characteristics of drainage and tube patency

Complications

- None known

✛ INTERPRETATION

Normal findings

- The kidneys are located between the superior iliac crests and the diaphragm.
- The renal capsule should be outlined sharply; the cortex should produce more echoes than the medulla.
- In the center of each kidney the renal collecting systems appear as irregular areas of higher density than surrounding tissue.

Abnormal results

- Fluid-filled, circular structures that don't reflect sound waves suggest cysts.
- Multiple echoes appearing as irregular shapes suggest tumor
- Fluid-filled structures with slightly irregular boundaries that don't reflect sound waves well suggest abscesses
- A renal capsule that appears irregular and a kidney that appears smaller than normal and is associated with an increased number of echoes arising from the parenchyma because of fibrosis may suggest acute pyelonephritis and glomerulonephritis.
- A large, echo-free, central mass that compresses the renal cortex may indicate hydronephrosis.
- After kidney transplantation, compensatory hypertrophy of the transplanted kidney is normal but an acute increase in size indicates rejection of the transplant.
- Abnormal accumulations of fluid within or around the kidneys may suggest an obstruction.
- Increased urine volume or residual urine postvoiding may indicate bladder dysfunction.

Ultrasonography, liver

● OVERVIEW

- Cross-sectional images of the liver produced by channeling high-frequency sound waves into the right upper quadrant of the abdomen; resultant echoes are converted to electrical energy, amplified by a transducer, and displayed on a monitor
- Different shades of gray depict various tissue densities
- Can show intrahepatic structures as well as organ size, shape, and position
- Indicated for patients with jaundice of unknown etiology, unexplained hepatomegaly and abnormal biochemical test results, suspected metastatic tumors and elevated serum alkaline phosphatase levels, and recent abdominal trauma
- When used to complement liver-spleen scanning, can define cold spots—focal defects that fail to pick up the radionuclide—as tumors, abscesses, or cysts; also provides better views of the periportal and perihepatic spaces than liver-spleen scanning

Purpose
- To distinguish between obstructive and nonobstructive jaundice
- To screen for hepatocellular disease
- To detect hepatic metastases and hematoma
- To define cold spots as tumors, abscesses, or cysts

Patient preparation
- Make sure the patient has signed an appropriate consent form.
- Note and report all allergies.
- Fasting is required for 8 to 12 hours before the test.
- Warn the patient that mild pressure may be felt as the transducer presses against the skin.
- Stress the need to remain as still as possible during the procedure and hold his breath when requested.

TEACHING POINTS
Be sure to cover:
- the purpose of the study and how it's done
- who will perform the test and where
- that the test takes 15 to 30 minutes
- that the test isn't harmful or painful.

▶ PROCEDURE

- The patient is placed in a supine position.
- A water-soluble gel is applied to the face of the transducer, and transverse scans are taken at ⅜" (1-cm) intervals, using a single-sweep technique between the costal margins.
- Sector scans are taken through the intercostal spaces to view the remainder of the right lobe.
- Scans are taken longitudinally, from the right border of the liver to the left.
- Oblique cephalad-angled scans may be taken beneath the right costal margin for better demonstration of the right lateral dome.
- Scans are then taken parallel to the hepatic portal, at a 45-degree angle toward the superior right lateral dome, to examine the peripheral anatomy, portal venous system, common bile duct, and biliary tree.
- During each scan the patient is asked to hold his breath briefly in deep inspiration.
- Clear images are recorded for later study.

Postprocedure care
- Remove gel from the patient's skin.
- Resume a usual diet as ordered.

Complications
- None known

✛ INTERPRETATION

Normal findings
- The liver demonstrates a homogeneous, low-level echo pattern, interrupted only by the different echo patterns of its vascular channels.
- Intrahepatic biliary radicles and hepatic arteries aren't apparent, but portal and hepatic veins, the aorta, and the inferior vena cava appear on ultrasound.
- Hepatic veins appear completely sonolucent; portal veins have margins that are highly echogenic.

Abnormal results
- Dilated intrahepatic biliary radicles and extrahepatic ducts suggest obstructive jaundice.
- Variable liver size, dilated, tortuous portal branches associated with portal hypertension, and an irregular echo pattern with increased echo amplitude, causing overall increased attenuation suggest possible cirrhosis.
- Hepatomegaly and a regular echo pattern that, although greater in echo amplitude than that of normal parenchyma, don't alter attenuation suggest possible fatty infiltration of the liver.
- Hypoechoic or echogenic and either poorly defined or well defined areas suggest possible metastasis in the liver.
- Sonolucent masses with ill-defined, slightly thickened borders and accentuated posterior wall transmission suggest possible abscesses.
- The presence of fluid lacking internal echoes with a more regular border suggests possible ascitic fluid.
- Spherical, sonolucent areas with well-defined borders and accentuated posterior wall transmission suggest possible cysts.
- Poorly defined, relatively sonolucent masses, with possible scattered internal echoes caused by clotting suggest possible intrahepatic hematomas.
- A focal, sonolucent mass on the periphery of the liver or a diffuse, sonolucent area surrounding part of the liver suggests possible subcapsular hematoma.

Ultrasonography, pancreas

● OVERVIEW

- Cross-sectional images of the pancreas produced by channeling high-frequency sound waves into the epigastric region, converting the resultant echoes to electrical impulses, and displaying them as real-time images on a monitor; pattern varies with tissue density and represents the size, shape, and position of the pancreas and surrounding viscera
- Can't provide a sensitive measure of pancreatic function, but useful in detecting anatomic abnormalities, such as pancreatic carcinoma and pseudocysts, and to guide the insertion of biopsy needles
- Doesn't expose the patient to radiation, so this procedure has largely replaced hypotonic duodenography, endoscopic retrograde cholangiopancreatography, radioisotope studies, and arteriography

Purpose
- To aid diagnosis of pancreatitis, pseudocysts, and pancreatic carcinoma

Patient preparation
- Make sure the patient has signed an appropriate consent form.
- Note and report all allergies.
- Fasting is required for 8 to 12 hours before the test to reduce bowel gas, which hinders transmission of ultrasound.
- Instruct the patient to abstain from smoking before the test to eliminate the risk of swallowing air while inhaling, which interferes with test results.
- Provide reassurance that this study isn't harmful or painful, although the patient may experience mild pressure.
- Instruct the patient to inhale deeply during scanning, when requested.
- Stress the need to remain as still as possible during imaging.

TEACHING POINTS
Be sure to cover:
- the purpose of the study and how it's done
- who will perform the test and where
- that the test takes 30 minutes.

▶ PROCEDURE

- The patient is placed in a supine position.
- A water-soluble gel or mineral oil is applied to the abdomen and, with the patient at full inspiration, transverse scans are taken at 1-cm intervals, starting from the xiphoid and moving caudally.
- Other scanning techniques include the longitudinal scan to view the head, body, and tail of the pancreas in sequence; the right anterior oblique view for the head and body of the pancreas; the oblique sagittal view for the portal vein; and the sagittal view for the vena cava.
- Good images are recorded for later study.

Postprocedure care
- Remove the lubricating jelly from the patient's skin.
- Resume the patient's usual diet as ordered.

Precautions
- Factors that may affect test results include:
- failure to fast
- bowel gas
- dehydration
- barium from previous diagnostic tests
- obesity.

Complications
- None known

✛ INTERPRETATION

Normal findings
- The pancreas demonstrates a coarse, uniform echo pattern (reflecting tissue density) and usually appears more echogenic than the adjacent liver.

Abnormal results
- Alterations in the size, contour, and parenchymal texture of the pancreas suggest possible pancreatic disease.
- An enlarged pancreas with decreased echogenicity and distinct borders suggests pancreatitis.
- A well-defined mass with an essentially echo-free interior suggests pseudocyst.
- An ill-defined mass with scattered internal echoes, or a mass in the head of the pancreas (obstructing the common bile duct) and a large noncontracting gallbladder suggests pancreatic carcinoma.

Ultrasonography, pelvic area

- High-frequency sound waves reflected to a transducer, which converts sound energy into electrical energy and forms images of the interior pelvic area on a screen
- B-mode (brightness modulation), a two-dimensional or cross-sectional image; gray scale, a representation of organ texture in shades of gray on a monitor; and real-time imaging, instantaneous images of the tissues in motion
- Selected views recorded for later examination and to keep as a permanent record of the test
- Most common uses: to evaluate symptoms that suggest pelvic disease, confirm a tentative diagnosis, and determine fetal growth during pregnancy
- Commonly required during pregnancy for women with a history or signs of fetal anomalies or multiple pregnancies, a history of bleeding, inconsistency of fetal size and conception date, or indications for amniocentesis

Purpose

- To detect foreign bodies and distinguish between cysts and solid masses (tumors)
- To measure organ size
- To evaluate fetal viability, position, gestational age, and growth rate
- To detect multiple pregnancy
- To confirm fetal abnormalities (such as molar pregnancy, and abnormalities of the arms and legs, spine, heart, head, kidneys, and abdomen)
- To confirm maternal abnormalities (such as posterior placenta and placenta previa)
- To guide amniocentesis by determining placental location and fetal position

Patient preparation

- Make sure the patient has signed an appropriate consent form.
- Note and report all allergies.
- Instruct the patient to drink fluids and avoid urination before the test because pelvic ultrasonography requires a full bladder as a landmark to define pelvic organs.

TEACHING POINTS
Be sure to cover:
- the purpose of the study and how it's done
- that the test is safe, noninvasive, and painless
- who will perform the test and where
- that the test may take a few minutes to several hours
- that the test won't harm the fetus.

- With the patient in a supine position, the lower abdomen is coated with mineral oil or water-soluble gel to increase sound wave conduction.
- The transducer crystal is guided over the area, images are observed on the oscilloscope screen, and good images are photographed.

Postprocedure care

- Allow the patient to empty her bladder immediately after the test.
- Remove gel from patient's skin.

Precautions

- When the bladder is empty, the uterus is more difficult to see because it's farther down inside the pelvis. Bones disrupt ultrasound signals. Failure to keep the bladder full will interfere with the study results, making interpretation difficult.

Complications

- None known

Normal findings

- The uterus is normal in size and shape.
- The ovaries are normal in size, shape, and sonographic density.
- The body of the uterus lies on the superior surface of the bladder; the uterine tubes are attached laterally.
- The ovaries are located on the lateral pelvic walls, with the external iliac vessels above, the ureter, posteroinferiorly, and covered by the fimbria of the uterine tubes medially.
- No other masses are visible.
- If the patient is pregnant, the gestational sac and fetus are of normal size for date; the placenta is located in the fundus of the uterus.

Abnormal results

- Homogeneous densities suggest possible both cysts and solid masses; however, solid masses (such as fibroids) appear more dense on ultrasonography.
- Inappropriate fetal size suggests possible miscalculation of conception or delivery date.
- Abnormal echo patterns suggest possible foreign bodies (such as an intrauterine device), multiple pregnancy, placenta previa or abruptio placentae, or fetal abnormalities (such as molar pregnancy or abnormalities of the arms and legs, spine, heart, head, kidneys, and abdomen).
- Fetal abnormalities suggest possible malpresentation (such as breech or shoulder presentation) and cephalopelvic disproportion.

Ultrasonography, spleen

● OVERVIEW

- Focused beam of high-frequency sound waves that passes into the left upper quadrant of the abdomen, creating echoes that vary with changes in tissue density
- Echoes: converted to electrical energy, amplified by transducer, and displayed on a monitor as a series of real-time images representing size, shape, and position of spleen and surrounding viscera
- Indicated for patients with a left upper quadrant mass of unknown origin, with known splenomegaly to evaluate changes in the spleen's size, with left upper quadrant pain and local tenderness, and with recent abdominal trauma
- Can show splenomegaly, but usually doesn't identify the cause; computed tomography scanning possibly needed to obtain more specific information
- As a supplementary diagnostic procedure after liver-spleen scanning: can clarify the nature of cold spots or detect focal defects not infiltrated by tracer radioisotopes

Purpose
- To demonstrate splenomegaly
- To monitor progression of primary and secondary splenic disease
- To evaluate the effectiveness of therapy
- To evaluate the spleen after abdominal trauma
- To detect splenic cysts and subphrenic abscess

Patient preparation
- Make sure the patient has signed an appropriate consent form.
- Note and report all allergies.
- Fasting is required for 8 to 12 hours before the procedure.
- Inform the patient that he will feel only mild pressure during the procedure.
- Instruct the patient to remain as still as possible during the procedure and to hold his breath when requested.

TEACHING POINTS
Be sure to cover:
- the purpose of the study and how it's done

- who will perform the test and where
- that the test takes about 15 to 30 minutes.

▶ PROCEDURE

- Because the procedure for ultrasonography varies, depending on the size of the spleen or the patient's body habitus, the patient is usually repositioned several times; the transducer scanning angle or path is also changed.
- A water-soluble gel is applied to the face of the transducer, and transverse scans of the spleen are taken at 1- to 2-cm intervals, beginning at the level of the diaphragm and moving posteriorly while the transducer is angled anteromedially.
- After the patient is placed in right lateral decubitus position, additional transverse scans are taken through the intercostal spaces using a sectoring motion.
- A pillow may be placed under the patient's right side to help separate the intercostal spaces, making it easier to position the transducer face between them.
- For longitudinal scans, the patient remains in the right lateral decubitus position and scans are taken from the axilla toward the iliac crest.
- To prevent rib artifacts, oblique scans are taken by passing the transducer face along the intercostal spaces; this scan provides the best view of the splenic parenchyma.
- During each scan, the patient may be asked to hold his breath briefly at varying stages of inspiration.

Postprocedure care
- Resume the patient's usual diet as ordered.
- Remove the gel.

Precautions
- Factors that may affect test results include overlying ribs, failure to fast, bowel gas, dehydration, and barium from previous diagnostic tests.
- Patients with a splenic injury may be unable to tolerate the procedure because of pain.

Complications
- None known

✤ INTERPRETATION

Normal findings
- The splenic parenchyma shows homogeneous, low-level echo pattern.
- The superior and lateral splenic borders are clearly defined, each having a convex margin.
- The undersurface and medial borders, in contrast, show indentations from surrounding organs (stomach, left kidney, and pancreas).
- The hilar region, where the vascular pedicle enters the spleen, produces an area of highly reflected echoes.
- The medial surface is generally concave, which is particularly useful when differentiating between left upper quadrant masses and splenomegaly.
- Even when splenomegaly is present, the spleen usually remains concave medially, unless a space-occupying lesion distorts this contour.

Abnormal results
- Increased echogenicity and enlarged vascular channels, especially in the hilar region, suggest splenomegaly.
- Splenomegaly and an irregular, sonolucent area (the presence of free intraperitoneal fluid) suggest splenic rupture.
- Splenomegaly as well as the presence of a double contour (blood accumulation between the splenic parenchyma and the intact splenic capsule), altered splenic position, and a relatively sonolucent area on the periphery of the spleen suggest subcapsular hematoma.
- A sonolucent area beneath the diaphragm suggests possible subphrenic abscess.
- Spherical, sonolucent areas with well-defined, regular margins, with acoustic enhancement behind them suggest cysts.

Ultrasonography, thyroid

● OVERVIEW

- Pulses emitted from a transducer, directed at the thyroid gland, and reflected back to the transducer; pulses are converted electronically to produce structural visualization on a monitor
- Used to differentiate between a cyst and a tumor larger than 1 cm with about 85% accuracy when mass is located by palpation or by thyroid imaging
- Especially useful in evaluating thyroid nodules during pregnancy because it doesn't expose the fetus to radioactive iodine used in other diagnostic procedures
- Can also be performed on parathyroid glands (see *Parathyroid ultrasonography*)

Purpose
- To evaluate thyroid structure
- To differentiate between a cyst and a solid tumor
- To monitor the size of the thyroid gland during suppressive therapy
- To allow accurate measurement of a nodule's size
- To aid in performance of thyroid needle biopsy

Patient preparation
- Make sure the patient has signed an appropriate consent form.
- Note and report all allergies.
- Restriction of food and fluids before the test isn't necessary.

TEACHING POINTS
Be sure to cover:
- the purpose of the study and how it's done
- who will perform the test and where
- that the test takes approximately 10 minutes and the results are almost immediately available
- that the test is painless and safe.

▶ PROCEDURE

- The patient is placed in a supine position with a pillow under his shoulder blades to hyperextend his neck.
- The neck is coated with water-soluble gel.
- The transducer scans the thyroid, projecting its echographic image on the oscilloscope screen.
- The image on the screen is photographed for subsequent examination.

Postprocedure care
- Thoroughly clean the patient's neck to remove the gel.

Complications
- None known

✛ INTERPRETATION

Normal findings
- A uniform echo pattern is found throughout the gland.
- No anatomical abnormalities are present.

Abnormal results
- Smooth-bordered, echo-free areas with enhanced sound transmission suggest cysts.
- Solid and well-demarcated areas with identical echo patterns may suggest adenomas and carcinomas.

PARATHYROID ULTRASONOGRAPHY

On ultrasonography, the parathyroid glands appear as solid masses, 5 mm or smaller in size, with an echo pattern of less amplitude than thyroid tissue. Glandular enlargement is usually characteristic of tumor growth or of hyperplasia. Normally, on a scan, the parathyroid glands are indistinguishable from the nearby neurovascular bundle.

Ultrasonography, transvaginal

● OVERVIEW

- Uses high-frequency sound waves to produce images of the pelvic structures
- Allows evaluation of pelvic anatomy and diagnosis of pregnancy at an earlier gestational age
- Eliminates need for a full bladder and circumvents difficulties encountered with obese patients
- Also known as *endovaginal ultrasound*

Purpose

- To establish early pregnancy with fetal heart motion as early as the 5th to 6th week of gestation
- To identify ectopic pregnancy
- To monitor follicular growth during infertility treatment
- To evaluate abnormal pregnancy (such as blighted ovum, missed or incomplete abortion, or molar pregnancy)
- To visualize retained products of conception
- To diagnose fetal abnormalities, placental location, and cervical length
- To evaluate adnexal pathology, such as tubo-ovarian abscess, hydrosalpinx, and ovarian masses
- To evaluate the uterine lining (in patients with dysfunctional uterine bleeding and postmenopausal bleeding)

Patient preparation

- Note and report all allergies; screen patient for latex allergies if a condom will be used to protect the probe during the examination
- If the sonographer is a male, assure the patient that a female assistant will be present during the examination
- Inform the patient that self-insertion of the vaginal probe may be possible

TEACHING POINTS

Be sure to cover:
- purpose of the test and how it's done.
- that no dietary restrictions are required
- that the test takes about 30 minutes.

▶ PROCEDURE

- Patient is placed in the lithotomy position.
- Water-soluble gel is placed on the transducer tip to allow better sound transmission, and a protective sheath is placed over the transducer.
- Additional lubricant is placed on the sheathed transducer tip, which is gently inserted into the vagina by the patient or the sonographer.
- The pelvic structures are observed by rotating the probe 90 degrees to one side and then the other.

Postprocedure care

- Help the patient remove gel.
- Provide the patient with privacy.
- Assist with perineal cleaning, as needed.

Complications

- None known

✥ INTERPRETATION

Normal findings

- The uterus and ovaries are normal in size and shape.
- The body of the uterus lies on the superior surface of the bladder; the uterine tubes are attached laterally.
- The ovaries are located on the lateral pelvic walls, with the external iliac vessels above and the ureters posteroinferior, and are covered by the fimbria of the uterine tubes medially.
- In pregnancy, the gestational sac and fetus are of normal size for the gestational period.

Abnormal results

- Free peritoneal fluid in the pelvic cavity suggests possible peritonitis.
- A tubal mass suggests possible ectopic pregnancy.
- Structural abnormalities in a nonpregnant woman may indicate cancer of the uterus, ovaries, vagina, and other pelvic structures; noncancerous growths of the uterus and ovaries; ovarian torsion; areas of infection, including pelvic inflammatory disease; and congenital malformations.
- Structural abnormalities in a pregnant woman may suggest threatened abortion; multiple pregnancies; fetal death; placental abnormalities, including placenta previa and placental abruption; and tumors of pregnancy, including gestational trophoblastic disease.

Upper GI and small-bowel series

● OVERVIEW

- Involves fluoroscopic examination of esophagus, stomach, and small intestine after ingestion of barium sulfate, a contrast agent
- As barium passes through digestive tract, fluoroscopy shows peristalsis and the mucosal contours of organs; spot films record significant findings
- Indicated for patients who have upper GI symptoms (difficulty swallowing, regurgitation, burning or gnawing epigastric pain), signs of small-bowel disease (diarrhea, weight loss), and signs of GI bleeding (hematemesis, melena)
- Can be used to detect various mucosal abnormalities; many patients need biopsy afterward to rule out cancer or distinguish specific inflammatory diseases
- Oral cholecystography, barium enema, and routine X-rays: should always precede this test because retained barium clouds anatomic detail on X-ray films

Purpose
- To detect hiatal hernia, diverticula, and varices
- To aid diagnosis of strictures, ulcers, tumors, regional enteritis, and malabsorption syndrome
- To detect motility disorders

Patient preparation
- Make sure the patient has signed an appropriate consent form.
- Note and report all allergies.
- Have patient remove all jewelry and metal objects.
- Withhold oral medications after midnight and anticholinergics and narcotics for 24 hours as ordered because these drugs affect small intestine motility.
- Withhold antacids, histamine-2–receptor antagonists, and proton pump inhibitors as ordered if gastric reflux is suspected.
- Instruct the patient to maintain a low-residue diet for 2 or 3 days before the test and to fast and avoid smoking after midnight before the test.

- Inform the patient that the barium mixture has a milkshake consistency and chalky taste; although flavored, the patient may find the taste unpleasant; 16 to 20 oz (480 to 600 ml) are needed for a complete examination.
- Warn the patient that the abdomen may be compressed to ensure proper coating of the stomach or intestinal walls with barium or to separate overlapping bowel loops.

TEACHING POINTS
Be sure to cover:
- the purpose of the study and how it's done
- who will perform the test and where
- that the test may take up to 6 hours to complete, so the patient should bring something to do.

▶ PROCEDURE

- After the patient is secured in a supine position on the X-ray table, the table is tilted until the patient is erect, and the heart, lungs, and abdomen are examined fluoroscopically.
- The patient is then instructed to take several swallows of the barium suspension and its passage through the esophagus is observed. (Occasionally, the patient is given a thick barium suspension, especially when esophageal pathology is strongly suspected.)
- During fluoroscopic examination, spot films of the esophagus are taken from lateral angles and from right and left posteroanterior angles.
- When barium enters the stomach, the patient's abdomen is palpated or compressed to ensure adequate coating of the gastric mucosa with barium.
- To perform a double-contrast examination, the patient is instructed to sip the barium through a perforated straw. As he does so, a small amount of air is also introduced into the stomach to allow detailed examination of the gastric rugae, and spot films of significant findings are taken.

- The patient is instructed to ingest the remaining barium suspension, and the filling of the stomach and emptying into the duodenum are observed fluoroscopically.
- Two series of spot films of the stomach and duodenum are taken from posteroanterior, anteroposterior, oblique, and lateral angles, with the patient erect and then in a supine position.
- The passage of barium into the remainder of the small intestine is then observed fluoroscopically, and spot films are taken at 30- to 60-minute intervals until the barium reaches the ileocecal valve and the region around it.
- If abnormalities in the small intestine are detected, the area is palpated and compressed to help clarify the defect and a spot film is taken.
- When the barium enters the cecum the examination is ended.

Postprocedure care
- Make sure additional X-rays haven't been ordered before allowing the patient food, fluids, and oral medications.
- Instruct the patient to drink plenty of fluid (unless contraindicated) to help eliminate the barium.
- Administer a cathartic or enema as ordered.
- Inform him that his stool will be light-colored for 24 to 72 hours.
- Because barium retention in the intestine may cause obstruction or fecal impaction, notify the doctor if the patient doesn't pass barium within 2 to 3 days.
- Tell the patient to advise the doctor of abdominal fullness or pain or a delay in return to brown stools.

MONITORING
- Vital signs
- Intake and output
- Bowel movements
- Abdominal distention
- Bowel sounds

(continued)

Precautions

- Upper GI and small-bowel series is contraindicated in patients with obstruction or perforation of the GI tract because barium may intensify the obstruction or seep into the abdominal cavity.
- If a perforation is suspected, Gastrografin (a water-soluble contrast medium) may be used instead of barium.
- Upper GI and small-bowel series is contraindicated in pregnant patients because of the possible teratogenic effects of radiation.

Complications

- Bowel obstruction
- Fecal impaction

✥ INTERPRETATION

Normal findings

- After the barium suspension is swallowed, it pours over the base of the tongue into the pharynx, and is propelled by a peristaltic wave through the entire length of the esophagus in about 2 seconds.
- The bolus evenly fills and distends the lumen of the pharynx and esophagus, and the mucosa appears smooth and regular.
- When the peristaltic wave reaches the base of the esophagus, the cardiac sphincter opens, allowing the bolus to enter the stomach; this is followed by closing of the cardiac sphincter.
- As barium enters the stomach, it outlines the characteristic longitudinal folds called rugae, which are best observed using the double-contrast technique.
- When the stomach is completely filled with barium its outer contour appears smooth and regular without evidence of flattened, rigid areas suggesting intrinsic or extrinsic lesions.
- After barium enters the stomach it quickly empties into the duodenal bulb through relaxation of the pyloric sphincter.

- Although the mucosa of the duodenal bulb is relatively smooth, circular folds become apparent as barium enters the duodenal loop; these folds deepen and become more numerous in the jejunum. Barium temporarily lodges between these folds, producing a speckled pattern on the X-ray film.
- As barium enters the ileum, the circular folds become less prominent and, except for their broadness, resemble those in the duodenum.
- The diameter of the small intestine tapers gradually from the duodenum to the ileum.

Abnormal results

- Structural abnormalities of the esophagus suggest possible strictures, tumors, hiatal hernia, diverticula, varices, and ulcers.
- Dilatation of the esophagus suggests possible benign strictures.
- Erosive changes in the esophageal mucosa suggest possible malignant strictures.
- Filling defects in the column of barium suggest possible esophageal tumors; malignant esophageal tumors change the mucosal contour.
- Narrowing of the distal esophagus strongly suggests achalasia (cardiospasm).
- Backflow of barium from the stomach into the esophagus suggests gastric reflux.
- Filling defects in the stomach, which usually disrupt peristalsis, suggest malignant tumors, usually adenocarcinomas.
- Outpouchings of the gastric mucosa that generally don't affect peristalsis suggest benign tumors, such as adenomatous polyps and leiomyomas.
- Evidence of partial or complete healing, characterized by radiating folds extending to the edge of the ulcer crater, suggests benign ulcers.
- Radiating folds that extend beyond the ulcer crater to the edge of the mass suggest malignant ulcers.

- Edematous changes in the mucosa of the antrum or duodenal loop, or dilation of the duodenal loop suggest possible pancreatitis or pancreatic carcinoma.
- Edematous changes, segmentation of the barium column, and flocculation in the small intestine suggest possible malabsorption syndrome.
- Filling defects of the small intestine suggest possible Hodgkin's disease and lymphosarcoma.

Urine culture and sensitivity test

● OVERVIEW

- Laboratory examination and culture of urine; necessary for evaluation of urinary tract infections (UTIs), most commonly bladder infections; urine in kidneys and bladder normally sterile, but small number of bacteria are usually present in urethra and may pass into urine
- Used to identify pathogenic fungi such as *Coccidioides immitis*
- Many laboratories perform quick and easy screen on urine submitted for culture to determine if urine contains high bacteria or white blood cell (WBC) counts; only urine with bacteria or WBCs is processed for culture; urine that doesn't contain either is classified negative by urine screen
- To distinguish between true bacteriuria and contamination: necessary to know the number of organisms in a milliliter of urine, estimated by a culture technique known as a "colony count"; additional quick centrifugation test used to determine where a UTI originates (see *Quick centrifugation test*)
- Clean-voided midstream collection, rather than suprapubic aspiration or catheterization, is the method of choice for obtaining a urine specimen
- Specimen collection possibly required on three consecutive mornings for patient with suspected urogenital tuberculosis

Purpose
- To diagnose UTI
- To monitor microorganism colonization after urinary catheter insertion

Patient preparation
- Confirm the patient's identity using two patient identifiers according to facility policy.
- Make sure the patient has signed an appropriate consent form.
- Note and report all allergies.
- Wash your hands thoroughly.
- Maintain asepsis throughout the procedure as indicated.
- Wear personal protective equipment throughout the procedure.
- Check the patient history for current use of antimicrobial drugs.

- Restriction of food and fluids isn't necessary.
- Explain that a urine specimen is required. Obtain the urine specimen before beginning antibiotic therapy.
- Instruct the patient to collect a clean-voided midstream specimen. Stress the importance of cleaning the external genitalia thoroughly.
- Warn of possible discomfort during specimen collection in catheterization.

TEACHING POINTS
Be sure to cover:
- the purpose of the study and how it's done
- who will perform the test and where
- that the test takes only a few minutes.

▶ PROCEDURE

- Collect a urine specimen as ordered.
- Use standard precautions when performing the procedure and handling specimens.
- Collect at least 3 ml of urine, but don't fill the specimen cup more than halfway.
- Seal the cup with a sterile lid and send it to the laboratory at once.
- Record the suspected diagnosis, the collection time and method, current antimicrobial therapy, and fluid- or drug-induced diuresis on the laboratory request.

Postprocedure care
- No specific posttest care is necessary.

Precautions
- If transport is delayed for more than 30 minutes, store the specimen at 39.2° F (4° C) or place it on ice unless a urine transport tube containing preservative is used.
- Antibiotics and diuretics may affect test results.

Complications
- Possible infection when specimens are obtained by catheterization

✦ INTERPRETATION

Normal findings
- Culture results of sterile urine are normally reported as "no growth," which usually indicates the absence of UTI.

Abnormal results
- Bacterial counts of 100,000 or more organisms of a single microbe species per milliliter suggest UTI; counts under 100,000/ml may be significant, depending on the patient's age, sex, history, and other individual factors.
- Counts under 10,000/ml usually suggest that the organisms are contaminants, except in symptomatic patients or those with urologic disorders.
- Isolation of *Mycobacterium tuberculosis* in a special test for acid-fast bacteria suggests tuberculosis of the urinary tract.
- Isolation of more than two species of organisms or of vaginal or skin organisms usually suggests contamination and requires a repeat culture.

QUICK CENTRIFUGATION TEST

The quick centrifugation test can be used to determine whether the source of a urinary tract infection (UTI) is in the lower tract (bladder) or the upper tract (kidneys). The test involves centrifugation of urine in a test tube, followed by staining of the sediment with fluorescein. If at least one-fourth of the bacteria fluoresce when viewed under a fluorescent microscope, an upper tract UTI is present; if bacteria don't fluoresce, a lower tract UTI is present.

Venography of the lower limb

- Radiographic examination of veins in the lower extremity
- Commonly used to assess the condition of the deep leg veins after injection of a contrast medium
- Not used for routine screening because it exposes the patient to relatively high doses of radiation and can cause complications, such as phlebitis, local tissue damage and, occasionally, deep vein thrombosis (DVT)
- Used in patients whose duplex ultrasound findings are equivocal
- Also known as ascending contrast phlebography

Purpose
- To confirm diagnosis of DVT
- To distinguish clot formation from venous obstruction (such as a large tumor of the pelvis impinging on the venous system)
- To evaluate congenital venous abnormalities
- To assess deep vein valvular competence (especially helpful in identifying underlying causes of leg edema)
- To evaluate chronic venous disease

Patient preparation
- Make sure the patient has signed an appropriate consent form.
- Note and report all allergies.
- Check the patient's history for and report hypersensitivity to iodine, iodine-containing foods, or contrast media.
- Reassure the patient that contrast media complications are rare, but tell him to report nausea, severe burning or itching, constriction in the throat or chest, or dyspnea at once.
- Discontinue anticoagulant therapy as ordered.
- Administer sedation if ordered.
- Instruct the patient to restrict food and drink only clear liquids for 4 hours before the test.
- Warn the patient that he might experience a burning sensation in the leg when the contrast medium is injected and some discomfort during the procedure.

TEACHING POINTS
Be sure to cover:
- the purpose of the study and how it's done
- who will perform the test and where
- that the test takes 30 to 45 minutes.

PROCEDURE

- The patient is positioned on a tilting X-ray table so that the leg being tested doesn't bear any weight.
- A tourniquet may be tied around the ankle to expedite venous filling.
- Normal saline solution is injected into a superficial vein in the dorsum of the patient's foot and contrast medium is injected after placement has been confirmed.
- Using a fluoroscope, the distribution of the contrast medium is monitored, and spot films of the thigh and femoroiliac regions are taken from the anteroposterior and oblique views.
- Overhead films are taken of the calf, knee, thigh, and femoral area.
- After filming, the patient is repositioned horizontally, the leg being tested is quickly elevated, and normal saline solution is infused to flush the contrast medium from the veins.
- Fluoroscope is checked to confirm complete emptying.
- The needle is removed.
- A dressing is applied to the injection site.

Postprocedure care
- Administer analgesics as ordered.
- Resume the patient's usual diet and medications as ordered.
- Encourage oral fluid intake as ordered.
- If DVT is documented, initiate therapy (heparin infusion, bed rest, leg elevation or support) as ordered.

MONITORING
- Vital signs
- Intake and output
- Injection site and dressing
- Bleeding
- Infection
- Hematoma
- Erythema
- Renal function
- Hydration

Precautions
- Improper needle placement in a superficial vein, weight bearing or muscle contraction, or use of tourniquets can produce artifacts of poor filling.
- Errors in diagnosis are commonly the result of incomplete filling of vessels.
- Fluoroscopy is essential for establishing that the contrast medium has reached the vessels being filmed and that opacification is adequate.

NURSING ALERT Because of the high volume of contrast used, especially if bilateral venography is necessary, monitor renal function and hydration status very carefully.

NURSING ALERT Because most allergic reactions to the contrast medium occur within 30 minutes of injection, carefully observe the patient for signs and symptoms of anaphylaxis, such as flushing, urticaria, and laryngeal stridor.

Complications
- Adverse reactions to contrast media or medications
- Thrombophlebitis
- Local tissue damage
- Renal insufficiency or failure

NURSING ALERT Small extravasations of contrast media (less than 10 ml) don't usually pose a problem. However, tissue necrosis and ulceration may occur, especially with larger extravasations and in patients with arterial insufficiency.

INTERPRETATION

Normal findings
- Test shows steady opacification of the superficial and deep vasculature with no filling defects.

Abnormal results
- Consistent filling defects, abrupt termination of a column of contrast material, unfilled major deep veins, or diversion of flow (through collaterals, for example) suggests DVT.

Vertebral radiography

- Used to visualize all or part of the vertebral column
- Films of bones used to determine bone density, texture, erosion, and changes in bone relationships
- Radiographs of cortex of bone: reveal any widening or narrowing and signs of irregularity
- Joint radiographs: may reveal fluid, spur formation, narrowing or widening of the cortex, and changes in joint structure
- Type and extent of vertebral radiography depend on patient's condition; for example, patient with lower back pain requires only study of the lumbar and sacral segments

Purpose

- To detect vertebral fractures, dislocations, subluxations, and deformities
- To detect vertebral degeneration, infection, and congenital disorders
- To detect disorders of the intervertebral disks
- To determine the vertebral effects of arthritic and metabolic disorders
- To follow progression of certain disorders (such as scoliosis in children)

Patient preparation

- Make sure the patient has signed an appropriate consent form.
- Note and report all allergies.
- Restriction of food and fluids isn't necessary.
- Inform the patient that positioning for the radiographic films may cause slight discomfort and that cooperation helps to ensure accurate results.
- Stress to the patient the importance of holding still and holding his breath for film exposure during the procedure.

TEACHING POINTS

Be sure to cover:

- the purpose of the study and how it's done
- who will perform the test and where
- that the test usually takes 15 to 30 minutes.

- The procedure varies considerably, depending on which vertebral segment is being examined.
- The patient is placed in a supine position on the X-ray table for an anteroposterior view.
- He may be repositioned for lateral or right and left oblique views; specific positioning depends on the vertebral segment or adjacent structures of interest.
- Radiographs are obtained as required.

Postprocedure care

- No specific posttest care is necessary.

Precautions

- Vertebral radiography is contraindicated during the first trimester of pregnancy unless the benefits outweigh the risk of fetal radiation exposure.
- Improper positioning may affect test results.

◆ NURSING ALERT Exercise extreme caution when handling trauma patients with suspected spinal injuries, especially of the cervical area. Such patients should be filmed while on the stretcher to avoid further injury during transfer to the X-ray table.

Complications

- Potential for spinal injury in a trauma patient

Normal findings

- Vertebrae are without fractures, subluxations, dislocations, abnormal curvatures, or other abnormalities.
- Specific positions and spacing of the vertebrae vary with the patient's age. In the lateral view, adult vertebrae are aligned to form four alternately concave and convex curves.
- The cervical and lumbar curves are convex anteriorly; the thoracic and sacral curves are concave anteriorly.
- Although the structure of the coccyx varies, it usually points forward and downward.

✳ AGE-RELATED CONCERN Neonatal vertebrae form only one curve, which is concave anteriorly.

Abnormal results

- Vertebral structural abnormalities suggest possible various disorders, including:
  - spondylolisthesis
  - fractures
  - subluxations
  - dislocations
  - wedging
  - deformities, such as kyphosis, scoliosis, and lordosis
  - congenital abnormalities
  - degenerative processes
  - tuberculosis
  - benign or malignant intraspinal tumors
  - ruptured disk
  - cervical disk syndrome.

Voiding cystourethrography

● OVERVIEW

- Involves use of contrast medium instilled by gentle syringe or gravity into the bladder through a urethral catheter
- Fluoroscopic films or overhead radiographs: demonstrate bladder filling and excretion of the contrast as the patient voids
- May be performed to investigate possible causes of chronic urinary tract infection
- Other indications: suspected congenital anomaly of the lower urinary tract, abnormal bladder emptying, and incontinence
- In males, used to assess hypertrophy of the prostatic lobes, urethral stricture, and the degree of compromise of a stenotic prostatic urethra

Purpose
- To detect abnormalities of the bladder and urethra, such as vesicoureteral reflux, neurogenic bladder, prostatic hyperplasia, urethral strictures, or diverticula

Patient preparation
- Make sure the patient has signed an appropriate consent form.
- Note and report all allergies.
- Check the patient's history for hypersensitivity to contrast media or iodine-containing foods such as shellfish; mark the chart and notify the doctor of sensitivities.
- Administer a sedative if ordered.
- Restriction of food and fluids before the test isn't necessary.
- Explain that the test requires a catheter to be inserted into the patient's bladder.
- Warn of a possible feeling of fullness and an urge to void when the contrast agent is instilled.

TEACHING POINTS
Be sure to cover:
- the purpose of the study and how it's done
- who will perform the test and where
- that the test takes 45 to 60 minutes.

▶ PROCEDURE

- The patient is placed in a supine position and an indwelling urinary catheter is inserted into the bladder.
- Contrast medium is instilled through the catheter until the bladder is full. The catheter is clamped and radiographic films are obtained, with the patient in supine, oblique, and lateral positions.
- The catheter is removed and the patient assumes the right oblique position — right leg flexed to 90 degrees, left leg extended, in males, penis parallel to right leg — and begins to void.
- High-speed exposures of the bladder and urethra, coned down to reduce radiation exposure, are obtained during voiding.
- If the right oblique view doesn't delineate both ureters, the patient is asked to stop urinating and to begin again in left oblique position.
- The most reliable voiding cystourethrograms are obtained with the patient recumbent.
- Patients who can't urinate in the recumbent position may do so standing (not sitting).

✸ **AGE-RELATED CONCERN** Young children who can't void on command may need to undergo expression cystourethrography under general anesthesia.

Postprocedure care
- Encourage oral fluid intake.
- Prepare the patient for surgery if indicated.
- Instruct the patient to report any fever, chills, or lower-abdominal pain.

MONITORING
- Vital signs
- Intake and output
- Bleeding
- Infection

◆ **NURSING ALERT** Observe and record the time, color, and volume of the patient's voidings. If hematuria is present after the third voiding, notify the doctor.

Precautions
- Voiding cystourethrography is contraindicated in patients with an acute or exacerbated urethral injury, or acute urethral or bladder infection
- Hypersensitivity to contrast medium may be a contraindication.
- Not recommended for a pregnant woman because of radiation exposure
- Factors that may affect test results include:
  - embarrassment at voiding in the presence of others
  - painful urination that may cause an interrupted or less vigorous stream, muscle spasm, or incomplete sphincter relaxation
  - previous X-ray study using dye
  - presence of feces or gas in the bowel.
- Difficulties encountered in bladder catheterization, especially in children, may prevent completion of the study.

Complications
- Bleeding
- Infection
- Adverse reaction to contrast media

✦ INTERPRETATION

Normal findings
- Delineation of the bladder and urethra shows normal structure and function, with no reflux of contrast medium into the ureters.

Abnormal results
- Structural and anatomical abnormalities suggest possible urethral stricture, vesical or urethral diverticula, ureterocele, prostatic enlargement, vesicoureteral reflux, or neurogenic bladder.

Wound culture

● OVERVIEW

- Microscopic analysis of a specimen from a lesion to confirm infection
- May be aerobic (for detection of organisms that usually require oxygen to grow and typically appear in a superficial wound) or anaerobic (for organisms that need little or no oxygen and appear in areas of poor tissue perfusion, such as postoperative wounds, ulcers, or compound fractures)

Purpose
- To identify an infectious microbe in a wound

Patient preparation
- Confirm the patient's identity using two patient identifiers according to facility policy.
- Make sure the patient has signed an appropriate consent form.
- Note and report all allergies.

TEACHING POINTS
Be sure to cover:
- the purpose of the study and how it's done
- who will perform the test and when
- that the test generally takes only a few minutes.

▶ PROCEDURE

- Wash your hands thoroughly.
- Maintain asepsis throughout the procedure.
- Wear personal protective equipment throughout the procedure.
- Prepare a sterile field.
- Clean the area around the wound with antiseptic solution.
- Record recent antimicrobial therapy, the source of the specimen, and the suspected organism on the laboratory request.
- Label the specimen container appropriately with the patient's name, doctor's name, hospital number, and wound site and time of specimen collection.

AEROBIC CULTURE
- Express the wound and swab as much exudate as possible, or insert the swab deep into the wound and gently rotate.
- Immediately place the swab in the aerobic culture tube.

ANAEROBIC CULTURE
- Insert the swab deep into the wound, gently rotate it, and immediately place it in the anaerobic culture tub. (See *Anaerobic specimen collector.*)

Postprocedure care
- Clean the area around the wound thoroughly to limit contamination of the culture by normal skin flora.
- Make sure no antiseptic enters the wound.
- Re-dress the wound, as ordered.

Precautions
- Obtain exudate from the entire wound using more than one swab.
- Because some anaerobes die in the presence of oxygen, place the specimen in the culture tube quickly; take care that no air enters the tube, and check that double stoppers are secure.
- Keep the specimen container upright and send it to the laboratory within 15 minutes to prevent growth or deterioration of microbes.

Complications
- Spread of any existing infection

✛ INTERPRETATION

Normal findings
- No pathogenic organisms are present in the wound.

Abnormal results
- The presence of *Staphylococcus aureus*, group A beta-hemolytic streptococci, Proteus species, *Escherichia coli* and other Enterobacteriaceae, and some *Pseudomonas* species suggests an aerobic wound infection.
- The presence of *Clostridium, Bacteroides, Peptococcus* and *Streptococcus* species suggests an anaerobic wound infection.

ANAEROBIC SPECIMEN COLLECTOR

Some anaerobes die when they're exposed to the slightest bit of oxygen. To facilitate anaerobic collection and culturing, tubes filled with carbon dioxide (CO_2) or nitrogen are used for oxygen-free transport.

The anaerobic specimen collector shown here consists of a rubber-stoppered tube filled with CO_2, a small inner tube, and a swab attached to a plastic plunger. The drawing on the left shows the tube before specimen collection. The small inner tube containing the swab is held in place by the rubber stopper.

After specimen collection (right), the swab is quickly replaced in the inner tube and the plunger depressed. This separates the inner tube from the stopper, forcing it into the larger tube, and exposing the specimen to the CO_2-rich environment. Keep the tube upright.

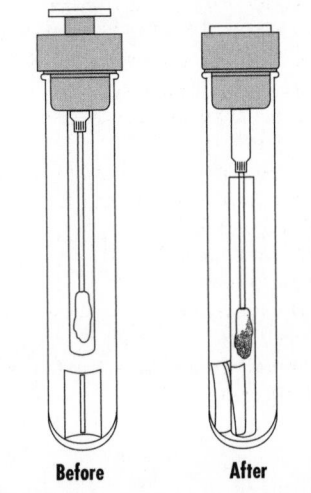

Before   **After**

APPENDIX
INDEX

RARE DISORDERS

Disease	Description	Cause	Treatment
Addison-Schilder disease: adrenoleukodystrophy	Adrenal atrophy and diffuse degeneration of the brain in infancy or adolescence; characterized by loss of myelin and progressive loss of cerebral function, leading to spasticity, optic neuritis, blindness, and dementia	Transmitted as X-linked recessive disorder	Symptomatic and supportive treatment; bone marrow transplant in boys; adrenal hormones, fatal in 1 to 10 years
African typanosomiasis: sleeping sickness	Febrile illness followed months or years after by progressive neurologic impairment and death; the Gambian form, found in west and central Africa, causes daytime drowsiness and nighttime insomnia and progresses to coma; the Rhodesian form, found in east Africa, can progress more rapidly and with more severe symptoms	*Trypanosoma brucei rhodesiense* and *T. brucei gambiense* transmitted by tsetse fly bite	Malarsoprol or pentamidine
Albers-Schönberg disease: osteopetrosis, marble bone disease	Rare heterogenous bone disorder marked by disorganization of bone structure that causes dense sclerotic bones vulnerable to recurrent fractures; in severe cases, the bone marrow cavity may be obliterated; malignant variant begins in utero and progresses rapidly to cause marked anemia, hydrocephalus, cranial nerve involvement, hepatosplenomegaly, and fatal infection; benign variant causes milder anemia and fewer neurologic abnormalities	Malignant variant transmitted as autosomal recessive trait, benign variant transmitted as autosomal dominant trait; increased bone mass secondary to defect in remodeling bone, resulting in thickened cortices; in the intermediate type, the disease is associated with renal tubular acidosis and cerebral calcification	Transfusion or nucleated marrow cells from a healthy, clinically normal donor (almost always a sibling); high doses of calcitriol have been used with some success in patients with lethal forms of the disease
Alport's syndrome	Hereditary nephritis characterized by recurrent gross or microscopic hematuria; associated with deafness, albuminuria, and progressive azotemia	Transmitted as X-linked autosomal trait	Supportive and symptomatic; antibiotic therapy for infection; antihypertensive therapy; protein-restricted diet; dialysis or renal transplant; avoidance of ototoxic drugs
American trypanosomiasis: Chagas' disease	Febrile parasitic illness prevalent in Central and South America; cardiomyopathy may occur; megaesophagus and megacolon may develop many years later; can be fatal in children	*Trypanosoma cruzi* transmitted by insect; can also be transmitted through the transfusion of blood donated by person who's infected	Nifurtimox or benznidazole in acute phase; supportive treatment in chronic phase
Arc-welders' disease: siderosis	Benign pneumoconiosis that can occur in iron ore miners, welders, metal grinders, and polishers from the inhalation and retention of iron	Inhalation and retention of iron after exposure to iron oxide fumes and dust	Supportive and symptomatic treatment; limiting or preventing exposure to iron dust or fumes with approved industrial respirators prevents progression
Armstrong's disease: lymphocyte choriomeningitis	Form of meningitis, usually occurring in adults age 20 to 40 during fall and winter; usually asymptomatic or mild, although myocarditis and severe meningoencephalitis can occur; can spread to fetus with congenital infection, resulting in hydrocephalus	Infection caused by lympthocytic choriomeningitis virus (a member of the family *Arenaviridae*) that follows exposure to food or dust contaminated by an infected common house mouse	Supportive and symptomatic treatment; infection can be prevented by careful hand washing (although mode of transmission may be airborne); corticosteroids and ribavirin may be considered in some cases
Ataxia telangiectasia: Louis-Bar's syndrome	Progressive, severe ataxia with telangiectasia of the face, earlobes, and conjunctivae; chronic recurrent sinopulmonary infections occur; ataxia usually occurs before age 2 but may not develop until as late as age 9; degree of immunodeficiency determines rate of deterioration	Transmitted as autosomal recessive disorder; a genetic mutation found in the ataxia telangiectasia mutated gene	Supportive treatment with early, aggressive antibiotic therapy to prevent onr control recurrent infections; immune globulin; fetal thymus transplant or histocompatible bone marrow transplant
Barometer-maker's disease: chronic mercury poisoning	Soreness of gums, loosening of teeth, salivation, fetid breath, abdominal cramping and diarrhea, weakness, ataxia, intention tremors, irritability and depression, birth defects, and death	Mercury poisoning resulting from chronic exposure to mercury or its vapors or to contaminated fish or fungicides used on seeds	Induce emesis or evacuate stomach, lavage with milk or sodium bicarbonate, and administer polythiol resins. Penicillamine is the chelating agent of choice; dimercaprol is also effective. Neurologic toxicity isn't considered reversible, although some practitioners recommend a trial dose of penicillamine.
Basal cell carcinoma of the eye	Common extraorbital cancer affecting the eyelid, conjunctivae, and cornea	Unknown, but predisposing factors include exposure to sunlight, radiation, chemicals, and other carcinogens	Surgery, possibly radiation therapy

Disease	Description	Cause	Treatment
Bauxite workers' disease: bauxite pneumoconiosis, Shaver's disease	Occupational disorder causing rapid and progressive pneumoconiosis and leading to empyema; may be accompanied by pneumothorax; puts patient at increased risk for blood and bladder cancers	Inhalation of dust particles of alumina and silica (bauxite), the chief source of aluminum	Elimination of exposure to bauxite
Behr's disease: degeneration of the macula retinae	Familial spastic paraplegia with or without optic atrophy; hyperactive deep tendon reflexes and sensory disturbances in adolescents and adults	Hereditary form of cerebellar ataxia	No confirmed treatment; vitamin B therapy sometimes indicated
Berylliosis: beryllium poisoning and beryllium disease	Systemic granulomatous disorder that's a form of pneumociosis with dominant pulmonary manifestations; two forms: Acute nonspecific pneumonitis an dchronic noncaseating granulomatous disease with interstital fibrosis; death may result from respiratory failure and cor pulmonale	Inhalation of absorption of beryllium; severity depends on amount inhaled or absorbed	Beryllium ulcer requires excision or curettage; acute form requires prompt corticosteroid therapy, oxygen and, possible, mechanical ventilation; chronic form is treated with corticosteroids
Blinding filarial disease: onchocerciasis, river blindness	Invasion of eye tissues by the filarial worm, which is enclosed in fibrous cysts or nodules; lesions also developing on the skin and, in severe infection, leading to chronic pruritis and disfiguring skin lesions	*Onchocerca volvulus* transmitted by the blackfly (*Simulium* and *Eusimulium*)	Ivermectin (Stromectol) the drug of choice
Bouillaud's syndrome: rheumatic endocarditis	Manifests as a heart murmur of either mitral or aortic insufficiency; pericarditis and heart failure are seen in severe cases	Delayed sequel to pharyngeal infection by group B streptococci	Although no specific cure is available, a course of penicillin should still be given to eliminate group A streptococci; supportive therapy to reduce morbidity and mortality should be provided
Breisky's disease: kraurosis vulvae	Vulval atrophy and dryness of skin and mucous membranes, causing shrinkage of the vaginal outlet; histopathologically identical to lichen sclerosis	Probably hypoestrogen	Surgery
Brill's disease: Brill-Zinsser disease, latent or recrudescent typhus	Relapse of typhus, which can occur years after the primary attack	*Rickettsia prowazekii*	Tetracycline, chloramphenicol, analgesics, antipyretics
Brown-Symmers disease	Acute serous encephalitis in children	Viral pathogens (rabies, measles, mumps, rubella, influenza)	Supportive care; control of intracranial pressure; correction of metabolic problems, disseminated intravascular coagulation, bleeding, renal failure, pulmonary emboli, and pneumonia; invariably fatal
Budd-Chiari syndrome	Hepatic vein obstruction that impairs blood flow out of the liver, producing massive ascites and hepatomegaly	Any condition or medication that obstructs blood flow from hepatic veins	Symptomatic management with diuretics and sodium and fluid restriction; surgery to shunt hepatic blood flow and remove obstruction; liver transplantation may be recommended for patients with marked hepatocellular dysfunction
Burkitt's tumor: Burkitt's lymphoma	Undifferentiated malignant lymphoma that usually begins as a large mass in the jaw (African Burkitt's) or as an abdominal mass (American Burkitt's)	Unknown, but Epstein-Barr virus suspected in some cases	Chemotherapy; radiation therapy; surgical resection in extensive local disease; in patients with a relapse, autologous bone marrow transplantation
Cat-scratch fever: cat-scratch disease	Subacute self-limiting disease characterized by a primary local lesion and regional lymphadenopathy; more common in children and young adults in contact with cats and dogs; disseminated form, bacillary angiomatosis, found in immunocompromised persons such as those infected with the human immunodeficiency virus	*Bartonella henoele*	Symptomatic management; if patient is ill, can use co-trimoxazole, ciprofloxacin, erythromycin, cefoxitin, cefotaxime, mezlocilin, or the antipseudomonal aminoglycosides
Central core disease: Shy-Magee syndrome	Rare muscle disease in which severe hypotonia causes weakness and arrests motor development in infancy; lack of oxidative enzymes in central core of each muscle fiber is diagnostic	Transmitted as autosomal dominant trait	Symptomatic and supportive treatment; genetic testing is available; recognition of this disease is important because patients with it have a well-established predisposition for malignant hyperthermia during anesthesia
Charcot-Marie-Tooth disease	Neuropathic (peroneal) muscular atrophy characterized by progressive weakness of the distal muscles of the arms and feet; most common form of the muscular dystrophies	Transmitted as autosomal dominant trait	Supportive treatment, including counseling, braces for foot drop, or orthopedic surgery to stabilize the foot and treat fractures

Disease	Description	Cause	Treatment
Chediak-Higashi syndrome	Characterized by morphological changes in granulocytes that impair the ability to respond to chemotaxis and to digest or kill invading organisms; associated with partial albinism	Transmitted as autosomal recessive trait; mutations found in Chediak-Higashi syndrome gene	Vigorous early treatment with antimicrobials and surgical drainage; large doses of Vitamin C
Chester's disease: xanthomatosis	Excessive accumulation of lipids in the long bones, marked by the formation of foam cells in skin lesions; results in progressive cerebellar ataxia, dementia, subnormal intelligence, spinal cord paresis, tendon xanthomas, and cataracts	Inherited as an autosomal recessive trait that causes disturbances in lipid metabolism	Unknown
Chiari-Frommel syndrome	Postpartum condition marked by uterine atrophy, persistent lactation, galactorrhea, prolonged amenorrhea, and low levels of urinary estrogen and gonadotropin	Possibly pituitary dysfunction or tumor	Treatment of underlying illness and bromocriptine to prevent osteoporosis
Choriocarcinoma	Rapidly metastasizing malignant tumor of placental tissue that typically causes profuse vaginal and intra-abdominal bleeding	Possibly hydatidiform mole, abortion, fetal-maternal histoincompatibility, inherited factors, or infections	Chemotherapy, suction to empty uterine contents, hysterectomy; serial chest X-rays and monitoring for progressively decreasing B-hCG levels
Chromomycosis: chromoblastomycosis	Slowly spreading fungal infection of the skin and subcutaneous tissues; produces cauliflower-like lesions on the legs or arms and may spread to the brain, causing an abscess	*Phialophora verrucosa, Fonsecaea pedrosoi,* and *Cladosporium carrionii*	Lesion removal with liquid nitrogen, electrocoagulation, or surgery; flucytosine alone or with ketoconazole; itraconazole may also be effective
Cockayne's syndrome	Hereditary syndrome consisting of dwarfism with retinal atrophy and deafness; associated with progeria, prognathism, mental regardation, photosensitivity, and accelerated atherosclerosis	Transmitted as autosomal recessive trait	Effective treatment unknown; symptomatic treatent, establishment of protective environment
Concato's disease: Bamberger's disease	Progressive malignant polyserositis with large effusions into the pericardium, pleura, and peritoneum; associated with tuberculosis	*Mycobacterium tuberculosis*	Thoracentesis and parenteral or oral antitubercular antibiotics, such as para-aminosalicylate and ethionamide
Conradi-Hunermann syndrome: dysplasia epiphysealis punctata	Abnormal development of the secondary bone-forming center, marked by depressions or pinpoint structures	Transmitted as autosomal dominant and X-linked dominant trait	Supportive treatment ensuring adequate calcium intake
Contact ulcers	Erosions on the laryngeal mucosa over the vocal cords, producing hoarseness, mild dysphagia, and gradual tissue necrosis	Vocal strain, laryngeal trauma, or emotional stress	Supportive management with absolute voice rest, adequate humidification, and aerosol therapy
Copper deficiency anemia: hypocupremia	Nutritional deficiency that impairs hemoglobin synthesis and causes shortness of breath, pallor, fatigue, edema, poor wound healing, and anorexia; if prolonged, can cause poor mental development in infants and mental deterioration in adults	Diseases associated with low protein levels; substantial protein loss; decreased GI absorption of copper; total parenteral nutrition without copper supplement; or Wilson's disease	Copper sulfate, supportive management of associated symptoms, treatment of underlying cause
Crocq's disease: acrocyanosis, Cassirer syndrome	Symmetrical cyanosis of the hands and feet; distinguished from Raynaud's disease by persistent discoloration	Vasospastic disturbance of smaller arterioles of the skin; may be due to dysregulation of the nervous system; more prevalent in females than in males	Protection from exposure to cold, occasionally relieved by warmth
Csillag's disease, planus type: lichen planus sclerous atrophicus	Acute inflammatory dermatitis, such as heat rash, prickly heat, miliaria rubra; chronic atrophic and lichenoid dermatitis	Keratin obstruction of sweat ducts	Symptomatic management, including cool environment, application of calamine lotion, and desquamation by ultraviolet rays
Cystinuria	Inborn error of amino acid transport in the kidneys and intestine that allows excessive urinary excretion of cystine and other dibasic amino acids; results in recurrent cystine renal calculi	Transmitted as autosomal recessive trait	Supportive treatment, including increasing fluid intake, sodium bicarbonate administration, alkaline-ash diet, and penicillamine; surgical removal of calculi
Czerny's disease	Joint pain with swelling	Serous effusion in a joint space or cavity	Treatment of inflammation, aspiration of joint space

Disease	Description	Cause	Treatment
Dengue: breakbone fever, dandy fever	Acute febrile disease endemic during the warmer months in the tropics and subtropics; rarely fatal unless it progresses to hemorrhagic shock syndrome	Group B arborviruses transmitted by the female *Aedes* mosquito	Symptomatic management, nonaspirin analgesics, I.V. fluid replacement, complete bed rest
Dubois' disease: congenital syphilis	Bulbous eruptions or macular copper-colored rash on palms and soles, and papular lesions around the nose, mouth, and diaper area	*Treponema pallidum,* a spirochete obtained by venereal contact of the mother and transmitted from her to the fetus via the placenta	Penicillin; in allergic patients, either desensitize to penicillin or seek infectious disease consultation
Duhring's disease: dermatitis herpetiformis	Chronic inflammatory disease marked by erythematous, papular, vesicular, bulbous, or pustular lesions, with tendency toward grouping and associated with itching and burning; usually symmetrical, with eruptions on elbows, knees, sacrum, buttocks, and occiput	Unknown, but associated with transplantation antigens HLA-B8, HLA-DR3, and HLA-DQW2; most prevalent in males	Removal of sources of reflex irritation, application of antiseptic to excoriated areas, dapsone, avoidance of dietary gluten; sulfapyridine may be used as an alternative
Dukes' disease: fourth disease	Marked by myalgia, headache, fever, pharyngitis, conjunctivitis, generalized adenopathy, and desquamation following confluent raised erythema	Most likely a viral exanthema of the coxsackievirus or echovirus group	Symptomatic and supportive management
Durand's disease: Durand-Nicholas-Favie disease	Venereal disease marked by involvement of the inguinal gland with an extruding lesion; found worldwide, but incidence higher in tropical and subtropical regions	*Chlamydia trachomatis* (serologic type L_1-3)	Symptomatic and supportive treatment; antiviral agent specific to chlamydia
Duroziez's disease: congenital mitral stenosis	Narrowing orifice of the mitral valve that obstructs blood flow, from left atrium to left ventricle	Congenital	Surgery, if possible; otherwise, supportive management with medications to maintain blood flow
Eales disease: peripheral neovascular retinopathy	Condition marked by recurrent hemorrhages into the retina and vitreous; men in their teens and 20s; most cases spontaneous and unilateral; some cases associated with trauma or stress, but also occurs after awakening	Unknown	Treatment of underlying causes, if associated with trauma or stress
Economo's disease: lethargic encephalitis	Epidemic encephalitis marked by increasing languor, apathy, and drowsiness, progressing to lethargy; accompanied by ophthalmoplegia; usually occurs in winter	Pathogen not clearly identified, but may be arthropod-borne virus or sequela of influenza, rubella, varicella, or vaccinia	Symptomatic management, including appropriate antibiotics for secondary infection
Elevator disease	Form of occupational pneumoconiosis affecting people who work in grain elevators	Inhalation of dust particles, causing irritation and inflammation of respiratory tract	Avoidance of exposure to dust
Engel-Recklinghausen disease: hyperparathyroidism, osteitis fibrosa cystica generalisata	Fibrous degeneration of bone, with the formation of cysts and fibrous nodules on affected bone; effective monitoring and control of hyperparathyroidism have made disease even rarer	Marked osteoclastic activity secondary to parathyroid hyperfunction, with calcium and phosphorus metabolic disturbances	Control of parathyroid hyperactivity; may require surgery if patient develops impaired renal function, bone demineralization, or significant hypertension
Eosinophilic endomyocardial disease: Löffler's endocarditis, Loeffler's endocarditis	Form of progressive endocarditis denoted by a highly increased number of eosinophilic granulocytes in the blood; fibrosis and thickening of the endocardium occur; cardiomegaly and heart failure may be present	Unknown	Suppression of eosinophilia with prednisolone or hydroxyurea; digoxin; diuretics; medical and surgical therapy for cardiac complications as indicated
Epstein-Barr virus: mononucleosis	Classic heterophil-positive infectious mononucleosis, occasionally complicated by neurologic diseases, such as encephalitis or transverse myelitis	Infection with Epstein-Barr virus	Symptomatic treatment; generally benign course
Erysipeloid	Acute, self-limiting skin infection most common in butchers, fishermen, and others who handle infected material; may progress to infective endocarditis if primary lesions aren't treated	*Erysipelothrix insidiosa* transmitted by contact with infected meat, fish, poultry, or animal hides, bones, or manure	Penicillin G or erythromycin; cloxacillin or cephalexin for persistent cases
Erythrasma	Superficial, bacterial skin infection that usually affects the skin folds, especially in the groin, axillae, and toe webs	*Corynebacterium minutissimum*	Keratolytics, topical antibiotics; treatment with oral erythromycin or tetracycline commonly for quick resolution
Eulenberg's disease: paramyotonia congenita, Thomsen's disease	Slowly progressive disease of skeletal muscles; similar to muscular dystrophy; muscle stiffness in hands, legs, and eyelids most prominent manifestation	Transmitted as autosomal dominant trait	Treatment with quinine sulfare, procainamide, tocainide, mexiletine, or phenytoin

Disease	Description	Cause	Treatment
Fabry's disease	Extremely painful systemic disorder related to a deficiency of enzyme alpha-galactosidase; characterized by glycolipid accumulation in body tissues	Transmitted as X-linked recessive trait	Symptomatic management with low-dose phenytoin or carbamazepine; possibly kidney transplantation
Fanconi's syndrome: De Toni-Fanconi syndrome	Disorder of fat storage related to a deficiency of enzyme alpha-galactosidase A; characterized by glucolipid accumulation in body tissues; results in clouding of the cornea; burning sensations of hands and feet, small raised purple blemishes on the skin, impaired arterial circulation, and renal and GI involvement	If diagnosed as a child, may be congenital; if diagnosed as an adult, considered acquired and may be secondary to Wilson's disease, cystinosis, galectosemia, or exposure to toxins as in heavy metal poisoning	Symptomatic treatment with replacement therapy, vitamin D for rickets, and aluminum hydroxide for hyperphosphatemia; treatment of underlying cause for acquired form; dialysis as necessary
Fifth disease: erythema infectiosum	Contagious disease characterized by rose-colored eruptions diffused over the skin, usually starting on the cheeks; mainly affects children ages 4 to 10	Human parvovirus, probably transmitted via the respiratory tract	Symptomatic treatment; screening of donated blood might prevent transfusion-related transmission
File-cutters' disease	Lead poisoning from inhalation of lead particles that arise during file cutting	Inhalation of lead particles	Avoidance of exposure to lead; chelating agents for moderate to high-level poisoning
Fish-skin disease: ichthyosis vulgaris, ichthyosis lamellar	Condition of dry and scaly skin resembling fish skin; several forms, including vulgaris and lamellar	Hereditary form an autosomal dominant genetic disorder; acquired form seen in adults usually from internal disease such as malignancy	Alpha-hydroxy acids (lactic, glycolic or pyruvic acids) to help hydrate the skin; removal of scales by keratolytics; propylene glycol; topical retinoids; treatment of underlying systemic condition for acquired form
Flax-dresser's disease	Pulmonary disorder of flax-dressers	Inhalation of flax particles	Avoidance of exposure to flax
Flecked retina syndrome	Group of retinal disorders, including fundus flavimaculatus, fundus albipunctatus, drusen, and congenital macular degeneration, all of which may be primary abnormalities of retinal pigment epithelium	Congenital	Supportive and symptomatic treatment, such as medications for pain and anxiety
Fleischner's disease	Inflammation of bone and cartilage affecting the middle phalanges of the hand	Unknown	Anti-inflammatories (including steroids in severe cases); analgesics
Friedländer's disease: endarteritis obliterans	Chronic, progressive thickening of the intima, leading to stenosis or obstruction of the lumen	Trauma, pyogenic bacterial infection, infective thrombi, or syphilis	Endarterectomy
Friedreich's disease: paramyoclonus multiplex, Friedrich's ataxia	Ataxic gait, cerebellar dysfunction, leg weakness, sensory disturbances in the limbs, and depressed tendon reflexes	Central nervous system damage secondary to trauma or infection; may be hereditary	Treatment of underlying disease; no specific treatment for hereditary form
Geotrichosis	Fungal infection affecting the mouth, throat, lungs, or intestines	*Geotrichum candidum*	Gentian violet for oral, throat, or intestinal infections; oral potassium iodide for pulmonary infections
Gerlier's disease: endemic paralytic vertigo, paralyzing vertigo	Nervous system disorder marked by pain, vertigo, paresis, and muscle contractions	Disease of the internal ear from pressure of cerumen on the drum membrane	Symptomatic management, including scopolamine to combat nausea
Glioma of the optic nerve	Slow-growing tumor that causes progressive vision loss	Unknown	Surgical excision, radiation therapy
Glossopharyngeal neuralgia	Disease of the ninth cranial (glossopharyngeal) nerve that produces paroxysms of pain in the ear, posterior pharynx, base of the tongue, or jaws; sometimes accompanied by syncope	Unknown	Surgery, carbamazepine, phenytoin
Glucose-6-phosphate dehydrogenase (G6PD) deficiency	Deficiency of the red blood cell enzyme G6PD, which causes anemia; common in people of African or Mediterranean descent	Transmitted as an X-linked trait, so mostly seen in males	Avoidance of oxidant drugs, including primaquine, salicylates, sulfonamides, nitrofurans, phenacetin, naphthalene
Graefe's sign: ophthalmoplegia progressiva	Gradual paralysis of the eyes, affecting first one eye muscle, then the other	Usually brain lesions or mitochondrial disorders	Treatment of underlying disease; corrective lenses
Grinder's disease: pneumoconiosis	Permanent deposition of particles in the lungs	Inhalation of dust particles	Irreversible pulmonary disease; eliminating exposure to dust particles can prevent further irritation of tissues

Disease	Description	Cause	Treatment
Habermann's disease: acute lichenoid pityriasis	Sudden onset of a polymorphous skin eruption of macules, papules and, occasionally, vesicles, with hemorrhage	Virus resembling smallpox	Supportive management, possibly isolation
Hagner's disease	Obscure bone disease resembling acromegaly; associated with increased soft-tissue growth after puberty, increased metabolic rate, and increased sweating and sebaceous activity	Growth hormone-secreting tumors that develop after puberty	Treatment of cardiovascular complications; surgery and irradiation (proton beam or heavy particle treatment and supravoltage) for large tumors
Heavy chain diseases	Neoplasms of the lymphoplasmacytes, in which abnormal proliferation occurs among cells that produce immunoglobulins, causing incomplete heavy chains and no light chains in their molecular structure	Possibly microorganisms and immune deficiency syndrome due to malnutrition or genetic predisposition	Supportive and palliative management with chemotherapy, radiation therapy, antibiotics, and steroids
Heerfordt's syndrome: Heerfordt's disease, uveoparotid fever	Variant of sarcoidosis manifested by parotid swelling and single or multiple palsies of cranial nerves	Impaired regulation of thymus-derived lymphocytes (T cells) and bone-marrow-derived lymphocytes (B cells)	Adrenal corticosteroids to suppress inflammation and control symptoms
Hemangioma of the eye	In children, tumors not encapsulated, grow quickly in the first year, and then regress by about age 7; in adults, tumors encapsulated	Unknown	Surgical excision for adults; no treatment for children
Hemochromatosis: bronze diabetes, Recklinghausen-Applebaum disease	Disorder characterized by iron overload in parenchymal cells, leading to cirrhosis, diabetes, cardiomegaly with heart failure and arrhythmias, and increased skin pigmentation	Erythropoietic disorders, hepatic disorders that increase iron absorption, autosomal recessive inheritance	Phlebotomy to remove excess iron, chelating agents such as deferoxamine
Hemoglobin C–thalassemia disease	Simultaneous heterozygosity for hemoglobin C and thalassemia; characterized by mild hemolytic anemia and persistent splenomegaly	Hereditary and congenital	Supportive management, including transfusions for severe anemia and folate therapy
Henderson-Jones disease: osteochondromatosis	Presence of numerous benign cartilaginous tumors in the joint cavity or in the bursa of a tendon sheath	Irritation and trauma	Resection of tumor with curettage and bone grafts
Hereditary spherocytosis	Anemia resulting in increased red blood cell membrane permeability and intracellular hypetonicity; characterized by slight jaundice, splenomegaly, and cholelithiasis	Transmitted as autsomal dominant trait	Splenectomy; supplementation with folic acid
Heubner's disease: Heubner's endarteritis	Syphilitic inflammation of tunica intima of cerebral arteries	*Treponema pallidum*	Supportive management, including antibiotic therapy
Hoffa's disease	Proliferation of fatty tissue (solitary lipoma) in the knee joint	Tissue trauma	Aspiration or surgery
Hutchinson-Gilford syndrome: progeria	Premature old age marked by small stature, wrinkled skin, and gray hair, with attitude and appearance of old age in very young children	Unknown	None known
Hutinel's disease	Tuberculous pericarditis, with cirrhosis of the liver in children	*Mycobacterium tuberculosis*	Tuberculostatic agents
Hydatid disease, alveolar	Infection characterized by invasion and destruction of tissue by cysts, which undergo endogenous budding and form an aggregate of innumerable small cysts that honeycomb the affected organ – usually the liver – and may metastasize	Infection by *Echinococcus multilocularis* (larvae)	Symptomatic management and surgery; usually fatal; high-dose mebendazole may be used in patients with medical problems that preclude surgery or in cases where surgery wouldn't be indicated
Hydatid disease, unilocal	Infection causing marked formation of single or multiple unilocular cysts	Infection by *Echinococcus granulosis* (larvae); hydatid tapeworm in dogs and cats	Surgery, drug therapy with albendazole or mebendazole
Iceland disease: epidemic neuromyasthenia, benign myalgic encephalomyelitis	Marked by headaches, muscle pain, low-grade fever, lymphadenopathy, fatigue, and paresthesia; outbreaks occur in summer, usually in young women	Probably infection but possibly psychosocial phenomenon	Symptomatic treatment, such as analgesics and rest
Intestinal lymphangiectasia	Dilation and possible rupture of intestinal lymphatic vessels, resulting in hypoproteinemia and steatorrhea due to loss of fat and albumin into the intestinal lumen	Congenital or may be acquired when obstruction, valvular heart disease, or constrictive pericarditis increases pressure on the lymphatics	No-fat diet, replacement of dietary sources of long-chain triglycerides with medium-chain triglycerides

Disease	Description	Cause	Treatment
Interstitial cystitis	Inflammation of the bladder wall commonly occurring in women and marked by urinary frequency and urgency and abdominal, urethral, or vaginal pain; dyspareunia possibly also occurring; urine cultures and urinalysis are normal; cystoscopic examination revealing pinpoint hemorrhages on distended bladder wall	Unknown	Symptomatic treatment (anti-inflammatories, antispasmodics, antihistamines, and muscle relaxants); dimethyl sulfoxide, silver nitrate, or pentosan polysulfate sodium instilled into the bladder; surgical diversion last resort
Isambert's disease: tuberculosis laryngitis	Acute miliary tuberculosis of the larynx and pharynx	*Myobacterium tuberculosis*	Tuberculostatic agents
Jaffee-Lichtenstein disease: cystic osteofibromatosis	Form of polyostotic fibrous dysplasia marked by an enlarged medullary cavity with a thin cortex, which is filled with fibrous tissue (fibroma)	May be a lipoid granuloma	Symptomatic and supportive management; surgery
Jaksch's syndrome: anemia pseudoleukemia infantum, Jaksh's syndrome	Syndrome of anisocytosis, peripheral red blood cell immaturity, leukocytosis, and hepatosplenomegaly that usually occurs in children younger than age 3	Malnutrition, chronic infection, malabsorption, hemoglobinopathies	Treatment of underlying cuases
Jansen's syndrome: metaphyseal dysotosis	Skeletal abnormality with nearly normal epiphyses in which the metaphyseal tissues are replaced by masses of cartilage	Unknown	Surgery to remove skeletal abnormality
Jensen's disease: retinochoroiditis juxta-paplilaris	Inflammation of the retina and choroid marked by small inflammatory areas of the fundus close to the papilla	Unknown; probably an autoimmune process	Steroids may induce improvements
Juvenile angiofibroma	Highly vascular, nasopharyngeal tumor that causes nasal obstruction and severe recurrent epistaxis	Unknown	Surgery
Keratoconus	Degenerative eye disorder typified by thinning and anterior protrusion of the cornea, causing major changes in the refractive power of the eye and requiring frequent eyeglass changes	Transmitted as autosomal recessive trait	Hard contact lenses or glasses with high astigmatic correction; corneal graft or transplantation may be necessary
Keratosis pilaris: keratosis follicularis, Darier's disease	Any skin condition marked by formation of horny plugs in the orifices of hair follicles; lesions appearing primarily on the lateral aspects of the upper arms, thighs, and buttocks; may also occur on face	Unknown, but may be transmitted as an autosomal dominant trait	No specific therapy; keratolytic lotions to prevent cracking, drying, and skin breakdown useful
Kienböck's disease: lunatomalacia	Slowly progressive osteochondrosis of the semilunar (carpal lunate) bone from avascular necrosis	Degenerative process precipitated by trauma	Anti-inflammatories and immobilization of wrist for several months (if ineffective, surgery)
Köhler's bone disease: tarsal scaphoiditis, epiphysitis juvenilis	Osteochondrosis of the tarsal navicular bone in children, occurring at about age 5	Unknown, but trauma suspected	Protection of foot from excessive use or trauma; if pain severe, plaster cast for 6 to 8 weeks; oral analgesics as needed; complete spontaneous recovery possible
Krabbe's disease: globoid cell leukodystrophy	Rapidly progressive cerebral demyelination with large globoid bodies in the white matter; associated with irritability, rigidity, tonic-clonic seizures, blindness, deafness, and progressive mental deterioration	Familial	Symptomatic management; death occurs by age 2
Kugelberg-Welander syndrome: type III spinal muscular atrophy	Slowly progressive muscular atrophy resulting from lesions of the anterior horns of the spinal cord; usual onset in preschool or adolescent years	Transmitted as autosomal recessive or dominant trait	Supportive treatment with physical therapy; bracing or special appliances may help; normal life span probable
Kümmell's disease: Kümmell-Verneil disease, posttraumatic spondylitis	Intercostal neuralgia with spinal pain and motor disturbances in the legs	Compression fracture of the vertebrae	Management of fracture, extension of spine; pain relief
Kuru	Chronic, progressive, and fatal neurologic disease found only in New Guinea	Slow virus thought to be associated with cannibalism	No effective treatment; invariably fatal
Larsen's disease: Larsen-Johansson disease	Accessory center of ossification within the patella, associated with flat facies and short metacarpals	Unknown	Supportive management; surgery
Leiner's disease: erythroderma desquamativum	Generalized exfoliative dermatitis and erythroderma, chiefly affecting breast-fed neonates; probably identical to severe seborrheic dermatitis	Allergic, hereditary, and psychogenic causes suspected	Symptomatic management

Disease	Description	Cause	Treatment
Leishmaniasis	Group of infectious disorders; Old World and New World cutaneous forms are self-limiting; kala-azar and New World mucocutaneous forms are sometimes fatal	*Leishmania* transmitted by sand fly bites	Drug of choice sodium stibogluconate; alternative drugs are meglumine antimoniate, pentamidine, paromomycin, or interferon plus antimony; amphotericin B should be used for resistant cases
Lenègre's disease	Acquired complete heart block	Primary degeneration of the conduction system	Artificial pacemaker; supportive management
Leptospirosis	Infectious disease that causes meningitis, hepatitis, nephritis, or febrile disease; may be mild (anicteric) or severe (icteric or Weil's disease)	*Leptospira* transmitted by contact with water, soil, food, or vegetation contaminated with urine from an infected lower mammal	Penicillin G, doxycycline, or ampicillin
Lesch-Nyhan syndrome	Disorder of purine metabolism marked by behavioral problems that include cognitive dysfunction and aggressive and impulsive behaviors; also includes self-injurious behaviors, spasticity, hyperuricemia, and excessive uricaciduria	Defective enzyme transmitted by female carriers as X-linked recessive trait	Allopurinol to control urine and sedimentation; baclofen and benzodiazepines for spasticity; symptomatic and supportive treatment, such as behavioral modification and medications for behavior treatment; few patients live beyond age 40 and most die suddenly
Letterer-Siwe disease: nonlipid reticuloendotheliosis	Hemorrhagic tendency with eczematoid skin eruptions, lymph node enlargement, hepatosplenomegaly, and progressive anemia; occurs mainly in infants	Unknown; may represent an unusual form of malignant lymphoma	Symptomatic and supportive management of anemia. Local radiation effective for osseous lesions; corticosteroids should be used to treat lung involvement
Lewandowsky-Lutz disease: epidermodysplasia verruciformis	May manifest as flat-topped papules that vary in color from pink to brown, resembling verruca plana; have a tendency to become malignant; they increase in number and coalesce to form large paques or scales on the knees, elbows, and trunk; often associated with mental retardation	Autosomal recessive trait with impaired cell immunity; about 15 human papillomaviruses implicated	No effective treatment
Lichtheim's disease	Subacute degeneration of the spinal cord associated with pernicious anemia	Vitamin B_{12} deficiency	Correction of vitamin B_{12} deficiency
Li-Fraumeni syndrome	Inherited syndrome predisposing patient to lung, breast, and soft-tissue cancers	Inherited family trait, deletion of tumor-suppression gene (chromosome 17)	Treatment specific to cancer
Little's disease: spastic diplegia, cerebral palsy	Form of cerebral spastic paralysis and stiffness of the limbs associated with muscle weakness, seizures, bilateral athetosis, and mental deficiencies	Congenital, resulting from birth trauma, fetal anoxia, or maternal illness during pregnancy	Preventive measures and symptomatic management
Ludwig's angina	Infection of the sublingual and submandibular spaces characterized by brawny induration of the submaxillary region, edema of the sublingual floor of the mouth, and elevation of the tongue	Usually abscesses of the second and third mandibular molars	Significant airway obstruction may require tracheotomy; antibiotics, such as nafcillin, effective against streptococci and staphylococci; clindamycin may be used in patients allergic to penicillin; incision and drainage should be performed to relieve pressure in the affected tissues
Lung fluke disease: *Paragonimus westermani, Paragonimus heterotrema*	Parasitic hemoptysis, or oriental hemoptysis from pulmonary cysts	Infestation by trematodes or flukes	Praziquantel the drug of choice; symptomatic and supportive management of hemoptysis usually necessary
MacLean-Maxwell disease	Chronic condition of the calcaneus marked by enlargement of the posterior third and by sensitivity to pressure	Trauma	Supportive shoes; surgery; avoidance of prolonged standing; high-impact exercises
Macroglobulinemia: Waldenström's macroglobulinemia	Osteoporosis of the alveoli of the teeth	Usually secondary to gingivitis	Steroid therapy for extreme inflammation; antibiotics for secondary infection
Malibu disease: surfer's knots	Hyperplastic, fibrosing granulomas occurring over bony prominences of the feet and legs of surfers	Repeated trauma from surfboard	Supportive shoes, avoidance of prolonged standing
Malignant melanoma of the eye	Malignant tumor stemming from the melanocytes in the uvea, retina, or iris	Unknown	Surgical excision; eye enucleation

Disease	Description	Cause	Treatment
Maple syrup urine disease	Enzyme defect in the metabolism of the branched chain amino acids, resulting in mental and physical retardation, reflex changes, feeding difficulties, characteristic odor of urine and perspiration, seizures, and death	Transmitted as autosomal recessive trait	Supportive management; controlled intake of branched chain amino acids; peritoneal dialysis, hemodialysis, or both
Marburg disease: Marburg virus disease	Severe viral disease characterized by fever, malaise, myalgia, headache, pharyngitis, vomiting, diarrhea, and rash commonly accompanied by hepatic damage, renal failure, encephalitis, and multiorgan dysfunction	Exposure to African green monkeys	Symptomatic and supportive management; usually fatal
Medullary cystic disease: familial juvenile nephronophthisis	Congenital renal disorder marked by cyst formation, primarily in the medulla and the corticomedullary junction, with insidious onset of uremia	Transmitted as autosomal recessive or dominant trait	High sodium and water intake, alkali replacement, symptomatic management; dietary management with increased protein; dialysis or kidney transplantation if conventional therapy fails
Megaloblastic anemia	Folic acid or vitamin B_{12} deficiency that alters the nucleic acid production needed for erythrocyte maturation in bone marrow	Cobalamin (vitamin B_{12}) deficiency, secondary to pernicious anemia and folate deficiency, resulting from poor diet, sprue, pregnancy, or antifolate medication	Folic acid or vitamin B_{12}, supplementation
Meyer-Betz disease: idiopathic or familiar myoglobinuria	Myoglobinuria that may be precipitated by strenuous exertion or possibly by infection; marked by tenderness, swelling, and muscle weakness	Unknown; familial tendences possible	Bed rest; anti-inflammatories, steroids in extreme cases, analgesics for pain
Microdrepanocytic disease	Sickle-cell thalassemia; anemia involving simultaneous heterozygosity for hemoglobin S and thalassemia	Hereditary transmission	Management of anemia
Milroy's disease: congenital lymphedema	Chronic lymphatic obstruction causing lymphedema of the legs; sometimes associated with edema of the arms, trunk, and face	Congenital and hereditary; transmitted as an autosomal dominant trait	Microsurgery to rechannel lymph flow; supportive care, compression stockings
Minamata disease	Severe neurologic disorder characterized by peripheral and circumoral paresthesia, ataxia, mental disabilities, and loss of peripheral vision	Alkyl mercury poisoning	Avoidance of causative agents, supportive and symptomatic management; usually fatal
Minor's disease	Hematomyelia involving the central parts of the spinal cord; marked by sudden onset of flaccid paralysis, with sensory disturbances	Unknown	Treatment of underlying disease, supportive management
Morton's neuroma: metatarsalgia	Pain over the ball of the foot	Abnormality of the foot or osteochondrosis	Supportive shoes, analgesics; perineural injections of long-acting corticosteroids with local anesthetics; use of foot orthosis and surgical excision if needed
Mule-spinners' disease	Warts or ulcers, especially on the scrotum, that tend to become malignant; common among operators of spinning mules in cotton mills	Unknown	Surgery
Mushroom picker's disease	Allergic respiratory disease of persons working with moldy compost prepared for growing mushrooms	Airborne irritant, usually mold: *Micropolyspora faeni* or *Thermoactinomyces vulgaris*	Supportive and symptomatic management
Mycetoma: maduromycosis, Madura foot	Chronic infection of the skin, subcutaneous tissues, and bone, usually affecting the foot	*Allescheria boydii, Actinomycetales* bacteria, or *Nocardia*	Sulfonamides, penicillin, tetracycline, amphotericin B, or ketoconazole; terbinafine may also be effective for sensitive fungus; amputation of the affected limb may be necessary to prevent secondary bacterial infection and death
Myelosclerosis	Sclerosis of the spinal cord; obliteration of the normal marrow cavity by the formation of small spicules of bone	Unknown	Antibiotics for actinomycetoma (streptomycin, co-trimoxazole, amikacin, rifampin, minocycline); itraconazole or ketoconazole for eumycetoma from fungi surgery for affected tissue or amputation if bone involved

Disease	Description	Cause	Treatment
Nezelof syndrome	Primary immunodeficiency disease characterized by absent T-cell function and variable B-cell function, with fairly normal immunoglobulin levels and little or no specific antibody production; failure to thrive and increased susceptibility to infection typical; usually fatal as a result of sepsis	May be transmitted as autosomal recessive trait	Symptomatic treatment (usually includes antibiotics for infection and monthly treatment with immune globulin or fresh frozen plasma infusions); bone marrow transplantation
Niemann-Pick disease: sphingomyelin lipidosis	Metabolic disorder resulting in abnormal accumulation of sphingomyelin in reticuloendothelial cells; most common in people of Eastern European Jewish ancestry; occurs in five different phenotypes, each with slightly different symptoms, but characterized by pulmonary infiltrates, brownish skin, and sea blue histiocytes	Transmitted as autosomal recessive trait	Supportive and symptomatic management, possibly splenectomy
Norrie's disease: atrophia bulborum hereditaria	Bilateral blindness resulting from retinal malformation, with mental retardation and deafness due to failure of the brain to develop	Transmitted as X-linked trait	None known
Nystagmus	Recurring involuntary eyeball movement that may be jerking or pendular	May be congenital or acquired; jerking nystagmus results from excessive stimulation of the vestibular apparatus in the inner ear, lesions of the brain stem or cerebellum, drugs and alcohol toxicity, and congenital neurologic disorder; pendular nystagmus results from improper transmission of visual impulses to the brain in the presnce of corneal opacification, high astigmatism, congenital cataract, or congenital anomalies of optic disk or bilateral macular lesions	Correction of the underlying cause if possible; eyeglasses for vision disturbances
Olivopontocerebellar atrophy	Progressively deteriorating neurologic disease marked by ataxia, dysarthria, and an action tremor that develops late in middle life; commonly mistaken for mental illness; usually normal deep tendon reflexes; associated with occasional rigidity and other extrapyramidal signs	Transmitted as autosomal dominant trait	No effective treatment; death usually follows pneumonia secondary to loss of cough reflex
Opitz's disease	Thrombophlebitic splenomegaly	Thrombosis of the splenic vein	Symptomatic and supportive management, including anticoagulation
Osteitis pubis	Painful condition at the symphysis pubis characterized by bony resorption and spontaneous reossification; excruciating pain radiating along the adductor aspect of both thighs; pain intensified by movement, especially abduction	Unknown; usually develops postpartum or after trauma such as lower pelvic surgery	Symptomatic treatment, including injection of local anesthetics, bed rest, and opioid analgesics or nonsteroidal anti-inflammatory drugs
Otto's disease: arthrokatadysis	Osteoarthritic protrusion of the acetabulum	Degenerative changes, probably hereditary	Surgery if night traction and rest are ineffective
Owren's disease: parahemophilia	Rare hemorrhagic tendency resulting from deficiency of coagulation factor V	Transmitted as autosomal recessive trait	Supportive management
Paracoccidioidomycosis: South American blastomycosis	Fungal infection of the skin, lungs, mucous membranes, lymphatics, and viscera; seen primarily in the tropical forests of South America and Mexico	*Paracoccidioides brasiliensis*	Ketoconazole, itraconazole, fluconazole; amphotericin B given I.V. for extremely ill patients
Paroxysmal nocturnal hemoglobinuria	Acquired abnormality in red blood cell membrane that increases susceptibility to lytic action of normal plasma components; abdominal and lumbar pain may occur, with splenomegaly, hemoglobinemia, hemoglobinuria, and symptoms of normocytic normochromic anemia; venous or arterial thrombi may cause death	Acquired clonal stem cell disorder	Treatment symptomatic, with corticosteroids producing good results; transfusions with washed red blood cells may be used during crisis; androgen therapy; oral iron supplements should be used
Pelizaeus-Merzbacher disease: sudanophilic leukodystrophy	Hyperplastic centrolobular sclerosis marked by nystagmus, ataxia, tremors, choreoathetotic movements, parkinsonian facies, and mental deterioration; begins early in life and occurs primarily in males	Familial transmission as a sex-linked recessive trait	No effective treatment; invariably fatal in several years

Disease	Description	Cause	Treatment
Pellegrini's disease: Pellegrini-Stieda disease, Köhler-Pellegrini-Stieda disease	Semilunar bony formation in the upper portion of the medial lateral ligament of the knee	Trauma	Surgical correction, supportive management
Pemphigus	Chronic blistering disease that causes superficial and deep lesions; pemphigus vulgaris, the most common form of this disease, can be fatal	Unknown	Corticosteroids, immunosuppressants; antibiotics for secondary skin infections; methotrexate, cyclophosphamide, and azathioprine
Perrin-Ferraton disease	Snapping hip	Unknown	No effective treatment
Progressive multifocal leukoencephalopathy	Demyelination of the white substance of the brain, producing sensory aphasia, cortical blindess, deafness, weakness, spasticity of the limbs and, eventually, complete paralysis, dementia, and coma; primarily affects patients who are immunosuppressed	Common human polyomavirus, JC virus	Symptomatic and supportive treatment
Pulseless disease: Takayasu arteritis	Progressive changes of th aorta and its branches resulting in decreased or absent radial pulse bilaterally with pain in arm and forearm; inflammation of carotid arteries cause vision problems; dizziness, or stroke; aneurysms and hypertension occur	Unknown, but appears to be related to autoimmunity	Steroids, immunosuppressants, surgery, angioplasty, angiotensin-converting enzyme inhibitors for hypertension
Purtscher's disease: Purtscher's angiopathic retinopathy	Retinal angiopathy with edema, hemorrhage, and exudation	Trauma (usually a crushing injury to the chest)	Treatment of underlying injury and supportive management
Q fever	Acute systemic disease that strikes people exposed to cattle, sheep, or goats	*Coxiella burnetii*	Tetracycline (doxycycline, co-trimoxazole, rifampin, or chloramphenicol for endocarditis); possibly valve replacement
Rat-bite fever: sodoku	Gram-negative bacterial infection that occurs 1 to 3 weeks after bite from an infected rat or mouse, causing chills, fever, headache, muscle pain, and maculopapular rash on extremities	*Streptobacillus moniliformis* or *Spirillum minor*	Penicillin G procaine, tetracycline, or streptomycin
Refsum's disease	Defect in metabolism of phytanic acid, marked by chronic polyneuritis, retinitis pigmentosa, and cerebellar signs (mild ataxia) with persistent elevation of protein levels in cerebrospinal fluid	Transmitted as autosomal recessive trait	Symptomatic and supportive management, dietary restriction of phytanic acid (chlorophyll-free)
Retinoblastoma	Most common eye tumor in children, arising from retinal gum cells	Transmitted as autosomal dominant trait (chromosome 13)	Enucleation, radiation therapy, or cryotherapy; systemic chemotherapy may be helpful for disseminated disease.
Rhabdomyosarcoma	Malignant tumors of muscle; affects throat, bladder, prostate, or vagina in infants; affects large muscle groups of the arm or leg in elderly patients	Unknown	Radiation therapy, surgical excision
Rhinosporidiosis	Fungal infection producing painless, vascularized, friable, and often large tumorlike lesions; most common in Ceylon and India	*Rhinosporidium seeberi*	Electrocauterization or surgical excision, followed by dapsone
Richter's syndrome	Chronic lymphocytic leukemia that evolves into an aggressive lymphoma	Clonal evolution of original leukemia	Chemotherapy for the leukemia
Rickettsialpox	Mild self-limiting disease characterized by a disseminated vascular skin rash and fever	*Rickettsia akari* transmitted by bites of mites carried by infected mice	Tetracycline or chloramphenicol, antipyretics, analgesics, increased fluid intake
Robles' disease: onchocerciasis	Onchocerciasis of the fibroid nodules, lymph, subcutaneous connective tissue (severe dermatitis and depigmentation) and eyes (river blindness)	*Onchocerca volvulus* transmitted by the black fly	Ivermectin or diethylcarbamazine albendazole or mebenedazole; corticosteroids or antihistamines to relieve allergic reactions from microfilariae
Schanz's syndrome: sarcoidosis (also known as Schaumann's disease)	Inflammation of the Achilles tendon	Trauma	Symptomatic management with anti-inflammatories, steroids, analgesics; rest

Disease	Description	Cause	Treatment
Sever's disease	Epiphysitis of the calcaneus	Inflammation from trauma or irritation	Treatment of underlying cause, heel pads in the shoe, possibly immobilization in a cast
Silo filler's disease	Pulmonary inflammation often associated with acute pulmonary edema	Inhalation of oxides of nitrogen and other gases that collect in silos	Corticosteroids, supportive respiratory management; bronchodilators, mild sedation, I.V. fluids with antibiotics, and oxygen may be required; avoidance of exposure to silo gases
Smith-Strang disease	Defective methionine absorption, resulting in white hair, mental retardation, seizures, attacks of hyperpnea, and characteristic odor of urine	Transmitted as autosomal recessive trait	No effective treatment
Soft-tissue sarcoma	Soft-tissue malignancy of muscle, fat, connective tissue, blood vessels, and synovium; composed of tightly packed cells similar to embryonic connective tissue	Unknown	Surgical resection, radiation therapy, chemotherapy with doxorubicin or dacarbazine
Sponge-diver's disease: sponge dermatitis	Burning, itching, erythema, necrosis, and ulceration of skin; common in Mediterranean divers	Irritation by toxins of sea anemones of the *Sagartia* and *Actinia* genera	Symptomatic management, including local application of calamine lotion or glucocorticoids, dilute acetic acid; administration of antihistamines for hives and itching; oral steroids may be effective in severe cases
Stargardt's disease	Degeneration of the macula lutea marked by rapid loss of visual activity and abnormal appearance and pigmentation of the macular area	Hereditary transmission	Corrective lenses as symptomatic treatment; supportive management
Strabismus: squint, heterotropia, cross-eye	Eye malalignment due to the absence of normal, parallel or coordinated eye movement	May be inherited, nonhereditary risk factors include trauma and vision problems	Depends on type, but may include patching, prescriptive lenses, surgery, eye exercises
Swediaur's disease: Schwediauer's disease	Inflammation of the calcaneal bursa	Irritation of bursa	Symptomatic management, including application of warm, moist heat and administration of anti-inflammatories and analgesics; also injections of corticosteroids with local anesthetics
Tangier disease	Deficiency of high-density lipoproteins (HDLs) in the serum with storage of cholesterol esters in the tonsils, causing orange-yellow tonsillar hyperplasia, and in the liver and spleen, causing hepatosplenomegaly	Absence of HDLs in plasma	No known treatment
Toxocariasis: visceral larva migrans	Chronic, frequently mild syndrome common in children, involving roundworm migration from the intestine to various organs and tissues; characterized by hepatosplenomegaly and eosinophilia	Ingestion of *Toxicara* larvae, usually from dirt	Thiabendazole, mebendazole, albendazole, diethylcarbamazine, or ivermectin
Trench fever: Wolhynia fever, shin bone fever, His-Werner disease, quintan fever	Self-limiting illness occurring sporadically in Eastern Europe, Asia, North Africa, and Mexico and producing multiple symptoms	*Rochalimaea quintana* transmitted by body lice	Analgesics, antipyretics, delousing with lindane or other pediculocide; tetracyclines and chloramphenicol probably effective
Trevor's disease	Dysplasia epiphysealis hemimelica	Unknown	No known treatment
Trichuriasis: whipworm disease	Nematode infection of the caecum and the anterior parts of the large intestine, producing various GI effects	Ingestion of food contaminated with *Trichurus*	Mebendazole or albendazole
Tropical sprue	GI disorder that causes atrophy of the small intestine, resulting in malabsorption, malnutrition, and folic acid deficiency; characterized by bulky, pale, frothy stools with increased fecal fat and macrocytic anemia; occurs mainly in Puerto Rico, Cuba, Haiti, Hong Kong, and India	Unknown	Tetracycline or oxytetracycline, phthalylsulfathiazole, diphenoxylate with atropine sulfate, folic acid
Typhus, endemic: murine, rat, or flea typhus	Mild form of typhus causing systemic illness characterized by fever, headache, rash, and myalgia	*Rickettsia typhi* transmitted by bites of infected fleas or lice or by inhalation of contaminated flea feces	Tetracycline, doxycycline, or chloramphenicol; analgesics; antipyretics

Disease	Description	Cause	Treatment
Typhus, epidemic: European, classic, or louse-borne typhus	Acute systemic illness that may lead to death	*Rickettsia prowazekii* transmitted by *Pediculus humanus trichiura*	Tetracycline, doxycycline, or chloramphenicol; analgesics; antipyretics; delousing with lindane or other pediculocide
Typhus, scrub: Japanese river or flood fever, tsutsugamushi fever	Acute systemic disease occurring almost exclusively in the western Pacific, Japan, and Southeast Asia	*Rickettsia tsutsugamushi* transmitted by mite larvae	Chloramphenicol or tetracycline; resistance to doxycycline and chloramphenicol has appeared in northern Thailand
Tyrosinemia	*Hereditary form:* results in liver failure and renal tubular failure, hypoglycemia, rickets, darkening of the skin, and mild mental retardation; occasionally causes liver cancer *Transient form:* usually occurs in premature neonates; marked by elevation of blood tyrosine levels	Autosomal recessive trait resulting in excess of tyrosine in blood and urine	Tyrosine and phenylalanine restriction; fatal early in childhood unless liver transplantation successful
Verneuil's disease	Syphilitic disease of the bursae	*Treponema pallidum*	Early treatment of syphilis
***Vibrio vulnificus* septicemia**	Overwhelming sepsis in a cirrhotic patient who has ingested oysters; typically affects men over age 40 in coastal states between May and October	*Vibrio vulnificans*	Tetracycline or chloramphenicol
Volkmann's disease	Tibiotarsal dislocation causing deformity of foot	Congenital	Surgery
Von Hippel-Lindau disease: cerebroretinal hemangiomatosis	Phakomatosis characterized by angiomatosis of the retina, cerebellum, spinal cord and, less commonly, cysts of the pancreas, kidneys, and other viscera; onset usually in third decade and marked by symptoms of retinal or cerebral tumors	Transmitted as autosomal dominant trait	Early surgical intervention
Wegner's disease	Osteochondritic separation of the epiphyses	Congenital syphilis	Effective treatment of syphilis during pregnancy
Werdnig-Hoffmann disease: Werdnig-Hoffmann spinal muscular atrophy	Progressive degeneration of anterior horn cells and bulbar motor nuclei in a fetus or infant; onset marked by hypotonia with abducted and externally rotated hips, flexed knees, and absent reflexes; later stages marked by accessory use of respiratory muscles	Transmitted as autosomal recessive trait	Symptomatic supportive management; death usually occurs in a year, but progression slower if disease limited to legs
Whipple's disease: intestinal lipodystrophy, lipophagia granulomatosis	GI malabsorption disorder characterized by chronic diarrhea and progressive wasting, with skin pigmentation and polyarthralgia	*Tropheryma whippelii*	Co-trimoxazole, penicillin G procaine with streptomycin, chloramphenicol, tetracycline, ampicillin, sulfasalazine
Wilms' tumor: congenital nephroblastoma, embryonal adenomyosarcoma	Malignant mixed tumors of the kidneys, primarily affecting children; major signs—abdominal mass, enlarged abdomen, hypertension, vomiting, and hematuria	Wilms' tumor recessive oncogen WT 21 chromosome 11	Surgery, radiation therapy, chemotherapy
Wolman's disease: infantile form of acid lipase deficiency	Hepatosplenomegaly, steatorrhea, and adrenal calcification manifested in the first weeks of life; results from accumulation of large amounts of neutral lipids in the body tissue associated with a deficiency of acid lipase	Autosomal recessive transmission	No specific therapy; usually fatal by age 6 months
Yaws: frambesia tropica	Chronic relapsing infection characterized by highly contagious primary and secondary cutaneous lesions and noncontagious tertiary lesions and systemic signs and symptoms	*Treponema pertenue*	Penicillin in aluminum monostearate 2%, oxytetracycline, or chlortetracycline
Yellow fever	Flavivirus infection that causes sudden illness accompanied by fever, slow pulse rate, headache, nausea, and vomiting; endemic in tropical Africa and Central and South America	Flavivirus transmitted by the *Aedes* mosquito	High-protein, high-carbohydrate liquid diet; analgesics; sedatives; antipyretics; bed rest; fluids to maintain adequate blood volume
Zygomycosis: phycomycosis, mucomycosis	Fungal infection commonly seen in immunocompromised patients; several forms, including rhinocerebral, GI, pulmonary, and disseminated mucomycosis	Zygomycetes	Amphotericin B; surgical removal of necrotic tissue

Index

i refers to an illustration; t refers to a table.

i refers to an illustration; t refers to a table.

i refers to an illustration; t refers to a table.

i refers to an illustration; t refers to a table.

i refers to an illustration; t refers to a table.

i refers to an illustration; t refers to a table.

---

i refers to an illustration; t refers to a table.